D1418806

Practical Clinical Drug Dosing
By Karim Rafaat, MD

THE CLINICAL DRUG DOSING AND
INFORMATION CARD CAN BE DETACHED
FROM THIS BOOK FOR EASY REFERENCE

Doses on this card may differ slightly
from those listed in the appendix.

This reflects the Author's practical
approach to clinical drug dosing. The
author recognizes that a wide range
of valid drug doses exist and that each
patient's individual needs may differ.
Clinical judgement must be used in
determining the proper drug dosing for
each patient.

REFERENCES

1) Fuhrman BP, Zimmerman JJ, Pediatric Critical Care 3rd edition, Mosby-Elsevier 2006
2) Slonim AD, Pollack MM, Pediatric Critical Care Medicine, Lippincott Williams ans Wilkins, 2006
3) Cote CJ, Lerman J, Todres ID, A Practice of Anesthesia for Infants and Children, Elsevier Health Sciences, 2009
4) Miller RD, Eriksson LI, Fleisher LA, Wiener-Kronish JP, Young WL, Miller's Anesthesia, Churchill Livingstone/Elsevier, 2009
5) Lacy CF, Armstrong LL, Goldman MP, Lance LL, Lexi-Comp: Drug Information Handbook, 19th edition, Lexi-Comp 2009

STEROIDS

		GLUCO	MINERAL
DEXAMETHASONE	EXTUB: 0.25 mg/kg/dose q6 IV, **CROUP**: 0.6 mg/kg x1 IV, **MENINGITIS**: 0.6 mg/kg/day q6 x4day IV	25	0
FLUDROCORTISONE	0.005-0.2 mg/day IV	0	14
HYDROCORTISONE	**SHOCK**: 12.5 mg/m2 IV q6 (50mg q6)	1	1
METHYLPREDNISOLONE	**ASTHMA**: 2 mg/kg then 1 mg/kg q6 IV	4	0.8

ANTIARRHYTHMICS

ADENOSINE	0.1 mg/kg then 0.2 mg/kg fast IV (max 6 mg, then 12 mg IV)
AMIODARONE	5 mg/kg (mx x1) then 7-21 mg/kg/day IV (**ADULTS**: 150-300 mg IV then 1 mg/hr)
LIDOCAINE	0.5-1 mg/kg IV, **PREINTUB**: 1.5 mg/kg IV (max 3 mg/kg) (**ok via ETT**)
PROCAINAMIDE	5-10 mg/kg IV then 40-80 mcg/kg/min IV (max 100 mg, then 6 mg/min)

MISCELLANEOUS

ALBUTEROL	0.15 mg/kg/dose INH (2.5-5mg) **CONT**: 0.3-0.45 mg/kg/hr INH (10-15 mg/h)
DANTROLENE	1-2.5 mg/kg IV q10 IV, then 1 mg/kg IV q6 x1-2d
DIPHENHYDRAMINE	1-2 mg/kg IV q6 (**ADULTS**: 25-50 mg IV)
PROSTAGLANDIN E₁	0.05-0.2 mcg/kg/min IV
RACEMIC EPI	0.05 ml/kg/dose IV in 3cc NS

OPIOID CONVERSION — 1 MG MORPHINE EQUALS

FENTANYL	0.01 mg IV
HYDROMORPHONE	0.15 mg IV, 0.75 mg PO
METHADONE	1 mg IV, 1.5 mg PO
MEPERIDINE	10 mg IV
OXYCODONE	2-3 mg PO

MAXIMUM LOCAL ANESTHETIC DOSE

	Without Epi	With Epi
BUPIVICAINE	3 mg/kg	4 mg/kg
CHLOROPROCAINE	8 mg/kg	10 mg/kg
LIDOCAINE	5 mg/kg	7 mg/kg
ROPIVICAINE	2.3 mg/kg	3 mg/kg

CHILD'S ESTIMATED WEIGHT (kg) = (Age x 2) + 8 (up to 9 yrs old)

ETT SIZE BY WEIGHT <1000 g: 2.5, 1000-2000 g: 3.0, 2000-3000 g: 3.5, >3000 g: 4.0

ETT SIZE or Age = Age/4 + 4

ETT DEPTH = 3 x ETT size or Age + 10 (adults: M 23 cm; F 20 cm)

LMA SIZE = **1** 0-5 kg **1.5** 5-10 kg **2** 10-20 kg **2.5** 20-30 kg **3** 30-50 kg **4** 50-70 kg **5** 70-100kg

1 MAC

	NEO	1-6 MO	6-12 MO	12-24 MO	CHILD	ADULT
DESFLURANE	9.2%	9.4%	9.9%	8.7%	7.9%	6.3%
ISOFLURANE	1.6%	1.9%	1.8%	1.6%	1.6%	1.2%
N2O					109%	109%
SEVOFLURANE	3.2%	3.2%	2.5%	2.5%	2.5%	2%

q="every", h="hours", IV="intravenous", INH="inhaled", PO="oral", PR="rectal", mg="milligram", kg="kilogram", IM="intramuscular", gm="gram", cc="cubic centimeters", U="units", mr="may repeat", D25W="dextrose 25% in water"

BENZODIAZEPINES/BARBITURATES/SEDATIVES

DEXMEDETOMIDINE	**SED**: 0.1-0.7 mcg/kg/hr IV
DIAZEPAM	**SED**: 0.05-0.2mg/kg IV, **STATUS**: 0.5mg/kg PR, **PREMED**: 0.2-0.5 mg/kg PO
ETOMIDATE	**IND**: 0.2-0.3 mg/kg IV
FLUMAZENIL	**REVERSAL**: 0.01 mg/kg IV (titrate in 0.2 mg increments in adults)
KETAMINE	**PREMED**: 5-6 mg/kg PO, 0.1-0.5 mg/kg IV, **IND**: 1-2mg/kg IV, 3-5 mg/kg IM, **PAIN**: 0.1-0.5 mg/kg IV, **IM COCKTAIL**: ketamine 2-3 mg/kg IV versed 0.1mg/kg IV, glyco 0.01 mg/kg IV
LORAZEPAM	**PREMED**: 0.05 mg/kg IV (2mg), **SED**: 0.01-0.01mg/kg IV (2mg), 0.1 mg/kg IM (4mg)
MIDAZOLAM	**PREMED**: 0.4-0.8 mg/kg PO, **SED**: 0.01-0.01 mg/kg IV (2mg), 0.1 mg/kg IM (4mg), **STATUS**: 0.1-0.2 mg/kg IV
PROPOFOL	**IND**: 2-3 mg/kg IV (**ADULTS**: 1-2.5 mg/kg IV), **INF**: 50-200 mcg/kg/min IV
THIOPENTAL	**IND**: 3-6 mg/kg IV

OPIOIDS AND ANALGESICS

ACETAMINOPHEN	40mg/kg PR then 15mg/kg PO, PR q6h (max ~90 mg/kg/day)
HYDROMORPHONE	**PAIN**: 0.015 mg/kg IV (0.2-1mg)
FENTANYL	**IND**: 2-5 mcg/kg IV, **PAIN**: 0.5-2 mcg/kg IV
ALFENTANIL	**PAIN**: 5-10 mcg/kg IV (250-500 mcg), **IND**: 10-50 mcg/kg IV
IBUPROFEN	**PAIN**: 10mg/kg PO q6h (800-1000mg)
KETOROLAC	0.5 mg/kg q6h IV (max 15 mg <50 kg, 30 mg >50 kg)
MEPERIDINE	**SHIVERING**: 0.1-1 mg/kg IV
MORPHINE	**PAIN**: 0.02-0.1 mg/kg IV
NALOXONE	**FULL**: 0.01 mg/kg IV (0.4-0.8 mg), **PARTIAL**: 0.01 mg/kg IV (0.04 mg)
REMIFENTANIL	**IND**: 0.5-1 mcg/kg IV, **INF**: 0.1-0.3 mcg/kg/min IV
SUFENTANIL	**IND**: 0.3-1 mcg/kg IV, **INF**: 0.3 mcg/kg/hr IV (dc 40 min pre end)

NEUROMUSCULAR BLOCKING AGENTS (INTUBATING DOSE)

CISATRACURIUM	0.15-0.2 mg/kg IV
PANCURONIUM	0.05-0.1 mg/kg IV
ROCURONIUM	**NEO**: 0.3 mg/kg IV, **CHILDREN**: 0.6 mg/kg IV, **ADULTS**: 0.8 mg/kg IV, **RSI**: 1.2 mg/kg IV, 1.8-2 mg/kg IM
SUCCINYLCHOLINE	**NEO**: 2-3 mg/kg IV, **KIDS/ADULTS**: 1-2 mg/kg IV, 4-5 mg/kg IM, **SUX FOR LARYNGOSPASM**: 1/10th dose
VECURONIUM	0.1 mg/kg IV

FFP="fresh frozen plasma", DDAVP="desmopressin", IND="induction", INF="infusion", RSI="rapid sequence induction", SED="sedation", STATUS="status epilepticus", T3="triiodothyronine", PRBC="packed red blood cells"

MANUAL OF
Clinical
Anesthesiology

INCLUDING

Color Atlas of Regional Anesthesia
Color Atlas of Transesophageal Echocardiography
Color Atlas of Anesthesia Procedures
Crisis Management Cognitive Aids

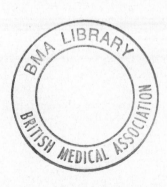

MANUAL OF
Clinical
Anesthesiology

EDITED BY

Larry F. Chu, MD, MS
Stanford University School of Medicine
Stanford, California

Andrea J. Fuller, MD
University of Colorado School of Medicine
Aurora, Colorado

ASSOCIATE EDITORS

Calvin Kuan, MD – Pediatric Anesthesia
Stanford University School of Medicine
Stanford, California

Danielle Ludwin, MD
Columbia University School of Medicine
New York, New York

Edward R. Mariano, MD – Regional Anesthesia
University of California – San Diego
San Diego, California

Nathaen Weitzel, MD – Cardiac Anesthesia
University of Colorado School of Medicine
Aurora, Colorado

 Wolters Kluwer | Lippincott Williams & Wilkins
Health

Philadelphia • Baltimore • New York • London
Buenos Aires • Hong Kong • Sydney • Tokyo

Acquisitions Editor: Brian Brown
Product Manager: Nicole Dernoski
Production Manager: Bridgett Dougherty
Senior Manufacturing Manager: Benjamin Rivera
Marketing Manager: Angela Panetta
Design Coordinator: Stephen Druding
Production Service: SPi Global

Printed in China

Library of Congress Cataloging-in-Publication Data
Manual of clinical anesthesiology / [edited by] Larry Chu, Stanford University School of Medicine; Department of Anesthesia, Stanford, CA 94305, aimlabstanford@gmail.com, Andrea Fuller, andisamf@aol.com.—First edition.
    p. ; cm.
Includes bibliographical references and index.
    ISBN 978-0-7817-7379-9 (alk. paper)
    1. Anesthesiology—Outlines, syllabi, etc. 2. Anesthesiology—Handbooks, manuals, etc. I. Chu, Larry, editor. II. Fuller, Andrea, editor.
    [DNLM: 1. Anesthesia—Outlines. 2. Anesthetics—Outlines.   WO 218.2]

    RD82.4.M36   2011
    617.9'6—dc22

                                                                                          2010048730

To purchase additional copies of this book, call our customer service department at (800) 638-3030 or fax orders to (301) 223-2320. International customers should call (301) 223-2300.

Visit Lippincott Williams & Wilkins on the Internet: at LWW.com. Lippincott Williams & Wilkins customer service representatives are available from 8:30 am to 6 pm, EST.

10 9 8 7 6 5 4 3 2 1

To Molly, Sherman, Anita, and Fred with much love (L.C.)

To all the anesthesia providers up in the middle of the night,
working to keep patients safe (A.F.)

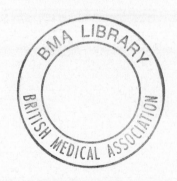

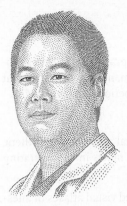

Larry F. Chu, MD, MS

Being the first to do something new is a uniquely terrifying experience. The concept of a practical book of anesthesiology, designed to be used at the point of care, is not new. However, my vision in creating this book was to offer a highly visual text, written in a rapid reference format that would bring the practice of anesthesiology alive to the reader in ways that have not been done before. My goal was to incorporate cognitive aids, clinical algorithms, and visual atlases of anesthesia practice into a single portable reference text that could be used at the point of care. I think this book has achieved these goals and offers something uniquely appealing to today's highly visual learners and practicing anesthesiologists.

Having a vision is an easy thing. To bring that vision to reality is the true challenge. I could not have asked for a better partner in this process than Dr. Andrea J. Fuller. Her intellect, dedication, and good humor throughout the five-year process of producing this book have been the primary reasons for its success. I also want to thank my Chairman, Dr. Ronald G. Pearl, for his mentorship and support during these years of work and, of course, Molly Chu without whose love and support this book would not have been possible.

Larry F. Chu, MD, MS
Stanford, California

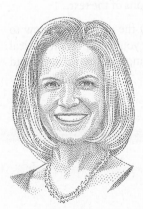

Andrea J. Fuller, MD

The practice of anesthesiology requires us to think "on the fly." We are often faced with clinical challenges late at night, emergently, and in patients with coexisting illnesses. The goal of this book was to provide a reliable place to turn at the point of care. We went to great lengths to recruit contributors and editors from every area of the country in an effort to reflect a broad view of the specialty and not just an institutional or regional approach. It is intended for anyone who practices general anesthesiology, whether he or she has been practicing for 3 days or 30 years.

I would like to thank Dr. Larry F. Chu for asking me to be involved in this project at a time when I was looking for academic challenges. I knew his unique ability to condense complex topics into visual resources would make this book special. I believe it has. I am sincerely grateful to my colleagues at the University of Colorado, many of whom have helped make this book a reality with contributions, time, and encouragement. Finally, I must thank my family—Sam, Brian, Henry, Norma, Bob, and John—for their unending love and support.

Andrea J. Fuller, MD
Aurora, Colorado

How to Use this Book

This book is designed to be used at the point of clinical care by practicing anesthesiologists. It is not a textbook of anesthesiology. There are already many excellent texts that provide detailed explanations of the principles and practice of perioperative medicine.

This is a **manual** of clinical anesthesiology.

We have designed it from the beginning to be a highly visual manual of anesthetic practice that brings practical information where it is needed most: in the operating room, on the wards, and at the patient bedside.

We have incorporated cognitive aids, clinical algorithms, and visual atlases of anesthesia practice into a single portable reference text that is intended to be used at the point of care.

In order to facilitate rapid reference of material, we have utilized several graphical conventions throughout this book.

You may already have noticed the use of color to provide emphasis to important ideas and information within the text.

Chapters are also easily identified by numbers that are printed in large, easy-to-read type at the top of each chapter heading.

Sections of the book are also immediately identified by color bars that are printed on the edge of the page, making it easy to rapidly reference sections of the text.

Finally, we have three main graphical enhancements: (1) the read more arrow to direct you to related material, (2) the skull and bones to alert you to important clinical information, and (3) pearls, which help highlight interesting and useful facts and information.

Monitoring Equipment and Procedures Subspecialty Anesthesia

Chapter numbers in large font with bold formatting. Size and color enhance rapid-reference readability.

READ MORE

Chp 74, Increased ICP, p214

These icons are used to link to other chapters in the book with related information. This helps direct readers to useful content quickly.

The needle used to treat a tension pneumothorax should be left in place until a tube thoracostomy is performed.

The Skull & Bones icon is meant to highlight extremely important clinical information that may help prevent adverse events.

Using clinical signs alone for placement of a Double-lumen endotracheal tube is an important clinical skill.

These icons are used to identify useful clinical pearls to the reader.

Color-coded heading bars bled to the edge of the page help readers quickly identify relevant sections of the book.

Contributors

Distinguished Contributors

Jay B. Brodsky, MD
Professor, Department of Anesthesia
Stanford University School of Medicine
Medical Director, Perioperative Services
Stanford University Medical Center
Stanford, California

Raymond Gaeta, MD
Associate Professor
Department of Anesthesia
Division of Pain Management
Stanford University School of Medicine
Stanford, California

Glenn P. Gravlee, MD
Professor
Director of Education
Department of Anesthesiology
University of Colorado School of
Medicine
Aurora, Colorado

Anita Honkanen, MD
Chief, Division of Pediatric Anesthesia
Clinical Associate Professor
Department of Anesthesia
Stanford University School of Medicine
Stanford, California

Ronald G. Pearl, MD, PhD
Dr. Richard K. and Erika N. Richards
Professor
Chairman
Department of Anesthesia
Stanford University School of Medicine
Stanford, California

Myer Rosenthal, MD
Professor Emeritus
Departments of Anesthesia, Medicine, and
Surgery
Stanford University School of Medicine
Stanford, California

Steven L. Shafer, MD
Professor of Anesthesiology, Columbia
University
New York, New York
Adjunct Professor of Anesthesia, Stanford
University
Stanford, California
Adjunct Professor of Bioengineering and
Therapeutic Sciences, UCSF
San Francisco, California
Editor-in-Chief, Anesthesia & Analgesia

Contributing Authors

Scott M. Ahlbrand, MD
Clinical Instructor (Affiliated)
Department of Anesthesia
Stanford University School of Medicine
Stanford, California

Bryan Ahlgren, DO
Resident Physician
Department of Anesthesiology
University of Colorado School of Medicine
Aurora, Colorado

Dondee Almazan, MD
Pediatric Anesthesia Fellow
Department of Anesthesia
Stanford University School of Medicine
Stanford, California

Leslie C. Andes, MD
Valley Anesthesiology Consultants
Barrow Neurological Institute
Phoenix, Arizona

Elisabeth A. Aron, MD, FACOG
Senior Clinical Instructor
Department of Obstetrics and Gynecology
University of Colorado School of Medicine
Aurora, Colorado

Arthur Atchabahian, MD
Associate Professor of Clinical Anesthesiology
The Hospital for Joint Diseases
NYU School of Medicine
New York, New York

Rachel L. Boggus, MD
Anesthesiology Resident
Department of Anesthesiology
University of Colorado School of Medicine
Aurora, Colorado

Jonathan T. Bradley, MD
Resident Physician
Department of Anesthesia
Stanford University School of Medicine
Stanford, California

Trent Bryson, MD
Resident Physician
Department of Anesthesiology
University of Colorado School of Medicine
Aurora, Colorado

Marek Brzezinski, MD, PhD
Associate Professor of Clinical Anesthesia
Department of Anesthesia
University of California – San Francisco
San Francisco, California

Scott W. Byram, MD
Assistant Professor
Department of Anesthesiology
Loyola University Medical Center
Maywood, Illinois

Divya Chander, MD, PhD
Instructor, Department of Anesthesia
Fellow, Department of Bioengineering
Stanford University School of Medicine
Stanford, California

Matthew T. Charous, MD
Regional Anesthesia and Acute Pain Medicine
    Fellow
Department of Anesthesiology
University of California – San Diego
San Diego, California

Sara S. Cheng, MD, PhD
Assistant Professor of Anesthesiology
Department of Anesthesiology
University of Colorado School of Medicine
Aurora, Colorado

Ellen Choi, MD
Pediatric Anesthesia Fellow
Department of Anesthesia
Stanford University School of Medicine
Stanford, California

Larry F. Chu, MD, MS
Associate Professor of Anesthesia
Department of Anesthesia
Stanford University School of Medicine
Stanford, California

Christopher L. Ciarallo, MD
Assistant Professor
Department of Anesthesiology
University of Colorado School of Medicine
Aurora, Colorado

Carlee A. Clark, MD
Assistant Professor
Department of Anesthesia and Perioperative
    Medicine
Medical University of South Carolina
Charleston, South Carolina

Rebecca Claure, MD
Clinical Assistant Professor
Department of Anesthesia
Stanford University School of Medicine
Stanford, California

Jeromy Cole, MD
Anesthesia Resident Physician
Department of Anesthesiology
University of Colorado School of Medicine
Aurora, Colorado

Matthew D. Coleman, MD
Assistant Professor
Department of Anesthesiology
College of Physicians & Surgeons of Columbia
    University
New York, New York

Christopher Cornelissen, DO
Division Head
Cardiovascular and Thoracic Anesthesia
Naval Medical Center, San Diego
San Diego, California

Tony Cun, BS
Research Assistant
Department of Anesthesia
Stanford University School of Medicine
Stanford, California

Brian M. Davidson, MD
Assistant Professor
Department of Anesthesiology
University of Colorado School of Medicine
Aurora, Colorado

Arjun Desai, MD
Resident Physician
Department of Anesthesia
Stanford University School of Medicine
Stanford, California

Laura Downey, MD
Resident Physician
Department of Anesthesia
Stanford University School of Medicine
Stanford, California

James C. Duke, MD, MBA
Associate Professor of Anesthesiology
Department of Anesthesiology
University of Colorado School of Medicine
Aurora, Colorado

Steven B. Edelstein, MD
Professor and Vice-Chairman
Department of Anesthesiology
Loyola University Medical Center
Maywood, Illinois

Brian J. Egan, MD, MPH
Assistant Professor of Anesthesiology
Department of Anesthesiology
Columbia University College of Physicians and
    Surgeons
New York, New York

Reuben L. Eng, MD
Resident Physician
Department of Anesthesia
University of Calgary
Calgary, Alberta, Canada

Amy R. Evers, MD
Obstetrical Anesthesia Associates
St. John's Mercy Medical Center
St. Louis, Missouri

Ruth Fanning, MB, MRCPI, FFARCSI
Clinical Assistant Professor
Department of Anesthesia
Stanford University School of Medicine
Stanford, California

**Ana Fernandez-Bustamante,
    MD, PhD**
Assistant Professor
Department of Anesthesiology
University of Colorado School of Medicine
Aurora, Colorado

Matthew J. Fiegel, MD
Assistant Professor; Director
Acute Pain Service
Department of Anesthesiology
University of Colorado School of Medicine
Aurora, Colorado

Andrea J. Fuller, MD
Assistant Professor of Anesthesiology
Department of Anesthesiology
University of Colorado School of Medicine
Aurora, Colorado

Amy J. Gagnon, MD
Fellow/Instructor of Maternal-Fetal Medicine
Department of Obstetrics and Gynecology
University of Colorado School of Medicine
Aurora, Colorado

Lisa Gramlich, MD
Associate Professor
Director of Pediatric Anesthesia
Loyola University Medical Center
Maywood, Illinois

Sara Goldhaber-Fiebert, MD
Clinical Instructor
Department of Anesthesia
Stanford University School of Medicine
Stanford, California

Anastassia Grigorieva, MD
Resident Physician
Department of Anesthesiology and Critical Care
    Medicine
Johns Hopkins University School of Medicine
Baltimore, Maryland

Eric Gross, MD
Resident Physician
Department of Anesthesia
Stanford University School of Medicine
Stanford, California

Cosmin Guta, MD
Clinical Assistant Professor
Department of Anesthesia
Stanford University School of Medicine
Stanford, California

Joyce Hairston, MD
Resident Physician
Department of Anesthesia
Stanford University School of Medicine
Stanford, California

Kellie Hancock, MD
Resident Physician
Department of Anesthesiology
University of Colorado School of Medicine
Aurora, Colorado

T. Kyle Harrison, MD
Clinical Assistant Professor of Anesthesia
(Affiliated)
Stanford University School of Medicine
Stanford, California
Staff Physician, VA Palo Alto Health Care System
Palo Alto, California

Jonathan Hastie, MD
Department of Anesthesiology
Columbia University College of Physicians and
Surgeons
New York, New York

Justin W. Heil, MD, PhD
Director, Acute Pain Service
Naval Medical Center – San Diego
San Diego, California

Peter M. Hession, MD
Resident Physician
Department of Anesthesiology
University of Texas Southwestern Medical Center
Dallas, Texas

Charles C. Hill, MD
Clinical Assistant Professor
Department of Anesthesia
Stanford University School of Medicine
Stanford, California

Camille Hoffman, MD
Fellow/Instructor of Maternal Fetal Medicine
Department of Obstetrics and Gynecology
University of Colorado School of Medicine
Aurora, Colorado

Steven K. Howard, MD
Associate Professor
Department of Anesthesiology
Stanford University School of Medicine
Stanford, California

Robert L. Hsiung, MD
Staff Anesthesiologist
Virginia Mason Medical Center
Seattle, Washington

Haley G. Hutting, MD
Resident Physician
Department of Anesthesiology
University of Colorado School of Medicine
Aurora, Colorado

Caleb Ing, MD
Assistant Professor
Department of Anesthesiology
College of Physicians and Surgeons of Columbia
University
New York, New York

Jerry Ingrande, MD, MS
Instructor
Department of Anesthesia
Stanford University School of Medicine
Stanford, California

Gillian E. Johnson, MB, Bchir
Anesthesiologist
Pike's Peak Anesthesia Associates
Colorado Springs, Colorado

Albert C. Ju, MD
Assistant Professor of Anesthesiology
Department of Anesthesiology
Columbia University College of Physicians and
Surgeons
New York, New York

Alma N. Juels, MD
Assistant Professor of Anesthesiology
Attending Physician
University of Colorado School of Medicine
Aurora, Colorado

Bronwen F. Kahn, MD
Fellow, Instructor of Maternal-Fetal Medicine
Department of Obstetrics and Gynecology
University of Colorado School of Medicine
Aurora, Colorado

Athina Kakavouli, MD
Fellow
Department of Anesthesiology
Columbia University College of Physicians and
Surgeons
New York, New York

Jack Kan, MD
Resident Physician
Department of Anesthesia
Stanford University School of Medicine
Stanford, California

Nicholette Kasman, MD
Pediatric Anesthesiologist
Children's Hospital and Research Center
  Oakland
Oakland, California

Shanthala Keshavacharya, MD
Anesthesiologist
Sequoia Hospital
Redwood City, California

Russell Kinder, MD
Resident Physician
Virginia Mason Medical Center
Seattle, Washington

Stephen M. Klein, MD
Associate Professor
Chief, Division of Ambulatory Anesthesiology
Department of Anesthesiology
Duke University Medical Center
Durham, North Carolina

Matthew S. Koehler, MD
Staff Anesthiologist
Kaiser Permanente
Denver, Colorado

Benjamin Kratzert, MD, PhD
Assistant Professor
Department of Anesthesiology and Critical Care
University of New Mexico
Albuquerque, NM

Calvin Kuan, MD
Clinical Assistant Professor
Department of Anesthesia
Stanford University School of Medicine
Stanford, California

Vivekanand Kulkarni, MD, PhD
Clinical Assistant Professor of Anesthesia
Department of Anesthesia
Stanford University School of Medicine
Stanford, California

Sunil Kumar, MD, FFARCS
Associate Professor of Anesthesiology
Department of Anesthesiology
University of Colorado School of Medicine
Aurora, Colorado

Shaun Kunnavatana, MD
Resident Physician
Department of Anesthesia
Stanford University School of Medicine
Stanford, California

Christopher Lace, MD
Clinical Faculty
Department of Anesthesiology
University of Colorado School of Medicine
Aurora, Colorado

Samsun (Sem) Lampotang, PhD
Professor of Anesthesiology
Director, Center for Simulation, Safety &
  Advanced Learning Technology
University of Florida College of Medicine
Gainesville, Florida

John S. Lee, MD
Anesthesia and Critical Care Fellow
University of California – San Francisco
San Francisco, California

Ray S. Lee, MD
Resident Physician
Department of Anesthesiology
Virginia Mason Medical Center
Seattle, Washington

Wesley Liao, MD
Resident Physician
Department of Anesthesiology and Critical Care
  Medicine
The Johns Hopkins Hospital
Baltimore, Maryland

Geoff Lighthall, MD
Associate Professor
Department of Anesthesia
Stanford University School of Medicine
Stanford, California

Ludwig H. Lin, MD
Clinical Associate Professor
Department of Anesthesia and Critical Care
Stanford University School of Medicone
Stanford, California

Linda L. Liu, MD
Professor of Clinical Anesthesia
Department of Anesthesia
UCSF School of Medicine
San Francisco, California

Vanessa J. Loland, MD
Assistant Clinical Professor of Anesthesiology
Fellowship Director, Regional Anesthesia and
    Acute Pain Medicine
University of California – San Diego
San Diego, California

Allison Long, MD
Clinical Faculty
Department of Anesthesiology
University of Colorado School of Medicine
Aurora, Colorado

Danielle B. Ludwin, MD
Assistant Professor of Anesthesia
Department of Anesthesiology
Columbia University College of Physicians and
    Surgeons
New York, New York

Alex Macario, MD, MBA
Professor of Anesthesia and (by courtesy) of
    Health Research & Policy
Residency Program Director
Department of Anesthesia
Stanford University School of Medicine
Stanford, California

Sarah J. Madison, MD
Regional Anesthesia and Acute Pain Medicine
    Fellow
Department of Anesthesia
University of California – San Diego
San Diego, California

Kevin Malott, MD
Clinical Assistant Professor
Department of Anesthesia
Stanford University School of Medicine and
    Lucile Packard Children's Hospital
Stanford, California

Edward R. Mariano, MD, MAS
Associate Professor of Anesthesia
Stanford University School of Medicine
Chief, Anesthesiology and Perioperative Care
    Service
Veterans Affairs Palo Alto Health Care System
Palo Alto, California

Bryan Maxwell, MD, MPH
Resident Physician
Department of Anesthesia
Stanford University School of Medicine
Stanford, California

Steve Melton, MD
Assistant Professor
Department of Anesthesiology
Duke University Medical Center
Durham, North Carolina

Julianne M. Mendoza, MD
Pediatric Anesthesia Fellow
Department of Anesthesia
Stanford University School of Medicine
Stanford, California

Samuel A. Mireles, MD
Clinical Assistant Professor
Department of Anesthesia
Stanford University School of Medicine
Stanford, California

Seshadri C. Mudumbai, MD
Instructor
Department of Anesthesia
Stanford University School of Medicine
Stanford, California

Jamie D. Murphy, MD
Assistant Professor of Anesthesia
Department of Anesthesiology
Johns Hopkins University School of Medicine
Baltimore, Maryland

Vladimir Nekhendzy, MD
Clinical Associate Professor
Department of Anesthesia
Stanford University School of Medicine
Stanford, California

Lynn Ngai, BS
Research Assistant
Department of Anesthesia
Stanford University School of Medicine
Stanford, California

John H. Nguyen, MD
Clinical Instructor
Department of Anesthesia
Stanford University School of Medicine
Stanford, California

Daryl A. Oakes, MD
Clinical Assistant Professor of Anesthesia
Department of Anesthesia
Stanford University School of Medicine
Stanford, California

Sabin Oana, MD
Assistant Professor
Department of Anesthesiology
Loyola University Hospital
Maywood, Illinois

Obianuju Okocha, MD
Instructor
Department of Anesthesiology
Northwestern University Feinberg School of
  Medicine
Chicago, Illinois

Amanda L. Peterson, MD
Regional Anesthesia and Acute Pain Medicine
  Fellow
Department of Anesthesiology
University of California – San Diego
San Diego, California

Rohith Piyaratna, MD
Resident Physician
Department of Anesthesia
Stanford University School of Medicine
Stanford, California

Tzevan Poon, MD
Resident Physician
Department of Anesthesia
Stanford University School of Medicine
Stanford, California

Chad Pritts, MD
Clinical Assistant Professor of Anesthesia and
  Critical Care
Department of Anesthesia
Stanford University School of Medicine
Stanford, California

Xiang Qian, MD
Resident Physician
Department of Anesthesia
Stanford University School of Medicine
Stanford, California

Karim Rafaat, MD
Fellow, Pediatric Anesthesia
Lucile Packard Children's Hospital
Palo Alto, California

Gurdev Rai, MD
Clinical Faculty
Department of Anesthesiology
University of Colorado School of Medicine
Aurora, Colorado

Jason G. Ramirez, MD
Private Practice
Denver, Colorado

Edward T. Riley, MD
Associate Professor – Med Center Line
Department of Anesthesia
Department of Obstetrics and Gynecology
  (By courtesy)
Stanford University School of Medicine
Stanford, California

Prairie Neeley Robinson, MD
Fellow
Department of Anesthesiology
University of Colorado School of Medicine
Aurora, Colorado

Echo V. Rowe, MD
Clinical Assistant Professor of Anesthesia
Department of Anesthesia
Stanford University School of Medicine
Stanford, California

Christie M. Sasso, MD
Resident Physician
Department of Anesthesia
Columbia University College of Physicians and
  Surgeons
New York, New York

Dominique H. Schiffer, MD
Assistant Professor
Department of Anesthesiology
University of Colorado School of Medicine
Aurora, Colorado

James Sederberg, MD
Clinical Faculty
Department of Anesthesiology
University of Colorado School of Medicine
Aurora, Colorado

Tamas Seres, MD, PhD
Assistant Professor
Department of Anesthesiology
University of Colorado School of Medicine
Aurora, Colorado

Evan Serfass, MD, PhD
Resident Physician
Department of Anesthesia
Stanford University School of Medicine
Stanford, California

Jeannie Seybold, MD
Clinical Assistant Professor
Department of Anesthesia
Stanford University School of Medicine
Stanford, California

Vikas Shah, MD, PhD
Resident Physician
Department of Anesthesia
Stanford University School of Medicine
Stanford, California

Marina Shindell, DO
Assistant Professor
Department of Anesthesiology
University of Colorado School of Medicine
Aurora, Colorado

Jessica Spellman, MD
Assistant Professor of Anesthesiology
Department of Anesthesiology
Columbia University College of Physicians and
    Surgeons
New York, New York

Quinn Stevens, MD
Resident Physician
Department of Anesthesiology
University of Colorado School of Medicine
Aurora, Colorado

Naiyi Sun, MD
Clinical Assistant Professor
Department of Anesthesia
Stanford University School of Medicine
Stanford, California

Pedro P. Tanaka, MD, PhD
Clinical Associate Professor
Department of Anesthesia
Stanford University School of Medicine
Stanford, California

Judy Thai, MD
Cardiac Anesthesia, Staff Anesthesiologist
Kaiser Permanente, Oakland
Oakland, California

Christopher Tirce, MD
Resident Physician
Department of Anesthesia
Stanford University School of Medicine
Stanford, California

Hien Nicole Tran, MD
Resident Physician
Department of Medicine
Kaiser Permanente Oakland Medical Center
Oakland, California

Andrew Wall, MD
Resident Physician
Department of Anesthesia
Stanford University School of Medicine
Stanford, California

Amy Wang, MD
Resident Physician
Department of Anesthesia
Stanford University School of Medicine
Stanford, California

Binbin Wang, MD
Anesthesia and Critical Care Fellow
University of California – San Francisco
San Francisco, California

Nathaen Weitzel, MD
Assistant Professor
Department of Anesthesiology
University of Colorado School of Medicine
Aurora, Colorado

Barbara J. Wilkey, MD
Resident Physician
Department of Anesthesiology
University of Colorado School of Medicine
Aurora, Colorado

Julie L. Williamson, DO
Clinical Assistant Professor
Department of Anesthesia and Pediatrics
Stanford University School of Medicine
Stanford, California

Gregory A. Wolff, MD
Resident Physician
Department of Anesthesiology
University of Colorado School of Medicine
Aurora, Colorado

Becky Wong, MD
Resident Physician
Department of Anesthesia
Stanford University School of Medicine
Stanford, California

Romy Yun, MD
Resident Physician
Department of Anesthesia
Stanford University School of Medicine
Stanford, California

Daniel Zaghi, MD
Clinical Research Fellow
Department of Dermatology
University of Utah
Salt Lake City, Utah

Consultants

Anita Y. Chu, BPharm, RPh, PharmD
Clinical Pharmacist and Instructor
University of Wisconsin Hospital and Clinics
Staff Pharmacist and Clinical Instructor
William S. Middleton Memorial Veterans Affairs
   Hospital
Madison, Wisconsin

Stanford Anesthesia Informatics and Media Lab

Major portions of this text were developed by
the Stanford Anesthesia Informatics and Media
Lab, specifically the visual atlases and cognitive
aids. We would like to recognize these important
contributors to this book.

Larry Chu, MD, MS
Director
Stanford AIM Lab

Dan Hoang, BA
Senior Production Assistant
Stanford AIM Lab

Anna Clemenson, BA
Production Assistant
Stanford AIM Lab

Tony Cun, BS
Production Assistant
Stanford AIM Lab

Lynn Ngai, BS
Production Assistant
Stanford AIM Lab

Reviewers

Tim Angelotti, MD

Associate Professor of Anesthesia
Department of Anesthesia
Stanford University School of Medicine

Jay Brodsky, MD

Professor, Department of Anesthesia
Stanford University School of Medicine
Medical Director, Perioperative Services
Stanford University Medical Center

Brenda Bucklin, MD

Professor
Department of Anesthesiology
University of Colorado School of Medicine

Sara S. Cheng, MD

Assistant Professor of Anesthesiology
Department of Anesthesiology
University of Colorado School of Medicine

Joy Hawkins, MD

Professor
Department of Anesthesiology
University of Colorado School of Medicine

John D. Mitchell, MD

Beth Israel Deaconess Medical Center
Department of Anesthesia
Critical Care and Pain Medicine
Harvard Medical School

Annette Mizuguchi, MD

Brigham and Women's Hospital
Department of Anesthesiology
Harvard Medical School

Contents

SECTION III

EQUIPMENT AND PROCEDURES 105

SECTION IV

INTRAOPERATIVE FLUID MANAGEMENT AND BLOOD COMPONENT THERAPY 193

SECTION V

NEURAXIAL AND REGIONAL ANESTHESIA 225

PART B - Immunology and Infectious Diseases

PART C - Respiratory Diseases

SECTION VIII

PEDIATRIC ANESTHESIA **751**

PART A - Diseases in Pediatric Patients

PART B - Anesthetic Concerns and Procedures in Pediatric Anesthesia

SECTION X

POSTOPERATIVE CONCERNS IN ANESTHESIA. 1069

SECTION XI

ATLAS OF ANESTHESIA PROCEDURES 1093

APPENDIX OF ANESTHESIA PHRASES IN FOREIGN LANGUAGES

APPENDIX OF ANESTHETIC DRUG INFORMATION

APPENDIX OF CRISIS MANAGEMENT ALGORITHMS IN ANESTHESIA

Advanced Cardiac Life Support

Crisis Management Algorithms in Anesthesia

1 The Anesthetic Plan and Induction of Anesthesia

Joyce Hairston, MD • Danielle B. Ludwin, MD • Larry F. Chu, MD, MS

ANESTHESIOLOGY

The anesthesiologist's role in the care of a patient for surgery begins with the preoperative assessment, continues with the induction and maintenance of anesthesia for the surgical procedure, and extends to the postoperative period until the effects of the anesthetic drugs and procedures have resolved and the patient has recovered. The anesthetic plan describes how the anesthesiologist and perioperative care team will approach their role to customize an individual care plan that is tailored to the patient and the surgeon's specific needs while also insuring a safe perioperative experience. This chapter discusses the development of an anesthetic plan and induction of anesthesia.

1) **Overview**
   a) The anesthetic plan is a guide to the perioperative care of patients undergoing anesthesia for surgery.
   b) The plan is customized to the individual patient so that both the patient's and the surgeon's preferences are considered in the development of a plan for the safe administration of anesthesia.
   c) Components of the anesthetic plan include the preoperative assessment and optimization, intraoperative management plan, and postoperative care plan.

2) **Preoperative assessment and optimization**
   a) A history and physical examination can help identify relevant coexisting diseases and allow the anesthesiologist to assess the patient's anatomy to determine if difficulty with certain anesthetic techniques such as endotracheal intubation should be anticipated.
   b) The anesthesiologist may choose to optimize certain coexisting diseases such as hypertension or heart disease prior to surgery.
   c) The needs of the patient and surgeon with regard to anesthesia for the procedure should be discussed.
   d) Selection of anesthetic technique
      An anesthetic technique should be selected during the preoperative assessment so that the risks and benefits can be discussed with both the patient and surgeon in order to ensure that the best technique is selected for the planned surgical procedure (Table 1-1).
      i) Types of anesthesia techniques. A combination of these techniques may also be used.
         (1) Local anesthesia
            (a) Infiltration or nerve block typically done by surgeons, with or without patient sedation
            (b) Many times, cases booked as "local anesthesia" without patient sedation are performed by surgeons without the involvement of an anesthesiologist.

READ
MORE

Difficult airway,
Chapter 210,
page 1326

Preoperative
assessment

Table 1-1

Anesthetic Plan Considerations

Perioperative Issue	Anesthetic Technique Considerations
Length of surgical procedure	Long surgical cases may require GA, even with neuraxial or PNB techniques, because of tourniquet pain and uncomfortable positioning.
Potential for blood loss and/or hemodynamic instability	Endotracheal intubation and mechanical ventilation may become necessary if a patient sustains loss of consciousness due to hemodynamic instability. Consider GA or plan for conversion to GA if necessary.
Patient position	Prone or lateral positioning is often uncomfortable for a patient and may require GA instead of RA or PNB techniques.
Airway anatomy	PNB and RA techniques may allow avoiding airway manipulation in patients with a difficult airway. Consider definitively securing the airway and GA in an elective and controlled manner if the potential for conversion to GA is likely.
Anticipated postsurgical pain	PNB and RA techniques are very effective in postoperative pain control, especially when high postoperative pain is anticipated (e.g., knee replacement surgery).
Requirement for surgical neuromuscular blockade	The need for neuromuscular blockade may require dense RA/PNB for extremity surgeries and GA and mechanical ventilation for abdominal surgeries.
Patient history of postoperative nausea and vomiting	RA/PNB techniques provide excellent analgesia and avoid the use of opioid narcotics and volatile anesthetic gases which are emetogenic.

(2) **Monitored anesthesia care (MAC)**

    (a) Anesthetic drugs are administered to varying levels of sedation, analgesia and anxiolysis as necessary for the procedure.

    (b) The provider must be prepared and qualified to convert to general anesthesia (GA) if necessary.

    (c) Loss of consciousness or the ability for purposeful response during MAC is GA, irrespective of whether the airway is instrumented. (1)

(3) **General anesthesia (GA)**

    (a) GA involves loss of consciousness and is induced by anesthetic drugs that can be given by inhalation or intravenous injection.

    (b) The airway is generally instrumented with an endotracheal tube, supraglottic airway device (e.g., laryngeal mask airway (LMA)) or can remain unsecured if the procedure is brief.

(4) **Peripheral nerve block (PNB)**

READ MORE

Overview of peripheral nerve blocks, Chapter 34, page 256

    (a) Anesthesia is provided by placing local anesthetic drugs near peripheral nerves using a needle.

    (b) Typically used for surgeries of the extremities, though truncal blocks such as TAP and paravertebral are also performed

    (c) May be used as the primary anesthetic or as postoperative analgesia when administered in conjunction with other techniques such as GA

(5) **Neuraxial anesthesia**
(a) Anesthesia is provided by placing local anesthetic within the cerebral spinal fluid (spinal) or epidural space (epidural).
(b) These techniques can provide dense surgical anesthesia for surgeries involving the abdomen and lower body.
(c) May be used as the primary anesthetic or for postoperative analgesia

3) **Intraoperative plan**
a) **Intravenous access**
i) Most anesthetics are done with IV access because of the need to rapidly administer medications and fluids during most surgical procedures.
(1) For healthy patients having procedures without the potential for blood loss (e.g., carpal tunnel, cataract surgery), one 20- or 22-G IV is likely adequate.
(2) For patients with comorbidities and/or having a more invasive procedure, one to two 18- to 20-G IVs is likely adequate.
(3) An additional IV can be placed intraoperatively, provided there is reasonable access to the patient's arms, legs, or neck.
(4) Large bore IV access (14 to 16-G) should be considered in situations with the potential for large blood loss or fluid shifts.
ii) Occasionally, it can be difficult to establish IV access in patients.
(1) Consider warming the extremity.
(2) Consider using ultrasound to assist in locating deeper veins.
(3) Consider establishing external jugular or central venous access.

b) **Selection of patient monitors**
i) Routine monitors
(1) ASA standard monitors should be used as minimum standards for all general, regional, and MAC anesthetic techniques.
ii) Special monitors
(1) Consider additional monitoring such as intra-arterial catheterization when consistent and continuous monitoring of blood pressure is needed (e.g., hemodynamic management during neurosurgery, patients at risk for myocardial or end-organ ischemia)
(2) Consider CVP monitoring in patients at risk for bleeding or in whom central venous pressures may be useful in guiding intraoperative fluid management.

READ MORE

Standard ASA monitors, Chapter 8, page 55

Intra-arterial monitoring, Chapter 29, page 220

Intravenous induction agents, Chapter 43, page 306

c) **Induction of GA**
i) Induction of anesthesia means administering anesthetic drugs to induce a state of anesthesia.
(1) Typically, induction of anesthesia implies GA and inducing a state of unconsciousness.
(2) Alternatively, induction of anesthesia may be qualified as induction of spinal anesthesia or induction of regional anesthesia, where surgical anesthesia is induced but the patient remains conscious.
ii) **Premedications prior to induction of GA**
Whenever premedications are given, the patient should be in a monitored setting with emergency airway equipment and reversal medications available.
(1) Anxiolytic drugs (e.g., benzodiazepines) can be administered to ease anxiety during transport to the operating room prior to induction.
(a) For pediatric patients, **oral midazolam** 0.5 mg/kg up to 20 mg. Some children may develop paradoxical hyperactivity.

        (b) For adults, starting doses of 0.5 to 2 mg **IV midazolam** can be titrated upward to effect. Chronic benzodiazepine or heavy alcohol users may require larger doses. Decrease or consider omitting benzodiazepines in the elderly patients with OSA or those with neurological impairment (2).

    (2) Antiemetic drugs (e.g., scopolamine) can be administered to prevent postoperative nausea and vomiting in at-risk patients.

        (a) **Scopolamine** transdermal patch (1.5 mg) is applied to the post-auricular area to prevent postoperative nausea and vomiting.

           (i) It is an anticholinergic agent and common side effects include dry mouth, drowsiness, blurred vision, sedation, and dilated pupils.

          (ii) It is contraindicated in patients <18 years of age and patients with glaucoma (3).

    (3) Antisialogogue drugs (e.g., glycopyrrolate) can be useful for patients undergoing fiberoptic bronchoscopy (FOB).

        (a) **Glycopyrrolate** is an anticholinergic (0.2 to 0.4 mg IV) used to decrease salivary, bronchial, and GI secretions.

        (b) Unlike scopolamine, it is a quaternary amine, so it does not cross the blood–brain barrier and cause central nervous system effects (2).

    (4) **Ketamine** can be used for its **bronchodilating properties** and therefore may be helpful for asthmatic patients.

    (5) **Dexmedetomidine** can cause significant bradycardia and hypotension but does not cause respiratory depression, so it can be a useful adjunct for an awake FOB.

    (6) Agents can be administered prior to induction of GA to **ablate the hemodynamic response to laryngoscopy (5,6).**

        (a) Opioids

           (i) Fentanyl: 1.5 to 5 μg/kg IV bolus (titrate dose upward for chronic opioid users)

          (ii) Remifentanil: 0.5 to 1 μg/kg IV bolus followed by infusion of 0.05 to 0.25 μg/kg/min

         (iii) Alfentanil: 10 to 50 μg/kg

        (b) Beta-adrenergic antagonists

           (i) Esmolol: 0.25 to 0.5 mg/kg IV bolus

  iii) **Induction of intravenous GA**

    (1) A wide variety of intravenous induction agents are available that each have advantages and disadvantages that depend on their unique pharmacokinetic and pharmacodynamic differences.

        (a) See chapter on Intravenous Induction Agents for a detailed discussion of these drugs.

    (2) **Standard induction of intravenous GA**

        (a) **Place standard ASA monitors,** special monitoring if indicated.

        (b) **Position patient in proper "sniffing position"**

        (c) **Baseline vital signs should be obtained prior to induction.** Consider measuring blood pressure every 1 minute during induction and intubation.

        (d) **Confirm MSMAIDS Algorithm (Table 1-2).**

READ MORE

Opioids,
Chapter 41,
page 299

Endotracheal
intubation,
Chapter 20,
page 137

Blood pressure should be measured every minute during induction to monitor for signs of hemodynamic instability.

ANESTHESIOLOGY

Table 1-2

MSMAIDS Algorithm Prior to Induction

Machine checked	Confirm high flow oxygen present Ambu Bag or device to provide positive pressure mask ventilation present Anesthesia machine functional
Suction on	Yankauer suction catheter at patient's head Audible and palpable suction present at catheter tip
Monitors on	Current vital signs are displayed Know patient's baseline vital signs Noninvasive blood pressure every 1 minute
Airway equipment	Oral airways immediately available Intubating equipment ready
IV access	IV runs freely to gravity into patient Adequate amount of IV fluid in bag
Drugs	Induction agent Neuromuscular blocking agent Narcotics Emergency drugs (e.g., ephedrine, phenylephrine)
Special	Any extra equipment that is anticipated for case

(e) **Preoxygenation** for 8 deep breaths over 60 seconds or 100% FiO_2 for 3 minutes is advisable (7,8).

(f) **Titrate IV induction agent to effect.**
  (i) Administer initial dose estimated based on weight and other factors such as age and amount of premedication.
  (ii) Administer additional small doses if the initial dose does not induce unconsciousness.
  (iii) Testing of eyelash reflex (reflex motion of the eyelid to stroking of the eyelash) can aid in assessing level of consciousness.

READ
MORE

Atlas of anesthe-
sia procedures:
mask ventilation,
Chapter 152,
page 1097

(g) **Administer neuromuscular blocking agent.**
  (i) Consider confirming the ability to ventilate the patient with positive pressure mask ventilation prior to administering neuromuscular blocking agent.
  (ii) Supraglottic airway devices such as LMAs do not usually require neuromuscular blocking agents for placement.

(h) **Mask ventilation**
  (i) Provide positive pressure mask ventilation to ensure adequate oxygenation and ventilation during induction.
  (ii) Please refer to mask ventilation cognitive aid for additional instruction.

(i) **Proceed with airway instrumentation**

(i) Once optimal intubating conditions have been achieved through adequate neuromuscular blockade, airway instrumentation and intubation can proceed.

(ii) Placement of supraglottic airway devices can proceed after adequate induction of anesthesia.

(3) **Rapid sequence induction (RSI)**

(a) A method of rapidly inducing GA and neuromuscular blockade to quickly provide optimal intubating conditions while minimizing risk of aspiration

(b) Indications for RSI include:

(i) Significant gastroesophageal reflux disease

(ii) Full stomach (Table 1-3)

(iii) Ileus or "acute abdomen"

(iv) Hiatal hernia

(v) Acute trauma

(vi) Pregnancy past first trimester

(vii) Diabetes mellitus

(c) **Performing RSI**

READ MORE

Endotracheal intubation, Chapter 20, page 137

(i) **Consider premedication for aspiration prophylaxis.**

　1. Nonparticulate antacid (e.g., 0.3 M Sodium citrate 30 cc)

　2. Metoclopramide 10 mg IV

　3. H_2 receptor antagonist (e.g., Ranitidine 50 mg IV)

(ii) Confirm **MSMAIDS** algorithm (Table 1-2).

(iii) **Place standard ASA monitors**, special monitoring if indicated.

(iv) Position patient in proper "sniffing position."

(v) **Baseline vital signs should be obtained prior to induction.** Consider measuring blood pressure every 1 minute during induction and intubation.

Table 1-3

ASA Fasting Guidelines to Reduce Risk of Pulmonary Aspiration (11)

Ingested Material	Minimum Fasting Period (h)
Clear liquids	2
Breast milk	4
Infant formula	6
Nonhuman milk	6
Light meal[a]	6
Heavy meal[b]	8

[a]Clear liquid and toast.
[b]Fried or fatty foods.

The 10N of force required for cricoid pressure is the amount of pressure required to depress the cartilage on the tip of your nose.

(vi) **Preoxygenation** for 8 deep breaths over 60 seconds or 100% FiO$_2$ for 3 minutes is advisable (7,8).

(vii) **Apply cricoid pressure**: a technique performed by an assistant that is used to occlude the esophagus during intubation to prevent passive regurgitation of gastric contents and to decrease the chance of pulmonary aspiration

   1. It has been suggested to apply 10 Newtons (N) of force to the awake patient and 30 N to the unconscious patient (9).

   2. If cricoid pressure obstructs the laryngoscopic view, pressure should be released.

(viii) **Administer precalculated dose of induction agent** (i.e., no titration).

   1. Suggested dosing for hemodynamically stable healthy adults includes propofol 2 to 3 mg/kg IV.

   2. For hemodynamically compromised patients, consider etomidate 10 mg IV.

(ix) **Follow immediately with neuromuscular blockade**: succinylcholine if not contraindicated 0.6 to 1 mg/kg (10) or Rocuronium 1.2 mg/kg IV.

   1. **Use of 1.5 to 2** times the effective intubating dose (ED$_{95}$) of a neuromuscular blocking agent can be used (at the risk/expense of prolonged paralysis—which may be an issue if the patient is difficult to intubate or mask ventilate).

(x) **No mask ventilation is performed prior to first laryngoscopy.**

(xi) **Cricoid pressure should not be released** until ETT placement is confirmed by auscultation and capnography.

(4) **Modified RSI**

  (a) The potential risks of RSI (inability to ventilate, hemodynamic instability, trauma to the airway) may not be warranted in patients who are at low risk for pulmonary aspiration.

  (b) In these cases, a modified RSI can be performed, which minimizes these risks to the patient.

  (c) The RSI technique is most commonly modified by

    (i) Performing gentle positive-pressure ventilation before tracheal intubation

    (ii) Ideally, peak pressures should be <20 mm Hg (closing pressure of the lower esophageal sphincter).

iv) **Inhalational induction**

  (1) Anesthesia is induced by inhalation of volatile anesthetic gases.

  (2) Commonly used in pediatric patients who cannot tolerate intravenous line placement prior to induction of anesthesia

  (3) May also be used in adult patients who present with

    (a) Difficult IV access

    (b) Severe anxiety and phobia of needles precluding IV placement

    (c) Airway anatomy such as airway tissues that may collapse and cause obstruction with loss of spontaneous ventilation

  (4) Cannot be used as the induction agent for RSI

  (5) **Technique**

    (a) Follow standard IV induction technique as described above.

        (b) Instead of administering IV induction agent, slowly administer an increasing dose of volatile anesthetic.

           (i) Sevoflurane is a desirable agent because it has a less pungent odor than other volatile anesthetics and decreases airway irritation.

           (ii) Increase dose until patient loses consciousness.

           (iii) It is advisable to maintain contact with vaporizer dial until GA is induced and then dial down anesthetic dose prior to removing your hand.

               1. This will reduce the chance of inadvertant overdose by forgetting to turn down anesthetic dose after induction.

           (iv) A N_2O/O_2/sevoflurane induction can be used, which will provide a more rapid inhalation induction due to the second gas effect, but this must be weighed against the benefit of inducing a patient on 100% FiO_2.

        (c) Once the patient is induced, you may establish intravenous access and proceed with your anesthetic plan.

    d) **Maintenance of anesthesia plan**

       i) Maintenance of anesthesia involves maintaining the state of surgical anesthesia for the duration of the procedure. Plans should be made for the maintenance of anesthesia during the surgical procedure.

       ii) This usually involves administration of volatile or intravenous anesthetic agents.

       iii) Different methods for maintenance of anesthesia have benefits and limitations that may be more ideally suited to certain patients and procedures. This topic is discussed in depth in the "Intraoperative Management and Maintenance of Anesthesia" of Chapter 3.

    e) **Emergence from anesthesia plan**

       i) Emergence from GA involves waking the patient up at the end of the procedure and removing the airway device in a manner that is safe and minimizes postoperative complications. Plans for the emergence from anesthesia should be discussed with the surgeon to minimize postoperative complications.

READ MORE
Postoperative nausea and vomiting, Chapter 7, page 47

           (1) Issues can include whether the patient should be extubated fully awake or unconscious during stage III anesthesia (deep extubation).

       ii) A detailed discussion of this topic is covered in Chapter 4, Emergence and Post-operative Issues in Anesthesia

       iii) PONV prophylaxis should be considered prior to emergence in at-risk patients.

  4) **Postoperative care plan**

    a) Postoperative care of a patient involves managing the patient's recovery from anesthetic drugs and procedures and managing postsurgical pain. Plans for postoperative care should be discussed with the surgeon and the postoperative care unit nursing staff.

       i) Issues can include treatment of postoperative anesthetic complications such as shivering or nausea and vomiting.

       ii) Pain control

       iii) Discharge to appropriate facilities based on the patient's condition (e.g., home, ward, monitored bed).

    b) A detailed discussion of this topic is covered in the chapter on "Emergence and Postoperative Issues in Anesthesia."

Chapter Summary for the Anesthetic Plan and Induction of Anesthesia

Anesthetic Plan	The **anesthetic plan** describes how the anesthesiologist will conduct an individual care plan that is tailored to the patient and surgeon's specific needs while also insuring a **safe perioperative experience.** **A successful anesthetic plan requires consideration of preoperative, intraoperative and postoperative management.**
Induction of Anesthesia	Induction of GA involves administering anesthetic drugs to induce a **state of unconsciousness.**
Induction Agents	**GA** can be induced using intravenous drugs or inhalational agents. IV agents are most commonly used for adults.
Induction Techniques	**Standard induction** techniques involve preoxygenation, administration of IV induction agent±neuromuscular blocking agents and ventilation of the patient prior to airway management. **Rapid sequence intubation** techniques are used to protect the patient from aspiration.

References

1. Position on Monitored Anesthesia Care. Committee on Economics. American Society of Anesthesiology. Approved October 21, 1986, amended on October 25, 2005 and last updated on September 2, 2008. http://www.asahq.org/publicationsAndServices/standards/23.pdf.
2. White PF, Eng MR. Intravenous anesthetics. In: Barash PG, Cullen BG, Stoelting RF, et al. eds. *Clinical Anesthesia*. 6th ed. Philadelphia, PA: Lippincott Williams & Wilkins; 2009:444–464.
3. Transdermal scopolamine [package insert]. Parsippany, NJ: Novartis; 2006.
4. Precedex [package insert]. Lake Forest, IL: Hospira, Inc.; 2008.
5. Johnson JO, Grecu L, Lawson NW. Autonomic nervous system. In: Barash PG, Cullen BG, Stoelting RF, et al. eds. *Clinical Anesthesia*. 6th ed. Philadelphia, PA: Lippincott Williams & Wilkins; 2009:326–368.
6. Coda BA. Opioids. In: Barash PG, ed. *Clinical Anesthesia*. 6th ed. Philadelphia, PA: Lippincott Williams & Wilkins; 2009:465–497.
7. Baraka AS, Taha SK, Aouad MT, et al. Preoxygenation: comparison of maximal breathing and tidal volume breathing techniques. *Anesthesiology* 1999;91:612–616.
8. Valentine SJ, Marjot R, Monk CR. Preoxygenation in the elderly: a comparison of the four-maximal breath and three-minute techniques. *Anesth Analg* 1990;71:516–519.
9. Vanner RG, Asai T. Safe use of cricoid pressure. *Anaesthesia* 1999;54:1–3.
10. Kopman AF, Zhaku B, Lai KS. The intubating dose of succinylcholine. *Anesthesiology* 2003;99:1050–1054.
11. ASA Taskforce on Preoperative Fasting. Practice guidelines for preoperative fasting and the use of pharmacologic agents to reduce the risk of pulmonary aspiration: application to healthy patients undergoing elective procedures. *Anesthesiology* 1999;90:896–905.

2 Preanesthesia Assessment

Jonathan Hastie, MD · Danielle B. Ludwin, MD

The preanesthesia assessment is an essential part of perioperative care. The anesthesiologist assesses the patient's medical history, performs a focused physical exam, and considers the nature of the proposed procedure in order to formulate an anesthetic plan. The patient's medical status should be optimized in order to provide safe and effective care. This may include immediate interventions such as anxiolysis, IV volume administration, or better control of blood pressure or blood glucose. Occasionally, the procedure must be delayed or postponed for further interventions or testing. The preanesthesia assessment is also an opportunity to educate the patient. This chapter reviews indications for preoperative testing, guidelines for the prevention of pulmonary aspiration, and the American Society of Anesthesiologists (ASA) physical status classification.

Formulating an anesthetic plan requires a history, physical exam, and consideration of the proposed procedure.

Consent for anesthesia care typically occurs during the preanesthesia assessment.

READ MORE

The anesthetic plan, Chapter 1, page 1

Allergy and anaphylaxis, Chapter 67, page 484

1) **Overview:** The ASA has published basic standards for a preanesthesia evaluation (1). These are considered to be minimal acceptable requirements and include:
   a) Determining the medical status of the patient
      i) Reviewing available medical records
      ii) Performing a history and physical exam
      iii) Pursuing further studies or consultations as indicated
   b) Developing an anesthesia plan, including the following:
      i) Ordering premedication
      ii) Obtaining consent for anesthesia care
      iii) Proper documentation in the medical record
2) **The medical history** allows the physician to assess the patient's current medical condition. Essential features include:
   a) Signs and symptoms related to the planned operation
   b) Surgical and anesthesia history, including personal and family history of anesthetic complications
   c) Focused review of systems (Table 2-1).
   d) Medications and allergies
      i) Inquiry should be complete and updated.
      ii) Strive to use generic names for clearer communication
      iii) Include both nonprescription and herbal therapies
      iv) Consider potential for drug interactions and side effects
      v) If the patient reports a history of allergic reaction, the type of reaction should be documented whenever possible.

Table 2-1
Basic Review of Systems

Neuromuscular: History of stroke or seizure. Alcohol or recreational drug use. History of weakness or nerve injury.

Respiratory: History of asthma, chronic obstructive pulmonary disease, snoring, or obstructive sleep apnea. History of recent respiratory tract infection. Tobacco use. Exercise tolerance.

Cardiac: History of hypertension or coronary artery disease. Heart failure symptoms: shortness of breath, orthopnea, paroxysmal nocturnal dyspnea. Palpitations, chest pain, or chest pressure. Exercise tolerance.

Endocrine: History of diabetes or high cholesterol.

Renal: History of kidney disease.

Liver: History of liver disease or hepatitis. History of pancreatic disease.

Gastric: History of gastroesophageal reflux disease (GERD) or hiatal hernia.

Hematologic: History of blood disorders or on anticoagulant medication.

Obstetric: For female patient, history of pregnancy, last menstrual period.

The physical examination should confirm and focus the information learned in the medical history.

3) **The physical examination** should generally confirm and focus the information learned in the medical history. It should include the following:
   a) Vital signs
   b) Global exam (Table 2-2)
   c) Comprehensive airway assessment (see 7.a. "Specific Considerations: Airway Examination").
   d) Neurological exam
      i) Mental status
      ii) Gross sensory and motor exam
      iii) Closer examination of focal neurological deficits
   e) Cardiac exam
      i) Auscultation for heart sounds
      ii) Quality of the heart sounds
      iii) Heart rate
      iv) Regularity
      v) Presence of subcutaneous pacemaker or other implantable cardiac device

READ
MORE

Cardiac arrhythmias and pacemakers, Chapter 57, page 412

Table 2-2
Global Exam

On entering a patient's room, the following things can often be assessed with a moment of observation
- General health and appearance
- Level of consciousness and state of distress
- Affect and posture
- Support of family, friends, or caretakers
- Accessory devices, such as a cane or wheelchair to assist ambulation

f) Pulmonary exam
  i) Auscultation for lung sounds
  ii) Assess respiratory effort
  iii) Respiratory rate
g) General exam *consider including the following:*
  i) Abdominal exam
    (1) Auscultation of bowel sounds
    (2) Assess for tenderness or guarding
    (3) Evaluate for the presence of ascites or distension
  ii) Extremity and skin exam
    (1) Signs of peripheral perfusion: temperature, capillary refill
    (2) Peripheral edema
    (3) Skin breakdown and rashes
    (4) Topical medications and patches
  iii) Musculoskeletal exam
    (1) Gait
    (2) Orthopaedic injuries or braces
    (3) Prosthetic devices

A chest radiograph should be considered for patients with cardiac or pulmonary disease.

4) Review any investigations that are available.
  a) None of the following is required for a generally healthy patient, but available studies should be noted.
  b) Table 2-3 contains ASA recommendations for ordering preoperative tests.
  c) Laboratory assessments that should be considered
    i) An electrolyte panel for patients on diuretics or angiotensin converting enzyme inhibitors
    ii) Electrolytes with blood urea nitrogen and creatinine for patients with cardiac, liver, or kidney disease
    iii) A complete blood count (CBC) for patients with hematologic disease or very old or very young patients
    iv) A basic metabolic panel, CBC, and coagulation studies for patients with liver disease
    v) Blood glucose level for patients with diabetes
  d) A chest radiograph should be considered for patients with acute or chronic pulmonary disease, as well as for patients with cardiac disease.
  e) An electrocardiogram (ECG) should be obtained for patients with a known history of cardiac disease or pulmonary disease and for patients with advanced age. An ECG should be considered for patients with coronary artery disease risk factors, such as hypertension, diabetes, or kidney disease.
    i) Other available imaging studies

An ECG should be obtained for patients with cardiac disease or pulmonary disease.

Every investigation should be guided by an analysis of the potential benefits of additional information while weighing the cost and possible risks of the investigation.

Always review any available anesthetic records for a history of difficult airway or other complications.

The urgency of a surgical procedure may preclude consultation with medical specialists.

5) **Review available prior anesthetic records** for the following:
  a) Airway complications
    i) Difficulty securing airway
    ii) Airway reactivity
  b) Anesthesia complications
    i) Allergies
    ii) Medication reactions
    iii) Hemodynamic instability
    iv) Postoperative nausea and vomiting
    v) Postoperative awareness
    vi) Delayed awakening
    vii) Postoperative delirium

   c) Surgical complications
      i) Bleeding
      ii) Infection
   d) Difficult postoperative pain management
6) Indications for additional information
   a) Further laboratory investigations, physiological tests, or imaging studies, should only be requested as guided by the history and physical examination.
   b) No specific study is required for every patient undergoing anesthesia care.
   c) Every investigation should be guided by an analysis of the potential benefits of additional information (Table 2-3). This is weighed against the cost and possible risks, such as delay of the procedure or hazards inherent to the study (1).

Table 2-3

Responders to a Survey of ASA Members Typically Consider Ordering Tests Based on the Indications Listed After Each Test

A. ECG
   1. Advanced age
   2. Known cardiac disease
   3. Known pulmonary disease
B. Chest radiograph
   1. Known pulmonary disease
   2. Smoking
   3. Recent respiratory tract infection
   4. Known cardiac disease
C. Pulmonary function test
   1. Reactive airway disease
   2. Chronic obstructive pulmonary disease
   3. Restrictive lung disease, such as scoliosis
D. Hemoglobin and hematocrit
   1. Extremes of age (very young or old)
   2. Anemia
   3. Liver disease
   4. Bleeding disorders
E. Coagulation studies
   1. Bleeding disorders
   2. Kidney disease
   3. Liver disease
   4. Anticoagulant medications
F. Serum electrolytes
   1. Endocrine disease
   2. Kidney disease
   3. Medications
G. Pregnancy test
   1. Consider for all female patients of childbearing age
   2. Unclear pregnancy history
   3. Pregnancy likely by history

The ASA Taskforce recommends testing based *only* on the **bolded** indications.
Adapted from Practice Advisory for Preanesthesia Evaluation. *Anesthesiology* 2002;96:485–496.

Consider a pregnancy test for all female patients of childbearing age.

The anesthesiologist is a perioperative medicine consultant who actively assesses disease severity, evaluates adequacy of management, and detects unrecognized disease.

d) Consider consultation with medical specialists if the adequacy of disease management is unclear. The urgency of a procedure may preclude consultation.

7) Specific considerations

a) Airway examination. This remains the most crucial component of the physical exam, because it determines how the airway is managed throughout the perioperative period.

    i) Components and predictors of difficult airway

        (1) High Mallampati classification (Fig. 2-1)

        (2) Small mouth opening

        (3) Prominent upper incisors

        (4) Thyromental distance <6 cm

        (5) Decreased neck extension

    ii) **Mallampati classification scheme (Fig. 2-1)**, which categorizes the approximate ratio of the size of the tongue to the oropharynx

    iii) The anesthesiologist should use these components to obtain a gestalt of the patient's airway anatomy. The composite impression is more predictive than any one component of the ease or difficulty in securing an endotracheal tube (2).

    iv) Other considerations

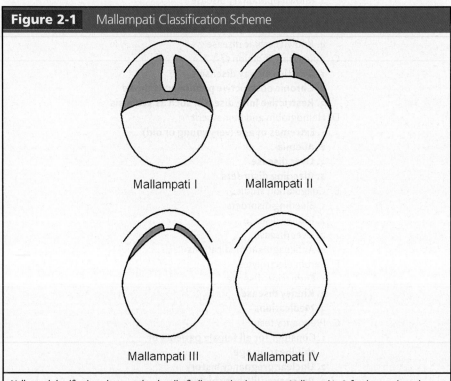

| **Figure 2-1** | Mallampati Classification Scheme |

Mallampati I

Mallampati II

Mallampati III

Mallampati IV

Mallampati classification scheme used to describe findings on the airway exam. Mallampati I - Soft palate, uvula, and tonsillar pillars seen. Mallampati II - Soft palate and uvula seen. Mallampati III - Soft palate and base of uvula seen. Mallampati IV - Hard palate only seen. Illustration by Jonathan Hastie.

Table 2-4

Nil Per Os (NPO) Guidelines and Pulmonary Aspiration Precautions, Summarized from ASA Published Practice Guidelines

Preanesthesia assessment: History, physical exam, review of available medical records. Screen for GERD, dysphagia, and diseases of gastric motility which may increase the risk of aspiration.

Fasting guidelines	
Clear fluids	At least 2 h for all patients
Breast milk	4 h for neonates and infants
Infant formula	6 h
Light food (toast, crackers, fruit)	6 h
Heavy food (fatty foods, meat)	8 h

Medications: Not recommended for routine use in patients with no increased risk of pulmonary aspiration.

Gastric motility agents	May reduce gastric volume, but not acidity
Inhibitors of acid secretion	Reduce gastric volume and acidity
Antacids	Reduce gastric acidity, but not volume. If indicated for other reasons, use nonparticulate antacids.

Adapted from practice guidelines for preoperative fasting and the use of pharmacologic agents to reduce the risk of pulmonary aspiration: application to healthy patients undergoing elective procedures. *Anesthesiology* 1999;90:896–905.

READ MORE

Difficult airway, Chapter 210, page 1326

If evidence of cervical spinal cord compromise— the spinal cord should be protected during manipulation of the airway with techniques such as manual in-line stabiliza- tion or fiberop- tic intubation or keeping a cervical spine collar in place.

(1)   Consider cervical spinal cord compromise based on history and physical examination. If evidence of spinal cord involvement exists, care should be taken to protect the spinal cord during manipulation of the airway, such as by cervical spine collar, manual in-line stabilization, or fiberoptic intubation.

(2)   In patients with preexisting airways (such as an endotracheal or tracheostomy tube), document the following:

   (a)   Indication and date of placement

   (b)   Ease of placement

   (c)   Size of device

   (d)   Presence of cuff

b)   Prevention of pulmonary aspiration

  i)   Pulmonary aspiration of gastric contents may lead to significant complications, including pneumonitis, superimposed infection, prolonged intubation, and death.

  ii)   The ASA has published guidelines to assist the perioperative physician in avoiding aspiration of gastric contents (Table 2-4) (3).

  iii)   In the context of urgent surgery, one should analyze the risks and benefits of proceeding with versus delaying surgery. In some cases, this may lead to the decision to modify or reject the recommendations.

  iv)   These guidelines are intended for healthy patients. Disease or physiological states that lead to increased gastric volume or acidity may prompt the anesthesiologist to practice with increased level of precaution.

Table 2-5

Screening Evaluation for the Cardiovascular System

Uncontrolled hypertension
Unstable cardiac disease
   Unstable angina
   Congestive heart failure
   Valvular heart disease
   Cardiac dysrhythmias
Auscultation of the heart
Carotid bruits
Peripheral pulses

Reproduced from Preoperative evaluation and management. In: Barash PG, Cullen BF, Stoelting RK, eds. *Handbook of Clinical Anesthesia*. 5th ed. Philadelphia, PA: Lippincott Williams & Wilkins; 2006:272–294, with permission.

8) Cardiac disease (Table 2-5)

READ MORE

Ischemic heart disease, Chapter 51, page 359

Valvular heart disease, Chapter 53, page 375

Heart failure, Chapter 60, page 436

Patients with unstable coronary syndrome, decompensated heart failure, significant arrhythmias, or severe valvular disease warrant further workup unless emergent surgery is indicated.

a) The American College of Cardiology (ACC) and American Heart Association (AHA) have jointly published guidelines for a perioperative cardiac examination for patients undergoing noncardiac surgery (4).

   i) Unless emergent surgery is indicated, patients with the following active conditions should have further testing and management prior to surgery, according to ACC/AHA guidelines (Fig. 2-2).

      (1) Unstable coronary syndrome (myocardial infarction within 1 month or unstable angina)

      (2) Decompensated heart failure

      (3) Significant arrhythmias

      (4) Severe valvular disease

   ii) The type of surgery must be considered in the cardiac risk assessment.

      (1) **Vascular surgery**

        (a) Reported cardiac risk >5%

        (b) Includes open aortic and other major vascular surgery

      (2) **Intermediate risk surgery**

        (a) Reported cardiac risk 1% to 5%

        (b) Includes intraperitoneal and intrathoracic surgery, head and neck surgery, carotid endarterectomy, and orthopaedic surgery

      (3) **Low risk surgery**

        (a) Includes superficial and endoscopic procedures, breast surgery, and most ambulatory surgery

   iii) In the absence of the aforementioned active conditions, most patients undergoing low-risk surgery may proceed.

   iv) **Exercise tolerance is a critical component of cardiac risk assessment** (Table 2-6).

      (1) One metabolic equivalent (MET) is approximately 3.5 mL/kg/min of oxygen, the amount an average size 40-year-old man uses at rest.

      (2) Patients who are able to perform >4 METs of exercise without symptoms may likely proceed to surgery.

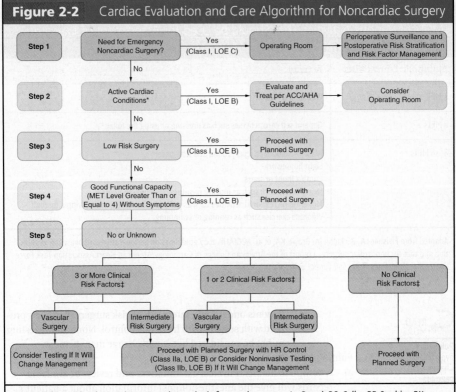

Figure 2-2   Cardiac Evaluation and Care Algorithm for Noncardiac Surgery

From Mantha S, Ochroch EA, Roizen MF, et al. Anesthesia for vascular surgery. In: Barash PG, Cullen BF, Stoelting RK, et al, eds. *Clinical Anesthesia*. 6th ed. Philadelphia, PA: Lippincott Williams & Wilkins/Wolters Kluwer Health; 2009:1113.

The planned operation is an important criterion for evaluating patients with poor exercise tolerance and three or more clinical risk factors.

v) Patients with poor exercise tolerance (<4 METs) and no clinical cardiac risk factors may proceed. Clinical risk factors include the following:
   (1) History of ischemic heart disease
   (2) Compensated or prior heart failure
   (3) History of cerebrovascular disease
   (4) Diabetes mellitus
   (5) Renal insufficiency

b) Patients with poor exercise tolerance and one or two clinical risk factors undergoing vascular or intermediate risk surgery may likely proceed with surgery. Noninvasive testing might be considered if it would change management.
   i) The planned operation is important for evaluating patients with poor exercise tolerance and three or more clinical risk factors.
      (1) Patients undergoing vascular surgery should have further testing if it would change management.

Table 2-6

METs of Various Activities That Should be Used for Assessment of Exercise Tolerance

Metabolic Equivalents	Activity
1 MET	Watching television
4 METs	General self care activities such as dressing or using the toilet
8–10 METs	Walk 1–2 blocks on level ground at a slow pace Light housework Climb a flight of stairs Heavy housework such as moving furniture or scrubbing floors Moderate recreational activities such as golf, doubles tennis, or throwing a football Vigorous exercise such as running or swimming

Adapted from Fleisher LA, Beckman JA, Brown KA, et al. ACC/AHA 2007 guidelines on perioperative cardiovascular evaluation and care for noncardiac surgery: a report of the American College of Cardiology/American Heart Association Task Force on Practice Guidelines. *J Am Coll Cardiol* 2007;50:e159–e242.

READ MORE

Pulmonary hypertension, Chapter 62, page 447

(2) Patients undergoing intermediate risk surgery may likely proceed with surgery with heart rate control. Noninvasive testing might be considered if it would change management.

9) Pulmonary disease

a) A complete history, physical examination, and review of available records will give the anesthesiologist information about a patient's pulmonary status (Table 2-7).

Table 2-7

Screening Evaluation for the Pulmonary System

History
  Shortness of breath (at rest or exertion)
  Cough
  Wheezing
  Stridor
  Snoring or sleep apnea
  Recent respiratory tract infection
Physical examination
  Respiratory rate
  Chest excursion
  Use of accessory muscles
  Nail shape and color
  Ability to walk or talk without dyspnea
  Auscultation

Reproduced from Preoperative evaluation and management. In: Barash PG, Cullen BF, Stoelting RK, eds. *Handbook of Clinical Anesthesia.* 5th ed. Philadelphia, PA: Lippincott Williams & Wilkins; 2006:275, with permission.

Pulmonary function tests are generally indicated for severe reactive airway disease or significant obstructive or restrictive pulmonary disease.

The ASA physical status classification is a general assessment of a patient's health that is useful for concise communication.

b) The anesthesiologist should form an independent assessment of the presence and severity of disease because patients may underestimate disease severity and may unintentionally minimize symptoms.

c) Evaluation for pulmonary disease often has significant implications for selection of anesthetic technique and counseling patients about their intraoperative risk and postoperative course.

d) A pulmonary function test is generally indicated for severe reactive airway disease or significant obstructive or restrictive pulmonary disease (1).

e) For compressing intrathoracic or mediastinal masses, further work-up is indicated, including a thoracic CT scan and flow-volume loops.

10) ASA physical status classification (7)

a) At the conclusion of the preanesthesia assessment, the anesthesiologist should classify the patient according to his or her ASA physical status.

   i) ASA 1 Normal, healthy patient
   ii) ASA 2 Patient with mild systemic disease
   iii) ASA 3 Patient with severe systemic disease
   iv) ASA 4 Patient with life-threatening systemic disease
   v) ASA 5 Patient not expected to survive without the operation
   vi) ASA 6 Brain-dead patient for organ harvest

11) Preoperative assessment of other medical diseases.

This chapter has focused mainly on the cardiac and pulmonary systems. The preanesthesia assessment must be thorough and tailored to the procedure. Each chapter in this book contains a perioperative approach to patients undergoing specific procedures or patients with coexisting disease. Additional information may be obtained throughout this book.

Chapter Summary for Preanesthesia Evaluation

General Principles	Even a generally healthy patient requires a comprehensive evaluation, including history, review of medications and allergies, review of systems, and focused physical exam. A standardized approach to a preanesthesia assessment allows for efficient and thorough evaluation. Actively screen for disease during the preanesthesia evaluation. In the presence of known disease, independently assess the adequacy of disease management. Investigations (labs, imaging) should be guided by an analysis of potential benefits and weighed against the cost and possible risks. Specific consideration must be made to the airway exam to anticipate difficulty with endotracheal intubation. Prevention of pulmonary aspiration requires consideration of NPO guidelines. Screening for and managing cardiac and pulmonary disease requires special attention. All patients should be categorized according to the ASA physical status classification.
Elective Procedures	Require a comprehensive preanesthesia assessment. The patient's medical status should be optimal.
Urgent Procedures	Anesthesia assessment may be more focused and management will require medical judgment.

References

1. ASA Taskforce on Pre-Anesthesia Evaluation. Practice Advisory for Preanesthesia Evaluation. *Anesthesiology* 2002;96:485–496.
2. Shiga T, Wajima Z, Inoue T, et al. Predicting difficult intubation in apparently normal patients. *Anesthesiology* 2005;103:429–437.
3. ASA Taskforce on Preoperative Fasting. Practice Guidelines for preoperative fasting and the use of pharmacologic agents to reduce the risk of pulmonary aspiration: application to healthy patients undergoing elective procedures. *Anesthesiology* 1999;90:896–905.
4. Fleisher LA, Beckman JA, Brown KA, et al. ACC/AHA 2007 guidelines on perioperative cardiovascular evaluation and care for noncardiac surgery: a report of the American College of Cardiology/American Heart Association Task Force on Practice Guidelines. *J Am Coll Cardiol* 2007;50:e159–e242
5. Fleisher LA, Beckman JA, Brown KA, et al. 2009 ACCF/AHA Focused update on perioperative beta blockade incorporated into the ACC/AHA 2007 Guidelines on perioperative cardiovascular evaluation and care for noncardiac surgery. *Circulation* 2009;120:e169–e276.
6. Hata TM, Moyers JR. Preoperative evaluation and management. In: Barash PG, Cullen BF, Stoelting RK, eds. *Handbook of Clinical Anesthesia*. 5th ed. Philadelphia, PA: Lippincott Williams & Wilkins; 2006:272–294.
7. ASA Physical Status Classification System. http://www.asahq.org/clinical/physicalstatus.htm

3

Intraoperative Management and Maintenance of Anesthesia

Arthur Atchabahian, MD

Intraoperative management occurs after induction and prior to emergence from anesthesia. The goals are to maintain surgical anesthesia and physiologic homeostasis. Multiple different techniques may be used and are discussed in this chapter.

1) **Overview**
   a) **Intraoperative management and maintenance** of anesthesia is defined as the management of physiological functions and the maintenance of surgical anesthesia following induction and until emergence.
   b) Several goals include
      i) Maintenance of surgical anesthesia
      ii) Maintenance of physiologic homeostasis
         (1) Hemodynamic parameters (BP, HR) are optimized to ensure adequate tissue perfusion
         (2) Patients under general anesthesia (GA) are unable to protect their airway, and an endotracheal tube or a supraglottic airway has been inserted during induction. Adequate ventilation and oxygenation must be ensured.
         (3) An adequate urine output is a surrogate for euvolemia and end-organ perfusion.
         (4) Plasma electrolytes and glucose levels must be maintained within physiological limits, especially in diabetics and patients undergoing large fluid shifts.
         (5) Temperature maintenance is of critical importance. Active warming is used to compensate for the loss of thermal homeostasis under GA.
      iii) Monitoring is needed to ensure that these goals are met.

2) **Maintenance of surgical anesthesia**
   a) **Maintenance of surgical anesthesia** can be accomplished by the intravenous (IV) and/or inhaled administration of medications in order to provide **unconsciousness** (hypnosis), **immobility**, **analgesia**, and, if needed, **muscle relaxation**. Table 3-1 compares balanced and total IV methods of anesthesia maintenance.
   b) **Hypnosis**
      i) Agents acting primarily at the thalamic and cortical levels and whose main activity is on the **GABA receptor** induce unconsciousness.
      ii) These include inhalation agents, benzodiazepines, propofol, and etomidate.

Maintenance of surgical anesthesia can be accomplished by the IV and/or inhaled administration of medications in order to provide unconsciousness (hypnosis), immobility, analgesia, and, if needed, muscle relaxation.

21

Table 3-1

Comparison of Balanced and IV Techniques of Maintenance of General Anesthesia

Balanced Anesthesia	Total Intravenous Anesthesia
Combines inhaled and IV agents	Only IV agents
Inhalation anesthetic elimination is independent of hepatic or renal function	Hepatic or renal insufficiency can significantly prolong drug effect
Easily adjustable, especially with newer poorly soluble agents (desflurane, sevoflurane)	More difficult to titrate, need to adjust infusion rate over time, occasional delayed awakening
Inhalation anesthetics do not provide postoperative analgesia	Postoperative analgesia by intermediate- or long-acting opioids
Higher incidence of PONV, emergence agitation, postoperative shivering	Recommended if history of PONV; smoother awakening
Low cost if low fresh gas flow is used	Higher cost
Potential for atmospheric pollution, destruction of the ozone layer	Potential for water pollution by phenol metabolites

iii) Amnesia accompanies unconsciousness, although benzodiazepines can provide amnesia while the patient is merely sedated.

c) **Analgesia**

i) Painful surgical stimuli have a number of physiological effects.

(1) They induce a neurohumoral response with activation of the sympathetic nervous system (hypertension, tachycardia), the coagulation cascade (hypercoagulable state), and the stress hormone release (hyperglycemia, protein catabolism, immunosuppression).

(2) Postoperative splinting and ileus are also among the side effects of inadequate analgesia.

Regional anesthesia is superior to opioid administration to block the neurohumoral response to surgical stress.

ii) **The blockade of nociception can be achieved by a conduction block** (peripheral nerve or central neuraxial blockade) **or, pharmacologically**, via agents acting primarily at the level of the spinal cord and the brainstem.

(1) Agents include opioids, nitrous oxide, central alpha-2 agonists, and ketamine.

(2) Regional anesthesia is superior to opioid administration to block the neurohumoral response to surgical stress.

iii) At this time, however, **there is no reliable monitor of the adequacy of analgesia provided during general anesthesia** (1), and clinicians have to rely on surrogates such as heart rate, blood pressure, patient movement, respiratory rate, pupillary size, and responsiveness.

Analgesic administration should take into account the fact that analgesia should extend into the postoperative period.

iv) Analgesic administration should take into account the fact that analgesia should extend into the postoperative period.

(1) Short-acting opioids such as remifentanil may be adequate intraoperatively, but medications with a longer half-life should be titrated at the end of the procedure, depending on how much postoperative pain is expected and on whether the patient is likely to be tolerant to opioids.

Table 3-2

Indications for Intraoperative Neuromuscular Blockade

Abdominal surgery, laparoscopic surgery, intrathoracic surgery
Open eye surgery
Orthopaedic surgery with the need for reduction of bone fragments on which powerful muscles insert
(e.g., femoral shaft fracture)
Facilitation of mechanical ventilation in patients with ALI or ARDS
Need for imaging while holding ventilation (e.g., angiography)

ALI, acute lung injury; ARDS, acute respiratory distress syndrome.

d) **Neuromuscular blockade (NMB)**

   i) Deeper planes of anesthesia cause a central decrease in muscle tone, but medications that block transmission at the neuromuscular junction are used to provide complete muscle relaxation.

   ii) NMB is useful for tracheal intubation and should be considered for any surgical procedure where movement of the patient could be detrimental (e.g., cerebral aneurysm surgery). Table 3-2 summarizes the main indications for NMB.

3) **Monitoring and maintenance of physiologic homeostasis**

   a) **Maintenance of hemodynamic parameters**

   Hypotension in patients on ACE inhibitors can be refractory to vasopressors.

   i) For normotensive patients, Euvolemia should be maintained, taking into account basic metabolism, blood loss, insensible fluid losses, and urine output.

   ii) Hypertensive patients tend to be volume depleted and become hypotensive as the vascular tone is reduced under general anesthesia.

      (1) In these patients, blood pressure is typically labile, and wide swings without clear triggering factors are common.

      (2) Diuretics should be held on the day of surgery to limit hypovolemia.

      (3) Hypotension in patients on ACE inhibitors can be refractory to vasopressors (2).

   iii) Controlled hypotension may be requested by the surgeon to reduce bleeding for procedures such as total hip replacement or extensive spine instrumentation.

      (1) Mean arterial pressure (MAP) should be decreased to a level compatible with adequate end-organ perfusion.

      (2) In young, healthy patients, a MAP of 50 mm Hg is generally safe, but in older, hypertensive patients, a higher MAP will be needed. Especially in the brain, the blood flow autoregulation range will be shifted to the right by chronic hypertension, and the blood flow will be pressure dependent.

   iv) In patients with CAD, the oxygen supply-demand balance should be optimized. ST-segment monitoring allows detection of myocardial ischemia.

   b) **Respiratory**

   i) Controlled ventilation is typically used under GA with endotracheal intubation.

      (1) Minute ventilation should be adjusted to maintain near-normal $PaCO_2$.

      (2) A high FiO_2 as well as PEEP may be needed to maintain oxygenation in the face of atelectasis in the dependent regions of the lungs.

ii) When possible, spontaneous ventilation is more physiologic, with less atelectasis and a better ventilation-perfusion matching.

(1) Analgesia can be titrated to the respiratory rate.

c) **Renal**

i) Urine output should be monitored for major procedures, as it is an excellent surrogate for end-organ perfusion.

ii) Patients with preexisting renal insufficiency and those who are hemodynamically unstable are at increased risk of renal failure.

iii) The kidney has a major role in maintaining electrolyte homeostasis.

Patients with preexisting renal insufficiency and those who are hemodynamically unstable are at increased risk of renal failure.

d) **Temperature**

i) Thermal control is impaired under GA, and patients will develop mild hypothermia unless active warming is instituted.

ii) Hypothermia has been shown to impair coagulation, causing increased blood loss and transfusion requirements, and to lead to a higher frequency of postoperative infection.

iii) In addition, hypothermia will cause shivering postoperatively, increasing severalfold the oxygen consumption and leading to myocardial ischemia in susceptible patients.

Hypothermia can impair coagulation causing increased blood loss and transfusion requirements.

e) **Endocrine**

i) Blood glucose should be measured periodically in diabetic patients, except for short procedures.

ii) Insulin should be administered if needed, either subcutaneously or as an IV infusion.

f) **Neurologic**

↪ READ MORE

Processed EEG and awareness monitoring, Chapter 15, page 96

i) **Monitoring of unconsciousness**

(1) Surface EEG signals processed via proprietary software are used by a number of monitors (e.g., BIS or entropy) to yield a number between 0 and 100.

(2) Maintenance between 40 and 60 should ensure an adequate depth of anesthesia and a rapid emergence.

(3) Numerous causes of errors have been described, the most prominent being the interference of muscular activity and a paradoxical increase in the presence of ketamine.

4) **Practical management**

a) The choice of agents is based on the personal preferences and experience of the anesthesiologist, the patient's comorbidities (especially cardiovascular function), the procedure type and anticipated duration, and the postoperative plan (extubation or not, analgesic requirements, ambulatory or inpatient).

i) Hypnotics are typically administered continuously, by inhalation or IV infusion.

ii) Analgesics and NMB agents can be administered intermittently or by continuous infusion.

The depth of hypnosis, analgesia, and NMB has to be adjusted based on surgical stimulus and patient response.

b) **The depth of hypnosis, analgesia, and NMB has to be adjusted based on surgical stimulus and patient response** (3), titrated up before laryngoscopy and intubation, skin incision, etc., and titrated down when surgical stimulation is low (e.g., draping, waiting for pathology). Figure 3-1 illustrates the variations in the intensity of stimulation and thus the need for anesthetic depth, during a generic surgical procedure.

i) Monitoring anesthesia depth may decrease the amount of hypnotics used, reducing side effects and recovery time while also preventing intraoperative awareness.

Figure 3-1	Schematic Representation of the Intensity of Stimulation and Need for Anesthetic Depth, During a Surgical Procedure

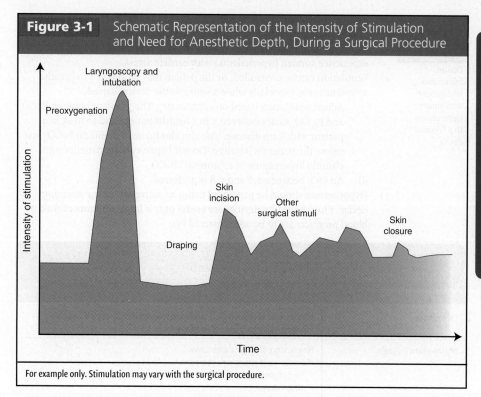

For example only. Stimulation may vary with the surgical procedure.

    ii) Analgesia titration currently relies on surrogate criteria such as hemodynamic response and respiratory rate in spontaneously ventilating patients.

c) Fluid and blood products should be administered to maintain euvolemia and the blood's oxygen-carrying capacity (4).

    i) The patient's baseline metabolic fluid requirement can be estimated using the 4-2-1 rule. Add 4 mL/kg/h for the first 10 kg of body weight, 2 mL/kg/h for the next 10 kg, and then 1 mL/kg/h for the remainder of the body weight. For example, a 70-kg patient needs (4 × 10) + (2 × 10) + (1 × 50) = 110 mL/h of crystalloids.

    ii) The fluid deficit due to the NPO period is estimated by multiplying the baseline requirement by the number of hours the patient has been NPO. Subtract any IV fluid administered. This deficit should be replenished using crystalloids over the first 3 hours, giving 50% in the first hour and 25% each of the next 2 hours.

    iii) Urine output should be replaced by crystalloids mL for mL.

    iv) Insensible fluid loss depends on the procedure and can vary from 0 (carpal tunnel release) to 12 mL/kg/h (open major abdominal surgery). It is due to evaporation and third-space fluid loss because of surgical trauma. It should be replenished mL for mL using crystalloids.

    v) Blood loss should be estimated and compensated, using 3 mL of crystalloid or 1 mL of colloid for each mL of blood loss.

    vi) These calculations should be adjusted based on clinical judgment and patient response (hemodynamics, urine output).

    vii) Red cell transfusion should be considered to maintain the hematocrit above 30% in patients with CAD. A lower hematocrit can be tolerated in healthy patients.

Do not hyperventilate patients with chronic hypercapnia to a "normal" PaCO$_2$.

d) As appropriate, plasma electrolytes and glucose levels should be monitored and corrected. Diabetic patients and those undergoing procedures with large fluid shifts are especially at risk. Transplant recipients can experience sudden hyperkalemia with cardiac arrest.

e) Ventilation can be controlled, or the patient may be allowed to breathe spontaneously, especially when a supraglottic device is used.

   i) Adjust ventilation based on capnometry. The gradient between PaCO$_2$ and P$_{ET}$CO$_2$ varies between 5 in a healthy patient and 10 to 15 in a patient with lung disease. The aim should be to maintain PaCO$_2$ just below the patient's baseline. Do not hyperventilate patients with chronic hypercapnia to a "normal" PaCO$_2$.

   ii) An FiO$_2$ between 0.6 and 0.8 is preferred.

f) Hypothermia should be prevented using an active forced-air warming device. Fluid-warming devices are useful only if large amounts of fluid or blood products are to be administered (5).

Chapter Summary for Intraoperative Management and Maintenance of Anesthesia

Definition	Management of physiological values and maintenance of surgical anesthesia following induction and until emergence.

Maintenance Goals	Maintenance of surgical anesthesia
	Maintenance of physiologic homeostasis
	   Hemodynamic parameters
	   Respiratory
	   Temperature
	   Renal and electrolytes
	Monitoring is needed to ensure that these goals are met.

Maintenance Strategies	IV and/or inhaled administration of medications in order to provide **unconsciousness** (hypnosis), **immobility, analgesia,** and, if needed, **muscle relaxation.** Balanced (combining inhaled and IV agents) or total IV methods of anesthesia maintenance can be used.
Intraoperative Management Issues	The depth of hypnosis, analgesia, and NMB has to be adjusted based on surgical stimulus and patient response. Analgesic administration should take into account the fact that analgesia should extend into the postoperative period. Fluid and blood products should be administered to maintain euvolemia and the blood's oxygen-carrying capacity. Plasma electrolytes and glucose levels should be monitored and corrected. Ventilation can be controlled, or the patient may be allowed to breathe spontaneously, especially when a supraglottic device is used. Hypothermia should be prevented using an active forced-air warming device.

References

1. Guignard B. Monitoring analgesia. *Best Pract Res Clin Anaesthesiol* 2006;20(1):161–180.
2. Rosenman DJ, McDonald FS, Ebbert JO, et al. Clinical consequences of withholding versus administering renin-angiotensin-aldosterone system antagonists in the preoperative period. *J Hosp Med* 2008;3(4):319–325.
3. Shafer SL, Stanski DR. Defining depth of anesthesia. *Handb Exp Pharmacol.* 2008;(182):409–423.
4. Prough DS, Mathru M. Fluid management in critically-ill patients. In: Murray MJ, Coursin DB, Pearl RG, Prough DS, eds. *Critical Care Medicine—Perioperative Management.* 2nd ed. Philadelphia, PA: Lippincott Williams & Wilkins; 2002:137–146.
5. Bissonnette B, Paut O. Active warming of saline or blood is ineffective when standard infusion tubing is used: an experimental study. *Can J Anaesth* 2002;49(3):270–275.

4

Emergence and Postoperative Issues in Anesthesia

Arthur Atchabahian, MD

Emergence is the transition process where a patient goes from general anesthesia to awake and spontaneously breathing. The patient's recovery in the postoperative care unit may also present challenges to the anesthesiologist.

1) **Overview**

a) **Emergence** from anesthesia is the critical period of recovery from general anesthesia, with the return of consciousness, neuromuscular conduction, and airway protective reflexes.

i) **Complications** can occur, for example, airway loss, bronchospasm, laryngospasm, aspiration of gastric contents.

b) A plan for emergence from anesthesia should be developed, considering the surgeon's needs and the patient's comorbidities.

Emergence from anesthesia is the critical period of recovery from general anesthesia, with the return of consciousness, neuromuscular conduction, and airway protective reflexes.

i) **Awake** extubation is the most common choice: the trachea is extubated only when the patient responds to simple commands and is breathing spontaneously.

ii) **Deep** extubation is chosen when the presence of an ETT is to be avoided during emergence, to prevent "bucking" (breathing out of phase with the ventilator such that the patient attempts to exhale when the ventilator is giving a breath) and straining, with the concomitant increase in intra-abdominal, intracranial, and intraocular pressures, and to decrease the risk of bronchospasm.

2) **Evaluation of the signs and stages of anesthesia during emergence**

a) It is important to be able to evaluate a patient's response to anesthetic drugs so that the patient's care may be appropriately managed during emergence from anesthesia.

i) Guedel defined four stages of anesthesia that occur in unpremedicated patients allowed to breathe spontaneously during ether anesthesia (1).

ii) The Guedel system described the respiratory changes, pupillary alterations, eye movements, and changes in vomiting and swallowing responses that occur at various depths of anesthesia.

(1) In modern practice, they are only seen during emergence, as intravenous or inhalation induction is too rapid. In addition, the use of medications such as opioids and neuromuscular blocking agents, as well as the use of mechanical ventilation, make the pupillar changes and the respiratory patterns described by Guedel unreliable.

    (2) Stage 1: Amnesia and analgesia

        (a) From the beginning of induction of anesthesia to loss of consciousness

    (3) Stage 2: Delirium

        (a) From the loss of consciousness to the onset of automatic breathing

        (b) The eyelash reflex disappears but other reflexes remain intact.

        (c) Coughing, vomiting, and struggling may occur.

        (d) Respiration can be irregular, with breath holding.

    (4) Stage 3: Surgical anesthesia

        (a) Plane I—sleep

Stage II is described as an excitement period with irregular breathing and possible agitation, laryngospasm, and regurgitation.

            (i) From the onset of automatic respiration to the cessation of eye movements

           (ii) Eyelid reflex is lost, swallowing reflex disappears, and marked eye movement may occur.

          (iii) The conjunctival reflex is lost at the bottom of the plane.

        (b) Plane II—sensory loss

             (i) From the cessation of eye movements to the beginning of **intercostal muscle paralysis**

           (ii) Laryngeal reflex is lost, although inflammation of the upper respiratory tract increases reflex irritability.

          (iii) Corneal reflex disappears

          (iv) Tear secretion increases

           (v) Respiration is automatic and regular

          (vi) Movement and deep breathing as a response to skin stimulation disappear

Extubation should be performed only once Stage I is reached, that is, eyes have returned to a central position, breathing is regular, and consciousness returns.

        (c) Plane III—loss of muscle tone

             (i) From the beginning to the completion of intercostal muscle paralysis

           (ii) Diaphragmatic respiration persists, but there is progressive intercostal paralysis.

          (iii) Pupils are dilated and light reflex is abolished.

          (iv) The laryngeal reflex lost in plane II can still be initiated by painful stimuli. This was the desired plane for surgery when muscle relaxants were not used.

        (d) Plane IV—intercostal paralysis

             (i) From complete intercostal paralysis to diaphragmatic paralysis (apnea)

    (5) Stage 4: Medullary paralysis

        (a) From the arrest of respiration until death

        (b) Anesthetic overdose causes medullary paralysis with respiratory arrest and vasomotor collapse.

        (c) Pupils are widely dilated and muscles are relaxed.

  b) **Stage II is described as an excitement period with irregular breathing and possible agitation, laryngospasm, and regurgitation.**

  c) **Extubation should be performed only once Stage I is reached, that is, eyes have returned to a central position, breathing is regular, and consciousness returns.**

    i) The main rationale is to keep the patient's airway secure and protected during Stage II, with its risk of laryngospasm and vomiting.

3) **Preparation for emergence**

  a) **Estimate remaining duration** of surgical procedure; decrease concentration of inhaled anesthetic and/or rate of intravenous agent.

b) Do not readminister muscle relaxants; give reversal medications.

c) **Titrate opioids to analgesia** (estimate requirements based on procedure, patient's weight, physiological status and opioid tolerance); if the patient is breathing spontaneously, the respiratory rate can be a useful indicator of adequate analgesia.

d) Administer a 5-HT3 antagonist if indicated to prevent PONV.

e) **Administer 100% oxygen** for 5 to 10 minutes, especially if N_2O used, to prevent hypoxemia.

　　i) If N_2O has been used and the patient is allowed to breathe room air, diffusion hypoxia can occur. N_2O has a low blood:gas partition coefficient and will diffuse rapidly from the blood into the alveoli once administration is discontinued, resulting in the displacement of oxygen in the alveoli.

f) **Return patient to supine or back-up position** prior to extubating. It is possible to extubate in the lateral or even prone position, but provisions should be made to be able to reposition the patient supine emergently if needed.

4) **Extubation criteria** (Table 4-1)

a) **Ensure that all the equipment to reintubate is available prior to extubating!**

b) **Assess the potential for airway obstruction**

　　i) Especially in a patient who has received massive amounts of fluids and/or was positioned head down or prone, significant airway edema can develop and cause airway closure once the ETT is removed, which can result in a difficult or impossible reintubation.

　　ii) Clinical inspection, possibly including direct laryngoscopy under GA to assess the feasibility of reintubation were the need to arise, should evaluate the degree of edema. Clinical judgment should be used to decide whether extubation should be delayed.

　　iii) A leak test can be performed by deflating the ETT cuff (after pharyngeal suctioning) and assessing the presence of a leak around the ETT, indicating the absence of significant airway edema; the predictive value of this test is unclear.

c) Suction pharynx; deflate ETT cuff and pull ETT; continue O_2 administration via nasal cannula or other appropriate device (e.g., face mask if nasal packing following sinus surgery).

d) Reassess consciousness, ventilation, and comfort (pain, shivering).

Ensure that all the equipment to reintubate is available prior to extubating.

Table 4-1
Extubation Criteria

Patient conscious and responding to simple commands ("open your eyes, squeeze my hand"). **If full stomach or high risk of regurgitation, or if difficult intubation, extubate patient only when fully awake.**

Patient hemodynamically stable, normothermic, not having received massive amounts of fluids

Adequate spontaneous ventilation with tidal volumes > 8 mL/kg, rate > 8

Adequate reversal of NMB; **hand strength or TOF not reliable**; sustained head lift or sustained tetanus (painful) for 5 s

5) **Deep extubation**

   a) Indications: Desire to avoid coughing, "bucking," straining, cardiovascular response to the ETT, or bronchospasm in a patient at low risk for aspiration of gastric contents.

   b) Contraindications

      i) Full stomach, severe GERD, other situations where aspiration of gastric contents is a concern

      ii) Difficult intubation

      iii) Obesity, as the redundant pharyngeal tissue may make it very difficult to maintain a patent airway until muscle tone has returned. This is a relative contraindication.

When performing a deep extubation technique, the goal is to extubate the patient during Stage III (surgical anesthesia), not during Stage II.

   c) Uses: Can be used in cases such as an unclipped intracranial aneurysm, reactive airway disease, open-globe eye surgery (1)

   d) Technique

      i) **The goal is to extubate the patient during Stage III (surgical anesthesia), not during Stage II.**

      ii) Face mask

         (1) The patient should not respond to stimulation and should be breathing spontaneously with a regular pattern.

         (2) After oropharyngeal suctioning, the ETT cuff is deflated and the tube is removed.

         (3) Ventilation is assisted as necessary via a facemask until the patient regains consciousness.

         (4) An oral or nasal airway can be placed (2).

      iii) Laryngeal mask: "Bailey maneuver" (3) (Fig. 4-1)

         (1) Following oropharyngeal suctioning, a laryngeal mask device is inserted behind the ETT and the cuff inflated.

         (2) The ETT cuff is deflated and the tube removed. The laryngeal mask is left in place until the patient regains consciousness.

Figure 4-1   Bailey Maneuver

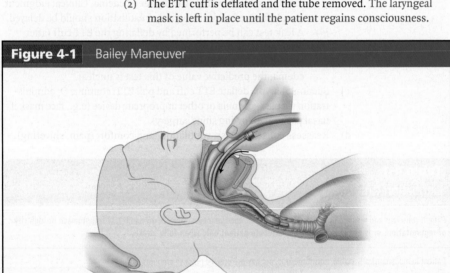

Insertion of a laryngeal mask device in stage 3 while the ETT is in place, prior to extubating the trachea, in order to maintain airway patency, yet avoid the stimulation caused by the presence of an ETT in the trachea during emergence. Adapted from airway challenge #1. Lma North America, www.lmana.com/docs/challenge1.pdf

6) Postoperative considerations

  a) **Respiratory failure**

READ MORE

The postanesthesia care unit, Chapter 147, page 1069

    i) Defined as the need to reintubate the trachea after extubation or the need for continued mechanical ventilation beyond 48 hours after the end of surgery

    ii) The most common causes are

      (1) Hypoventilation due to Surgical swelling or hematoma causing airway obstruction, laryngospasm, bronchospasm, central apnea (opioid overdose, stroke), residual neuromuscular blockade.

      (2) V/Q mismatch (aspiration of gastric contents, pulmonary edema, PE, atelectasis)

  b) **Delayed emergence**

READ MORE

Crisis management: delayed emergence, Chapter 223, page 1345

    i) Residual drug effects: hypnotic or opioid overdose, reduced metabolism, potentiation by other drugs, residual neuromuscular blockade

    ii) Respiratory failure with significant hypercarbia

    iii) Metabolic derangements: hypoglycemia, severe hyperglycemia, electrolyte imbalance, hypothermia, central anticholinergic syndrome

    iv) Neurological complications: cerebral hypoxia, CVA [hemorrhage, embolism or thrombosis]

  c) **Agitation and delirium**

Delayed emergence can be due to residual drug effects, respiratory failure, metabolic derangements, and/or neurological complications.

    i) Agitation upon awakening is not uncommon in children and young patients, especially when a balanced technique is used.

    ii) Patients are thrashing, crying, moaning, or incoherent.

    iii) Delirium usually resolves spontaneously within a few minutes.

    iv) Poor pain control may be implicated.

    v) Older patients can also experience emergence delirium, especially those who received anticholinergics that cross the blood–brain barrier, such as scopolamine.

    vi) Physostigmine (30 mg/kg) can be used to reverse anticholinergics.

    vii) Ketamine can cause hallucinations and delirium.

    viii) In one study, preoperative medication by benzodiazepines, breast surgery, abdominal surgery, and long duration of surgery increased the risk of delirium, while a previous history of illness and long-term treatment by antidepressants decreased the risk. Preoperative anxiety was not found to be a risk factor (4).

    ix) Hypoxia, severe hypercarbia, hypotension, hypoglycemia, increased intracranial pressure, as well as bladder distention can yield a similar clinical picture and should be excluded.

  d) **Inadequate postoperative analgesia**

    i) Besides the discomfort caused to the patient, postoperative pain can lead to severe complications such as myocardial ischemia and infarction.

    ii) Careful planning based on the patient's weight and history of opioid use as well as the procedure performed allows adequate analgesia upon emergence in most cases; in some patients, however, more analgesics will be needed.

    iii) Regional analgesia as well as multimodal pharmacologic analgesia (acetaminophen, NSAIDs, gabapentin or pregabalin, etc.) can reduce the risk of inadequate postoperative analgesia.

    iv) Pain is subjective and should be treated, especially if the patient complains of severe pain (VAS>7), by titrating strong opioids until the VAS is <4.

Shivering can significantly increase oxygen consumption, leading to myocardial ischemia in susceptible patients.

READ MORE

Postoperative Nausea and Vomiting Chapter 7, page 47

e) **Hypothermia and shivering**

   i) Postoperative hypothermia is best prevented by intraoperative active forced-air warming.

   ii) Hypothermia may lead to increased blood loss and transfusion requirements (because of platelet dysfunction) as well as poor wound healing and increased incidence of wound infection.

   iii) Shivering is a physiological response to hypothermia, using striated muscle contraction to produce heat. However, shivering is uncomfortable for the patient and can significantly increase oxygen consumption, leading to myocardial ischemia in susceptible patients.

   iv) Shivering can be treated with meperidine, 12.5 to 25 mg IV, and forced-air warming to correct hypothermia.

f) **PONV**

   i) Prophylaxis should be used, depending on the patient's risk factors.

   ii) Emptying the stomach with a gastric tube at the end of surgery, especially following ENT or oral surgery, where blood can be present in the stomach, also helps decrease the risk of PONV.

   iii) Treatment options include ondansetron (or another 5-HT3-antagonist), dopamine antagonists (metoclopramide, prochlorperazine, droperidol), and as a last resort a low-dose (0.1 mL/kg/h) propofol infusion (5).

Chapter Summary for Emergence and Postoperative Issues in Anesthesia

Definition	Emergence is the return of consciousness, neuromuscular conduction, and airway protective reflexes.
Preparing for Emergence	**Prior to extubation, ensure equipment to reintubate is available.** Decrease doses of inhaled anesthetics and/or intravenous agents. Give neuromuscular blockade reversal if appropriate. Titrate opioids to analgesia. Consider a 5-HT3 antagonist for PONV prophylaxis. Administer 100% FiO_2. Typically return patient supine/back-up position.
Technique of Routine Extubation	Confirm the patient conscious and responding to simple commands ("open your eyes, squeeze my hand"). Patient is hemodynamically stable, normothermic, not having received massive amounts of fluids leading to airway edema. Adequate spontaneous ventilation with tidal volumes >8 mL/kg, rate >8. Adequate reversal of NMB, sustained head lift or sustained tetanus (painful) for 5 s.
Technique of Deep Extubation	Used to avoid coughing, bucking, straining on extubation. **Prior to extubation, ensure equipment to reintubate is available.** Goal is to extubate the patient during Stage III of anesthesia.
Postoperative Complications	Delayed emergence is most commonly due to residual drug effects, respiratory failure, metabolic derangements, or neurologic complications.

References

1. Guedel AF. *Inhalational Anesthesia*. 2nd ed. New York, NY: The Macmillan Co., 1951:10–52.
2. Daley MD, Norman PH, Coveler LA. Tracheal extubation of adult surgical patients while deeply anesthetized: a survey of United States anesthesiologists. *J Clin Anesth* 1999;11(6):445–452.
3. Nair I, Bailey PM. Use of the laryngeal mask for airway maintenance following extubation. *Anaesthesia* 1995;50(2):174–175.
4. Lepousé C, Lautner CA, Liu L, et al. Emergence delirium in adults in the post-anaesthesia care unit. *Br J Anaesth* 2006;96(6):747–753.
5. Ewalenko P, Janny S, Dejonckheere M, et al. Antiemetic effect of subhypnotic doses of propofol after thyroidectomy. *Br J Anaesth* 1996;77(4):463–467.

5 Positioning of the Surgical Patient

Anastassia Grigorieva, MD • Jamie Murphy, MD

Proper positioning of the surgical patient is critical. Positioning injuries range in severity from minor skin abrasions to peripheral neuropathies, nonhealing pressure ulcers, and blindness.

1) **Overview**

   a) Proper positioning of the surgical patient requires a careful balance of optimal surgical field exposure without subjecting the patient to inappropriate positioning.

   b) Each surgical position (supine, prone, lithotomy, and lateral) presents its own unique risks and challenges.

   c) Knowledge of potential positioning complications and their timely recognition and management are critically important for a successful outcome of any surgical procedure.

Perioperative cigarette smoking is associated with an increased incidence of postoperative neuropathies, presumably because of the vasoconstrictive effects of nicotine.

2) Factors affecting positioning (Table 5-1)

   a) Complications arising from patient malpositioning during surgery depend on both non-patient and patient factors.

   b) While most of these factors (e.g., type of procedure, patient's age or gender) cannot be modified, recognition of patients who are at additional risk for positioning complications should alert the anesthesia provider to take extra precautions.

   c) These patients are typically 70 years of age or older; morbidly obese (BMI of > 40); thin, small in stature, have a poor preoperative nutritional status; or a history of diabetes or vascular disease.

3) **General positioning guidelines** (1–4)

   a) Proper patient positioning balances the need for adequate exposure of the surgical field and prevention of positioning injury.

Table 5-1

Risks Factors Affecting Positioning of Patient

Non-patient Factors	Patient Factors
Type of procedure	Patient's age
Length of procedure	Patient's height
Type of anesthesia	Patient's weight
Equipment affecting patient's position	Nutritional status Deconditioning Other preexisting conditions

ANESTHESIOLOGY

b) Optimal positioning is achieved when:

    i) Adequate arterial supply and venous outflow are maintained to all body parts

    ii) Nerves are protected from undue pressure or stretching

    iii) Bony prominences are padded

    iv) Circulatory and respiratory systems are minimally compromised

    v) Maximum surgical field exposure is achieved

It is the responsibility of the entire OR team to ensure proper patient positioning.

4) **Positioning guidelines**

  a) **Supine**

    i) Used for abdominal, pelvic, open-heart, head and neck, and most extremity surgery.

    ii) Padding should be applied to the heels, elbows, knees, spinal column, and occiput.

    iii) To avoid pressure alopecia, periodically rotate the patient's head, especially during prolonged cases.

    iv) To avoid brachial plexus injury, upper extremities should be abducted to <90 degrees with hands and forearms in a supinated or neutral position.

    vi) IV tubing and stopcocks touching the skin should be padded.

    vii) For the Trendelenburg position, a nonsliding mattress is recommended to prevent patients from sliding cephalad.

      (1) The Trendelenburg position may cause cardiovascular and/or respiratory compromise.

      (2) Patients may develop significant edema of the face and upper airway.

In the prone position, the eyes should be free of pressure and checked frequently.

  b) **Prone (Fig. 5-1)**

    i) Used for posterior spine, skull, buttocks, perirectal, and lower extremity surgery.

    ii) The patient is typically placed in this position by log-rolling after being anesthetized.

    iii) The patient's proper body alignment should be maintained while turning from supine to prone with special attention to breasts, male genitalia, arms, legs, and cervical spine.

    iv) The arms are usually kept <90 degrees.

    v) The eyes should be free of pressure and checked frequently.

    vi) To avoid stress on the cervical spine, there should be, at least, two fingerbreadths between the chin and the chest.

  c) **Lithotomy (Fig. 5-2)**

    i) Used for gynecologic and urologic surgery.

    ii) When placing the patient into and out of this position, both legs are moved simultaneously to prevent torsion of the lumbar spine.

    iii) The hips are flexed 80 to 100 degrees from the trunk, and the legs are abducted 30 to 45 degrees from the midline.

    iv) Lower extremities are padded to prevent compression against the stirrups and injury to the common peroneal nerve.

    v) Hands and arms should be positioned away from the bed to prevent crush injury during manipulation of the foot section of the OR table.

    vi) This position can increase intra-abdominal pressure resulting in impeded venous return to the heart.

| **Figure 5-1** | The Classic Prone Position |

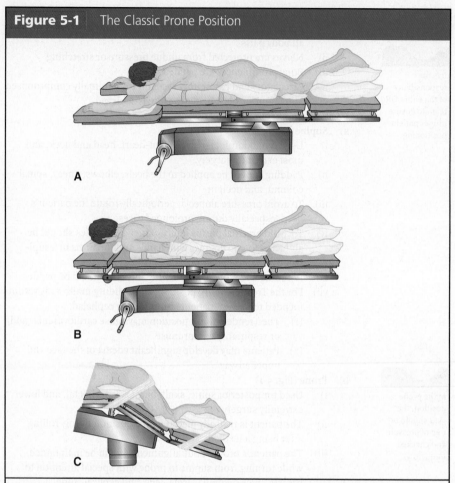

A: Flat table with relaxed arms extended alongside patient's head. Parallel chest rolls extended from just caudad of clavicle to just beyond inguinal area, with pillow over pelvic end. elbows and knees are padded, and legs are bent at the knees. head is turned onto a C-shaped foam sponge that frees the down-side eye and ear from compression. **B:** Same posture with arms snugly retained alongside torso. **C:** Table flexed to reduce lumbar lordosis; subgluteal area straps placed after the legs are lowered to provide cephalad thrust and prevent caudad slippage. Reproduced from Warner MA. Patient positioning and related injuries. In: Barash PG, Cullen BF, Stoelting RK, eds. *Clinical Anesthesia*. 6th ed. Philadelphia, PA: Lippincott Williams & Wilkins, 2009:793–814, with permission.

d) **Lateral (Fig. 5-3)**
   i) Used for thoracic, retroperitoneal, and hip surgery.
   ii) The patient is typically placed in this position after being anesthetized in the supine position.
   iii) The patient's head and neck should be maintained in neutral position to prevent injury to the cervical spine and brachial plexus.

ANESTHESIOLOGY

Figure 5-2 Standard Lithotomy Position with "Candy Cane" Extremity Support

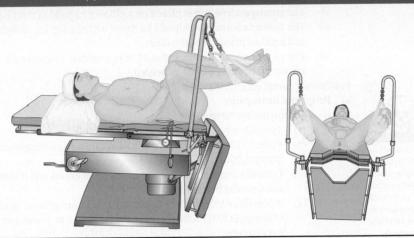

Thighs are flexed approximately 90 degrees on abdomen; knees are flexed enough to bring lower legs grossly parallel to the torso section of the tabletop. Arms are retained on boards, crossed on the abdomen, or snugged at the sides of patient. From Warner MA. Patient positioning and related injuries. In: Barash PG, Cullen BF, Stoelting RK, eds. *Clinical Anesthesia.* 6th ed. Philadelphia, PA: Lippincott Williams & Wilkins, 2009:793–814, with permission.

Figure 5-3 The Standard Lateral Decubitus Position

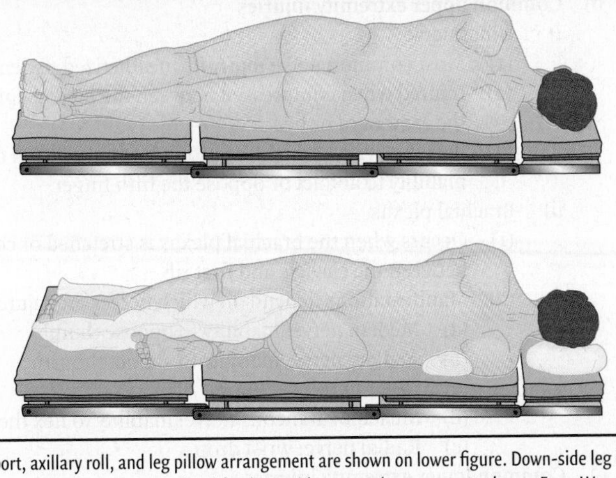

Proper head support, axillary roll, and leg pillow arrangement are shown on lower figure. Down-side leg is flexed at hip and knee to stabilize torso. Retaining straps and pad for down-side peroneal nerve are not shown. From Warner MA. Patient positioning and related injuries. In: Barash PG, Cullen BF, Stoelting RK, eds. *Clinical Anesthesia.* 6th ed. Philadelphia, PA: Lippincott Williams & Wilkins, 2009:793–814, with permission.

      iv) To prevent injury to the brachial plexus, an "axillary roll" is placed just caudad to the dependent axilla with the dependent arm perpendicular to the torso on a padded arm board.

      v) The nondependent arm is placed on a pillow or a padded armrest.

      vi) The patient's bottom leg should be flexed with the top leg straight and a pillow placed between them.

      vii) The patient's head and neck should be in a neutral position with additional padding placed as needed.

5) Positioning complications (6)

  a) **Peripheral neuropathy**

    i) Sensory/motor neuropathy

For patients with postoperative peripheral neuropathy exclude any correctable causes such as vascular injury, hematoma, and cast compression.

      (1) Typically transient, especially if sensory only.

      (2) Patient follow-up is important to determine improving/worsening symptoms.

      (3) Consider neurology consultation for serial exams and if symptoms persist beyond 5 days.

      (4) A baseline EMG can help determine a preexisting nerve injury. Changes in EMG activity do not appear until 2 to 3 weeks after a nerve injury.

      (5) Exclude any correctable causes: for example, vascular injury, hematoma, cast compression.

      (6) Consider physical therapy early for the best outcome.

      (7) Patients with symptoms for 6 to 8 weeks or progressive deficits need a neurosurgical consult.

    ii) Other etiologies

Ulnar nerve injury is the most common nerve injury in an anesthetized patient.

      (1) Other neurologic disorders such as stroke, spinal injury, disc herniation

      (2) Musculoskeletal injury

      (3) Autoimmune neurologic disorder

  b) **Common upper extremity injuries**

    i) Ulnar nerve

      (1) Most common nerve injury in anesthetized patient

      (2) Injured when compressed between the medial epicondyle and the armboard or bed

      (3) Presents with loss of sensation of lateral portion of hand and inability to abduct or oppose the fifth finger

    ii) Brachial plexus

      (1) Occurs when the brachial plexus is stretched or compressed between the clavicle and first rib

      (2) Manifestations depend on which nerves are injured

        (a) Median nerve: inability to oppose thumb

        (b) Axillary nerve: inability to abduct the arm

        (c) Ulnar nerve: see above

        (d) Musculocutaneous nerve: inability to flex the forearm

        (e) Radial nerve: wrist drop

  c) **Common lower extremity injuries**

    i) Common peroneal nerve

      (1) Most common injury in lithotomy position when lateral aspect of knee is compressed against stirrup

      (2) Results in foot drop and a loss of dorsal extension of toes

  ii) Sciatic nerve
    (1) Injured from excessive flexion of hips
    (2) Results in weakness in all muscles below the knee and foot drop
  iii) Femoral nerve
    (1) Injured from trapping under inguinal ligament from extreme flexion and abduction of thighs
    (2) Results in decreased knee jerk, loss of flexion of hip and extension of knee
  iv) Saphenous nerve
    (1) Injured when the medial tibial condyle is compressed by leg support in lithotomy position
    (2) Paresthesia along medial and anteriomedial aspect of the calf
  v) Anterior tibial nerve
    (1) Injured when feet are plantar flexed for extended periods of time (sitting or prone)
    (2) Manifests as foot drop
  vi) Obturator nerve
    (1) Damaged during excessive flexion of the thigh to the groin or during difficult forceps delivery
    (2) Results in inability to adduct the leg and diminished sensation along medial aspect of the thigh

6) **Eye injury (4,5)**
  a) Corneal abrasion
    i) Most common type of eye injury
    ii) Eyes should be protected and frequently checked during anesthesia.
    iii) Patients are also at risk in the PACU.
    iv) Treated with antibiotic ointment, patching; usually resolves without any sequelae in several days
    v) Consult ophthalmologist if persistent eye discharge or "foreign body" sensation.

Postoperative blindness requires **immediate consultation** by ophthalmologist.

  b) Postoperative blindness
    i) Risk factors for blindness include intraoperative hypotension, prone position, and anemia
    ii) Requires **immediate consultation** by ophthalmologist
    iii) Etiology includes ischemic optic neuropathy and/or retinal vessel occlusion
      (1) Ischemic optic neuropathy
        (a) Bilateral blindness
        (b) Anterior optic nerve ischemia can result in
          (i) Initial optic disc edema
          (ii) Occasional improvements in vision
        (c) Posterior optic nerve ischemia can result in
          (i) Initially normal fundoscopic exam
          (ii) Delayed optic disc edema
          (iii) Vision which seldom improves
      (2) Retinal artery or vein occlusion
        (a) Usually unilateral vision loss
        (b) Cherry red spot with retinal edema is observed on examination
        (c) Associated with carotid disease and atherosclerosis
        (d) Vision occasionally improves

        (3) Cortical blindness

           (a) Total or partial loss of vision in one or both eyes with normal fundoscopic and papillary reflex

           (b) Associated with ischemia to the occipital visual cortex

           (c) Vision frequently improves

7) **Summary of perioperative neuropathy task force consensus** (7)

  a) **Perioperative assessment.** When judged appropriate, it is helpful to ascertain that patients can comfortably tolerate the anticipated operative position.

  b) **Upper extremity positioning**

    i) Arm abduction should be limited to 90 degrees in supine patients.

      (1) Patients who are positioned prone may comfortably tolerate arm abduction >90 degrees.

    ii) Arms should be positioned to decrease pressure on the postcondylar groove of the humerus (ulnar groove).

      (1) When arms are tucked at the side, a neutral forearm position is recommended.

      (2) When arms are abducted on arm boards, either supination or a neutral forearm position is acceptable.

      (3) Prolonged pressure on the radial nerve in the spiral groove of the humerus should be avoided.

      (4) Extension of the elbow beyond a comfortable range may stretch the median nerve.

  c) **Lower extremity positioning**

    i) Lithotomy positions that stretch the hamstring muscle group beyond a comfortable range may stretch the sciatic nerve.

    ii) Prolonged pressure on the peroneal nerve at the fibular head should be avoided.

    iii) Neither extension nor flexion of the hip increases the risk of femoral neuropathy.

  d) **Protective padding**

    i) Padded arm boards may decrease the risk of upper extremity neuropathies.

    ii) The use of chest rolls in laterally positioned patients may decrease the risk of upper extremity neuropathies.

    iii) Padding at the elbow and at the fibular head may decrease the risk of upper and lower extremity neuropathies, respectively.

A simple postoperative assessment of extremity nerve function may lead to early recognition of peripheral neuropathies.

  e) **Equipment**

    i) Properly functioning automated blood pressure cuffs on the upper arms do not affect the risk of upper extremity neuropathies.

    ii) Shoulder braces in steep head-down positions may increase the risk of brachial plexus neuropathies.

  f) **Postoperative assessment**

    i) A simple postoperative assessment of extremity nerve function may lead to early recognition of peripheral neuropathies.

  g) **Documentation**

    i) Charting specific positioning actions during the care of patients may result in improvements of care by helping practitioners focus attention on relevant aspects of patient positioning.

    ii) Providing information that continues improvement processes can use to lead to refinement in patient care.

Chapter Summary for Positioning of the Surgical Patient

General Considerations	Proper patient positioning balances the need for adequate exposure of the surgical field and prevention of positioning injury. It is the responsibility of the entire OR team to ensure proper patient positioning.
Specific Considerations Eyes	Eyes should be frequently checked to make sure that they are free from pressure, especially in the prone position. Corneal abrasion is the most common type of eye injury and is typically treated with antibiotic ointment. An ophthalmologist should see patients with postoperative blindness immediately.
Upper Extremity	Arms should be abducted <90 degrees in the supine position. Avoid pressure on the ulnar groove by the elbow.
Lower Extremity	Avoid overstretching the hamstring, which can cause sciatic nerve injury. The common peroneal nerve can be compressed against the fibula below the knee in the lithotomy position.

References

1. Faust RJ, Cucchiara RF, Bechtle PS. Patient positioning. In: Miller, RD, ed. *Miller's Anesthesia*. 6th ed. Philadelphia, PA: Elsevier Churchill Livingstone; 2004:1151–1167.
2. Graling, P, Tea C. Intraoperative nursing management. In: Smeltzer SC, Bare B, eds. *Brunner and Suddarth's Textbook of Medical-Surgical Nursing*. 10th ed. Philadelphia, PA: Lippincott Williams & Wilkins; 2003:432–434.
3. Winfree CJ, Kline DG. Intraoperative positioning nerve injuries. *Surg Neurol* 2005;63(1):5–18.
4. Warner MA. Patient positioning and related injuries. In: Barash PG, ed. *Clinical anesthesia*. 6th ed. Philadelphia, PA: Lippincott Williams & Wilkins; 2009:793–814.
5. Hebl JR. Peripheral nerve injury. In: Neal JM, Rathmell JP, eds. *Complications in Regional Anesthesia and Pain Medicine*. 1st ed. Philadelphia, PA: Saunders Elsevier; 2007:136–139.
6. Roth S. Perioperative blindness. In: Miller, RD, ed. *Miller's Anesthesia*. 6th ed. Philadelphia, PA: Elsevier Churchill Livingstone; 2004: 2991–3020.
7. American Society of Anesthesiologists Task Force on Prevention of Perioperative Peripheral Neuropathies: practice advisory for the prevention of perioperative peripheral neuropathies. *Anesthesiology* 2000; 92:1168.

6

Hazards of the Operating Room

Albert Ju, MD

Hazards of the operating room (OR) include occupational exposure to volatile anesthetics, electrical hazards, the potential for drug addiction, fall hazards and blood-borne pathogens exposure.

Occupational exposure to volatile anesthetics can be caused by inhalational inductions, poorly fitting masks, leaky endotracheal tube cuffs, and malfunctioning scavenging systems.

1) **Occupational exposure to volatile anesthetics**
   a) Anesthesiologists are exposed to trace amounts of anesthetic gas when working in the operating room.
      i) Exposure can be caused by inhalational inductions, poorly fitting masks, leaky endotracheal tube cuffs, and malfunctioning scavenging systems.
      ii) Some retrospective studies show associations between trace anesthetic gas exposure and spontaneous abortion, cancer, and congenital abnormalities. However, the results were mixed and susceptible to recall bias.
   b) It is difficult to separate exposure to anesthetic gases from other risk factors such as work stress and radiation.
      i) The only prospective study studied 11,500 female British physicians and showed no difference as far as spontaneous abortion, infertility, or miscarriage between anesthesiologists and their peers (1).
      ii) Based on this information and a review of the literature, the ASA Task Force on Trace Anesthetic Gases concluded that no definite relationship has been shown between trace anesthetic gas exposure and adverse health outcomes (2).
   c) Although the ASA recommends that anesthetic gases be scavenged, no recommendation has been made for routine monitoring of levels.
      i) The National Institute of Occupational Safety and Health recommends no more than 25 ppm nitrous oxide or 2 ppm volatile anesthetic.
      ii) Some countries have much higher thresholds (up to 100 ppm nitrous, and 50 ppm volatile agent).
   d) **If gas can be smelled, the exposure limit has been exceeded.**
      i) Steps should be taken to ensure adequate scavenging as well as the eliminating of other sources of gas leak.

Electrical current running through the body can lead to physical damage, including burns, seizures, and ventricular fibrillation.

2) **Electrical OR safety (3,4)**
   a) The OR contains many pieces of equipment in an environment that is frequently "wet" with fluid, leading to a potential for electric shock.
   b) Electrical current running through the body can lead to physical damage, including burns, seizures, and ventricular fibrillation.
      i) For current to flow, a circuit must be created.
         (1) Electrical current is supplied via a high-voltage "hot wire" and a low-voltage neutral wire, which is grounded.

(2)   Touching a hot wire can lead to a shock, since current can flow from the hot wire through the victim into the ground, which then flows back into the neutral wire, completing a circuit.

  ii)   To decrease the risk of a shock, modern OR power is electrically isolated from the ground by use of a **transformer**.

    (1)   Even if a person touches a hot wire, there is no circuit completed. Thus, no shock occurs.

c)   Line isolation monitor (LIM)

  i)   If the hot wire short circuits with a device chassis, the system is no longer isolated from the ground as all devices have a ground plug.

  ii)   While touching this device alone will not deliver a shock, the system is less safe, for if the neutral wire becomes grounded, now a circuit between the two lines and the ground has been created, creating a shock risk. This is detected by a LIM.

    (1)   LIMs are designed to detect whether the electrical power system is still isolated from the ground.

  iii)   Failures of grounding can occur from faulty OR devices or faulty wiring.

    (1)   To determine if an OR device is the problem, **unplug each device in the order they were plugged in**.

    (2)   If the alarm stops, then the device may be the cause of the problem, and should be replaced.

    (3)   If the LIM continues to alarm after all devices have been unplugged, then the problem may lie in the OR wiring.

    (4)   If one device can be identified as a problem, it should be replaced as soon as possible.

      (a)   However, if the use of the device cannot be interrupted without compromising patient safety, then it may be acceptable to continue using the device, as a second fault is required to create a shock hazard.

If the line isolation monitor alarms, unplug each device in the order they were most recently plugged in.

d)   **Ground fault circuit interrupters (GFCI)**

  i)   A GFCI immediately shuts off current to a device if it becomes grounded.

  ii)   Compared to using a LIM, the GFCI provides better shock protection as the device creating the shock risk is turned off quickly before a second fault can occur.

    (1)   The disadvantage is that the GFCI will automatically switch off power to any device, including those whose function cannot be interrupted without risk to the patient.

  iii)   To troubleshoot the GFCI, first reset the GFCI as temporary current surges can activate the GFCI in the absence of an increased shock risk.

    (1)   If the GFCI still triggers, then unplug each device one at a time, resetting the GFCI after each time.

    (2)   If the GFCI stops triggering after the device is unplugged, then replace the device.

e)   **Macroshock/microshock**

  i)   **Macroshock** refers to shocks applied to the outside of the body.

    (1)   Minimum perceptible macroshock occurs around 1 mA.

    (2)   At 10 mA, involuntary muscle contractions can occur.

    (3)   At 100 mA, ventricular fibrillation can occur.

  ii)   **Microshock** refers to current applied directly to the heart.

    (1)   Much lower levels of current are needed to induce microshock—as little as 10 µA can induce ventricular fibrillation.

(2) Neither LIMs nor GFCIs protect against microshock, as the amount of current needed to cause microshock is too low to trigger those devices.

(3) Devices in direct contact with the heart, including central venous pressure catheters and transcutaneous pacing leads, can increase the risk of microshock.

    (a) It is important not to touch electrical equipment and objects in contact with the heart at the same time as small amounts of charge on the casing can create microshock.

    (b) Temporary pacemakers should only be powered by battery to avoid connections to the ground that can create a circuit (4).

f) **Bovie safety**

    i) Bovie electrocautery uses high frequency electrical current to cauterize and cut tissue.

    (1) A high-voltage tip is applied to the patient.

    (2) A large flat return pad is placed on the patient, which connects back to the electrocautery unit, creating a circuit by allowing current to flow back to the device.

    (3) At the tip of the Bovie, the current density is very high, causing localized heating and tissue damage. The return pad's large size leads to lower current density, which causes no local damage.

      (a) Pads should be inspected before use.

        (i) If the pad is dry or improperly applied, then the total surface area of current return may decrease, leading to an increased risk of burns.

        (ii) Likewise, if the patient touches an OR table that has become ungrounded, burns can occur.

    (4) The high frequencies (500,000 to 2,000,000 Hz) used by electrocautery are too high to fibrillate the heart from electrical current.

    (5) The predominant concern with Bovie safety is burn prevention.

3) **Addiction**

a) Drug addiction is a serious problem in anesthesiology.

b) Causes include stress, access to drugs, curiosity, and genetic susceptibility.

c) Although the Medical Association of Georgia Disabled Doctors Program identified an increased proportion of anesthesiologists reporting substance abuse (5), not all studies have shown an increased risk of drug addiction compared to other specialties.

    i) However, due to the access to addictive controlled substances such as opiates and benzodiazepines, anesthesiologists have an increased relative risk of drug fatality compared to internists (6).

d) Signs of addiction include increasing amount of opioids used during cases, volunteering for extra work, frequent bathroom breaks, being slow to answer pages, and changes in behavior. Sadly, the first sign of drug addiction is often sudden death.

e) Anyone with suspected drug use should be reported to the proper authorities, both for the user's sake as well as for their patients' sake.

f) Treatment includes both inpatient and outpatient therapies.

g) **Recovery is possible**, although relapse is frequent.

h) The American Disabilities Act provides some protection for patients recovering from addiction, although it does not protect active drug users. **The ASA Executive Office provides a hotline that provides information for state programs that serve impaired physicians (847-825-5586).**

Drug addiction is a serious problem in anesthesiology and may be due to stress, access to drugs, curiosity, and genetic susceptibility.

The ASA Executive Office provides a hotline that provides information for state programs that serve impaired physicians (847-825-5586).

4) **Fall hazards**
   a) Anesthetized patients are not able to protect themselves from falls.
   b) It is important to make sure that the patient is strapped in at all times unless someone is directly next to the patient and watching for falls.
   c) Fall risks are also increased among OR personnel. The floor should be kept clean to reduce the risk of slipping.

5) **Blood exposure (7)**
   a) Due an increased exposure to patient blood, anesthesiologists are at increased risk for acquiring blood borne diseases.

READ MORE

Needlestick injury, Chapter 69, page 493

   i) All anesthesiologists should wear gloves whenever any risk of patient blood exposure exists.
   ii) Needles should not be recapped and should be disposed of carefully.
      (1) Accidental needlesticks increase the risk of developing infections.
         (a) The risk of contracting HIV with a single needlestick with HIV infected blood is 0.3%.
         (b) By contrast, the risk of contracting Hepatitis C with an infected needlestick is 1.8%.
         (c) Although the risk of developing Hepatitis B with accidental exposure is the highest (between 23% and 62%), immunization significantly decreases this risk.
   iii) Anesthesiologists who sustain a needlestick should report immediately to occupational health for evaluation and possible prophylaxis.

Chapter Summary for Hazards of the OR

Types of OR Hazards	Occupational exposure to volatile anesthetics, electrical OR safety, the potential for drug addiction, fall hazards and blood borne pathogens exposure.
Volatile Anesthetics	Exposure to volatile anesthetics can be caused by inhalational inductions, poorly fitting masks, leaky endotracheal tube cuffs, and malfunctioning scavenging systems.
Electrical Safety	If the line isolation monitor alarms, unplug each device in the order they were most recently plugged in. Macroshock refers to shocks applied to the outside of the body and microshock refers to shocks applied directly to the heart. Both can cause arrhythmias. For Bovie safety, a grounding pad is placed on the patient to prevent burns.
Impaired Physicians	The ASA executive office provides a hotline for information for state programs that serve impaired physicians (847-825-5586).
Blood Borne Pathogens Exposure	Anesthesiologists who sustain a needlestick should report immediately to occupational health for evaluation and possible prophylaxis.

ANESTHESIOLOGY

References

1. Maran NJ, Knill-Jones RP, Spence AA. Infertility among female hospital doctors in the UK. *Br J Anaesth* 1996;76:581P.
2. Waste Anesthetic Gases: Information for Management in Anesthetizing Areas and the Postanesthetic Care Unit (PACU). Task Force on Trace Anesthetic Gases, American Society of Anesthesiologists, 2004. http://www.asahq.org/publicationsAndServices/wastanes.pdf
3. Gross JB. ASA Refresher Course in Anesthesiology 2005;33(1):101–114.
4. Ehrenwerth J, Seifert HA. Electrical and fire safety. In: Barash PG Cullen BF, Stoelting RK, eds. *Clinical Anesthesia*. 6th ed. Philadelphia, PA: Lippincott Williams &Wilkins; 2009:165–191.
5. Talbott DG, Gallegos KV, Wilson PO, et al. The Medical Association of Georgia's impaired physicians program review of the first 1000 physicians: analysis of specialty. *JAMA* 1987;257:2927–2930.
6. Alexander BH, Checkoway H, Nagahama SI, et al. Cause-specific mortality risks of anesthesiologists. *Anesthesiology* 2000;93:922–930.
7. Berry AJ, Katz JD. Occupational health. In: Barash PG, Cullen BF, Stoelting RK, eds. *Clinical Anesthesia*. 6th ed. Philadelphia, PA: Lippincott Williams & Wilkins; 2009:57–81.

7

Postoperative Nausea and Vomiting

T. Kyle Harrison, MD • Bassam Kadry, MD

Postoperative nausea and vomiting (PONV) is a common problem in patients recovering from surgery and anesthesia. Several risk factors have been associated with increased risk of PONV. Having an effective strategy to prevent PONV is vitally important in today's modern anesthetic practice.

1) Pathophysiology
   a) **Prevalence and risk stratification**
      i) Estimated to occur in 30% of all anesthetics
         (1) In high-risk patients, the prevalence approaches 80% (1).
      ii) PONV can adversely affect patient satisfaction and lead to
         (1) Increased cost in extended PACU times
         (2) Unplanned admission to the hospital
         (3) Increased drug use to treat it once it develops (2)
   b) **Molecular mechanism** (Fig. 7-1)
      i) Etiology of PONV is multifactorial.
      ii) The emetic center of the brain
         (1) Located in the lateral reticular formation of the medulla
             Receives input from (1,2)
            (a) Chemoreceptor trigger zone
            (b) Vestibular apparatus
            (c) Cerebellum
            (d) Solitary tract nucleus
            (e) Cerebral cortex
         (2) Receptors that are related to and serve as a basis for the
             treatment and prevention of PONV include (1)
            (a) Dopamine (D_2)
            (b) Acetylcholine (M_1)
            (c) Histamine (H_1)
            (d) Serotonin ($5HT_3$)
            (e) Neurokinin (NK_1) receptors
   c) **Risk factors** (2,3)
      i) Surgery related:
         (1) Prolonged surgical duration
         (2) Procedure type (neurological, ENT, breast, strabismus, abdominal, and laparoscopic surgeries)
      ii) Anesthesia related:
         (1) **Nitrous oxide**
         (2) **Volatile anesthetic**
         (3) **Opioids**

Figure 7-1 Mechanisms for PONV and Recommended Strategies for Minimizing the Incidence of PONV

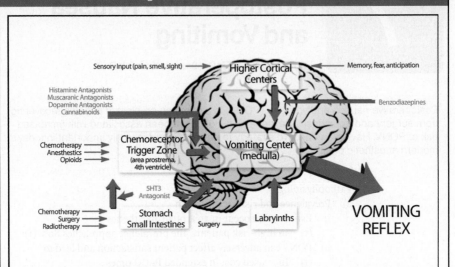

Sensory Input (pain, smell, sight) → **Higher Cortical Centers** ← Memory, fear, anticipation

Histamine Antagonists
Muscaranic Antagonists
Dopamine Antagonists
Cannabinoids

Benzodiazepines

Chemotherapy → **Chemoreceptor Trigger Zone** (area prostrema, 4th ventricle)
Anesthetics →
Opioids →

Vomiting Center (medulla)

5HT3 Antagonist

Chemotherapy → **Stomach Small Intestines**
Surgery →
Radiotherapy →

Surgery → **Labrynths**

VOMITING REFLEX

Recommended Strategies for Minimizing the Incidence of PONV

1. Identify high-risk patients
2. Avoid emetogenic stimuli
   Etomidate
   Inhalational Anesthetics
   Opioids*
3. Multimodal Therapy
   Antiemetics (consider combination therapy)
   TIVA with Propofol
   Adequate Hydration
   Effective Analgesia with local anesthetics and Cox-2 inhibitors
   Anxiolytics
   Intraop O₂ (FiO2 0.8)
   Nonpharmacologic techniques

* Although opioids are emetogenic, optimal analgesia should be the goal and can be achieved by incorporating preop education, local anesthetics, and Cox-2 inhibitors. Optimal analgesia may include an opioid.

Risk Factors for PONV and Guidelines for Prophylactic Antiemetic Therapy

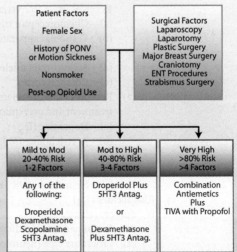

Patient Factors	Surgical Factors
Female Sex	Laparoscopy
History of PONV or Motion Sickness	Laparotomy, Plastic Surgery, Major Breast Surgery, Craniotomy, ENT Procedures, Strabismus Surgery
Nonsmoker	
Post-op Opioid Use	

Mild to Mod 20-40% Risk 1-2 Factors	Mod to High 40-80% Risk 3-4 Factors	Very High >80% Risk >4 Factors
Any 1 of the following: Droperidol Dexamethasone Scopolamine 5HT3 Antag.	Droperidol Plus 5HT3 Antag. or Dexamethasone Plus 5HT3 Antag.	Combination Antiemetics Plus TIVA with Propofol

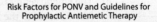

(4)   General anesthesia

(5)   Anitcholinesterase (e.g., neostigmine)

(6)   Dehydration

(7)   Anxiety

(8)   Pain

iii)   Patient related:

   (1)   **Woman**

   (2)   **History of PONV/motion sickness**

   (3)   **Nonsmoker**

   (4)   Young age

   (5)   Anxiety

   (6)   Disease with GI involvement, like ileus

2)   **Treatment and Prevention of PONV (5–10)**

   a)   Pharmacology

      i)   Several classes of drugs have been studied for the prevention and/or treatment of PONV:

         (1)   Corticosteroids (e.g., Dexamethasone)

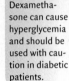

Dexamethasone can cause hyperglycemia and should be used with caution in diabetic patients.

            (a)   Dexamethasone

               (i)   Should be administered at induction of anesthesia to have maximal effect.

               (ii)   Recommended prophylactic dose is 4 to 5 mg IV for patients at increased risk of PONV.

               (iii)   A 4-mg IV dose has similar efficacy to ondansetron 4 mg IV and droperidol 1.25 mg IV.

               (iv)   Doses <8 mg have not been shown to have significant side effects.

               (v)   Use with caution in diabetic patients.

         (2) D_2-Antagonists

Droperidol is associated with prolonging QTc interval and possible fatal cardiac arrhythmias.

            (a)   Droperidol

               (i)   Recommended prophylactic dose is 0.625 to 1.25 mg IV.

               (ii)   Similar efficacy as ondansetron for PONV prophylaxis

               (iii)   Most effective when administered at the end of surgery

               (iv)   FDA black box warning

                  1.   Associated with prolonging the QTc interval

                  2.   Possible fatal cardiac arrhythmias

                  3.   Unlikely to occur at the extremely low dosing levels used of PONV prophylaxis

            (b)   Phenothiazines

            (c)   Haloperidol

               (i)   Has been used as an alternative to droperidol.

               (ii)   Meta-analysis shows doses of 0.5 to 2 mg IM or IV reduces PONV risk.

                  1.   Sedation and cardiac arrhythmias were not reported at these doses.

         (3) H_1-Antagonists

            (a)   Dimenhydrinate

               (i)   Antihistamine with antiemetic effects

               (ii)   Antiemetic efficacy may be similar to $5HT_3$ receptor antagonists.

               (iii)   Recommended dose is 1 mg/kg IV.

      (4) NK$_1$-Antagonist

        (a) Aprepitant

          (i) 40-mg PO dose equivalent to 4 mg ondansetron IV in incidence of nausea during initial 24 hours

          (ii) Better than ondansetron in preventing vomiting 24 to 48 hours postoperatively

      (5) M$_1$-Antagonist

        (a) Transdermal scopolamine

          (i) Useful adjunct to other antiemetic treatments

          (ii) Onset of effect is 2 to 4 hours.

            1. Apply in evening prior to surgery or 4 hours prior to end of anesthesia.

          (iii) Adverse effects are mild and can include

            1. Visual disturbances

            2. Dry mouth

            3. Dizziness

      (6) Serotonin (5HT$_3$) receptor antagonists

        (a) Favorable side-effect profile

        (b) All considered equally safe and antiemetic for the treatment of established PONV

        (c) 5HT$_3$ receptor antagonists used in clinical practice

          (i) Ondansetron

            1. Recommended prophylactic dose is 4 mg IV.

            2. Most effective when given at the end of surgery

          (ii) Dolasetron (Table 7-1)

          (iii) Granisetron (Table 7-1)

          (iv) Tropisetron (Table 7-1)

   b) Approaches to PONV Prophylaxis (2,8)

      i) Once PONV develops, it can be difficult to treat. Therefore, an effective preventive strategy should be employed for patients most at risk of developing PONV.

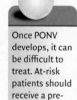

Once PONV develops, it can be difficult to treat. At-risk patients should receive a preventive strategy for PONV.

      ii) Identify patients at risk for PONV

        (1) Apfel's risk score can be used to quantify a patient's risk profile based on a point system for each of the following risks:

          (a) Female gender

          (b) History of PONV

          (c) Nonsmoking status

          (d) Use of postoperative opioids

          (e) For points 0, 1, 2, 3, or 4, adults have a PONV risk of 10%, 20%, 40%, 60%, and 80% risk of PONV, respectively (3).

        (2) Low risk

          (a) Wait and see (2).

        (3) Medium risk

          (a) Select one to two interventions for adults.

        (4) High risk

          (a) Select two or more interventions for adults.

          (b) Consider multimodal approach.

      iii) Reduce baseline risk of PONV

        (1) Several factors reduce risk, including avoiding volatile anesthetic agents, nitrous oxide, general anesthesia, and emetogenic drugs such as etomidate and neostigmine (Table 7-2).

Table 7-1
PONV Treatment Options (4–11)

Drug Name	Adult Dose	Cost	Time of Dosing	Receptor Site
Ondansetron (QT)	4–8 mg IV	$$	Emergence	5HT$_3$
Dolasetron (QT)	12.5 mg IV	$$	Emergence	5HT$_3$
Granisetron	0.35–1 mg IV	$$$	Emergence	5HT$_3$
Palonosetron	0.075 mg IV	$$$$	Induction	5HT$_3$
Droperidol^a (QT)	0.625–1.25 mg IV	$	Emergence	D$_2$
Prochlorperazine^b	2.5–10 mg IV	$	Emergence	D$_2$
Metoclopramide^b	10–20 mg IV	$	Induction	D$_2$
Promethazine^c	12.5–25 mg IV	$	Emergence	D$_2$, H$_1$, M$_1$
Diphenhydramine (QT)	25–50 mg IV	$	Induction	H$_1$, M$_1$
Scopolamine	0.4 mg patch	$$	Before surgery	M$_1$
Aprepitant	40–125 mg PO	$$$$	Before surgery	NK$_1$
Fosaprepitant	115–150 mg IV	$$$$	Before surgery	NK$_1$
Propofol	5–15 µg/kg/min	$$$	Emergence	?
Dexamethasone^d	4–8 mg IV	$	Induction	?
Ephedrine	35–50 mg IM	$	Emergence	?

Alternative therapies: adequate hydration, isopropyl alcohol vapor, supplemental oxygen; aroma therapy—peppermint, acupressure.
QT, risk of QT prolongation.
5HT$_3$, serotonin; D$_2$, dopamine; H$_1$, histamine; M$_1$, muscarinic; NK$_1$, neurokinin; ?, exact mechanism unknown.
^{a}Black box warning for QT prolongation.
^{b}Risk of extrapramidal reaction. Reverse with diphenhydramine.
^{c}Do not give IV push. Must be diluted.
^{d}Can cause severe perineal burning and pain.

    iv) Administer PONV prophylaxis when appropriate.
      (1) Single-agent therapy (see Section A above)
      (2) Combination therapy (Table 7-3)
        (a) Consider for adults at moderate risk for PONV.
        (b) Combine treatment using drugs from different classes.
        (c) Generally, combination therapy has superior efficacy compared with monotherapy for PONV prophylaxis.

ANESTHESIOLOGY

Table 7-2

Strategies to Reduce Baseline PONV Risk (2)

1. Avoidance of general anesthesia if regional anesthetic reasonable alternative
2. Use of propofol for induction and maintenance (TIVA) of anesthesia
3. Avoidance of nitrous oxide
4. Avoidance of volatile anesthetic
5. Minimization of intraoperative/postoperative opioids
6. Minimization of neostigmine
7. Adequate hydration

        (d) Optimal antiemetic dosing with combination therapy needs to be established.

    (3) Failed prophylaxis

        (a) If prophylaxis fails or was not received, use drug from different class than prophylactic agent (2).

        (b) Redose antiemetic only after more than 6 hours in PACU.

            (i) Do not redose dexamethasone or scopolamine

c) Nonpharmacologic approaches to PONV prophylaxis

    i)   Acupuncture (P_6 acupuncture point)

    ii) Transcutaneous electrical nerve stimulation

    iii) Acupoint stimulation (Korean hand acupoint)

    iv) Acupressure

d) Appropriate treatment depends on a careful assessment of risk versus benefit for each treatment modality (Table 7-4).

    i)   Some risks of treatment depending on the medication include

    ii) QT prolongation (Table 7-4)

    iii) Drug reactions (metoclopramide)

    iv) Perineal burning (dexamethasone)

    v) Thrombophlebitis (promethazine, hydroxyzine)

e) Ineffective therapies for PONV

Some therapies have been studied and found to be ineffective for PONV prophylaxis. These include

    i)   Metoclopramide when used in standard 10-mg IV doses

    ii) Ginger root

    iii) Cannibinoids

    iv) Hypnosis

Metoclopramide when used in standard 10-mg IV doses is ineffective for PONV prophylaxis.

Table 7-3

Combination Therapy for PONV Prophylaxis in Adults (2)

1. Droperidol + dexamethasone
2. $5HT_3$ receptor antagonist + dexamethasone
3. $5HT_3$ receptor antagonist + droperidol
4. $5HT_3$ receptor antagonist + dexamethasone + droperidol

Table 7-4

Risks Associated with Treating PONV

1. Droperidol has black box warning for QTc prolongation.
2. Other drugs with QTc prolongation (see Table 7-1 for QT).
3. Metoclopramide has extrapyramidal side effects reversed with diphenhydramine.
4. Dexamethasone can cause perineal burning and pain.
5. Do not administer promethazine via IV push.

Chapter Summary for PONV

General Considerations	PONV is a common problem that is best treated with prevention. It is important to understand the side-effect profile for each drug.
Approach	1. Identify patients' risk for PONV 2. Reduce baseline risk for PONV 3. Administer PONV prophylaxis when appropriate

Risk Factors	Risk factors can be surgery related, anesthesia related, or patient related.
	Most important risk factors include
	    History of PONV/motion sickness
	    Nitrous oxide
	    Opioids
	    Volatile anesthetic
	    Female gender
	    Nonsmoker

Treatment	The drug classes used to treat PONV include dopamine, serotonin, muscarinic, histamine, and neurokinin receptor antagonists. Appropriate treatment depends on a careful assessment of risk versus benefit for each treatment modality.
Prevention Strategy	For patients at moderate risk, use 1–2 interventions. For patients at high risk, use a multimodal approach

References

1. Gan TJ. Postoperative nausea and vomiting-can it be eliminated? *JAMA* 2002;287:1233–1236.
2. Gan TJ, Meyer TA, Apfel CC, et al. Society for Ambulatory Anesthesia guidelines for the management of postoperative nausea and vomiting. *Anesth Analg* 2007;105(6):1615–1628, table of contents.
3. Apfel CC, Korttila K, Abdalla M, et al. A factorial trial of six interventions for the prevention of postoperative nausea and vomiting. *N Engl J Med* 2004;350:2441–2451.
4. Watch MF, White PF. Post operative nausea and vomiting: its etiology, treatment, and prevention. *Anesthesiology* 1992;77:162–184.
5. Gan TJ. Mechanisms underlying postoperative nausea and vomiting and neurotransmitter receptor antagonist-based pharmacotherapy. *CNS Drugs* 2007;21(10):813–833.
6. Habib AS, White WD, Eubanks S, et al. A randomized comparison of a multimodal management strategy versus combination antiemetics for the prevention of postoperative nausea and vomiting. *Anesth Analg* 2004;99(1):77–81.
7. Gan TJ, Apfel CC, Kovac A, et al. A randomized, double-blind comparison of the NK₁ antagonist, aprepitant, versus ondansetron for the prevention of postoperative nausea and vomiting. *Anesth Analg* 2007;104(5):1082–1089.
8. Scuderi PE, James RL, Harris L, et al. Multimodal antiemetic management prevents early postoperative vomiting after outpatient laparoscopy. *Anesth Analg* 2000;91(6):1408–1414.

9. Gan TJ. Mechanisms underlying postoperative nausea and vomiting and neurotransmitter receptor antagonist-based pharmacotherapy. *CNS Drugs* 2007;21(10):813–833.
10. Habib AS, Gan TJ. The use of droperidol before and after the Food and Drug Administration black box warning: a survey of the members of the Society of Ambulatory Anesthesia. *J Clin Anesth* 2008;20(1):35–39.
11. Zarate E, Mingus M, White PF, et al. The use of transcutaneous acupoint electrical stimulation for preventing nausea and vomiting after laparoscopic surgery. *Anesth Analg* 2001;92(3):629–635.

8 Standard ASA Monitors

Trent Bryson, MD

In 1986 the American Society of Anesthesiologists (ASA) approved the first edition of *Standards for Basic Anesthetic Monitoring.* Periodically these standards are updated according to advances in technology and practice, the most recent being in 2005 (1). The standards are to be considered a minimum during **all general, regional, and monitored anesthetic care** and may be exceeded at any time as deemed necessary. These measures are to only be suspended when interfering with emergent life supportive measures or in the rare instance when they are impractical or failing to detect clinical developments.

Continuous presence of a qualified anesthesia provider is a standard set by the ASA.

1) **Overview of required elements**—Published standards address broad elements instead of specific devices and are broken down into two required standards (2).

   a) **Standard I**

      i) The **presence of a qualified anesthesia provider is continuously required** throughout the duration of all anesthetic care due to the rapidity with which physiologic derangements may occur during surgical intervention.

   b) **Standard II**

      i) Continual monitoring of **oxygenation, ventilation, circulation, and temperature.**

      ii) Frequency of mandatory monitoring varies between each category, but never exceeds five minutes.

         (1) If not used, a reason should be recorded on the patient record.

      iii) The following are all specifically mandated.

         (1) **Oxygen analyzer** with a low inspired concentration limit alarm during general anesthesia

         (2) Quantitative assessment of **blood oxygenation**

         (3) Ensuring adequate ventilation during all anesthetic care including **verification of expired oxygen** (when possible), quantitative **measurement of tidal volume,** and **capnography** in all general anesthetics.

         (4) Qualitative evaluation of ventilation is required during all other care.

         (5) Ensure correct placement of endotracheal tube or laryngeal mask airway via **expired carbon dioxide (CO_2).**

         (6) **Alarms for disconnects** when a mechanical ventilator is used

         (7) Continuous display of **ECG**

         (8) Determination of **arterial BP and heart rate** at least every 5 minutes.

         (9) Adequacy of circulation is to be determined by **quality of pulse** either electronically, through palpation, or auscultation

         (10) The means to determine **temperature** must be available and should be employed when changes in temperature are anticipated or intended.

MONITORING

55

An audible alarm should be set to notify the anesthesia provider of a hypoxic gas mixture.

2) **Oxygen analyzer**
    a) Most modern anesthesia machines monitor both inspired and expired concentrations of O_2.
    b) This is essential during anesthesia because it is possible to deliver a hypoxic gas mixture when mixing O_2, air, nitrous oxide, and/or volatile anesthetic agents.

3) **Pulse oximetry**
    a) Provides quantitative analysis of the patient's saturation of hemoglobin with O_2.

4) **Carbon dioxide (CO_2)**
    a) Inspired and expired CO_2 should be monitored.
    b) Expired CO_2 is frequently displayed through capnography with a displayed value correlating to the peak expired CO_2 of each breath.
    c) **Capnography**
        i)   Provides qualitative and quantitative information regarding expired CO_2.
        ii) Quantitatively, this is **useful to ensure the endotracheal tube is within the respiratory tract** as well as to ensure adequate cardiac output.
    d) Inspired CO_2
        i)   Monitored to ensure that the CO_2 absorber of the anesthesia machine is adequately removing all CO_2 from the circuit.
        ii) **If inspired CO_2 is greater than zero, changing of the absorbent should be considered.** The color of absorbent turns blue when its capacity is exhausted.

 READ MORE

Pulse oximetry
Chapter 9
page 61

Capnography
Chapter 10
page 65

EKG leads are color-coded to assist placement. RA and LA leads are easily remembered: imagine the LA becomes sun-tanned (black) driving a car with the window open, while the RA remains untanned (white) inside the car.

5) **Multiple expired gas analysis**
    a) While not an essential monitor according to the ASA, this allows determination of the percent inspired and expired of the volatile agents and nitrous oxide.
    b) This allows the ability to better determine the delivery of an adequate anesthetic without over or under dose.

6) **ECG**
    a) The minimum of three leads is to be used, although five leads are used for most adults (3).
    b) Consideration must be taken for the surgical field and patient positioning.
        i)   Lead placement is commonly altered for cases involving the chest, shoulders, back, and neck.
    c) Five Lead ECG
        i)   Includes the right arm (**RA**), left arm (**LA**), right leg (**RL**), left leg (**LL**), and **V**.
        ii) The five lead arrangement can be used to display **I, II, III, aVR, aVL, aVF, and/or V** (Fig. 8-1).
    d) Three lead ECG
        i)   Includes the **RA, LA, and LL** leads and can be used to display leads **I, II, and/or III** (Fig. 8-2).
            (1) A three lead ECG can be modified to display V5 by moving the LA lead to the V5 position in the fifth intercostal space at the anterior axillary line (Fig. 8-3).
    e) The **most commonly monitored leads are II and V5.**
        i)   II is best used to monitor rhythm because it provides the best visibility of the P wave.
        ii) V5 monitors for anterior and lateral ischemic events.

| **Figure 8-1** | Normal Five Lead ECG Lead Placement |

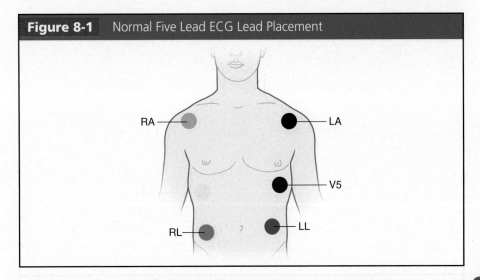

| **Figure 8-2** | Normal Configuration of a Three Lead EKG |

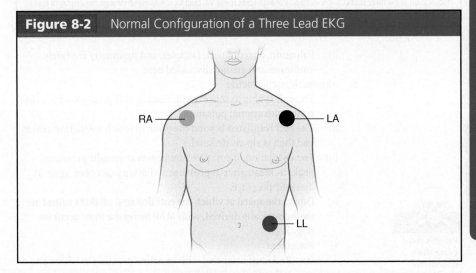

MONITORING

For most patients, printing the ECG tracing at the beginning of the case allows for later comparison should an intraoperative event occur.

iii) Most anesthesia machines will allow you to change how many and which leads are displayed.

(1) Some will show all leads simultaneously, although this often removes all other monitors from the display while viewing all leads.

(2) If an arrhythmia or ischemic event appears to be present, temporarily viewing all leads simultaneously may be helpful for diagnostic purposes.

7) **Arterial blood pressure (BP)**

a) BP can be monitored invasively or non-invasively.

b) Non-invasive methods

i) Include palpation, auscultation, Doppler probe, oscillometric cuff, or tonometry.

Figure 8-3	Modification of Three Lead ECG

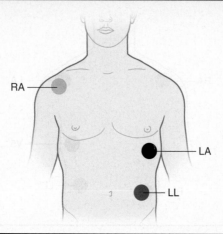

Modification of the three lead ECG allows display of both leads II and V5. Lead V5 is monitored through the display of lead I in this configuration.

        ii)   Palpation, auscultation, Doppler, and tonometry are rarely employed and are not discussed here.

    c)   Automatic oscillometric

        i)   The cuff is able to sense oscillations in cuff pressure which correlate with arterial pulsation.

        ii)   The cuff is inflated beyond the point at which oscillation ceases and then is slowly deflated.

        iii)   The oscillation in cuff pressure begins at systolic pressure, peaks at mean arterial pressure and disappears once again at diastolic pressure.

        iv)   **Due to the speed at which the cuff deflates, all three values are mathematically derived, with MAP being the most accurate** (Fig. 8-4).

Patients in the beach chair position are especially prone to cerebral ischemia even with "normal" brachial BPs.

        v)   Placement

            (1)   Each cuff is labeled with an arrow pointing to where arterial pulsation is felt best.

            (2)   The cuff is then placed on the arm over the brachial artery, forearm over the radial artery, or thigh/calf over the popliteal artery.

READ MORE

Invasive arterial blood pressure monitoring, Chapter 11, page 70

        vi)   Patient positioning

            (1)   When monitoring non-invasive pressure, consideration must be taken of patient position.

        vii)   Invasive BP monitoring

8)   **Temperature**

    a)   Temperature changes should be anticipated and expected under any general anesthetic and therefore **any general anesthetic requires temperature measurement.**

        i)   Very brief procedures may be an exception, but the availability of temperature monitoring should be recorded.

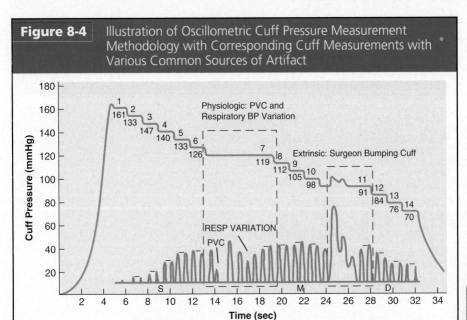

Figure 8-4 Illustration of Oscillometric Cuff Pressure Measurement Methodology with Corresponding Cuff Measurements with Various Common Sources of Artifact

Reproduced from Greenberg SB, Murphy GS, Vender JS. Standard monitoring techniques. In: Barash PG, Cullen BF, Stoelting RK, et al., eds. *Clinical Anesthesia*. 6th ed. Philadelphia, PA: Lippincott Williams & Wilkins; 2009:702, with permission.

b) The temperature may be measured from many locations including skin, nasopharynx, esophageal, bladder, rectal, or a pulmonary arterial catheter.

c) Core temperatures obtained from a pulmonary catheter, esophageal stethoscope, or rectal probe are preferable sources.

Chapter Summary for Standard Monitors

Definition	ASA standard monitors are to be considered a minimum during **all general, regional, and monitored anesthetic care** and may be exceeded at any time as deemed necessary. *These measures are to only be suspended when interfering with emergent life supportive measures or in the rare instance when they are impractical or failing to detect clinical developments.*

Function	Physical Signs	Monitor	Equipment Alarms and Monitoring
Oxygenation	Color of skin and mucous membranes	Pulse oximeter, Inhaled oxygen concentration	Low limit alarms
Ventilation	Breath sounds, chest excursion	Ventilator, End-tidal CO_2 analysis	Disconnect alarm, tidal volume measurement, $ETCO_2$ alarms
Circulation	Pulse palpation, auscultation of heart sounds	ECG BP Heart rate	ECG, BP cuff, arterial line, pulse oximeter
Temperature	Skin	Temperature probe	Low temperature alarm

References

1. "Standards for Basic Anesthetic Monitoring," last amended October 25, 2005. http://www.asahq.org
2. Greenberg SB, Murphy GS, Vender JS. Standard monitoring techniques. In: Barash PG, Cullen BF, Stoelting RK, et al., eds. *Clinical Anesthesia.* 6th ed. Philadelphia, PA: Lippincott Williams & Wilkins, 2009:702.
3. Morgan GE, Mikhail MS, Murray MJ, eds. Patient monitors. In: *Clinical Anesthesiology.* 4th ed. New York, NY: McGraw Hill, 2006:117–154.

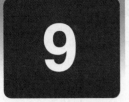

9

Pulse Oximetry

Rachel Boggus, MD

Pulse oximetry is one of the most commonly employed monitoring modalities in anesthesia. It is a non-invasive way to monitor the oxygenation of a patient's hemoglobin. A sensor with both red and infrared wavelengths is placed on the patient. Absorption of these wavelengths by the blood is measured and oxygen saturation (SpO_2) can be calculated.

1) Basic Concepts
   a) Pulse oximetry measures the amount of oxyhemoglobin using the **Lambert-Beer law**
      i) The Lambert-Beer law is a mathematical means of expressing how light is absorbed by matter
   b) There are two main types of oximetry. **Fractional oximetry** and **functional oximetry**
      i) **Fractional oximetry.** Oxyhemoglobin/(oxyhemoglobin + deoxyhemoglobin + methemoglobin + carboxyhemoglobin)
      ii) Fractional oximetry measures the arterial oxygen saturation (SaO_2)
         (1) Can only be measured by an **arterial blood sample**
      iii) **Functional oximetry**

      oxyhemoglobin/(oxyhemoglobin + deoxyhemoglobin) = SpO_2

         (1) Functional **oximetry** gives you the **SpO_2**
         (2) Can be measured noninvasively by a **standard pulse oximeter**
2) How pulse oximetry works
   a) A pulse oximeter emits two wavelengths of light: red (660 nm) and infrared (940 nm)
      i) **Deoxyhemoglobin** absorbs more light in the **red band**
      ii) **Oxyhemoglobin** absorbs more light in the **infrared band**
   b) Sensors in the oximeter detect the amount of red and infrared light absorbed by the blood
   c) **Photoplethysmography** is then used to identify **pulsatile arterial flow (alternating current [AC])** and **non-pulsatile flow (direct current [DC])**
   d) The ratio of AC/DC at both 660 and 940 nm is measured using the equation: $(AC/DC)_{660}/(AC/DC)_{940}$
   e) The pulse oximeter calculates the SpO_2 by taking the above equation and using an algorithm built into the software to derive the SpO_2
      i) The calibration to derive SpO_2 from the $(AC/DC)_{660}/(AC/DC)_{940}$ ratio was made from studies of **healthy volunteers**
3) Accuracy of the pulse oximeter

SpO_2 measurements are not accurate below 70%.

   a) If the SpO_2 is between **70% and 100%** the pulse oximeter is **accurate to within 5%**
      i) It is not accurate below 70% because calibration of the pulse oximeter involved healthy volunteers whose SpO_2 did not routinely reach levels <70%

MONITORING

61

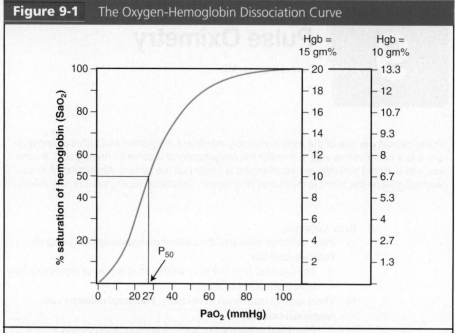

Figure 9-1   The Oxygen-Hemoglobin Dissociation Curve

The oxygen dissociation curve showing the relationship between SpO_2 and PaO_2. P_{50} is the PaO_2 at which hemoglobin is 50% saturated with oxygen. The normal value is 27 mmHg. Adapted from Martin L. *All you really need to know to interpret arterial blood gases*. 2nd ed. Philadelphia: Lippincott Williams & Wilkins; 1999.

SpO₂ of 90% correlates to a PaO₂ of 60 mm Hg.

ii)   For the relationship between SaO_2 and PaO_2 (see Fig. 9-1) (7)

iii) It is also not as accurate below 70% because there is more **deoxyhemoglobin present**

   (1)   The absorption spectrum of deoxygenated hemoglobin is **very steep at 600 nm in the red range** so **small changes in the amount of deoxyhemoglobin can cause very wide variances in SpO_2** (Fig. 9-2)

b)   **Ear probes** may be **more accurate** than finger probes because the probe is closer to the heart

c)   Pulse oximetry is not as accurate in low amplitude states (Table 9-1)

   i)   **Low perfusion** makes it difficult for the pulse oximeter to distinguish a true signal from background noise

4)   Dyshemoglobinemias

a)   Pulse oximetry only accurately measures oxyhemoglobin and deoxyhemoglobin—all other forms of hemoglobin are not accurately measured

   i)   **Carboxyhemoglobin is measured as 90% oxyhemoglobin and 10% deoxyhemoglobin**

      (1)   Thus, when there are high amounts of carboxyhemoglobin it will **overestimate** the SpO_2

      (2)   This is an important consideration in patients exposed to smoke or fires

   ii)   **Methemoglobin absorbs equal amounts of red and infrared light so the SpO_2 will read 85%**

      (1)   Methemoglobin is formed when iron goes from it's **+2 ferrous form to the +3 ferric state**

      (2)   The **ferric state** of iron displays a **left shift on the oxygen dissociation curve** and releases oxygen less easily

Figure 9-2   Light Absorption with Oxygenated and Deoxygenated Hemoglobin

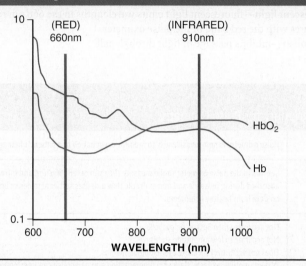

Oxygenated hemoglobin (*red line*) absorbs more infrared light and allows more red light (*vertical red line*) to pass through. Deoxygenated hemoglobin (*purple line*) absorbs more red light and allows more infrared light (*vertical purple line*) to pass through. Adapted from red and infrared light absorption. http://www.oximeter.org/pulseox/principles.htm accessed March 8, 2010

      (3) Methemoglobinemia can be caused by many drugs (Table 9-2)
      iii) **Patients with sickle cell anemia presenting in a vasoocclusive crisis** can have an inaccurate SpO_2 reading
      iv) **High levels of bilirubin** do not alter SpO_2 readings
5) **Other Limitations**
    a) **IV dyes**
      i) **Methylene blue, indocyanine green, and indigo carmine** all cause transient decreases in the SpO_2 lasting anywhere from 30 seconds to 20 minutes

Table 9-1
Low Amplitude States
Hypovolemia
Hypothermia
Cardiac arrest
Arrhythmias
Cardiac bypass
Vasoconstriction
Tourniquet
BP cuff inflation

Table 9-2
Causes of Methemoglobinemia
Nitrates/Nitrites
Local anesthetics (e.g., Benzocaine or Hurricaine Spray)
Chlorates
Antimalarials
Antineoplastics
Sulfonamides
Dapsone
Metoclopramide

MONITORING

b) **Dark skin pigmentation**—melanin inhibits passage of light through tissue
c) **Motion artifact**—pulse oximeter unable to measure peaks and troughs of waveform correctly
d) **Fluorescent light**—fluorescent light emits wavelengths in the 660 nm region which interferes with the red band of the pulse oximeter
e) **Nail polish**—inhibits passage of light through nail.

Chapter Summary for Pulse Oximetry

Definition	Pulse oximetry is non-invasive way to monitor oxygenation of a patient's hemoglobin using light.
How it Works	Sensors in the pulse oximeter probe measure the ratio of red (660 nm) and infrared (940 nm) light absorbed during pulsatile and non-pulsatile flow and uses software to derive an SpO_2 value based on data from healthy volunteers.
Limitations	Not accurate when SpO_2 is below 70% Not accurate in low amplitude states Does not accurately measure dyshemoglobinemias. IV dyes, motion artifacts, dark skin pigmentation and nail polish can interfere with measurement.

References

1. Huch A, Huch R, Konig V, et al. Limitations of pulse oximetry. *Lancet* 1988;1:357–358.
2. Juban, A. Pulse Oximetry. *Crit Care*. 1999;3(2):R11–R17.
3. Schnapp LM, Cohen NH. Pulse oximetry-uses and abuses. *Chest* 1990;98:1244–1250.
4. Tremper KK, Barker SJ. Pulse oximetry. *Anesthesiology*.1989;70:98–108.
5. Welch JP, DeCesare MS, Hess D. Pulse oximetry: instrumentation and clinical applications. *Respir Care*. 1990;35:584–601.
6. Wukitisch MW, Peterson MT, Tobler DR, et al. Pulse oximetry: analysis of theory, technology, and practice. *J Clin Monit*. 1988;4:290–301.
7. Martin, Lawrence. *All you really need to know to interpret arterial blood gases*. 2nd ed. Lippincott Williams & Wilkins, 1999.
8. "Red and infrared light absorption." *Oximetry.org*. Web. Mar 8, 2010. http://www.oximeter.org/pulseox/principles.htm.

10 Capnography

Jessica Spellman, MD

Monitoring of CO_2 through capnometry and capnography can be a valuable tool in detecting acute alterations in ventilation, metabolism, and circulation. Continuous monitoring of CO_2 is an American Society of Anesthesiology (ASA) standard for basic monitoring in all patients receiving general anesthesia (unless invalidated by the nature of the patient, procedure, or equipment) and for confirming proper endotracheal tube and LMA placement (1).

Capnography is continuous monitoring of a patient's capnogram during the respiratory cycle.

1) **Definitions (2)**
   a) **Capnometry**
      i) Measurement and numeric representation of CO_2 concentration or partial pressure in respiratory gases during inspiration and expiration
   b) **Capnogram**
      i) Concentration time display of CO_2 concentration sampled at a patient's airway
   c) **Capnography**
      i) Continuous monitoring of a patient's capnogram during the respiratory cycle
2) **Methods of capnometry (3)**
   a) **Sidestream capnometers**
      i) Sample tubing connected to the airway that continually aspirates respiratory gases at a rate of 50 to 400 mL/min to a measurement chamber
      ii) Advantages
         (1) Allows for accurate capnography when attached as close as possible to the patient
         (2) Lightweight
         (3) Can be used to measure CO_2 and anesthetic gases
      iii) Disadvantages
         (1) Condensation of humidified gases may cause frequent clogging of the tubing (water traps and filters must be used to prevent condensation from reaching the measuring chamber)
         (2) Delay in measurement response time depending on the size and length of the tubing
   b) **Mainstream capnometers**
      i) Light absorption chamber directly attached to the airway
      ii) Advantages
         (1) Direct measurement allows for fast response time
      iii) Disadvantages
         (1) Bulky equipment placed directly in endotracheal tube
         (2) Does not allow for measurement of anesthetic gases

3) Techniques of CO_2 measurement (4)
   a) **Infrared spectrography**
      i) Employed by most operating rooms
      ii) In the measuring chamber, gases are exposed to an infrared light beam
      iii) Each molecule (CO_2, anesthetic gases) has a specific absorbance spectrum of the infrared beam that can be quantified
   b) Mass spectrography
      i) Measurement of CO_2 and other gas concentrations on the basis of differing molecular weights
   c) **Raman spectrography**
      i) Use of spectral analysis of scattered light energy that results from an argon laser light source exposed to a gas mixture
   d) **Colorimetric CO_2 analysis (5)**
      i) pH sensitive test paper
      ii) When in the presence of CO_2, color change occurs
      iii) Often used to confirm CO_2 and endotracheal intubation outside of the operating room

4) Normal capnogram (6) (Fig. 10-1)
   a) **Phase I**
      i) Initiation of expiration
      ii) CO_2-free gas from anatomic dead space
   b) **Phase II**
      i) Expiration of **mixture of dead space and alveolar gas**
   c) **Phase III**
      i) **Alveolar plateau**
      ii) CO_2-rich gas from alveoli
   d) Phase IV or 0 (7)
      i) **Inspiration**

5) Clinical uses of capnography (4)
   a) **Confirmation of endotracheal intubation**

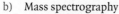

Colorimetric CO_2 analysis is often used to confirm CO_2 and endotracheal intubation outside of the operating room.

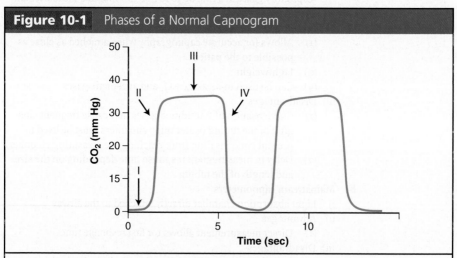

| **Figure 10-1** | Phases of a Normal Capnogram |

Reproduced from Eisenkraft JB, Leibowitz AB. Hypoxia and equipment failure. In: Yao FS, ed. *Yao & Artusio's Anesthesiology: Problem-Oriented Patient Management.* 6th ed. Philadelphia, PA: Lippincott Williams & Wilkins; 2008:1185, with permission.

Capnography can be used to monitor the adequacy of ventilation in controlled or spontaneously ventilating patients.

Causes of increased CO_2 production include: fever, sepsis, malignant hyperthermia, shivering.

Causes of decreased CO_2 production include: decreased cardiac output, hypovolemia, pulmonary embolism, hypothermia, hyperventilation.

b) **Monitoring** of adequacy of ventilation in controlled or spontaneously ventilating patients

c) Noninvasive **estimate of $PaCO_2$**
   i) Assumes the normal 2 to 5 mm Hg difference between expired ($PETCO_2$) and arterial ($PaCO_2$) that exists in the awake state is present
   ii) The gradient between $PETCO2$ and $PaCO2$ may be increased with age, pulmonary disease, pulmonary embolus, low cardiac output, and hypovolemia

d) **Detection of patient disease**
   i) Causes of increased CO_2 production
      (1) Fever
      (2) Sepsis
      (3) Malignant hyperthermia
      (4) Hyperthyroidism
      (5) Shivering
   ii) Causes of decreased $PETCO_2$
      (1) Decreased cardiac output
      (2) Hypovolemiaism
      (3) Pulmonary embolism
      (4) Hypothermia (6)
      (5) Hyperventilation (6)
   iii) Airway obstruction may be detected due to abnormalities in the capnography tracing

e) **Detection of problems with the anesthetic breathing system**
   i) Rebreathing
   ii) Incompetent valves
   iii) Circuit disconnect
   iv) Circuit leak

6) **Interpretation of abnormal capnograms (3,4,6) (Fig. 10-2)**
   a) **Rebreathing of CO_2**
      i) Elevation in baseline CO_2 and Phase I
      ii) Can eliminate by increasing fresh gas flow or changing CO_2 absorber
   b) **Obstruction** to expiratory gas flow
      i) Prolonged Phase II and steeper Phase III slope
      ii) Occurs with bronchospasm, COPD, kinked endotracheal tube
   c) **"Curare Cleft"**
      i) Dip in Phase III
      ii) Indicates return of spontaneous respiratory efforts
   d) **Cardiogenic oscillations**
      i) Oscillations of small gas movements during phase III and IV (or 0)
      ii) Produced by aortic and cardiac pulsations
   e) **Increased CO_2**
      i) Elevated plateau height
      ii) Indicates increased CO_2 production states (see above), other source of CO_2 (as in laparoscopic surgery), or inadequate minute ventilation
   f) **Decreased measured CO_2**
      i) Decreased plateau height
      ii) May indicated decreased CO_2 production state (see above) or increased minute ventilation

MONITORING

g) **Incompetent inspiratory valve**
   i)   Prolonged Phase III with elevation of baseline CO_2 and plateau height
   ii) Results in rebreathing
   iii) May be difficult to detect without simultaneous analysis of flow waveforms (7)
h) **Esophageal intubation**
   i)   Initial presence of CO_2 followed by no CO_2 detection

Figure 10-2	Abnormal Capnograms

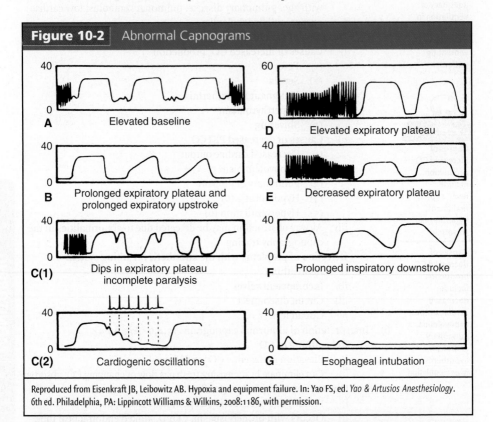

A — Elevated baseline
B — Prolonged expiratory plateau and prolonged expiratory upstroke
C(1) — Dips in expiratory plateau incomplete paralysis
C(2) — Cardiogenic oscillations
D — Elevated expiratory plateau
E — Decreased expiratory plateau
F — Prolonged inspiratory downstroke
G — Esophageal intubation

Reproduced from Eisenkraft JB, Leibowitz AB. Hypoxia and equipment failure. In: Yao FS, ed. *Yao & Artusios Anesthesiology*. 6th ed. Philadelphia, PA: Lippincott Williams & Wilkins, 2008:1186, with permission.

Chapter Summary for Capnography

Definition	Capnography is the continuous monitoring of a patient's CO_2 during the respiratory cycle.
Intraoperative Use	Basic standard for ASA monitoring in general anesthesia and to confirm endotracheal intubation.
Techniques for CO_2 Measurement	Most operating rooms utilize sidestream capnometers and infrared spectrography to sample and measure CO_2.
Clinical Applications	Continuous monitoring for alterations in the CO_2 waveform may be useful for detecting esophageal intubation, rebreathing, hypermetabolic or low cardiac output states, obstruction, and return of spontaneous respiratory efforts.

References

1. American Society of Anesthesiology. *Standards for Basic Anesthetic Monitoring*. [Internet]. Park Ridge, IL: American Society of Anesthesiology, 2005 Oct 25, c2008. [cited 2010 Jul 7].
2. Greenberg SB, Murphy GS, Vender JS. Standard monitoring techniques. In: Barash PG, ed. *Clinical Anesthesia*. 6th ed. Philadelphia, PA: Lippincott Williams & Wilkins; 2009:697–700.
3. Szocik JF, Barker SJ, Tremper KK. Fundamental principles of monitoring instrumentation. In: Miller RD, ed. *Miller's Anesthesia*. 6th ed. Philadelphia, PA: Elsevier, 2005:1213.
4. Bhivani-Shankar K, Moseley H, Kumar AY, et al. Capnometry and anaesthesia. *Can J Anaesth*. 1992;39:617–632.
5. Moon RE, Camporesi EM. Respiratory monitoring. In: Miller RD, ed. *Miller's Anesthesia*. 6th ed. Philadelphia, PA: Elsevier; 2005:1454.
6. Eisenkraft JB, Leibowitz AB. Hypoxia and equipment failure. In: Yao, FS, ed. *Yao & Artusio's Anesthesiology: Problem-Oriented Patient Management*. 6th ed. Philadelphia, PA: Lippincott Williams & Wilkins; 2008:1184–1187.
7. Bhavani-Shankar K, Philip JH. Defining segments and phases of a time capnogram. *Anesth Analg* 2000;91:973–977.

MONITORING

Invasive Arterial Blood Pressure Monitoring

Quinn Stevens, MD • Nathaen Weitzel, MD

Invasive arterial blood pressure monitoring allows for continuous, beat to beat monitoring of arterial blood pressure (BP) displayed as a waveform and provides access for arterial blood sampling.

1) **Indications**
   a) Need for instantaneous analysis of BP
      i) Patients with end organ disease or procedures prone to wide and rapid changes in BP, such as trauma, cardiac, vascular, chest, spine, craniotomies, or monitored hypotension.
      ii) Procedures with anticipated fluid shifts where multiple blood samples for arterial blood gas analysis may be needed.
      iii) Long procedures to reduce risk of noninvasive blood pressure–related nerve damage.

2) **Mechanics**
   a) Arterial lines utilize saline filled tubing, which is connected directly into the artery via a catheter, to transmit pressure waves to a transducer.
   b) Transducers consist of a diaphragm in the base of a plastic dome that converts pressure changes into the arterial pressure tracing.
      i) As the diaphragm moves, a silicon crystal is stretched and its resistance changes.
      ii) Changes in resistance are interpreted as voltage changes, which are amplified and filtered into a tracing.
      iii) This is based upon the strain gauge principle, where stretching a wire or silicon crystal changes its resistance (1).
   c) In the supine patient, the transducer should be placed at the midaxillary line, corresponding to the level of the right atrium, and must be readjusted with patient level adjustments.
   d) When patients are in the sitting position, cerebral pressure can also be determined by placing the transducer at the level of the external auditory meatus, which approximates the level of the circle of Willis.
   e) The transducer must be zeroed to create a reference point, most commonly to atmospheric pressure. This is accomplished by opening the line to room air via a stopcock.
   f) **Due to hydrostatic pressure, every 1 cm change in height of the transducer correlates with a 0.75 mm Hg pressure difference.** Thus, raising a zeroed transducer 20 cm from the right atrium will lower the systolic and diastolic pressure reading by 15 mm Hg.
   g) The fluid column between the catheter and transducer has no effect on the pressure reading. Thus, raising or lowering a patient's arm with a radial catheter will not affect the reading from a stationary transducer.

Raising or lowering the transducer will alter the BP reading, but changes in position of the patient's arm where the arterial catheter is located will not change the reading.

3) Arterial access sites

a) **Radial artery**

   i) Commonly cannulated due to its superficial location and good collateral flow, using a 20- or 22-gauge catheter (22 to 24-gauge for children and infants)

   ii) While 5% of individuals have an incomplete palmar arch, far fewer patients develop complications from vascular compromise following arterial cannulation.

   iii) The Allen test, doppler probe, or pulse oximetry are all proposed methods to evaluate collateral flow, although none have been clinically proven to improve outcomes.

The ulnar artery can be cannulated; however, it is technically more difficult and should be avoided once attempts on the radial artery have been made.

b) **Brachial artery**

   i) The brachial artery is large and easily identifiable.

   ii) The artery's proximity to aorta reduces waveform distortion.

   iii) Brachial artery cannulation was traditionally avoided because hematoma formation or injury could potentially threaten the vascular supply to the entire forearm and risk injury to the adjacent median nerve.

   iv) Evidence suggests that the complication rate following brachial arterial cannulation is lower than previously reported, making this site an acceptable alternative for cannulation (3,4).

   v) Ultrasound use during placement may reduce the incidence of injury to adjacent structures.

c) **Axillary artery**

   i) Generally avoided because it is adjacent to the axillary plexus, making nerve injury a concern.

   ii) The artery is also much closer to the cerebral circulation, potentially increasing the risk of cerebral embolism during flushing.

d) **Femoral artery**

   i) The femoral artery provides rapid and accurate access using a long 18 or 20-gauge catheter.

   ii) Prone to pseudoaneurysm and atheroma formation.

   iii) Aseptic necrosis of femoral head in children is a rare but reported complication.

   iv) Infection rates are generally higher than radial cannulation, although some evidence suggests comparable rates of infection (5–7).

READ
MORE

Atlas of anesthesia procedures, Radial artery catheterization, Chapter 158, page 1112

e) **Other**

   i) **Dorsalis pedis** and **posterior tibial** arteries form an anastamotic arch in the foot analogous to the hand.

   ii) They are appropriate alternatives in situations of difficult upper extremity access such as trauma or neurosurgery.

   iii) Theses arteries are far from the aorta and therefore prone to more distortion and systolic pressure exaggeration (1).

f) **Cannulation technique**

   i) Multiple techniques for placement exist and are largely determined by practitioner familiarity.

   ii) In general, the catheter can be advanced directly off the needle or using the "through and through" artery technique. Either technique can be performed using a Seldinger technique by first threading a wire.

Increasing use, familiarity, and availability make ultrasound a viable option when difficulty during placement is either encountered or anticipated.

4) **Interpretation**

   a) **Waveform**

   i) The rate of upstroke generally correlates with contractility, and downstroke rate indicates peripheral vascular resistance.

   ii) As the arterial lumen decreases in size, velocity increases, leading to a peaked but shorter wave.

   iii) The systolic BP and pulse pressures are falsely elevated while the diastolic pressure and mean pressures are lower when the distal arterial system is cannulated. This is often clinically evident by a lack of congruency between NIBP and the arterial line measurements. A transducer in the aortic root theoretically provides the most accurate measurement (2).

   iv) **Systolic pressure variation during the respiratory cycle >8 mm correlates strongly with hypovolemia.** This is a particularly useful tool during mechanical ventilation when variables that affect systolic pressure variation including tidal volume, frequency, and PEEP can be held constant (8).

   b) **Dampening of the arterial tracing**

   i) Underdampening

   (1) Refers to a system that resonates when the frequency of the pressure waveform approaches the frequency of the system

   (2) This can be thought of as a diaphragm within the transducer that vibrates for a prolonged period of time in relation to a single pressure wave.

   (3) **Underdampened systems overestimate systolic pressure by 15 to 30 mm Hg and amplify catheter artifact or catheter whip.** This occurs with very small tubing (<1.5 mm diameter), or long connection lines (>1.5 m), stiff tubing, or large catheters (18 G)(2).

A common cause of BP exaggeration is when extra tubing is in use, such as for a dorsalis pedis arterial line. A common cause of BP underestimation is when an arm is tucked and the catheter is kinked.

   ii) **Overdampening**

   (1) Refers to a transducer diaphragm or measuring system that is too rigid

   (2) **Overdampened systems underestimate systolic pressure** and occur with high viscosity, soft tubing, air bubbles, blood clots, and kinked catheters (2). Mean pressures are typically less affected.

   iii) **Optimization**

   (1) The system is optimized by minimizing tubing length (<120 cm), eliminating stopcocks and air bubbles, using low compliance tubing with internal diameter 1.5 to 3.0 mm, and using continuous flush with heparinized saline 1 to 3 mL/h (1 unit of heparin per mL saline).

   iv) **Assessment of dampening**

   (1) The engineering and in vitro laboratory gold standard for assessing the accuracy of the damping coefficient is the square wave test.

   (2) The fast flush test is a clinical equivalent of this method, where the system is flushed and the subsequent oscillations from the system are observed (9).

   (3) Several oscillations following a flush occur in underdampened systems, whereas fewer than 1.5 oscillations following a flush will occur in overdampened systems.

   (4) The amplitude ratio between any two oscillating peaks can also be measured, which can be extrapolated graphically to determined dampening coefficient (1,2). As natural frequency increases, broader ranges of dampening coefficients become allowable (Fig. 11-1).

Place padding between the stopcock and the patient's arm when tucking to avoid bruising or skin excoriation.

Figure 11-1 Parameters that Enable a System to have an Adequate Dynamic Response

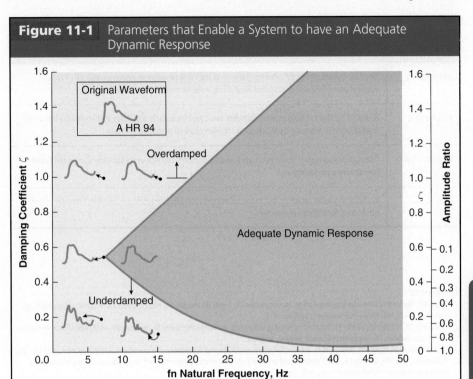

As natural frequency increases, the range of allowable damping coefficients increases. The right hand side of the figure enables a quick determination of damping coefficient based upon amplitude ratio that is determined from the fast flush technique. Reproduced from Greenberg SB, Murphy GS, Vender JS. Standard monitoring techniques. In: Barash PG, Cullen BF, Stoelting RK, et al., eds. *Clinical Anesthesia.* 6th ed. Philadelphia, PA: Lippincott Williams & Wilkins; 2009:704, with permission.

5) **Complications of arterial cannulation** (Table 11-1)
   a) Risks are minimized with small catheters, heparinized saline continuously infused slowly (2 to 3 mL/h), flushing is minimized, aseptic technique utilized, and pulse oximetry is utilized to continuously assess perfusion.

Table 11-1

Complications from Arterial Cannulation (1,2)

Vascular insufficiency and vasospasm
Hematoma
Blood loss
Arterial thrombosis
Air or thrombotic embolic
Nerve damage
Infection
Intra-arterial drug injection

MONITORING

Chapter Summary for Arterial BP Monitoring

Indications	Need for instantaneous BP reading: Patients at high risk for adverse outcomes with BP changes, surgical procedure with anticipated fluid shifts, need for multiple blood gas analyses.
Mechanics	Based on pressure in fluid column therefore must zero transducer and place at mid-axillary line or at level of brain in neurologic procedures to monitor cerebral perfusion pressure.
Clinical Pearls	Overdampened system underestimates systolic pressure and vice versa for underdampened system (see square wave testing 4b.)
Access Site	Radial artery most common, but many alternatives including brachial are possible. Consider use of ultrasound for difficult placements.

References

1. Spiess BD, Gomez MN. Hemodynamic monitoring. In: Longnecker DE, Tinker JH, Morgan GE, eds. *Principles and Practice of Anesthesiology.* 2nd ed. St. Louis, MO: Mosby-Year Book Inc.; 1998:802–825.
2. Greenberg SB, Murphy GS, Vender JS. Standard monitoring techniques. In: Barash PG, Cullen BF, Stoelting RK, et al., eds. *Clinical Anesthesia.* 6th ed. Philadelphia, PA: Lippincott Williams & Wilkins; 2009:704.
3. Alvarez-Tostado JA, Moise MA, Bena JF, et al. The brachial artery: a critical access for endovascular procedures. *J Vasc Surg* 2009;49(2):378–385.
4. Bazaral MG, Welch M, Golding LA, et al. Comparison of brachial and radial arterial pressure monitoring in patients undergoing coronary artery bypass surger. *Anesthesiology* 1990;73:38–45.
5. Lorente L, Santacreu R, Martín MM, et al. Arterial catheter-related infection in 2949 catheters. *Crit Care* 2006;10(3):R83.
6. Koh DB, Gowardman JR, Rickard CM, et al. Prospective study on peripheral artery catheter and comparison with concurrently sited central venous catheters. *Crit Care Med* 2008;36(2):397–402.
7. Thomas F, Burke JP, Parker J, et al. The risk of infection related to radial vs femoral sites of arterial catheterization. *Crit Care Med* 1983;11(10):807–812.
8. Rooke GA, Schwid HA, Shapira Y. The effect of graded hemorrhage and intravascular volume replacement on systolic pressure variation in humans during mechanical and spontaneous ventilation. *Anesth Analg* 1995;80:925–932.
9. Kleinman B, Powell S, Gardner RM. Equivalence of fast flush and square wave testing of blood pressure monitoring systems. *J Clin Monit* 1996;12:149–154.

Central Venous Monitoring

Quinn Stevens, MD • Nathaen Weitzel, MD

Central venous catheterization involves placement of a sterile catheter into one of the large central veins and allows for multiple modalities of intervention along with the option of monitoring central venous pressure (CVP). CVP monitoring can be a useful tool for evaluating intravascular volume and preload in the absence of left ventricular (LV) dysfunction (ejection fraction <40%), severe mitral valve disease, pulmonary hypertension, or significant reduction in LV compliance (ischemia/diastolic dysfunction).

1) **Indications**
   a) Need for IV access, when peripheral access cannot be obtained or if prolonged IV access is anticipated.
   b) Rapid fluid administration can be achieved when an 8.5 to 9 Fr side port introducer, or "cordis" is placed. Flow rates through a triple lumen catheter are significantly less than through a large peripheral IV (18 g or greater).
   c) Measurement of fluid status and filling pressures via CVP (see 7a).
   d) Central access is indicated for the administration of medications such as inotropes, electrolytes, and total parenteral nutrition.
   e) Transvenous pacing electrodes can be introduced.
   f) Treatment of air embolism via aspiration
      i) Aspiration via a single lumen Cook Bunegin–Albin air aspiration catheter has been shown to be more effective than a triple lumen or Swan-Ganz catheter.
      ii) Little evidence exists regarding success of emergent catheter placement during hemodynamic compromise from venous air embolism (1).
   g) Insertion of pulmonary artery (PA) catheter.
2) **Mechanics of CVP monitoring**
   a) CVP monitoring is accomplished with saline filled tubing connected to a transducer system, such as with arterial lines.
   b) The transducer should be placed at the level of the right atrium and must be readjusted with patient level adjustments.
   c) The transducer must be zeroed to create a reference point, most commonly to atmospheric pressure. This is accomplished by opening the line to room air, via a stopcock and then pressing the zero function on the machine.
3) **Cannulation sites**
   a) **Internal jugular (IJ)**
      i) The IJ vein lies within the carotid sheath along with the carotid artery and vagus nerve.
      ii) **The IJ is usually located lateral to the carotid artery (Fig. 12-1).**
         (1) Anatomic variation where the vein lies more anterior to the carotid artery is not uncommon.

READ MORE

Invasive arterial blood pressure monitoring, Chapter 11, page 70

MONITORING

| Figure 12-1 | Anatomy for a Right Sided Internal Jugular Vein Puncture |

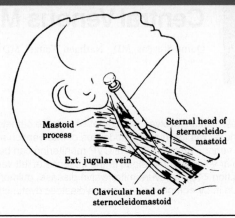

Mastoid process

Sternal head of sternocleido- mastoid

Ext. jugular vein

Clavicular head of sternocleidomastoid

Note the triangle formed by the two heads of the sternocleidomastoid muscle indicating the typical site of access. Reproduced from Chatburn J, Sandberg WS. Monitoring. In: Levine WC, ed. *Handbook of Clinical Anesthesia Procedures of the Massachusetts General Hospital.* 8th ed. Philadelphia, PA: Lippincott Williams & Wilkins; 2010:136, with permission.

Left-sided IJ cannulation has been associated with chylothorax due to injury of the thoracic duct.

    iii) The right IJ vein is commonly preferred, as left-sided cannulation has been associated with chylothorax due to injury of the nearby thoracic duct.

    iv) Carotid puncture can occur on either side.

        (1) A relative contraindication to IJ cannulation is a previous ipsilateral carotid endarterectomy.

        (2) Carotid puncture with large bore needle or catheter may cause rapid hematoma formation and represents a stroke risk in certain patients.

        (3) Management includes removal of the needle or catheter with direct pressure application.

        (4) The patient may require vascular repair.

        (5) In the anticoagulated patient, carotid catheters should be left in place until coagulation status is normal or repair can be performed.

  b) **Subclavian vein**

    i) Subclavian vein cannulation offers the benefit of patient comfort in awake patients.

    ii) Historically, the risk of pneumothorax was considered higher than the IJ approach, but the majority of evidence suggests rates are similar, around 1% (2).

    iii) The risk of pneumothorax varies considerably with practitioner expertise.

    iv) Occasionally, subclavian catheters will advance in a retrograde fashion into the IJ vein. Distal resistance when advancing a wire may be an indicator that this is occurring.

  c) **Femoral vein**

    i) The femoral vein lies medial to the femoral artery and provides relatively rapid and technically straightforward access.

    ii) Precautions should be taken to avoid femoral artery puncture or cannulation.

    iii) Although evidence is conflicting, most studies suggest that femoral line infection rates are higher than either IJ or subclavian cannulation (3,4).

d) **Antecubital veins**
   i) Antecubital veins can be cannulated with a long catheter.
   ii) Referred to as a peripheral intravenous central catheter, or PICC line. PICC lines are particularly suited for long-term venous access and patient comfort.
   iii) Relatively high resistance makes them poorly suited for volume administration and CVP measurements can be inaccurate.

e) **External jugular**
   i) External jugular vein cannulation is an alternative to IJ access but is technically challenging due to the vein's small diameter and tortuous course.

4) **Technique**
   a) **Placement of central venous catheters can be performed either by direct cannulation, by using a catheter over a needle or by a catheter over a guidewire, referred to as a Seldinger technique. Using a guidewire is by far the most common technique (see Cognitive aid for further details).**
   b) **Several methods to avoid or rule out inadvertent arterial catheterization exist:**
      i) Ultrasound

⌐ READ
→ MORE
─────────
Atlas of anesthe-
sia procedures,
central venous
catheterization,
Chapter 159,
page 1114

(1) Becoming a widely incorporated technique, particularly for IJ catheterization (Fig. 12-2).
(2) Allows for real-time observation of cannulation and is particularly useful when aberrant anatomy or difficult placement is encountered.
(3) Ultrasound use does not guarantee that arterial cannulation has not occurred, particularly in scenarios where the artery and vein lie in the same plane as the needle (5).

Figure 12-2 Ultrasound Image Demonstrating Typical Relationship of Right Internal Jugular Vein and Carotid Artery

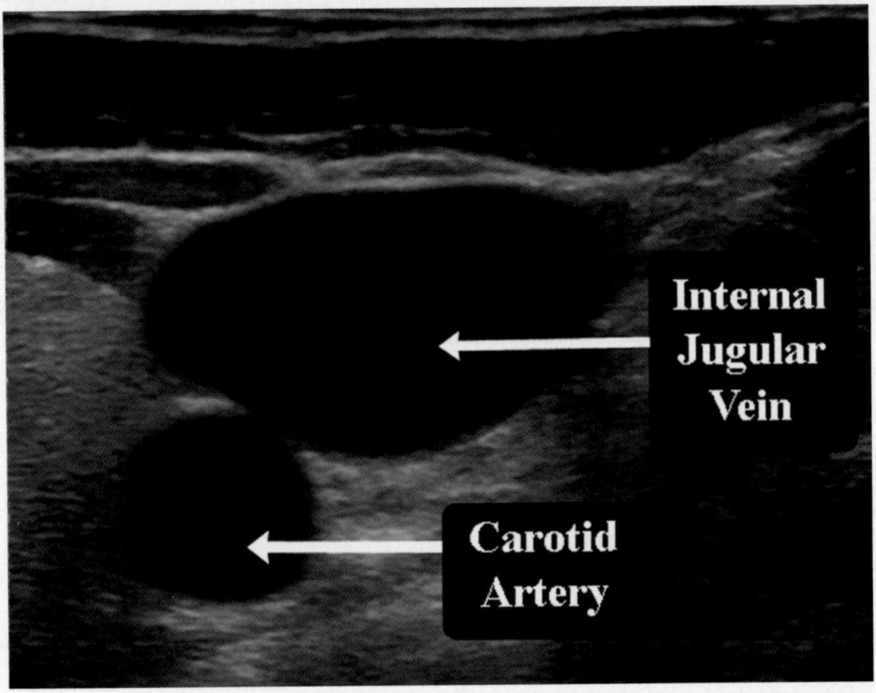

Internal
Jugular
Vein

Carotid
Artery

MONITORING

    (4) **Ultrasound equipment.** Multiple display platforms are available, but commonly GE or Sonosite machines are used.

        (a) A linear probe is ideal for vascular access techniques. High frequency transducers (10 to 15 mHz) give the best resolution, but with a limitation of reduced imaging depth. Sterile probe sheaths are needed for real time imaging on the sterile field.

  ii) Transducing the system during cannulation

    (1) Reliable and simple.

    (2) Attach tubing from a transducer to the end of the needle, or to a small catheter placed over a wire.

    (3) Inspecting the resulting waveform and pressures easily delineates arterial versus venous placement.

    (4) Alternatively, this can be performed manually by allowing blood to rise up the catheter to a level corresponding to either CVP or arterial pressure.

    (5) It is important to note that transducing the system should be performed before the vein or artery is dilated, lowering the risk for vascular injury requiring operative repair.

    (6) Care should be taken to avoid entrainment of air.

  iii) Arrhythmias elicited in the right ventricle during wire advancement are common. The wire should be withdrawn to avoid hemodynamic compromise.

READ MORE

Transesophageal echocardiography basic views, Chapter 162, page 1123

  iv) A sample of blood may be sent for blood gas analysis, which allows for easy differentiation between arterial and venous access.

    (1) This is often performed once a catheter is already in place, and there is a question regarding the catheter location.

  v) If TEE is used, consider examining the heart during line placement using the midesophageal bicaval view, which allows visualization of the wire in the superior vena cava (SVC), ruling out arterial puncture.

5) Complications

  a) Pneumothorax: Pneumothorax is a collection of air in the pleural cavity between the chest wall and the lung. Risk is greatest for subclavian lines, as needle placement is in close proximity to the pleura.

    i) All central venous catheter placements should be followed up with a chest x-ray looking for absence of peripheral lung markings or a lung edge that has receded from the chest wall on the ipsilateral side.

    ii) Diagnosing a pneumothorax radiographically can be subtle and the radiologist's official read should be followed up. Further, a pneumothorax can expand over time, particularly with aggravating risk factors such as positive pressure ventilation or CPAP.

  b) Thrombus formation

    i) Incidence of right heart thromboembolism or pulmonary embolism in patients with a central venous catheter is likely several times higher than the general population.

    ii) Occurrence of upper extremity DVT should be evaluated further with ultrasound imaging (6).

  c) Infection

    i) Infected central venous catheters carry a significant risk of bacteremia, sepsis, and overall mortality.

    ii) Reported incidence of infection varies but is generally <3%.

       iii)   Infection has historically been considered to be more common for femoral lines; however, a recent study examining 831 catheters in 657 patients demonstrated no appreciable difference in infection rates between IJ, subclavian, and femoral lines (3,4).

       iv)   Decreased rates may be achieved with antibiotic coated lines and full sterile technique/draping.

   d) Chylothorax

       i)   Risk is greatest with left IJ line placement.

   e) Arrhythmias

       i)   Typically occur during wire advancement, although can be caused by the catheter alone.

   f) Others include atrial/ventricular perforation, air embolism, vascular erosion.

6) **Interpretation of CVP**

   a) **Waveform analysis**

       i)   **The "a" wave** correlates with atrial contraction.

           (1) Absence of **a** wave suggests lack of contraction, as in atrial fibrillation.

           (2) The **a** wave is enlarged when atrial pressure increases abnormally during systole.

               (a) This occurs if the atrium contracts against a closed tricuspid valve, as in heart block when the atrium and ventricle contracts dyssynchronously, or in conditions such as tricuspid stenosis or pulmonary hypertension (7).

       ii)   **The "c" wave** corresponds to ventricular contraction, tricuspid closure, and the slight elevation of pressure caused by tricuspid bulging into the right atrium.

Enlarged **"a"** waves on the CVP waveform that occur irregularly, as a result of arrhythmia, are referred to as canon **a** waves.

MONITORING

Figure 12-3   Diagram of Normal CVP Waveforms Along with Corresponding ECG Tracing

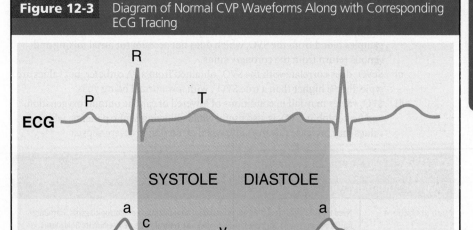

Reproduced from Greenberg SB, Murphy GS, Vender JS. Standard monitoring techniques. In: Barash PG, Cullen BF, Stoelting RK, et al., eds. *Clinical Anesthesia*. 6th ed. Philadelphia, PA: Lippincott Williams & Wilkins; 2009:705, with permission.

- iii) The "x" descent occurs between the c and v waves and correlates with atrial relaxation.
- iv) The "v" wave correlates with atrial filling against a closed tricuspid valve, during diastole.
- v) The "y" descent correlates with tricuspid valve opening in early diastole and passive flow from RA to RV (Fig. 12-3).

7) **CVP and intravascular volume**
   a) CVP is considered to reflect right ventricular filling pressure, or right ventricular end-diastolic pressure. Considerations when using CVP are as follows (8):
      i) **CVP may correlate with left sided filling pressures in the absence of LV dysfunction (EF < 40%), pulmonary hypertension, or severe valvular dysfunction.**
      ii) Normal values vary but are generally <10 mm Hg.
      iii) Elevations of CVP can indicate volume overload or right heart failure.
      iv) The high degrees of compliance in the right atrium and ventricle suggest that changes in volume may not accurately or appropriately reflect as changes in CVP.
      v) Changes in extrathoracic pressure or the presence of PEEP during ventilation will increase transmural pressure, altering CVP, and ultimately ventricular filling.
      vi) CVP monitoring is often used to assess fluid status and subsequent volume administration. This may be most useful in terms of monitoring trends in CVP values over time, as opposed to using absolute values to guide intervention. Evidence evaluating the relationship between CVP values and blood volume, or CVP and fluid responsiveness has failed to demonstrate a causal relationship (8).

8) Mixed Central Venous Oxygen Saturation (ScVO$_2$)
   a) An additional value which may be obtained from a central venous monitor
   b) ScVO$_2$ is not a true mixed venous (SVO$_2$) measurement because it typically samples blood from the SVC, which does not account for atrial mixing and venous return from the coronary sinus.
   c) ScVO$_2$ does correlate with the SVO$_2$ obtained from a PA catheter, but values are typically 5% higher than a true SVO$_2$, with low normal being 70%.
   d) SVO$_2$ values may fall in conditions of lowered of cardiac output, oxygenation, and hemoglobin. SVO$_2$ is also useful while following septic patients, where values may increase due to poor oxygen extraction in severe sepsis.

V waves on the CVP waveform become enlarged with tricuspid regurgitation.

Use of CVP for assessment of volume status is probably best done by following trends rather than absolute values.

Chapter Summary for CVP Monitoring

Main Indications	Need for IV access/rapid fluid administration, administration of inotropic agents, introducer for PA catheter or pacing wires, need to measure central pressure to estimate fluid status.
Risks	Carotid puncture, pneumothorax, arrhythmias, infection, thrombus formation.
Access Site	Internal Jugular preferred due to ease of access, followed by subclavian as most common.
Interpretation	*a, c,* and *v* waves along with *x/y* descent correlate to cardiac cycle and valve closures. Consider measuring **ScVO**$_2$ in sepsis. CVP is a reasonable measure of fluid status/left sided filling in a normal heart.

References

1. Mirski MA, Lele AV, Fitzsimmons L, et al. Diagnosis and treatment of vascular air embolism. *Anesthesiology* 2007;106:164–177.
2. Ruesch S, Walder B, Tramer MR. Complications of central venous catheters: internal jugular versus subclavian access—a systematic review. *Crit Care Med* 2002;30:454–460.
3. Lorente L, Henry C, Martin MM, et al. Central venous catheter related infection in a prospective and observational study of 2595 catheters. *Crit Care* 2005;9:631–635.
4. Deshpande KS, Hatem C, Ulrich HL, et al. The incidence of infectious complications of central venous catheters at the subclavian, internal jugular, and femoral sites in an intensive care unit population. *Crit Care Med* 2005;33:13–20.
5. Feller-Kopman D. Ultrasound-guided internal jugular access: a proposed standardized approach and implications for training and practice. *Chest* 2007; 132:302–309.
6. Burns KE, McLaren A. A critical review of thromboembolic complications associated with central venous catheters. *Can J Anaesth* 2008; 55:532–541.
7. Greenberg SB, Murphy GS, Vender JS. Standard monitoring techniques. In: Barash PG, Cullen BF, Stoelting RK, et al., eds. *Clinical Anesthesia*. 6th ed. Philadelphia, PA: Lippincott Williams & Wilkins; 2009:705.
8. Marik PE, Baram M, Vahid B. Does central venous pressure predict fluid responsiveness? A systematic review of the literature and the tale of seven mares. *Chest* 2008;134:172–178.

MONITORING

13 Pulmonary Artery Catheter

Quinn Stevens, MD · Nathaen Weitzel, MD

The pulmonary artery (PA) catheter is a controversial but potentially powerful tool, offering information about cardiac filling pressures, cardiac output (CO), derived parameters of cardiac performance, and mixed venous oxygen saturation (SvO_2). ASA consensus opinion is that "PA catheter monitoring may reduce perioperative complications if critical hemodynamic data obtained are accurately interpreted and appropriate treatment is instituted." (1).

1) **Technical considerations**
   a) A PA catheter is a long multiport catheter inserted into a central vein through the right ventricle (RV) and into the PA (Fig. 13-1).
   b) The PA catheter is inserted using sterile technique through a side port introducer, commonly referred to as a cordis, which can be inserted via Internal Jugular (IJ), subclavian, or femoral veins.
   c) The typical PA catheter is 7 Fr, 110 cm, with—two to three lumens: the PA lumen at the tip, the proximal injectate port (PIP) at 26 cm, and optionally the venous infusion port (VIP) at 30 cm.
      i) At the tip of the PA catheter is a small balloon with 1.5 mL capacity for "floating."
      ii) Additional capabilities include a fiberoptic tip for calculation of SvO_2 and a thermistor for determination of CO.
      iii) Some PA catheters are enabled for pacing via bipolar electrodes or an additional port for advancement of pacing wires.
2) **Catheter placement**
   a) Catheter placement can be performed in the awake or anesthetized patient.
   b) Under any circumstance, ECG, pulse oximetry, and BP monitoring are mandatory during placement.
   c) Using sterile technique, with the balloon deflated and PA lumen attached to a pressure transducer, the catheter should be advanced until past the end of the sideport introducer. The balloon is inflated, and the catheter is advanced further. See Figures 13-2 and 13-3 for waveforms.
      i) Superior vena cava and right atrium reveal a low pressure CVP waveform under normal circumstances.
      ii) RV pressure waveform demonstrates wide pressure swing, from RV systolic pressure, normally 15 to 30 mm Hg to RV diastolic pressure, or right atrial pressure.
         (1) The RV is typically reached by 25 to 30 cm from the right IJ.
      iii) Attainment of the PA is characterized by diastolic rise, normally 6 to 12 mm Hg, while the systolic pressure is unchanged.
         (1) Elevation of diastolic pressure is due to closure of the pulmonic valve.
         (2) The PA is typically entered approximately 10 cm from entry in the RV (Fig. 13-2).

Unlike CVP monitoring, understanding of waveform analysis is crucial to correct placement of the PA catheter and must be done in real-time.

Figure 13-1   Typical Oximetric PAC*

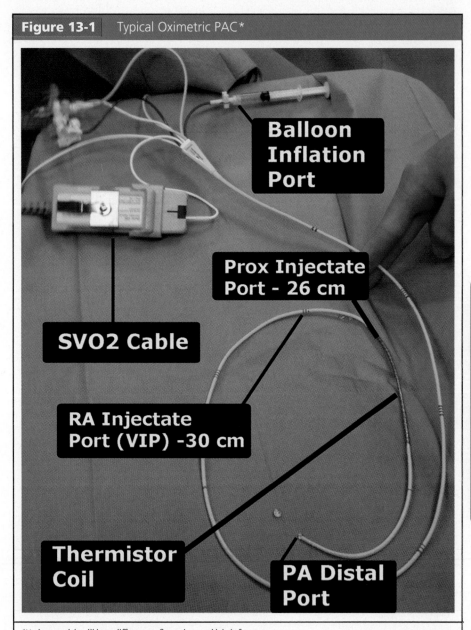

Balloon Inflation Port

Prox Injectate Port - 26 cm

SVO2 Cable

RA Injectate Port (VIP) -30 cm

Thermistor Coil

PA Distal Port

*Various models will have different configurations and labels for ports.

Figure 13-2   Typical PAC Waveform Pressure Tracing

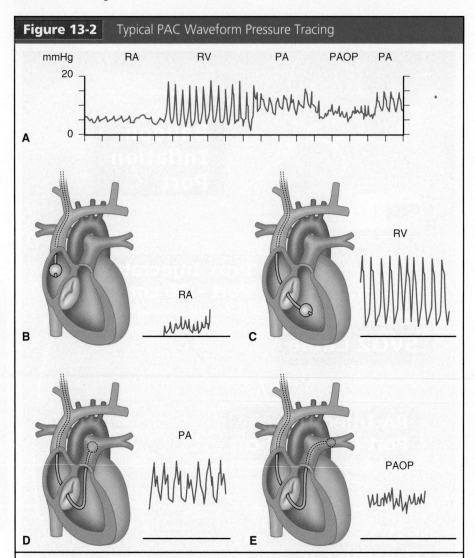

As the PA catheter is advanced from the right atrium to the pulmonary capillary wedge. **A:** Entire PAC Series; **B–E:** Sequential tracings expected as the catheter is advanced from the right atrium through to the PA wedge. Reproduced from Mihm FG, Rosenthal MH. Pulmonary artery catheterization. In: Benumof JL, ed. *Clinical procedures in anesthesia and intensive care.* Philadelphia, PA: Lippincott Williams & Wilkins, 1992:416, with permission.

Placement of PAC in patients with severe mitral stenosis, aortic stenosis, or severe cardiac dysfunction carries significant risk of lethal arrhythmias.

The sideport introducer is larger and more rigid than a typical central line—which makes vascular injury more likely.

iv) The wedge or PA occlusion pressure generally correlates with PA diastolic pressure and is observed with transition from the more pulsatile PA waveform to the pulmonary capillary wedge pressure (PCWP) waveform (Fig. 13-2). The balloon is then deflated (3).

v) The PA catheter can also be viewed using transesophageal echocardiography and is most easily visualized in the midesophageal RV inflow-outflow view.

3) **Indications for PAC placement**

a) **General indications** (Table 13-1)

i) Significant variation exists among institutional and practitioner indications for the use of PA catheters.

ii) The PA catheter can be useful and should be considered when determination of intracardiac pressures and hemodynamic parameters will potentially change management (1).

b) **PAC in cardiac surgery**

i) Indications are listed in Table 13-2.

ii) Consider inserting catheter to approximately 18 to 20 cm until sternotomy and aortic cannula placed for patients who may not tolerate significant arrhythmias (severe AS, severe MS, severe congestive heart failure [CHF]) (2).

iii) Suggested indications for placement of PAC for cardiac surgery may also apply to other high-risk surgery.

c) **Relative contraindications to PAC placement** (Table 13-3)

4) **Complications**

a) All the potential complications of establishing central venous access are also present with PA catheter insertion.

i) Accidental arterial dilation is a traumatic complication, and case reports of injury to the inominate vein also exist (4).

MONITORING

Figure 13-3 PA Waveform Diagram

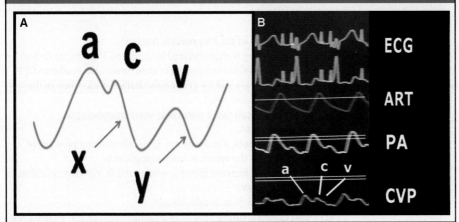

(**A**) depicts the waveform expected when the PAC is in the wedge position. (**B**) is a screen shot of a typical hemodynamic series. Note the CVP tracing has similar waveform characteristics of the PCWP in (**A**). The PA tracing below is a PA tracing, not the PCWP tracing. Also note that the waveform timing is slightly delayed from the CVP compared to the PA due to timing of flow from the right and left heart.

Table 13-1
General Indications for PAC (1)
Assessment of volume status, particularly when right and left filling pressures do not correlate
Can assist in complex fluid management during conditions of renal failure or shock
Diagnosis and management of CHF and differentiation between RV and LV failure
Diagnosis of valvular heart disease
Diagnosis and management of pulmonary hypertension

Table 13-2
Indications for PAC in Cardiac Surgery (1)
Surgical patient with an EF < 40%
Severe Aortic or Mitral valve disease
Patient with severe angina or recent myocardial infarction
Patients with moderate or severe pulmonary hypertension

READ MORE

Central venous monitoring, Chapter 12, page 75

b) Other complications include arrhythmias including ventricular tachycardia, damage to the valves, endocarditis, cardiac perforation, thrombus formation, and PA rupture.

c) The PA catheter is generally pulled back after the wedge during cardiac surgery in anticipation of sternal retraction causing further advancement of the catheter and potential PA rupture.

d) Cooling of the heart during bypass can cause the PA catheter to become very stiff, increasing the likelihood of injury from a deeply advanced catheter.

e) If the catheter is persistently wedged following balloon deflation, the catheter should be retracted several centimeters and refloated.

f) Balloon inflation should be done cautiously, due to risk of PA rupture if the catheter migrates distally to a smaller caliber of the vessel.

g) A knot can develop from over advancement of the catheter without appropriate tip migration (5).

5) **Waveform interpretation**
   a) **Normal characteristics of the PA pressure tracing**
      i) PA pressure tracing is characterized by A, C, and V waves, as well as X and Y descent on PCWP tracing. Note these waves are similar to CVP waveform (Figs. 13-2 and 13-3) but only characteristic when in the wedge position (Table 13-4).
   b) **Pathologic conditions can cause particular wave morphologies**
      i) Myocardial ischemia
         (1) Can distort both a and v waves, generally causing peaking of each wave as the ventricle loses compliance.
         (2) Ischemia can increase filling pressures and PCWP as systolic function deteriorates.
      ii) Pericardial constriction or tamponade
         (1) End diastolic filling pressures equalize between PA, wedge pressure (WP), and CVP (7).
      iii) Large a waves
         (1) May be associated with mitral stenosis, complete heart block, atrial myxoma, and acute heart failure.

Table 13-3	
Relative Contraindications to PA Catheters (2)	
Presence of mechanical heart valve	Wolf-Parkinson-White syndrome
Left bundle branch block (placement can induce right bundle branch block)	Hypercoagulable state
Bacteremia	Recent transvenous pacing wire placement

Consideration should be made in patients with the above risks regarding risk-benefit ratio in placing PAC. Consider TEE as a possible alternative.

Table 13-4	
Events Characterized by PCWP Waveform	
PAC Wave Tracing Characteristics	
A wave	Left atrial systole
C wave	Mitral valve closure
X descent	Left atrial diastole
V wave	LV contraction/atrial filling (MV closed)
Y descent	LV diastole (mitral valve opening)

(2) With mitral stenosis, the PAWP will be artificially elevated and the Y descent more gradual, a reflection of slower atrial emptying.

iv) Large **v** waves
  (1) May be associated with mitral regurgitation, CHF, and ventricular septal defect.
  (2) With mitral regurgitation, large v waves occur during systole, creating fusion of the c and v waves.
  (3) The mean wedge will overestimate left ventricular filling pressure. To approximate the left ventricular end-diastolic pressure (LVEDP) most closely, the wedge just prior to the v wave should be taken.

6) **Pulmonary capillary wedge pressure**
  a) In normal patients, the PCWP = left atrial pressure = LVEDP.
    i) LVEDP can be extrapolated to represent left ventricular end-diastolic volume, or preload.
    ii) Normal values are typically <15 mm Hg.
  b) PCWP is generally a better representation of LVEDP than CVP.
  c) Differences in CVP and PCWP are useful clues in diagnosing heart failure and ischemia.
  d) The relationship between LVEDP and PCWP is altered by changes in pulmonary vascular resistance (PVR), alveolar–PA relationships, and intracardiac factors.
    i) Conditions in which PCWP is lower than LVEDP include premature closure of the mitral valve, as occurs with a noncompliant ventricle, aortic insufficiency, or aortic regurgitation.
    ii) The catheter tip should be in west zone III, or below the level of the left atrium, to meet criteria for uninterrupted blood flow.
      (1) In zones I and II, alveolar pressure exceeds the PA or capillary pressure.
      (2) Fluoroscopy or lateral chest film can be useful in determining PA position (5).

Conditions in which PCWP is greater than LVEDP include mitral stenosis, mitral regurgitation and atrial myxoma.

↳ READ MORE

Thoracic anesthesia, Chapter 140, page 999

MONITORING

  iii) Increases in PVR also raise PCWP as a reflection of capillary hydrostatic pressure. Increases in PVR are commonly seen in lung disease, PE, hypoxia, acidosis, hypoxemia, and the use of vasoactive drugs.

  iv) Spontaneous or mechanical ventilation exerts negative or positive pulmonary pressures, respectively. PCWP is best measured at end expiration.

7) CO, SvO_2, and hemodynamic parameters

 a) **Cardiac output (CO)**

  i) Determined by Fick method, indicator dilution, thermodilution, Doppler ultrasound, and/or echocardiography.

   (1) Continuous CO can be obtained if PAC has thermal filament capability, which is more accurate than a standard injectate method.

   (2) Intermittent method: inject known volume into RA, measure change in temperature at catheter tip. Based on assumption that flow is constant, blood volume is constant, and no significant venous pooling.

   (3) Sources of error include inaccurate temperature or volume of injectate and intracardiac shunts (2).

 b) **Derived parameters**

  i) A number of derived hemodynamic parameters can be obtained from the PA catheter, including PVR, systemic vascular resistance, cardiac index, stroke volume, left ventricular stroke work index, and right ventricular work index.

 c) SVO_2

  i) **One of the most easily interpreted parameters provided by the PAC is the mixed SVO_2.**

  ii) Continuous SvO_2 monitoring can provide information about oxygen supply and demand in terms of the patient's hemoglobin level, oxygen saturation (SaO_2), and CO.

  iii) The Fick equation defines the relationship between CO, oxygen consumption (VO_2), and arterial and venous oxygen content (C_a and C_v).

$$CO = VO_2/C_a - C_v$$

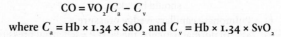

$$\text{where } C_a = Hb \times 1.34 \times SaO_2 \text{ and } C_v = Hb \times 1.34 \times SvO_2$$

By rearranging the Fick equation, it becomes apparent that the SvO_2 is dependent upon SaO_2, O_2 consumption, CO, and hemoglobin.

PA catheters by definition are not therapeutic, and offer only data.

$$SvO_2 = SaO_2 - [VO_2/(CO \times Hb \times 13.4)]$$

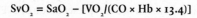

  iv) Increasing SaO_2, CO, and Hb increases SvO_2, while increasing O_2 consumption decreases SvO_2.

8) **Evidence**

 a) Sparse data exist to support the vast majority of commonly employed monitoring devices.

 b) Recent studies have shown increased mortality or lack of mortality benefit in patients receiving PA catheters.

 c) Studies of PA catheters have been hindered by low power and are not effectively randomized and blinded.

  i) Proper patient selection is an issue, as likely only critically ill patients can benefit from PA catheters, placed early in the patient's course (8). On the other hand, terminally ill patients with end organ disease are unlikely to derive benefit. More clinical trials would be helpful to determine ideal patient selection; however, these are difficult to conduct due to issues listed above regarding critically ill patients.

Chapter Summary for PA Catheters

Indications in Surgery	Severe systolic dysfunction, severe valve disease, pulmonary hypertension, complex fluid management combined with CHF or renal failure
Contraindications	LBBB or significant conduction abnormalities, mechanical valves, bacteremia, hypercoagulable state.
Risks and Complications	Risk of central line placement, arrhythmias, vascular injury, PA rupture
Equipment	Introducer required, PA catheter either with SVO_2 capabilities or not. Can either use manual CO catheters or automatic CO catheter.

References

1. Gerhardt MA, Skeehan TM. Monitoring the cardiac surgical patient. In: *A Practical Approach to Cardiac Anesthesia*. Philadelphia, PA: Lippincott Williams & Wilkins, 2008:104–141.
2. Marino, PM. The pulmonary artery catheter. In: *The ICU Book*. 3rd ed. Philadelphia, PA: Lippincott Williams & Wilkins; 2007:163–179.
3. Murphy GS, Vender JS. Monitoring the anesthetized patient. In: Barash PG, Cullen BF, Stoelting RK, eds. *Clinical Anesthesia*. 5th ed. Philadelphia, PA: Lippincott Williams & Wilkins; 2006:668–687.
4. Chen CY, Chen KY, Taso SL, et al. Perforation of right innominate vein by pulmonary artery introducer sheath: a case report. *J Clin Anesth.* 2009;3:206–208.
5. Spiess BD, Gomez MN. Hemodynamic monitoring. In: Longnecker DE, Tinker JH, Morgan GE, eds. *Principles and Practice of Anesthesiology*. 2nd ed. St. Louis, MO: Mosby-Year Book, Inc.; 1998:802–825.
6. Mihm FG, Rosenthal MH. Pulmonary artery catheterization. In: Benumof JL, ed. *Clinical Procedures in Anesthesia and Intensive Care*. Philidelphia, PA. Lippincott Williams & Wilkins; 1992:416.
7. Schroeder RA, Barbeito A, Bar-Yosef S. Pulmonary Artery Catheter Monitoring. In: Miller RD, ed. *Miller's Anesthesia*. 7th ed. Philadelphia, PA: Churchill Livingstone/Elsevier; 2010:1297–1314.
8. Greenburg SB, Murphy GS, Vender JS. Current use of the pulmonary artery catheter. *Curr Opin Criti Care* 2009;15:249–253.

MONITORING

14 Transesophageal Echocardiography: Indications as a Monitoring Tool

Peter M. Hession, MD • Nathaen Weitzel, MD

Transesophageal echocardiograpy (TEE) is a monitoring modality gaining popularity in the field of anesthesiology due to its versatility, reliability, and safety. It was initially used as a diagnostic tool primarily by cardiologists but has become a mainstay in intraoperative cardiac anesthesia and its utility is extending into other arenas as well. This chapter provides an overview of the indications and contraindications for TEE, the risks and complications associated with its use, as well as the training and credentialing requirements currently in place.

1) **General indications**
   a) TEE is a relatively safe monitoring technique, though it is not without its complications. Therefore, clearly defined indications must be documented prior to its use.
   b) **Evaluation** of hemodynamic instability in which ventricular function, volume status, or other factors are indeterminate.
      i) Refractory hypotension is an intraoperative complication that every anesthesiologist encounters on a regular basis, but the cause is not always clear.
         (1) **Sources of hypotension**
             (a) Hypovolemia
             (b) Myocardial dysfunction
             (c) Valvular abnormality
             (d) Left ventricular outflow obstruction
             (e) Cardiac tamponade
             (f) Pulmonary embolism
             (g) Ventricular septal defect
             (h) Decreased systemic vascular resistance
             (i) Aortic dissection
         (2) All sources of hypotension must be detected early and treated aggressively.
         (3) The treatment of each diagnosis differs greatly and inappropriate interventions may worsen the clinical scenario.
      ii) Left ventricular end diastolic volume can be determined, providing an accurate assessment of volume status (1).
      iii) Wall motion abnormalities resulting from coronary ischemia can be detected before EKG changes are evident (2).
2) **Guidance of surgical intervention for a variety of cardiac complications**

In the setting of refractory hypotension without a clear underlying cause, TEE is an appropriate and effective tool that can reliably diagnose and guide therapy.

a) **Valvular repair**
  i) Mitral valve regurgitation is frequently treated with either repair or replacement.
    (1) The intraoperative TEE exam can accurately assess the severity of disease and help the surgeon determine if a repair is feasible or if replacement is necessary.
      (a) It is also crucial for evaluating the success of the procedure immediately following intervention.
  ii) Complications of mitral valve repair/replacement can be diagnosed immediately with TEE and direct additional surgical repair if necessary.
    (1) **Complications include**
      (a) New mitral stenosis
      (b) Perivalvular leak
      (c) Residual mitral regurgitation
      (d) Obstruction of the left ventricular outflow tract due to systolic anterior motion of the mitral leaflet.
b) **Aortic dissection**
  i) Emergent repair of an ascending aortic dissection requires accurate assessment of the location and extent of the dissection.
    (1) TEE can accurately and quickly provide this information to the surgical team.
c) **Congenital heart lesions**
  i) This is primarily necessary in the neonatal and pediatric population where detailed information about the anomalous cardiac anatomy is required.
  ii) The population of adults with congenital heart disease, repaired or uncorrected, is growing.
    (1) The anesthetic management of these patients can often be assisted by TEE.
d) **Endocarditis repair**
  i) TEE exam of patients with suspected endocarditis can play a major role in the surgical plan.
    (1) Identification of valvular abscesses may direct early surgical intervention.
e) **Placement of intracardiac devices**
  i) During minimally invasive, port-access cardiac surgery, TEE is useful in identifying cardiac structures and guiding placement of the coronary sinus catheter, venous cannula, and endoaortic clamp.
f) **Pericardial window procedures**
  i) In skilled hands, pericardial window procedures can be positively impacted by a thorough exam.
  ii) Posterior or loculated pericardial effusions may be missed by the surgeon but are identified by TEE.
g) **Aortic cross-clamp**
  i) Cross-clamping of the aorta is frequently necessary as part of cardiopulmonary bypass.
    (1) Calcification or atheroma of the ascending aorta can be dislodged by the cross-clamp placing the patient at risk of embolic stroke.
    (2) Accurate assessment of the aorta prior to cross-clamp helps reduce this risk and allows the surgeon to place the clamp at a safe location (3).
3) **Other indications**
  a) **Management of the ICU patient**
    i) **Transthoracic echocardiography (TTE) is commonly used to guide therapy in the critically ill patient, but TEE offers advantages over TTE in a variety of scenarios:**
      (1) Mechanical ventilation
      (2) Cardiac tamponade
      (3) Diagnosis of vegetations and complications of endocarditis

MONITORING

(4) Central pulmonary emboli

(5) Exclusion of a cardiac source of embolism

(6) Evaluation of a mediastinal hematoma

(7) Diagnosis of ascending or descending thoracic aortic dissection

(8) Structural and functional evaluation of native valves

(9) Acute hemodynamic instability

ii) TEE may also be left in place for several hours, allowing the intensivist to assess the patient's response to therapy.

READ MORE

Pulmonary artery catheter, Chapter 13, page 82

iii) TEE offers additional benefit above the capability of a pulmonary artery catheter.

(1) PA catheters rely on occlusion pressures to estimate LV volume.

(a) This value can be affected by things such as PEEP, mitral valve abnormalities, and changes to LV compliance leading to over or underestimated data (4).

b) **Assessment of intracardiac masses and embolic sources**

i) TTE can falsely identify normal intra-atrial structures such as a pectinate muscle or Coumadin ridge as a thrombus or tumor.

ii) TEE provides further information to accurately diagnose intra-atrial pathology, which may help to guide therapy (4).

4) **Contraindications**

a) There is some debate about the classification of certain scenarios as relative or absolute contraindications.

i) Ultimately, the clinician must take into consideration the entire clinical situation and weigh the potential risks and benefits of TEE.

Esophageal spasm, stricture, laceration, perforation, and diverticular are all absolute contraindications to TEE.

(1) **Absolute**

(a) Esophageal spasm

(b) Stricture

(c) Laceration

(d) Perforation

(e) Diverticula

(2) **Relative**

(a) Unstable neck injuries

(b) Esophageal trauma

(c) Varices

(d) Cancer

(e) Dysphagia

(f) Active upper gastrointestinal bleeding

(g) History of chest radiation

(h) Hiatal hernia (5–7).

5) **Risks and complications**

a) TEE complications are extremely rare, especially in the hands of a trained clinician, but there are risks associated with the modality (5,6,8).

i) **Incorrect interpretation**

(1) Can lead to improper surgical or medical interventions just as proper interpretation can correctly guide therapy.

ii) **Probe placement can result in**

(1) Oral trauma

(2) Pharyngeal, esophageal or gastric perforation

(3) Dysphagia

(4) Esophageal or gastric bleeding

          (5)   Thermal injury

          (6)   Transient bacteremia

          (7)   Displacement of the endotracheal tube

          (8)   Hemodynamic changes

  b) **Avoid injury**

      i)   To avoid oropharyngeal trauma, probe placement must be done by a skilled clinician using the proper technique.

          (1)   Generous lubrication with ultrasonic gel is placed in the mouth, and the probe is then guided to the posterior oropharynx.

          (2)   A jaw lift followed by gentle posterior and caudal pressure on the probe usually results in a loss of resistance as it passes through the upper esophageal sphincter.

          (3)   When resistance is experienced, it is best to redirect the probe rather than force it in the same direction.

              (a)   If resistance is still encountered, aborting the procedure should be considered.

          (4)   With adequate depths of anesthesia, a direct laryngoscopy can help displace oropharyngeal structures and assist with probe placement.

  6) Equipment

READ MORE

Placement and management of TEE probe, Chapter 167, page 1160

  a) **TEE Probe**

      i)   The two-dimensional (2D) TEE probe consists of an ultrasound transducer, which is fixed at one end of a flexible rod.

      ii)   The handle consists of a series of controls allowing manipulation of the transducer in a variety of planes.

      iii) The probe can be retro and ante flexed, flexed to the right or the left, turned right or left, advanced and withdrawn and rotated 180 degrees.

      iv) By obtaining 2D images of the heart in multiple planes, a 3D understanding of the heart is obtained.

  b) **TEE transducer**

      i)   Functions by transmitting ultrasound through the esophagus and into the heart.

          (1)   These ultrasound waves are then reflected back to the transducer.

              (a)   Because the speed of sound is constant in tissue, the time it takes for the sound waves to return to the transducer from different structures is extrapolated into a visual image in real time (4).

The Doppler effect states that ultrasound waves directed at a moving object will compress as the object moves toward the source and expand as it moves away.

  c) **Color flow Doppler**

      i)   This is a modality that provides invaluable information during a TEE exam.

      ii)   It is based on the principle of the Doppler Effect, which states that the ultrasound waves, directed at a moving object (in this case, red blood cells), will be compressed as the object moves toward the source and expanded as it moves away.

      iii) The color flow Doppler function assigns the color red to ultrasound waves returned at a higher frequency, that is, blood flow toward the transducer and blue to waves returned at a lower frequency, that is, blood flow away from the transducer.

          (1)   This allows for analysis of the severity of valvular disease, detection of a patent foramen ovale, identification of the true and false lumens of an aortic dissection, and many others (4).

    d) **Pulsed wave Doppler**
      i) This is a function that utilizes a single vibrating crystal to emit an ultrasound wave and focus it on a specific point of interest in the 2D image and calculate blood velocity at that point.
        (1) Continuous wave Doppler differs in that it uses one crystal to continuously emit an ultrasound signal and another to continuously receive.
          (a) This modality is used to measure blood flow velocity along the entire path of the ultrasound beam rather than at a discrete point.
    e) **Tissue Doppler**
      i) This uses the same Doppler principles and applies it to the myocardium itself.
        (1) This allows for assessment of myocardial movement and contractility.
    f) **3D echocardiography**
      i) This is among the newest advances for cardiac imaging. There are two ways of obtaining 3D images.
        (1) Gated reconstruction
          (a) A series of 2D images obtained simultaneously, which are then reconstructed to produce a 3D image.
        (2) Real Time 3D
          (a) Requires a special transducer that emits a pyramidal shaped sector and produces a real time 3D image (4).

7) **Credentialing**
    a) **National Board of echocardiography (NBE)**
      i) Began offering board certification in TEE in 2004 as a way to recognize those clinicians completing special training in intraoperative TEE.
    b) **PTEeXAM**
      i) The Special Competence in Perioperative Transesophageal Echocardiography (PTEeXAM) is offered once a year for eligible physicians.
    c) **Board certification**
      i) Two pathways exist for certification.
        (1) **Practice experience pathway**
          (a) Exists for physicians who did not complete a cardiothoracic anesthesia fellowship but have participated in cardiac anesthesia in private practice
            (i) **Requirements**
              1. Medical licensure
              2. Board certification
              3. A passing score on the PTEeXAM
              4. 24 months of clinical experience dedicated to the care of surgical patients with cardiovascular disease.
              5. Documented care of 150 patients per year for 2 years immediately preceding application.
              6. Completion of 300 complete transesophageal echocardiograms in the past 4 years.
            (ii) Not available for physicians who completed their training after June 30, 2009.
        (2) **Training program pathway**
          a) Available for physicians who have completed or are currently enrolled in ACGME accredited cardiothoracic anesthesia fellowship programs.
            (i) Requirements
               1. Medical licensure
              2. Anesthesiology board certification

3. A passing score on the PTEeXAM
4. 300 complete transesophageal echocardiograms under direct supervision.
    a. 150 of these must be performed, interpreted, and reported by the trainee directly.

d) **Testamur**

i) Physicians who do not qualify for board certification may still take the PTEeXAM and with a passing score, obtain the title of "testamur" (9).

Chapter Summary for TEE as a Monitoring Tool

Indications	Assessment of hemodynamic instability, guidance of cardiac surgical therapy, evaluation of intracardiac masses as well as others.
Contraindications	Absolute contraindications include esophageal spasm, stricture, laceration, perforation, and diverticula. All others are relative and the risks and benefits must be weighed by the clinician.
Risks and Complications	Rare but include oropharyngeal and esophageal trauma and postoperative dysphagia.
Equipment	2D TEE includes a semiflexible probe, ultrasound source and hand controls. Multiple modalities are available to acquire specific anatomical and physiologic information.
Credentialing	Board certification is available through the NBE and requires a passing score on the PTEeXAM as well as documentation of extensive TEE experience.

MONITORING

References

1. Clements FM, Harpole DH, Quill T, et al. Estimation of left ventricular volume and ejection fraction by two-dimensional transeophageal echocardiography: comparison of short axis imaging and simultaneous radionuclide angiography. *Br J Anaesth* 1990;64:331–336.
2. Smith JS, Cahalan MK, Benefiel DJ, et al. Intraoperative detection of myocardial ischemia in high-risk patients: electrocardiography versus two-dimensional transesophageal echocardiography. *Circulation* 1985;72(5):1015–1021.
3. Marschall K, Kanchuger M, Kessler K, et al. Superiority of transesophageal echocardiography in detecting aortic arch atheromatous disease: identification of patients at increased risk of stroke during cardiac surgery. *J Cardiothorac Vasc Anesth* 1994;8(1):5–13.
4. Perrino, Albert MD Jr, Reeves ST. *A practical approach to tranesophageal echocardiography*. 2nd ed. Philadelphia, PA: Lippincott Williams & Wilkins; 2008.
5. Marymont J, Murphy GS. Intraoperative monitoring with transesophageal echocardiography: indications, risks, and training. *Anesthesiol Clin* 2006;24(4):737–753.
6. Spier BJ, Larue SJ, Teelin TC, et al. Review of complications in a series of patients with known gastro-esophageal varices undergoing transesophageal echocardiography. *J Am Soc Echocardiogr* 2009;22(4):396–400.
7. Mathew JP, Glas K, Troianos CA, et al. American Society of Echocardiography/Society of Cardiovascular Anesthesiologists recommendations and guidelines for continuous quality improvement in perioperative echocardiography. *J Am Soc Echocardiogr* 2006;19(11):1303–1313.
8. Min JK, Spencer KT, Furlong KT, et al. Clinical features of complications from transesophageal echocardiography: a single-center case series of 10,000 consecutive examinations. *J Am Soc Echocardiogr* 2005;18(9):925–929.
9. National Board of Echocardiography website. http://www.echoboards.org/pte/comboapp2009.pdf

15

Processed EEG and Awareness Monitoring

Arjun Desai, MD • Alex Macario, MD, MBA

Intra-operative awareness with recall involves explicit recall of sensory perceptions during general anesthesia including aspects of their surgical environment, procedure, and even pain related to the intervention. Intra-operative awareness with recall is defined as a patient having an unexpected and undesirable recall of wakefulness. Processed EEG analysis has been developed as a method to monitor depth of anesthesia intraoperatively and can be used as an effect-site monitor to aid in titration of anesthetic drugs and may be useful in reducing the incidence of intra-operative awareness with recall.

Targeting a range of BIS values between 40 and 60 is marketed to help prevent anesthesia awareness while allowing for minimizing the anesthetic dose to the patient.

1) **Intraoperative awareness**
   a) **Symptoms**
      i) The most common symptoms reported by patients suggesting awareness with recall are auditory perceptions such as voices or noises, followed by loss of motor function (inability to move, sensation of weakness, or paralysis), pain, and feelings of helplessness, anxiety, panic, impending death, or catastrophe.
      ii) Awareness with recall can lead to anxiety, sleep difficulties, insomnia, irritability, nightmares, and posttraumatic stress disorder.
   b) **Incidence of awareness**
      i) The incidence of awareness with recall varies among studies, countries, anesthetic techniques, patient characteristics, and types of surgery.
      ii) The most commonly cited rate of intra-operative awareness is 0.2% (1). This figure is thought to reflect the incidence in routine cases but not including cardiac or obstetric surgeries. When further stratified, awareness occurs in approximately 1.14% to 1.5% of cardiac surgery cases, 0.4% of obstetric cases, and 11% to 43% of trauma surgeries (6). Awareness with recall associated with pain is estimated to occur in 0.01% to 0.03% of cases.
   c) **Risk factors for awareness** Factors associated with increased risk of awareness with recall include
      i) "light" anesthesia (e.g., delivering a low level of inhaled anesthetic minimum alveolar concentration),
      ii) specific surgeries,
      iii) history of intra-operative awareness,
      iv) chronic use of central nervous system depressants,
      v) younger age,
      vi) obesity, and
      vii) inadequate or misused anesthesia delivery systems.
   d) **Detecting episodes of intra-operative awareness**
      i) Often it is difficult to know for sure that intra-operative awareness with recall occurred. For example, if the patient is not asked

specifically about it they may not report it voluntarily. Or, the patient may recollect hearing sounds during surgery, when in fact they are remembering something that occurred in the recovery room.

ii) One accepted method to assess intra-operative awareness with recall is to conduct three structured interviews with open ended questions at intervals of 24 hours, between 24 and 72 hours, and at 30 days after surgery (awareness may not arise until days to weeks postoperatively).

iii) It is important to note that bispectral index (BIS) monitoring (see below) is a probability distribution where a measure of 40 does not provide a 100% guarantee of no awareness.

2) **Prevention or vigilance for detecting intraoperative awareness**

a) **Monitor delivered volatile anesthetic levels**

The unintended inadequate delivery of volatile anesthetic agents ("light anesthesia") during maintenance of anesthesia may be avoided by the addition of a low alarm limit to end-tidal gas monitoring settings, as well as use of a "near empty" alarm in anesthetic vaporizers.

b) **Monitor processed EEG signals**

Depth of anesthesia monitoring, via the processed EEG, has proved useful in reducing the amount of anesthetic drugs, optimizing extubation times, and in some studies reducing awareness with recall. Although most anesthesiologists in the UK, USA, and Australia accept that clinical signs are unreliable indicators of awareness, few believe that monitors of anesthetic depths should be used for all routine cases (9).

i) **Depth of anesthesia monitors**

Several brain-function monitors based on the processed electroencephalogram (EEG) or evoked potentials have been developed to assess anesthetic depth.

(1) **BIS (Aspect Medical Systems).** The most widely used monitor is the BIS monitor. This device integrates several parameters of an EEG into a calculated, dimensionless variable (0 to 100). The BIS calculations are derived from large patient databases that incorporate recorded EEG waveforms as they relate to anesthetic drug concentration data, memory, and awareness (5). The term bispectral applies because it incorporates both power and phase spectrums of an EEG into the calculated 0 to 100 value. BIS values between 40 and 60 purportedly indicate adequate general anesthesia for surgery, and values below 40 indicate a deep hypnotic state. Targeting a range of BIS values between 40 and 60 is marketed to help prevent anesthesia awareness while allowing for minimization the anesthetic dose.

(2) **SNAP II (Everest Biomedical Instruments).** An index derived from low frequency (0.1 to 18 Hz) and high frequency (80 to 420) EEG frequency analysis. SNAP II is also calculated into a dimensionless variable (0 to 100). High frequency EEG wave forms are thought to be more sensitive to vigilant states and anesthetics.

(3) **Narcotrend Index Monitor (MonitorTechnik).** This technology also uses a dimensionless index (0 to 100). However, calculations represent visual stages of the EEG which were previously defined to describe changes recorded during sleep. These stages (A-F) were later refined to represent depth of anesthesia (A=awake and F=very deep level of anesthesia) (6). These stages are then quantified into the numerical index on the display screen.

(4) **M-Entropy Module (GE-Healthcare).** A mathematical approach that quantifies EEG using non-linear dynamics. This mode measures spectral entropy and

MONITORING

applies it to the power spectrum of EEGs. Two variables, state and response entropy, which measure EEG and combined EEG/EMG activity respectively, are displayed on the awareness monitor as a dimensionless unit (0 to 100) (2).

(5) **Mid-latency auditory evoked potentials (MLAEPs).** This method is thought to be an alternative to the use of EEG monitoring. MLAEP are electroencephalographic responses to auditory stimuli.

ii) **Measurement errors and artifacts associated with depth of anesthesia monitors.**

(1) Depth of anesthesia monitors have built-in mechanisms that detect external artifacts (electrocautery, pacemakers, ECG monitoring), increases in beta EEG activity from anesthetics, and burst suppression patterns.

(2) Clinical situations that falsely increase depth of anesthesia monitoring include: excessive facial muscle tone, electrocautery, pacemaker, twelve lead ECG monitoring, movement, surgical drilling, and agents that may produce anesthesia without a reduction in the awareness monitor index (nitrous oxide, xenon, ketamine).

(3) A subdural hematoma—via reduced voltage at the scalp—may falsely decrease depth of anesthesia recordings (5).

3) Using processed EEG as a depth of anesthesia monitor

a) Depth of anesthesia monitoring may be especially useful as an effect-site monitor during total intravenous anesthetic (TIVA) and especially in patients who are paralyzed during TIVA. Unlike volatile anesthetics in which there is a real time metric to assess end-tidal concentrations of the anesthetic, TIVA procedures are limited to ED50 values that do not translate as well to depth of anesthesia.

b) Furthermore, if a patient's IV is not under direct visualization it is difficult to assess if the IV has dislodged. In such a scenario, the IV pump will not alarm and the anesthesia provider may believe that the patient is receiving the anesthetic. This can be especially troubling if the patient received neuromuscular blockade. Use of a depth of anesthesia monitor may help prevent such a scenario.

c) Titration of an anesthetic to an adequate depth based on hemodynamic parameters and depth of anesthesia monitors can also help limit the negative impact of excessive anesthesia. In addition, in the ICU, depth of anesthesia monitoring may help reduce total ventilation time as well as hypotension related to chronic sedation.

4) Postoperative outcomes

While BIS monitoring provides a more accurate way gauge of depth of anesthesia than hemodynamic monitoring alone, recent studies have found correlations between deep hypnotic states as recorded by BIS and increased post operative mortality.

a) In a trial of adults undergoing non-cardiac surgery, deep hypnotic time under anesthesia was determined to be a BIS <45. This was deemed a significant independent predictor of post-operative mortality.

b) Some data indicate BIS can play a role in reducing adverse neurocognitive outcomes. For, example, BIS-guided anesthetic care (BIS 40 to 60) resulted in less neurocognitive distortion in patients three months post-operatively as compared with non-BIS guided anesthetic care. In contrast, BIS guided trials in elderly patients show no statistical difference in neuropsychological outcomes between BIS guided groups and non-BIS guided control populations. Further research studies to explore these relationships are ongoing.

Chapter Summary: Processed EEG and Awareness Monitoring

Awareness	Intraoperative awareness with recall involves explicit recall of sensory perceptions during general anesthesia including aspects of the surgical environment, procedure, and even pain related to the intervention.
Incidence	The most cited rate of intraoperative awareness is 0.2%.
Goals	Targeting a BIS range of 40–60 is marketed to help prevent anesthesia awareness while allowing for minimization of anesthetic dose.
False ↑ DOA	Excessive facial muscle tone, electrocautery, pacemaker, ECG monitoring, movement, surgical drilling, agents that may produce anesthesia without a reduction in the awareness index (N_2O, xenon, ketamine).
False ↓ DOA	Subdural hematoma, which causes reduced voltage at the scalp.
Other Uses	Titration using DOA monitors may help limit the negative effects of excessive anesthesia and detect inadvertent light anesthesia during TIVA.

BIS, bispectral index; DOA, depth of anesthesia; ECG, electrocardiogram; N_2O, nitrous oxide; TIVA, total intravenous anesthesia.

References

1. Liu WHD, Thorp T, Graham SG, Aitkenhead AR. Incidence of awareness with recall during general anaesthesia. *Anesthesia* 1991;46:435–437.
2. Ghoneim MM. Incidence of and risk factors for awareness during anaesthesia. *Best Pract Res Clin Anaesthesiol* 2007;21(3):327–343.
3. Lennmarken C, Sydsjo G. Psychological consequences of awareness and their treatment. *Best Pract Res Clin Anaesthesiol* 2007;21:357–367.
4. Ranta S, Jussila J, Hynynen M. Recall of awareness during cardiac anesthesia: influence of feedback information to the anaesthesiologist. *Acta Anaesthesiol Scand* 1996;40:554–560.
5. Rampil IJ. Monitoring depth of anesthesia. *Curr Opin Anaesthesiol* 2001;14:649–653.
6. Ghoneim MM, Block RI. Learning and memory during general anesthesia: An update. *Anesthesiology* 1997;87:387–410.
7. Bogetz MS, Katz JA. Recall of surgery for major trauma. *Anesthesiology* 1984;61:6–9.
8. Jones JG. Perception and memory during general anesthesia. *Br J Anaesth* 1994;73:31–37.
9. Lau L, Matta B, Menon DK, et al. Attitudes of anesthetists to awareness and depth of anesthesia monitoring in the UK. *Eur J Anaesthesiol* 2006;23(11):921–930.

MONITORING

16 Neurophysiologic Monitoring and Anesthetic Management

Obianuju Okocha, MD

Neurophysiologic monitoring or neuromonitoring allows early detection of events that may increase postoperative neurological morbidity. The aim of monitoring is to identify changes in brain, spinal cord, and peripheral nerve function prior to irreversible damage. Neuromonitoring is also useful in identifying anatomical structures.

1) **Overview of neurophysiologic monitoring in anesthesia**
   a) Neurophysiologic monitoring is becoming the standard of care in all cases where the potential exists for damage to the brain and spinal cord due to surgical manipulation of the tissue or its blood supply.
   b) **Basic concepts**
      i) Evoked potentials (responses recorded from the nervous system following electrical stimulation) are described in terms of **latency and amplitude.** (Fig. 16-1)
      ii) Intraoperative changes in either parameter may result from surgical injury or ischemia of the specific neural pathway, or they may be due to nonspecific physiologic or pharmacologic influences.
      iii) Physiologic factors that influence evoked potentials include **temperature, BP, hematocrit, acid-base balance, and O_2 and CO_2 tensions.**
      iv) **Anesthetic drugs are the most common pharmacologic causes of nonspecific changes in evoked potentials (1).**

2) **Techniques**

Physiologic factors that influence evoked potentials include temperature, BP, hematocrit, acid-base balance, and O_2 and CO_2 tensions.

   a) **Electromyography (EMG)**
      i) EMG is the recording of electrical activity of muscle and therefore an indirect indicator of function of the innervating peripheral nerve.
      ii) This technique is also used to identify and verify the integrity of a peripheral nerve, including cranial nerves as well as pedicle screw testing during spine surgery.
      iii) EMG is only sensitive to neuromuscular blocking agents.
   b) **Somatosensory evoked potentials (SSEP)**
      i) SSEP are the recording, usually at the cerebral cortex, of responses from electrically stimulated peripheral afferent nerves.
         (1) The most commonly used peripheral nerves are median, ulnar, posterior tibial, and common peroneal nerves.
      ii) Significant changes in SSEP are as follows:
         (1) **A decrease in amplitude of $\geq 50\%$**
         (2) **An increase in latency of $\geq 10\%$**
         (3) Both of the above reflect loss of integrity of a neural pathway, provided these changes are not caused by physiologic or pharmacologic factors (2).

| **Figure 16-1** | Schematic of Evoked Potential in Terms of Latency and Amplitude |

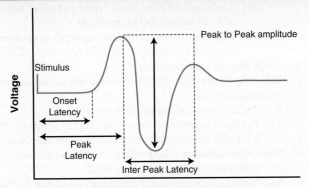

Time after Stimulation in msecs

Reproduced from Banoub M, Tetzlaff JE, Schubert A. Pharmacologic and physiologic influences affecting sensory evoked potentials: Implications for perioperative monitoring. *Anesthesiology* 2003; 99(3):717, with permission.

iii) SSEP are sensitive to volatile anesthetics in a dose-dependent manner (3). Certain anesthetics (etomidate and ketamine) increase SSEP amplitude (4).

c) **Brainstem auditory evoked potentials (BAEP)**
  i) BAEP are the recording of brainstem responses to auditory stimuli.
  ii) Other acronyms include brainstem auditory evoked responses (BAER) and auditory brainstem responses.
  iii) BAEP monitors the function of the entire auditory pathway along the acoustic nerve, through the brain stem to the cerebral cortex.
  iv) BAEP is **insensitive to both volatile anesthetics and neuromuscular blocking agents (5).**

d) **Motor evoked potentials (MEP)**
  i) MEP is the recording obtained from electrical stimulation of the motor cortex, which elicits potentials in the spinal cord or (myogenic) potentials from the innervated muscle.
  ii) Monitors motor pathway function
  iii) **MEP is sensitive to both volatile anesthetics and neuromuscular blocking agents.**
  iv) MEP is almost always performed in conjunction with SSEP. These techniques function as complementary tests (6).

e) **Electroencephalography (EEG)**
  i) EEG monitoring can be a useful supplement to surgery when
    (1) Seizure foci need to be identified
    (2) The general state of cerebral metabolism needs monitoring
    (3) Cerebral ischemia can occur
  ii) EEG is a standard of care in many institutions for carotid endarterectomy.
  iii) EEG is the recording of brain electrical activity and is highly dependent on anesthetic depth.
    (1) Alpha waves are rhythmically regular waves of 8 to 12 Hz seen in a lightly anesthesized patient.
    (2) A faster, disorganized beta (>12 Hz) rhythm is seen upon awakening.
    (3) Slower theta waves (4 to 8 Hz) are seen with deep inhalational or moderate dose narcotic anesthesia.
    (4) Slow delta waves (<4 Hz) indicate deep anesthesia, or ischemia if the amplitude is low.

(5) Burst suppression represents bursts of EEG activity with alternating periods of inactivity.

(6) Under special conditions, "spike and wave" seizure activity identify seizure foci for resection.

(7) EEG also allows for monitoring depth of anesthesia using mathematical processing of the EEG (processed EEG).

3) **Anesthetic management strategies**

a) **EEG only:** moderately sensitive to volatile anesthetic, insensitive to neuromuscular blockade

   i) Induction and maintenance as usual

   ii) Balanced maintenance using inhalational agents (≤1 MAC) with propofol, opioids, and neuromuscular blockade as needed

b) **BAER only:** insensitive to both volatile anesthetics and neuromuscular blockade

   i) Induction and maintenance as usual

c) **SSEP only:** sensitive to volatile anesthetic, insensitive to neuromuscular blockade

   i) Induction and maintenance as usual

   ii) Balanced maintenance using inhalational agents (½ to 1 MAC), ketamine, propofol, and/or dexmedetomidine

   iii) Opioids and neuromuscular blockade as needed

d) **MEP only:** very sensitive to volatile anesthetic and neuromuscular blockade

   i) Induction as usual (neuromuscular blockade as needed for induction or as needed for surgical exposure)

   ii) TIVA: Opioids, propofol, and ketamine

      (1) Use of dexmedetomidine is controversial in this setting as MEP may not be reproducible.

   iii) In some cases, inhalational agents (<½ MAC) could be used if the MEP responses remain intact.

e) Multiple techniques

   i) Often, multiple techniques are used simultaneously. The **technique with the most anesthetic restriction dictates anesthetic management.**

   ii) When EMG is used in combination with any of the techniques above, neuromuscular blockade should be avoided.

   iii) Communication between the surgical, anesthesia and the neuromonitoring teams is essential (6).

> Avoid NMB when EMG or MEP is being monitored because neuromuscular transmission is inhibited.

Chapter Summary for Neurophysiologic Monitoring and Anesthetic Management

Definition	Neuromonitoring during anesthesia measures electrical activity in various parts of the nervous system, including the brain, spinal cord and peripheral nerves.
Goals	The goal of neuromonitoring is to identify changes in neurologic function during surgery in order to prevent irreversible damage.
Physiologic Effects	Neuromonitoring affected by temperature, BP, hematocrit, acid–base balance, and O_2 and CO_2 tensions
Volatile Effects	↓EEG, ↓SSEP, ↓↓MEP, ↔BAER
NMB	↓↓MEP, ↔EEG, ↔BAER, ↔SSEP

BAER, brainstem auditory evoked response; EEG, electroencephalogram; MEP, motor evoked potential; NMB, neuromuscular blockade; SSEP, somatosensory evoked potential.

References

1. Banoub M, Tetzlaff JE, Schubert A. Pharmacologic and physiologic influences affecting sensory evoked potentials: Implications for perioperative monitoring. *Anesthesiology* 2003;99(3):716–737.
2. Faberowski LW, Black S, Trankina MF, et al. Somatosensory evoked potentials during aortic coarctation repair. *J Cardiothorac Vasc Anesth* 1999;13:538–543.
3. Porkkala T, Kaukinen S, Hakkinen V, et al. Median nerve somatosensory evoked potentials during isoflurane anaesthesia. *Can J Anaesth* 1997;44:963–968.
4. Koht A, Schutz W, Schmidt G, et al. Effects of etomidate, midazolam, and thiopental on median nerve somatosensory evoked potentials and the additive effects of fentanyl and nitrous oxide. *Anesth Analg* 1988;67:435–441.
5. Schwender D, Klasing S, Conzen P, et al. Midlatency auditory evoked potentials during anaesthesia with increasing end expiratory concentrations of desflurane. *Acta Anaesthesiol Scand* 1996;40:171–176
6. Husain, AM, ed. *A Practical Approach to Neurophysiologic Intraoperative Monitoring*. New York, NY: Demos; 2008.

MONITORING

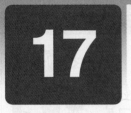

The Anesthesia Machine

Chad Pritts, MD · Samsun (Sem) Lampotang, PhD

The anesthesia machine is a vital component to the safe and reliable delivery of anesthesia and provides oxygenation, ventilation, and anesthetic gases to the patient. Anesthesia machines have become increasingly complex; however, they all employ the same fundamental functions.

1) **Overview of anesthesia machine elements.** In order to understand the anesthesia machine, it helps to divide it into four component subsystems (Fig. 17-1).

   a) **The high-pressure system**
      i) Receives connections from the hospital pipeline gas supply and includes the cylinder gas supplies

   b) **The low-pressure system**
      i) Blends oxygen and anesthetic gases according to the control settings

   c) **Breathing system**
      i) Delivers the fresh gas mixture from the low-pressure system to the patient and provides ventilation

   d) **Scavenging system**
      i) Collects excess gas from the breathing system and delivers it to the waste gas evacuation system

2) **The high-pressure system**

   a) **Gas sources**
      i) Central or pipeline supply
         (1) The primary gas source for the anesthesia machine
         (2) There is a central piping system in most hospitals that delivers medical gases (oxygen, nitrous oxide, and air) to the operating room.
         (3) For the anesthesia machine to work properly, the correct gas must be delivered to its corresponding inlet port at an appropriate pressure.
         (4) **Inadequate oxygen pressure** is the most common reported problem.
         (5) The most devastating problem is accidental delivery of hypoxic gases from the oxygen pipeline, which has resulted in hypoxic deaths (e.g., crossover of oxygen and nitrous oxide).
            (a) **If pipeline crossover is suspected**, two steps must be taken.
               (i) The backup oxygen cylinder should be turned on.
               (ii) The pipeline supply must be disconnected.
                  1. This step is essential because the machine uses the inappropriate pipeline gas at 45–55 psi instead of the lower-pressure 40–45 psi oxygen cylinder.

For the anesthesia machine to work properly, the correct gas must be delivered at an appropriate pressure into the corresponding inlet port of the anesthesia machine.

EQUIPMENT AND PROCEDURES

105

Figure 17-1 — A Typical Layout for A Bellows Anesthesia Machine with the Four Component Subsystems Depicted

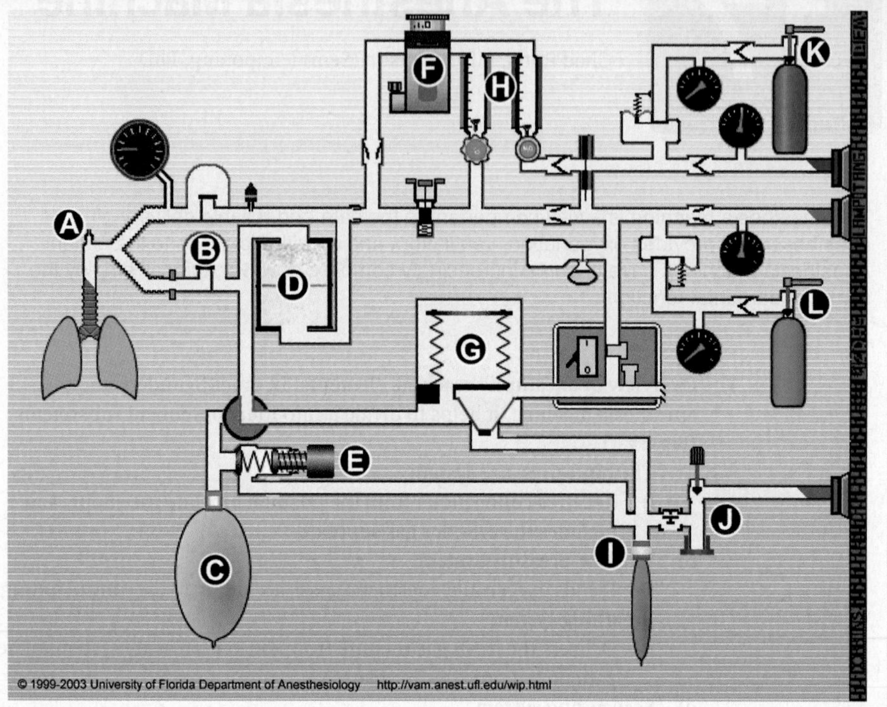

© 1999-2003 University of Florida Department of Anesthesiology   http://vam.anest.ufl.edu/wip.html

(A) Anesthesia breathing circuit, (B) Unidirectional flow valve, (C) Reservoir bag, (D) CO_2 Absorber, (E) APL "Pop Off" valve, (F) Anesthetic vaporizer, (G) Ventilator, (H) Flowmeters, (I) Scavenging bag, (J) Scavenging manifold, (K) Nitrous oxide cylinder, (L) Oxygen cylinder. From the virtual anesthesia machine simulation http://vam.anest.ufl.edu/wip.html, with permission.

If pipeline crossover is suspected, the backup oxygen cylinder should be turned on and the oxygen pipeline supply must be disconnected.

(6) The pipeline inlet fittings are gas specific
    (a) The Diameter Index Safety System provides threaded body fittings that are noninterchangeable to minimize the risk of misconnection

ii) **The cylinder supply**
    (1) Reserve **E cylinders are for use if a pipeline source is not available** or if the pipeline fails.
    (2) **Color-coded cylinders** are attached to the anesthesia machine through a hanger yoke assembly.
        (a) In the United States, the color coding is green for oxygen, blue for nitrous oxide, and yellow for air.
        (b) The international color code is white for oxygen, blue for nitrous oxide, and white and black for air.
    (3) **Hanger yoke assembly**
        (a) Orients and supports the cylinder and provides a gas tight seal to the machine

(b) It is equipped with a **Pin Index Safety System**, which is a safeguard to eliminate accidental cylinder misconnection.

(i) Each gas has a specific pin arrangement.

(4) **Check valve located downstream**

(a) It minimizes gas transfer from a cylinder with high pressure to one with low pressure.

(b) It allows an empty cylinder to be exchanged for a full one while gas flow continues into the machine.

(5) The **cylinder gauge indicating supply pressure** is located downstream or upstream from the check valve.

(a) Newer machines have an electronic pressure sensor instead of a gauge, and the measured pressure is displayed on the display panel.

(6) Each cylinder has a **pressure regulator** that reduces the high and variable storage pressure to a more constant pressure.

(7) The **oxygen cylinder pressure regulator** reduces the cylinder pressure from a high of 2,200 to 40–45 psi.

(8) The **nitrous oxide cylinder pressure regulator** reduces the cylinder pressure from a high of 745 to 40–45 psi.

(9) If both the cylinder and the pipeline are open and connected, gas flows preferentially from the pipeline because the pressure is slightly higher than the cylinder's regulated pressure.

(10) **Cylinders should be turned off except during the preoperative machine check.**

(a) They can become depleted if open and the pressure in the pipeline falls below 45 psi.

b) **Pneumatic and electronic alarm devices**

i) Many older machines have a **pneumatic alarm device** that sounds a warning when the oxygen supply pressure falls below a threshold value.

(1) A commonly used mechanism employs a pressurized canister that is filled with oxygen.

(2) When the machine is turned on, a stream of oxygen passes through a whistle.

(3) If the oxygen pressure drops below a certain value, the canister will empty and a reverse stream of oxygen will flow through the whistle.

ii) Electronic alarms are used to meet this requirement on newer machines.

c) **Oxygen flush valve**

i) It provides a high flow directly to the common gas outlet.

ii) The **oxygen flush** can be used even when the **machine is not turned on.**

iii) It bypasses the flow meters and vaporizers.

iv) The flow is at **35 to 75 L/min.**

(1) Because of this, there is a real potential for barotrauma.

v) If the oxygen flush valve is used during the expiratory phase of mechanical ventilation, the bellows will fill to their maximum capacity.

(1) After the maximum capacity is reached, any excess will be vented through the ventilator pressure relief valve.

vi) During inspiration, the ventilator pressure release valve is closed, so there is no outlet for the excess gas.

(1) If the oxygen flush valve is pressed during mechanical inspiration, dangerously high pressures can be transmitted to the lungs, if the high pressure limit is improperly set.

EQUIPMENT AND PROCEDURES

d) **Oxygen pressure failure** devices

    i) **Fail-safe system**

        (1) As oxygen supply pressure decreases below a preset level, the supply of gases other than oxygen is shut off and an alarm goes off.

        (2) This **prevents the delivery of a hypoxic gas mixture.**

        (3) An oxygen analyzer in the inspiratory arm is mandated to insure that a hypoxic mixture is detected.

3) **Low-pressure system**

  a) The flow meter assembly **precisely controls and measures the gas flow to the common gas outlet.**

    i) Gas flows continuously from the anesthesia machine to the breathing circuit.

    ii) The **gas flow rate** is determined by the **flow control valves** and is measured by the flow meters.

    iii) Many anesthesia machines have a **mandatory minimum oxygen flow rate of 200 mL/min when the machine is turned on.**

        (1) In these machines, the bobbin in the oxygen flowmeter will not completely return to zero.

  b) **Flow control valves**

    i) The high-pressure system is separated from the low-pressure system by the flow control valves.

    ii) There is a substantial **pressure drop as gas passes through the flow control valve.**

    iii) The flow control valves are variable-orifice needle valves.

        (1) When the knob of the flow control valve is turned counterclockwise, a pin is disengaged, allowing gas to flow through the valve

    iv) The knobs are touch and color coded to make it more difficult to turn on or off the wrong gas.

  c) **Flow meters**

    i) There are two types of flow meters, **constant pressure and variable orifice.**

    ii) With the constant pressure flow meter, the pressure decrease remains constant across the float at all positions of the tube.

    iii) The variable orifice flow meter has a tapered tube with the largest diameter at the top. These tapered, transparent, glass tubes are also known as *Thorpe tubes.*

    iv) The bobbin **floats at a point of equilibrium**, where the downward force of gravity is equal to the upward force generated by gas flow.

    v) **Flow is read at the top of plumb bob** and at the center of ball type floats.

    vi) Flow meters are calibrated to a specific gas density and viscosity and can't be interchanged.

    vii) **Many newer machines have** conventional control knobs and flow control valves but have **digital flow meters (see Fig. 17-3).**

    viii) The oxygen flow meters should be positioned downstream from the other medical gas flow meters to lessen the risk of delivering a hypoxic gas mixture.

d) **Vaporizers**

   i) Volatile anesthetics **must be vaporized before being delivered to the patient.**

   ii) Modern vaporizers are agent specific and capable of delivering a constant concentration of agent even at different temperatures and flows.

   iii) Agent-specific vaporizers are also known as variable-bypass vaporizers; some of the entering gas is never exposed to (bypasses) the anesthetic liquid.

   iv) Variable-bypass vaporizers should be located outside of the circle system, between the flowmeters and the common gas outlet.

   v) **Desflurane requires a special vaporizer called the Tec 6.**

      (1) Desflurane's vapor pressure is so high that it almost boils at room temperature, and it has a potency that is only one fifth that of the other volatile agents.

   vi) Machines have interlock devices that prevent the use of more than one vaporizer at a time.

4) **Breathing system**

   a) **Traditional circle breathing system**

     i) Circle system prevents rebreathing of carbon dioxide by use of CO_2 absorbents but allows partial rebreathing of other exhaled gases.

     ii) **Unidirectional valves** are used to ensure that gas flows in the proper direction.

       (1) The **inspiratory valve prevents backflow** through the inspiratory limb during expiration, and the expiratory valve prevents backflow through the expiratory limb during inspiration.

     iii) **Types of circle systems**

       (1) **Semiopen**

         (a) No rebreathing and requires a very high flow of fresh gas

       (2) **Semiclosed**

         (a) Associated with rebreathing of gases and is the most commonly used system in the United States

       (3) **Closed**

         (a) The inflow gas exactly matches that being consumed by the patient.

         (b) There is complete rebreathing of exhaled gases after the absorption of CO_2.

         (c) No excess gas flows into the scavenging system.

     iv) The circle system consists of seven components (Fig. 17-2):

       (1) Fresh gas inflow source

       (2) Inspiratory and expiratory unidirectional valves

       (3) Inspiratory and expiratory corrugated tubing

       (4) Y-piece connector

       (5) Overflow or pop-off valve; (APL-adjustable pressure limiting) valve

       (6) Reservoir bag

       (7) Canister with CO_2 absorbent

The circle system prevents rebreathing of CO_2 but allows partial rebreathing of other exhaled gases.

EQUIPMENT AND PROCEDURES

Figure 17-2   The Circle System with Relevant Parts Labeled

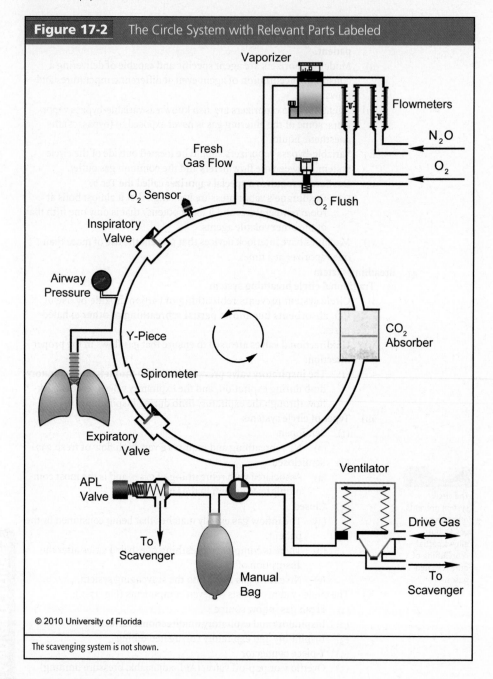

Vaporizer

Flowmeters

N₂O

O₂

Fresh
Gas Flow

O₂ Flush

O₂ Sensor

Inspiratory
Valve

Airway
Pressure

Y-Piece

CO₂
Absorber

Spirometer

Expiratory
Valve

Ventilator

APL
Valve

Drive Gas

To
Scavenger

Manual
Bag

To
Scavenger

© 2010 University of Florida

The scavenging system is not shown.

5) Scavenging system
   a) Classification of scavenging systems
      i) **Active scavenging systems**
         (1) Vacuum source, vacuum hose, and vacuum control
         (2) The negative pressure, vacuum, source actively pulls the excess gas from the anesthesia machine, transports it through the hospital's gas disposal system, and typically releases it through the roof.

Figure 17-3 A Typical Layout for an Anesthesia Workstation with a Piston Ventilator

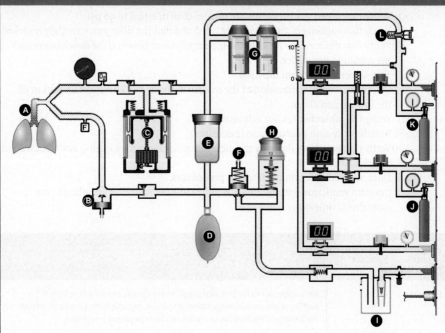

(A) Anesthesia breathing circuit, **(B)** Active exhalation/peep valve, **(C)** Piston ventilator, **(D)** Reservoir bag, **(E)** CO_2 absorber, **(F)** Manual/automatic ventilation selection actuator, **(G)** Anesthetic vaporizers, **(H)** APL valve, **(I)** Bag-less active scavenger system, **(J)** Nitrous oxide cylinder, **(K)** Oxygen cylinder, **(L)** Oxygen flush valve. Adapted from the virtual Fabius GS simulation - http://www.simanest.org/vfgs3.html

   ii) **Passive scavenging system**
      (1) Waste gas evacuation hose
      (2) Does not require a vacuum source
      (3) Relies on a slight positive pressure difference to push waste gas through the evacuation hose
6) **Preanesthesia machine checkout**
   a) In 1993, a preanesthesia checkout was developed and widely accepted.
   b) Anesthesia delivery systems have evolved (most notably with the addition of piston ventilators—Fig. 17-3) and the 1993 PreAnesthesia Checkout is not applicable to all machines on the market.
   c) In 2008, the ASA Committee on Equipment & Facilities made recommendations for new checkout procedures.
      i) Their document was meant to be a template for developing checkout procedures for individual machines and practice settings.
   d) **Checkout steps**
      i) Verify auxiliary oxygen cylinder and self-inflating manual ventilation device are available and functioning.
      ii) **Verify patient suction** is adequate to clear the airway.
      iii) Turn on the anesthesia delivery system and confirm that AC power is available.

EQUIPMENT AND PROCEDURES

    iv) Verify availability of required monitors and check alarms.

    v) Verify that pressure is adequate on the spare oxygen cylinder mounted on the anesthesia machine.

    vi) Verify that piped gas pressures are greater than or equal to 50 psi.

    vii) Verify that vaporizers are adequately filled and that the filler ports are tightly closed.

    viii) Verify that there are no leaks in the gas supply lines between the flow meters and the common gas outlet.

    ix) Test scavenging system function.

    x) Calibrate or verify calibration of the oxygen monitor and check the operation of the low oxygen alarm.

    xi) Verify CO_2 absorbent is not exhausted.

    xii) Breathing system pressure and leak testing

    xiii) Verify that gas flows properly through the breathing circuit during both inspiration and exhalation.

    xiv) Document completion of checkout procedures.

    xv) Confirm ventilator settings and evaluate readiness to deliver anesthesia care (anesthesia time out).

Chapter Summary for Anesthesia Machines

Definition	The anesthesia machine is a vital component to the safe and reliable delivery of anesthesia and provides oxygenation, ventilation, and anesthetic gases to the patient. The anesthesia machine can be divided into four component subsystems.
High-pressure System	Receives connections from the hospital pipeline gas supply and includes the cylinder gas supplies.
Low-pressure System	Blends oxygen and anesthetic gases according to the control settings.
Breathing System	Delivers the fresh gas mixture from the low-pressure system to the patient and provides ventilation.
Scavenging System	Collects excess gas from the breathing system and delivers it to the waste gas evacuation system.
Anesthesia Machine Checkout	The ASA Committee on Equipment & Facilities made new recommendations for anesthesia machine check out practices prior to administration of anesthesia. These should be reviewed and adopted to individual machines and practice settings.

References

1. Brockwell CB, Andrews JJ. Inhaled anesthetic delivery systems, In: *Miller RD, Anesthesia*. 6th ed. Philadelphia, PA:. Elsevier Churchill Livingstone, 2005:273–316.

2. Lampotang S, Good ML. The anesthesia machine, anesthesia ventilator, breathing circuit, and scavenging system. In: Kirby RR et al., eds. *Clinical anesthesia practice*. 2nd ed. Philadelphia, PA: WB Saunders, 2002:277–302.

3. Virtual Anesthesia Machine, http://vam.anest.ufl.edu/wip.html

4. Virtual Fabius GS, http://www.simanest.org/vfgs3.html

Anesthesia Breathing Circuits

Vivekanand Kulkarni, MD, PhD • Romy Yun, MD

The anesthesia breathing circuit creates a local environment surrounding the patient within which respiratory gas exchange occurs. The circuit is vital for ventilation of the patient undergoing anesthesia and provides a conduit through which anesthetic gases can be administered.

1) Overview
   a) Most modern circuits incorporate 22 mm corrugated breathing tubes with one end (elbow) linked to the patient's airway via a mask/laryngeal mask airway (LMA)/endotracheal tube (ETT) and a fresh gas inlet (FGI) at the other.
   b) A spring-loaded pop-off valve/adjustable pressure-limiting (APL) valve and a reservoir breathing bag (RBB) are also included.
   c) With most circuits, there is a general increase in *dead space* so that V_d/V_t increases from 0.33 to 0.46 if intubated and to 0.66 with a mask.
   d) The *resistance* to breathing depends on the presence of valves and the diameter of the tubing.
   e) The positions of the elements of these circuits determine their functional characteristics.
   f) When there is no CO_2 absorber present, they constitute **nonrebreathing systems**, which were classified by Mapleson into A, B, C, D, E, and F.
   g) When unidirectional valves and a CO_2 absorber are included, the resistance to breathing is greater, and these circuits constitute **rebreathing Systems**.

2) Nonrebreathing systems—Mapleson circuits (Fig. 18-1)
   a) Nonrebreathing systems work by using fresh gas flow (FGF) to push the patient's exhaled gas down the expiratory limb of the circuit.
      i) The exhaled gases collect in the RBB, and some escapes through an expiratory (APL) valve.
         (1) The remaining exhaled gas is diluted by FGF
      ii) The patient draws his next breath through the expiratory limb and RBB.
         (1) Some rebreathing of the previous breath may occur depending upon the degree of dilution (from FGF rate, patient's tidal volume (TV), and length of expiratory pause).
   b) Mapleson in 1954 classified the circuits into five groups depending on the position of the FGI, RBB, and APL in the circuit.
   c) The F system, as described by Willis, was later added to the original group of five.
   d) **Gas is expelled through the APL.**

Incorporation of unidirectional valves and a CO_2 absorber into an anesthesia circuit allows rebreathing of some exhaled gases and constitutes rebreathing systems.

Circuits classified as nonrebreathing systems are not intended to allow rebreathing of exhaled gases, but rebreathing can still occur.

113

Figure 18-1 Mapleson Circuits

	Spontaneous	Controlled
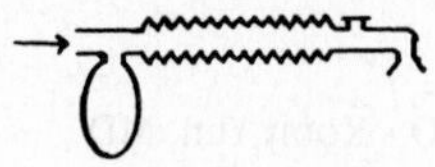 A	1 x MV	>3 x MV
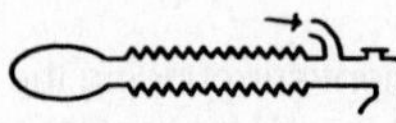 B	2 x MV	2.5 x MV
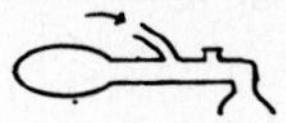 C	2 x MV	2.5 x MV
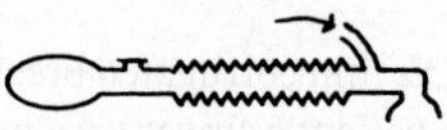 D	2–3 x MV	1–2 x MV
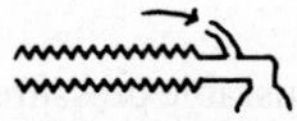 E	2–3 x MV	3 x MV
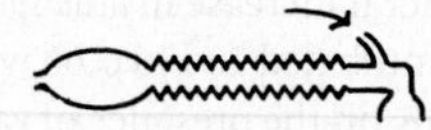 F	2–3 x MV	3 x MV

The FGF necessary to prevent rebreathing is represented as a function of the patient's minute ventilation. MV, minute ventilation. Adapted from Dorsch JA, Dorsch SE. *Understanding Anesthesia Equipment.* 5th ed. Philadelphia, PA: Lippincott Williams & Wilkins, 2008.

    i) In the **A, B, and C classes**, expired gas leaves the circuit close to the patient.

    ii) The **D, E, and F are T-piece systems**, and expired gas leaves the circuit away from the patient.

  e) Since there is no CO_2 absorber, there is always potential for rebreathing some amount of exhaled gases using Mapleson circuits.

    i) The amount of rebreathing depends on the following:

      (1) The circuit elements and their position.

      (2) Minute ventilation (MV)

      (3) The pattern of breathing (TV, respiratory rate, peak inspiratory flow rate, Expiratory pause duration, and I:E ratio)

      (4) The FGF

        (a) The FGF needed to prevent significant rebreathing depends also on the mode of ventilation.

          (i) **Spontaneous**

          (ii) **Controlled**

    ii) The efficiency with respect to FGF needed to prevent rebreathing is

      (1) During Spontaneous Ventilation A > D,F,E > C,B

      (2) During Controlled Ventilation D,F,E > B,C > (Table 18-1)

  f) Mapleson circuits

    i) **Mapleson A—Magill circuit**

Table 18-1
The Advantages and Disadvantages of Mapleson Circuits

Advantages of Mapleson Circuits	• Inexpensive, lightweight, simple to use, disassemble, and sterilize. • Rugged, no moving parts except APL, and low resistance to flow. • Changes in FGF result in rapid changes in inspiratory gas concentrations. • Since there is no absorber, there are no toxic products of agent breakdown. • In Coaxial systems, inspiratory gas is heated by the warm exhaled gas.
Disadvantages of Mapleson Circuits	• Higher flows are needed to prevent CO_2 rebreathing, hence more expensive. • Because of higher flows, there is loss of heat and humidity. • Scavenging is more difficult in some circuits, and environmental pollution is greater. • In some circuits, the APL is close to the patient and more difficult to access. • Assembly errors can cause significant CO_2 rebreathing.

FGF, fresh gas flow; APL, adjustable pressure limiting valve.

(1) It has a single breathing tube with the FGI and RBB close to the machine, while the APL is close to the patient connector or elbow.

(2) A drawback of Mapleson A is that waste gas is released close to the patient, which makes scavenging difficult.

(3) **Spontaneous ventilation (Fig. 18-2)**

    (a) During expiration, the corrugated breathing tube is filled first by dead space gas, which is CO_2 free, followed by Alveolar gas from the patient end of the circuit and simultaneously by FGF from the FGI.

    (b) The flow from the FGI continues during the expiratory pause.

    (c) If the FGF is high enough, pressure in the circuit rises, the APL opens and expels CO_2 containing expired Alveolar gas.

    (d) During the next inspiration, the FGF and some dead space gas will be inhaled.

    (e) **When the FGF is above 70% of MV during Spontaneous Ventilation, rebreathing is prevented as long as breathing is regular.**

(4) **Controlled ventilation**

    (a) The inspiratory force is provided by the anesthesiologist who squeezes the RBB after partially closing the APL.

    (b) During inspiration, therefore, some fresh gas is vented via the APL.

    (c) During expiration, expired gas fills the RBB. This is mixed with the FGF during the expiratory pause, so that rebreathing CO_2 containing gas is inevitable.

    (d) Now the system is inefficient because the FGF needs to be more than three times MV to prevent CO_2 buildup from rebreathing.

    (e) The Miller modification of the Magill system keeps the APL closed during inspiration thus decreasing FGF requirements.

(ii) **Lack system (Coaxial Mapleson A)**

(1) The Lack coaxial system has two tubes.

    (a) The outer tube is similar to that of the Mapleson A with FGI and RBB close to the machine end.

    (b) The expired gases from the patient are, however, conducted by the inner tube to the machine end so that the APL is closer to the machine end.

EQUIPMENT AND PROCEDURES

Figure 18-2   Mapleson A (Magill Circuit) During Spontaneous Ventilation MV

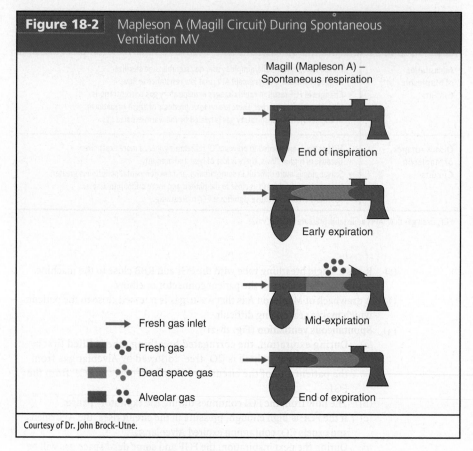

Magill (Mapleson A) –
Spontaneous respiration

End of inspiration

Early expiration

Mid-expiration

→ Fresh gas inlet

Fresh gas

Dead space gas

Alveolar gas

End of expiration

Courtesy of Dr. John Brock-Utne.

(2) **Functionally similar to the Mapleson A, the arrangement allows for easier scavenging and manipulation of the APL.**

iii) **Mapleson B and C systems**

   (1) In these systems, the APL and FGI are close to the patient connector.

   (2) The RBB and corrugated tubing when present (Mapleson B) form a blind end where mixed expired and fresh gases collect.

   (3) A FGF >2×MV is needed to prevent rebreathing in both spontaneous and controlled modes.

   (4) The C system is also called Waters to & fro system without absorber.

   (5) These systems are rarely used today.

iv) **Mapleson D system**

   (1) This system is basically a T-tube system with the FGI close to the patient forming one limb of the T-tube.

   (2) Expired gases flow through the other limb of the T, which is a long corrugated tube with a reservoir bag and a pop-off valve.

   (3) **Spontaneous Ventilation**

      (a) In expiration, the dead space gas, alveolar gas and FGF mix in the corrugated tubing and the RBB.

      (b) When the bag fills, the pressure in the system rises and the APL opens to vent the mixture.

Figure 18-3   Mapleson D Used in Transporting Intubated Patients

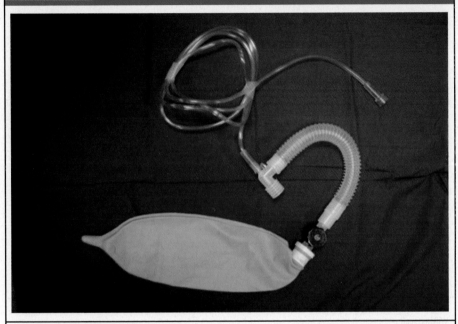

Courtesy of Dr. John Brock-Utne.

    (c)   In the expiratory pause, the FGF continues to push the expired Alveolar gas toward the RBB and APL.

    (d)   **During spontaneous breathing, 2×MV of FGF is needed to prevent rebreathing.**

    (e)   It is less efficient than Mapleson A but more efficient than Mapleson B and C.

    (4)   **Controlled ventilation**

        (a)   On expiration, the corrugated tubing and RBB fill up with a mixture of FGF, Dead Space and Alveolar gas.

        (b)   In the expiratory pause, the FGF pushes the expired gas toward the RBB and APL.

        (c)   Compressing the bag manually allows this FGF in the corrugated tubing to enter the lungs, whereas the higher pressure opens the APL to vent the FGF expired gas mixture from the bag.

        (d)   **During controlled ventilation, 1 to 2×MV of FGF is needed to prevent rebreathing.**

        (e)   The circuit is often used for manual ventilation during transport of patients (Fig. 18-3).

  v) **Bain System (Co-axial Mapleson D)**

    (1)   Fresh gas enters the inner small-bore tube and is delivered to the patient connection.

    (2)   **Expired gases go into the outer corrugated tubing to the RBB and APL close to the machine end** (Fig. 18-4).

EQUIPMENT AND PROCEDURES

Figure 18-4 | Bain Circuit

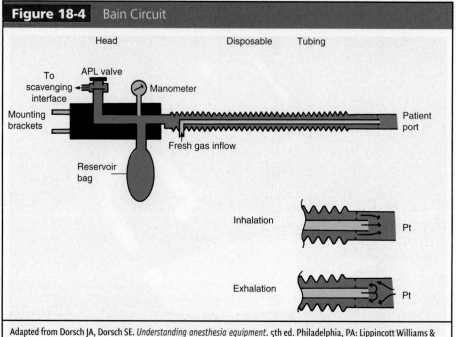

Head   Disposable   Tubing

To scavenging interface

APL valve

Manometer

Mounting brackets

Patient port

Fresh gas inflow

Reservoir bag

Inhalation   Pt

Exhalation   Pt

Adapted from Dorsch JA, Dorsch SE. *Understanding anesthesia equipment*. 5th ed. Philadelphia, PA: Lippincott Williams & Wilkins, 2008.

    (a) **Spontaneous ventilation**
        (i) During expiration, dead space and alveolar gas enter the outer corrugated tubing and RBB.
        (ii) During the expiratory pause, FGF from the inner tube fills the outer tube, pushing the expired gas to the RBB and APL.
        (iii) **Keeping the FGF adequate (2.5 to 3 × MV) prevents rebreathing.**
    (b) **Controlled ventilation**
        (i) **During controlled ventilation, 70 mL/kg/min or 1 to 2 × MV prevents rebreathing.**
        (ii) For controlled ventilation, the reservoir bag can be removed for ventilator attachment.
  (3) **Pethick test**
    (a) If the inner tube that delivers FGF gets disconnected or kinked at the proximal end, the entire corrugated tubing becomes additional dead space, which is difficult to compensate for, leading to respiratory acidosis.
        (i) Prevention by checking for the patency of the inner tube connection uses the Pethick Test.
            1. Occlude the patient end and close the APL valve.
            2. Fill the circuit with the Oxygen Flush button, distending the RBB.
            3. Release the patient end.
            4. The resulting Venturi effect flattens the RBB confirming inner tube connection patency.

(4) **CPAP system**
   (a) Occasionally, during one-lung-ventilation, a modified Mapleson D system can be attached to the nonventilated lung and a secondary O_2 source.
   (b) This provides CPAP to the nonventilated lung and decreases the shunt fraction, thus improving oxygenation.

vi) **Mapleson E and F systems**
   (1) These are valveless T-piece systems, which have low resistance.
   (2) Ayre's original T-piece system with additional expiratory limb of open corrugated tube (which acts as a reservoir) forms the E-system.
   (3) Loss of moisture because of the high FGF can be significant.
   (4) Partial occlusion of the expiratory limb opening (Mapleson E) or the RBB (Mapleson F) during manual ventilation can lead to high pressures.
      (a) A pressure relief mechanism is necessary to prevent barotrauma.
   (5) **Spontaneous ventilation**
      (a) The Mapleson E is similar to the D system.
      (b) During inspiration, no rebreathing occurs if there is no expiratory limb.
         (i) With an expiratory limb, however, rebreathing is avoided if the FGF is adequate.
            1. If the volume of the expiratory limb is less than the TV of the patient, air dilution can occur.
         (ii) **A FGF of 2 to 3× MV prevents rebreathing** (Fig. 18-5).
   (6) **The Mapleson F**
      (a) **The Jackson-Rees'** modification has a RBB with an open end attached to the expiratory limb of the Mapleson E.

Figure 18-5   Mapleson F: The Jackson-Rees Circuit

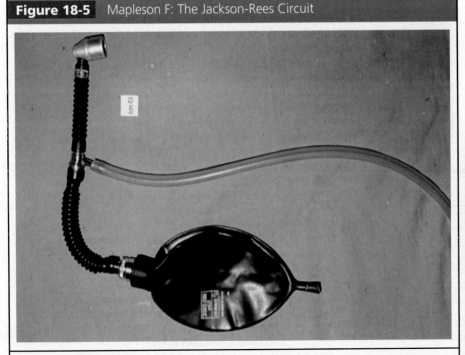

Courtesy of Dr. John Brock-Utne.

Table 18-2

The Advantages and Disadvantages of Circle Systems

Advantages of circle systems	a) Lower gas flows are economical. b) Reduced environmental pollution. c) Conservation of heat and humidity. d) More stable anesthetic gas concentrations and less chance of barotraumas due to sudden rise in circuit pressure.
Disadvantages of circle systems	a) Greater attention required to prevent hypercarbia from exhaustion of the CO_2 absorber. b) Decreased ability to alter anesthetic concentrations rapidly with low flows. c) Accumulation of small quantities of undesirable compounds from breakdown by dessicated absorbent.

(b) The addition of a bag acts as a reservoir to prevent dilution with air and allows manual ventilation when necessary.

(c) FGF requirements are similar to that of the Mapleson E.

3) Nonrebreathing systems

   a) **Circle system**

      i) This is currently the most popular system in the United States.

      ii) The system was first described by Brian Sword in 1926.

        (1) It allows low FGF.

        (2) It conserves heat and humidity.

        (3) It decreases pollution by allowing efficient scavenging.

The circle system is the most popular system in the United States. It allows low FGF, conserves heat and humidity, and allows efficient scavenging.

      iii) The earlier problem of predicting inspired gas composition is no longer an issue because gas concentrations are sampled for measurement at the patient yoke (Y-connector).

      iv) There is no further increase in patient dead space compared to other systems since gas sampling begins at the patient yoke.

      v) The resistance in the circle is <3 cm of water.

      vi) Rebreathing of CO_2 is prevented by absorption of CO_2 from the exhaled gas using the carbon dioxide absorber.

        (1) The position of components of the circle is also important in this respect.

      vii) **Classical circuit configuration**

        (1) Vaporizer is outside the circle.

        (2) Unidirectional valves lie between the patient yoke and the RBB in both inspiratory and expiratory limbs.

        (3) Two additional requirements are that the FGI, APL, and RBB should all be in between the two valves and not on the patient side of the circle.

        (4) **Spontaneous ventilation**

          (a) **Inspiration**

            (i) The unidirectional expiratory valve closes.

            (ii) Gas flows to the patient from the RBB (via the absorber) and the FGI through the inspiratory limb and the open unidirectional inspiratory valve.

          (b) **Expiration**

            (i) The unidirectional inspiratory valve closes.

Figure 18-6   Classic Circle System

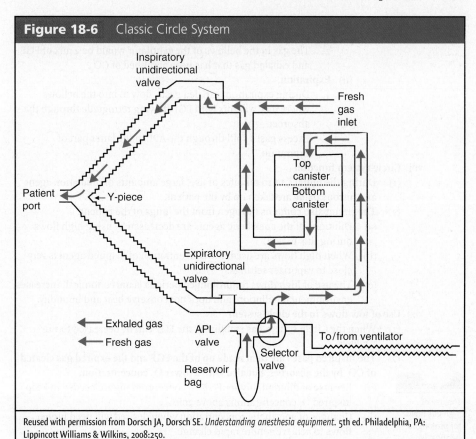

Reused with permission from Dorsch JA, Dorsch SE. *Understanding anesthesia equipment.* 5th ed. Philadelphia, PA: Lippincott Williams & Wilkins, 2008:250.

    (ii) Expired gas flows through the open unidirectional expiratory valve in the expiratory limb to the RBB and to the CO_2 absorber.

    (iii) The APL is positioned just before the CO_2 absorber in the expiratory limb.

    (iv) When flows are high CO_2 rich expired gas is the first to spill out of the circle thus conserving the CO_2 absorber.

(5) **Manual ventilation**

  (a) **Inspiration**

    (i) Excess gases are vented through the partially open APL valve during inspiration.

    (ii) The gas flowing through the absorber to the patient will be a mixture of FGF and expired gases.

    (iii) The composition of the mixture depends on the FGF.

  (b) **Expiration**

    (i) Exhaled gases flow into the RBB.

    (ii) There may be some retrograde flow of fresh gas through the absorber depending on FGF rate.

  (c) **Mechanical ventilation**

    (i) **Inspiration**

1. During inspiration, gas flows from the ventilator through the absorber and unidirectional inspiratory valve to the patient.
2. The gas in the bellows of the ventilator would be a mix of FGF and exhaled gas that has been scrubbed of CO_2.

(ii) **Expiration**

1. During expiration, exhaled gases flow to into the bellows where they will mix with FGF flowing retrograde through the absorber.
2. Excess gases spill through the APL in the latter part of expiration.

viii) **Circle system function**

(1) During the initial 5 to 10 minutes of use, large amounts of inhalation agent and nitrous oxide are taken up by the patient.

(2) The circuit also contains nitrogen from the lungs of the patient.

  (a) Dilutions of the anesthetic agents are decreased by using high flows during this period.

  (b) When high flows are used, the concentration of inspired agent is very close to vaporizer settings.

  (c) The use of high flows for prolonged periods is uneconomical, increases environmental pollution, and does not conserve heat and humidity.

ix) **Use of low flows in the circle system**

(1) When the Circle system has stabilized, the FGF can be decreased to 1 to 1.5 liters.

(2) **The inspired gases are then made up of the FGF and the expired gas cleared of CO_2 by the absorber, but also with a lower O_2 concentration.**

  (a) Because of dilution, higher FGF O_2 concentrations are needed to keep inspired O_2 concentrations above 30%.

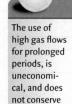

  (b) Changes of anesthetic concentration when desired will need **higher flows** to achieve a more rapid change.

The use of high gas flows for prolonged periods, is uneconomical, and does not conserve airway heat and humidity.

    (i) Advantages of **low flows** include economy, decreased environmental pollution, and conservation of heat and humidity.

    (ii) Disadvantages include greater use of the absorber and possible accumulation of undesired breakdown products from the absorber.

x) **Closed circle system**

(1) In this system, the APL is completely closed, and the minimum FGF flow should be equivalent to the oxygen consumption (250mls/min in the average 70kg patient).

xi) **CO_2 absorber**

(1) **Soda Lyme and BaraLyme are the most commonly used absorbers.**

  (a) Small amounts of Silica or Kieselguhr are added for hardening to reduce dust formation.

  (b) The absorptive efficiency is inversely related to hardness.

  (c) Absorptive surface area depends on granule size.

    (i) Smaller granules increase the absorptive surface but also increase resistance to flow of gas, while larger granules decrease the absorptive surface and decrease resistance leading to **channeling** of gas flow.

    (ii) The usual mesh size is therefore 4–8 mesh (1/4" to 1/8").

  (d) Up to 26L of CO_2 can be absorbed by 100g of absorbent.

(e) Composition of Soda Lyme: NaOH 4%; KOH 1%; H_2O 15%; 80% $Ca(OH)_2$.

(f) Composition of Bara Lyme: $Ba(OH)_2$ 20%; $Ca(OH)_2$ 80%; plus KOH indicator

(g) **The moisture or water content of the absorbent forms carbonic acid with CO_2, which reacts with alkali forming carbonate and generating heat.**

(h) $H_2O + CO_2 \Leftrightarrow H_2CO_3 \Leftrightarrow H^+ + HCO_3^-$

$NaOH + H_2CO_3 \Leftrightarrow NaHCO_3 + H_2O$

$2NaHCO_3 + Ca(OH)_2 \Leftrightarrow 2\,NaOH + CaCO_3 + H_2O$

(2) **Amsorb is a new CO_2 absorbant. It contains $Ca(OH)_2$ and $CaCl_2$. The hardening agents are $CaSO_4$ and Polyvinylpyrrolidine.**

(a) Since it does not contain NaOH or KOH, there is no CO or Compound-A production.

(b) It is more expensive, and the CO_2 absorption capacity is less.

(3) **Indicators**

(a) These are pH sensitive and added to the granules to show when they are exhausted

(i) Phenlophthalein: White when fresh and pink when exhausted

(ii) Ethyl Violet: White when fresh and purple when exhausted

(iii) Clayton yellow: Red when fresh and yellow when exhausted

(4) **Interactions with anesthetic agents**

(a) **Carbon monoxide**

(i) When the absorbents become dry and desiccated, they can react with anesthetic agents containing the CHF_2-O functional group resulting in **carbon monoxide** production.

1. CO production can be significant with Sodalyme and Baralyme leading to carboxyhemoglobin concentrations of up to 30%.

2. CO production increased by dehydrated absorbent, higher temperatures, lower FGF, and higher anesthetic agent concentration.

3. CO production is also dependent on anesthetic agent
   a. Desflurane > Enflurane > Isoflurane > halothane = sevoflurane

4. CO production is dependent on absorbent
   a. BaraLyme > SodaLyme

(ii) The production of CO can be decreased by decreasing the drying of absorbent by shutting off gas flow after cases, changing the absorbent if gas flow had not been shut off, rehydrating the absorbent, and using absorbents such as Amsorb that do not contain NaOH and KOH.

(b) **Other Breakdown compounds**

(i) **Compound-A**

1. Sevoflurane reacts with dry absorbent to produce an Olefin compound called Compound A (Fluoromethyl-2–2-difluoro-1-trifluoromethyl vinyl ether).

   a. The production is worse in dehydrated Baralyme with higher concentrations of Sevoflurane, low FGF, and higher absorbent temperatures.

   b. The concentration is low and is not known to cause toxic effects in humans.

EQUIPMENT AND PROCEDURES

  (ii) Other compounds produced in small quantities include **Acetone, methane, hydrogen, and ethanol.**

 (c) Fire

  (i) There is a small risk of fire within the absorber and breathing circuit with high temperatures and dry absorbents when Sevoflurane is used.

Chapter Summary for Anesthesia Breathing Circuits

Overview	The anesthesia breathing circuit creates a local environment surrounding the patient within which respiratory gas exchange occurs.
Nonrebreathing Systems	Nonrebreathing systems do not have the ability to absorb exhaled CO_2 gas. There are 6 main types of Mapleson circuits: A, B, C, D, E, and F. Each differs based on the position of the FGI, RBB, and APL valve in the circuit. The Bain circuit is a modification of the Mapleson D.
Rebreathing Systems	Rebreathing systems incorporate unidirectional valves and CO_2 absorbent to allow rebreathing of some exhaled gases. The circle system is currently the most popular rebreathing system used in the United States. It has methods for both spontaneous and manual ventilation.

RBB, reservoir breathing bag; APL, adjustable pressure-limiting; FGI, fresh gas inflow.

References

1. Mapleson WW. The elimination of rebreathing in various semiclosed anaesthetic systems. *Br J Anaesth.* 1954;26:323–332.
2. Dorsch JA, Dorsch SE. *Understanding anesthesia equipment.* 5th ed. Philadelphia, PA: Williams and Wilkins, 2008.

19 Mechanical Ventilation

Scott Ahlbrand, MD

Mechanical ventilation is considered by some to be one of the most influential discoveries of modern medicine. Defined as a method to mechanically assist or replace spontaneous breathing by the application of positive airway pressure, it has allowed critically ill patients to survive at increasing rates, surgeries of greater complexity to be performed, and those with neuromuscular disease are living longer, more fruitful lives. This artificial means of lung ventilation has come a long way since its inception in 1550 when Paracelsus used "fire bellows" connected to a tube inserted into a patient's mouth as a device for assisted ventilation. Modern mechanical ventilators are subtly tuned to each patient's ventilatory needs.

1) **Indications for mechanical ventilation**
   a) To support ventilation and oxygenation of the lungs
   b) **Failure to ventilate**
      i) Reduced alveolar ventilation whereby a $PCO_2 > 50$ mm Hg is produced
      ii) There are many different clinical situations that can cause ventilatory failure.
         (1) Neurologic, muscular, anatomic, or gas exchange abnormalities
      iii) Origin of **neurologic causes** of ventilatory failure
         (1) Centrally from the brain, such as oversedation
         (2) Narcosis secondary to elevated PCO_2 levels
         (3) Stroke
            (a) Ischemic or hemorrhagic
         (4) Any other general cause of brain injury
         (5) Can also originate from the spine or spinal cord
            (a) Any injury to the spinal cord near levels C3, C4, or C5 is associated with the potential loss of diaphragmatic function.
            (b) An injury to the thoracic spine may be associated with loss of intercostal muscle function and associated weakness.
            (c) Injury to peripheral nerves can also be associated with ventilatory failure as is the case when phrenic nerve loss occurs following certain surgical procedures.
            (d) Additionally, any lower motor neuron disease such as Guillain-Barre, poliomyelitis, or amylotrophic lateral sclerosis can contribute to muscle weakness and impending ventilatory failure.
      iv) **Muscular causes** of ventilatory failure are less common but no less life threatening.

(1) Autoimmune diseases such as myasthenia gravis can create a state of increasing muscle weakness that can lead to the inability to expire CO_2.

(2) Other entities such as steroid-induced myopathy or protein malnutrition, more commonly seen in the critically ill patient, are all associated with an increased likelihood of ventilatory failure.

v) **Anatomic causes** of ventilatory failure

(1) Can occur almost anywhere throughout the chest or the thorax

(2) Damage to structures of the chest wall such as rib fractures or flail chest may impair adequate ventilation

(3) Any clinical situation that increases transthoracic pressure can have deleterious effects on ventilation.

(4) Morbid obesity, abdominal hypertension, or the presence of restrictive dressing (abdominal binders) can all bring about this effect.

vi) **Disorders of the pleura**

(1) Pleural effusions, pneumothoraces, and hemothoraces

(a) Make it difficult for patients to fully inspire, thereby decreasing their minute ventilation

vii) **Any obstruction to the free passage of air** through the upper airways

(1) Results in more difficult ventilation, which increases the risk of hypercapnia.

(a) Therefore, any patient with evidence of laryngeal edema, bronchospasm, laryngospasm, or the presence of a foreign body is at an increased risk for ventilatory failure.

viii) **Gas exchange** abnormalities can cause significant ventilatory failure.

(1) Gas exchange abnormalities most commonly caused by the presence of a ventilation/perfusion mismatch

(2) "V/Q" mismatch results from inequality between the amount of ventilation and the amount of perfusion in a specific part of the lung.

(a) This can result from many clinical situations including an increase in alveolar deadspace where a decrease in the functional residual capacity (FRC) is produced.

(b) Any kind of injury to the lung as would occur from hyperinflation, pulmonary contusion, acute lung injury (ALI), or a pulmonary embolism.

ix) It is important to realize that ventilatory failure can occur in the presence of normal oxygenation.

(1) Therefore, adequate ventilation cannot be assessed solely by pulse oximetry.

c) **Failure to oxygenate**

i) Another common indication for mechanical ventilation

ii) Defined as any impairment in the ability to oxygenate as to produce a PO_2 < 60 mm Hg

iii) As is the case with ventilatory failure, failure to oxygenate, or hypoxic respiratory failure, can arise from many different clinical situations.

iv) The two main causes of respiratory failure are diffusion defects and V/Q mismatching.

(1) **Diffusion defects**

(a) Any process that thickens the alveolar membrane where gas exchange occurs

Ventilatory failure can occur in the presence of normal oxygenation and cannot be assessed solely by pulse oximetry.

(b) **Thickened alveolar membranes** can be the result of pulmonary fibrosis, where an abnormal and excessive amount of fibrotic tissue is deposited in the pulmonary interstitium.

(c) Thickened alveolar membranes can also be the result of the accumulation of fluid in the area of gas exchange, as in the case of pulmonary edema.

v) **Ventilation/perfusion (V/Q) mismatching**

(1) Can result in hypercapneic or hypoxic respiratory failure

(2) One can think of V/Q mismatch as involving a spectrum of gas exchange abnormalities.

(3) At one end is pure **dead space ventilation.**

(a) Alveoli are ventilated but not perfused.

Dead space ventilation occurs when alveoli are ventilated but not perfused.

(4) Dead space ventilation can be divided into anatomic or physiologic.

(a) **Anatomic deadspace**

(i) An example would be something as simple as rapid, shallow breathing.

(ii) Since the conducting airways typically occupy 150 mL or 1 to 2 mL/kg, when one takes breaths of 150 to 200 mL, these small tidal volumes do not reach the alveoli.

1. This leads to decreased gas exchange and results in hypercapnia and hypoxia.

(b) **Physiologic deadspace**

(i) An example would be a pulmonary embolus (PE).

(ii) In the case of a PE, there is no blood flow to an area or normal ventilated lung.

Shunting occurs when alveoli are normally perfused but are not ventilated.

(5) At the other end of the spectrum is **shunt.**

(a) An example is alveoli that are normally perfused, but are not ventilated.

(b) Shunt results in the admixture of well-oxygenated blood (that which went around the shunt) with deoxygenated blood (that which passed through the shunt)

(i) Dilutes the resultant partial pressure of oxygen and creating hypoxic blood

(c) Examples of shunt include acute respiratory distress syndrome (ARDS)/ALI, airway collapse, pneumonia, or pulmonary contusion.

2) There are no absolute contraindications to mechanical ventilation.

a) However, it is important to remember that there are relative contraindications to different modes of mechanical ventilation.

3) Modes of ventilation

a) Two primary modes of noninvasive positive-pressure ventilation (NPPV) and three primary modes of invasive positive-pressure ventilation (IPPV) (Table 19-1)

Table 19-1
Modes of Ventilation

Non-Invasive Positive-Pressure Ventilation	Invasive Positive-Pressure Ventilation
BiPAP ventilation	VCV
CPAP ventilation	PCV PSV

EQUIPMENT AND PROCEDURES

b) **Noninvasive positive-pressure ventilation**

    i) The application of **positive airway pressure** using a mechanical ventilator, without the presence of an endotracheal tube.

    ii) **History**

        (1) NPPV was first developed by Professor Colin Sullivan at the Royal Prince Alfred Hospital in 1981.

    iii) **Modes of NPPV**

        (1) Bilevel positive airway pressure (**BiPAP**)

            (a) A noninvasive form of positive-pressure ventilation that is used to increase oxygenation by providing high-flow positive airway pressure

            (b) Cycles between high positive pressure and a lower positive airway pressure depending on its timing in the respiratory cycle

        (2) Continuous positive airway pressure (**CPAP**)

            (a) Another form of NPPV that is used for increasing ventilation by providing **CPAP**

    iv) **Indications for NPPV**

        (1) Any condition where reversible respiratory failure is present and there is concern for alveolar collapse, merits consideration of NPPV

        (2) Examples of clinical situations (1)

            (a) An exacerbation of congestive heart failure

            (b) Obstructive sleep apnea

            (c) Asthma

            (d) COPD exacerbation (2)

    v) **Advantages of NPPV (1)**

        (1) Reduced cost

        (2) Avoidance of intubation-related trauma

        (3) Shorter duration on a ventilator

        (4) Enhanced patient comfort

        (5) Shorter hospital stay

        (6) Decreased incidence of nosocomial pneumonias

    vi) **Disadvantages of NPPV (1)**

        (1) **Difficult to tolerate**

            (a) **20%** intolerance rate in patients who are started on NPPV

            (b) May be due to a preexisting anxiety disorder or an uncomfortable fit on the face

        (2) **Unsuitable for patients with neuromuscular disease**

            (a) They may lack the strength and endurance to expire against the positive pressure.

c) **Invasive positive-pressure ventilation**

    i) The application of positive airway pressure using a mechanical ventilator, with the **presence of an endotracheal tube**

    ii) **Indications for IPPV**

        (1) When mechanical ventilation is required but NPPV is not tolerated, indicated, or adequate for the patient

    iii) **Modes of IPPV**

        (1) **Volume-cycled, pressure-cycled, and pressure support ventilation (PSV)**

        (2) **Volume-cycled ventilation (VCV)** (Fig. 19-1)

Consider NPPV in cases of reversible respiratory failure where there is a concern for alveolar collapse.

IPPV applies positive airway pressure through an endotracheal tube using a mechanical ventilator and is indicated when mechanical ventilation is required and NPPV cannot be used.

Figure 19-1   Volume Control for VCV

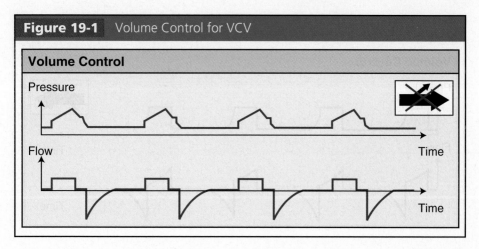

(a) Ventilator will deliver a set tidal volume irrespective of the pressure that it generates.

(b) Can be divided into assisted, controlled, assist-controlled, and intermittent mechanical ventilation (IMV)

(c) **Assisted VCV**
   (i) Mode of ventilation where the ventilator is triggered by an initiated breath from the patient
   (ii) The ventilator will not generate a breath without the patient's effort.

(d) **Controlled VCV**
   (i) Requires the operator to assign a set minute ventilation by determining an appropriate tidal volume and respiratory rate
   (ii) This mode will generate breaths whether the patient is spontaneously breathing or not.

(e) **Assist-controlled (ACV) volume-cycled ventilation**
   (i) Combination of the aforementioned two
   (ii) The ventilator will generate breaths whenever triggered by the patient's spontaneous breathing.
   (iii) Will also deliver set tidal volumes to make sure the predetermined minute ventilation is achieved

(f) **Intermittent Mandatory Ventilation (IMV)**
   (i) Essentially ACV + spontaneous ventilation (SV)
   (ii) The ventilator will allow SV, assist with spontaneous breaths, and generate its own breaths.
   (iii) **Advantage of IMV**
      1. When SV occurs, muscle atrophy is reduced.
      2. Risk of lung hyperinflation and the generation of intrinsic PEEP is minimized.
   (iv) **Disadvantage of IMV**
      1. Spontaneously breathing through a breathing circuit and mechanical ventilator is difficult.
         a. A patient typically requires a pressure support of 10 cm H_2O to overcome that resistance.
         b. Because of this, IMV becomes much more similar to ACV, as there is no longer any truly SV occurring.

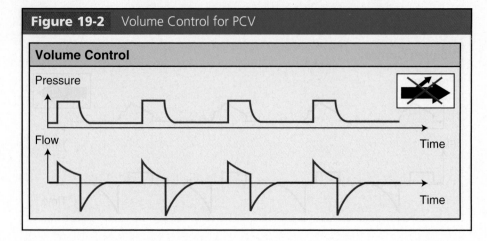

Figure 19-2   Volume Control for PCV

(3) **Pressure-cycled ventilation (PCV)** (Fig. 19-2)

    (a) Indicates that the ventilator generates a constant pressure that is applied to inflate the lungs

        (i) This principle is important to remember anytime someone is on PCV, as one can see variability in the inflation volumes depending on the patient's lung compliance.

> PCV generates a constant pressure to inflate the lungs, but the delivered tidal volume varies depending upon lung mechanics.

    (b) **Advantages of PCV**

        (i) Generates a decelerating inspiratory flow pattern

            1. This effectively decreases the peak inspiratory pressure (PIP) and can thereby improve gas exchange.

    (c) **Disadvantages of PCV**

        (i) Changes in lung mechanics will change the resultant inflation volumes

            1. Therefore, it is imperative that the delivered tidal volumes are monitored to prevent the occurrence of volutrauma.

(4) **Pressure support ventilation (PSV)**

    (a) The spontaneously ventilating patient has each tidal volume "supported" with a set pressure.

    (b) When the patient initiates a spontaneous breath, the ventilator is triggered to apply a positive pressure and augment each tidal volume.

    (c) **Pressure support settings**

        (i) Typically range from 5 to 20 cm H_2O depending on the patient's needs.

    (d) **Common indications for PSV**

        (i) Weaning a patient from ventilatory support

            1. This can be particularly beneficial when a patient has a minimal oxygen requirement but may be deconditioned and require additional pressure support for adequate ventilation.

        (ii) The amount of pressure support can be reduced on a regular basis until the patient is then able to ventilate without the need for pressure support and possibly ready for discontinuation of mechanical ventilation.

        (iii) **Contraindication to PSV**

            1. A patient receiving neuromuscular blocking agents

                a. Since PSV has no backup set respiratory rate, ventilating a paralyzed patient with this mode would be catastrophic.

4) **Ventilator settings**

a) Typically include a combination of settings.

i) The fraction of inspired oxygen (FiO_2)

ii) Tidal volume

iii) Peak airway pressure

iv) Respiratory rate

v) Inspiratory to expiratory ratio

vi) Positive end-expiratory pressure (PEEP)

b) **Fraction of inspired oxygen**

PSV cannot be used to ventilate a paralyzed patient because the patient must trigger a breath. There is no backup set respiratory rate.

i) The concentration of oxygen in the gas mixture with which the patient is ventilated

ii) Immediately following an endotracheal intubation and the initiation of mechanical ventilation, most patients should be placed on 100% inspired oxygen.

iii) A FiO_2 of 1.0 should be used until adequate arterial oxygenation is documented

iv) **A short period of ventilation with a FiO_2 of 1.0 is not dangerous** to the patient and offers some **clinical advantages** (3).

(1) **Protects the patient against hypoxemia** if unrecognized problems occur as a result of the endotracheal intubation

(2) Using the PaO_2 measured with a FiO_2 of 1.0, a clinician can more easily **estimate the shunt fraction** and calculate the next desired FiO_2 (4).

(a) The degree of shunt while receiving a FiO_2 of 1.0 can be estimated by applying the rule **700—PaO_2**.

(b) **For each difference of 100 mm Hg, the shunt fraction is 5%.**

(i) For example, if the PaO_2 is 500 mmHg while receiving a FiO_2 of 1.0, then the shunt fraction is estimated at 10%.

(ii) **A shunt fraction of 25% should remind the clinician to consider the use of PEEP.**

(iii) A low PaO_2, despite a FiO_2 of 1.0, should prompt a search for complications related to endotracheal intubation and positive-pressure ventilation.

(c) **Complications**

(i) Mainstem bronchial intubation

(ii) Presence of a pneumothorax

(iii) If such complications are not present, PEEP may be needed to treat some common causes of intrapulmonary shunt pathology.

(iv) Common causes of intrapulmonary shunt pathology

1. Atelectasis

2. Pneumonia

3. ARDS

4. Congestive heart failure

5. Hemorrhage

c) **Tidal volume**

i) The volume of gas the ventilator will deliver to the patient with each breath.

ii) For a patient **without preexisting lung disease**, 10 to 12 mL/kg is a commonly used tidal volume for the assist-control mode.

        iii)   For patients with a history of obstructive pulmonary disease, such as COPD, a smaller tidal volume of 8 to 10 mL/kg is commonly used.

        iv)   In the setting of **ARDS**, it is suggested that the lungs may function best, and volutrauma may be minimized, with a lower tidal volume of 6 to 8 mL/kg in the assist-control mode (5).

           (1)   These lower volumes may lead to slight hypercarbia.

           (2)   However, this elevated PCO_2 is typically recognized and accepted without correction, leading to the term **permissive hypercapnia** (5).

    d)   **Peak airway pressure**

        i)   The pressure measured by the ventilator in the major airways

           (1)   Strongly reflects airway resistance

        ii)   As the tidal volume increases, so too does the pressure required to drive that volume into the lung.

Keep plateau pressures <30 cm H_2O to minimize barotraumas to the lungs.

        iii)   Persistent peak pressures higher than 45 cm H_2O are a risk factor for barotraumas and should be avoided.

           (1)   Therefore, **tidal volumes suggested by the above rules are only estimates** (6).

           (2)   May need to be decreased in some patients in order to keep peak airways pressures < 45 cm H_2O

    e)   **Plateau pressures**

        i)   Pressures measured at the end of the inspiratory phase of a volume-cycled tidal volume.

        ii)   Most modern ventilators are programmed not to allow expiratory airflow for a set time, typically a half of a second.

        iii)   The pressure measured to maintain this lack of expiratory airflow is the plateau pressure.

        iv)   It has been suggested that the plateau pressure should be monitored as a means to prevent barotraumas in patients with ARDS.

           (1)   **Barotrauma can be minimized when the plateau pressure is maintained < 30 cm H_2O (5).**

    f)   **Respiratory rate**

        i)   The frequency of breaths delivered per minute during mechanical ventilation

        ii)   Minute ventilation (MV), by definition, is set by the tidal volume (TV) and respiratory rate (RR) by an equation.

           (1) $MV = RR \times TV$

        iii)   **Typical respiratory rates**

           (1)   Range from 8 to 16 breaths/min but really depend on the desired PCO_2

              (a)   Higher respiratory rate decreases PCO_2.

              (b)   Lower respiratory rate increases PCO_2

           (2)   A situation where a higher-than-normal PCO_2 may be desired is in the case of weaning a patient from mechanical ventilation.

              (a)   The higher PCO_2 is required for the patient's drive to breathe.

           (3)   A situation when one may desire a lower-than-normal PCO_2 is in the case of elevated intracranial pressure.

              (a)   The low PCO_2 causes cerebral vasoconstriction and a decrease in cerebral blood flow and a theoretical decrease in intracranial pressure.

              (b)   **If a respiratory rate is too** high, the risks include the following:

(i) Inadequate expiratory time

(ii) **"breath stacking"**

(iii) The development of **intrinsic PEEP** can occur.

(iv) In order to **minimize this risk**, the **I:E ratio can be adjusted** to allow more expiratory time and completion of the expiratory phase.

g) **I:E ratio**

i) Defined as inspiratory time + inspiratory pause time:expiration

ii) This ratio is usually set to 1:2 or 1:2.5 in an attempt to mimic the usual pattern of spontaneous breathing.

iii) A **higher I:E ratio** is the equivalent to a longer inspiratory time.

   (1) This adjustment may improve oxygenation by increasing the mean airway pressure and allowing redistribution of gas from more compliant alveoli to less compliant alveoli.

   (2) However, this also **increases the risk** of "**breath stacking**" (leading to intrinsic PEEP), and **barotrauma** by reducing the expiratory time (6).

   (3) It is important to keep in mind, however, that a higher I:E ratio is generally less well tolerated by the patient and typically **necessitates a deeper level of sedation.**

iv) A **lower I:E ratio** is the equivalent to a longer expiratory time.

   (1) This can be particularly **useful** when obstructive pulmonary disease is present such as asthma or **COPD.**

   (2) It is also useful in settings where **high minute ventilation is required**, necessitating a higher-than-normal respiratory rate

      (a) The risk of breath stacking must be minimized.

h) **Positive end-expiratory pressure**

i) A positive pressure applied at the end of the expiratory cycle

ii) PEEP is generally effective when used in patients with diffuse lung disease that results in a decrease in FRC.

iii) PEEP works by increasing end-expired lung volume and preventing airspace closure at the end of expiration.

   (1) Essentially "splinting" the alveoli open

iv) **Most patients who require mechanical ventilation may benefit from the application of 5 cm H_2O of PEEP.**

   (1) It can limit the amount of atelectasis that frequently accompanies endotracheal intubation and mechanical ventilation in the supine position.

v) More importantly, PEEP can be **utilized to permit lower levels of FiO_2**, while preserving adequate oxygenation.

   (1) This is important in limiting lung injury that may result from prolonged exposure to high inspired oxygen concentrations (FiO2 > 0.6).

   (2) **Higher levels of PEEP**, in the range of 5 to 15 cm H_2O, have been shown to **improve oxygenation in more severe alveolar filling disorders** such as cardiogenic pulmonary edema in ARDS (5,7,8).

      (a) The mechanism behind this is likely redistribution of fluid from the alveoli to the interstitium and opening up collapsed alveoli.

vi) With all the benefits of PEEP, it is important to keep in mind that PEEP is **not a benign mode of therapy.**

   (1) In the **hypovolemic patient**, PEEP increases intrathoracic pressure and can impede venous return.

   (2) This commonly results in hypotension and hemodynamic instability. **PEEP** also increases intra-alveolar pressures and thus places patients at increased risk for barotrauma.

EQUIPMENT AND PROCEDURES

(3)   The addition of PEEP is typically justified when a PaO_2 of 60 mm Hg cannot be achieved with a FiO_2 of 0.6 (8).

(4)   The addition of PEEP is also justified when the estimated initial shunt fraction is >25% (7).

(5)   Therefore, the use of PEEP should have a well-defined indication.

5)   Sedation

a)   Sedation is defined as depression of a patient's awareness to the environment and reduction of his or her responsiveness to external stimulation

b)   The level of sedation required by a patient receiving mechanical ventilation depends not only on the mode of ventilation but also on other variables.

   i)   Patient's respiratory status

   ii)   Hemodynamic profile

   iii)   Drug sensitivities

c)   As such, various levels of sedation have been defined to allow clinicians to describe not only patient clinical states but also patient needs.

d)   **Minimal sedation**

   i)   Defined as a drug-induced relief of apprehension with minimal effect on sensorium

   ii)   Equivalent to anxiolysis

e)   **Moderate sedation**

   i)   A depression of consciousness in which the patient can respond to external stimuli but airway reflexes, spontaneous ventilation, and cardiovascular function are maintained.

f)   **Deep sedation**

   i)   A depression of consciousness in which the patient cannot be aroused but responds purposefully to painful stimuli

   ii)   When patients are deeply sedated, they may not be able to maintain airway reflexes or spontaneous ventilation, but cardiovascular function is preserved.

g)   **General anesthesia**

   i)   A drug-induced loss of consciousness during which patients are not arousable, even by painful stimulation

   ii)   Under general anesthesia, cardiovascular function and the ability to independently maintain ventilatory function are often impaired.

h)   **Dissociation**

   i)   A drug-induced disconnect between the thalamoneocortical system and the limbic systems where airway reflexes, spontaneous ventilation, and cardiovascular function are all maintained

i)   Typically, patients requiring invasive mechanical ventilation in the operating room undergoing a surgical procedure require general anesthesia.

   i)   The patient in the intensive care unit requiring invasive mechanical ventilation for respiratory failure requires only moderate to deep sedation.

6)   Medications

a)   Commonly used to allow patients to tolerate invasive mechanical ventilation

b)   Typically fall into two broad categories: analgesics and sedatives

c)   The most frequently used class of **analgesic** medication to augment sedation is the opioids.

d)   **Opioids**

   i)   Induce systemic analgesia, some anxiolysis, and mild sedation by binding to specific opioid receptors in the central nervous system

READ MORE

Opioid analgesics and antagonists, Chapter 41, page 299, Opioids Appendix B, Chapter 194, page 1278

ii) **Morphine**

   (1) The oldest and most established agent in the opioids class

   (2) Possesses a relatively rapid onset of action

     (a) Duration of action can last as long as 3 to 4 hours

   (3) **Adverse effects** of morphine

     (a) Hypotension, primarily due to histamine release

     (b) Respiratory depression

iii) **Fentanyl**

   (1) A newer, more potent synthetic opioids

   (2) Rapidly crosses the blood–brain barrier and has an even faster onset of action (<90 seconds)

     (a) It has a duration of action of 30 to 40 minutes.

   (3) Can be administered as a bolus or in the form of an infusion

e) Although analgesics are commonly used as adjuvants, **sedative hypnotics**, as a class, are the mainstay of sedation regimens.

READ MORE

Intravenous induction agents, Chapter 43, page 306

i) **Propofol**

   (1) May be the most widely used agent for sedation of mechanically ventilated patients

   (2) Propofol works by modulating the GABA receptor.

     (a) Ideal for patients who are expected to have a short need for mechanical ventilation

   (3) **Advantages of propofol**

     (a) Short onset

     (b) Short duration of action

   (4) **Disadvantages of propofol**

     (a) Respiratory depression

     (b) Cardiovascular depression

     (c) Relative contraindication to patients with allergies to eggs.

READ MORE

Benzodiazepines, Chapter 40, page 296

ii) **Benzodiazepines**

   (1) Benzodiazepines are arguably the most commonly used class of drugs for sedation.

   (2) **Diazepam**

     (a) The first benzodiazepine developed for intravenous use

     (b) Has a relatively rapid onset of action

     (c) Duration of action of 2 to 4 hours

     (d) Metabolized almost exclusively by the liver

   (3) **Lorazepam**

     (a) Another benzodiazepine commonly used for sedation

     (b) Onset of action between 3 and 5 minutes

     (c) Duration of action of 1 to 4 hours

     (d) Metabolized by means of conjugation.

       (i) This makes lorazepam a more attractive alternative in the setting of renal or hepatic dysfunction.

   (4) **Midazolam**

     (a) Shorter-acting benzodiazepine

       (i) Commonly used as an infusion because of this reason

     (b) Onset of action of <5 minutes

     (c) Duration of action of 30 minutes

     (d) Like diazepam, is metabolized by the liver

EQUIPMENT AND PROCEDURES

7) **Conclusions**
   a) Mechanical ventilation can sometimes be a confusing and overwhelming topic.
   b) The best way to approach a patient who has a need for mechanical ventilation is to identify the specific needs of the patient, and decide how you will support him/her.
      i) Create ventilator settings to accomplish this goal, and follow up on how well that goal is being achieved.
   c) Similarly, sedation should also be directed by a specific need, in an attempt to realize a certain goal.
   d) Daily re-evaluation of those goals is important and adjustments to regimens should be made accordingly.

Chapter Summary for Mechanical Ventilation

Indications for Mechanical Ventilation	Typically either failure to oxygenate or failure to ventilate.
Modes of Mechanical Ventilation	Various different modes can be used to achieve the same goal but have unique advantages and disadvantages. NPPV includes BiPAP and CPAP. Various modes of IPPV include volume-cycled, pressure-cycled, and pressure support ventilation.
Ventilator Settings	Be aware that proper ventilator settings not only provide safety but also minimize risk. Certain modes of ventilation cannot be used in certain patients, such as PSV in the paralyzed patient.
Sedation	Always ensure adequate and appropriate sedation for the patient undergoing mechanical ventilation. Inappropriate use of sedation can frequently lead to unnecessary tests, monitoring, and interventions.

References

1. Keenan SP, Kernerman PD, Cook DJ, et al. Effect of noninvasive positive pressure ventilation on mortality in patients admitted with acute respiratory failure: a meta-analysis. *Crit Care Med* 1997;25(10):1685–1692.
2. Khan NA, Palepu A, Norena M, et al. Differences in hospital mortality among critically ill patients of Asian, Native Indian, and European descent. *Chest* 2008;134(6):1217–1222.
3. Spearman CB, Egan DF, Egan J. *Fundamentals of Respiratory Therapy.* 4th ed. St. Louis, MO: Mosby; 1982.
4. Marino PL. *The ICU Book.* 3rd ed. Philadelphia, PA: Lippincott Williams &Wilkins; 2007.
5. Acute Respiratory Distress Syndrome Network. Ventilation with lower tidal volumes as compared with traditional tidal volumes for acute lung injury and the acute respiratory distress syndrome. *N Engl J Med* 2000;342(18):1301–1308.
6. Andrews P, Azoulay E, Antonelli M, et al. Year in review in intensive care medicine. 2005. I. Acute respiratory failure and acute lung injury, ventilation, hemodynamics, education, renal failure. *Intensive Care Med* 2006;32(2):207–216.
7. Apostolakos MJ, Levy PC, Papadakos PJ. New modes of mechanical ventilation. *Clin Pulm Med* 1995;2:121–128.
8. Briel M, Meade M, Mercat A, et al. Higher vs lower positive end-expiratory pressure in patients with acute lung injury and acute respiratory distress syndrome: systematic review and meta-analysis. *JAMA* 2010;303(9):865–873.

20 Endotracheal Intubation

Arthur Atchabahian, MD

Intubation of the trachea using a cuffed tube is the gold standard to ensure airway patency and protection. Endotracheal intubation allows for the provision of positive-pressure ventilation to patients receiving general anesthesia or experiencing respiratory failure. This chapter discusses elective endotracheal intubation in adults using direct laryngoscopy (DL).

Endotracheal intubation consists of inserting a tube into a patient's trachea in order to ensure airway patency and protection and to provide positive-pressure ventilation.

READ MORE

Difficult airway management, Chapter 21, page 150

1) **Overview**
   a) Endotracheal intubation consists of inserting a tube into a patient's trachea in order to ensure airway patency and protection and to provide positive-pressure ventilation.
   b) Magill developed this technique after World War I because of the difficulty of administering chloroform by mask to patients with facial injuries.
   c) It is typically performed using direct laryngoscopy (DL), but alternative techniques such as fiberoptic intubation or retrograde intubation are used in specific settings
   d) **Indications**
      i) To ensure airway patency in an unconscious patient
      ii) To protect the lungs from the aspiration of gastric contents
      iii) To provide positive-pressure ventilation, in the setting of respiratory failure or of general anesthesia
   e) Contraindications to DL for endotracheal intubation
      i) Predictable difficult DL due to abnormal anatomy or trauma to the airway
      ii) Contraindication to extending the head because of trauma to the cervical spine
   f) **Complications**
      i) Inability to intubate the trachea in a patient who cannot ventilate spontaneously
      ii) Incorrect endotracheal tube (ETT) placement (esophageal or bronchial intubation)
      iii) Trauma to the airway during ETT insertion
      iv) Aspiration of gastric contents prior to intubation
2) **Anatomy**
   a) Airway anatomy (Fig. 20-1)
   b) Anatomical considerations for endotracheal intubation
      i) The ETT will have to be guided through the oral or the nasal conduits through the pharynx, under the epiglottis and through the larynx and the vocal cords into the trachea.

EQUIPMENT AND PROCEDURES

137

Figure 20-1 The Major Landmarks of the Upper Airway

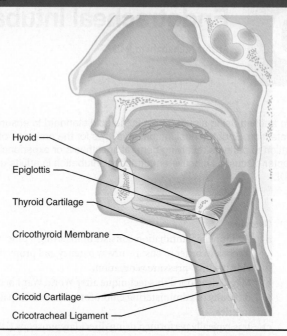

Hyoid

Epiglottis

Thyroid Cartilage

Cricothyroid Membrane

Cricoid Cartilage

Cricotracheal Ligament

Note that the cricoid cartilage is <1 cm in height in its anterior aspect but may be 2 cm in height posteriorly. Reproduced from Rosenblatt WH, Sukhupragarn W. Airway Management. In: Barash PG, Cullen BF, Stoelting RK, et al., eds. *Clinical Anesthesia*. 6th Ed. Philadelphia, Pa: Lippincott Williams & Wilkins, 2009:752, with permission.

READ MORE

Difficult intubation, Chapter 21, page 150

The anesthesiologist should be familiar with evaluation of the airway to assess the likelihood of difficulty with intubation.

READ MORE

Atlas of anesthesia procedures: Endotracheal intubation, Chapter 154, page 1101

    ii)   The oral and nasal axes are not aligned with the laryngeal axis (Fig. 20-1). Therefore, careful positioning and instrumentation is needed to allow direct visualization of the glottis, the uppermost laryngeal opening.

3)   **Preoperative assessment**

    a)   **Predictors of difficulty with airway management**

    b)   The anesthesiologist should be familiar with evaluation of the airway to assess the likelihood of difficulty with intubation.

4)   **Equipment for endotracheal intubation**

    a)   Endotracheal tubes

        i)   An ETT is a tube inserted into a patient's trachea, allowing positive-pressure ventilation and typically isolating the airway from the oroesophageal tract by means of an inflatable cuff, thus preventing aspiration of gastric contents. The components of a typical ETT are as follows:

           (1) A clear curved PVC tube, allowing visualization of condensation of secretions; ETT sizes are based on the internal diameter (ID) in mm.

           (2) A standard 15-mm ISO connector that adapts to the breathing circuit at the proximal end of the tube

           (3) An inflatable cuff (for ETT above 5 or 6 mm ID) at the distal end of the tube. Modern ETTs have high-volume low-pressure cuffs to prevent tracheal wall injury.

Figure 20-2 Types of ETTs

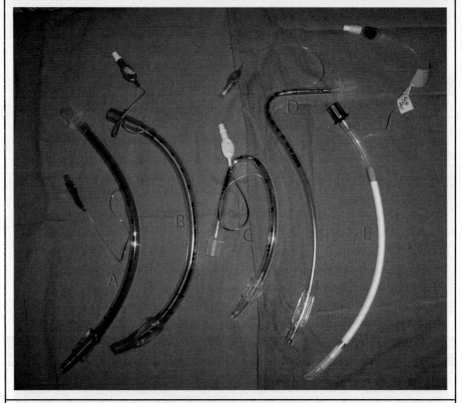

(A) Standard, **(B)** Reinforced or "anode", **(C)** Oral RAE, **(D)** Nasal RAE, **(E)** Laser ETT.

        (4)   The tip of the ETT is beveled and has an additional small side opening known as the *Murphy eye*.
    ii) **Types of Endotracheal Tubes** (Fig. 20-2). ETTs are designed in a plethora of forms and materials to accommodate a wide range of anesthetic and surgical situations.
        (1)   Standard (A)
        (2)   Reinforced or "anode" (B)
           (a)   Used in situations where a standard tube would be likely to kink
        (3)   Oral RAE, taped to the lower lip (C)
           (a)   Used in ENT surgery to provide full access to the face
        (4)   Nasal RAE (D)
           (a)   Used in oral surgery
        (5)   Laser ETT (E)
           (a)   Covered with nonflammable material; some laser ETTs are made out of metal.
  b) **Laryngoscope blades** (Fig. 20-3)
    i) A laryngoscope blade is a metallic curved or straight blade, fitted with a light source, which is used to lift the tongue and allow direct visualization of the vocal cords through the patient's mouth.
    ii) Several types of laryngoscope blades are used for endotracheal intubation. They differ in shape and design, and a number of modified blades have been designed to facilitate DL.

EQUIPMENT AND PROCEDURES

iii) The MacIntosh blade is inserted in the glossoepiglottic fold. The flange is used to hold the tongue to the left side, out of the field of vision.

iv) A lifting motion in the axis of the handle elevates the epiglottis and uncovers the vocal cords.

v) The Miller blade is used to lift the epiglottis.

c) Other equipment

i) A means to provide mask ventilation should be available in order to maintain oxygenation after apnea has been induced, until full muscle relaxation is reached and provides optimal laryngoscopy conditions

(1) This can be an anesthesia machine or a bag-valve–mask device, also known as an *Ambu bag*.

ii) Oral and nasal airways should also be available in case of difficult mask ventilation.

iii) Magill forceps are occasionally used to maneuver the ETT.

iv) A functioning suction catheter with a Yankauer-type tip to clear secretions or gastric contents

v) A malleable stylet to facilitate guiding the tube; the tip of the stylet should not extend beyond the Murphy eye of the ETT, to avoid airway trauma.

vi) ETTs of various sizes should be available.

vii) Tape or a commercially available securing device for the ETT

viii) Lubricant and mucosal local anesthetic can be used if desired.

ix) Gloves and face-shield should be worn to minimize exposure to body fluids.

During intubation, oral and nasal airways should be available in case of difficult mask ventilation.

DL is performed in order to insert the ETT into the trachea under direct vision and avoid airway trauma that could be caused by blind ETT insertion.

Figure 20-3 Laryngoscope Blades

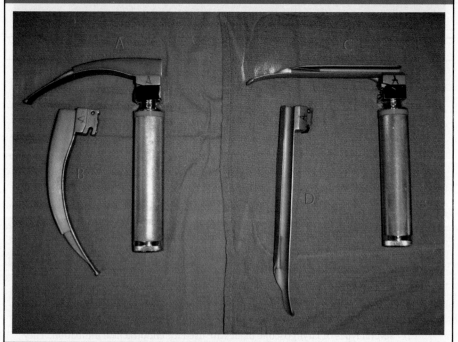

Macintosh 3 **(A)**, Macintosh 4 **(B)**, Miller 2 **(C)**, Miller 3 **(D)**.

5) **Principles of DL**
   a) DL consists in visualizing the glottic opening directly by means of positioning the patient's head and using a laryngoscope to lift the tongue and the epiglottis.
   b) It is performed in order to insert the ETT into the trachea under direct vision and avoid airway trauma that could be caused by blind ETT insertion.
   c) Positioning for DL
      i) **Appropriate elevation**
         (1) The table's height should be adjusted so that the patient's face is at the level of the operator's xiphoid.
      ii) **Sniffing position**
         (1) The sniffing position consists in flexing the cervical spine over the trunk by means of a small pillow placed under the head and extending the head over the neck (Fig. 20-4C).
      iii) **Three-axes theory**
         (1) The three-axes theory postulates that, in order to facilitate DL, the oral, pharyngeal, and laryngeal axes should be aligned through patient positioning.
      iv) The classic "sniffing position" aims at aligning oral, pharyngeal, and laryngeal axes by flexing the neck over the trunk and extending the head.

Patient positioning is paramount for optimizing laryngoscopic view.

         (1) One study showed that the DL view is mostly improved with this maneuver in morbidly obese patients and patients with reduced neck mobility.
         (2) In 11% of the patients, the sniffing position actually worsened the laryngoscopy view (2).
      v) Head-elevated laryngoscopy position (HELP)
         (1) HELP is a position used to facilitate DL in morbidly obese patients.
         (2) These patients typically have a "buffalo hump," and positioning them flat on a bed will force the head backward, hyperextending the neck and making DL very difficult.

In case of cervical spine trauma with suspected or confirmed cervical spine instability, head hyperextension is contraindicated as it could lead to spinal cord compression.

         (3) In addition, morbidly obese patients have a large chest that renders laryngoscope blade insertion difficult (a short-handle laryngoscope can facilitate insertion).
         (4) Position the patient, using pillows, such that the patient's sternum is level with the external auditory meatus (Figs. 20-5 and 20-6).
      vi) In-line stabilization for cervical spine trauma
         (1) In case of cervical spine trauma with suspected or confirmed cervical spine instability, head hyperextension is contraindicated as it could lead to spinal cord compression.
         (2) Two operators are needed to use this technique.
         (3) One operator holds the head and stabilizes it, minimizing cervical spine motion.
         (4) The other operator performs DL without extending the head.
         (5) While this technique allows vocal cord visualization and tracheal intubation in most cases, having a videolaryngoscopy device as backup is recommended.
6) **Performing DL for orotracheal intubation**
   a) DL for orotracheal intubation requires general anesthesia.

READ MORE

Preoperative assessment and anesthetic plan, Chapter 1, page 1

      i) Induction of anesthesia should be performed after a thorough preoperative assessment and preoxygenation, using either normal tidal ventilation for about 3 minutes or 4 forced vital capacity breaths; adequate denitrogenation is achieved when the expired FiO_2 is above 0.8.
      ii) An appropriate dose of an induction agent and a muscle relaxant should be administered.

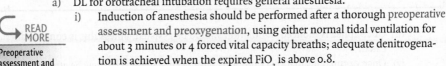

Figure 20-4 Understanding Aligning the Oral Axis, Pharyngeal Axis, and Laryngeal Axis

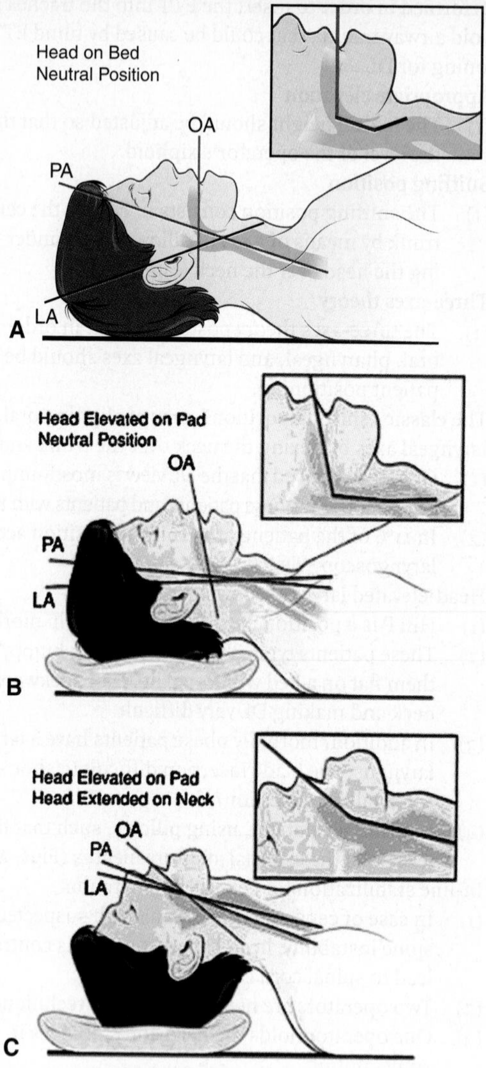

Head on Bed
Neutral Position

OA
PA
LA

A

Head Elevated on Pad
Neutral Position

OA
PA
LA

B

Head Elevated on Pad
Head Extended on Neck

OA
PA
LA

C

A: Anatomical neutral position. The Oral Axis (OA), Pharyngeal Axis (PA), and Laryngeal Axis (LA) are at greater angles to one another. **B:** Head, still in neutral position, has been lifted by a pillow flexing the lower cervical spine and aligning the PA and the LA. **C:** The head has been extended on the cervical spine, aligning OA with the PA and the LA creating the optimum sniffing position for intubation. Reproduced from Murphy MF, Barker TD, Schneider RE. Endotracheal Intubation. Reproduced from Walls RM, Murphy MF, Eds. *Manual of Emergency Airway Management*. 3rd ed. Philadelphia, PA: Lippincott Williams & Wilkins; 2008:66, with permission.

      iii) Once apnea is induced, ventilation should be assisted, unless this is contraindicated.

      iv) Once optimal intubation conditions have been achieved, DL may be attempted.

   b) Place patient in proper "sniffing" or "HELP" (Head Elevated Laryngoscopy Position) positions (obese patients).

Figure 20-5 The Patient Positioned Flat on the OR Bed

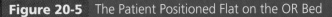

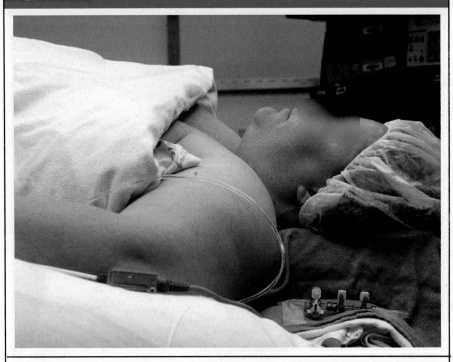

The head and neck are hyperextended, making DL challenging. Photo Courtesy of Dr. Jay Brodsky.

Do not use a lever motion with a laryngoscope—this motion could lead to dental trauma.

After ETT placement, confirm placement in the trachea by waveform capnography for at least 3 breaths.

c) Open patient's mouth, typically using a scissoring motion of the thumb and the index finger of the right hand.

d) Insert laryngoscope blade into the right corner of the mouth, and "load" the tongue on the flange using a sweeping motion, as the blade is inserted deeper around the tongue.

e) Once the epiglottis is visualized, the laryngoscope should be lifted in the axis of the handle.

   i) Do not use a lever motion, as that might lead to dental trauma.

   ii) This will uncover the glottic opening.

f) When using a straight blade, insert the blade under the epiglottis prior to lifting (Fig. 20-7).

g) Insert the ETT, held in the right hand, through the vocal cords until about 1 to 2 cm beyond the passage of the cuff through the cords.

h) Confirm endotracheal position by waveform capnography for at least three breaths.

i) Laryngoscopic views are graded according to Cormack and Lehane (Fig. 20-8).

   i) If visualization of the glottis is suboptimal, a BURP (backward-upward-rightward pressure) maneuver may improve the view.

   ii) If the vocal cords are not seen, it is preferable to insert an Eschmann stylet (gum elastic bougie) blindly and use it as a guide to insert the ETT, rather than attempting to insert the ETT blindly.

EQUIPMENT AND PROCEDURES

Figure 20-6 The Patient Positioned in the Head Elevated Laryngoscopy Position (HELP), Flexing the Neck and Allowing Head Extension

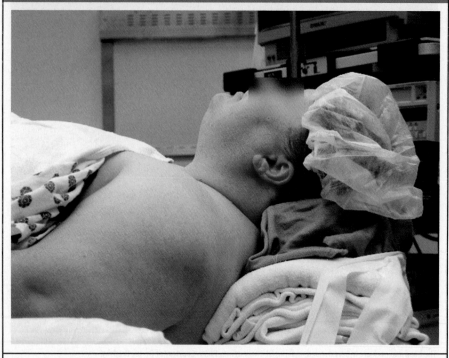

Photo courtesy of Dr. Jay Brodsky.

Figure 20-7 Use of a Mac Versus Miller Blade

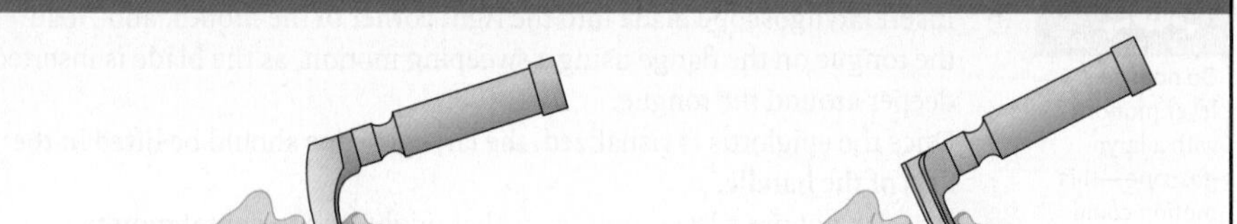

Epiglottis

Epiglottis

A

B

When a curved laryngoscope blade is used, the tip of the blade is placed in the vallecula, the space between the base of the tongue and the pharyngeal surface of the epiglottis (**A**). The tip of a straight blade is advanced beneath the epiglottis (**B**). Reproduced from Rosenblatt WH, Sukhupragarn W. Airway Management. In: Barash PG, Cullen BF, Stoelting RK, et al, eds. *Clinical Anesthesia*. 6th Ed. Philadelphia, PA: Lippincott Williams & Wilkins, 2009:765, with permission.

Figure 20-8   Cormack and Lehane Laryngoscopic Views

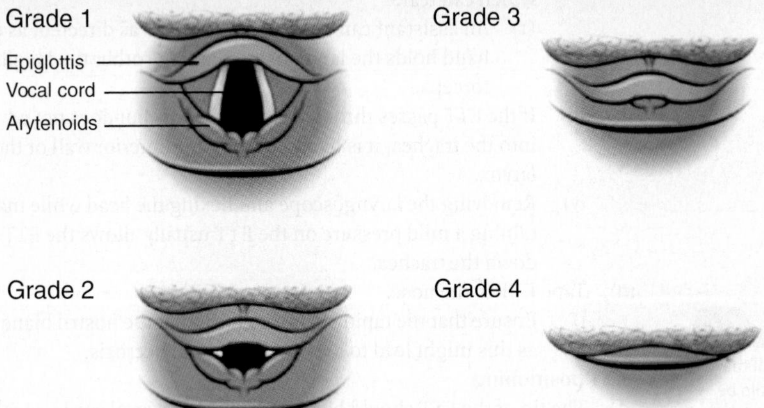

Grade 1

Epiglottis
Vocal cord
Arytenoids

Grade 3

Grade 2

Grade 4

Reproduced from Murphy MF, Barker TD, Schneider RE. Endotracheal Intubation. In: Walls RM, Murphy MF, eds. *Manual of Emergency Airway Management*. 3rd ed. Philadelphia, PA: Lippincott Williams & Wilkins, 2008:72, with permission.

7) **Technique of nasotracheal intubation**
   a) **Indications**
      i) Oral surgery, to provide full access for the surgeon
      ii) Limited mouth opening (e.g., tempromandibular joint stiffness) that will allow inserting a straight laryngoscope blade but not provide enough space for orotracheal intubation
   b) **Contraindications**
      i) Increased potential for bleeding: nasal polyps, coagulation disorder
      ii) Very limited mouth opening: a fiberoptic technique should then be used.
      iii) Likelihood of prolonged intubation, as a nasal ETT will lead to sinus obstruction and infection within a few days
      iv) Presence of a basilar skull fracture
   c) Prepare both nostrils with two puffs of a decongestant, for example, oxymetazoline (Afrin), in the holding area prior to bringing the patient to the OR, and two more puffs once in the OR.
   d) Assess which nostril is larger; consider septum deviation.
   e) Preoxygenate
   f) Induce GA and administer muscle relaxation.
   g) Insert soft nasal trumpet lubricated with lidocaine ointment to ensure easy passage of the ETT.
   h) The trumpet/ETT should be inserted perpendicular to the face.
   i) Remove nasal trumpet; use larger size if needed.
   j) Insert nasal RAE ETT until the tip reaches the oropharynx.
      i) Do not force if resistance is felt!
   k) Perform DL; visualize vocal cords and ETT.
   l) Advance ETT into the trachea.

Nasotracheal intubation is used for oral surgery and/or patients with limited mouth opening.

EQUIPMENT AND PROCEDURES

    i)   Use Magill forceps if needed.

    ii)   Take care not to use the forceps to grasp the ETT by the cuff, which can tear.

       (1)   An assistant can push or pull the ETT as directed, as one hand holds the laryngoscope and the other the Magill forceps.

    iii) If the ETT passes through the vocal cords but does not advance into the trachea, it is likely abutting the anterior wall of the larynx.

    iv) Removing the laryngoscope and flexing the head while maintaining a mild pressure on the ETT usually allows the ETT to go down the trachea.

  m) Tape ETT to the nose.

    i)   Ensure that the taping is not so tight that the nostril blanches, as this might lead to local ischemia and necrosis.

The tip of the ETT should be placed below the vocal cords, ideally 4 cm (and at least 3 cm) above the carina.

8) **ETT positioning**

  a) The tip of the ETT should be placed below the vocal cords, ideally 4 cm (and at least 3 cm) above the carina (Fig. 20-9).

    i)   However, this is difficult to assess without a chest radiograph or a fiberoptic bronchoscopy.

    ii)   In most patients, a position of 21 cm at the lips for women and 23 cm for men will provide correct positioning.

Figure 20-9   Position of the ETT in the Trachea and Distance of the Tip of the ETT from the Carina

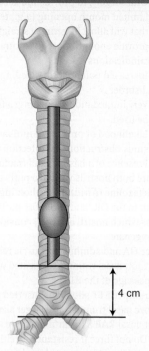

4 cm

Position of the tip of the ETT above the carina. It should ideally be 4 cm.

b) Auscultation should confirm bilateral breath sounds and the absence of epigastric sounds.

READ MORE

Difficult airway management, Chapter 21, page 150

c) The cuff of the ETT can be palpated in most patients in the suprasternal notch.

d) The ETT position in the trachea will change with head motion and should be verified after repositioning the patient.

   i) The rule is that "the ETT follows the nose, except when it is in the nose."

9) **Video Laryngoscopy**

a) Videolaryngoscopes, for example, the GlideScope, offer an improved view of the vocal cords in the following cases:

   i) Limited mouth opening

   ii) Impossibility to extend the neck or the anterior larynx

Videolaryngo-scopes can offer an improved view of the vocal cords for patients with limited mouth opening or inability to extend the neck or an anterior larynx.

10) **Complications**

a) **Dental injury**

   i) DL can lead to dental injury, especially of the upper incisors, as it is very easy to apply force on those teeth when lifting the blade to improve glottic visualization.

   ii) Teeth can be chipped or dislodged, occasionally leading to aspiration of dental fragments; it is very important to ascertain preoperatively which teeth are loose or in such poor state that they may be easily dislodged.

      (1) Preexisting chipping, missing teeth, etc. should be documented preoperatively.

   iii) In case of dental injury, ensure to recover all tooth fragments and obtain dental consult as soon as possible. Dislodged teeth can be reinserted.

b) **Esophageal intubation**

Undetected esophageal intubation can lead to rapid hypoxemia with a potential for cardiac arrest and hypoxic brain injury unless rapidly recognized and treated.

   i) Insertion of the ETT into the esophagus instead of the trachea

   ii) Confirm endotracheal placement with **end-tidal CO_2 monitoring** and **auscultation.**

   iii) Undetected esophageal intubation will prevent effective gas exchange and lead to rapid hypoxemia, with a potential for cardiac arrest and hypoxic brain injury unless recognized and treated.

c) **Aspiration of gastric contents**

   i) Passive regurgitation of gastric contents with subsequent aspiration into the lungs can lead to **severe chemical pneumonitis** even in a patient who was NPO for an appropriate duration.

   ii) Administer a **nonparticulate antacid** (Bicitra) preoperatively to patients at risk for aspiration of gastric contents.

   iii) **A working suction should always be available and ready to use.**

   iv) Cricoid pressure has become controversial and is probably of limited efficacy to limit passive regurgitation (4).

During intubation, a working suction should always be available and ready to use.

      (1) Patients at risk for regurgitation probably benefit more from **mild reverse Trendelenburg** (head-up) positioning.

   v) In case of aspiration

      (1) Intubate trachea

      (2) Suction trachea vigorously **prior to** applying PPV, which may push aspirated gastric contents into the bronchi

   vi) In case of vomiting rather than passive regurgitation

      (1) Turn patient to the side

EQUIPMENT AND PROCEDURES

(2) Suction pharynx as thoroughly as possible

(3) Return to supine position once vomiting has stopped

(4) Intubate trachea

(5) Suction trachea vigorously **prior to** applying PPV

d) **Endobronchial intubation**

i) Typically in the right mainstem bronchus, leading to substantial shunt and arterial hypoxemia

ii) This is detected by auscultation, with decreased breath sounds on the left. If auscultation is inconclusive, fiberoptic bronchoscopy can be needed to ascertain ETT tip position.

iii) The ETT should be withdrawn into correct position.

e) **Airway trauma**

i) The tip of the ETT can injure larynx and trachea, especially if a rigid stylet is used.

ii) Mild trauma will lead to edema and bleeding and can be diagnosed post-operatively by indirect laryngoscopy. Severe trauma can disrupt the airway, perforate the trachea, and lead to pneumomediastinum and mediastinal infection, necessitating surgery.

iii) Trauma prevention consists of performing DL and intubation under direct vision rather than blindly, in using smooth motions and avoiding excessive force, and in sliding the ETT on the stylet once the tip is beyond the vocal cords, rather than inserting the rigid ETT-stylet assembly down the trachea.

f) **Compression of the tracheal wall** may be caused by **overinflation of the cuff.**

i) **This can lead to the following complications:**

READ MORE

Crisis management: Bronchospasm, Chapter 222, page 1344

(1) Tracheitis

(2) Pressure necrosis of the tracheal wall

(3) Tracheal rupture

ii) Patients requiring prolonged intubation are most at risk, although it can occur in a long case, especially when nitrous oxide is used.

(1) Cuff pressure should be checked periodically using an adapted device and **maintained below 25 mm Hg.**

g) **Bronchospasm (5)**

i) Bronchospasm is defined as a reflex narrowing of the small airways (bronchioles) through a combination of smooth muscle contraction and, secondarily, inflammation with edema.

ii) Endotracheal intubation can cause severe bronchospasm, such that no $ETCO_2$ will be detected and no breath sounds will be heard, despite the ETT being correctly positioned.

Endotracheal intubation can cause severe bronchospasm, such that that no $ETCO_2$ will be detected and no breath sounds will be heard, despite the ETT being correctly positioned.

(1) Perform DL again to ensure correct ETT position through the vocal cords.

(2) Ensure that the ETT is not **kinked** or **too deep**, against the carina.

(3) Continue ventilation using 100% O_2.

(4) **Deepen anesthesia** using IV anesthetics, ideally bronchodilators such as propofol, ketamine.

(5) Consider low-dose epinephrine (10 mcg subcutaneously) or terbutaline (0.2 mg subcutaneously).

(6) **Inhaled beta-2 agonists** and volatile anesthetics can be used as bronchodilators if the patient can be ventilated.

Chapter Summary for Endotracheal Intubation

Definition	Endotracheal intubation consists of inserting a tube into a patient's trachea in order to ensure airway **patency** and **protection** and to provide **positive-pressure ventilation.**
Positioning for Endotracheal Intubation	The sniffing position consists of flexing the cervical spine over the trunk by means of a small pillow placed under the head and extending the head over the neck. For morbidly obese patients, the HELP position consists of positioning the patient such that the patient's sternum is level with the external auditory meatus.
Technique of Orotracheal Intubation	Preoxygenate, induce general anesthesia and muscle relaxation, mask ventilate, open mouth, insert laryngoscope blade, visualize glottic opening, insert ETT, confirm proper positioning by capnography and chest auscultation, secure ETT.
Technique of Nasotracheal Intubation	Prepare nostrils with a decongestant, preoxygenate, induce general anesthesia and muscle relaxation, insert soft nasal trumpet lubricated with lidocaine ointment, mask ventilate, insert ETT into nostril until the tip reaches the oropharynx, open mouth, insert laryngoscope blade, visualize glottic opening, place ETT, using Magill forceps if needed, confirm proper positioning by capnography and chest auscultation, secure ETT.
ETT Positioning	The tip of the ETT should be placed 4 cm below the vocal cords and 3 cm above the carina.
Complications	Major complications are due to esophageal intubation, aspiration of gastric contents, endobronchial intubation, airway trauma, compression of the tracheal wall, and bronchospasm.

References

1. Kheterpal S, Han R, Tremper KK, et al. Incidence and predictors of difficult and impossible mask ventilation. *Anesthesiology* 2006;105(5):885–891.
2. Adnet F, Baillard C, Borron SW, et al. Randomized study comparing the "sniffing position" with simple head extension for laryngoscopic view in elective surgery patients. *Anesthesiology* 2001;95(4):836–841.
3. Levitan RM, Mechem CC, Ochroch EA, et al. Head-elevated laryngoscopy position: improving laryngeal exposure during laryngoscopy by increasing head elevation. *Ann Emerg Med* 2003;41(3):322–330.
4. Ellis DY, Harris T, Zideman D. Cricoid pressure in emergency department rapid sequence tracheal intubations: a risk-benefit analysis. *Ann Emerg Med* 2007;50(6):653–665.
5. Leibowitz A, Atchabahian A. Asthma. In Reed AP, ed. *Clinical Cases in Anesthesia.* 3rd ed. New York, NY: Churchill Livingstone; 2005:495–501.

EQUIPMENT AND PROCEDURES

21 Difficult Airway Management

Vladimir Nekhendzy, MD

Every general anesthetic begins and ends with airway management. It constitutes the true cornerstone of our specialty. Difficult tracheal intubation, unrecognized esophageal intubation, inadequate ventilation/oxygenation, and premature extubation account for 60% of all perioperative events associated with the patient's death or permanent brain damage (1). No two difficult airways are alike, and providing the cookbook recipe on "how to" deal with difficult airway situations is unrealistic and may be counterproductive. Competent difficult airway management will depend on successful integration of one's knowledge, clinical judgment, and technical skills—factors that are constantly evolving throughout one's clinical career.

1) Overview
   a) **Definition**
      i) The American Society of Anesthesiologists (ASA) Task Force on Difficult Airway Management defines a difficult airway as "**the clinical situation in which a conventionally trained anesthesiologist experiences difficulty with face mask ventilation of the upper airway, difficulty with tracheal intubation, or both**" (2).
   b) **Incidence of difficult airway and management outcomes (3–5) (Table 21-1)**

Honing the technical skills and proficiency with difficult airway devices and techniques should constitute a life-long goal of every anesthesiologist.

Table 21-1
The Incidence of Difficult Airway (3–5)

	EMV	DMV	IMV
Overall incidence	98%	1.4%	0.15%
Difficult DL/intubation	8%	3–4 times higher	
Failed DL/intubation	0.5%	10–12 times higher	
Successful DL	99.5%	94%	86%
Overall success (DL + alternative techniques)	(100%)	? (~100%)	97%
CVCI	(0%)	? (0%)	1:50,000

CVCI, "cannot ventilate-cannot intubate"; DL, direct laryngoscopy; DMV, difficult mask ventilation; EMV, easy mask ventilation; IMV, impossible mask ventilation.

One should practice difficult airway management techniques in the airway workshop or simulator setting, and electively in the operating room on a regular basis.

If DMV is encountered, immediate preparations should be made for alternative airway management.

The first attempt at direct laryngoscopy is always the best. Positioning and oxygenation should be optimized from the beginning.

When tracheal intubation is difficult, the primary focus should be ventilation of the lungs. Repeated attempts at direct laryngoscopy should be discouraged, as this is the primary reason for airway related morbidity and rapid progression to the "cannot ventilate—cannot intubate" situation (6).

i)   The vast majority (98%) of patients are easy to mask (EMV).

ii)   Difficult mask ventilation (DMV) may be encountered slightly more frequently than 1:100 patients.

iii) Impossible mask ventilation (IMV) may be expected to happen once in approximately 700 patients.

iv)   Should mask ventilation prove to be difficult or impossible after induction of anesthesia, the incidence of difficult and failed tracheal intubation increases dramatically.

v)   Although the majority (94%) of patients in DMV group can still be intubated conventionally, the success rate in IMV group decreases significantly (86%). Nevertheless, the 86% success rate is still sufficiently high to suggest that, patient's condition permitting, a single attempt at direct laryngoscopy (DL) may be feasible if IMV is encountered in anesthetized patient.

vi)   The majority of patients (97%) with IMV can still be intubated with the use of alternative airway management techniques, highlighting the crucial role of the anesthesiologist's familiarity and proficiency with different difficult airway management devices.

vii) The most feared situation, "cannot ventilate—cannot intubate" (CVCI), fortunately is extremely rare.

2) Approach to the difficult airway

a) **The ASA difficult airway algorithm**

i)   Has been associated with significantly decreased airway management–related morbidity and mortality (6)

ii)   Despite some limitations (e.g., primary focus on tracheal intubation), the updated ASA guidelines (2) continue to provide rational and effective framework for the anesthesiologist's approach to difficult airway (Fig. 21-1).

iii) As a general rule, when difficult tracheal intubation is anticipated, it is safest to secure the patient's airway awake (Fig. 21-1).

(1) Almost all intubation techniques can be performed in an awake patient.

(2) For the majority of cases of **anticipated difficult airway**, awake flexible fiberoptic intubation (FOI) remains the gold standard of management (7).

b) **Predicting Difficult Airway**

i)   It is difficult to precisely predict patients with difficult airways in the absence of gross anatomical problems.

ii)   The majority of standard airway assessment tests suffer from at least one of the following shortcomings:

(1) Low to modest sensitivity, specificity, positive and negative predictive values, large interobserver variability, failure to account for aspiration risk, lower airway problems, and inability to evaluate unsuspected base of the tongue pathology (e.g., lingual tonsillar hypertrophy)

(2) Sole reliance on these tests may lead to overprediction of airway difficulty and choosing an unindicated awake approach to tracheal intubation, resulting in permanently labeling a patient as "difficult airway" for the future.

Figure 21-1 The ASA Difficult Airway Algorithm (2)

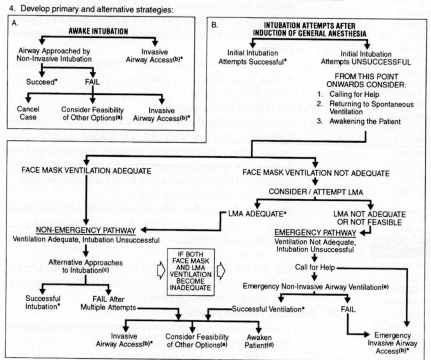

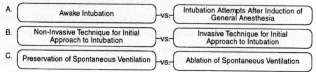

DIFFICULT AIRWAY ALGORITHM

1. Assess the likelihood and clinical impact of basic management problems:
   A. Difficult Ventilation
   B. Difficult Intubation
   C. Difficulty with Patient Cooperation or Consent
   D. Difficult Tracheostomy

2. Actively pursue opportunities to deliver supplemental oxygen throughout the process of difficult airway management

3. Consider the relative merits and feasibility of basic management choices:

   A. Awake Intubation —vs.— Intubation Attempts After Induction of General Anesthesia

   B. Non-Invasive Technique for Initial Approach to Intubation —vs.— Invasive Technique for Initial Approach to Intubation

   C. Preservation of Spontaneous Ventilation —vs.— Ablation of Spontaneous Ventilation

4. Develop primary and alternative strategies:

A. AWAKE INTUBATION

Airway Approached by Non-Invasive Intubation — Invasive Airway Access(b)*

Succeed* / FAIL

Cancel Case — Consider Feasibility of Other Options(a) — Invasive Airway Access(b)*

B. INTUBATION ATTEMPTS AFTER INDUCTION OF GENERAL ANESTHESIA

Initial Intubation Attempts Successful* — Initial Intubation Attempts UNSUCCESSFUL

FROM THIS POINT ONWARDS CONSIDER:
1. Calling for Help
2. Returning to Spontaneous Ventilation
3. Awakening the Patient

FACE MASK VENTILATION ADEQUATE — FACE MASK VENTILATION NOT ADEQUATE

CONSIDER / ATTEMPT LMA

LMA ADEQUATE* — LMA NOT ADEQUATE OR NOT FEASIBLE

NON-EMERGENCY PATHWAY
Ventilation Adequate, Intubation Unsuccessful

EMERGENCY PATHWAY
Ventilation Not Adequate, Intubation Unsuccessful

Alternative Approaches to Intubation(c)

IF BOTH FACE MASK AND LMA VENTILATION BECOME INADEQUATE

Call for Help

Emergency Non-Invasive Airway Ventilation(e)

Successful Intubation* — FAIL After Multiple Attempts — Successful Ventilation* — FAIL

Invasive Airway Access(b)* — Consider Feasibility of Other Options(a) — Awaken Patient(d) — Emergency Invasive Airway Access(b)*

* Confirm ventilation, tracheal intubation, or LMA placement with exhaled CO_2

a. Other options include (but are not limited to): surgery utilizing face mask or LMA anesthesia, local anesthesia infiltration or regional nerve blockade. Pursuit of these options usually implies that mask ventilation will not be problematic. Therefore, these options may be of limited value if this step in the algorithm has been reached via the Emergency Pathway.

b. Invasive airway access includes surgical or percutaneous tracheostomy or cricothyrotomy.

c. Alternative non-invasive approaches to difficult intubation include (but are not limited to): use of different laryngoscope blades, LMA as an intubation conduit (with or without fiberoptic guidance), fiberoptic intubation, intubating stylet or tube changer, light wand, retrograde intubation, and blind oral or nasal intubation.

d. Consider re-preparation of the patient for awake intubation or canceling surgery.

e. Options for emergency non-invasive airway ventilation include (but are not limited to): rigid bronchoscope, esophageal-tracheal combitube ventilation, or transtracheal jet ventilation.

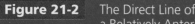

| **Figure 21-2** | The Direct Line of Sight to the Vocal Cords may be Blocked by a Relatively Anterior Larynx (*1*), Prominent Upper Incisors (*2*), and a Large and Posteriorly Located Tongue (*3*) |

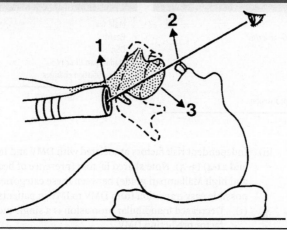

Reproduced from Cormack RS, Lehane J. Difficult tracheal intubation in obstetrics. *Anaesthesia* 1984;39(11):1105–1111.

The ASA difficult airway algorithm is intended for use during administration of anesthesia care; the approaches to difficult airway may be different in emergency settings.

iii) Routine and thorough preoperative airway exam is always warranted to try to detect the most common problems that may impede the laryngeal exposure (8,9) (Fig. 21-2)

b) **Face mask ventilation**

i) Devastating complications of unsuccessful tracheal intubation can be avoided if the ability to ventilate the patient's lungs by face mask is preserved.

ii) As with the recognition of a difficult airway, predicting difficulty with face mask ventilation can be relatively easy when significant anatomical abnormalities are present (**Table 21-2**).

Table 21-2

Anatomic Abnormalities Predictive of Difficult or Impossible Face Mask Ventilation

Standard approach to upper airway and airway opening maneuvers not possible
    Wired jaws
    Facial trauma
    Cervical rigidity
    Halo fixation
Poor seal between the face and a mask
    Facial abnormalities
    Facial trauma
Airway narrowing
    Laryngospasm
    Upper and lower airway tumors, especially mobile, and those associated with respiratory systems
    Narrowed pharyngeal space that cannot be easily modified (pharyngeal edema, copious amount of blood, pus or secretions)
    Upper and/or lower airway collapse

EQUIPMENT AND PROCEDURES

Table 21-3

Predictors of Difficult Face Mask Ventilation (3,4)

Age > 55–57 y.o.
Body mass index $\geq$ 26–30 kg/m^2
Beard
Snoring
Lack of teeth
Mallampati III or IV
Limited mandibular protrusion

Table 21-4

Predictors of Impossible Face Mask Ventilation (5)

Male sex
Beard
OSA
Mallampati III or IV
Neck radiation changes

The presence of three or more standard abnormal airway assessment tests should raise the anesthesiologist's level of suspicion for difficult airway.

READ MORE

Atlas of anesthesia procedures: mask ventilation, Chapter 152, page 1097

The transition from DMV to IMV may be sudden, especially if previous repeated attempts on DL were present.

iii) Independent risk factors associated with DMV and IMV (**Tables 21-3 and 21-4**) (3–5). Note shared factors (presence of beard, snoring/OSA and high Mallampati grade) between these categories, pointing to a possible easy transition from DMV to IMV in patients at risk.

(1) Decreased mandibular protrusion is a single most significant factor predicting DMV.

(2) The presence of **neck radiation changes is the single most significant factor predicting IMV (4,5), and therefore these patients shall be given special consideration.**

(3) Moderate to severe, obstructive sleep apnea (OSA) requiring either the use of CPAP/BiPAP or a history of OSA surgery (Table 21-6)

(4) Of particular interest are the findings predicting both DMV and IMV *and* difficult tracheal intubation (**Table 21-5**). The overall incidence of this event in patient population is 0.37% (5).

(a) One may consider an inhalation induction in these patients, therefore preserving spontaneous ventilation, but this approach does not exclude possible loss of airway.

(b) Appreciate that patients with DMV and IMV are at high risk for iatrogenic complications associated with difficult airway management. Keep in mind that the transition from DMV to IMV may be sudden, especially if previous repeated attempts on DL were present.

(c) Almost 15% of patients with IMV will be difficult to intubate, which places them at highest risk for CVCI situation.

(d) Note that **limited mandibular protrusion** (Tables 21-3 and 21-5) constitutes a single most important predictor for both DMV *and* difficult intubation, and therefore this test **should become an essential part of preoperative airway assessment.**

Table 21-5

Predictors of Difficult and IMV and Difficult Intubation (5)

Body mass index $\geq$ 30 kg/m^2
Snoring
OSA
Thick/obese neck
Limited mandibular protrusion

c) **Deciding on awake versus asleep airway management**
   i) **An awake intubation should be considered** if difficulty with ventilation by both—mask and supraglottic airway device—is anticipated.
   ii) Given the very low incidence of IMV, it would be difficult to justify a conservative awake approach in all patients (5).
   iii) Risk stratification for anticipated difficult ventilation
      (1) **Consider the presence of at least three factors predictive of DMV, IMV** (see Tables 21-3 and 21-4), and their combination with difficult tracheal intubation, to assure appropriately high "likelihood" (odds ratio) of encountering these events (4,5).
      (2) Anatomical features most commonly associated with unanticipated difficult intubation may include the following (8):
         (a) Anterior larynx (most common)
         (b) Abnormal neck anatomy (poor neck mobility and short neck)
         (c) Decreased mouth opening
      (3) It is an opinion of this author that coexistence of these factors with the clear predictors of DMV or IMV may warrant an awake approach to tracheal intubation.
   iv) **If an asleep approach is chosen,** *several* **preformulated alternative airway management plans for tracheal intubation must be devised, and necessary assistance (equipment, personnel) shall be in place before induction of anesthesia.**

d) **Difficult tracheal intubation in the anesthetized patient.** If difficulty in tracheal intubation is encountered after induction of general anesthesia (**unanticipated difficult airway**), or **asleep** approach to the recognized difficult airway was intentionally chosen (e.g., uncooperative patient), a variety of techniques can be employed (see **Table 21-6**).
   i) **Overview**
      (1) The nonemergency pathway of the algorithm implies that the patient's lungs can be adequately ventilated through face mask or laryngeal mask airway (LMA).
      (2) If this ventilation becomes inadequate or fails, and tracheal intubation proves unsuccessful—**"cannot ventilate-cannot intubate"** situation—management approaches for salvaging the airway will be severely limited (**emergency pathway** of the algorithm) (see **Table 21-7**).
   ii) **Avoid direct laryngoscopy**

READ
MORE

Atlas of anesthesia procedures: awake fiberoptic intubation, Chapter 155, page 1103

Awake intubation should be strongly considered if the predictors of DMV and IMV coincide with the factors predicting difficult intubation, and difficulty with the placement of a supraglottic device (e.g., LMA) to provide rescue ventilation is anticipated.

Table 21-6
Alternative Difficult Airway Management Devices and Techniques: Nonemergency Pathway
Simple intubating aids (gum-elastic bougie, introducers, Trachlight, video laryngoscopy)
Blind intubation (largely superseded by FOI)
LMA techniques (use as a rescue aid, a guide for intubation, or as ultimate ventilatory device)
Fiberoptic techniques (flexible and rigid)
Transtracheal techniques (retrograde intubation and cricothyrotomy)

EQUIPMENT AND PROCEDURES

Table 21-7

Devices and Techniques for Managing "Cannot Ventilate-Cannot Intubate" Situation: Emergency Pathway

Combitube
Transtracheal jet ventilation
Rigid bronchoscope
Transtracheal techniques (cricothyrotomy, tracheostomy)

(1) If difficulty in tracheal intubation is anticipated, consider instituting an initial alternative airway approach, therefore avoiding direct laryngoscopy completely. The use of the intubating laryngeal mask (ILMA), video laryngoscopy, and fiberoptic bronchoscopy will be associated with 95–100% success rate (10–13).

iii) **Perform direct laryngoscopy**

(1) If DL is chosen as an initial approach, it is important to remember that **the first attempt will always be the best** (14). **The patient's head position should be carefully optimized for laryngoscopy, and full preoxygenation should precede the induction of anesthesia.**

iv) **Use of neuromuscular blockade**

(1) **The data does not support avoidance of muscle relaxants for managing anticipated difficult tracheal intubation under general anesthesia** (3,5,15) and demonstrate possible preference for depolarizing agents over nondepolarizing neuromuscular blockers (15).

3) **Specialized airway devices and techniques**

a) **Introducer stylets (Bougies)**

i) Solid or hollow semimalleable stylets

(1) Solid: Portex tracheal tube guide (Smith), coude tip bougie 15 Fr × 7 cm (SunMed) (Fig. 21-3)

(2) Hollow: Frova intubating introducer (Cook)

(a) Allows insufflation of oxygen and detection of CO_2

"Clicks" are felt as the bougie passes under the epiglottis and into the trachea. An endotracheal tube (ETT) can then be advanced into the trachea over the bougie.

ii) Can be used to assist with tracheal intubation when the glottic opening is not adequately visualized with direct laryngoscopy

iii) Manipulate angled segment anteriorly under the epiglottis

iv) "Clicks" are felt as the angulated tip of the bougie slides against the tracheal rings, and the "distal hold up" sign is elicited when the angulated tip of the bougie lodges in small bronchus.

v) ETT can be guided into trachea over the bougie device

b) **Supraglottic airway devices in difficult airway management**

i) **General advantages**

(1) Placement of the LMA-Classic results in a 94% success rescue ventilation rate in patients with unanticipated difficult airway (16).

(2) Successful placement of the LMA-Classic (and other types of the LMA) in patients with abnormal and/or difficult airway is probably independent of factors used to predict or score difficult intubation (17,18).

| **Figure 21-3** | Examples of Solid Bougies, Coude Tip from SunMed (**Top**) and Portex Tracheal Tube Guide (**Bottom**) |

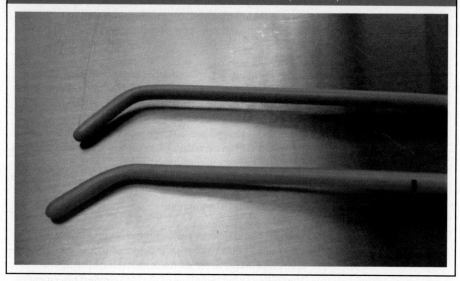

ii) **Limitations**
   (1) Failures of the LMA and Combitube may occur, and they cannot be considered fail-safes for the difficult airway, particularly when an infraglottic obstruction is present (6).
   (2) Some of the problems common to both these devices that may preclude their use are as follows (19):
      (a) Inability to insert the device (e.g., restricted mouth opening)
      (b) Inability to properly position the device in the hypopharynx, (e.g., when cricoid pressure is applied or with upper airway pathology)
      (c) Inability to maintain a seal or to ventilate (e.g., disrupted trachea, decreased lung compliance, or obstructing pathology either at, or below the cords).
iii) **Flexible FOI through the LMA-Classic**
   (1) Offers the advantage of direct visualization of the laryngeal structures and carries minimal risk of intubation trauma and esophageal intubation
   (2) Use of the standard LMA insertion technique will maximize chances for obtaining a clear view of the vocal cords while performing the flexible FOI through the LMA.
   (3) Success rate
      (a) The true success rate of this technique in patients with **unanticipated** difficult airway is unknown. The technique, however, offers 96% to 100% success rate in patients with **anticipated** difficult airway (20,21).
      (b) Troubleshooting
         (i) Should the advancement of the ETT over the fiberoptic bronchoscope (FOB) placed inside the LMA-Classic prove to be difficult secondary to the S-bend in the FOB, or impaction of the ETT with the LMA aperture bars, the glottic inlet or the anterior tracheal wall (20), advanced flexible FOI techniques employing the use of the gum elastic bougie (GEB), guidewire or the Aintree intubation catheter can be attempted.

EQUIPMENT AND PROCEDURES

iv) **Intubating LMA (ILMA, LMA-Fastrach)**

    (1) Advantages

        (a) Prospectively documented 100% success rate in providing **adequate ventilation and oxygenation,** even during prolonged intubation attempts; however, several insertion attempts and repositioning maneuvers may be required (10,21,22).

    (2) Troubleshooting

        (a) Use of the manufacturer's supplied straight silicone ETT is important to increase a success rate for the blind endotracheal intubation and to minimize the incidence of airway trauma.

    (3) Success rates

        (a) Use of an ILMA *in patients with different types of the difficult airway* is associated with an overall 96.5% success rate of blind intubation, and it may increase to 100% with the use of the FOB (10,22).

        (i) Several intubating attempts may be required, which predictably prolongs the intubation time.

v) **The LMA-ProSeal and the LMA-Supreme**

    (1) Advantages

        (a) Superior seal and better airway protection port for gastric access allows quick and reliable detection of malposition of the device and access to the gastrointestinal tract (23,24).

        (b) The GEB-assisted technique of the LMA-ProSeal placement is probably superior to the finger- and metal introducer-guided techniques and assures that the LMA will be optimally positioned against the upper esophageal sphincter (24).

        (c) Can be used for the airway exchange with the aid of the Aintree catheter

vi) **Contraindications to the LMA**

    (1) Relative contraindications include supraglottic pathology, glottic or subglottic airway obstruction, and in patients with bleeding diatheses.

    (2) Airway obstruction caused by collapsible airways or pathology at the glottic and subglottic level cannot be prevented with the LMA.

    (3) Patients at risk for aspiration, patients with low chest wall/lung compliance, and high airway resistance comprise the categories of patients in whom the use of the LMA would most likely be contraindicated.

The risk for aspiration of gastric contents is the single most limiting factor of the LMA use (24).

vii) **Combitube**

    (1) The Combitube is a rescue supraglottic ventilatory device, which can be used to ventilate the patient's lungs in the esophageal as well as the tracheal position.

    (2) Though designed to be inserted blindly, concomitant use of the laryngoscopic blade helps to minimize the incidence of the upper airway trauma.

    (3) In a recent retrospective study (25), the Combitube reliably provided rescue ventilation in emergency airway management, when the GEB and LMA had failed.

    (4) **Advantages**

        (a) Rapid and easy airway control

        (b) No need for patient's neck and head movement (implications for patients with neck injury)

        (c) Effective protection against aspiration

The rescue ability of the LMA or Combitube may be reduced by the effects of multiple preceding attempts at conventional intubation (6).

If ventilation is not possible through either lumen of the Combitube, it is likely inserted too deep.

(d) Special benefit in patients with limited access to the airway and massive upper airway bleeding or regurgitation (26).

(5) **Placement of Combitube device**

(a) Insert Combitube into the oropharnyx according to the manufacturer's recommendations.

(b) After insertion, inflate the esophageal (10 to 12 mL) and oropharyngeal (60 to 100 mL) cuffs and attach the ventilator bag to lumen No. 1.

(c) Ventilation should be possible in the vast majority of cases (esophageal position). If ventilation is impossible, switch over to lumen No. 2 (Combitube is in the trachea—tracheal position) (Fig. 21-4).

(d) If ventilation not possible through either lumen, the Combitube is likely inserted too deep (Fig. 21-5).

(e) Switch the ventilation back to lumen No. 1 and slowly withdraw the Combitube until ventilation becomes possible.

c) **Video laryngoscopic techniques**

i) **General overview**

(1) Major technological innovation in difficult airway management

(2) Airway is visualized by high-resolution digital imager within the oropharynx

(3) Captures glottis through a wide angle of view (Fig. 21-6)

(4) Transmits image to video monitor

(5) Unlike conventional DL, it is unnecessary to align laryngeal, pharyngeal, and oral axes to visualize the glottis (11).

| Figure 21-4 | Combitube in Esophageal ("Normal") |

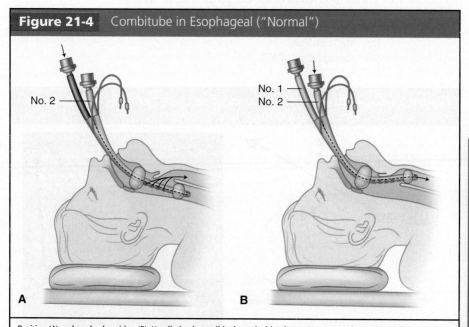

Position (A) and tracheal position (B). Ventilation is possible through either lumen No. 1 (A) or lumen No. 2 (B).
Adapted from Ovassapian A, ed. *Fiberoptic Endoscopy and the Difficult Airway.* 2nd ed. Philadelphia, PA: Lippincott-Raven, 1996.

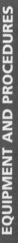

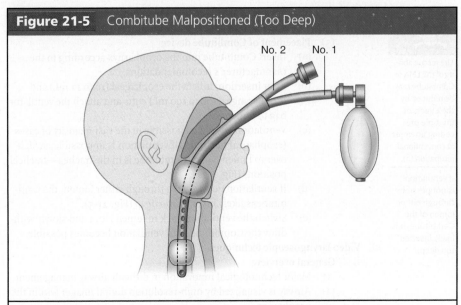

Figure 21-5 Combitube Malpositioned (Too Deep)

Ventilation is impossible through either lumen. Ventilation should be switched over back to lumen No. 1, and the Combitube slowly withdrawn until the chest rise is observed. Adapted from Green KS, Beger TH. Proper use of the Combitube. *Anesthesiology* 1994;81:513–514.

ii) **Types of video laryngoscopes (VLs)**
  (1) VLs are represented by five categories of the devices:
    (a) Glidescope (GVL)
    (b) VideoMac (or CMac)
    (c) McGrath VLs
    (d) Airway scope (AWS)

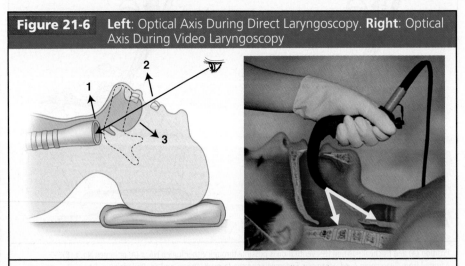

Figure 21-6 **Left**: Optical Axis During Direct Laryngoscopy. **Right**: Optical Axis During Video Laryngoscopy

Modified from http://www.verathon.com/canada_products.htm, Verathon Medical Canada ULC.

Figure 21-7	Example of Steering (GlideScope) and Channeled (Airtraq) Video Laryngoscopic Devices

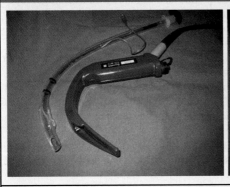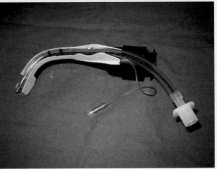

Left: The Glidescope VL with tracheal tube and rigid stylet. **Right:** The airtraq optical laryngoscope with tracheal tube inserted in the adjacent channel. Reproduced from Lange M, Frommer M, Redel A, et al. Comparison of the glidescope and airtraq optical laryngoscopes in patients undergoing direct microlaryngoscopy. *Anaesthesia* 2009;64:323–328.

(e) Airtraq (although, strictly speaking, Airtraq is an optical laryngoscope). Some of these devices are shown in Figure 21-7.

iii) **Proper use of video-laryngoscopes**

(1) **Placement of VL**

(a) All VLs require adequate mouth opening to accommodate the device in the patient's oropharynx.

(b) Standard cross-finger technique is used to open the mouth with the right hand, and the laryngoscope is introduced into the oropharynx in the midline axis with the left hand.

(c) The intubation should proceed in a step-wise fashion, by moving from one anatomical landmark to another.

Continuously alternate attention between the video monitor/ eyepiece and the styletted ETT when attempting to advance ETT through the glottic opening to avoid damaging airway soft tissues.

(i) The first landmark is the uvula, and the edge of the epiglottis usually comes in the view within 2–2.5 cm upon further advancement of the blade.

(ii) The intubation sequence should alternate the operator's view between the manipulations in the patient mouth and the monitor screen: eyes in the mouth upon blade introduction – eyes on the screen immediately after the blade is in – eyes in the mouth for ETT introduction (for steering technique) – eyes on the screen.

(iii) Compared to other devices, the tip of the Pentax AWS blade is lodged under the epiglottis, as opposed to the advancement in the vallecula.

(iv) With either technique, it is utterly important to not advance the tip of the blade too close to the vallecula or too deep under the epiglottis, in order not to obscure the wide angle view of the glottis.

(2) Placement of the ETT

(a) With the steering technique, care must be taken to avoid damaging the tonsilar pillars, soft palate, or palatoglossal arch when advancing the ETT, especially since the attention may be focused on the video screen during this time.

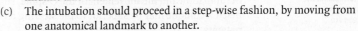

EQUIPMENT AND PROCEDURES

(b) Steering technique. With the use of the GVL (Fig. 21-5), VideoMac (CMac), and McGrath VLs, the ETT is introduced in the regular fashion—that is, independent of the laryngoscope through the patient's mouth—and typically requires the use of the ETT stylet to overcome steep angulation of the blade.

    (i) Adjustment of the stylet angle or withdrawing/advancing the VL may assist with advancing the ETT through the glottic opening.

(c) **Channeled technique.** The AWS and Airtraq (Fig. 21-5) possess the integrated ETT channel guide system, where the stylet use is usually unnecessary: the ETT is advanced through the channel directly into the glottis.

    (i) Advancement of the ETT through the glottic opening can sometimes be difficult even with excellent visualization of the glottis.

    (ii) Advancement of a bougie through the ETT can help guide the ETT through the glottic opening.

iv) **Steering versus channeled VL (11,12,27)**

    (1) Irrespective of which technique is used, all VLs effectively improve the Cormack-Lehane grade by 2 (or at least 1).

    (2) There is less interference of blood and secretions with visualization, and OR personnel are better able to provide airway assistance by observing the intubation procedure on the video monitor.

    (3) Both steering and channeled techniques offer similar intubation success rates in anticipated difficult airway (overall success of 98% to 99% steering versus 95% to 99% channeled) (Table 21-8).

    (4) Substantial differences between techniques in patients with simulated c-spine injuries have been found (28–30), related to the speed of intubation and the movement of the C-spine, suggesting the channeled technique may be superior to the steering technique in these patients.

Channeled devices may be superior to the steering technique in patients with unstable c-spine injuries.

READ MORE

Atlas of anesthesia procedures: wire cricothroidotomy, Chapter 157, page 1110

Table 21-8
Differences in Video-laryngoscope Techniques

	Steering	Channeled
Stylet use	Yes	No
Use of adjuncts (e.g., GEB)	No	Yes
ETT maneuverability	More	Less
Intubation time *vs.* DL	Longer	Equal or faster
Potential for upper airway trauma	More	Less
Learning curve	May be better for channeled	

GEB, gum elastic bougie; DL, direct laryngoscopy; ETT, endotracheal tube.

d) **Cricothyroidotomy**
   i) Most commonly performed airway rescue procedure in "cannot ventilate–cannot intubate" scenario
   ii) Can be achieved through surgical incision, followed by insertion of a cannula or an ETT or a wire-guided (Seldinger) technique

Chapter Summary for Difficult Airway Management

Overview	Expertise in managing patients with difficult airway anatomy is critical for safe anesthesia practice. Approaches to difficult airway management are outlined in the ASA difficult airway algorithm. The anesthesiologist should be familiar with specialized airway management devices that may assist management of patients with difficult airways.
Incidence	98% Patients have EMV 1:100 have DMV 1:700 have IMV The majority (97%) of patients can be intubated, even if they have IMV. To achieve this high success rate, the use of alternative airway management devices and techniques may be required in at least 10% of these patients.
Approach	As a general rule, when difficult tracheal intubation is anticipated, it is the safest to secure the patient's airway awake, with FOI remaining the gold standard of care. Consider specialized equipment and alternative airway techniques where appropriate.
Specialized Equipment/ Alternative Techniques	Intubation aids such as bougie-type devices. Supraglottic airway devices: LMA-Classic (Unique), ILMA, and LMA-Proseal (Supreme) for rescue ventilation, airway exchange, and the use in lieu of the ETT. Video laryngoscopy devices Crichothyroidotomy (Seldinger technique)

References

1. Cheney FW, Posner KL, Lee LA, et al. Trends in anesthesia-related death and brain damage: a closed claims analysis. *Anesthesiology* 2006;105:1081–1086.
2. American Society of Anesthesiologists Task Force on Management of the Difficult Airway. Practice guidelines for management of the difficult airway: an updated report by the American Society of Anesthesiologists Task Force on Management of the Difficult Airway. *Anesthesiology* 2003;98:1269–1277.
3. Langeron O, Masso E, Huraux C, et al. Prediction of difficult mask ventilation. *Anesthesiology* 2000;92:1229–1236.
4. Kheterpal S, Han R, Tremper KK, et al. Incidence and predictors of difficult and impossible mask ventilation. *Anesthesiology* 2006;105:885–891.
5. Kheterpal S, Martin L, Shanks AM, et al. Prediction and outcomes of impossible mask ventilation: a review of 50,000 anesthetics. *Anesthesiology* 2009;110:891–897.
6. Peterson GN, Domino KB, Caplan RA, et al. Management of the difficult airway: a closed claims analysis. *Anesthesiology* 2005;103:33–39.
7. Popat M. The airway. State of the art. *Anaesthesia* 2003;58:1166–1171.
8. Connelly NR, Ghandour K, Robbins L, et al. Management of unexpected difficult airway at a teaching institution over a 7-year period. *J Clin Anesth* 2006;18:198–204.
9. Benumof JL. Management of the difficult adult airway: with special emphasis on awake tracheal intubation. *Anesthesiology* 1991;75:1087–1110.
10. Ferson DZ, Rosenblatt WH, Johansen MJ, et al. Use of the intubating LMA-Fastrach™ in 254 patients with difficult-to-manage airways. *Anesthesiology* 2001;95:1175–1181.
11. Cooper RM, Pacey JA, Bishop MJ, et al. Early clinical experience with a new videolaryngoscope (GlideScope) in 728 patients. *Can J Anaesth* 2005;52:191–198.
12. Asai T, Liu EH, Matsumoto S, et al. Use of the Pentax-AWS in 293 patients with difficult airways. *Anesthesiology* 2009;110:898–904.
13. Heidegger T, Gerig HJ, Ulrich B, et al. Validation of a simple algorithm for tracheal intubation: daily practice is the key to success in emergencies—an analysis of 13,248 intubations. *Anesth Analg* 2001;92:517–522.
14. Benumof JL. Difficult laryngoscopy: obtaining the best view. *Can J Anaesth* 1994;41:361–365.

EQUIPMENT AND PROCEDURES

15. Lundstrom LH, Moller AM, Rosenstock C, et al. and the Danish Anaesthesia Database. Avoidance of neuromuscular blocking agents may increase the risk of difficult tracheal intubation: a cohort study of 103 812 consecutive adult patients recorded in the Danish Anaesthesia Database. *Br J Anaesth* 2009;103:283–290.

16. Parmet JL, Colonna-Romano P, Horrow JC, et al. The laryngeal mask airway reliably provides rescue ventilation in cases of unanticipated difficult tracheal intubation along with difficult mask ventilation. *Anesth Analg* 1998;87:661–665.

17. Brimacombe J. Analysis of 1500 laryngeal mask uses by one anaesthetist in adults undergoing routine anaesthesia. *Anaesthesia* 1996;51: 76–80.

18. Brimacombe J, Berry A. Mallampatti classification and laryngeal mask insertion. *Anaesthesia* 1993;48:347.

19. Hung O, Adam LJ. Advances in airway management. *Can J Anesth* 2006;53:628–631.

20. Benumof J. Laryngeal mask airway and the ASA difficult airway algorithm. *Anesthesiology* 1996;84:686–696.

21. Silk JM, Hill HM, Calder I. Difficult intubation and the laryngeal mask. *Eur J Anaesthesiol Suppl* 1991;4:47–51.

22. Joo HS, Kapoor S, Rose DK, et al. The intubating laryngeal mask airway after induction of general anesthesia versus awake fiberoptic intubation in patients with difficult airways. *Anesth Analg* 2001;92:1342–1346.

23. Brimacombe J, Keller C. The ProSeal laryngeal mask airway. A review. *Anesthesiol Clin North America* 2002;20:871–891.

24. Brimacombe JR, Berry A. The incidence of aspiration associated with the laryngeal mask airway: a meta-analysis of published literature. *J Clin Anesth* 1995;7:297–305.

25. Mort TC. Laryngeal mask airway and bougie intubation failures: the Combitube as a secondary rescue device for in-hospital emergency airway management. *Anesth Analg* 2006;103:1264–1246.

26. Agro F, Frass M, Benumof JL, et al. Current status of the Combitube™: a review of the literature. *J Clin Anesth* 2002;14:307–314.

27. Jungbauer A, Schumann M, Brunkhorst V, et al. Expected difficult tracheal intubation: a prospective comparison of direct laryngoscopy and video laryngoscopy in 200 patients. *Br J Anaesth* 2009;102:546–550.

28. Turkstra TP, Pelz DM, Jones PM. Cervical spine motion: a fluoroscopic comparison of the AirTraq Laryngoscope versus the Macintosh laryngoscope. *Anesthesiology* 2009;111:97–101.

29. Liu EH, Goy RW, Tan BH, et al. Tracheal intubation with videolaryngoscopes in patients with cervical spine immobilization: a randomized trial of the Airway Scope and the GlideScope. *Br J Anaesth* 2009;103:446–451.

30. Turkstra TP, Craen RA, Pelz DM, et al. Cervical spine motion: a fluoroscopic comparison during intubation with lighted stylet, GlideScope, and Macintosh laryngoscope. *Anesth Analg* 2005;101:910–915.

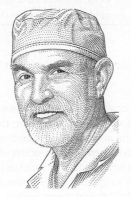

22

Challenges in Anesthesia: The Patient Requiring Reliable Separation of the Lungs

Jay B. Brodsky, MD

Clinical Vignette

A 16-year-old, 5' tall female patient presents urgently to the emergency room after suffering traumatic injury to her chest when her bicycle collided with a tree. On clinical examination, the patient was pale and tachypneic and had an oxygen saturation level of 92% on room air. Air entry on the right side of the chest was absent. She was hemodynamically stable, and the remainder of the examination was unremarkable. A radiographic image of the chest showed complete opacification of the right hemithorax, with right-to-left mediastinal shift. The trauma surgery team requests that she be brought emergently to the operating room for thoracotomy.

Using clinical signs alone for placement of a double-lumen endotracheal tube is an important clinical skill.

Every anesthesiologist should be able to isolate and collapse a lung when requested to do so. The methods currently used to accomplish this are blockade with a bronchial blocker (BB) or by endobronchial intubation with a double-cuffed, double-lumen tube (DLT). A BB is advanced alongside or through an endotracheal tube (ETT) into the bronchus of the lung, and when the blocker's balloon is inflated, lung tissue distal to the obstruction will collapse. Since a BB can be used once an ETT is in place, it is a good option for a patient with a "difficult airway" and in pediatric patients too small for the smallest DLT. However, for most patients a DLT offers many more advantages than a BB (Table 22-1). This chapter will discuss the use of DLTs for separation of the lungs.

The first rubber DLTs (1950s) were difficult to position. The introduction of the plastic DLTs (1980s) coupled with the intraoperative use of fiberoptic bronchoscopes (FOBs) improved the safety and reliability of DLT placement, although the potential for airway trauma still exists (Table 22-2) (1).

Clinical Signs for Placement of DLT

This chapter will focus on the use of clinical signs for DLT placement. Why not just use a FOB from the start? I believe it is essential to be familiar with other methods. A clean, functioning FOB may not always be available, especially during an emergency. Should the case then be delayed or cancelled? Many pediatric FOBs are too large for small DLTs. Blood or mucus can obstruct the endoscopist's ability to identify the carina or visualize the blue bronchial cuff. A FOB remains an extremely useful adjunct for confirmation of DLT placement, especially for residents in training and for clinicians who use a DLT infrequently. As one gains experience with clinical DLT placement there is less need for absolute reliance on a FOB (2).

The clear plastic material of disposable DLTs allows observation of moisture during ventilation and/or the presence of secretions or blood in either lumen. The blue bronchial cuff is easily visualized with a FOB. The high volume/low pressure bronchial cuffs reduce the danger of ischemic pressure damage to airway, and the large lumens allow easy passage of a FOB or suction catheter with less resistance to gas flow during one-lung ventilation (OLV) (3).

Table 22-1
Advantages of DLTs

1. Easy to position
2. Less likely to be displaced than BB
3. Each lung protected from contamination
4. Either lung can be collapsed and re-expanded at will
5. Suction of operated lung
6. FOB inspection of either lung
7. CPAP to operated lung
8. Split-lung ventilation (ICU)

Selection of DLT

A right- or a left-DLT can be used for either a right or a left thoracic procedure (4), but the "margin of safety" is greater with a left-DLT (5). Human airways are asymmetric; the right bronchus is very short (average 2.3 cm in males, average 2.1 cm in females) compared to the left bronchus (average 5.4 cm in males, average 5.0 cm in females). There is a greater risk of malposition with a right-DLT. As many as 10% of normal adults have a carinal or even tracheal origin of their right upper-lobe bronchus, so correct placement of a right-DLT is even more difficult in these patients. Therefore, unless contraindicated, a left-DLT should always be chosen. A right-DLT is indicated when a left-DLT cannot be used, as with obstruction of the proximal left-main bronchus or when placement would interfere with the planned surgical procedure (Table 22-3).

It is important to select the largest DLT that can be atraumatically introduced into the left bronchus (6). A large DLT cannot be advanced as far as a thinner one so there is less chance of left upper-lobe obstruction when a larger tube is used. In addition, the bronchial cuff requires

Table 22-2
Risk Factors for Airway Rupture with DLTs

1. Trauma during insertion
2. Too large a tube
3. Tube advanced with stylet in place
4. Overinflation of tracheal or bronchial cuff
   - Rapid inflation
   - Large volume
   - Nitrous oxide
5. Asymmetric cuff distention pushing distal tip into airway wall
6. Movement of the tube with cuffs inflated
7. Preexisting airway pathology
   - Congenital airway wall abnormalities
   - Airway wall weakness (tumor infiltration, infection, steroids)
   - Airway distortion from mediastinal lymph nodes, tumors

less air to seal the airway reducing the risk of trauma from overinflation. Larger internal lumens offer less resistance to airflow during OLV so less auto-PEEP develops (Table 22-4).

Although some select DLT size based on patient height and gender—tall men get larger tubes, small women get smaller tubes—this method is relatively inaccurate since bronchial diameter is not proportional to height or gender (7). Prior to intubation left bronchial width or tracheal width should be measured from the patient's chest radiograph or chest CT scan. Although average tracheal diameter varies (average 20.6 mm, range 16.0 to 29.0 mm for men, average 17.0 mm, range 13.0 to 22.0 mm for women), the diameter of the left bronchus is directly proportional (~70%) to tracheal diameter (8). Therefore, if tracheal width is known then left bronchial width can be estimated and an appropriate (large) DLT selected (Table 22-5) (9).

Table 22-3
Indications for Right DLTs

1. Obstruction of left-bronchus
   - Intrinsic—tumor, stenosis
   - Extrinsic—tumor, adenopathy, aortic aneurysm
2. Unilateral left lung transplant
3. Sleeve resection left-bronchus
4. Left broncho-pleural fistula

Design of DLTs
Plastic DLTs are molded ("memory" of the plastic) to conform to the shape of the airway. The tube is straight for most of its length (for the trachea) and then the distal endobronchial portion curves to the left. Since the distal end of the tube is inserted into the patient's mouth under direct vision and the bronchial cuff is seldom torn; it is the fragile tracheal cuff that is damaged by the upper teeth if the glottis is anterior and laryngoscopy is attempted with an unbent tube directly from its package. The tube has to be bent into a "hockey stick" shape prior to laryngoscopy to avoid tearing the tracheal cuff. A Miller blade obstructs the view needed for DLT placement; a MacIntosh blade should always be used (10). Special adjuncts like the Bullard or Glidescope laryngoscopes and the Airtraq will help if a difficult airway is encountered.

After placement of a right-sided chest tube, the 16-year-old female trauma patient is brought to the operating room and ASA standard monitors are placed. A chest radiograph confirmed re-expansion of the right lung and a tracheal width of 15 mm was noted. Clinical examination reveals a Mallampati class I airway with normal neck anatomy, and cervical spine that has been cleared by radiologic and clinical exams. A rapid sequence induction is performed and direct laryngoscopy with a Mac 3 blade reveals a grade I view of the glottic opening.

Table 22-4
Advantages of Large DLTs

1. Cannot be advanced as deeply—fewer positioning problems
2. Large lumens
   - Less resistance to airflow during OLV
   - Less auto-PEEP during OLV
   - Easier passage of FOB or suction catheter
3. Tighter bronchial fit
   - Less air in bronchial cuff—potential for less trauma
   - Less unintentional intubation of right bronchus with left-DLT

DLT, double-lumen endotracheal tube; FOB; fiberoptic bronchoscope; OLV, one-lung ventilation; PEEP, positive end-expiratory pressure.

Table 22-5
Guidelines for Left-DLT Selection

Tracheal Width (mm)	Recommended Size
>18	41 Fr (M,R,S,P)
>17	41 Fr (M,S) 39 Fr (R,P)
>16	39 Fr (M,S) 37 Fr (R,P)
>15.5	37 Fr (M,S) 35 Fr (R,P)
>15	35 Fr (M,R,S,P)
>14	32 Fr (M)
>13	32 Fr (M)
>12	28 Fr (M)
>11	26 Fr (R)

Manufacturer: M, Mallinckrodt (St. Louis, MO); R, Rusch (Duluth, GA); S, Sheridan (Argyle, NY); P, Portex (Keene, NH).

Placement of DLTs

The DLT can be advanced into the trachea once laryngoscopy has established a view of the glottic opening. Initially, the tube should be held vertically at the "12 noon" position. Once the distal tip of the DLT is past the vocal cords the stylet in the bronchial lumen should be withdrawn. The tube should be rotated 90 to 180 degrees counter-clockwise until the distal tip is directed towards the left before advancing it further down the trachea.

With bulky rubber DLTs the conventional teaching was to advance the tube until moderate resistance to further advancement was encountered. With thinner plastic DLTs, especially if a small tube is selected, resistance as an end-point will result in the tube being inserted too deeply into the bronchus where it can obstruct the left-upper lobe bronchus (11). The depth of placement of left-DLTs for both men and women is highly correlated with patient height (12), and is easily expressed as $DLT_{cm} = 12 + 0.1$ (Height cm) (13).

Once in the bronchus, both the bronchial and tracheal cuffs should be inflated. If an appropriate (large) left-DLT has been selected, the bronchial cuff should require <3 mL air to seal the airway. If >3 mL of air is needed, the cuff is most likely in the trachea and the tube should be advanced further into the bronchus. The exception is the patient with a very large airway since a 41-Fr is the largest size DLT available and for some the left-bronchus may be large enough to accommodate a larger DLT. The volume of air needed in the bronchial cuff to seal the airway and the tension in its pilot balloon should be noted. If the DLT is subsequently displaced, the pilot balloon will soften. At this point both lungs should be ventilated.

The 16 year-old trauma patient now has a 35 Fr Mallinckrodt left-DLT inserted into her trachea and advanced to 27 cm. The tracheal and bronchial cuffs are inflated and the patient is ventilated through both the tracheal and bronchial lumens. The chest is auscultated and bilateral breath sounds are detected. However, when a FOB is advanced through the tracheal lumen, blood and secretions obscure the view. Despite multiple attempts, you are unable to confirm proper placement of the DLT using direct visualization with FOB.

Troubleshooting and Confirming Proper Position Using Clinical Signs
Assess with Both Tracheal and Broncheal Lumens Open

A capnograph will demonstrate a wave-form and the appearance of end-tidal-CO_2. If both lumens are open to lung tissue water vapor should be visible in both lumens, bilateral chest wall excursion should occur, and bilateral breath sounds should be heard (Fig. 22-1A). If water vapor is seen in only one lumen (with both cuffs inflated) it is usually the bronchial lumen, and it often signals that the bronchial lumen has unintentionally entered the right-bronchus. It is also possible, although unlikely, that the tube is so deep into the left bronchus that the tracheal cuff is at the carina obstructing any ventilation of the right-bronchus.

Assess with Tracheal (Right) Lumen Closed

The next step is to clamp the tracheal (right) lumen while ventilating the left (bronchial) lumen (14). Breath sounds should be heard only over the (intubated) left lung (Fig. 22-1B). If breath sounds are present only over the right lung the DLT is in the right-bronchus (Fig. 22-1C). When this occurs, both cuffs should be deflated and the tube withdrawn several centimeters until its tip is above the carina. While bending and turning the patient's head and neck to the right shoulder with the chin pointed to the left, the tube is re-rotated to the left and re-advanced (15). This maneuver usually redirects the tube into the left-bronchus. If the head-turn maneuver is unsuccessful after several attempts, a FOB should be inserted down the bronchial lumen, the left bronchus identified, and the FOB is used as a stylet to advance the DLT into the left-bronchus.

If while ventilating only the left lumen, breath sounds are heard bilaterally (with both cuffs inflated) the DLT is either not deep enough into the left bronchus (bronchial cuff not sealing the bronchus, Fig. 22-1D) or the tube is in correct position but the bronchial cuff has an inadequate amount of air to seal the bronchus.

Assess with Bronchial (Left) Lumen Closed

Once the DLT is in the left-bronchus, the left lumen should be clamped and the patient should be ventilated through the tracheal lumen. Breath sounds should now be heard only over the right lung (Fig. 22-1E).

If the DLT is still not in satisfactory position (with both cuffs inflated), ventilation through only the right (tracheal) lumen will be difficult or impossible because of very high resistance. The tracheal lumen's orifice will be obstructed by the inflated tracheal cuff (above) and the inflated bronchial cuff (below). In this situation only the bronchial cuff should be deflated while ventilation through the tracheal lumen continues.

If the DLT is not deep enough bilateral breath sounds will immediately be present (Fig. 22-1F). If the tube is too deep breath sounds will be heard only over the left-lung (Fig. 22-1G).

Assessing Peak Inspiratory Pressures

While ventilating both lungs the peak inspiratory pressure should be noted. The bronchial lumen should be clamped and only the right lung ventilated, then the tracheal lumen should be clamped and the left lung is ventilated. If both lungs are relatively equal in volume, that is, in the absence of a pleural effusion, large mass or previous pulmonary resection, sequential ventilation of each lung should produce almost identical peak inspiratory pressures and end-tidal CO_2 waveforms.

If ventilation of the left lung (with a left-DLT) produces significantly higher peak pressures than with identical tidal volume ventilation to the right, the endobronchial lumen is probably partially obstructing the left-upper lobe bronchus and the tube should be withdrawn in 0.5 cm

EQUIPMENT AND PROCEDURES

| **Figure 22-1** | Double-lumen ETT Placement by Clinical Signs |

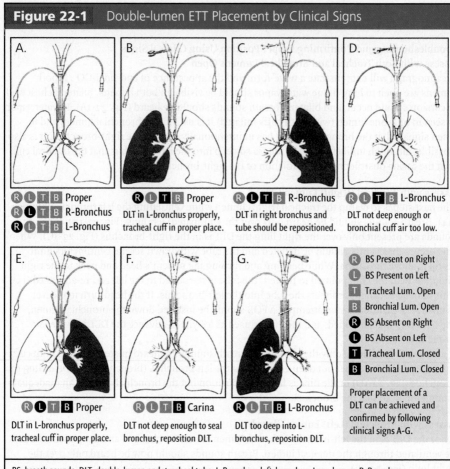

A. Ⓡ ⬤L ⬤T ⬤B Proper
    ⬤R ⬤L ⬤T ⬤B R-Bronchus
    Ⓡ ⬤L ⬤T ⬤B L-Bronchus

B. Ⓡ ⬤L ⬤T ⬤B Proper
    DLT in L-bronchus properly, tracheal cuff in proper place.

C. Ⓡ ⬤L ⬤T ⬤B R-Bronchus
    DLT in right bronchus and tube should be repositioned.

D. Ⓡ ⬤L ⬤T ⬤B L-Bronchus
    DLT not deep enough or bronchial cuff air too low.

E. Ⓡ ⬤L ⬤T ⬤B Proper
    DLT in L-bronchus properly, tracheal cuff in proper place.

F. Ⓡ ⬤L ⬤T ⬤B Carina
    DLT not deep enough to seal bronchus, reposition DLT.

G. Ⓡ ⬤L ⬤T ⬤B L-Bronchus
    DLT too deep into L-bronchus, reposition DLT.

Ⓡ BS Present on Right
Ⓛ BS Present on Left
Ⓣ Tracheal Lum. Open
Ⓑ Bronchial Lum. Open
⬤R BS Absent on Right
⬤L BS Absent on Left
⬤T Tracheal Lum. Closed
⬤B Bronchial Lum. Closed

Proper placement of a DLT can be achieved and confirmed by following clinical signs A-G.

BS, breath sounds; DLT, double-lumen endotracheal tube; L-Bronchus, left-bronchus; Lum, lumen; R-Bronchus, right-bronchus.

increments. If ventilation through the tracheal lumen (left-DLT) produces higher pressures than ventilation to the left, the bronchial cuff is probably herniating into the carina partially obstructing ventilation into the right bronchus. In this situation the tube is advanced in 0.5 cm increments until the peak pressures and waveforms become similar.

Reconfirm Position of DLT after Patient Repositioning

Once the patient is turned to the lateral position it is mandatory to reconfirm DLT position. A DLT is never advanced deeper into the airway but is frequently pulled out. The very first thing to do after turning the patient is to feel the tension in the bronchial cuff's pilot balloon. If it is no longer as tense as when it was with the patient supine, the cuff is no longer completely in the bronchus. Do not add more air to the bronchial cuff, rather, both cuffs should be deflated and the tube should be advanced in 0.5 to 1.0 cm increments into the airway. The bronchial cuff should be re-inflated with the same volume of air that was initially used when the patient was supine; the pilot balloon should once again be tense.

Use of a FOB initially with the patient supine only serves to identify which bronchus has been intubated. Tube position changes with turning, so once the patient is in position for

Table 22-6
Clinical Signs for Reliable Placement of Left DLTs

1. Select a left-DLT whenever practical
2. Measure left bronchus or trachea to determine size, select a large DLT
3. Remove DLT from package, bend into "hockey stick" shape
4. Direct laryngoscopy (use MacIntosh blade)
5. Remove bronchial stylet once tip past vocal cords
6. Then turn tube counter-clockwise until distal tip is pointed towards left
7. Advance down airway into bronchus
   - Depth based on height [$\text{depth}_{cm} = 12 + 0.1\ (\text{height}_{cm})$]
8. Inflate both cuffs slowly
   - Use 3 mL syringe for bronchial cuff. Note volume used
   - Note tension in pilot balloon to bronchial cuff
   - <3 mL air should be adequate if appropriate (large) DLT selected
   - If >3 mL air needed, reassess tube position
9. Confirm tube placement (clinical signs) with patient supine
10. Turn patient; confirm tube placement (clinical signs, FOB) with patient lateral
11. If using N_2O—periodically relieve cuff pressure; deflate bronchial cuff to original inflation volume
12. Deflate bronchial cuff when lung isolation or selective ventilation not needed.

DLT, double-lumen endotracheal tube; FOB, fiberoptic bronchoscope; N_2O, nitrous oxide.

surgery a FOB should then be used to confirm DLT position. The FOB should be advanced down the tracheal lumen; the right-main bronchus should be open and a rim of blue from the bronchial cuff should be visible just below the carina in the appropriate (left) bronchus (16). If the bronchial cuff is fully visible, the tube can be advanced further into the bronchus. If the bronchial cuff is not visible the tube can be slowly withdrawn under direct FOB vision until a rim of blue is seen. Although seldom performed, the FOB should also be advanced down the bronchial lumen to demonstrate a patent upper-lobe bronchus.

Using clinical signs alone (Table 22-6), more than 98% of the left-DLTs functioned with appropriate lung collapse and satisfactory oxygenation during OLV (17).

References

1. Fitzmaurice BG, Brodsky JB. Airway rupture from double-lumen tubes. *J Cardiothorac Vasc Anesth* 1999;13:322–329.
2. Brodsky JB, Macario A, Cannon WB, et al. "Blind" placement of plastic double-lumen tubes. *Anaesth Intens Care* 1995;23:583–586.
3. Burton NA, Watson DC, Brodsky JB, et al. Advantages of a new polyvinyl chloride double-lumen tube in thoracic surgery. *Ann Thorac Surg* 1983;36:78–84.
4. Campos JH, Massa C. Is there a better right-sided tube for one-lung ventilation? A comparison of the right-sided double lumen tube with the single-lumen tube with right-sided enclosed bronchial blocker. *Anesth Analg* 1998;86:696–700.
5. Benumof JL, Partridge BL, Salvatierra C. Margin of safety in positioning modern double-lumen endotracheal tubes. *Anesthesiology* 1987;67:729–738.
6. Hannallah M, Benumof JL, Silverman PM, et al. Evaluation of an approach to choosing a left double-lumen tube size based on chest computed tomographic scan measurement of left mainstem bronchial diameter. *J Cardiothor Vasc Anesth* 1997;11:168–171.
7. Brodsky JB, Mackey S, Cannon WB. Selecting the correct size left double-lumen tube. *J Cardiothorac Vasc Anesth* 1997;11:924–925.
8. Brodsky JB, Malott K, Angst M, et al. The relationship between tracheal width and left bronchial width: implications for left-sided double-lumen tube selection. *J Cardiothorac Vasc Anesth* 2001;15:216–217.
9. Brodsky JB, Macario A, Mark JBD. Tracheal diameter predicts double-lumen tube size: a method for selecting left double-lumen tubes. *Anesth Analg* 1996;82:861–864.
10. Gaeta RR, Brodsky JB. A new laryngoscopy blade to facilitate double-lumen tube placement. *J Cardiothorac Vasc Anesth* 1991;5:418–419.
11. Brodsky JB, Shulman MS, Mark JBD. Malposition of left-sided double-lumen endobronchial tubes. *Anesthesiology* 1985;62:667–669.

EQUIPMENT AND PROCEDURES

12. Brodsky JB, Benumof JL, Ehrenwerth J. Depth of placement of left double-lumen endobronchial tubes. *Anesth Analg* 1991;73:570–572.
13. Takita K, Morimoto Y, Kemmotsu O. The height-based formula for prediction of left-sided double-lumen tracheal tube depth. *J Cardiothorac Vasc Anesth* 2003;17:412–413.
14. Brodsky JB, Mark JBD. A simple technique for accurate placement of double-lumen endobronchial tubes. *Anesth Review* 1983;10:26–30.
15. Neustein SM, Cohen E, Kirschner PA. Intraoperative left endobronchial tube positioning. *J Cardiothorac Vasc Anesth* 1991;5:101–102.
16. Slinger PD. Fiberoptic bronchoscopic positioning of double-lumen tubes. *J Cardiothorac Anesth* 1989;3:486–496.
17. Brodsky JB, Lemmens HJ. Left double-lumen tubes: clinical experience with 1,170 patients. *J Cardiothorac Vasc Anesth* 2003;17:289–298.

23 Laryngeal Mask Airway

Brian Egan, MD • Reuben L. Eng, MD

The laryngeal mask airway (LMA) is a supraglottic airway device that sits above the glottic opening to facilitate ventilation of patients under general anesthesia. The device is placed blindly into the airway and seals the laryngeal inlet to allow easy ventilation of the patient.

1) Overview
   a) The LMA is a supraglottic airway device that consists of a tube connected to an inflatable cuff; this cuff is inserted into the pharynx to permit ventilation of a patient under general anesthesia.
   b) It was invented by British anesthesiologist Archie Brain and introduced to clinical practice in Britain in 1983 and the United States in 1991.
   c) Today, the LMA remains one of the most commonly used supraglottic airway devices.
   d) Function of the LMA
      i) The LMA cuffed mask seals off the laryngeal inlet from the gastrointestinal inlet (Fig. 23-1).
      ii) The tip of the mask sits in the hypopharynx, at the level of the upper esophageal sphincter (UES), with the lateral aspects of the mask spreading into the pharynx, and the superior component displacing the base of the tongue forward.
      iii) The glottic opening and epiglottis sit within the "bowl" formed by this chamber; spontaneous ventilation (SV) or positive pressure ventilation (PPV) is effectively channeled via the bowl and into the respiratory tract (1).

2) Advantages of LMAs
   a) A supraglottic airway offers several advantages over an endotracheal tube (ETT) or mask ventilation, including
      i) Minimal hemodynamic changes with placement due to decreased stimulation with LMA placement
      ii) Low risk of dental/perioral trauma
      iii) First-pass success rates of up to 89%, and successful use in up to 98% of patients appropriately selected for LMA use (2)
      iv) Minimal airway reactivity upon placement, assuming appropriate anesthetic depth
      v) Low incidence of postoperative sore throat
      vi) Compared to a mask general anesthetic, the LMA frees the anesthesiologist's hands from having to hold a mask
      vii) Minimizes coughing/pharyngeal irritation on emergence
      viii) Avoids tracheal intubation in special patient populations (e.g., singers)

| **Figure 23-1** | Dorsal View of the LMATM Cuff Showing Position in Relation to Pharyngeal Anatomy |

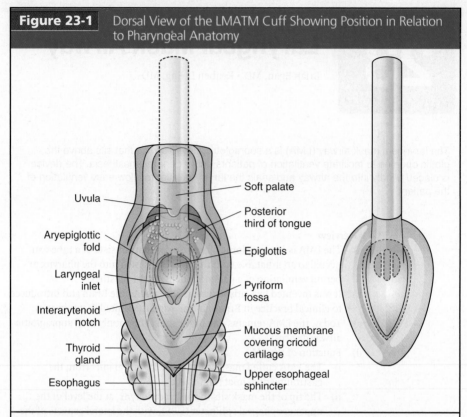

The LMA consists of an inflatable cuff connected to a tube. This figure shows the final position of the LMA in the airway after correct placement. The tip of the mask sits in the hypopharynx at the level of the UES with the lateral aspects spreading into the pharynx and the superior component displacing the base of the tongue forward. Adapted from http://www.lmana.com/docs/LMA_Airways_Manual.pdf

3) **Disadvantages of LMAs**

   a) PPV is limited to peak airway pressures of 20 cm H_2O with the Classic LMA, and 30 cm H_2O with the ProSeal and Supreme LMAs.

      i) This limitation is due to the fact that the pressure at the lower esophageal sphincter (LES) is approximately 20 cm H_2O.

      ii) Ventilation with airway pressures >20 cm H_2O carries the risk of gastric insufflation.

   b) Although the aspiration risk is reported as <0.02% (3), the airway is not completely protected from aspiration of gastric contents.

Patients at high risk of aspiration may not be good candidates for LMA.

      i) Patients at high risk of aspiration (e.g., obese, pregnant, gastroesophageal reflux disease, full stomach) may not be good candidates for LMA.

   c) Adequate function of the LMA is dependent on appropriate position in the hypopharynx.

      i) It is susceptible to displacement with changes in patient position and/or manipulation of the head and neck.

    d) Reported rare, but severe, neurovascular complications due to trauma secondary to LMA use include
        i) Lingual nerve injury (4)
        ii) Recurrent laryngeal nerve injury (5)
        iii) Hypoglossal nerve injury (6)
        iv) Tongue cyanosis (7)

4) **Description of different types of LMAs**

a) **Classic LMA and Unique LMA**
    i) The Classic
        (1) The original LMA
        (2) Reusable for 40 uses
    ii) The Unique
        (1) The disposable version of the Classic
    iii) All versions are **latex-free**.
    iv) Designed for SV, though PPV to a maximum of 20 cm H_2O has been safely utilized without any sequelae of gastric insufflation
    v) Can be used as a rescue airway device for difficult intubation/ventilation scenarios (8)

The LMA can be used as a rescue airway device for situations where difficult intubation and/or ventilation occur.

b) **ProSeal LMA**
    i) The cuff of the ProSeal rests deeper in the hypopharynx, thus improving the seal and permitting PPV up to 30 cm H_2O.
    ii) A gastric drainage conduit was added to allow contents of the gastrointestinal tract to be safely suctioned, bypassing the mouth and respiratory tract.
        (1) A 14-French orogastric tube can be placed through the drainage tube to decompress the stomach.

c) **Flexible LMA**
    i) Designed to optimize LMA use in shared airway cases in which surgeons operate in close proximity to the airway
        (1) The Flexible LMA can be easily positioned out of the surgeon's working space.
    ii) Wire-reinforced, flexible breathing tube
        (1) Allows maintenance of proper mask position in the hypopharynx while the tube is proximally displaced at extreme angles.
    iii) The tube is longer and of smaller diameter.
        (1) Increases resistance to air flow through the LMA.

d) **Supreme LMA**
    i) Like the ProSeal, a "drain tube" terminates in the tip of the mask and should sit in the UES.
    ii) Has a built-in bite block, a more rigid breathing tube facilitates non-digital placement, and a fixation-tab and dual tube configuration that minimizes rotational displacement.

e) **Intubating LMA and LMA C-trach**
    i) Designed to facilitate tracheal intubation
    ii) The basic components of the Classic LMA are retained but modified to achieve both blind and videoscope-guided placement of an ETT.
    iii) After successful ETT placement, they are typically removed from the airway.
        (1) However, they can remain in situ when conditions make removal prohibitive.

5) **Placement of an LMA—Standard technique**

   a) **Preparation of the LMA**

↪ READ
MORE
Atlas of anesthe-
sia procedures:
Laryngeal mask
airway insertion,
Chapter 153,
page 1099

   i) Completely deflate the cuff of the mask with a syringe into a flat, smooth, wedge-shaped tip to minimize down-folding of the epiglottis on placement.

   ii) Place water-soluble lubricant on the posterior surface of the cuff only.

      (1) Placement on the ventral surface could cause airway obstruction and aspiration of lubricant, as well as laryngospasm secondary to vocal cord irritation by lubricant.

      (2) Lubricant should be placed right before LMA insertion to minimize drying.

   b) **Patient positioning**

   i) LMA placement is facilitated by neck flexion and head extension (i.e., the "sniffing" position).

      (1) Grasp and push the head with the nondominant hand during insertion to place the patient's head in the "sniffing position".

   c) **Insertion** (Fig. 23-2) (9)

   i) **LMA Classic, Unique, and Flexible**

      (1) Grasp the tube in the dominant hand, and place the index finger in the space between the tube and the deflated cuff of the mask.

      (2) Use the nondominant hand to place the patient's head in the "sniffing" position.

      (3) With the flat side of the cuff facing the patient's head, place the tip of the mask firmly against the hard palate and advance the LMA along the palate, above the tongue, and into the posterior pharynx in a smooth continuous motion; the initial direction of force should be directed toward the operator's umbilicus.

      (4) The nondominant hand is then used to push the LMA further into the hypopharynx until resistance is encountered at the UES; 7 to 10 cm of LMA should protrude from the oral cavity.

         (a) Withdraw the index finger while stabilizing the LMA with the opposite hand.

   d) **Completion**

   i) Inflate the mask with just enough air to create a seal.

      (1) Maximum inflation volumes (to keep the pressure <60 cm H_2O) are printed on each device.

   ii) A slight rise (1 to 2 cm) of the LMA out of the mouth on inflation suggests that the LMA is appropriately positioned.

   iii) Connect the circuit, and confirm proper placement by gentle manual ventilation.

      (1) Observe for chest rise, presence of $ETCO_2$, and listen for an audible leak, evidence of airway obstruction, and bilateral breath sounds.

   e) **Troubleshooting**

   i) Difficulty ventilating through the LMA

      (1) Possible etiologies:

         (a) Inadequate anesthetic depth

         (b) Epiglottis has folded over during insertion, thus obstructing the airway

Figure 23-2	Technique for Insertion of LMA

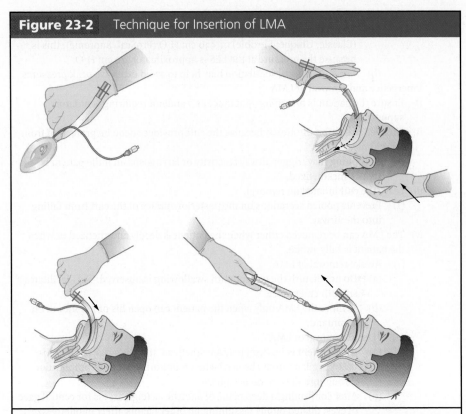

Top Left: Grasp the airway tube in the dominant hand and place the index finger between the tube and the deflated cuff of the mask. **Top Right:** with the nondominant hand adjusting the head into the "sniffing" position, place the tip of the mask firmly against the palate and advance the LMA along the palate and into the posterior pharynx with the initial direction of force directed toward the operator's umbilicus. **Lower Left:** The nondominant hand is then used to push the LMA further into the hypopharynx until resistance is encountered at the UES. **Lower Right:** Once inserted, the cuff of the LMA is insufflated with just enough air to create a seal. Adapted from Walls RM, Murphy MF. *Manual of Emergency Airway Management.* 3rd ed. Philadelphia, PA: Lippincott Williams & Wilkins; 2008:125–127.

(c) Tip has migrated into the airway rather than the esophageal inlet, thus malpositioning the LMA

ii) With correct placement, an ovoid swelling in the anterior of the neck is often visible.

iii) **When in doubt, take it out, ensure adequate depth, and reinsert.**

f) **Ventilation**

i) Spontaneous ventilation is preferred for the Classic LMA and Unique LMA.

(1) Well tolerated when anesthetic depth is appropriate for the level of stimulation.

(2) Changes in respiratory pattern (e.g., sudden increase in tidal volume or respiratory rate) suggest inadequate depth of anesthesia.

When in doubt of LMA proper positioning, take it out, ensure adequate depth, and reinsert.

EQUIPMENT AND PROCEDURES

      (3) Positive pressure ventilation can be done safely, with some caveats.

          (a) To avoid gastric insufflation, keep peak airway pressures <20 cm H_2O (Classic, Unique, Flexible) or <30 cm H_2O (ProSeal, Supreme); this is because the pressure at the LES is approximately 20 cm H_2O.

          (b) Pressure-control ventilation may help to avoid excessive peak pressures.

g) **Emergence and removal of LMA**

    i) Ensure the patient is breathing spontaneously and not requiring ventilatory support.

    ii) No need to suction the airway because the cuff provides adequate protection from secretions.

      (1) Suctioning may trigger airway reactivity or laryngospasm if the patient is lightly anesthetized.

    iii) Leave the cuff inflated on removal.

      (1) Prevents pooled secretions on the posterior surface of the cuff from falling into the airway.

    iv) The LMA can be removed either when the patient is deeply anesthetized or when the patient is fully awake.

      (1) Awake removal of LMA

          (a) Do not disturb the patient until swallowing is observed. This facilitates a smooth emergence.

          (b) Remove the LMA only when the patient can open his or her mouth on command.

      (2) "Deep" removal of LMA

          (a) If the patient is inadequately anesthetized, there is a risk of laryngospasm; vigilance must be used when monitoring for this complication throughout the emergence phase.

          (b) After confirming a deep plane of anesthesia (e.g., assess for central gaze of eyes, dilated pupils [assuming no other factors affect pupillary size]), remove the LMA from the oral cavity.

          (c) Consider 100% oxygen for a brief period before removing LMA to optimize apneic time in the event of transient upper airway obstruction after LMA removal.

          (d) Consider placing the patient in a lateral decubitus position after removal of LMA to facilitate outward drainage of oral secretions.

h) **Complications associated with LMA use**

    i) **Aspiration**

      (1) Regurgitation of gastric contents occurs rarely, and aspiration of gastric contents even more rarely, in part because of LMA design and appropriate patient selection for LMA use.

      (2) If regurgitation does occur, place the patient in the head-down (Trendelenburg) position.

          (a) This encourages gastric contents to flow out the mouth.

      (3) Leave the LMA in place.

      (4) Suction down the airway tube with a soft suction catheter.

          (a) If secretions are aspirated from the airway, consider suctioning via fiberoptic scope or replacing the LMA with an ETT.

ii) **Cuff trauma**
   (1) The cuff of the LMA can place traumatic pressure on vulnerable anatomic structures, including the
      (a) Mucosa
      (b) Hypoglossal nerve
      (c) Lingual and superior laryngeal nerves
   (2) Avoiding cuff trauma
      (a) Use the minimal amount of air to create a good seal.
         (i) Do not exceed the recommended maximum cuff volumes.
         (ii) Additional air rarely improves a poorly ventilating LMA.
            1. It is better to remove and replace the LMA.
      (b) Avoid any tension on the airway tube (e.g., via the anesthetic circuit) because it may be translated distally to the cuff, and thus to the tissues against which the cuff approximates.

iii) **Laryngeal injuries**
   (1) There are rare cases of arytenoid cartilage dislodgement, vocal cord injury, and/or paralysis.
   (2) Proper placement of the LMA obviates direct contact with glottic structures.
   (3) The period of greatest resistance to LMA advancement occurs when the tip slides behind the tongue.
      (a) Typically, there is a notable decrease in resistance once this is achieved.
      (b) Persistent resistance to advancement should be treated with caution.
         (i) Removing the LMA to the level of the palate and readvancing is advised.

iv) **Other uses**
   (1) Airway emergencies
      (a) The LMA Classic, Unique, ProSeal, and Supreme are part of the ASA difficult airway algorithm.
         (i) May be used in situations of difficult mask ventilation and/or intubation (8).
         (ii) Depending on the clinical scenario, the availability and use of a rescue airway with gastric decompression capability may be favored.
      (b) Fiberoptic conduit
         (i) The exit point of the LMA airway tube through which the fiberoptic scope emerges from the LMA permits good visualization of the glottic opening or epiglottis.
            1. This allows examination of vocal cord function during certain surgeries (e.g., thyroid procedures).
            2. Also provides a conduit for fiberoptic intubation.
         (ii) Modifications of the disposable Unique have been suggested to facilitate fiberoptic intubation.
            1. Removing the airway bars at the distal end of the airway tube (5–9) and shortening the tube to ensure complete passage of the ETT balloon after rail-roading.
            2. Use of an Aintree Intubating Catheter can also facilitate fiberoptic intubation through an LMA (10).

EQUIPMENT AND PROCEDURES

Chapter Summary for Laryngeal Mask Airway

Definition	Seals off the laryngeal inlet from the gastrointestinal inlet using a cuffed mask connected to a tube.
Insertion	Place the tip of the mask firmly against the palate. Advance the LMA along the palate and into the posterior pharynx with the initial direction of force directed toward the operator's umbilicus. Keep advancing until resistance is encountered at the upper esophageal sphincter.
Completion	Reinflate the mask with just enough air to create a seal. A slight rise of the LMA out of the mouth on inflation suggests good position.
Emergence	Avoid suctioning the airway. Leave the cuff inflated on removal. If removing with the patient awake, leave the patient undisturbed until swallowing is observed. Remove the LMA only when the patient opens his or her mouth on command.

References

1. http://www.lmana.com/docs/LMA_Airways_Manual.pdf. Accessed June 2009.
2. Wakeling HG, Butler PJ, Baxter PJ. The laryngeal mask airway: a comparison between two insertion techniques. *Anesth Analg* 1997;85: 687–690.
3. Brimacombe JR, Berry A. The incidence of aspiration associated with the laryngeal mask airway: a meta-analysis of published literature. *J Clin Anesth* 1995;7:297–305.
4. Foley E, McDermott TED, Shanahan E, et al. Transient isolated lingual nerve neuropraxia associated with general anesthesia and laryngeal mask use: two case reports and a review of the literature. *Ir J Med Sci* 2010;179:297–300.
5. Endo K, Okabe Y, Maruyama Y, et al. Bilateral vocal cord paralysis caused by laryngeal mask airway. *Am J Otolaryngol* 2007;28:126–129.
5. Ianchulev SA. Letter to the editor. *Anesth Analg* 2005;101:1882–1883.
6. Stewart A, Lindsay WA. Bilateral hypoglossal nerve injury following the use of the laryngeal mask airway. *Anaesthesia* 2002;57:264–265.
7. Wynn JM, Jones KL. Tongue cyanosis after laryngeal mask insertion. *Anesthesiology* 1994;80:1403–1404.
8. www.asahq.org/publicationsAndServices/Difficult%20Airway.pdf. Accessed June 2009.
9. Walls RM, Murphy MF. *Manual of Emergency Airway Management.* 3rd ed. Philadelphia, PA: Lippincott Williams & Wilkins; 2008:125–127.
10. Blair EJ, Mihai R, Cook TM. Tracheal intubation via the classic and proseal laryngeal mask airways: a manikin study using the Aintree Intubating Catheter. *Anaesthesia* 2007;62:385–387.

24 Fiberoptic Intubation

Marina Shindell, DO

Fiberoptic intubation is a technique for establishing placement of an endotracheal tube through the oropharynx or the nasopharynx with the aid of a small, flexible fiberoptic device. The key to successful airway management with fiberoptic intubation techniques depends upon a careful examination of the airway, good knowledge of airway anatomy, sound knowledge of pharmacology of local anesthetics, a cooperative patient (if done awake), and a patient surgeon.

1) Indications for fiberoptic intubation
   a) Prior history of difficult intubation either related by the patient or found in the chart review
   b) Mandibular hypoplasia
   c) Fixed cervical spine disease (e.g., ankylosing spondylitis)
   d) Acromegaly
   e) **Awake intubation should be considered in the following situations**
      i) Patients with a high risk of aspiration
      ii) Undesirable neck movement (unstable or uncleared cervical spine)
      iii) When self-positioning for surgery is desirable
      iv) Inability to ventilate patient, predicted or unpredicted (e.g., "cannot intubate, cannot ventilate")
      v) Morbid obesity
      vi) Lower and/or upper airway obstruction (e.g., tracheal compression, foreign body, laryngeal or pharyngeal tumors, neck masses, hematomas, Ludwig's angina, airway burns)
      vii) Radiation to the neck after cancer surgery
      viii) Facial trauma
      ix) Congenital syndromes (e.g., Pierre Robin syndrome)

2) Contraindications to fiberoptic intubation

As soon as the decision is made to proceed with awake airway management, patient must be prepared both physically (pharmacologically) and psychologically.

   a) **Lack of time is an absolute contraindication**, as this technique requires time to set up. However, one must carefully weigh the extremely serious, and potentially deadly, risk of an airway with the benefit of saving time.
   b) Necessity to rapidly secure an airway precludes asleep (anesthetized) approach in patients with the following conditions:
      i) Full stomach
      ii) Potential for gastric reflux
      iii) Morbid obesity
   c) Adults or children with mental incapacitations are extremely difficult to perform awake FOI on due to their inability to cooperate.
   d) Bleeding from upper or lower airway which is not relieved (or sometimes made worse) by suction, strong potential for bleeding in patients with coagulopathy
   e) Heavy airway secretions not relieved by suction or antisialagogues

3) **Preparation for fiberoptic intubation**
   a) **Checklist for fiberoptic cart**
      i)   Fiberoptic bronchoscope (FOB) and light source
      ii)   Endotracheal or nasotracheal tube and air syringe
            (1) **Have various sizes available, if patient has any tracheal obstruction a smaller ETT may be necessary.**
      iii) A bottle of warm water may be used to soften the ETT, so it is less likely to cause mucosal damage.
      iv)   **Intubating/endoscopic oral airway**
            (1) **Berman**
                (a) Tubular along the entire length
                (b) Available in different sizes, but FOB cannot be maneuvered by bending its tip once it has been placed through the airway
            (2) **Ovassapian**
                (a) Designed to provide an open air space in the oropharynx, to protect the FOB from being bitten by the patient
                (b) Available in one size
                (c) Accommodates an ETT up to 8.5 mm in inner diameter
                (d) **Best suited and specifically designed for fiberoptic intubation**
            (3) **Williams**
                (a) Designed for "blind" orotracheal intubation
                (b) Available in two sizes, 90 and 100 mm
                (c) Due to its design, the tip of FOB cannot be maneuvered in AP or lateral direction.
                (d) At times, this airway must be partially withdrawn to allow better exposure of the vocal cords
      v)   Tongue depressor
      vi)   Gauze (4″ × 4″)
      vii) Lubricant
      viii) Suction
      ix)   Auxiliary source of oxygen
      x)   Emergency airway equipment, including criocothyroidotomy kit and/or a surgeon who can perform a surgical airway expeditiously
   b) **Preparation and inspection of the fiberoptic scope**
      i)   Place the scope and all the necessary equipment on the cart next to the patient's bed, so it is easily accessible.
      ii)   Test the adjustment focus against any writing (e.g., back of the alcohol pad).
      iii) Test all the operator's functions on the scope: anteflexing and retroflexing.
      iv)   **Choose and attach appropriate size endotracheal tube (ETT) to the scope.**
            (1) Generally, the ETT is at least 1.5 mm larger in internal diameter than the diameter of FOB (the fiberoptic shaft diameters are approximately 3.5 to 5.5 mm).
            (2) Remove the connector from ETT prior to doing so, as it gives you more length on the scope and more maneuverability (do not lose the connector).
            (3) Lubricate the shaft of the scope prior to attaching the tube.
      v)   Turn on the light source.
      vi)   **Connect the port to the oxygen.**
            (1) This improves oxygenation and displaces some secretions during fiberoptic intubation.
            (2) It is also possible to connect the suction to the appropriate port on the scope, but it is not very powerful.

Placing an ETT in a warm solution prior to intubation softens the tube, and it is less likely to cause mucosal damage.

Figure 24-1   Overview of a Fiberoptic Bronchoscope

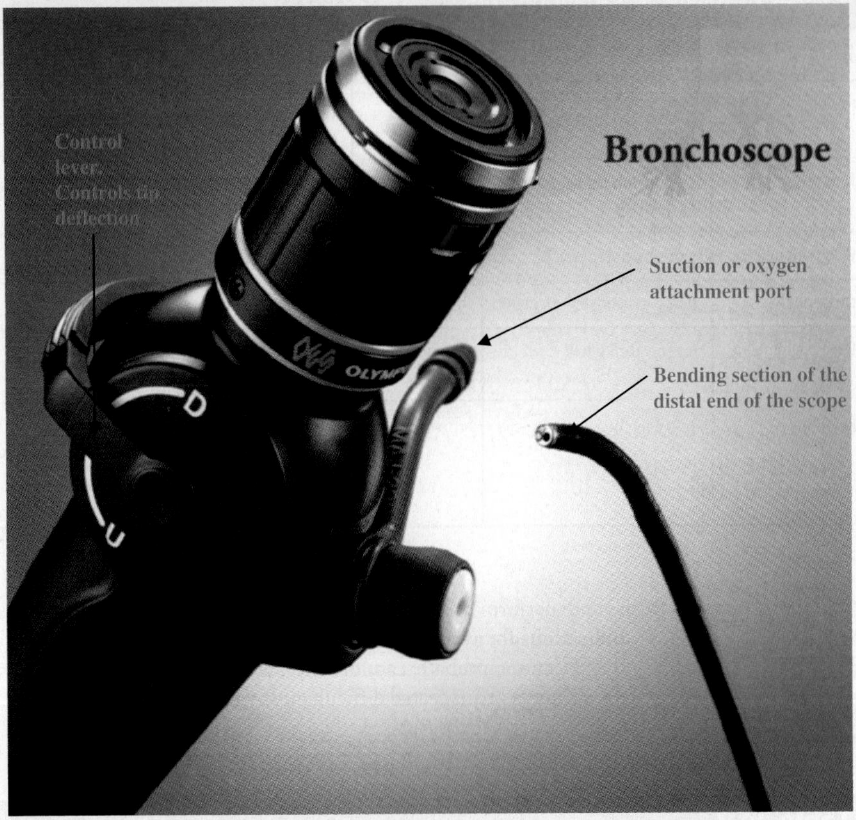

Control lever. Controls tip deflection

Bronchoscope

Suction or oxygen attachment port

Bending section of the distal end of the scope

4) Operation of a fiberoptic scope
  a) Overview of device (Fig. 24-1)
  b) **Manipulation of scope tip (for a right-handed individual)**
    i) The head of the fiberoptic scope is held in the right hand, with the right thumb on the control lever.
      (1) Alternatively, FOB could be held in the nondominant hand, if it is more comfortable for the operator.
    ii) Anteroflexion
      (1) Pull the right thumb down, to curve the distal end of the scope upwards.
    iii) Retroflexion
      (1) Push the right thumb up, to curve the distal end of the scope downwards.
  c) **Directing movement of fiberoptic scope**
    i) While the right hand is positioned at the control section of the fiberoptic scope, hold the bronchoscope shaft in the left hand about 15 cm from the distal tip.
      (1) It is crucial to keep bronchoscope taut between the right and the left hands so that the orientation of the tip is the same as that of the control lever.

EQUIPMENT AND PROCEDURES

Table 24-1
Profiles of Available Sedation Drugs

Drug	Dose	Frequency	Side Effects	Reversal Agents
Midazolam	0.25–4 mg IV	1–5 min	Respiratory depression	Flumazemil, 0.2 mg IV q1min up to 1 mg
Fentanyl	Load up to 1 µg/kg, then 12.5–50 µg IV	5–10 min	Respiratory depression	Naloxone, 40–400 µg IV q5–10min
Remifentanil	0.01–0.5 µg/kg/min IV	Infusion	Respiratory depression	
Droperidol	0.625–1.25 mg up to 5 mg IV	5–10 min	Torsades de points	
Dexmedetomidine	0.2–0.7 µg/kg/h IV	Infusion	Hypotension and bradycardia	
Ketamine	10–50 mg IV		Hallucinations which can be attenuated with midazolam administration, arrhythmias	

READ MORE

Difficult airway management, Chapter 21, page 150

5) Decision to perform awake fiberoptic intubation
   a) **Indications for awake FOI**
     i) "Cannot intubate, cannot ventilate" scenario
     ii) Known or suspected difficult airway as mentioned in Section 1.c.

Table 24-2
Profiles of Available Anesthetics

Drug	Maximum Dose	Additives	Route	Contraindications	Complications
Cocaine 4%	1.5 mg/kg		Nasal	Patients with ischemic heart disease, preeclampsia, on monoamine oxidase inhibitors	Tachycardia, hypertension
Benzocaine spray	100 mg		Oral	Local anesthetic allergy	Methemoglobinemia. Caution not to exceed recommended dose of a single 0.5–2 s spray.
Lidocaine • 4% • 2% viscous • 5% jelly	5 mg/kg with epinephrine or 7 mg/kg without epinephrine	• Afrin spray (oxymetazoline) • 1% Phenylphrine	Oral	Local anesthetic allergy (although extremely rare in amide category)	CNS toxicity Cardiovascular toxicity

b) **Indications for asleep FOI**
   i) Patient's comfort
   ii) Uncooperative patient
6) Preparation of the patient for awake fiberoptic intubation
   a) Premedication
      i) Glycopyrrolate 0.2 to 0.3 mg IV can be administered 15 to 20 minutes prior to FOI as an antisialogogue.
         (1) It is important to administer the drug early in order for it to be effective during the FOI attempt.
   b) Explain to the patient the reason for the awake intubation and how it will proceed.
   c) Sedate the patient, being careful not to oversedate him/her.
      i) **There are multiple techniques for sedation; choose one that is most comfortable (Table 24-1).**
   d) Apply anesthesia to the airway.
      i) **The airway can be anesthetized by topicalization or nerve blocks, or combination of both (Table 24-2).**
         (1) Topicalization of oral pharynx can be done with atomizers, nebulizers, or direct application of lidocaine or with aerosol benzocaine.
         (2) For nasal route, cocaine can be used to topicalize the nasal passages, as well as cause vasoconstriction to decrease the possibility of epistaxis.
            (a) Phenylephrine or afrin spray can be mixed with lidocaine for vasoconstriction.
   e) **Common airway nerve blocks**
      i) **Glossopharyngeal nerve (CN IX) and lingual branch block**
         (1) Carries the sensory innervation of the pharynx, tonsils, and posterior third of the tongue

---

Figure 24-2   The Palatoglossal Arch (Arrow). Intraoral Approach to the Glossopharyngeal Nerve

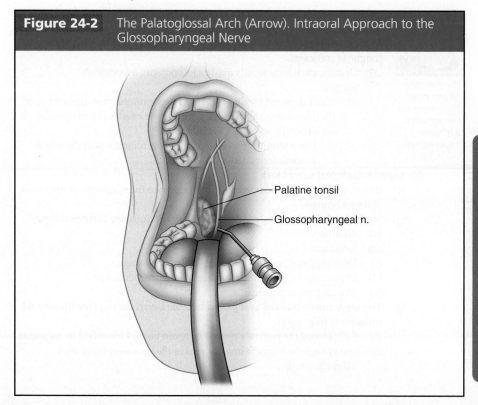

Palatine tonsil

Glossopharyngeal n.

EQUIPMENT AND PROCEDURES

Figure 24-3	Superior Laryngeal Nerve Block

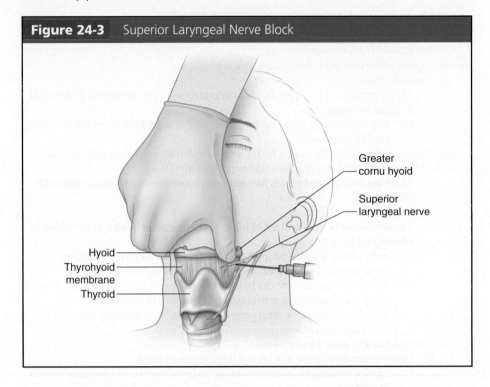

Greater
cornu hyoid

Superior
laryngeal nerve

Hyoid
Thyrohyoid
membrane
Thyroid

(2) The block of this nerve depresses the gag reflex during the awake fiberoptic intubation.

(3) **In most patients, the local anesthetic applied topically to the back of the tongue is sufficient.**

(a) Usually, 5% lidocaine jelly used as lollipop can accomplish the goal.

(i) If this does not produce satisfactory anesthesia, injection of 2 cc of 1% lidocaine with 25-gauge needle at the caudal part of tonsillar pillar bilaterally will block the nerves.

1. Use a tongue depressor to move the tongue out of the way in anteroinferior direction (Fig. 24-2).

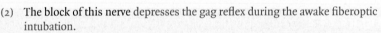

The glossopharyngeal nerve block depresses the gag reflex during the awake fiberoptic intubation.

iii) **Superior laryngeal nerve block**

(1) Innervates larynx (provides sensory innervation to the epiglottis, arythenoids, and vocal cords)

(2) **Methods of anesthetizing the distribution of the Superior Laryngeal Nerve**

(a) Atomizer

(b) Nebulizer

(c) Trickling local anesthetic down the posterior tongue

(d) Depositing local anesthetic through the fiberoptic scope

(e) Blocking the nerve directly

(3) **The nerve can be blocked as it passes into the larynx through the thyrohyoid membrane (Fig. 24-3).**

(a) Fully extend the patient's neck. The hyoid bone is identified by palpation.

(b) Use syringe with approximately 3 ml of 1% lidocaine, fitted with 25-gauge needle.

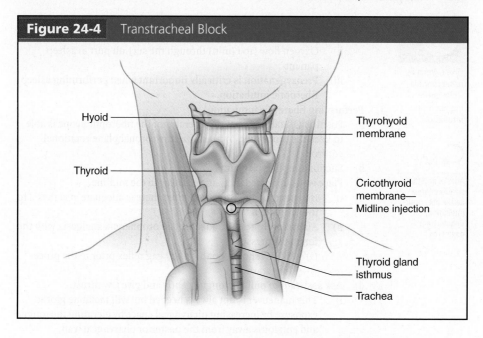

Figure 24-4 | Transtracheal Block

Hyoid

Thyrohyoid
membrane

Thyroid

Cricothyroid
membrane—
Midline injection

Thyroid gland
isthmus

Trachea

    (c)   Insert the needle until it rests on the lateral portion of hyoid bone.

    (d)   Withdraw it slightly and walk it off the hyoid bone in caudad direction and advance couple of millimeters until it passes though the thyrohyoid membrane (slight resistance should be felt).

    (e)   After negative aspiration for air and blood, and inject 2 to 3 ml. Repeat on the other side.

  iv) **Transtracheal nerve block**

    (1)   Provides anesthesia to the area between carina and vocal cords.

    (2)   The block should be performed about 1 minute prior to the start of bronchoscopy.

    (3)   Use 10-cc syringe, filled with 3 cc of 4% lidocaine with 22- or 23-gauge needle.

    (4)   Place patient in the supine position with neck extended (Fig. 24-4).

    (5)   Introduce the needle at the level of crycothyroid membrane, directed posteriorly, perpendicular to the skin, continuously aspirating.

    (6)   Once you have positive air aspiration, inject local anesthetic, as the patient inhales and remove the needle quickly. The patient will cough.

    (7)   **Differences in method**

        (a)   Some advocate using a catheter technique and advancing the catheter once positive aspiration is achieved and leaving it in to later inject local anesthetic through the catheter.

        (b)   Others advocate avoiding transtracheal block and spraying local anesthetic through the fiberoptic scope as the scope is advanced through the airway.

  f) **Patient positioning**

    i) Supine position

      (1)   Endoscopist is at the head of the table.

    ii) Sitting position

      (1)   Endoscopist faces the patient.

EQUIPMENT AND PROCEDURES

g) **Oxygenation and Suction**

    i)   Oxygen via nasal cannula in spontaneously breathing patient

    ii)   Oxygen flow (10 L/min) through the suction port in asleep patient

    iii) **Preoxygenation is critically important when performing asleep fiberoptic intubation.**

Give oxygen by nasal cannula while performing fiberoptic intubation.

7) **Performing fiberoptic intubation**

  a) Position OR table so that the operator of the fiberoptic scope is able to keep the scope taut, to maximize the coronal plane rotational control.

  b) Suction oropharynx gently.

  c) Place well-lubricated intubating airway in the midline.

    i)   If patient tolerates this well, then there is adequate anesthesia to the oropharynx.

    ii)   Alternatively, test the adequacy of oropharynx analgesia with the tongue depressor

        (1)   Patient should not have any gag reflex prior to the procedure start.

  d) Ask assistant to pull the tongue gently and give jaw thrust.

    i)   This maneuver is not always needed but will facilitate glottic exposure by increasing pharyngeal space by elevating the tongue and epiglottis away from the posterior pharyngeal wall.

  e) Insert the fiberoptic scope through the ETT.

  f) Secure the tube with the tape at the proximal portion of the flexible portion of the scope.

  g) Insert the distal tip of the scope in the middle of the patient's mouth or in the nostril (if using nasal approach).

    i)   Once the FOB is inserted into the patient, look though the eyepiece or watch the video monitor.

    ii)   As the FOB is advanced, the tip of the airway and the patient's soft palate and uvula will come in view.

    iii) Slowly anteflex (thumb down) the tip of the scope until you visualize the epiglottis or the glottis.

    iv) Advance the tip under the epiglottis until cords come into the view.

    v)   Once the vocal cords are identified, keep them in the middle of the screen by fine adjustments of rotation of the body of FOB and manipulations of the tip control lever as FOB is being advanced through the cords.

    vi) Advance the scope until you see carina.

    vii) **Do not advance the scope further.**

    viii) Loosen the ETT from the proximal end of the fiberoptic scope and advance it carefully over the shaft of the FOB into the airway.

    ix) Stop advancing once the ETT is 22 to 24 cm at the teeth or about 3 to 4 cm above the carina.

    x)   Withdraw the FOB.

    xi) Inflate the cuff.

    xii) Connect ventilator circuit.

    xiii) Reconfirm the correct placement by presence of end-tidal CO_2.

⟲ READ
➤ MORE

Atlas of anesthesia procedures: awake fiber optic intubation, Chapter 155, page 1103

Nasal fiberoptic intubation may be easier because the pathway to the airway is more direct.

Jaw thrust will improve your view. Keeping the scope "taut" at all times will improve the maneuverability.

    h) Induce general anesthesia if patient is awake.

    i) If positioning a double-lumen endotracheal tube, it is essential to identify tracheal rings
        i) They will be complete anteriorly, to guide to left or right main bronchus.

8) **Difficulties and troubleshooting**

    a) **Inability to advance FOB into the trachea**

        i) **Uncooperative patient**

            (1) Consider optimizing sedation and topical analgesia.

            (2) Consider if this could be done with the patient anesthetized.

        ii) **Poor visualization**

            (1) **Scope is foggy**

                (a) Prior to starting, put FOB into the warm solution (use the same warm bottle as for your ETT).

                (b) Use commercially available defogging solution.

                (c) Touch the distal end of the scope to buccal or other mucosa to clear it.

            (2) **Too many secretions or blood**

                (a) Administer antisialogogue early.

                (b) Suction the mouth prior to inserting the FOB.

                (c) Clean tip as necessary.

                (d) Secretions can be suctioned through the working channel of the FOB.

                    (i) Alternatively, one can insufflate oxygen through the suction channel to help keep secretions away and improve exposure.

                    (ii) Be aware of possible baroutrauma to lungs if FOB advanced through a narrowed airway, limiting the oxygen escape from the lungs.

Figure 24-5 Aintree Intubation Catheter

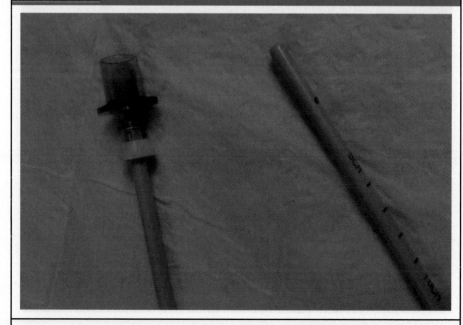

Proximal and distal ends of Aintree intubation catheter. Proximal end has a removable piece (shown attached), which allows for ventilation if necessary during exchange procedure. Catheter is usually 56 cm in length and has 4.7 mm internal diameter, which allows for a passage of small fibertoptic scope.

EQUIPMENT AND PROCEDURES

Figure 24-6 Using Aintree Intubation Catheter with Fiberoptic Scope

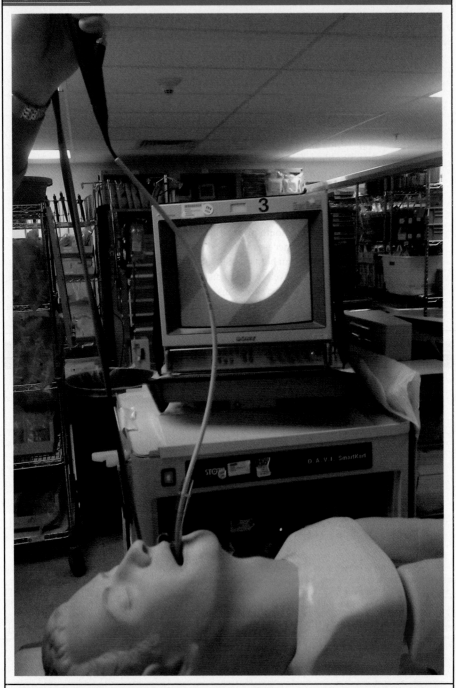

Aintree intubation catheter is inserted with fiberoptic bronchoscope (FOB) guidance through a laryngeal mask airway (LMA). After Aintree is placed in trachea, FOB and LMA are removed and endotracheal tube is inserted over Aintree. Placement is confirmed again with FOB through Aintree and then Aintree removed and circuit is connected to endotracheal tube.

iii)   Presence of a large, floppy epiglottis interferes with passage of FOB to the trachea.

(1)   Ask assistant to provide jaw thrust or pull the tongue forward to move epiglottis away from the posterior pharyngeal wall.

Assemble airway equipment in one place prior to starting fiberoptic intubation. Familiarize yourself with all the necessary equipment and its location during elective cases, so you are prepared in case of emergency.

b)   **Inability to advance ETT into the trachea over FOB**

i)   Too tight of a fit between FOB and ETT

(1)   Consider using larger ETT or smaller FOB.

(2)   Consider better lubrication.

ii)   Consider using a smaller ETT, as patient's airway might be too narrow.

iii)   Consider removing intubating airway.

iv)   Consider rotating ETT 90 degrees counterclockwise, as the most common site of ETT being caught is on right arytenoid cartilage.

v)   FOB is not taut.

(1)   Always keep FOB straight (one hand on proximal end of the scope with the thumb on the plane control lever and the other hand on the distal end of the scope, with hands maximally apart).

vi)   Consider using fiberoptic intubation in an Aintree ETT (Figs. 24-5 and 24-6).

c)   **Inability to remove FOB**

i)   Tip of the FOB gone through the Murphy's eye of the ETT.

(1)   Withdraw FOB and ETT together.

(a)   Take out FOB.

(b)   Repeat the procedure.

(2)   Pass the scope through the ETT under direct vision prior to initiation of intubation.

ii)   Not a straight insertion of the vocal cord (see Section 8.b.v.1)

iii)   Too tight of a fit of an unlubricated ETT.

Chapter Summary for Fiberoptic Laryngoscopy

Indications	History of difficult intubation, "cannot intubate, cannot ventilate" scenario, facial abnormalities, compromised airway (upper or lower obstruction), undesirable neck movement, high risk of dental injury
Contraindications	Lack of time if doing awake fiberoptic intubation, bleeding or secretions obstruct airway visualization or an uncooperative patient.
Equipment	Fiberoptic scope, light source, endotracheal tube and airway cart.
Complications	Damage to vocal cords (as ETT is inserted blindly over the FOB), failure to withdraw FOB due to tight fit, passage of FOB through Murphy's eye. Agitation and/or labile hemodynamic response due to inadequately prepared patient.

EQUIPMENT AND PROCEDURES

References

1. Rosenblatt WH, Sukhupragarn W. Airway management. In: Barash PG, ed. *Clinical Anesthesia*. 6th ed. Philadelphia, PA: Lippincott Williams & Wilkins; 2009: 773–782.
2. Wheeler M, Ovassapian A. Fiberoptic endoscopy-aided techniques. In: Hagberg CA, ed. *Benumof's Airway Management: Principles and Practice*. 2nd ed. Philadelphia, PA: Mosby, Inc.; 2007:399–433.
3. Simmons ST, Schleich AR. Airway regional anesthesia for awake fiberoptic intubation. *Reg Anesth Pain Med* 2002;27:180–192.
4. Stackhouse RA. Fiberoptic airway management. *Anesthesiol Clin North America* 2002;20: 933–951.
5. Unger RJ, Gallagher CJ. Dexmedetomidine sedation for awake fiberoptic intubation. *Semin Anesth Periop Med Pain* 2006;25:65–70.
6. Gil KSL. Fiber-optic intubation: tips from the ASA workshop. *Anesthesiol News Guide Airway Manag* 2009;35:8:91–98.
7. Johnson DM, From AM, Smith RB, et al. Endoscopic study of mechanisms of failure of endotracheal tube advancement in the trachea during awake fiberoptic orotracheal intubation. *Anesthesiology* 2005;102:910–914.
8. OLYMPUS BF TYPE 3C40 brochure from www.olympusamerica.com

MANAGEMENT AND THERAPY

25 Perioperative Fluid Management

Tzevan Poon, MD

Competent perioperative fluid management is of the utmost importance because intravascular fluids affect all physiological and biochemical processes essential for life. The goals of fluid management are to provide adequate delivery of oxygen to tissues (Fig. 25-1) and to maintain the environment necessary for proper function of cells and organ systems (Table 25-1).

Inadequate or inappropriate fluid therapy can lead to poor perfusion, tissue hypoxia, and worsening acidosis.

1) Determinants of O_2 delivery to tissue
   a) Generation of flow (cardiac output)
   b) O_2 content of blood
   c) **Preload** and **hemoglobin (Hb)** are most often manipulated by intravascular fluid therapy (Fig. 25-1).
      i) **A Key assumption is that the vascular system (i.e., vascular autoregulation and normal endothelial permeability) is intact.**

2) **Fluid compartments**
   a) Circulating blood volume makes up a small percentage of body weight and total body water (Fig. 25-2).
      i) Yet, one should appreciate the profound influence this small fraction has on homeostasis.
   b) Estimated circulating blood volume should be compared with blood loss during surgery or trauma.
   c) The type and amount of fluid therapy used to treat blood/fluid loss have a greater physiologic effect as the proportion of fluid therapy to circulating blood volume increases.

3) **Classical calculation of fluid requirements**

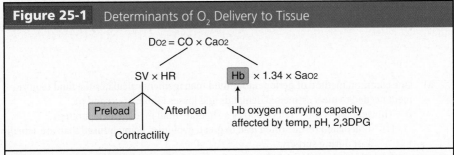

Figure 25-1 Determinants of O_2 Delivery to Tissue

$$D_{O2} = CO \times Ca_{O2}$$

$$SV \times HR \qquad \boxed{Hb} \times 1.34 \times Sa_{O2}$$

Preload — Afterload
Contractility

Hb oxygen carrying capacity affected by temp, pH, 2,3DPG

Ca_{O_2}, O_2 content of arterial blood; CO, cardiac output; DO_2, delivery of O_2; Hb, hemoglobin; HR, heart rate; Sa_{O_2}, arterial oxygen saturation; SV, stroke volume.

193

Table 25-1

Physiologic Variables and Blood Components Affected by Fluid Administration

Factors Affected by Fluid Therapy	Comments
Temperature	Patients are often hypothermic on arrival to the operating room. Fluid administration can cause or exacerbate hypothermia and acidosis. Hypothermia and acidosis significantly decrease platelet function and coagulation factor activity. Moderate to severe hypothermia in severely injured trauma patients is associated with higher morbidity and mortality, independent of other risk factors (1).
pH	NS has an average pH of 5.6 but can have a pH as low as 4.5. Large infusions of NS lead to hyperchloremic metabolic acidosis. LR has less effect on pH, but large volumes can also lead to acidosis.
Electrolytes	Electrolyte derangements occur with changes in pH, temperature, and large volume administration of crystalloid, colloid, and blood products.
RBC	Hemodilution, temperature, and pH affect RBC concentration and function. Stored PRBCs have lower pH and 2,3-DPG levels (decreased O_2 delivery) and have higher ammonia, PCO_2, and microaggregate levels. Massive transfusion of PRBCs can lead to hypocalcemia (due to citrate additive, though this is relatively transient) and hyperkalemia (due to RBC cell lysis).
Platelets and Coagulation factors	Hypothermia and acidosis often seen with massive fluid infusions can cause or further exacerbate platelet dysfunction and coagulopathy. Certain disease states may cause baseline platelet dysfunction (e.g., uremia, liver failure, preeclampsia/HELLP syndrome, massive trauma), and patients with these diseases may be more affected by fluid therapies.
Albumin	Albumin has important drug interactions and oncotic pressure effects. Preexisting hypoalbuminemia and concomitant third-spacing is worsened by the hemodilution effects of large infusions.
WBC	Artificial colloids (e.g., hetastarch) and LR significantly activate neutrophil activity and may play a pivotal role in resuscitation injury.
Inflammatory cytokines	Blood products and artificial colloids increase inflammatory cytokines. The effect is unclear but is an area of active research.

HELLP, hemolysis, elevated liver enzymes, low platelets; LR, lactate Ringer's; NS, normal saline; (P)RBC, (packed) red blood cell; WBC, white blood cells.

a) One common method of perioperative fluid management calculates the fluid requirement needed to meet estimated demands and losses (Table 25-2a and b).
    i) This method is often referred to as a "liberal" fluid management strategy.
        (1) Calculated results often lead to greater volumes being infused than are actually lost during surgery.
        (2) This approach can help one gain a sense of the magnitude of fluids needed during a case.

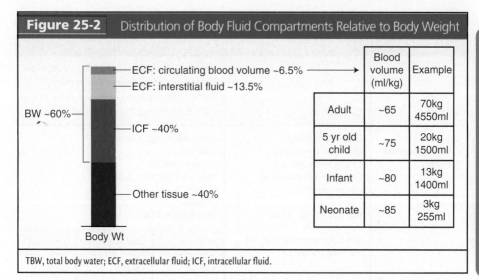

Figure 25-2 Distribution of Body Fluid Compartments Relative to Body Weight

	Blood volume (ml/kg)	Example
Adult	~65	70kg 4550ml
5 yr old child	~75	20kg 1500ml
Infant	~80	13kg 1400ml
Neonate	~85	3kg 255ml

ECF: circulating blood volume ~6.5%
ECF: interstitial fluid ~13.5%
BW ~60%
ICF ~40%
Other tissue ~40%
Body Wt

TBW, total body water; ECF, extracellular fluid; ICF, intracellular fluid.

MANAGEMENT AND THERAPY

(a) However, evidence from many different surgical populations suggests that following a "liberal" fluid infusion strategy may lead to higher cardiac, pulmonary, renal, gut, and wound complications than more "restrictive" fluid strategies (2).

(b) Thus, the use of classical fluid management results should be done with caution.

4) **Modern perioperative fluid management**

a) The current intraoperative environment requires a sophisticated, individualized approach to fluid management.

b) Clear goals should be used to determine the type of fluid, the amount, and the method in which it should be given (Fig. 25-3 and Table 25-3).

c) Fixed and dynamic variables influence fluid requirements and include:
   i) Patient
   ii) Anesthetic technique and intraoperative course
   iii) Type of surgery

d) Different data streams should be used as necessary to gather information.
   i) Functional reserve
   ii) Tissue oxygenation
   iii) Fluid responsiveness
   iv) Other hemodynamic variables

e) One must learn the strengths and weaknesses associated with each monitor.
   i) Avoid over reliance on any one.

f) Taken together, "goal-directed," patient and procedure-oriented fluid management approaches have been shown to decrease morbidity and mortality in a wide range of populations (2–6).

5) **Types of IV fluids**

a) See next chapter "Crystalloids and Colloids".

6) **Pearls and pitfalls for select surgical populations**

a) **Neonates**
   i) Require dextrose (D5) and should go no more than 3 to 4 hours without fluids.
   ii) Monitor blood glucose levels.
   iii) Limit fluids with a mini-infusion device.
   iv) Remove all air bubbles from lines to prevent any possibility of air emboli.

Table 25-2a

Intraoperative Fluid Requirements based on Classical Physical Indexes

Factors	Calculation	Example: Richard is a 65-y.o., 70 kg Man Undergoing Small Bowel Resection, NPO for 10 h with 24-h Bowel Prep. (all Values for Crystalloid Administration)		
Step 1 Calculate preoperative fluid deficit	Use the "4-2-1 rule" = 4 mL/kg for the 1st 10 kg 2 mL/kg for the 2nd 10 kg 1 mL/kg for the remaining kg × no. of hours NPO (shortcut: wt + 40 = mL/h)	4(10) + 2(10) + 1(50) = 110 mL/h or via shortcut 70 + 40 = 110 mL/h Thus, 110 × 10hr NPO = *1,100 mL* GI losses from bowel prep ~**900 mL** **Total deficit = 2,000**		
	Give ½ of volume in 1st hour, and 2nd ½ over the next 2 h.	**1st hour**	**2nd hour**	**3rd hour**
		1,000 mL	500 mL	500 mL
Step 2 Estimate compensatory volume expansion from anesthetic technique	6–8 mL/kg	~500	~500	~500
Step 3 Calculate maintenance	Use the "4-2-1 rule"	110	110	110
Step 4 Calculate insensible, third space losses	Minimal tissue trauma = 0–2 mL/kg/h Moderate tissue trauma = 2–4 mL/kg/h Severe tissue trauma or large exposed surface area = 4–8 mL/kg/h	4 × 70 = 280	6 × 70 = 420	6 × 70 = 420
Step 5 Estimate blood loss	1:3 ratio replacement for blood: crystalloid 1:1 ratio replacement for blood: colloid	0	~100 EBL = 300	~200 EBL= 600
Step 6 UOP		100	110	75
	Totals (mL/h)	1,990	1,940	2,205

EBL, estimated blood loss; GI, gastrointestinal; MAP, mean arterial pressure; NPO, nothing per os; NS, normal saline; UOP, urine output.

MANAGEMENT AND THERAPY

Table 25-2b

Intraoperative Fluid Requirements based on Classical Physical Indexes

Guidelines to Consider if Giving Fluid Therapy Based on Calculated Fluid Requirements

Use sound medical judgment regarding the patient's current condition, medical history, and type of surgery and anesthetic when considering the type and amount of fluid to give.

In general, try to maintain MAP within ±20% of baseline; UOP 0.5 mL–1 mL/kg/h; core temperature 36°C–37°C.

Be aware that even if vital signs continue to be around normal limits, this may not fully account for blood or insensible losses, especially in healthy patients with robust compensatory mechanisms

Use fluids that can be used for volume expansion for intraoperative maintenance. Do not use 1/2NS or other fluids with less osmolarity as it will further increase interstitial fluid gain with little or no addition to effective intravascular circulating volume.

↳ READ
MORE

Pregnancy and
HTN, Chapter 98,
page 701

Dextrose
containing
fluids should
be avoided
in patients
with neuro-
logic injury or
undergoing
intracranial
neurosurgical
procedures.

b) **Preeclampsia**
  i) Patients usually have notable fluid deficits and decreased uretoplacental blood flow (9).
  ii) Despite intravascular volume depletion, these patients **are at risk for pulmonary edema**.
  iii) Randomized-controlled trials to guide fluid management are lacking.
  iv) Most practitioners limit crystalloid administration to 1 to 2 L.
     (1) Some use colloid prior to spinal anesthesia.
     (2) Arterial BP monitoring should be considered in patients with severe preeclampsia.
     (3) Other invasive monitoring (e.g. PA catheter, TEE) may be helpful to guide fluid management in patients with renal failure in the setting of severe preeclampsia.

c) **Cerebral edema and/or intracranial neurosurgical patients**
  i) Dextrose containing fluids are contraindicated because of worse neurological outcome (10).
     (1) Hyperglycemia and oxidative stress leads to increased glycolytic metabolism and toxic derivative production
     (2) The optimal level of glucose is unknown, but it is generally accepted that values >180 mg/dL should be treated with insulin.

d) **Congestive heart failure (CHF)**
  i) Judicious fluid management should be the rule in CHF patients.
  ii) Expect third space redistribution to stress the heart in the first 24 to 96 hours post surgery.
  iii) Consider invasive monitoring and Intensive Care Unit (ICU) post-operative care.

e) **Acute respiratory distress syndrome (ARDS)**
  i) Patients with ARDS may need emergency surgical services.
  ii) Fluid restrictive therapy has been shown to reduce morbidity in these patients in the ICU setting (10). However, this study had goals of CVP < 4 mm Hg or PAOP < 8 mmHg, which may be difficult to achieve.
  iii) A fluid restrictive approach may be beneficial, but this may be complicated by other factors and conditions.
     (1) For example, a septic patient with ARDS who needs an emergent exploratory laparotomy due to necrotic bowel may necessitate more fluid resusciation.
  iv) Invasive monitoring should be considered to guide fluid therapy.

| **Figure 25-3** | The Feedback Loop of Continuous Goal-Directed Fluid Management |

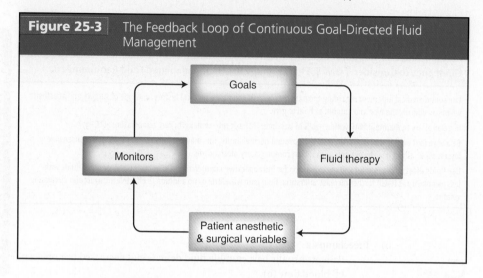

   f) **Lung resection**

      i) Although multifactorial in origin, postpneumonectomy pulmonary edema (PPE) rates increase with excessive fluid therapy (3).

      ii) Minimize fluids to approximately 1.5 L for an entire case.

        (1) Use vasopressors intraoperatively as needed.

      iii) Fluid restriction may also be beneficial during the first 72 hours post-operatively.

      iv) Blood transfusion should be avoided.

        (1) It is linked to worse perioperative pulmonary inflammatory changes and increased risk for PPE (3).

   g) **Anuric renal failure**

      i) These patients are unable to compensate for fluid overload and are often challenging.

      ii) Consider invasive BP monitoring with an arterial line.

      iii) Central venous access

READ MORE

Diseases of the liver and biliary tract, Chapter 77, page 551

        (1) If deemed necessary, consider consultation with a vascular surgeon before cannulating upper body central veins as these may be sites for future arteriovenous fistulae (AVF).

        (2) No IV catheters or BP cuffs on should be placed on same side as an arteriovenous fistula unless absolutely necessary.

          (a) Every effort should be made to protect patients' fistula when anesthetized.

   h) **Liver failure/hepatic transplantation**

      i) Patients often have multisystem organ dysfunction.

      ii) A wide variety of possible complications and comorbidities may be present (11).

        (1) Cerebral edema

        (2) Hyperdynamic ventricular function

        (3) Cardiomyopathy

        (4) Pulmonary hypertension

        (5) Hepatopulmonary syndrome

        (6) Hepatorenal syndrome

Table 25-3

Continuous Goal-Directed Fluid Management: Expanded View of Factors Involved in Decision Making

Fixed and Dynamic Variables	Monitors and Other Data Streams	Overall Goals of Fluid Management	Fluid Therapies

• Cardiac function
• Vascular function
• Pulmonary function
• Renal function
• Preoperative intra-vascular volume depletion
• Anesthetic plan: technique and phar-macologic agents
• Type of IV access and other resources avail-able (fluid warmers, rapid infusers, etc.)
• Patient positioning
• Type of surgery
• Anatomic changes during surgery (e.g., thoracotomy, pneu-moperitoneum, etc.)
• Duration of surgery
• Outcomes data from prior studies per-taining to patient or surgery.
	• Preoperative studies
	• Preoperative functional status
	• Physical exam findings
	• NIBP
	• Dynamic A-line BP and respiratory variability (7)
	• Pulse oximetry respi-ratory variability (8)
	• UOP
	• Temperature probes
	• Intraoperative lab data
	  ○ ABG
	  ○ MVO2 saturation
	  ○ Electrolytes
	  ○ Lactate
	  ○ Coagulation labs/TEG
	• CVP
	• PAC
	• Continuous MVO$_2$ sat
	• Continuous pulse Hb monitoring
	• TEE
		• Adequate deliv-ery of oxygen (DLO2)
		  ○ Preload
		  ○ Adequate Hb
		  ○ Cardiac indices
		  ○ SvO$_2$ sat >65%
		• Normothermia
		• Acceptable:
		  ○ pH
		  ○ coagulation
		  ○ electrolyte
		  ○ environment
		  ○ glucose levels
		• Unique require-ments of surgery or patient.
		• Prevention of fluid excess (possibly leading to pulmonary edema or CHF)
			• Crystalloids
			• Colloids
			• PRBCs
			• FFP
			• Platelets
			• Fibrinogen
			• Electrolyte replacements
			• Choice of IV access
			• Rapid infusers/warmers

Accounting for and synthesizing the issues in this table enable a global perspective on the patient, the procedure, monitors, and the goals of fluid therapy.

ABG, arterial blood gas; A-line, arterial line; BP blood pressure; CHF, congestive heart failure; FFP, fresh frozen plasma; Hb, hemoglobin; NIBP, noninvasive blood pressure; MVO$_2$, mixed venous oxygen; PRBCs, packed red blood cells; TEE, transesoph-ageal echocardiogram; TEG, thromboelastogram; UOP, urine output.

(7) Effective circulating volume depletion
(8) Electrolyte perturbations
(9) Anemia
(10) Coagulopathy

READ MORE

Burn Injuries, Chapter 91, page 657

i) **Burns**

  i) These patients often have massive fluid requirements due to wide-spread loss of epidermal barrier and circulating oncotically active proteins

    ii)   The Parkland formula is frequently used as an *initial guide* for fluid requirements for burns >30% total body surface area:

        (1) **BSA (use % as whole number not as fraction) × wt (kg) × 4 = total mL over 24 hours.**

            (a) Give ½ of volume over 8 hours and second ½ over next 16 hours.

        (2) More importantly, titrate infusions to hemodynamic parameters or to a urine output of 0.5-1ml/kg/h or more.

    iii) Albumin is often given to replace large intravascular protein losses from injury after the first 24 hours.

        (1) However, timing and amount vary widely among institutions.

  j) **Liposuction**

    i)   The "tumescent technique" consists of infiltration of the surgical region with very dilute lidocaine (1 mg/ml) and very dilute epinephrine (1:1,000,000 = 1 mg/L) in large volumes of saline.

    ii) The area becomes swollen (tumescent) which helps minimize bleeding, decreases lidocaine absorption, and achieves effective local anesthesia in the surgical region.

    iii) Maximum lidocaine dose for this technique is up to 55 mg/kg versus 7 mg/kg maximum for 1% to 2% lidocaine with 1:100,000 epinephrine (12).

    iv) **Minimize any additional fluids that may be given intravenously**

    v)   Cardiopulmonary complications may be increased when liposuction volumes exceed 5 L due to large fluid shifts.

  k) **Laparoscopic gastric bypass surgery**

    i)   Transient intraoperative oliguria frequently develops due to increased SVR and compression of intra-abdominal renal cortices and the inferior vena cava secondary to pneumoperitoneum (13)

        (1) Effects are reversed when pneumoperitoneum is abolished.

    ii) A liberal management strategy is often used for these patients. However, care must be taken to avoid perioperative cardiopulmonary complications.

  l) **Massive trauma**

    i)   Patients require close attention in order to avoid the "Lethal Triad" of acidosis, hypothermia, and coagulopathy.

↳ READ
MORE

Trauma,
and massive
transfusion,
Chapter 29,
page 220

Chapter Summary for Perioperative Fluid Management

Overview	Management of perioperative fluid infusions is often best served by a goal directed approach. This may be straightforward or highly complex depending on the patient and the procedure.
Key Points	Classical calculations on fluid requirements may be helpful in giving an overall sense of the volume needed, but strict adherence with less regard to the other physiologic variables (e.g., respiratory variation in pulse pressure, arterial blood gas results, type of surgery, etc.) may lead to over-infusion.
	The timing of when to give fluids, how much, and how fast to give it should be the primary concern. Choosing the type of fluid among the various volume replacements available is important; however, all intravenous infusions can adversely affect homeostatic variables when given in excessive amounts (Table 25-1).

References

1. Beekley AC. Damage control resuscitation: A sensible approach to the exsanguinating surgical patient. *Crit Care Med* 2008;36(7 Suppl):S267–S274.
2. Holte K, Sharrock NE, Kehlet H. Pathophysiology and clinical implications of perioperative fluid excess. *Br J Anaesth* 2002;89:622–632.
3. Parquin F, Marchal M, Mehiri S, et al. Post-pneumonectomy pulmonary edema: analysis and risk factors. *Eur J Cardiothorac Surg* 1996;10:929–933.
4. Josh GP. Intraoperative fluid restriction improves outcome after major elective gastrointestinal surgery. *Anesth Analg* 2005:101;601–605.
5. Rosenthal MH. Intraoperative fluid management—what and how much? *Chest* 1999;115:106S–112S.
6. Wiedemann HP, Wheeler AP, Bernard GR, et al. Comparison of two fluid-management strategies in acute lung injury. *N Engl J Med* 2006;354(24):2564–2567.
7. Michard F, Teboul JL. Using heart-lung interactions to assess fluid responsiveness during mechanical ventilation. *Crit Care* 2000;4:282–289.
8. Desebbe O, Cannesson M. Using ventilation-induced plethysmographic variations to optimize patient fluid status. *Curr Opin Anaesthesiol* 2008;21(6):772–778.
9. Farragher R, Datta S. Recent advances in obstetric anesthesia. *J Anesth* 2003;17(1):30–41.
10. Prakash A, Matta BF. Hyperglycemia and neurological injury. *Curr Opin Anaesthesiol* 2008;21(5):565–569.
11. Ozer Y, Klink JR. Anesthetic management of hepatic transplantation. *Curr Opin Anaesthesiol* 2008;21:391–400.
12. Kacuera IJ, Lambert TJ, Klein JA, et al. Liposuction: contemporary issues for the anesthesiologist. *J Clin Anesth* 2006;18(5):379–387.
13. McGlinch BP, Que FG, Nelson JL. Perioperative care of patients undergoing bariatric surgery. *Mayo Clinic Proc* 2006;81(10 Suppl):S25–S33.

MANAGEMENT AND THERAPY

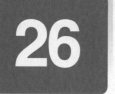

Crystalloids and Colloids

Tzevan Poon, MD

Crystalloids and colloids should be thought of not only as volume replacements but also as pharmacologic agents, each with a different composition and physiological effects. It is these unique properties that have led to decades of research and often heated debates.

1) Crystalloids
   a) **Crystalloids commonly used for resuscitation (Tables 26-1 and 26-2).**
      i) **Normal saline (NS)**
         (1) Lower pH, higher osmolarity, and higher chloride content than plasma
            (a) Large volume administration (>2 to 3 L) leads to hyperchloremic metabolic acidosis.
               (i) This can take hours to days to resolve in patients with acute and/or chronic renal failure.
               (ii) Lactated Ringers (LR) and Normosol cause less perturbation to chloride and acid-base homeostasis.
      ii) **Lactated Ringers (LR)**
         (1) The lactate in LR is rapidly converted into pyruvate and shuttled into the Krebs cycle mostly by liver cells.
            (a) During severe liver failure or overwhelming lactic acidosis, *net* conversion is diminished.
         (2) LR contains a small amount of potassium.
      iii) **Normosol**
         (1) Currently, more expensive than other crystalloids but less expensive than colloids.
         (2) A reasonable, balanced choice for resuscitation crystalloid for critically ill patients who have severely diminished compensatory mechanisms
         (3) Normosol also contains a small amount of potassium.
      iv) **Replacement of intravascular volume with crystalloid**
         (1) Classically, it has been taught that approximately three to four liters of crystalloid (versus only one liter of colloid) should be replaced for every liter of blood loss (1).
         (2) Recent human data has shown that tissue equilibration may be slower than previously thought (20 to 30 minutes after infusion) and that this process is complex and dynamic (2).
         (3) Furthermore, robust clinical trial data have shown that titrating crystalloids and colloids to similar hemodynamic goals leads to a crystalloid:colloid ratio of only 1.3 to 1.6:1.0.
            (a) This ratio is stable over hours to days (3,4)

Table 26-1

Characteristics of Commonly Used Crystalloids by pH, Osmolarity, and Ion Content

Crystalloid	pH	mOsm/L	Na$^+$	Cl$^-$	Ca^{2+}	lactate$^-$	K$^+$	Mg^{2+}	gluconate$^-$	acetate$^-$
NS (0.9% Saline)	5.6 (4.5–7.0)	308[a]	154[b]	154						
LR	6.6 (6.0–7.5)	274	130	109	3	28	4			
Normosol	7.4 (6.5–7.6)	295	140	98			5	3	23	27

[a]Normal range of human plasma osmolarity is approximately 275 to 295 mOsm/L, whereas, at the extremes of overhydration and dehydration, plasma osmolarity can reach limits of 260 and 310 mOsm/L, respectively.
[b]All units of ions are mEq/L.
LR, lactated Ringers; NS, normal saline.

b) **Additional forms of crystalloid** are available and have a diverse array of uses.
   i) Various mixtures of ½ NS
      (1) D5 or 20 mEq/L of KCl may be added.
      (2) Used as maintenance fluids before and after surgery
      (3) These hypotonic forms provide minimal intravascular volume effect and are usually not used intraoperatively
   ii) Isotonic sodium bicarbonate (300 mEq/L) in D5W plus n-acetylcysteine.
      (1) May be used to prevent contrast-induced nephropathy
      (2) May be superior to saline plus n-acetylcysteine (5).
   iii) Hypertonic 3% or 7.5% Saline
      (1) Commonly administered to patients with brain injury to decrease intracranial pressure (ICP).
      (2) Thought to osmotically promote outflow of brain interstitial fluid from the enclosed calvaria.
      (3) May be more effective than mannitol and has a good safety profile (6).
         (a) Imaging and autopsy studies have not shown evidence of central pontine myelinolysis from this therapy (7,8).
      (4) Hypertonic saline may be given through a central line as a 250 mL bolus every 6 hours as needed.
         (a) Gradually achieve a plasma sodium goal of 145 to 155 mEq/L and an osmolarity of 310 to 320 mOsm/L.
            (i) Increase plasma sodium no more than 10 to 20 mEq/L/24 h.
   iv) Highly concentrated 23.4% sodium chloride
      (1) May emergently reverse transtentorial herniation and temporize the situation until more invasive interventions can be performed (e.g., craniectomy).
      (2) Mechanism of action is similar to lower concentration hypertonic saline administration.
      (3) May lead to transient hypotension after initial bolus (i.e., seconds to minutes).
         (a) However, heart rate, mean arterial pressure, and cerebral perfusion pressure generally remain stable.
         (b) ICP may continue to decrease for up to 24 hours (9).
      (4) Given centrally in 30 or 60 mL boluses over 15 to 20 minutes.

Table 26-2

Characteristics of Commonly Used Crystalloids by Chemical Components

Crystalloid	Composition by Compound and Mass				
Normal Saline (NS) (0.9% Saline)	Sodium chloride NaCl 900 mg[a]				
Lactated Ringers (LR)	Sodium chloride NaCl 600 mg	Potassium chloride KCl 30 mg	Sodium lactate[b] $NaC_3H_5O_3$ 310 mg	Calcium chloride dihydrate $CaCl_2 \cdot H_2O$ 20 mg	
Normosol	Sodium chloride NaCl 526 mg	Potassium chloride KCl 30 mg		Sodium gluconate[c] $Na C_6H_{11}O_7$ 502 mg	Sodium acetate[d] $Na C_2H_3O_2$ 222 mg	Magnesium chloride hexahydrate $MgCl_2 \cdot 6H_2O$ 30 mg

LR, lactated Ringers; NS, normal saline.

[a] All masses given are per 100 mL of sterile water.

[b] Under normal circumstances, lactate is converted to pyruvate and shuttled back into the Krebs cycle by lactate dehydrogenase (LDH), an enzyme predominantly found in the liver. There are also other isoenzymes in organs such as the kidneys, striated muscle, lungs, and heart.

[c] The majority of parenteral gluconate is excreted unchanged by the kidneys (60% to 80%), with much of the rest converted into CO_2 during the production of adenosine triphosphate (ATP) or into glucose through gluconeogenesis.

[d] Acetate is mostly oxidized by the liver into CO_2 by way of acetyl-CoA during ATP production (~70%), while a lesser percentage is recycled into ketone bodies or glucose through gluconeogenesis.

2) Colloids
   a) **Provides** oncotic pressure **effects in addition to volume.**
   b) **Can be further classified as protein or nonprotein colloids.**
      i) **Protein colloids**
         (1) Human serum albumin
         (2) Modified gelatin solutions
      ii) **Nonprotein colloids**
         (1) Dextrans
         (2) Hydroxyethyl starches (HES)
   c) **Colloids commonly used for resuscitation (Table 26-3)**
      i) **Albumin**
         (1) The most expensive resuscitation fluid with the exception of blood products.
         (2) Well tolerated, and not associated with anaphylaxis, increased infection, or coagulopathy (aside from hemodilution effects) even at high volumes
      ii) **Gelatins**
         (1) Not sold in the United States
         (2) Similar in safety to albumin but with much shorter effects (3-6 hours) (10,11).
      iii) **Dextrans**
         (1) Have plasma expanding volume effects.
            (a) Also have robust anticoagulant properties.
         (2) They have a low but relatively higher association with anaphylactoid reactions than other colloids (12).
         (3) Currently not used for resuscitation
         (4) Dextrans may be used during vascular cases such as free muscle flap transfers to potentially improve perfusion and decrease risk of graft thrombosis.
      iv) **Hydroxyethyl Starch**
         (1) Available in the United States as medium molecular weight pentastarch (200 kDa) and high molecular weight hetastarch (450 kDa).
         (2) Pentastarch is less commonly available due to concerns regarding increased risk of acute kidney injury in diabetic patients (4).

Doses of hydroxyethyl starch in excess of 20 mL/kg/d may have an anticoagulant effect.

         (3) Hetastarch
            (a) Generally safe for most patients, although there have been some safety concerns
            (b) Clinically idiosyncratic anticoagulant effects may occur in some patients receiving hetastarch in **doses >20 mL/kg/d (approximately 1.5 L for a 75 kg patient)** (12, 13).
            (c) Hetastarch molecules are thought to bind to factor VIII, von Willebrand factor, and fibrinogen.
               (i) This leads to decreased function among these factors and a reduction in platelet aggregation
      v) **Blood products**
         (1) Have oncotic effects that expand intravascular volume similar to colloids
   d) **Possible benefits of colloids**
      i) Require less volume than crystalloids to maintain the same effective arterial circulating volume.
      ii) Remain intravascularly for a much longer time period than crystalloids
      iii) May lead to less total body and organ edema
      iv) Possible greater improvement than crystalloids in myocardial contractility, tissue oxygen tension, and microcirculation in organs such as bowel after anastomosis (15,16).
      v) Possible better clinical outcomes during resuscitation, although demonstrating a beneficial effect of colloids on morbidity and mortality has proven difficult (11).

Table 26-3

Characteristics of Commonly Used Perioperative Colloids for Resuscitation

Colloid	Description	Content	Intravascular Half-life (12)	Comments
Albumin	Human serum albumin, 584 amino acids. Average MW = ~690 kDa Pasteurized through alcohol fractionation and heat treated at 60°C for 10 h	**Albumin 5%** albumin 12.5 g in 250 mL Contains Na ~145 mEq/L; K content <2 mEq/L. 5% is isotonic to plasma	~16 hours	Generally safe at any volume infused (outside of dilution effects). No clear link between albumin transfusion and infection risk. Albumin 25% comes as 12.5 g in 50 mL. It expands circulating plasma volume 4–5 times its volume but is not commonly used due to its unpredictable volume and electrolyte effects, especially in hypovolemic patients.
Hetastarch	Multipolymer chain polysaccharide that differs in C2, C3, or C6 position. Average MW = ~450 kDa $(C_6H_{10}O_5)_m(C_2H_4O)_n$	**Hespan 6%** pH 5.5; hetastarch 3 g in 500 mL NS: Na 154 mEq/L, Cl 154 mEq/L **Hextend 6%** pH 5.9; hetastarch 3 g in 500 mL solution similar to LR In mEq/L: Na 143, Cl 124, K 3, lactate 28, Ca 5, Mg 0.9. Excreted mainly by kidneys	~10 hours to days (?)	Higher doses to lead to decreased factor VIII, vWF, and fibrinogen, as well as reductions in platelet aggregation. Limit use to ~20 mL/kg/24 h, especially in patients at risk for coagulopathy or in those whom bleeding would be poorly tolerated (patients with coronary artery disease, diabetes, vasculopathies). Hextend may have less coagulopathic side effects than Hespan.[15]
Blood Products	Blood products have similar volume effects in the intravascular space as colloids. Blood products should be used to treat blood component deficits and should not be given purely for volume expansion purposes due to scarcity, high cost, side effects, and risk of adverse reactions.			

HES, hydroxyethyl starch; LR, lactated Ringers; vWF, von Willebrand factor.

3) **Crystalloids versus colloids in primary resuscitation**
   a) **Controversy and the emergence of meta-analyses**
      i) Risk and benefit analyses regarding crystalloids vs. colloids are controversial despite more than sixty clinical trials over three decades (18).
      ii) Three issues stand out from the key meta-analyses of trial data (10,18–22).
         (1) The majority of trials available for analysis were of poor methodological quality. Most are underpowered, poorly randomized, lacking allocation concealment, and/or not double-blinded.
         (2) A large percentage of trials analyzed from the literature were performed before 1980 and used outmoded fluid resuscitation strategies. For example, titrating albumin boluses to plasma albumin levels.
         (3) Different meta-analyses authors reached different conclusions and recommendations despite overall similar findings.

4) **The saline versus albumin fluid evaluation (SAFE) trial**
   a) High quality, well powered, multicenter, double-blinded randomized, controlled study.

Consider caution in using albumin in patients with traumatic brain injury.

   i) Designed to address the safety of albumin administration (3).
   ii) Albumin did not confer overall mortality benefit or harm to a large representative group of critically ill patients.
      (1) Did not increase or decrease the risk of organ failure, duration of mechanical ventilation, or duration of renal replacement therapy.
   iii) A statistically significant increase in mortality in traumatic brain injury patients was observed.
      (1) An ad hoc follow-up study showed that this increase involved only the most severely injured (GCS 3-8) patients (23).

5) **Rational use of crystalloids and colloids**
   a) Crystalloids should usually be the initial fluids used for resuscitation.

READ MORE

Perioperative fluid management, Chapter 25, page 193

      i) They are inexpensive, readily available, safe, and effective for intravascular volume replacement in a wide variety of surgical and critically ill populations.
   b) Nonprotein colloids may be considered second line volume agents due to cost and possible anticoagulant effects.
   c) Albumin may be considered a third-line agent.
   d) Despite being equivalent in terms of mortality and other major endpoints, there continues to be a large gap in our knowledge on what indication is best suited for colloid.

Surgeries involving large (and sometimes unexpected) amounts of blood loss will often use not just one type of fluid but a combination of crystalloids and colloids, including blood products.

      i) Colloid may be considered if a large amount of crystalloid (>3 to 4 L) has already been given and the patient still appears intravascularly depleted.
      ii) Elderly or extremely frail patients (with plasma albumin <2.5 g/dL) might not tolerate large volumes of fluid resuscitation and may benefit from early colloid administration.
      iii) Giving albumin in special situations may provide benefits to certain patients such as:
         (1) After paracentesis with >4 L of ascites removed.
         (2) After plasmapheresis
         (3) Resuscitation in the setting of nephrotic syndrome or severe diarrhea with albumin <2 g/dL
   e) The choice to give crystalloid or colloid is only one factor among many other considerations when administering fluid therapy.

Chapter Summary for Crystalloids and Colloids

Crystalloids	Crystalloids are solutions of salts and electrolytes that are commonly used for intravascular volume expansion. Classically, 3–4 L crystalloid are administered for every liter of blood loss, although new data suggests this might be excessive.
Colloids	Colloids are solutions that contain large molecules and provide oncotic pressure in addition to intravascular volume. Colloids are categorized as protein (albumin or gelatin solutions) and nonprotein (dextrans or HES). Usually, 1 L of colloid is administered for every liter of blood loss.
Key Points	The pharmacologic properties of crystalloids and colloids are important to consider in addition to their volume effects. Rigorous randomized controlled evidence suggests that the ratio of the volume effects for blood to albumin to crystalloid is not 1:1:3 as has been traditionally taught, but approximately 1:1:1.4. Normal saline and albumin have been shown to be essentially equally safe from a mortality standpoint in wide variety of critically ill populations. In reality, many complex surgical cases involve large fluid requirements to maintain adequate flow and vascular homeostasis may require a combination of crystalloid and colloid (including blood products). Areas of uncertainty remain on the use of colloids in special populations.

References

1. Lamke LO, Liljedahl SO. Plasma volume changes after infusion of various plasma expanders. *Resuscitation* 1976;5:93–102.
2. Svensen CH, et al. Arteriovenous differences in plasma dilution and the distribution kinetics of lactated ringer's solution. *Anes Analg* 2009;108:128–133.
3. The SAFE Study Investigators. A comparison of albumin and saline for fluid resuscitation in the intensive care unit. *N Engl J Med* 2004;350:2247–2256.
4. Brunkhorst FM, et al. Intensive insulin therapy and pentastarch resuscitation in severe sepsis. *N Engl J Med* 2008;358(2):125–139.
5. Meier P, et al. Sodium bicarbonate-based hydration prevents contrast-induced nephropathy: a meta-analysis. *BMC Med* 2009;7:23.
6. Wakai A, Roberts IG, Schierhout G. Mannitol for acute traumatic brain injury. *Cochrane Database Syst Rev* 2007;1:CD001049.
7. Khanna S, et al. Use of hypertonic saline in the treatment of severe refractory posttraumatic intracranial hypertension in pediatric traumatic brain injury. *Crit Care Med* 2000;28: 1144–1151.
8. Peterson B, et al. Prolonged hypernatremia controls elevated intracranial pressure in head-injured pediatric patients. *Crit Care Med* 2000;28:1136–1143.
9. Koenig MA, et al. Reversal of transtentorial herniation with hypertonic saline. *Neurology* 2008;70:1023–1029.
10. Perel P, Roberts IG. Colloids versus crystalloids for fluid resuscitation in critically ill patients. *Cochrane Database Syst Rev* 2007;4:CD000567.
11. Rizoli SB. Crystalloids and colloids in trauma resuscitation: a brief overview of the current debate. *J Trauma* 2003;54:S82–S88.
12. Boldt J. Fluid choice for resuscitation of the trauma patient: a review of the physiological, pharmacological, and clinical evidence. *Can J Anesth* 2004;51(5):500–513.
13. Warren BB, Durieux ME. Hydroxyethyl starch: safe or not? *Anesth Analg* 1997;84:206–212.
14. Gan TJ, et al. Hextend, a physiologically balanced plasma expander for large volume use in major surgery: a randomized phase III clinical trial. *Anesth Analg* 1999;88:992–998.
15. Hankeln K, et al. Comparison of hydroxyethyl starch and lactated Ringer's solution on hemodynamics and oxygen transport of critically ill patients in prospective crossover studies. *Crit Care Med* 1989;17:133–135.
16. Kimberger O, et al. Goal-directed colloid administration improves the microcirculation of healthy and perianastomotic colon. *Anesthesiology* 2009;110:496–504.
17. Yim JM, et al. Albumin and nonprotein colloid solution use in US academic health centers. *Arch Intern Med* 1995;155:2450–2455.
18. Velanovich V. Crystalloid versus colloid fluid resuscitation: a meta-analysis of mortality. *Surgery* 1989;105:65–71.
19. Bisonni RS, Holtgrave DR, Lawler F, Marley DS. Colloids versus crystalloids in fluid resuscitation: an analysis of randomized controlled trials. *J Fam Pract* 1991;32:387–390.
20. Schierhout G, Roberts I. Fluid resuscitation with colloid or crystalloid solutions in critically ill patients: a systematic review of randomised trials. *BMJ* 1998;316:961–964.
21. Choi PTL, et al. Crystalloids vs. colloids in fluid resuscitation: a systematic review. *Crit Care Med* 1999;27(1):200–210.
22. Wilkes MM, Navickis RJ. Patient survival after human albumin administration: a meta-analysis of randomized, controlled trials. *Ann Intern Med* 2001;135:149–164.
23. The SAFE Study Investigators. Saline or albumin for fluid resuscitation in patients with traumatic brain injury. *N Engl J Med* 2007;357(9): 874–884.

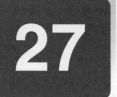

27 Blood Component Therapy

Andrea J. Fuller, MD

Administration of blood components is often necessary in the perioperative period. Blood component therapy should be used to treat specific indications, bearing in mind the potential complications associated with transfusion. Vigilance is absolutely critical as complications are most often due to human error.

1) Pretransfusion testing
   a) When preparing to transfuse blood, draw a blood sample from the patient and send it to the blood bank.
   b) **Type and screen**
      i) Determines the ABO type and Rhesus (Rh) factor and screen the **sample for** common antibodies.
      ii) **ABO type**
         (1) Determined by cell surface glycoprotein antigens present on the RBC surface
         (2) Patients may be type A, B, AB, or O.
         (3) Type O patients lack type A and B antigens.
      iii) **Rh factor**
         (1) 85% of patients have the D antigen from the Rh group and are Rh positive.
         (2) Patients who are Rh negative are at risk of alloimmunization (synthesis of antibodies against foreign antigens) when exposed to the D antigen.
      iv) **Antibody screen**
         (1) Commercially available RBC are mixed with the patient's blood in order to detect antibodies with the potential to cause hemolysis.
   c) **Type and cross**
      i) Cross-matching the blood involves mimicking the transfusion by mixing the donor's RBC with the recipient's blood.
         (1) Ensures compatibility of donor and recipient blood samples.
   d) **Time to obtain blood**
      i) Type and screen can usually be done within 45 minutes and the cross-match within an additional 15 minutes.
      ii) If antibodies are present, these steps can take much longer, especially if the antibodies are uncommon.
   e) **Autologous blood donation**
      i) If time permits, patients may donate their own blood preoperatively.
      ii) Patients who elect to do autologous blood donation may become anemic and require iron and erythropoietic agents.
      iii) Autologous blood should be meticulously handled as human errors still occur with its administration.

If a patient requires emergent blood transfusion Type O, Rh negative blood can be given.

f) **Directed donor blood donation**
  i) A family member or friend may be designated by the patient to donate blood which may be used if needed, provided compatibility can be assured.
  ii) This technique does not decrease the incidence of transfusion-transmitted infection as the patient may not be aware of the donor's infection status.

2) **Packed red blood cells (PRBCs)**
  a) The purpose of PRBC transfusion is to increase the O_2 carrying capacity of the blood.
  b) The decision whether to transfuse PRBC is multifactorial. The patient's coexisting disease and risk of ongoing blood loss should be considered.
    i) For example, a patient with coronary artery disease will likely require transfusion at a lower threshold due to the need to maintain myocardial oxygen delivery.

The decision to transfuse PRBC depends on the potential for ongoing blood loss and the patient's coexisting medical conditions.

  c) **PRBC transfusion parameters**
    i) **There is no absolute laboratory value that necessitates blood transfusion.**
    ii) Transfusion is rarely indicated for hemoglobin concentrations >10 g/dL (1).
    iii) Transfusion is usually indicated for hemoglobin concentrations <6 g/dL (1).
    iv) Within the range of 6 to 10 g/dL, the risk of ongoing blood loss and patient's coexisting disease must be considered. For example, patients with coronary artery disease probably should be transfused at a higher hemoglobin than a young, healthy patient.
  d) In the absence of continued blood loss, one unit of PRBC should increase the hemoglobin concentration by 1 g/dL and the hematocrit by 3%.
  e) **ABO compatibility**
    i) ABO blood type is determined by the presence or absence of A and/or B antigens on the surface of the RBC.
      (1) Patients who lack either antigen are Type O.
      (2) Patients have circulating antibodies to RBC antigens that they lack.
        (a) For example, Type O patients have circulating anti-A and anti-B antigens and Type A patients have anti-B antibodies.
      (3) Type specific transfusion is essential. This is because ABO incompatibility leads to immediate and potentially life-threatening hemolysis.
        (a) Type AB patients are universal recipients, and type O donors are universal donors (2).
        (b) If type specific blood is not available, Type O, usually Rh negative, blood may be given.

Transfusion of the wrong blood type leads to serious hemolytic transfusion reactions.

3) **Fresh frozen plasma (FFP)**
  a) FFP contains all plasma proteins and clotting factors.
  b) Stored at −18°C to −30°C and must be thawed prior to administration
  c) **Indications for FFP**
    i) Rapid reversal of warfarin therapy
    ii) Correction of known coagulation factor deficiencies when factor concentrates are unavailable
    iii) Antithrombin III deficiency in patients receiving heparin
    iv) Correction of microvascular bleeding in patients who have been transfused greater than one blood volume
    v) Correction of microvascular bleeding in patients with abnormal coagulation parameters (PT > 1.5 times normal, INR > 2.0, aPTT > 2 times normal) (1)

d)   Recent studies in trauma patients who require massive transfusion have shown decreased morbidity and mortality with earlier administration of FFP (3).

e)   The goal of FFP administration is to achieve 30% of clotting factor concentration. The starting dose is 10-15 mL/kg.

f)   ABO compatibility

   i)   Compatibility requirements are different than with RBC because the plasma contains anti-A and/or anti-B antibodies in patients who lack these antigens.

   ii)   FFP should be ABO compatible.

   iii)   For instance, a patient with type AB blood should receive only type AB plasma, but a patient with type O blood can receive types O, A, B, or AB plasma (2).

In patients with bleeding, the surgical field should be scanned and discussions should be had with the surgeon regarding the presence of microvascular bleeding indicative of coagulopathy.

4)   Platelets

a)   Platelets are usually available in 6 to 9 unit equivalents from pooled donors or from apheresis from a single donor.

b)   Must be stored at room temperature, which increases the likelihood of bacterial contamination and decreases shelf life

c)   One unit usually increases the patient's platelet count by 5 to 10,000 cells/mm³, while one single donor aphoresis unit increases the platelet count by 30 to 60,000 cells/mm³ in the absence of platelet destruction (4).

d)   Indications

   i)   Platelets are rarely indicated if a patient's platelet count exceeds 100,000 cells/mm³.

   ii)   Platelet transfusion should be considered in the presence of excessive microvascular bleeding with platelet counts <50,000 cells/mm (1,4).

   iii)   May also be necessary in the presence of platelet dysfunction (anti-platelet therapy, uremia, post-cardiopulmonary bypass) and microvascular bleeding.

   iv)   ABO compatibility

      (1)   Although you can transfuse ABO-incompatible platelets, these cells may have a shorter lifespan than ABO-compatible platelets (2).

When transfusing blood products in women of childbearing age, either give Rh negative products or ensure Rh compatibility (2).

5)   **Cryoprecipitate**

a)   Made from slowly thawing FFP

b)   Contains high levels of Factor VIII, von Willebrand factor, and fibrinogen

c)   **Indications**

   i)   Treatment of microvascular bleeding in the presence of fibrinogen deficiency, which most commonly occurs due to disseminated intravascular coagulation (DIC) or massive transfusion

   ii)   Treatment of congenital fibrinogen deficiencies or bleeding in patients with Von Willebrand disease, where factor concentrates are unavailable (1)

   iii)   Ideally, a fibrinogen level should be obtained before administering cryoprecipitate.

      (1)   Patients whose fibrinogen concentrations exceed 150 mg/dL usually do not require cryoprecipitate.

      (2)   When fibrinogen concentrations are <80 to 100 mg/dL, cryoprecipitate is usually indicated (1).

d)   ABO compatibility

   i)   Because cryoprecipitate has only a small amount of plasma, ABO compatibility is not necessary (2).

6) **Complications of transfusion**

a) **Human error**

Vigilance is essential when transfusing blood products.

    i) Due to recent advances in detecting potentially infectious agents, complications due to human error are significantly more common than transfusion-related infections.

    ii) Catastrophic outcomes during blood product administration are usually associated with multiple errors during the process (5,6).

    iii) In order to prevent errors, it is critical that all persons involved in administering blood products exercise extreme caution, including verifying blood samples sent to the lab against a patient's armband and verifying blood prior to transfusion.

b) **Acute hemolytic reaction**

Prior to transfusing blood products, always check the patient's armband. Verify that the unit is the correct blood type and intended for that patient.

    i) The most serious complication of blood product administration

    ii) Usually caused by ABO incompatibility, resulting in an immune reaction by the recipient to the transfused RBC

    iii) Signs/symptoms of acute hemolytic reaction

       (1) Anxiety, fever, urticaria, nausea, chest and flank pain, hyperkalemia, hypotension, DIC, hemoglobinemia, and acute renal failure (4)

       (2) Many symptoms are masked by general anesthesia.

    iv) If you suspect an acute hemolytic reaction

       (1) Immediately stop the transfusion

       (2) Begin supportive care, which includes

READ MORE

Crisis management: Transfusion reaction, Chapter 219, page 1341

          (a) BP support with pressors and inotropes as needed

          (b) Preservation of renal function with fluid administration and diuresis

          (c) Alkalinize the urine with sodium bicarbonate (4)

       (3) Obtain urine and plasma hemoglobin, an antibody screen, coagulation parameters, and blood counts (4)

       (4) Send the blood being infused to the blood bank with a sample of the patient's blood to confirm or rule out incompatibility

c) **Delayed hemolytic reaction**

If you suspect a transfusion reaction, immediately STOP the transfusion.

    i) Caused by extravascular hemolysis of donor erythrocytes

    ii) Due to the presence of antibodies from previous transfusions or pregnancy in recipient serum at levels too low to be detected during the cross-match (4)

    iii) **Signs/symptoms of delayed transfusion reaction**

       (1) Occur approximately one week after a seemingly compatible transfusion

       (2) Include anemia, mild fever, increased unconjugated bilirubin, jaundice, hemoglobinuria, decreased haptoglobin, and spherocytosis on the blood smear (4)

    iv) Because the hemolysis is extravascular, the reaction is much less severe than in an acute hemolytic reaction, and the symptoms are self-limited (4).

d) **Transfusion related acute lung injury (TRALI)**

    i) An acute respiratory distress syndrome occurring within 2 to 6 hours after transfusion (7–9)

ii) Characterized by noncardiogenic pulmonary edema manifesting as hypoxia and bilateral infiltrates on chest radiograph (7–10)

iii) Its true incidence is unknown, because it is difficult to distinguish from other forms of acute lung injury, and it often occurs in patients with multiple coexisting illnesses (9).

    (1) TRALI is not rare; its estimated occurrence is 1 in 2,000 to 1 in 5,000 transfusions of blood or blood products (9).

iv) According to the Food and Drug Administration, TRALI is the leading cause of death from transfusions in the United States (9).

v) Treatment

    (1) Supportive care with most patients requiring mechanical ventilation. Small tidal volumes are recommended.

    (2) Hypotension is generally responsive to IV fluid.

    (3) Despite the presence of pulmonary edema, diuretic administration can worsen the patient's condition (8).

e) **Infectious risks**

  i) **Bacterial contamination**

    (1) Bacterial contamination of blood products is most common with **platelets** because platelets are stored at room temperature.

      (a) Incidence of 1 in 12,000 platelet transfusions (11)

    (2) The most frequent contaminating organism is *Yersinia entercolitica* for RBC and *Staphylococcus aureus* for platelets.

    (3) The clinical presentation ranges from mild fever to acute sepsis leading to death.

    (4) Suspect bacterial contamination and consider antibiotic therapy in patients who develop a fever within 6 hours after platelet transfusion (11).

  ii) **Viral transmission**

    (1) The incidence of viral transmission has decreased substantially over the past 20 years.

    (2) Currently, the estimated risk per unit of blood transfused of acquiring human immune deficiency virus is 1 in 1,780,000 and 1 in 1,600,000 for hepatitis C virus (3,12).

    (3) Other viral pathogens that can be transmitted via transfusions are cytomegalovirus, B19 parvovirus, human T-lymphotrophic virus, West Nile virus, and hepatitis B virus.

  iii) **Other**

    (1) Other potentially transmissible infectious diseases include malaria, variant Creutzfeldt-Jakob disease, and Chagas disease (7).

When administering blood products, urine output and color and peak airway pressures should be periodically assessed for signs and symptoms of transfusion reaction (1).

Chapter Summary for Blood Component Therapy

Blood Component/ Contents	Indication/Guidelines	Complications/ Warnings
PRBC (Red Blood Cells)	Increase O_2 carrying capacity Almost always indicated for Hgb < 6 Almost always not indicated with Hgb > 10 1 unit pRBC $\rightarrow \uparrow$ HCT 3%, Hgb 1 g/dL	Warm blood ABO compatibility essential
FFP (Plasma Lotting Factors)	Treatment of microvascular bleeding in the setting of coagulopathy (INR > 2.0; aPTT > two times normal) Reversal of specific agents such as warfarin For trauma, evidence supports earlier FFP administration	May require time to thaw ABO compatibility essential
Cryoprecipitate (Factor VIII and Fibrinogen)	Treatment of fibrinogen deficiency (usually <80–100 mg/dL) Commonly used in the setting of DIC	
Platelets	Treatment of severe thrombocytopenia in the setting of bleeding, surgery, or platelet destruction Usually not required with platelet counts >100,000 cells/mm³ Usually given for platelets <50,000 cells/mm³, especially in surgical patients	Single donor aphresis unit most common Potential for bacterial contamination

Blood components should be given to treat specific indications and not for volume replacement.
Extreme vigilance is required by all persons involved in blood product replacement to prevent errors.

References

1. Practice guidelines for perioperative blood transfusion and adjuvant therapies: an updated report by the American Society of Anesthesiologists Task Force on Perioperative Blood Transfusion and Adjuvant Therapies. *Anesthesiology* 2006;105:198–208.
2. Yazer MH. The blood bank "black box" debunked: pretransfusion testing explained. *Can Med Assoc J* 2006;174:29–32.
3. Holcomb JB, Wade CE, Mitchalek JE, et al. Increased plasma and platelet to red cell ratios improves outcome in 466 massively transfused civilian trauma patients. *Ann Surg* 2008;248:447–458.
4. Drummond JC, Petrovich CT, Lane TA. Hemostasis and transfusion medicine. In: Barash PG, Cullen BF, Stoelting RK, Cahalan MK, Stock MC, eds. *Clinical Anesthesia*. 6th ed. Philadelphia, PA: Lippincott-Raven Publishers; 2009:369–412.
5. Linden JV, Wagner K, Voytovich AE, Sheehan J. Transfusion errors in New York State: an analysis of 10 years' experience. *Transfusion* 2000;40:1207–1213.
6. Stainsby D. Errors in transfusion medicine. *Anesth Clin North America* 2005;23:253–261.
7. Goodnough LT. Risks of blood transfusion. *Anesth Clin North America* 2005;23:241–252.
8. Moore SB. Transfusion-related acute lung injury (TRALI): Clinical presentation, treatment, and prognosis. *Crit Care Med* 2006;34(Suppl):S114–S117.
9. Toy P, Popovsky MA, Abraham E, et al. Transfusion-related acute lung injury: Definition and review. *Crit Care Med* 2005;33:721–726.
10. Nathens AB. Massive transfusion as a risk factor for acute lung injury: Association or causation? *Crit Care Med* 2006;34(Suppl):S144–S150.
11. Goodnough LT, Brecher ME, Kanter MH, et al. Transfusion Medicine: first of two parts. *New Engl J Med* 1999;340:438–447.
12. Dodd RY, Notari EP IV, Stramer SL. Current prevalence and incidence of infectious disease markers and estimated window-period risk in the American Red Cross blood donor population. *Transfusion* 2002;42:975–979.

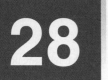

Alternatives to Blood Product Replacement

Andrea J. Fuller, MD

There are occasions where transfusion of blood products is not possible or practical due to extreme difficulty in obtaining blood or patient refusal. Alternative techniques may be employed bearing in mind that these may only be temporizing measures. The inability to treat coagulopathy and/or increase oxygen carrying capacity when indicated may result in life-altering morbidity and/or death.

1) **Overview**

   a) Difficult cross-match

      i) Occasionally, the situation arises where obtaining cross-matched blood is difficult or nearly impossible due to the development of anti–red blood cell (RBC) antibodies (alloimmunization).

      ii) Patients at risk for alloimmunization (1).

         (1) Alloimmunization in transfusion medicine refers to the development of antibodies to human RBC antigens.

         (2) Patients who are at high risk are those who have had multiple blood transfusions or pregnancies.

   b) **Patient refusal of blood products**

      i) **Informed consent**

         (1) Patients should be informed about blood transfusion when appropriate and the consequences (including death) of blood product refusal.

         (2) A thorough discussion of alternatives to blood transfusion, including the limitations of each technique, should be undertaken.

         (3) The alternatives that are acceptable to patient should be clearly documented.

2) **Maintenance of normovolemia**

   a) One of the primary goals of any anesthetic should be maintenance of normovolemia.

   b) IV crystalloid or colloid should be given as volume replacement, using urine output or possibly central venous pressure as a guide.

3) **Intraoperative cell salvage ("Cell Saver")**

   a) **Procedure (1,2)**

      i) Blood is suctioned from the operative field and usually is then anticoagulated.

      ii) RBCs are separated from other elements by centrifuge.

      iii) Cells are then washed, suspended in saline, and **reinfused to the patient**

         (1) Reinfusion is usually via bagged aliquots with a hematocrit of 45% to 65%.

Patients should always be informed that a possible consequence of blood product refusal is extreme anemia resulting in death.

READ MORE

Crystalloids and colloids, intravenous fluid therapy, Chapter 26, page 202

The efficiency of RBC recovery with cell salvage is approximately 30%.

215

b) **Indications (3)**
  i) Procedures where blood loss is expected to be high
  ii) Common procedures include cardiovascular surgeries, liver transplantation, spinal instrumentation, joint arthroplasty, and aortic reconstruction.
c) **Contraindications (3)**
  i) Generally related to the presence of cells or other substances that have the potential to cause harm if reinfused to the patient. They include
    (1) Malignancy
    (2) Infection
    (3) Pharmacologic agents such as methyl methacrylate or clotting agents
    (4) Urine, bone chips, fat, or bowel contents in surgical field
    (5) Presence of amniotic fluid (relative)
      (a) Cell salvage has been used for cesarean section without complications and may be considered in certain high risk situations (2).
  ii) **Potential complications (1,2)**
    (1) Coagulopathy from the anticoagulants used during blood processing
      (a) Substantially reduced with modern cell salvage equipment
    (2) Dilution of clotting factors and platelets can occur since only RBC are returned to the patient.
    (3) Contamination of the cell salvage device with bacteria or debris from the surgical field resulting in systemic infection
    (4) Air embolism if blood is directly returned from the machine or a rapid infusion device and not properly monitored
  iii) **Advantages**
    (1) Compatiblity testing not required
    (2) Little risk for human error, unless the machine is not properly operated
  iv) **Disadvantages**
    (1) Requires specialized equipment and trained personnel
    (2) Not applicable in all surgeries
4) **Normovolemic hemodilution (1,4)**
  a) Involves collection of **autologous blood** immediately prior to surgery and maintenance of normovolemia by IV fluid administration with colloid or crystalloid.
    i) The volume of colloid administered should be equal to the volume of blood withdrawn.
    ii) When crystalloid is administered, the volume should be three times the volume of blood removed (3,4).
  b) When blood is subsequently lost, it has less RBC mass, and the blood removed can be returned to the patient as needed.
  c) **Candidates for this procedure include (4)**
    i) Patients who have a high likelihood of transfusion
    ii) Preoperative Hgb of at least 12 g/dL
    iii) Absence of coronary, pulmonary, renal, or liver disease
    iv) Absence of severe hypertension
    v) Absence of infection and low risk of bacteremia
  d) **Advantages**
    i) Virtually, no potential for ABO incompatibility, provided that the blood does not leave the operating room
    ii) No need for compatibility testing
    iii) Lower cost than banked blood.
  e) **Disadvantages (4)**
    i) Decreased oxygen delivery may result in organ ischemia, although this is very unlikely in patients without cerebrovasuclar or coronary artery disease.

5) Pharmacologic alternatives
  a) **Erythropoietic agents (5,6)**
    i) **Recombinant human erythropoietin** (Procrit or Epogen) with folate and iron supplementation can be used preoperatively or postoperatively to increase RBC production.
    ii) Advantages
      (1) May be used in patients at high risk for anemia and blood loss
        (a) Examples include chronic renal failure and anemia.
      (2) Accepted by many patients who otherwise refuse blood transfusion
    iii) Disadvantages
      (1) Effect takes approximately 2 weeks.
        (a) Not helpful in the acute situation or when blood loss is unexpected
      (2) Expensive
  b) **Recombinant activated factor VII (rFVIIa) (7–9)**
    i) rFVIIa is identical in structure and function to human factor VIIa.
    ii) Developed to prevent or control bleeding in patients with Hemophilia A or B with inhibitors to factors VIII and IX
    iii) rFVIIa acts by binding with tissue factor to augment the intrinsic clotting pathway by directly activating factors IX and X.
    iv) It is now used in many different clinical situations and is effective for treatment of life-threatening hemorrhage.
    v) There are no specific guidelines for rFVIIa therapy, but it is often given for life-threatening coagulopathy when other measures have failed.
      (1) The dose is 50 to 100 mg/kg IV, with most patients responding to the drug within 30 minutes.
        (a) It can be repeated every 2 hours until hemostasis is achieved, but the vast majority of patients require only one dose.
        (b) Less effective in the presence of acidosis, hypothermia, and inadequate clotting factors (9).

rFVIIa may be beneficial in cases of intractable hemorrhage complicated by coagulopathy.

    vi) **Advantages**
      (1) rFVIIa is a pharmacologic agent and not a blood product.
      (2) Does not carry risk of transfusion-transmitted disease.
      (3) Accepted by many patients who object to blood transfusion
    vii) Disadvantages
      (1) Thrombotic events are the most commonly reported problems associated complications and include cerebrovascular accidents, myocardial infarction, pulmonary embolism, and clotting of indwelling devices (10).
      (2) Very expensive
6) Management strategies for patients who refuse blood transfusion
  a) Minimize blood loss
    i) **Meticulous surgical technique** should be discussed with the physician performing the procedure.
    ii) **Minimizing phlebotomy** and using point-of-care laboratory testing can significantly reduce blood loss.
  b) **Minimize O_2 consumption**
    i) **Mechanical ventilation** with or without muscle paralysis reduces the work of breathing (11).
    ii) Other strategies include **hypothermia, analgesics,** and **sedation (5,11).**
  c) **Maximize O_2 delivery**

One of the most common perioperative situations where patients refuse blood products is the care of the Jehovah's Witness.

i)   Tissue O_2 delivery can be increased by **increasing inspired oxygen** (FiO_2), **maintaining normovolemia**, and **increasing cardiac output**, using inotropes if necessary (5).

   (1)   A pulmonary artery catheter with the capability to measure cardiac output and mixed venous SpO_2 can be helpful (5).

ii)   **Hyperbaric O_2** can also be used to increase blood O_2 content if available (12).

7)   **The Jehovah's Witness (JW)**

a)   **Definition**

   i)   JW are patients who object to receiving blood or blood products on religious grounds.

   ii)   There are over one million JW in the United States and over six million worldwide (13)

b)   **Preoperative informed consent**

   i)   Whenever possible, discuss patient's wishes **alone** (i.e., without the presence of family or religious personnel).

   ii)   Patients should be informed about blood transfusion when appropriate and the consequences (including death) of blood product refusal.

   iii)   Some patients will accept intraoperative cell salvage, normovolemic hemodilution, or fractionated products.

   iv)   These options need to be discussed thoroughly and the patient's wishes understood prior to the operative procedure.

c)   **Alternative techniques and the JW patient (Table 28-1)**

   i)   Many techniques have variable acceptance in JW patients.

   ii)   Therefore, preoperative discussion and documentation of acceptance or refusal of various techniques is absolutely essential.

Table 28-1

Alternatives to Blood Transfusion and the JW Patient[a]

Alternative Technique	Acceptance by JW Patients	Comments
Crystalloid	Generally accepted	May be used for volume expansion
Hetastarch	Generally accepted	May be used for volume expansion
Albumin	Acceptance varies	Derived from human sources
Cell salvage Normovolemic hemodilution	Acceptance varies	Pt may desire continuous circuit with his/her body
Cryoprecipitate	Generally refused but may vary with the patient	Use has been reported, discuss with patient
Erythropoietic agents	Acceptance varies	May contain small amounts of human albumin
Recombinant factor VIIa	Generally accepted	Should be discussed in cases where risk of coagulopathy is high

[a]Patients vary widely with their acceptance of techniques. Whenever possible, ALWAYS confirm the patient's wishes prior to administration.

Chapter Summary for Alternatives to Blood Transfusion

General Principles	Patients may refuse blood product transfusion based on religious grounds. Rarely, cross-matched blood is difficult to obtain
Intraoperative Cell Salvage	Requires specialized equipment Blood suctioned from operative field, processed, and reinfused to the patient Contraindications include malignancy, bacterial contamination, urine and bowel contents in the surgical field
Normovolemic Hemodilution	Blood is removed from the patient and reinfused after most blood loss has occurred Blood removed must be replaced with colloid or crystalloid
Pharmacologic Agents	Include erythropoietin and rFVIIa
Management Strategies to Minimize Need for Blood Transfusion	Minimize phlebotomy, notify surgeon of need for minimizing blood loss with surgical technique, controlled ventilation, increase FiO_2
Jehovah's Witness	Patients who object to blood transfusion on religious grounds Discuss patient's wishes alone if possible Clearly explain the risks associated with blood product refusal, including death Understand and document the patient's wishes

MANAGEMENT AND THERAPY

References

1. Drummond JC, Petrovich CT, Lane TA. Hemostasis and transfusion medicine. In: Barash PG, Cullen BF, Stoelting RK, Cahalan MK, Stock MC, eds. *Clinical Anesthesia.* 6th ed. Philadelphia, PA: Lippincott-Raven Publishers; 2009:369–412.
2. Allam J, Cox M, Yentis SM. Cell salvage in obstetrics. *Int J Obstet Anesth* 2008;17:37–45.
3. Waters JH. Indications and contraindications of cell salvage. *Transfusion* 2004;44:40S–44S.
4. Monk TG. Acute normovolemic hemodilution. *Anesthesiol Clin North America* 2005;23:271–281.
5. Kulvatunyou N, Heard SO. Care of the injured Jehovah's Witness patient: case report and review of the literature. *J Clin Anesth* 2004;16(7):548–553.
6. Remmers PA, Speer AJ. Clinical strategies in the medical care of Jehovah's Witnesses. *Am J Med* 2006;119(12):1013–1018.
7. Hedner U, Erhardtsen E. Potential role for rFVIIa in transfusion medicine. *Transfusion* 2002;42:114–124.
8. Biss TT, Hanley JP. Recombinant activated Factor VII (rFVIIa/novoseven) in intractable haemorrhage: use of a clinical scoring system to predict outcome. *Vox Sang* 2006;90:45–52.
9. Martinowitz U, Kenet G, Segal E, et al. Recombinant activated Factor VII for adjunctive hemorrhage control in trauma. *J Trauma* 2001;51(3):431–439.
10. OConnell KA, Wood JJ, Wise RP, et al. Thromboembolic adverse events after use of recombinant human coagulation factor VIIa. *J Am Med Assoc* 2006;295:293–298.
11. Mann MC, Votto J, Kambe J, et al. Management of the severely anemic patient who refuses transfusion: Lessons learned during the care of a Jehovah's Witness. *Ann Intern Med* 1992;117:1042–1048.
12. McLoughlin PL, Cope TM, Harrison JC. Hyperbaric oxygen therapy in the management of severe acute anaemia in a Jehovah's Witness. *Anaesthesia* 1999;54(9):891–895.
13. http://www.watchtower.org/statistics/worldwide_report.htm,Statistics. 2005 report of Jehovah's Witnesses worldwide, 2006.

29 Massive Transfusion and Resuscitation

Andrea J. Fuller, MD

Massive bleeding in the operating room can be expected, as in the case of liver transplant or abdominal aortic aneurysm repair, or unexpected, as in the case of trauma, vascular injury or postpartum. Hemorrhage can cause decreased tissue perfusion, cellular injury, and death if not treated appropriately. Significant bleeding may result in the need for transfusion of large amounts of blood products.

1) **Definition**
    a) Massive hemorrhage has been described as the loss of one's entire blood volume in a 24-hour period or half of the entire blood volume in a 3-hour period (1).
    b) Massive transfusion is defined as transfusion of 10 units of PRBC or blood products in 24 hours (2).
2) **Causes (Table 29-1)**
    a) Causes of massive hemorrhage requiring massive transfusion are variable. Any time of the day or night one can be faced with the potential for massive bleeding in most major centers and community hospitals.
3) **Management goals in massive hemorrhage**
    a) The primary goal is maintenance of adequate perfusion and cellular function. Prevention of microvascular bleeding is a secondary goal.
    b) **Lines and monitors**
        i) Standard ASA monitors plus invasive monitors are usually required.
        ii) **Central venous access**
            (1) Large bore central lines are extremely beneficial for volume replacement and can be used in conjunction with a rapid infusion device.
            (2) Central venous pressure can be used as a guide for volume replacement.
            (3) Ultrasound guidance should be used when placing central venous lines whenever possible.
            (4) While placement of central access can aid in management, it can also draw attention and personnel resources away from treatment of the patient. Ensure that the patient is being adequately resuscitated while the line is being placed, or defer placement to focus on volume replacement.
        iii) **Intra-arterial blood pressure monitoring**
            (1) Offers the ability for close monitoring of BP and frequent blood draws for laboratory analysis
            (2) Should be placed early in a hemorrhagic emergency because placement may be difficult once significant peripheral vasoconstriction is present

READ MORE
Central venous monitoring, Chapter 12, page 75

MANAGEMENT AND THERAPY

Table 29-1
Causes of Massive Hemorrhage

Cause of Massive Hemorrhage	Example
Obstetric hemorrhage	Placenta accreta
Trauma	Motor vehicle accident, gunshot wound
Surgical	Liver transplant, aortic surgery
Coagulopathy	Von Willebrand disease, factor deficiency

In cases of hemorrhage, an arterial line is extremely helpful for BP monitoring and blood draws and should be placed as early as possible.

Temperature monitoring is **vital** in patients with massive hemorrhage. Every effort should be made to maintain normothermia.

READ MORE

Alternatives to blood product replacement, Chapter 28, page 215

    (3) Radial artery is the most common cannulation site, but femoral is often used in emergent or difficult situations.

iv) Adequate IV access is essential in the bleeding patient. The flow of a fluid through a catheter is proportional to the fourth power of the radius, so large bore peripheral IV access allows for rapid transfusion.

    (1) Recommended IV access includes two large bore (14 to 16 g) IV cannulae.

v) **Urine output**

    (1) Monitoring urine output is an effective indicator of the patient's intravascular volume status.

        (a) Urine output <15 mL/kg/h is indicative of severe volume depletion (3).

vi) **Temperature monitoring**

    (1) Monitoring core temperature is essential in patients with hemorrhage.

    (2) Hypothermia is extremely problematic in the massively bleeding patient because acidosis and coagulopathy are worsened by decreased temperature.

vii) **Airway management and maintenance**

    (1) Massively bleeding patients may arrive in the operating room or emergency department with an endotracheal tube in place.

    (2) Severe blood loss significantly alters consciousness. The airway should be protected and managed by endotracheal intubation and ventilation.

c) **Maintenance of adequate perfusion**

i) In order to assure organ perfusion, intravascular volume must be maintained by large amounts of IV fluid, appropriate amounts of colloid, and potentially blood products.

ii) Blood products should be replaced with appropriate indications.

4) **Mobilization of resources**

a) Call for help of anesthesia technicians and additional anesthesia personnel.

b) Mobilize necessary equipment.

c) Notify blood bank and clinical laboratory.

d) Activate massive transfusion protocol (MTP), if applicable.

The purpose of IV crystalloid and/or colloid in massive hemorrhage is to maintain adequate organ perfusion and blood flow. The purpose of RBC transfusion is to increase oxygen delivery.

READ MORE

Blood component therapy, Chapter 27, page 209

In an emergency where blood is required and not available, Type O blood may be transfused.

5) **Massive transfusion protocol (4)**

  a) **Clear communication among all parties involved in caring for the massively bleeding patient is essential.**

  b) A MTP that gives clear directions on laboratory data, blood product availability and transport, as well as equipment and personnel is extremely helpful.

  c) Instituting a MTP should be seriously considered in every institution where the potential to treat massive hemorrhage exists.

6) **Blood product replacement specific to massive transfusion**

  a) **Packed red blood cells (PRBC) (5)**

    i) Given to increase oxygen carrying capacity

    ii) Estimated blood loss is a reasonable guide to PRBC replacement, although in a massive hemorrhage, estimating blood loss is often difficult. In this situation, RBC are often given in response to clinical events or laboratory values such as hemoglobin with consideration of the patient's acid/base status.

    iii) Often in a hemorrhagic emergency, type-specific, cross-matched blood is not available.

      (1) Type specific, un–cross-matched blood may be given in an emergency as the risk of a hemolytic transfusion reaction with un–cross-matched blood in patients who have not been previously transfused or pregnant is very low (6).

      (2) If no blood is available and the patient requires blood emergently, type O blood can be given.

      (3) Type O, Rh negative, blood is preferred, especially in women of childbearing age.

      (4) Once a large volume of Type O blood is given in an emergency, caution must be taken when subsequently administering type specific blood due to the presence of anti-A and anti-B antigens in the circulating Type O blood leading to hemolysis in the type-specific blood.

      (5) Although the exact amount of transfused Type O blood that may cause this problem is unknown, it is prudent to consider avoiding type specific-blood when approximately one blood volume of Type O blood has been given (6).

    iv) Large volume PRBC administration is associated with coagulopathy due to dilution of clotting factors and platelets (dilutional thrombocytopenia).

  b) **Fresh frozen plasma (FFP)**

    i) Current ASA guidelines state that FFP should be given in the presence of microvascular bleeding in patients who have been transfused one blood volume or when INR is >2.0 (5).

    ii) Recent data suggest that early transfusion of FFP and platelets aids in prevention of coagulopathy associated with trauma-related massive transfusion (7–9).

    iii) It is unclear if this data can be extrapolated to other situations. This is an active area of research.

  c) **Platelets**

    i) Current guidelines recommend a platelet count prior to platelet transfusion and state that platelet transfusion is typically not indicated for platelet counts >50,000 cells/mm^3 (5).

In massively bleeding patients, blood product replacement ratios that approximate whole blood may improve patient outcome and should be considered.

READ MORE

Alternatives to blood component therapy, Chapter 28, page 215

READ MORE

Water, electrolytes, and acid/base disorders, Chapter 80, page 576

MANAGEMENT AND THERAPY

ii)   Recent information in massively bleeding trauma patients suggests that platelet and plasma transfusion early in resuscitation with an attempt to approximate whole blood is associated with lower mortality (7).

7)   **Complications of massive transfusion**

a)   Complications associated with blood component therapy also apply to massive transfusion.

   i)   These include acute and delayed hemolytic reactions, transfusion-related acute lung injury (TRALI), transfusion-transmitted infectious disease.

b)   Other complications are more specific to large volume transfusion.

c)   **Hypothermia**

   i)   **Hypothermia with a core temperature <35°C significantly affects coagulation.**

      (1)   The more hypothermic the patient becomes, the higher the risk of microvascular bleeding.

      (2)   Every effort should be made to prevent the lethal triad of hypothermia, acidosis, and coagulopathy.

   ii)   In trauma patients, hypothermia is associated with an increased risk of developing disseminated intravascular coagulation.

      (1)   Trauma patients often arrive in the OR hypothermic. Rewarming requires substantial effort, but the difference in outcome can be significant.

   iii)   Every effort to maintain normothermia, including using warming devices for all IV fluids and blood products and forced-air heating devices if possible (8)

d)   **Hypocalcemia (2,8)**

   i)   Due to citrate anticoagulant in the blood products binding calcium.

   ii)   May manifest as decreased cardiac contractility and ECG abnormalities.

   iii)   Contributes to coagulopathy (calcium is Factor IV in the clotting cascade).

   iv)   Carefully monitor calcium levels and treat hypocalcemia with IV calcium chloride.

e)   **Hyperkalemia (8)**

   i)   Increased potassium is due to RBC lysis during storage.

   ii)   Potassium should be carefully monitored and hyperkalemia treated appropriately.

f)   **Volume overload (10)**

   i)   Care must be taken to avoid excess volume replacement as circulatory overload can lead to pulmonary edema and other potential complications.

   ii)   Furthermore, excessive crystalloid administration may lead to abdominal compartment syndrome and potentially other cardiopulmonary complications.

g)   **Dilutional coagulopathy (2,7,11)**

   i)   Administration of large volumes of products that do not contain clotting factors or platelets results in decreased circulating clotting factors and platelets, which may result in coagulopathy.

   ii)   Clotting factors and platelets should be administered either based on an MTP that attempts to approximate whole blood, laboratory values, or microvascular bleeding in the situation of large volume resuscitation.

h) **Decreased 2,3-diphosphoglycerate (6,8)**
  i) 2,3-Diphosphoglycerate is a compound that binds deoxyhemoglobin and increases oxygen delivery to cells.
  ii) Transfusion of large volumes of stored RBCs can lead to decreased 2, 3-Diphosphoglycerate thereby decreasing oxygen delivery to tissues.

i) **Disruptions in acid base balance (6,8)**
  i) The addition of citrate-phosphate-dextrose solution during RBC storage decreases the pH to approximately 7.0.
  ii) In the normally perfused liver, the citrate is metabolized to bicarbonate, which should mitigate the acidic pH of the transfused blood.
  iii) In situations where the liver is not adequately perfused, this process may be altered, which the potential for exacerbation of metabolic acidosis.
  iv) The clinical significance of the low pH associated with stored RBC is unclear, but it is possible that transfusion of large volumes may significantly contribute to metabolic acidosis.

Chapter Summary for Massive Transfusion

Causes	May be surgical, trauma, or obstetric
Definition	Massive transfusion is the administration of 10 or more units of blood products in 24 h
Goals	Adequate tissue perfusion, oxygen delivery, and prevention of coagulopathy
Blood Product Replacement	Should be based on specific indications Consider ratio of PRBC:FFP:platelets of 1:1:1, which closer approximates whole blood, especially in massively bleeding trauma patients
Complications	Risks associated with blood product replacement apply Specific risks for massive transfusion included hypothermia, hyperkalemia, hypocalcemia, dilutional coagulopathy, volume overload, and decreased 2,3-diphosphoglycerate

References

1. Gutierrez G, Reines HD, Wulf-Gutierrez ME. Clinical review: hemorrhagic shock. *Crit Care* 2004;8:373–381.
2. Shaz BH, Dente CJ, Harris RS, et al. Transfusion management of trauma patients. *Anesth Analg* 2009;108:1760–1768.
3. Shock. American College of Surgeons Committee on Trauma. *Advanced Trauma Life Support for Doctors*. Chicago, IL: American College of Surgeons; 2004:69–102.
4. Nunez TC, Young PP, Holcomb JB, et al. Creation, implimention, and maturation of a massive transfusion protocol for the exsanguinating trauma patient. *J Trauma* 2010;68:1498–1505.
5. Practice guidelines for perioperative blood transfusion and adjuvant therapies: an updated report by the American Society of Anesthesiologists Task Force on Perioperative Blood Transfusion and Adjuvant Therapies. *Anesthesiology* 2006;105:198–208.
6. Drummond JC, Petrovich CT, Lane TA. Hemostasis and transfusion medicine. In: Barash PG, Cullen BF, Stoelting RK, Cahalan MK, Stock MC, eds. *Clinical Anesthesia*. 6th ed. Philadelphia, PA: Lippincott-Raven Publishers; 2009:369–412.
7. Holcomb JB, Wade CE, Mitchalek JE, et al. Increased plasma and platelet to red cell ratios improves outcome in 466 massively transfused Civilian trauma patients. *Ann Surg* 2008;248:447–458.
8. Perkins JG, Cap AP, Weiss BM, et al. Massive transfusion and nonsurgical hemostatic agents. *Crit Care Med* 2008;36:S325–S339.
9. Johansson PI, Stensballe J. Effect of haemostatic control resuscitation and mortality in massively bleeding patients: a before and after study. *Vox Sang* 2009;96:111–118.
10. Cotton BA, Guy JS, Morris JA Jr, et al. The cellular, metabolic, and systemic consequences of aggressive fluid resuscitation strategies. *Shock* 2006;26:115–121.

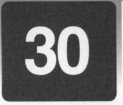

Spinal Anesthesia

Ray S. Lee, MD • Robert L. Hsiung, MD

Injection of local anesthetic into the subarachnoid space produces rapid onset of surgical anesthesia. When coadministered with local anesthetics, intrathecal opioids may enhance the quality of spinal anesthesia and provide postoperative analgesia (1).

1) Indications and contraindications
   a) **Indications**
      i) Spinal anesthesia is generally performed for surgical procedures involving the lower abdomen, perineum, and lower extremities.
      ii) It is the preferred anesthetic technique for Cesarean delivery due to decreased morbidity and mortality (2).
   b) **Contraindications**
      i) **Absolute contraindications**
         (1) Language or consent barrier
         (2) Increased intracranial pressure
         (3) Coagulopathy
      ii) **Relative contraindications**
         (1) Systemic infection
         (2) Inability to position
         (3) Hemodynamic profile that would not tolerate a decrease in systemic vascular resistance (e.g., shock or aortic stenosis)

2) **Anatomy**
   a) Spinal cord
      i) 31 pairs of spinal nerves consisting of paired ventral motor roots and paired dorsal sensory roots
      ii) The area of skin innervated by the cutaneous branches from a single spinal nerve is called a *dermatome* (Fig. 30-1) (3).
      iii) In term infants, the caudal extent of the spinal cord, known as the *conus medullaris*, normally ends at L2 (4).
      iv) In adults, the mean level at which the conus medullaris ends is L1, with a range between T11 and L3 (5).
      v) Spinal anesthesia should not be performed above the L2-3 interspace due to the increased potential for mechanical injury to the spinal cord.
   b) Potential anatomical paths for the spinal needle
      i) Midline approach: Skin, subcutaneous tissue, supraspinous ligament, interspinous ligament, ligamentum flavum, dura mater, arachnoid mater, and subarachnoid space
      ii) Paramedian approach: Bypasses the supraspinous and the interspinous ligaments

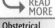

READ MORE

Obstetrical anesthesia, chapter 144, page 1047

Spinal anesthesia should not be performed above the L2-3 interspace due to risk of injuring the spinal cord.

NEURAXIAL AND REGIONAL ANESTHESIA

225

Figure 30-1   Sensory Dermatomes

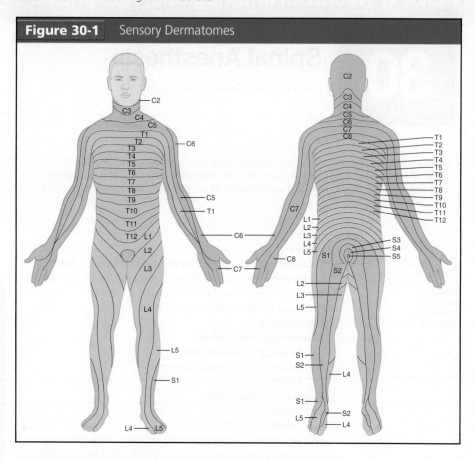

3) **Pharmacology**
   a) Determinates of block height
      i) Baricity and patient position are the two major factors
      ii) Baricity is defined as the density of the local anesthetic solution relative to the density of CSF at 37°C.
         (1) Hyperbaric solutions have a density greater than CSF.
             (a) Usually prepared by mixing local anesthetic in 5% to 8% dextrose (e.g., bupivacaine 0.75%)
             (b) In the supine position, hyperbaric solutions distribute by way of gravity toward the thoracic and sacral concavities, producing an average block height at the midthoracic level.
             (c) Block height may be affected by solution volume and duration of time spent in block position (e.g., sitting or lateral decubitus) prior to assuming the supine position.
         (2) Isobaric solutions have a density equal to CSF.
             (a) Positioning does not affect the distribution of local anesthetic, and the average block height is at the low thoracic level (e.g., lidocaine 2%).
         (3) Hypobaric solutions have a density lower than CSF (e.g., bupivacaine 0.5%).
   b) **Determinates of block duration**
      i) **Local anesthetic selection (Table 30-1) (6)**

Table 30-1

Local Anesthetics Used for Spinal Anesthesia

Local Anesthetic	Dose (mg)	Mean Peak Block	Complete Regression (min) (SD)
Short duration			
2-Chloroprocaine, 2%*	40	T7	114 (14)
Intermediate duration			
Lidocaine, 5%	50	T6	130 (18)
Long duration			
Bupivacaine, 0.5%*	10	T7	178 (20)
Bupivacaine, 0.75%	15	T4	360

*Not FDA approved for spinal anesthesia. Considered "off label" use.

READ MORE

Local anesthetics, Chapter 37, page 282

Add opioids to local anesthetics administered intrathecally to enhance block quality and prolong analgesia.

ii) **Local anesthetic dose**
  (1) Increasing the dose results in an increased duration of spinal anesthesia.
iii) Elimination of local anesthetic occurs through vascular absorption from the subarachnoid space and the epidural space.

c) **Differential block**
  i) Sympathetic blockade often occurs a few dermatomes higher than sensory blockade, which in turn, occurs higher than motor blockade.
  ii) This effect may be secondary to local anesthetic action on the differing fiber sizes and degree of myelination (7).

d) **Site of action**
  i) Local anesthetics deposited in the subarachnoid space are thought to act primarily on the spinal nerve rootlets.

e) **Adjuvants**
  i) Opioids (e.g., fentanyl, sufentanil, morphine) may be added to local anesthetics to enhance the quality of block or prolong analgesia (1,8,9).
  ii) Clonidine may extend the duration of sensory and motor block (10).
  iii) Epinephrine added to local anesthetics may produce untoward side effects such as flu-like symptoms (11).

4) **Equipment**
  a) Common equipment for all regional anesthetic techniques includes a marking pen and an appropriate volume of local anesthetic solution.
  b) Spinal anesthesia should be performed with meticulous sterile technique with sterile skin cleansing solution, sterile gloves, hat, mask, and large clear sterile fenestrated drape.
  c) Spinal needle and introducer, if desired

NEURAXIAL AND REGIONAL ANESTHESIA

Meticulous sterile technique should always be used when performing spinal anesthesia.

i)   Small gauge, pencil-point (Whitacre, Sprotte) spinal needles are recommended due to the decreased incidence of postdural puncture headache (PDPH) (12).

ii)   Most practitioners use 24 to 26-G pencil-point needles.

iii)   Occasionally, 22-G needles may be useful during difficult blocks (e.g., elderly patients with arthritic changes in the spine). The potentially higher incidence of PDPH should be weighed against the benefit of easier placement.

d)   A prepackaged custom tray with all anticipated equipment and labeled syringes will save time during the procedure.

5)   **Technique**

a)   **Monitoring**

i)   Spinal anesthetics should be performed in a location where the patient's noninvasive BP, SpO_2, and EKG may be monitored.

ii)   Supplemental O_2 should be provided *via* a face mask or nasal cannulae especially if sedation is to be administered.

iii)   Emergency airway equipment and resuscitation drugs should be immediately available.

b)   **Positioning and preparation**

i)   Apply monitors and supplemental O_2 prior to administering IV sedation.

ii)   Patients are typically positioned lateral decubitus or sitting.

(1)   Lateral decubitus (Fig. 30-2) (3)

(a)   The patient's back should be at the edge of the bed, while keeping the shoulders and the hips perpendicular to the bed to prevent rotation of spine.

(b)   The knees are drawn upward toward the chest, with forward neck flexion, and active protrusion of the lower back.

(2)   Sitting (Fig. 30-3) (13)

(a)   May help identify midline, particularly in obese patients.

(b)   The knees are drawn upward toward the chest, with forward neck flexion, and active protrusion of the lower back.

iii)   The anticipated injection site is prepped with appropriate antiseptic solution and draped in a sterile fashion.

(1)   It is beneficial to prepare a wide area to facilitate any subsequent attempt at a different level.

(2)   If using povidone-iodine, allow the antiseptic solution to dry and wipe away any excess.

c)   **Identification of surface anatomy**

i)   A line drawn between the tips of the scapula estimates T7, while one drawn between the iliac crests (Tuffier's line) estimates L4 (Fig. 30-4).

ii)   Using the index and the middle finger side by side, palpate the spinous processes by sliding side to side and up and down the midline.

iii)   The target interspace for spinal anesthesia is L4-5 or L3-4.

d)   **Midline approach**

i)   Identify the middle of the target interspace.

ii)   After warning the patient, infiltrate the skin and intended path of the spinal needle with local anesthetic.

iii)   Insert the introducer needle at the infiltration site with a 10 to 15 degree angulation in the cephalad direction until it engages the interspinous ligament.

| **Figure 30-2** | Lateral Decubitus Position for Spinal Anesthesia |

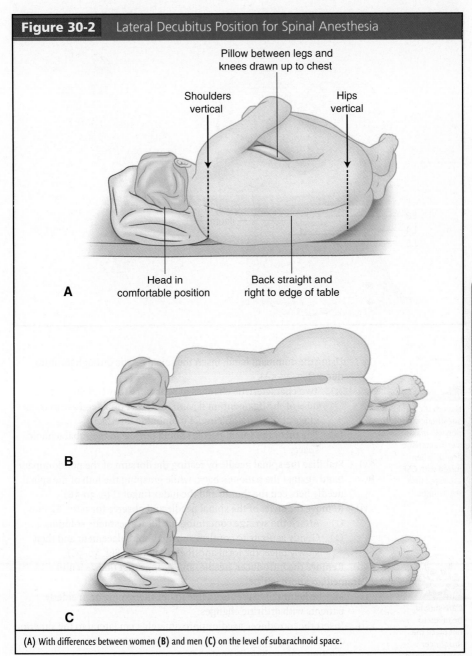

(**A**) With differences between women (**B**) and men (**C**) on the level of subarachnoid space.

Figure 30-3	Correct Sitting Position Demonstrated for Spinal Anesthesia

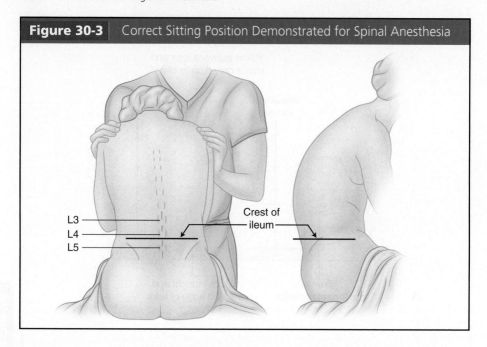

L3
L4
L5

Crest of ileum

Hyperbaric local anesthetic solution will make a characteristic "swirl" when mixed with CSF aspirated into the syringe.

Care should be taken to not place the introducer needle beyond interspinous ligaments in an effort to avoid dural puncture with a large bore needle.

iv) Using the dominant hand, insert the spinal needle through the introducer (Fig. 30-5A).
   (1) Two characteristic changes in resistance may be felt: the firmness of the ligamentum flavum, followed by a decrease in resistance at the dura-arachnoid membrane interface.
   (2) The tip of the spinal needle should now be in the subarachnoid space.

v) Stabilize the spinal needle by resting the dorsum of the nondominant hand against the patient's back, while grasping the hub of the spinal needle between the thumb and the index finger (Fig. 30-5B).

vi) Remove the stylet of the spinal needle and observe for free CSF flow.
   (1) Attach the syringe containing the local anesthetic solution.
   (2) Gently aspirate to confirm subarachnoid placement and then slowly inject the local anesthetic solution (Fig. 30-5C).

vii) Remove the introducer, needle, and syringe together as a unit.

e) **Paramedian approach**

i) May be helpful in patients unable to flex their spine or in elderly patients with arthritic changes.

ii) Insert the introducer needle approximately 1 cm lateral to the superior aspect of the inferior spinous process and angle 15 degrees toward midline and 45 degrees cephalad.

iii) Insert the spinal needle through the introducer.
   (1) The first resistance encountered should be the ligamentum flavum.
   (2) If bone is contacted past the estimated depth of the spinous process, this is most likely the lamina.
   (3) Proceed to locate the interlaminar space by "marching" off the lamina cephalad or caudad.

iv) Once free-flowing CSF is achieved, proceed as above.

Figure 30-4   A Line Drawn Between the Iliac Crests Approximates L4

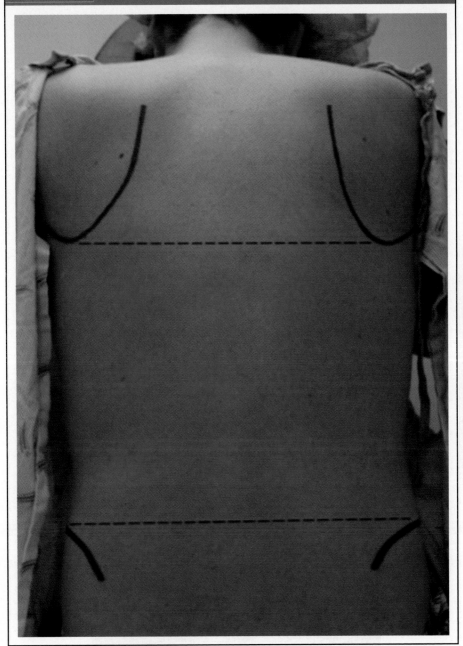

Figure 30-5   Spinal Needle Insertion Techniques

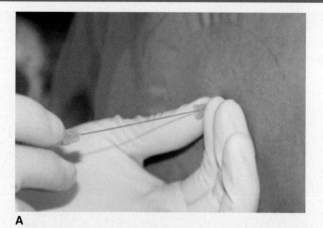

A

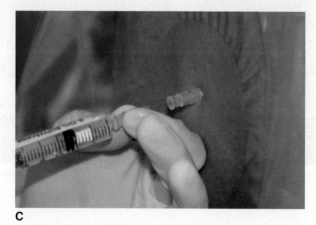

B

C

(A) Using the dominant hand, insert the spinal needle through the introducer (B) Stabilize the spinal needle by resting the dorsum of the nondominant hand against the patient's back, while grasping the hub of the spinal needle between the thumb and the index finger (C) Attach syringe with desired spinal medication, aspirate to confirm intrathecal location, and inject.

f) **Troubleshooting**

   i) Bony contact

     (1) It is important to have a working 3D mental image of the spine.

     (2) Adjustments of the needle angle must first be preceded by withdrawing the introducer and spinal needle to the subcutaneous tissue and should be made in small increments.

     (3) In the midline approach, note the depth at which bone is contacted and redirect slightly cephalad.

       (a) If bone continues to be contacted at a shallower depth, the needle is likely marching up the inferior aspect of the superior spinous process, and a more caudad angle is warranted.

       (b) If bone continues to be contacted at a deeper depth, the needle is likely marching down the superior aspect of the inferior spinous process, and a more cephalad angle is warranted.

       (c) If bone is contacted repeatedly at the same depth, the needle is likely contacting lamina and not in the midline.

   ii) **No CSF flow**

     (1) It is unlikely that the spinal needle is in the subarachnoid space although low CSF pressure is another possible etiology.

     (2) The needle may still be in the epidural space, and further advancement is warranted.

     (3) Otherwise, rotation of the needle may result in more brisk flow.

     (4) If these measures fail, then the needle should be removed and reinserted.

   iii) **Paresthesia**

     (1) Immediately stop needle advancement, and remove the spinal needle stylet.

     (2) If CSF flow is obtained, the needle may have encountered a cauda equina nerve root in the subarachnoid space (14).

     (3) Paresthesia is frequently transient, and injection of local anesthetic may proceed after needle repositioning and only if the paresthesia resolves.

     (4) If no CSF flow occurs, remove the needle and attempt reinsertion.

6) **Risks and complications**

   a) **Pulmonary function changes that occur due to spinal anesthesia**

     i) Usually not clinically significant in healthy patients because the diaphragm is innervated by the phrenic nerve (C3-5)

     ii) Respiratory rate and tidal volumes remain unchanged, though a high thoracic level block can result in decreased expiratory reserve volume from deafferentation of the abdominal wall and intercostal muscles (15).

     iii) Caution is advised in performing neuraxial blocks in patients with limited respiratory reserve, who may be dependent on these muscles for active respiration and clearing of secretions.

     iv) Respiratory arrest associated with high spinal is attributed to hypoperfusion of the medullary respiratory neurons, rather than phrenic nerve block. Prompt hemodynamic resuscitation is associated with immediate return of spontaneous respiration (3).

If a paresthesia is elicited, ensure that it has resolved prior to injection of local anesthetic solution.

Spinal anesthesia can cause symptomatic bradycardia and even lead to cardiac arrest, especially in young patients with high parasympathetic tone.

v) Complaints of dyspnea in an otherwise healthy patient who is able to vocalize normally should be addressed with supportive feedback, supplemental O_2 if needed, and continued vigilance for a total spinal.

b) **Hypotension** is a frequently encountered physiologic effect of spinal anesthesia.

READ MORE

Post-dural puncture headache and epidural blood patch, Chapter 32, page 247

i) Sympathetic efferent blockade results in arterial and venous dilation, causing a decrease in afterload and preload, respectively.

ii) Treatment involves IV fluid resuscitation and vasoactive agents (e.g., ephedrine or phenylephrine) (16–18).

c) **Bradycardia** may result from blockade of T1-4 sympathetic cardioaccelerator fibers and decreased venous return (19).

i) Treatment is recommended when the heart rate is <50 to 60 bpm or dysrhythmia is observed, since sudden asystole and cardiovascular collapse may follow especially in young patients with high parasympathetic tone (20).

ii) If this occurs, external chest compressions and fluid resuscitation are necessary to maintain coronary perfusion and circulation of medications.

iii) Pharmacologic resuscitation includes atropine, ephedrine, and epinephrine.

Patients with hand numbness and decreased grip strength following spinal anesthesia are at risk for total spinal and should be closely monitored for respiratory depression.

d) **Postdural puncture headache**

i) May occur within 12 to 48 hours

ii) Characterized by a severe fronto-occipital headache in the upright position and improves with recumbency (21)

iii) PDPH is more common in women, younger patients, and use of larger gauge needles.

iv) Severe cases may be treated with 12 to 20 mL of autologous blood injected into the epidural space under sterile conditions (i.e., epidural blood patch) (21).

e) **Total spinal**

i) May occur when the block rises past the cervical region, potentially involving the brainstem

ii) Symptoms include a rapidly ascending motor-sensory block, hypotension, bradycardia, and possible respiratory arrest.

iii) Management includes hemodynamic and airway support and administration of an amnestic/anxiolytic agent until the block resolves.

iv) Most commonly seen as a result of inadvertent injection of an epidural dose of local anesthetic into the subarachnoid space

TNS have been associated with lidocaine spinal anesthesia, typically presenting the day following surgery, and resolve without sequelae.

Any patient with persistent or recurrent neurologic deficits and/or back pain after neuraxial block resolution should be immediately examined for signs and symptoms of spinal or epidural hematoma.

f) **Transient neurologic symptoms (TNS)**

i) Characterized by low back pain that radiates to the buttocks and lower extremities

ii) Is primarily associated with the use of lidocaine for spinal anesthesia but has been reported with other local anesthetics (22)

iii) Usually occurs the day following spinal anesthesia

iv) Risk factors include lithotomy position, obesity, and outpatient surgery.

v) Treatment is supportive since TNS usually resolves within 72 hours.

g) **Spinal or epidural hematoma** is extremely rare but often devastating.

i) Patients with pathologic defects in hemostasis or those pharmacologically anticoagulated are most at risk.

      ii) **Signs and symptoms**
- (1) May include persistent or residual weakness or numbness, back pain, or bladder dysfunction
- (2) Most importantly, the reappearance of anesthesia or neurologic deficits after block regression must be investigated.

      iii) Diagnostic MRI scan and neurosurgical consultation must be obtained immediately because prognosis is poor, especially for those with symptoms greater than 8 hours.

  h) **Persistent neuropathy** is extremely rare.
- i) For spinal anesthesia, the incidence is estimated at 3.8/10,000 with permanent neurological injury estimated from 0 to 4.2/10,000 (23).
- ii) In contrast, an epidural's estimated rate of neuropathy is 2.2/10,000 with permanent injury at 0 to 7.6/10,000 (23).

READ MORE

Epidural anesthesia, Chapter 31, page 237

  i) **Infection**
- i) Epidural abscess
- ii) Meningitis
  - (1) Rare complication
  - (2) Risk is significantly decreased by using meticulous sterile technique, including the use of masks (24).

Chapter Summary for Spinal Anesthesia

Definition	Placement of local anesthetic into the subarachnoid space.
Indications	Surgical anesthesia for procedures involving the lower abdomen, perineum, and lower extremities.
Advantages	Technically easy to perform, rapid onset of dense neural blockade, small volume of local anesthetic required.
Disadvantages	Limited duration unless catheter-based technique employed.
Potential Complications	Hemodynamic perturbations, PDPH, total spinal, hematoma, infection (rare).

NEURAXIAL AND REGIONAL ANESTHESIA

References
1. Cardoso MM, Carvalho JC, Amaro AR, et al. Small doses of intrathecal morphine combined with systemic diclofenac for postoperative pain control after cesarean delivery. *Anesth Analg* 1998;86:538–41.
2. Hawkins JL. Anesthesia-related maternal mortality. *Clin Obstet Gynecol* 2003;46:679–87.
3. Cousins MJ, Bridenbaugh PO. Neural Blockade In *Clinical Anesthesia and Management of Pain*. Philadelphia: Lippincott Williams & Wilkins, 1998.
4. Kesler H, Dias MS, Kalapos P. Termination of the normal conus medullaris in children: a whole-spine magnetic resonance imaging study. *Neurosurg Focus* 2007;23:1–5.
5. Soleiman J, Demaerel P, Rocher S, et al. Magnetic resonance imaging study of the level of termination of the conus medullaris and the thecal sac: influence of age and gender. *Spine* (Phila Pa 1976) 2005;30:1875–80.
6. Mulroy MF, Bernards CM, McDonald SB, et al. *A Practical Approach to Regional Anesthesia.* 4th Ed. Philadelphia: Lippincott Williams & Wilkins, 2009.
7. Fink BR. Mechanisms of differential axial blockade in epidural and subarachnoid anesthesia. *Anesthesiology* 1989;70:851–8.
8. Hamber EA, Viscomi CM. Intrathecal lipophilic opioids as adjuncts to surgical spinal anesthesia. *Reg Anesth Pain Med* 1999;24:255–63.
9. Vath JS, Kopacz DJ. Spinal 2-chloroprocaine: the effect of added fentanyl. *Anesth Analg* 2004;98:89–94.
10. Davis BR, Kopacz DJ. Spinal 2-chloroprocaine: the effect of added clonidine. *Anesth Analg* 2005;100:559–65.
11. Smith KN, Kopacz DJ, McDonald SB. Spinal 2-chloroprocaine: a dose-ranging study and the effect of added epinephrine. *Anesth Analg* 2004;98:81–8, table of contents.

12. Vallejo MC, Mandell GL, Sabo DP. Postdural puncture headache: a randomized comparison of five spinal needles in obstetric patients. *Anesth Analg* 2000;91(4):916–20.

13. Lund, P.C. Principles and Practice of Spinal Anesthesia. Springfield, IL, Charles C. Thomas, 1971.

14. Pong RP, Gmelch BS, Bernards CM. Does a paresthesia during spinal needle insertion indicate intrathecal needle placement? *Reg Anesth Pain Med* 2009;34:29–32.

15. Egbert LD, Tamersoy K, Deas TC. Pulmonary function during spinal anesthesia: the mechanism of cough depression. *Anesthesiology* 1961;22:882–5.

16. Carvalho B, Mercier FJ, Riley ET, et al. Hetastarch co-loading is as effective as pre-loading for the prevention of hypotension following spinal anesthesia for cesarean delivery. *Int J Obstet Anesth* 2009;18:150–5.

17. Riley ET. Editorial I: Spinal anaesthesia for Caesarean delivery: keep the pressure up and don't spare the vasoconstrictors. *Br J Anaesth* 2004;92:459–61.

18. Riley ET, Cohen SE, Rubenstein AJ, et al. Prevention of hypotension after spinal anesthesia for cesarean section: six percent hetastarch versus lactated Ringer's solution. *Anesth Analg* 1995;81:838–42.

19. Salinas FV, Sueda LA, Liu SS. Physiology of spinal anaesthesia and practical suggestions for successful spinal anaesthesia. *Best Pract Res Clin Anaesthesiol* 2003;17:289–303.

20. Pollard JB. Cardiac arrest during spinal anesthesia: common mechanisms and strategies for prevention. *Anesth Analg* 2001;92:252–6.

21. Candido KD, Stevens RA. Post-dural puncture headache: pathophysiology, prevention and treatment. *Best Pract Res Clin Anaesthesiol* 2003;17:451–69.

22. Freedman JM, Li DK, Drasner K, et al. Transient neurologic symptoms after spinal anesthesia: an epidemiologic study of 1,863 patients. *Anesthesiology* 1998;89:633–41.

23. Brull R, McCartney CJ, Chan VW, et al. Neurological complications after regional anesthesia: contemporary estimates of risk. *Anesth Analg* 2007;104:965–74.

24. Hebl JR. The importance and implications of aseptic techniques during regional anesthesia. *Reg Anesth Pain Med* 2006;31:311–23.

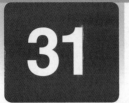

Epidural Anesthesia

Ray S. Lee, MD • Robert L. Hsiung, MD

Injection of local anesthetic solution with or without opioids into the epidural space produces various degrees of anesthesia and analgesia. Potential advantages over spinal anesthesia include the ability to perform an epidural at almost any level of the spine to target specific dermatomes, and the established practice of placing a catheter into the epidural space to allow titration of the block and continuous postoperative analgesia. Disadvantages include a longer time to perform the technique, slower onset, and a potentially less dense block.

1) **Indications and contraindications**
   a) **Indications**
      i) Epidural anesthesia or analgesia is generally performed for surgical procedures involving the chest, abdomen, pelvis, and lower extremities.
      ii) It can be used intraoperatively as the primary or the adjunct anesthetic or postoperatively as a continuous infusion with or without patient-controlled epidural analgesia.
   b) **Contraindications**
      i) Absolute contraindications
         (1) Language or consent barrier
         (2) Increased intracranial pressure
         (3) Coagulopathy
      ii) Relative contraindications
         (1) Systemic infection
         (2) Inability to position
         (3) Hemodynamic profile that would not tolerate a decrease in systemic vascular resistance (e.g., shock or aortic stenosis)

2) **Anatomy**
   a) The epidural space is located between the dura and the walls of the vertebral canal and extends from the foramen magnum down to the sacrococcygeal ligament (1).
   b) It is bound anteriorly by the posterior longitudinal ligament, laterally by the vertebral pedicles, and posteriorly by the ligamentum flavum and vertebral lamina.
   c) Unlike the subarachnoid space, the epidural space is not a closed space.
      i) It communicates with the paravertebral spaces through the intervertebral foramina.
      ii) In addition, it becomes a series of discontinuous compartments when the dura intermittently abuts the ligamentum flavum or pedicles.

The site of injection, volume, and dose are the major factors that determine spread of epidural block.

The choice of medication administered in the epidural space depends on whether the catheter is used for **anesthesia** or **analgesia** and the side effect profile tolerated by the patient.

    iii) Injection of liquid or air may open up the potential space connecting these compartments.

  d) The epidural space contains lymphatics, epidural fat pads, and a network of valveless veins known as *Baston's plexus*.

3) **Pharmacology**

 a) **Determinates of block spread**

  i) **Site of injection**

    (1) Thoracic injection produces symmetrical spread of anesthetic solution.

      (a) A reduced volume of local anesthetic solution should be used at this level because of the potential for higher block and resultant hemodynamic perturbations.

    (2) Lumbar injection produces a preferential cephalad spread due to the narrowing of the epidural space at the lumbosacral junction.

      (a) The larger diameter of the L5-S1 nerve roots may delay the onset or result in patchy anesthesia.

    (3) Caudal injection predominantly results in sacral and low lumbar anesthesia, except in young children (2).

  ii) **Volume and dose**

    (1) Volume and dose are independent variables in predicting the spread of anesthetic solution.

    (2) Increasing the injected volume will increase the extent of epidural block.

 b) **Determinates of block duration**

  i) Local anesthetic selection (3) (Table 31-1)

    (1) There are many different options for epidural medication dosing. Most include a local anesthetic and/or opioid.

Table 31-1

Local Anesthetics Commonly Used for Epidural Anesthesia

Local Anesthetic	Complete Resolution (min)
Short Duration	
2-Chloroprocaine 3%	100–160
Intermediate Duration	
Lidocaine 2%	160–200
Mepivacaine 2%	160–200
Long Duration	
Ropivacaine 0.5%–1.0%	240–420
Bupivacaine 0.5%–0.75%	300–460

Adapted from Mulroy MF, Bernards CM, McDonald SB, et al. *A Practical Approach to Regional Anesthesia.* 4th ed. Philadelphia, PA: Lippincott Williams & Wilkins; 2009.

(2) The selection of local anesthetic depends on the desired duration of the anesthetic, which in large part depends on the surgical procedure.

(3) For postoperative analgesia, dilute solutions (0.08% to 0.15%) of ropivacaine or bupivacaine (0.08% to 0.15%) with or without opioids such as morphine or hydromorphone are commonly used.

(4) Bupivacaine 0.75% solution was historically used for epidural anesthesia but is no longer available due to the potential for severe local anesthetic toxicity (i.e., cardiac arrest) with inadvertent intravascular injection.

ii) **Volume**

(1) For lumbar injections, a recommended bolus volume of 15 to 20 mL will, on average, produce a midthoracic block.

(2) For thoracic injections, a starting bolus volume of 5 mL is reasonable.

(3) The use of an epidural catheter allows titration of the epidural block.

(4) All dosing should be incremental and performed only after a negative aspiration for CSF and blood.

iii) **Adjuvants**

(1) The addition of epinephrine prolongs the duration of epidural anesthesia during bolus injection.

(a) The precise mechanism is unknown but may be attributed to decreased clearance of the local anesthetic due to vasoconstriction.

(b) Epinephrine is not recommended as an adjuvant for continuous infusions.

(2) Opioids (e.g., fentanyl, sufentanil) improve the quality of sensory blockade, depending on dose and lipid solubility (4,5).

iv) **Site of action**

(1) Local anesthetic solutions injected into the epidural space are thought to act on the spinal nerves traversing the epidural space and the spinal nerve rootlets in the subarachnoid space.

4) **Equipment**

a) Common equipment for all regional anesthetic techniques includes a marking pen and an appropriate volume of local anesthetic solution.

b) Epidural anesthesia should be performed with meticulous sterile technique with sterile skin cleansing solution, sterile gloves, hat, mask, and large clear sterile fenestrated drape.

c) Epidural needle and catheter

i) Epidural needles typically have a blunt tip (e.g., Tuohy tip).

ii) Needles are usually large enough to pass a catheter, most commonly 17 to 18 G.

iii) Epidural catheters may be single- or multiorifice.

d) Low-friction syringe filled with preservative-free saline, air, or a combination of both.

e) A prepackaged custom tray with all anticipated equipment and labeled syringes will save time during the procedure.

5) **Technique**

a) **Monitoring**

i) Epidural anesthetics should be performed in a location where the patient's noninvasive BP, SpO_2, and EKG may be monitored.

READ MORE

Obstetrical anesthesia, Chapter 144, page 1047

ii) Supplemental O_2 should be provided *via* a face mask or nasal cannulae, especially if sedation is to be administered.

iii) **For labor analgesia**

(1) Sedation is not usually administered.

(2) The ASA recommends that the parturient's vital signs and the fetal heart rate be monitored and documented, with additional monitoring based on the clinical condition of the patient or fetus (6).

    a) Practically speaking, BP is typically monitored during the procedure and for the duration of analgesia.

    b) SpO_2 is often monitored during the procedure and when indicated (e.g., maternal sleep apnea).

    c) ECG is frequently not monitored but should be immediately available and used for any maternal indications.

iv) Emergency airway equipment and resuscitation drugs should be immediately available.

b) **Positioning and preparation**

    i) Patients are typically positioned lateral decubitus or sitting.

      (1) Lateral decubitus

READ MORE

Spinal anesthesia, Chapter 30, page 225

        (a) The patient's back should be at the edge of the bed, while keeping the shoulders and hips perpendicular to the bed to prevent rotation of the spine.

        (b) The knees are drawn upward toward the chest, with forward neck flexion, and active protrusion of the lower back.

      (2) Sitting

        (a) May help identify midline, particularly in obese patients

    ii) The anticipated injection site is prepared with appropriate antiseptic solution and draped in sterile fashion.

      (1) It is beneficial to prepare a wide area to facilitate any subsequent attempt at a different level.

      (2) If using povidone-iodine, allow the antiseptic solution to dry and wipe away any excess.

c) **Identification of surface anatomy**

    i) The most prominent spinous process at the cervical level is C7.

    ii) A line drawn between the tips of the scapula estimates T7, while one drawn between the iliac crests (Tuffier's line) estimates L4 (Fig. 31-1 A).

    iii) Using the index and middle finger side by side, palpate the spinous processes by sliding side to side and up and down the midline.

d) **Paramedian approach**

    i) May be used for any level but commonly applied to thoracic epidurals

    ii) Palpate the desired interspace and after warning the patient, infiltrate the skin with local anesthetic approximately 1 cm lateral to the inferior aspect of the superior spinous process (Fig. 31-1B).

    iii) To help determine the location and depth, inject along the desired pathway of the epidural needle to the lamina.

    iv) Insert the epidural needle perpendicular to the skin at the infiltration site until lamina is contacted.

      (1) Direct the needle medially along the lamina by intermittently withdrawing the needle and redirecting it towards midline (Fig. 31-2).

      (2) If the depth decreases, this likely represents the juncture between the lamina and the lateral aspect of the spinous process.

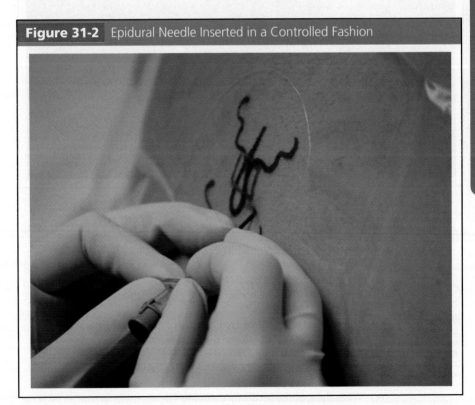

Figure 31-1 Landmarks for Placement of Epidural Anesthesia

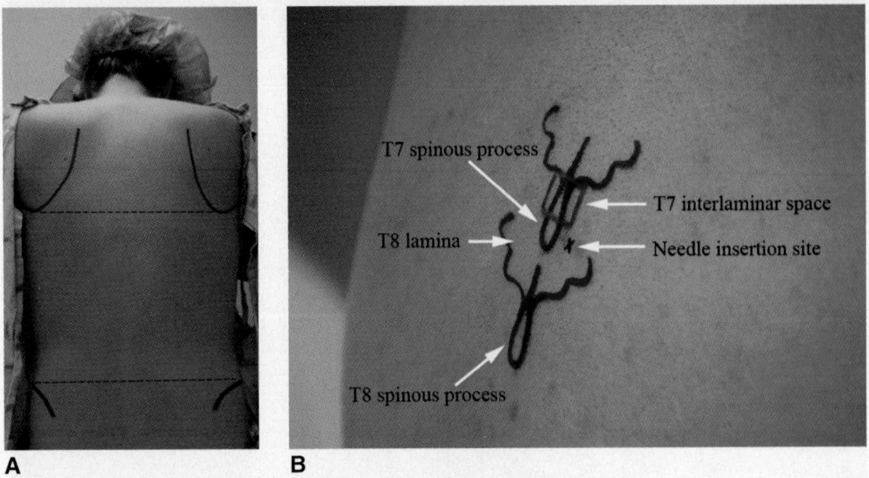

T7 spinous process

T7 interlaminar space

T8 lamina

Needle insertion site

T8 spinous process

A   **B**

A: A Line drawn between the tips of the scapula estimates T7. **B.** Thoracic epidural landmarks.

Figure 31-2 Epidural Needle Inserted in a Controlled Fashion

Figure 31-3 Loss-of-Resistance Technique with Saline and Air

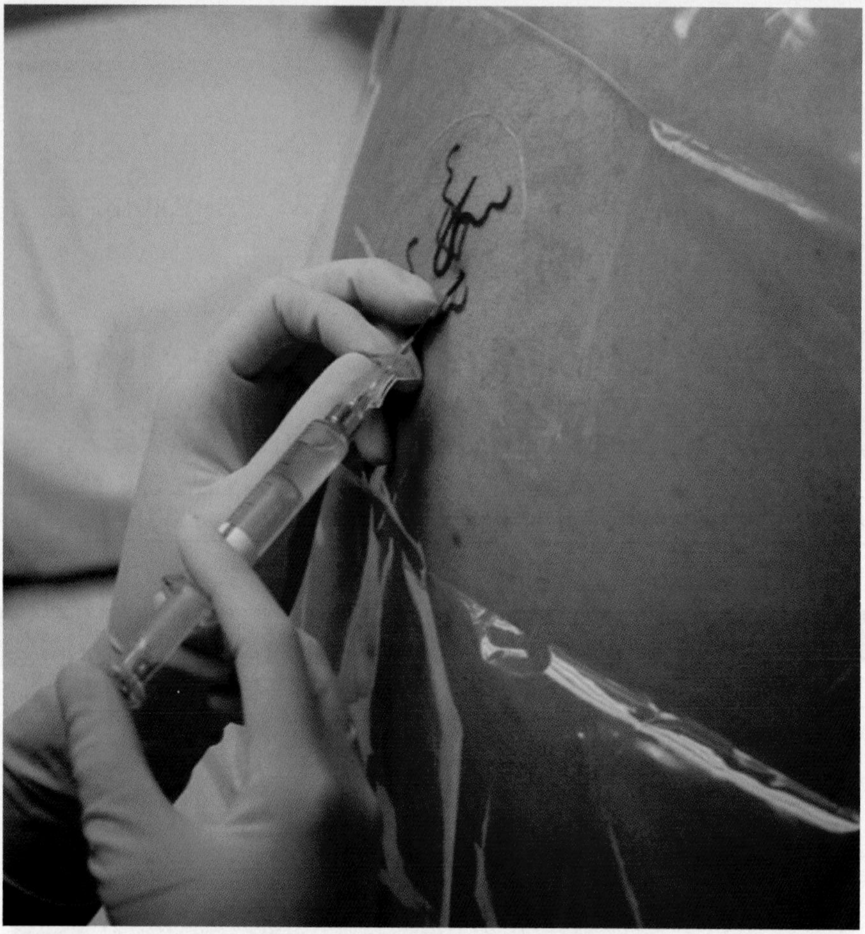

v) **Loss-of-resistance technique with saline (author's preferred technique)**
(1) Remove the stylet and attach a low-friction syringe containing preservative-free saline with or without a small visible air bubble (Fig. 31-3).
(2) Stabilize the epidural needle by resting the dorsum of the nondominant hand against the patient's back, while grasping the needle between the thumb and the index finger.
(3) The epidural needle is then redirected in the cephalad direction and "marched" off the lamina into the ligamentum flavum.
(4) Apply continuous pressure on the syringe plunger with the dominant hand, while carefully advancing the epidural needle shaft with the non-dominant hand.
(5) When the epidural needle tip encounters ligamentum flavum, **an increase in resistance is felt.**

READ
MORE

Atlas of anesthe-
sia procedures:
lumbar epidural
placement,
Chapter 161,
page 1118

It is important to note and document the depth of the epidural space, which can be determined by noting the location on the needle where loss of resistance is encountered.

(6) When the epidural needle tip subsequently enters the epidural space, a **decrease or a loss of resistance is felt as saline is injected into the space.**

(7) Stop advancement of the needle.

(8) For a continuous catheter technique, disconnect the syringe and thread the epidural catheter 3 to 5 cm into the epidural space.

(9) Stabilize the catheter while withdrawing the epidural needle.

e) **Median or midline approach**

i) Commonly performed for lumbar epidurals

ii) The target interspace is identified, and the approach is similar to the midline spinal anesthetic technique.

iii) The epidural needle is inserted in the midline of the target interspace and carefully advanced through the interspinous ligament.

iv) Attach the low-friction syringe containing preservative-free saline and proceed with the loss-of-resistance technique as described previously.

f) Alternative techniques may be used for identification of the epidural space such as loss of resistance to air or the "hanging drop" method, although an increased incidence of accidental dural puncture has been associated with the air technique (7).

g) **Test dose**

i) The use of an epinephrine-containing test dose to assess catheter position is controversial, especially for obstetrical patients (8).

ii) Aspirate prior to injecting the test dose to check for CSF or blood.

iii) Injection of up to 3 mL of 1.5% lidocaine with 1:200,000 epinephrine may help detect subarachnoid injection (rapid onset of spinal anesthesia) or intravascular placement (increased HR by ~30 bpm in <1 minute) (9).

6) **Troubleshooting**

a) False loss of resistance

Epidural catheters should always be aspirated to rule out intrathecal or intravascular location prior to injection.

i) When the characteristic loss of resistance is not felt, the epidural needle may have passed obliquely through the ligamentum flavum and into the paraspinous muscle.

ii) Using the low-friction syringe, injection of a small amount of air (0.5 mL) can help differentiate between these two scenarios.

iii) Almost no resistance will be felt in the epidural space, while resistance can be felt in the paraspinous muscles.

iv) Furthermore, a loss of resistance may represent any change in tissue interface, including fascial layers, pleural lining, and bone.

v) Passage of a small gauge spinal needle *via* the epidural needle through the dura and observation of free CSF flow may be a useful confirmatory test of proper epidural needle placement.

READ MORE

Combined spinal-epidural technique, Chapter 33, page 252

b) Difficulty threading the catheter

i) The needle may either be partially in the epidural space, occluded by epidural fat, or incorrectly positioned.

ii) First, confirm appropriate needle placement with loss of resistance to air or saline.

iii) Often, additional fluid or air creates a potential space for catheterization.

iv) Only when the epidural needle is properly positioned in the epidural space should epidural needle rotation or slight advancement be considered.

NEURAXIAL AND REGIONAL ANESTHESIA

c) Obesity

    i) The optimal position for obese patients is sitting, knees suspended on a support, and arms and neck embracing a stand.

    ii) A special apparatus like a massage chair is helpful, but an assistant to prevent falls and provide patient encouragement is essential.

    iii) Location of interspaces may be estimated, but depth to the spinous process and lamina may be determined by separate insertion of "finder" spinal needles or needles used for local anesthetic infiltration.

        (1) The key is to direct the needles perpendicular, or even caudad, to skin to avoid accidental insertion into the intrathecal space and spinal cord.

    iv) Alternatively, ultrasound can also help determine vertebral interspaces, depth of spinous and transverse processes, and depth to the ligamentum flavum and the posterior longitudinal ligaments for both spinal and epidural placements (10).

7) **Risks and complications**

a) The incidence and variety of complications related to epidurals are similar to those associated with spinal anesthesia.

READ MORE

Spinal anesthesia, Chapter 30, page 225

b) **Hypotension**

    i) Generally, slower onset and more gradual than encountered in spinal anesthesia

    ii) Management includes IV fluids and vasoactive agents

c) **Unilateral epidural anesthesia**

    i) Despite attempts at directing epidural catheters during placement, they are rarely found in the midline position (11).

    ii) Epidural injectate spread is highly variable (12).

    iii) A unilateral block may occur if the epidural catheter tip enters an intervertebral foramen or is positioned in the anterior epidural space, especially when inserted more than 5 cm.

    iv) Uniform anesthesia may sometimes be achieved by increasing the volume of local anesthetic solution, increasing the dosing frequency, or withdrawing the catheter so that only 3 to 5 cm remains in the epidural space.

    v) When these maneuvers fail, the epidural catheter should be removed and a replacement catheter offered.

The risk of unilateral epidural blockade is higher when the catheter is inserted >5 cm.

d) **Dural puncture**

    i) Given the larger diameter of the epidural needle, inadvertent subarachnoid puncture increases the likelihood of postdural puncture headache (13).

    ii) If free-flowing CSF appears after removal of the stylet, options include

        (1) Remove the epidural needle and reattempt placement at a different level

        (2) Placement of an intrathecal catheter, using doses appropriate for intrathecal administration

            (a) May decrease the incidence of postdural puncture headache (14)

            (b) Only recommended at the lumbar level

If an epidural catheter is not functioning properly and appropriate measures to correct problems have been taken, it is appropriate to offer the patient a replacement catheter.

e) **Intravascular injection of local anesthetics**

    i) Epidural catheters, especially when used for surgical anesthesia, may require large volumes of concentrated local anesthetic that may be toxic if injected intravascularly.

READ MORE

Postdural puncture headache and epidural blood patch, Chapter 32, page 247

Local anesthetics,
Chapter 37,
page 282

Spinal anesthesia,
Chapter 30,
page 225

    ii)   Catheters may migrate intravascularly at any time and must always be aspirated for blood prior to injection.

f) **Epidural hematoma**

    i)   This rare complication can lead to permanent paralysis and requires immediate diagnosis and intervention.

    ii)   Avoid performing epidural anesthesia in patients receiving anticoagulants (15).

g) **Epidural abscess**

    i)   Rare complication that may be associated with prolonged epidural catheter duration (16).

    ii)   Symptoms

        (1) Usually presents several days after the epidural catheter is removed

        (2) Severe backache with tenderness, fever, headache, sensory and motor deficits, and bladder incontinence

        (3) Erythema at catheter site and increased white blood cell count may be observed.

        (4) Symptoms should prompt rapid diagnostic MRI scan.

    iii) Treatment

        (1) Surgical decompression *via* laminectomy

        (2) Must be initiated as soon as possible for optimal outcome

h) **Persistent neurologic symptoms (see Chapter 30, Spinal Anesthesia, for more information)**

i) **Block failure**

    i)   Unlike spinal anesthetics, epidurals have a higher rate of not working, possibly from needle misplacement or inadvertent catheter dislodgement (17).

    ii)   Furthermore, they are sometimes discontinued postoperatively due to side effects from drugs.

        (1) Opioids may cause pruritis, nausea and vomiting, sedation, and respiratory depression.

        (2) Local anesthetics produce hypotension and may cause lower extremity weakness, thereby increasing the risk of falls.

Chapter Summary for Epidural Anesthesia

Definition	Placement of medications and or an indwelling catheter in the epidural space, which is between the ligamentum flavum and the dura.
Indications	Postoperative analgesia, labor analgesia, and surgical anesthesia.
Advantages	Long duration, especially with catheter-based technique; may be used at any level in the spine for more precise location of analgesia; allows the avoidance or reduction of IV narcotics.
Disadvantages	Longer time to perform the technique, slower onset, and a potentially less dense block; potential for unilateral block, and motor blockade.
Potential Complications	Hemodynamic perturbations, dural puncture, epidural hematoma or infection (rare).

NEURAXIAL AND REGIONAL ANESTHESIA

References

1. Barash PG, Cullen BF, Stoelting RK. *Clinical Anesthesia*. Philadelphia, PA: Lippincott Williams & Wilkins; 2009.
2. Hong JY, Han SW, Kim WO, et al. A comparison of high volume/low concentration and low volume/high concentration ropivacaine in caudal analgesia for pediatric orchiopexy. *Anesth Analg* 2009;109(4):1073–1078.
3. Mulroy MF, Bernards CM, McDonald SB, et al. *A Practical Approach to Regional Anesthesia*. 4th ed. Philadelphia, PA: Lippincott Williams & Wilkins; 2009.
4. Scott DA, Blake D, Buckland M, et al. A comparison of epidural ropivacaine infusion alone and in combination with 1, 2, and 4 microg/mL fentanyl for seventy-two hours of postoperative analgesia after major abdominal surgery. *Anesth Analg* 1999;88:857–864.
5. Polley LS, Columb MO, Wagner DS, et al. Dose-dependent reduction of the minimum local analgesic concentration of bupivacaine by sufentanil for epidural analgesia in labor. *Anesthesiology* 1998;89:626–632.
6. American Society of Anesthesiologists Task Force on Obstetric Anesthesia. Practice guidelines for obstetric anesthesia: an updated report by the American Society of Anesthesiologists Task Force on Obstetric Anesthesia. *Anesthesiology* 2007;106(4):843–863.
7. Evron S, Sessler D, Sadan O, et al. Identification of the epidural space: loss of resistance with air, lidocaine, or the combination of air and lidocaine. *Anesth Analg* 2004;99:(1):245–250.
8. Norris MC, Ferrenbach D, Dalman H, et al. Does epinephrine improve the diagnostic accuracy of aspiration during labor epidural analgesia? *Anesth Analg* 1999;88:1073–1076.
9. Moore DC, Batra MS. The components of an effective test dose prior to epidural block. *Anesthesiology* 1981;55(6):693–696.
10. Carvalho JC. Ultrasound-facilitated epidurals and spinals in obstetrics. *Anesthesiol Clin* 2008;26:145–158, vii–viii.
11. Asato F, Goto F. Radiographic findings of unilateral epidural block. *Anesth Analg* 1996;83:519–522.
12. Hogan Q. Epidural catheter tip position and distribution of injectate evaluated by computed tomography. *Anesthesiology* 1999;90:964–970.
13. Kuczkowski KM. Post-dural puncture headache in the obstetric patient: an old problem. New solutions. *Minerva Anestesiol* 2004;70:823–830.
14. Dennehy KC, Rosaeg OP. Intrathecal catheter insertion during labour reduces the risk of post-dural puncture headache. *Can J Anaesth* 1998;45(1)42–45.
15. Horlocker TT, Wedel DJ, Rowlingson JC, et al. Regional anesthesia in the patient receiving antithrombotic or thrombolytic therapy: American Society of Regional Anesthesia and Pain Medicine Evidence-Based Guidelines (Third Edition). *Reg Anesth Pain Med* 2010;35:64–101.
16. Grewal S, Hocking G, Wildsmith JA. Epidural abscesses. *Br J Anaesth* 2006;96(3):292–302.
17. Pan PH, Bogard TD, Owen MD. Incidence and characteristics of failures in obstetric neuraxial analgesia and anesthesia: a retrospective analysis of 19,259 deliveries. *Int J Obstet Anesth* 2004;13(4):227–233.

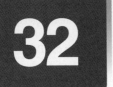

32

Postdural Puncture Headache and Epidural Blood Patch

Andrea J. Fuller, MD

When the dura is punctured for diagnostic or anesthetic purposes, loss of cerebral spinal fluid (CSF) occurs. In some patients, this results in a postdural puncture headache (PDPH), the symptoms of which range from mild to debilitating. It is important for the anesthesia provider to consider the differential diagnosis of headache when evaluating a patient with a suspected PDPH.

1) Pathophysiology (1,2)
   a) **Dural puncture results in loss of CSF**
   b) The pathophysiology and mechanism of PDPH is poorly understood.
   c) Commonly accepted theories
      i) Traction on pain-sensitive structures due to pressure changes in the cranium
      ii) Cerebral venous dilation (1,2)

2) Symptoms (2)

The symptoms of a PDPH sometimes are not a classic headache but are instead dizziness, auditory changes, visual disturbances, or neck pain that are positional in nature.

   a) **Characteristics**
      i) Onset is usually 12 to 48 hours after dural puncture.
      ii) PDPH is located in the **frontal or occipital** region.
      iii) Accompanying symptoms include **neck pain, visual disturbances** (which may be due to cranial nerve palsies), **photophobia, nausea and vomiting, dizziness, and auditory changes.**
         (1) Double vision is possible due to traction on the VI cranial nerve.
   b) **Positional changes**
      i) The classic symptom of PDPH is that the headache (HA) is relieved upon assuming the supine position and worsened in the upright position.

3) Incidence of HA with dural puncture depends on several variables.
   a) **Needle size**
      i) In general, the larger the needle, the higher the incidence of HA.
   b) **Needle type**
      i) Pencil-point needles (Whitacre, Sprotte, and Gertie-Marx) have a lower incidence of HA than cutting-point needles (Quincke).
         (1) For example, a 26-g Quincke needle has a PDPH incidence of 5%, while a 25-g Whittacre needle has an incidence of approximately 1% (3).
   c) **Bevel direction**
      i) If a Quincke needle is used, care should be taken to orient the bevel of the needle with the longitudinal axis of the spine as this decreases the incidence of headache.

d) **Patient characteristics**
  i) Female patients and/or those younger than 40 years have a higher incidence of PDPH than male patients and those over 60 years old.
  ii) Morbidly obese patients have a lower incidence of PDPH.

4) **Patient evaluation**
  a) The patient must have a thorough history and physical examination.
  b) The onset, characteristics, severity, and exacerbating factors should be determined.
  c) A thorough chart review should focus on coexisting disease, vital signs (especially temperature and blood pressure), and laboratory evaluations such as the white blood cell count.
  d) Physical exam should be focused on ruling out neurologic deficits.

5) **Differential diagnosis**
  a) **Preeclampsia**
    i) Hypertensive disorders of pregnancy are often accompanied by HA.
  b) **Musculoskeletal HA**
    i) Patients may have muscle tension headaches from lying in bed.
    ii) Postpartum patients may experience muscle tension due to breast-feeding.
  c) **Caffeine withdrawal**
    i) Patients who regularly consume caffeine may experience HA when caffeine is withheld.
  d) **Pneumocephalus**
    i) Immediate onset of severe HA can be associated with pneumocephalus due to use of the loss of resistance to air technique for localizing the epidural space and subsequent unintended dural puncture.
      (1) High inspired O_2 concentration can result in improvement of symptoms (2).
  e) **Subarachnoid hematoma**
    i) Sudden onset of severe HA and/or accompanying neurological deficits may be the result of a ruptured of cerebral aneurysm and/or arteriovenous malformation (2).
  f) **Venous sinus thrombosis**
    i) Peripartum patients are at higher risk for this condition, and many will have undergone dural puncture for labor analgesia or cesarean delivery.
    ii) In these patients, the HA loses its positional nature and/or other neurologic signs/symptoms are present over time (4).
  g) **Subdural hematoma**
    i) Decreased CSF volume from dural puncture rarely may result in bleeding from cerebral vessels.
  h) **Migraine**
    i) In patients with a history of migraine HA, it is important to differentiate between his/her typical symptoms and PDPH.
  i) **Meningitis**
    i) The presence of fever and nuchal rigidity is an ominous sign in a patient with HA.
      (1) Antibiotic therapy must be started in a timely manner.

In postpartum patients with PDPH, patient safety is an important concern as they often are sleep deprived and have children to care for at home.

6) Conservative treatment
   a) **IV and/or oral hydration**
      i) While widely prescribed for treatment of PDPH, there is no evidence supporting the benefit of hydration for PDPH (2).
   b) **Caffeine**
      i) The effectiveness of caffeine has been debated, but studies have shown a modest benefit to oral and IV caffeine (5,6).
         (1) Caffeine is a central nervous stimulant with side effects of insomnia, arrhythmias, and seizures and should not be used for long-term therapy.
   c) **Supine position**
      i) Maintaining the supine position after dural puncture is not effective in preventing or treating PDPH (2).
   d) **Other treatments**
      i) **The most consistently effective and well-studied treatment for PDPH is an epidural blood patch (EBP).**

7) Natural course of PDPH
   a) In most patients, the HA resolves after 1 to 2 weeks.
   b) However, performance of daily activities is impaired in many patients and can last up to 1 month. Rarely, symptoms can last much longer (years in some patients) (2).
      i) The importance of this in parturients cannot be emphasized enough, as this patient population expects to care for an infant and often other children.

READ MORE

Epidural anesthesia, Chapter 31, page 237

Lumbar epidural placement, Chapter 161, page 1118

8) **Epidural blood patch**
   a) **Effectiveness**
      i) The reported success rate of EBP varies significantly. In one study, the success rate of EPB in a heterogeneous population that included parturients was 75% (7).
      ii) The rate of success depends on the type of needle used for dural puncture, with large bore needles resulting in lower success rates.
      iii) When the EBP is delayed for 24 hours after the dural puncture, it is more effective (8).
   b) **Informed consent**
      i) The patient should be counseled about the **possibility of repeat dural puncture and worsening HA.**
      ii) The most common complaint after EBP is back pain lasting up to 1 week.
      iii) Otherwise, the risks are equivalent to the risks of epidural placement.

Patient follow-up after PDPH diagnosis is essential.

   c) **Performing EBP**
      i) **Meticulous sterile technique** must be maintained.
      ii) Many patients are not comfortable in the upright position, so the lateral position may be used.
         (1) However, especially in patients with potentially difficult EBP, the upright position can be used, with care taken to minimize the time the patient spends in this position.
      iii) The epidural space is localized.
      iv) Blood is obtained under sterile conditions by an assistant and passed to the person performing the epidural.

         v)   After aspiration for blood and CSF, the blood should be injected in 5-ml increments to a total of 20 mL or until the patient experiences pressure in his/her head or back.

         vi)   The patient should then lie flat for approximately one hour, after which he or she is reassessed for resolution of HA (9).

         vii)   In the days following the procedure, the patient should be advised against heavy lifting and valsalva maneuvers, which may dislodge the clot.

         viii) Patient follow-up is extremely important in order to monitor for complications and ensure resolution of the HA.

   d) **EBP through an epidural catheter**

         i)   The effectiveness of EBP performed through an epidural catheter in parturients with unintended dural puncture was recently examined. In this study, the **duration of the HA was shortened, but the incidence and severity were unchanged** (10).

         ii)   Given this information, this author recommends EBP through an epidural catheter only for patients whose epidural catheters were extremely difficult to place and are at high risk for repeat dural puncture with EBP.

 9) **Contraindications to EBP**

   a) Immunosuppression, systemic infection, coagulation disorder, and patient refusal

10) **Other treatments**

   a) **Intrathecal catheter**

         i)   Recent evidence in parturients suggests that when an unintended dural puncture occurs and the anesthetic plan included an epidural catheter, placing the catheter in the intrathecal space may reduce the incidence of PDPH.

         ii)   HA incidence is reduced most in patients whose catheter is left in place for 24 hours after delivery (11).

         iii)   **Extreme caution must be taken when an intrathecal catheter is in place.**

             (1)   Communication to all staff (nursing, obstetrics, and anesthesia) about the presence of an intrathecal catheter is paramount.

             (2)   Clearly label the catheter as **intrathecal** in order to prevent administration of medications intended for intravascular or epidural administration.

             (3)   Care must also be taken to prevent infection.

Patients with a perioperative or postpartum HA require a thorough evaluation to eliminate causes other than CSF leak from dural puncture.

11) **Managing a patient with a PDPH in whom EBP has been ineffective**

   a) In the vast majority of patients with PDPH, two blood patches will result in resolution symptoms.

   b) **Indications for imaging studies and/or consultation with a neurologist include unresolved headache after two EBP, worsening HA severity, changing characteristics (including loss of positional nature), fever, and associated sensory or motor deficits.**

Chapter Summary for PDPH and Epidural Blood Patch

Patient Characteristics	↑ risk in women, age < 40 ↓ risk with obesity
Signs and Symptoms	Positional (improved with supine position) Frontal/occipital Throbbing Associated photophobia, double vision, nausea/vomiting
Differential Diagnosis	Must always be considered and patient thoroughly evaluated Includes musculoskeletal headache, caffeine withdrawal, migraine, meningitis, subarachnoid hemorrhage, and subdural hematoma
Treatment	Conservative measures include caffeine and hydration and have limited effectiveness EBP most effective

References

1. Gaiser R. Postdural puncture headache. *Curr Opin Anaesthesiol* 2006;19:249–253.
2. Weeks SK. Postpartum headache. In: Chestnut DH, ed. *Obstetric Anesthesia: Principles and Practice*. 3rd ed. Philadelphia, PA: Elsevier Mosby; 2004:562–578.
3. Lambert DH, Hurley RJ, Hertwig L, et al. Role of needle gauge and tip configuration in the production of lumbar puncture headache. *Reg Anesth* 1997;22(1):66–72.
4. Lockhart E, Baysinger C. Intracranial venous thrombosis in the parturient. *Anesthesiology* 2007;2007(4):652–658.
5. Halker RB, Demaerschalk BM, Wellik KE, et al. Caffeine for the prevention and treatment of postdural puncture headache: debunking the myth. *Neurologist* 2007;13(5):323–327.
6. Camann WR, Murray RS, Mushlin PS, et al. Effects of oral caffeine on postdural puncture headache. A double-blind, placebo-controlled trial. *Anesth Analg* 1990;70(2):181–184.
7. Safa-Tisseront V, Thormann F, Malassine P, et al. Effectiveness of epidural blood patch in the management of post-dural puncture headache. *Anesthesiology* 2001;95(2):334–339.
8. Vilming S, Kloster R, Sandvik L. When should an epidural blood patch be performed in postlumbar puncture headache? A theoretical approach based on a cohort of 79 patients. *Cephalgia* 2005;25:523–527.
9. Martin R, Jourdain S, Clairoux M, et al. Duration of decubitus position after epidural blood patch. *Can J Anaesth* 1994;41(1):23–25.
10. Scavone BM, Wong CA, Sullivan JT, et al. Efficacy of a prophylactic epidural blood patch in preventing post dural puncture headache in parturients after inadvertent dural puncture. *Anesthesiology* 2004;101(6):1422–1427.
11. Ayad S, Demian Y, Narouze S, et al. Subarachnoid catheter placement after wet tap for analgesia in labor: Influence on the risk of headache in obstetric patients. *Reg Anesth Pain Med* 2003;28:512–515.

33 Combined Spinal-Epidural Technique

Andrea J. Fuller, MD

The combined spinal-epidural (CSE) technique involves administering a dose of medication in the intrathecal space and also placing an epidural catheter. It is widely used for labor analgesia and may be utilized for nonobstetric procedures.

1) Indications
   a) **Labor analgesia**
      i) Rapid onset of analgesia
      ii) Improved patient satisfaction in some studies (1)
      iii) Lower incidence of motor block, especially if intrathecal opioids are given without local anesthetic (e.g., "walking epidural" [1])
   b) **Operative procedure of uncertain duration**
      i) A CSE can be placed in patients who strongly desire a regional anesthetic but whose procedure length may exceed the duration of the local anesthetic chosen for a single injection spinal (1).
   c) **Administration of long-acting epidural medication**
      i) The CSE technique may be used when one prefers the rapid onset of a spinal anesthetic but would like to have an epidural in place for administration of long-acting epidural medications, such as sustained-release epidural morphine (DepoDur) (2).
2) Technique
   a) **Needle-through-needle** (Fig. 33-1)
      i) **Most common CSE technique**
      ii) The epidural space is localized with the loss of resistance to saline or air technique.
      iii) A spinal needle is placed through the epidural needle.
      iv) A characteristic "pop" is felt and free flow of cerebrospinal fluid (CSF) observed.
      v) Spinal medication is administered and the spinal needle removed.
      vi) The epidural catheter is then placed and secured.
   b) **Separate procedures**
      i) When the epidural and spinal are performed separately, they can be done at the same or different interspinous spaces.
      ii) It is advisable to place the spinal portion first as it is theoretically possible to traumatize a previously placed epidural catheter when the spinal needle passes through the epidural space.
3) Failures with the CSE technique (Fig. 33-2)
   a) **Failure of spinal portion of block**
      i) "Tenting" of the dura—low dural pressure (3)
         (1) More likely when the procedure is done in the lateral position due to lower CSF pressure

When saline is used for the epidural portion of CSE, it is important to confirm free flow of CSF to avoid the possibility of mistaking saline for CSF, resulting in failed spinal block.

Figure 33-1   Needle-Through-Needle Technique for CSE

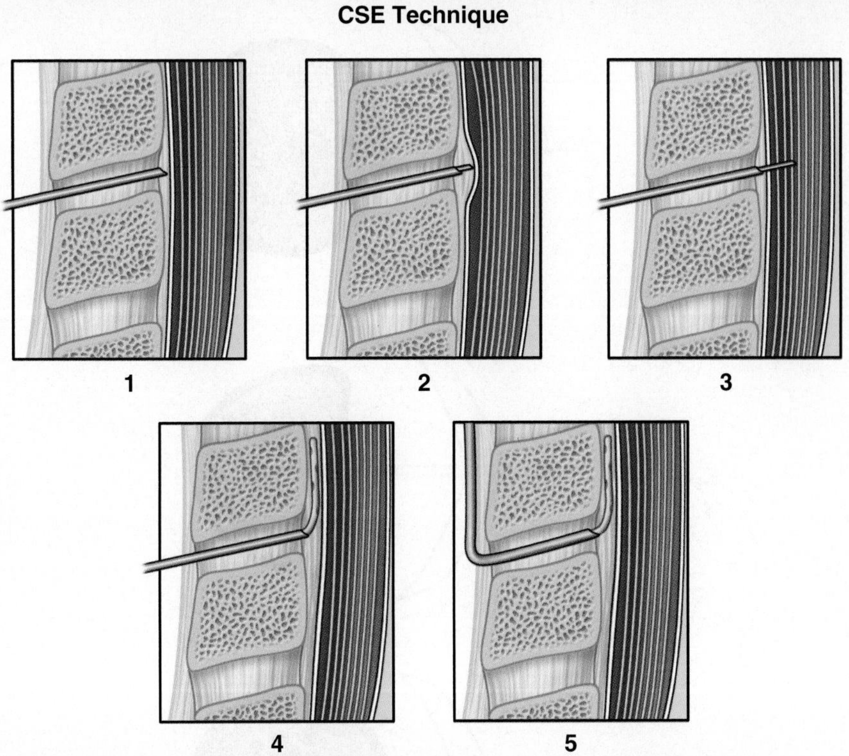

CSE Technique

1. Epidural space is located with standard techniques; **2.** Spinal needle is inserted through epidural needle and may cause tenting of the dura prior to puncture; **3.** Dura is punctured and free flow of CSF confirmed. Intrathecal injection is now administered; **4.** Epidural catheter is placed; **5.** Epidural needle is removed and catheter is secured. Modified from Eisenach JC. Combined spinal-epidural analgesia in obstetrics. *Anesthesiology* 1999;91(1):299–302.

For patients for whom the reliability of an epidural catheter is extremely important (severe preeclampsia, difficult airway, nonreassuring fetal heart rate tracing), it may be advisable to avoid the CSE technique in favor of epidural placement.

    ii) Off midline
        (1) When the needle is not in the midline, it is possible for the spinal needle to be lateral to the dural sac (3).
    iii) Spinal needle not long enough to puncture dura (3,4)
    iv) Mistaken saline for CSF when LOR to saline technique is used
        (1) Must confirm free flow of CSF in spinal needle before injection
  b) **Failure of epidural**
    i) **Untested catheter**
        (1) It is advisable to avoid CSE in patients with a difficult airway if one must rely on the epidural catheter for surgery (e.g., cesarean section)
4) **Complications**
  a) **Fetal bradycardia**
    i) Association of fetal bradycardia with CSE labor analgesia is controversial and likely related to rapid onset of analgesia resulting in excess maternal circulating catecholamines affecting uterine tone (5).

NEURAXIAL AND REGIONAL ANESTHESIA

Figure 33-2 Possibilities for CSE Block Failure

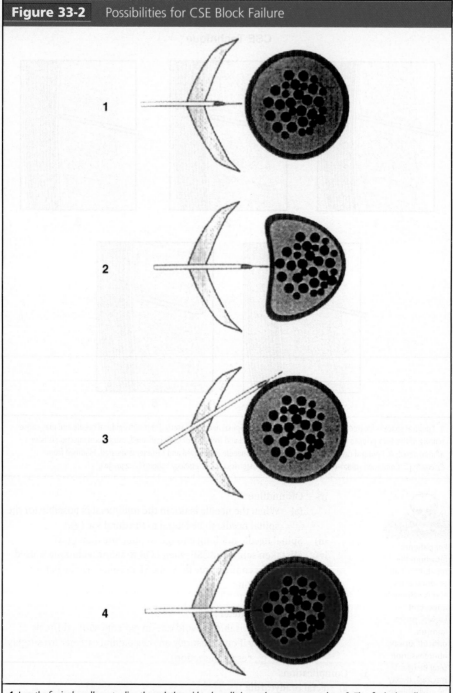

1. Length of spinal needle protruding through the epidural needle is too short to puncture dura; **2.** Tip of spinal needle "tents" the dura but fails to pierce it; **3.** Malposition of the epidural needle away from midline causing the spinal needle to miss the dural sac; **4.** Correct position of epidural and spinal needles. Adapted from Hughes SC. Intraspinal analgesia in obstetrics, Part II: Clinical applications. In: Hughes SC, Levinson G, Rosen MA, eds. *Shnider and Levinson's anesthesia for obstetrics*. 4th ed. Philadelphia, PA: Lippincott Williams & Wilkins, 2002:161.

    ii)   **Hypotension**

    iii)   **Respiratory depression**

        (1)   Estimated incidence of 0.01% to 0.1% with intrathecal fentanyl and/or sufentanil

        (2)   Higher incidence with higher doses

  b) Rates of other complications associated with neuraxial analgesia are similar (6,7).

    i)   Postdural puncture headache

    ii)   Intravascular catheter

    iii)   Intrathecal catheter

        (1)   Concerns regarding epidural catheter migration through the dural hole have not been substantiated when studied (8).

    iv)   Infection

        (1)   The incidence of infection is so low that the relative risk of meningitis for CSE versus epidural is unclear, but it appears to be similar with CSE as with other neuraxial techniques (7).

    v)   Bleeding

> **ALL** epidural catheters should be aspirated for blood or CSF prior to dosing at any time.

Chapter Summary for CSE

Indications	Labor analgesia, long surgical procedure where neuraxial anesthesia or postoperative epidural catheter desired
Complications	May be associated with increased fetal bradycardia, rate of complications similar to other neuraxial techniques
Considerations	Epidural catheter is untested; potential for spinal portion to be unsuccessful due to technical issues

NEURAXIAL AND REGIONAL ANESTHESIA

References

1. Collis RE, Davies DW, Aveling W. Randomised comparison of combined spinal-epidural and standard epidural analgesia in labour. *Lancet* 1995;345:1413–1416.
2. Carvalho B, Riley ET, Cohen SE, et al. Single-dose, sustained-release epidural morphine in the management of postoperative pain after elective cesarean delivery: Results of a multicenter randomized controlled study. *Anesth Analg* 2005;100(4):1150–1158.
3. Hughes SC. Intraspinal analgesia in obstetrics, part II: clinical applications. In: Hughes SC, Levinson G, Rosen MA, eds. *Shnider & Levinson's Anesthesia for Obstetrics*. 4th ed. Philadelphia, PA: Lippincott Williams & Wilkins; 2002:155–188.
4. Riley ET, Hamilton CL, Ratner EF, et al. A comparison of the 24-gauge sprotte and gertie marx spinal needles for combined spinal-epidural analgesia during labor. *Anesthesiology* 2002;97(3):574–577.
5. Eisenach JC. Combined spinal-epidural analgesia in obstetrics. *Anesthesiology* 1999;91(1):299–302.
6. Norris MC, Fogel ST, Conway-Long C. Combined spinal-epidural versus epidural labor analgesia. *Anesthesiology* 2001;95(4):913–920.
7. Rawal N, Holmstrom B, Crowhurst JA, et al. The combined spinal-epidural technique. *Anesth Clin North America* 2000;18(2):267–295.
8. Holmstrom B, Rawal N, Axelsson K, et al. Risk of catheter migration during combined spinal epidural block: percutaneous epiduroscopy study. *Anesth Analg* 1995;80(4):747–753.

34 Overview of Peripheral Nerve Blocks

Russell Kinder, MD • Robert L. Hsiung, MD

A peripheral nerve block (PNB) involves the injection of local anesthetic medication in the vicinity of a target nerve to inhibit neural transmission, producing surgical anesthesia in the distribution of the peripheral nerve and/or postoperative analgesia in the same distribution. Excluded from the definition are neuraxial blocks and intravenous regional anesthesia techniques. Specific nerve block techniques are described in detail in their respective chapters.

READ MORE

Atlas of Peripheral Nerve Block Procedures
Section 13
page 1171

1) **Basics of peripheral nerve blocks**
    a) Basic peripheral nerve anatomy
        i) The upper extremity is innervated by the branches of the brachial plexus, formed from the anterior rami of the C5-T1 nerve roots (Figs. 34-1 and 34-2).
            (1) Proximal blocks of the brachial plexus include the interscalene and supraclavicular approaches.

Figure 34-1 Illustration of the Brachial Plexus from Roots to Branches

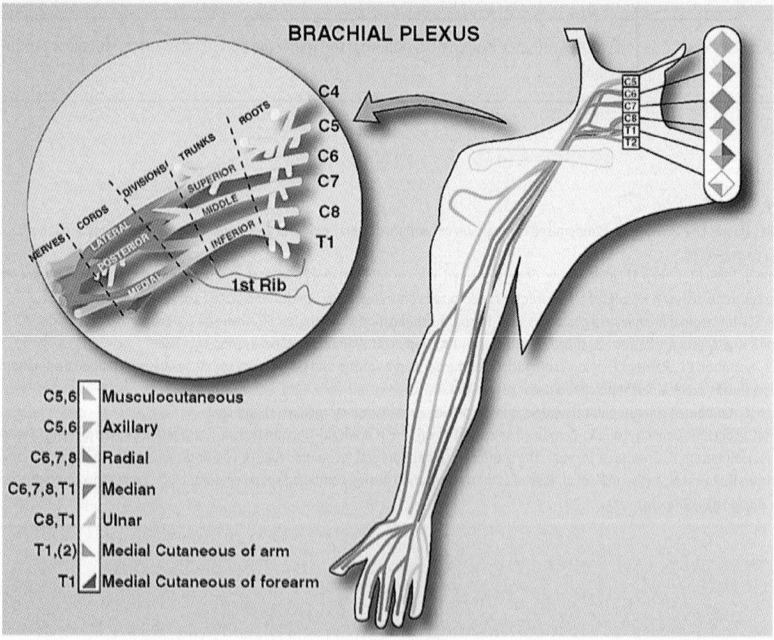

BRACHIAL PLEXUS

C4
C5
C6
C7
C8
T1

ROOTS
TRUNKS
SUPERIOR
MIDDLE
INFERIOR
DIVISIONS
CORDS
LATERAL
POSTERIOR
MEDIAL
NERVES
1st Rib

C5,6   Musculocutaneous
C5,6   Axillary
C6,7,8   Radial
C6,7,8,T1   Median
C8,T1   Ulnar
T1,(2)   Medial Cutaneous of arm
T1   Medial Cutaneous of forearm

From Chelly JE, ed. *Peripheral Nerve Blocks: A Color Atlas.* 2nd ed. Philadelphia, PA: Lippincott Williams & Wilkins; 2009:20.

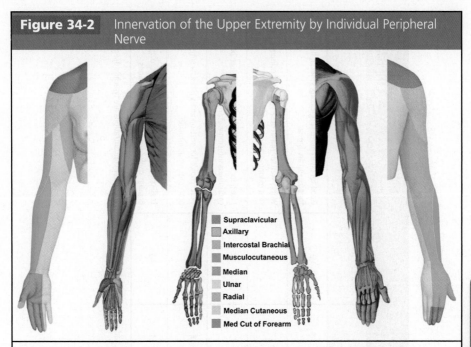

| **Figure 34-2** | Innervation of the Upper Extremity by Individual Peripheral Nerve |

Supraclavicular
Axillary
Intercostal Brachial
Musculocutaneous
Median
Ulnar
Radial
Median Cutaneous
Med Cut of Forearm

From Chelly JE, ed. *Peripheral Nerve Blocks: A Color Atlas*. 2nd ed. Philadelphia, PA: Lippincott Williams & Wilkins; 2009:32.

NEURAXIAL AND REGIONAL ANESTHESIA

   (2) Distal blocks of the brachial plexus include the infraclavicular and axillary approaches.

  ii) The lower extremity is innervated by branches of the lumbar plexus (L1-4) (Figs. 34-3 and 34-4) and sacral plexus (L5-S3) (Fig. 34-5).

   (1) The lumbar plexus and branches may be blocked posteriorly or anteriorly.

   (2) The major branch of the sacral plexus, the sciatic nerve, may be blocked in a number of locations along its course.

 b) Local anesthetics and adjuncts used for peripheral nerve blockade (Table 34-1)

  i) Many local anesthetics can be used for peripheral nerve blocks with differing concentrations and volumes in order to achieve the anticipated density, onset, and duration of the block.

  ii) Individual characteristics are discussed in the local anesthetic chapter.

  iii) Vasoconstrictors such as epinephrine prolong block duration and delay systemic absorption of local anesthetics as well as help identify intravascular injection, but its addition may increase the risk of neuronal injury (1).

  iv) Sodium bicarbonate has been used to hasten block onset for intermediate-acting local anesthetics (2).

  v) Clonidine added to local anesthetics can prolong block duration for single-injection blocks only (2,3).

 c) Contraindications

  i) Absolute contraindications (4)

   (1) Active skin infection over the site of planned needle placement

   (2) Severe coagulopathy

   (3) Allergy to local anesthetic medication

   (4) Patient refusal

Table 34-1

Table of Common Local Anesthetics (LA) Used for Peripheral Nerve Blocks

	Common Local Anesthetics	Concentrations[a] (%)	Onset (min)[b]	Block Duration (h)[b]	Max Dose w/epi (mg/kg)[c]	Comments and Recommendations
Short-acting	Chloroprocaine	1–3	7–15	0.5–1.5	15	Good for short-term surgical anesthesia, but not for post-op analgesia.
Intermediate-acting	Lidocaine	1.5–2	10–20	1–4	7	Works well for initial dose when a continuous infusion of long-acting LA is planned.
	Mepivacaine	1.5–2	10–20	2–5	7	Like lidocaine, can be used as initial dose before a continuous infusion is started.
Long-acting	Bupivacaine	0.25–0.5	10–30	10–14	3	Good choice for post-op analgesia as a single dose or a continuous infusion.
	Ropivacaine	0.2–0.5	10–30	10–14	2.5	Less-potent alternative to bupivacaine. 0.2% is a popular choice for continuous infusions.

[a]Concentration and volumes used depend on desired effect (e.g., anesthesia vs. analgesia), location of the block, and nerve localization technique used. The lower concentrations are typically used for continuous infusions.
[b]Onset time and block duration depend on dose of LA, block location, and the use of adjuncts.
[c]Actual plasma concentration can vary greatly, with toxicity being possible at much lower doses.

Figure 34-3   Branches of the Lumbar Plexus Important in Lower Extremity Innervation

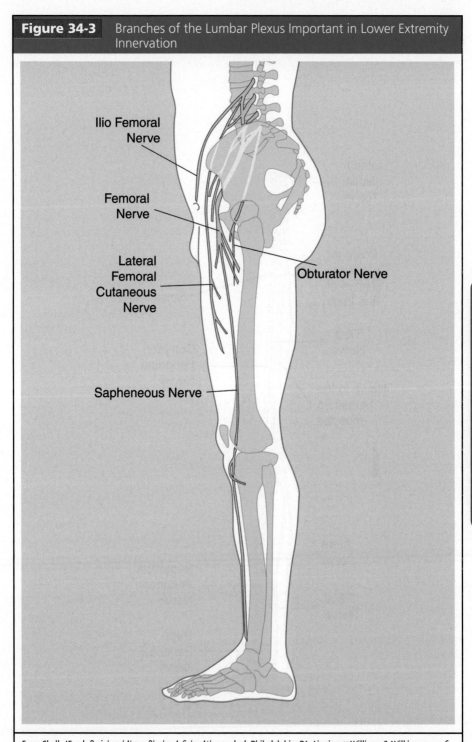

From Chelly JE, ed. *Peripheral Nerve Blocks: A Color Atlas*. 2nd ed. Philadelphia, PA: Lippincott Williams & Wilkins; 2009:76.

Figure 34-4   Branches of the Sacral Plexus Important in Lower Extremity Innervations

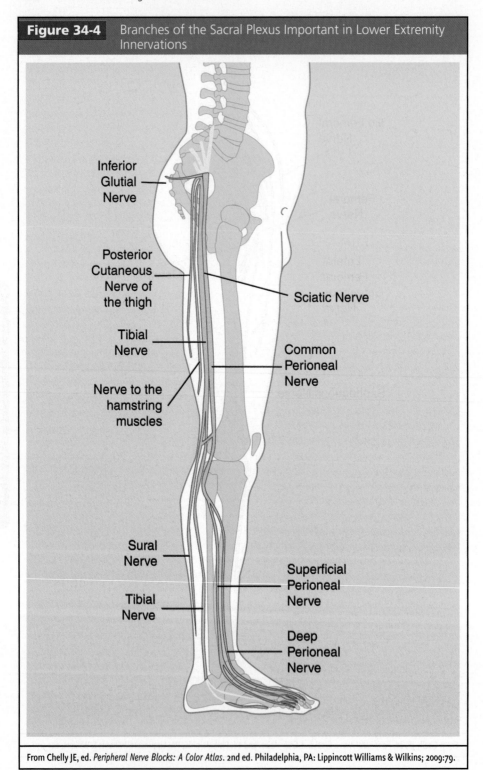

From Chelly JE, ed. *Peripheral Nerve Blocks: A Color Atlas*. 2nd ed. Philadelphia, PA: Lippincott Williams & Wilkins; 2009:79.

| Figure 34-5 | Innervation of the Lower Extremity by Individual Peripheral Nerve |

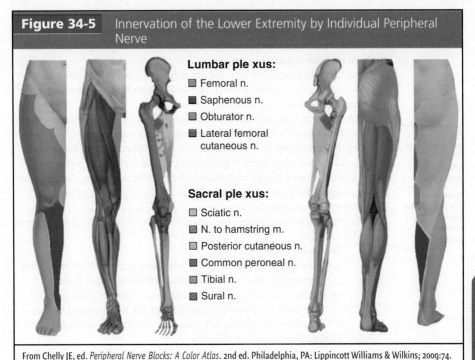

Lumbar ple xus:

☐ Femoral n.
■ Saphenous n.
☐ Obturator n.
■ Lateral femoral cutaneous n.

Sacral ple xus:

☐ Sciatic n.
■ N. to hamstring m.
☐ Posterior cutaneous n.
■ Common peroneal n.
■ Tibial n.
■ Sural n.

From Chelly JE, ed. *Peripheral Nerve Blocks: A Color Atlas.* 2nd ed. Philadelphia, PA: Lippincott Williams & Wilkins; 2009:74.

NEURAXIAL AND REGIONAL ANESTHESIA

(5) Coagulopathy
  (a) The American Society of Regional Anesthesia has not released specific guidelines on peripheral nerve blocks in anticoagulated patients (5).
  (b) Certain peripheral nerve blocks in noncompressible areas (e.g., paravertebral and lumbar plexus blocks) should be considered high risk for bleeding complications and are best avoided in the anticoagulated patient.
  ii) Adverse outcomes have been reported from peripheral nerve blocks performed under general anesthesia, and this practice in adults remains controversial (6).

2) **Benefits of peripheral nerve blocks**
  a) Peripheral nerve blocks can be used by themselves as an anesthetic technique or in conjunction with general anesthesia.
    i) As a primary anesthetic technique, peripheral nerve blockade may bypass many of the potential dangers of general anesthesia such as difficult airways, nausea and vomiting, hemodynamic instability, and malignant hyperthermia.
    ii) Studies suggest that the use of peripheral nerve blocks, especially continuous peripheral nerve catheters, provides better analgesia compared to opioids, greater patient satisfaction, decreased pruritus, decreased nausea vomiting, improved sleep, and decreased length of hospitalization (4).
    iii) To date, however, no mortality studies have demonstrated a conclusive advantage in favor of peripheral nerve block (PNB) anesthesia, nor has there been convincing evidence that suggests perioperative peripheral nerve blocks improve quality of life and rehabilitation (7).

b) Placement of a peripheral nerve catheter can allow for continuous perineural infusion or repeated boluses of local anesthetic, providing a longer duration of analgesia than can be obtained with a single-shot nerve block

3) **Risks of peripheral nerve blocks**

a) Specific risks associated with axillary, infraclavicular, interscalene, distal elbow and wrist, supraclavicular, popliteal, femoral, sciatic, and ankle blocks are discussed in their respective chapters

b) These risks may include infection, neurologic injury, local anesthetic toxicity, pneumothorax, and ipsilateral diaphragmatic paralysis.

c) General techniques to decrease the risks of peripheral nerve blocks (discussed individually), include performing a good history and physical, performing these blocks only when indicated, checking coagulation status or assessment for bacteremia when indicated, using sterile technique, performing incremental injection and aspiration, and using a "test dose" of epinephrine-containing local anesthetic to avoid intraneural or intravascular injection.

READ MORE

Continuous peripheral nerve blocks, Chapter 35, page 256

Overview of Peripheral Nerve blocks, Chapter 34, page 256

   i) **Preventing infection**

      (1) The risk of infection from a peripheral nerve block (PNB) is low but may be increased with the use of indwelling catheters.

      (2) Infection rate is decreased by the use of sterile technique, and the risks and benefits of performing the block should be reassessed in the setting of bacteremia or overlying skin infection.

   ii) **Minimizing neurological injury**

      (1) A meta-analysis of 32 studies over a 10-year period found 3% rate of any neurological event after peripheral nerve blocks (interscalene > axillary > femoral nerve blocks) and only one case of permanent neuropathy (8).

      (2) There have been no randomized clinical studies that clearly demonstrate nerve stimulation or ultrasound-guided peripheral nerve block (PNB) to have lower complication rates compared to transarterial or paresthesia techniques.

      (3) However, many practitioners believe that direct visualization under ultrasound may minimize needle-to-nerve trauma, as motor response may not be elicited even if the needle is intraneural (9).

      (4) Other possible factors that may lead to increased neurologic injury are the injection of local anesthetics after paresthesia elicitation and injection of local anesthetics under high pressure or resistance (10,11).

   iii) **Detecting systemic toxicity**

      (1) Toxicity from local anesthetics primarily affects the central nervous system (CNS) and the cardiovascular system.

         (a) CNS toxicity symptoms progress from oral numbness, dizziness, and visual disturbances to seizures and coma.

         (b) If allowed to evolve unimpeded, local anesthetic systemic toxicity may progress to cardiovascular toxicity, manifesting as an arrhythmia or a complete cardiovascular collapse.

      (2) Most cases of systemic toxicity have been attributed to inadvertent intravascular injection of local anesthetic.

      (3) The maximum doses of specific local anesthetics with and without epinephrine are discussed separately

Local anesthetics,
Chapter 37,
page 282

Avoid peripheral nerve blocks in noncompressible areas (e.g., paravertebral and lumbar plexus blocks) in the anticoagulated patient as these sites should be considered high risk for bleeding complications.

iv)   **Minimizing the risk of bleeding**

    (1)   Unlike the risk of anticoagulation in neuraxial blocks, the risk of vascular injury for peripheral nerve blocks in anticoagulated patients is not well defined (5).

    (2)   While placement of nerve blocks in severely coagulopathic patients should be avoided, peripheral nerve blocks are generally considered relatively safe compared to neuraxial blocks.

    (3)   Hematomas may be more common with the use of continuous catheters than with single-injection techniques due to the larger gauge catheter-introducing needle (2).

4)   **Nerve localization techniques in peripheral nerve blockade (2)**

a)   **Paresthesia-seeking technique**

    i)   Success depends on a good understanding of the relevant block anatomy.

    ii)   The needle insertion site is identified based on surface anatomic landmarks (e.g., muscles, tendons, bones, arteries) to estimate the course of the target nerve.

    iii)   The nerve is localized after needle insertion by eliciting a paresthesia in the distribution desired, which indicates that the needle is in close proximity to the target nerve.

    iv)   There is concern about paresthesias leading to long-term sequelae (12), and use of this technique has declined with the advent of alternative techniques that typically avoid elicitation of painful paresthesias altogether.

b)   **Nerve stimulation technique**

    i)   Similar to the paresthesia-seeking technique, the site for needle insertion is determined based on surface anatomic landmarks based on the most likely location of the target nerve.

    ii)   Following needle insertion, the nerve stimulator technique relies on the use of electrical current through a special insulated nerve stimulator needle to identify nerves by eliciting evoked motor responses (EMRs) in the distribution of the nerve(s) to be blocked.

        (1)   Strength of the motor response, however, does not necessarily correlate with proximity to the nerve although maintenance of a desired EMR at a current level <0.05 mA is a commonly accepted endpoint prior to local anesthetic injection.

        (2)   A positive "Raj test" occurs when EMR cessation immediately follows initial injection of local anesthetic, which is thought to be due to increasing the conductive surface area and decreasing the current density at the stimulating needle tip (13).

c)   **Ultrasound-guided technique** (Fig. 34-6)

    i)   The goal of using ultrasound is to directly visualize the target nerve and the needle placement.

    ii)   Target nerves can be imaged in short-axis (cross-sectional) or long-axis (longitudinal) views (14).

    iii)   Needle guidance can be performed using one of the two approaches: *in-plane* allowing for visualization of the entire needle shaft or *out-of-plane* with cross-sectional imaging of the needle (14).

Figure 34-6 Illustration Depicting the Various Methods Available to Perform Ultrasound-Guided Peripheral Nerve Blocks

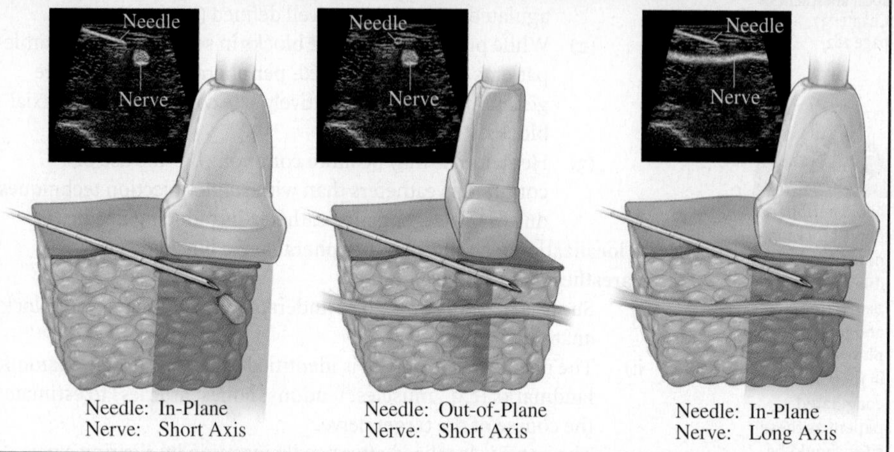

Needle: In-Plane
Nerve: Short Axis

Needle: Out-of-Plane
Nerve: Short Axis

Needle: In-Plane
Nerve: Long Axis

A: Nerve in short axis with the needle guided in-plane. **B:** Nerve in short axis with the needle guided out-of-plane. **C:** Nerve in long axis with the needle guided in-plane. From Ilfeld BM, Fredrickson MJ, Mariano ER. Ultrasound-guided perineural catheter insertion: Three approaches but few illuminating data. *Reg Anesth Pain Med* 2010;35:123–126; Fig. 1, p. 124.

(1) While proponents of each technique discuss theoretical advantages, differences in success of block or outcomes have yet to be shown.

(2) The use of ultrasound-guided blocks is increasing in popularity with many studies suggesting possible advantages of ultrasound-guided techniques compared to other traditional techniques (15,16).

(3) Less passes of the needle are often necessary with ultrasound guidance compared to other techniques (17).

iv) Due to the high cost of equipment, ultrasound equipment is not universally available. Therefore, performance of ultrasound-guided blocks is not always feasible.

v) Learning ultrasound-guided nerve block techniques

(1) Data regarding the learning curve for learning interventional ultrasound-guided tasks are based on studies involving inexperienced anesthesia residents (18).

(a) The most common error is failure to accurately image the needle during advancement, resulting in inadvertent excessive depth of penetration of the needle.

(b) Inability to visualize the needle may result in unintentional iatrogenic injury in the form of vascular or neural placement and/or injection.

(c) The learning curve is steep, and inexperienced practitioners are able to rapidly learn and improve and their speed and accuracy during simulated procedures.

(2) The American and European Societies of Regional Anesthesia have published a suggested training curriculum for ultrasound-guided regional anesthesia (19).

Table 35-1

Recommended Catheter Locations and Infusion Regimens for Common Surgical Procedures

Catheter Location	Planned Surgical Site
Interscalene	Shoulder, humerus
Supraclavicular/infraclavicular	Elbow and distal upper extremity
Lumbar plexus	Hip, thigh
Femoral	Thigh, knee, leg
Sciatic (including popliteal)	Ankle, foot
Paravertebral	Breast, thorax, abdomen

Figure 35-1 ◦ Example of a Properly Dressed Perineural Catheter Employing Liquid Adhesive, Clear Occlusive Dressings, and an Anchoring Device

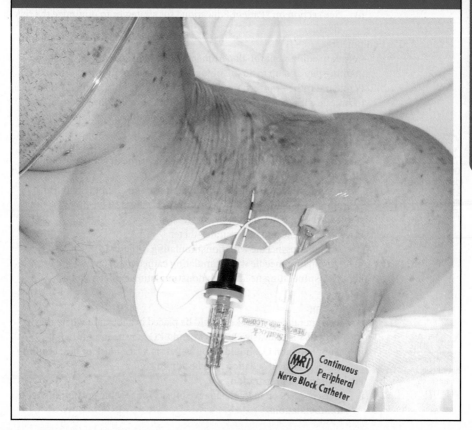

       i) Dependent upon many factors, including the experience of the practitioner, equipment and technique, as well as patient factors such as body habitus

       ii) The use of ultrasound may improve catheter insertion success rates (10,11).

   c) Nerve injury is a potential complication following performance of both single-injection and CPNB, presumably related to needle trauma and/or subsequent local anesthetic or adjuvant neurotoxicity.

       i) Prospective clinical evidence from human subjects suggests that the incidence of neural injury from a perineural catheter and ropivacaine (0.2%) infusion is no higher than following single-injection regional blocks (12–14).

Patients with lower extremity perineural catheters and continuous local anesthetic infusions should be considered HIGH FALL RISK.

   d) Infection

       i) Catheter site bacterial colonization is relatively common, but clinically relevant infection is not (15,16).

   e) Catheter knotting and retention (17) or shearing

       i) Avoid advancing the catheter >5 cm past the needle tip.

       ii) Once the catheter is past the needle tip, do not withdraw the catheter back into the needle unless the placement needle design is approved for this maneuver.

   f) Fall risk during postoperative period

       i) Efferent motor nerve fibers, as well as afferent sensory and proprioception fibers, are potentially anesthetized resulting in undesirable side effects such as muscular weakness.

       ii) See section on "Patient Education" for strategies to minimize the risk of falls.

3) **Equipment**

   a) Common equipment for all peripheral nerve block techniques include a marking pen and up to 40 mL of local anesthetic solution.

   b) Perineural catheter insertion should be performed with meticulous sterile technique with sterile skin cleansing solution, sterile gloves, hat, mask, gown, large clear sterile fenestrated drape, and dressing supplies (Fig. 35-2) (18).

READ MORE

Overview of peripheral nerve blocks, Chapter 34, page 256

   c) A nerve stimulator technique may be employed and requires an electrical nerve stimulator with a compatible needle/catheter set and grounding electrode.

   d) Ultrasound guidance requires portable ultrasound equipment and an appropriate transducer (see chapters on "Individual Nerve Block") with sterile ultrasound gel and probe cover.

   e) Placement needle and perineural catheter

       i) Stimulating needle with nonstimulating catheter (3)

       ii) Stimulating needle with stimulating catheter (19)

       iii) Nonstimulating needle with nonstimulating catheter (10,11)

4) **Technique**

   a) **Monitoring**

       i) Peripheral nerve blocks should be placed in a location where the patient's noninvasive BP, SpO$_2$, and EKG may be monitored.

READ MORE

Atlas of regional anesthesia, Chapter 172, page 1171

       ii) Supplemental O$_2$ should be provided *via* a face mask or nasal cannulae especially if sedation is to be administered.

   b) **Positioning and preparation**

       i) See chapters on individual nerve blocks for specific positioning recommendations.

Figure 35-2	Popliteal-Sciatic Perineural Catheter Insertion Demonstrating Proper Sterile Technique

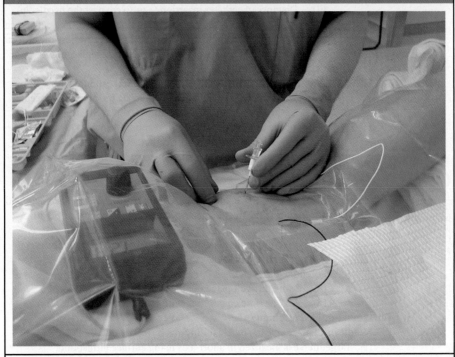

Note the use of a clear fenestrated drape that allows the practitioner to operate the nerve stimulator and observe the distal extremity for evoked motor responses.

    ii)   Apply monitors and supplemental O$_2$ prior to administering IV sedation.
- c) **Identification of surface anatomy**
  - i) See chapters on individual nerve blocks for surface anatomic landmarks specific to each approach.
- d) **Stimulating technique**
  - i) Target nerve or plexus is localized using electrical stimulation that is transmitted *via* an insulated needle.
    - (1) An evoked motor response from muscles innervated by the target nerve is sought.
    - (2) Sustained motor response at <0.5 mA of stimulating current suggests appropriate needle position.
  - ii) Once appropriate placement needle position is inferred as above, one of two methods of catheter insertion may be implemented:
    - (1) Nonstimulating catheter (3)
      - (a) The total planned volume of local anesthetic solution is injected incrementally *via* the placement needle.
      - (b) The perineural catheter is subsequently advanced past the needle tip (1 to 3 cm recommended).
      - (c) Potential advantages
        - (i) Ease of placement
        - (ii) Efficiency

(d) Potential disadvantages
   (i) It is possible to provide a successful surgical block with inaccurate catheter placement.
   (ii) Distance of catheter insertion (4 to 10 cm past the needle tip) greatly increases the variability in catheter tip-to-nerve distance.
   (iii) A misplaced catheter will decrease the effectiveness of the local anesthetic infusion and will likely require replacement.

(2) Stimulating catheter (19)
   (a) Prior to local anesthetic bolus, the perineural catheter with a stimulating lead connected to its tip is inserted *via* the placement needle.
   (b) As the catheter is advanced 3 to 5 cm past the needle tip, maintenance of the desired evoked motor response provides feedback on the positional relationship of the catheter tip to the target nerve.
   (c) The local anesthetic bolus is then injected incrementally *via* the perineural catheter.

READ MORE

Overview of peripheral nerve blocks, Chapter 34, page 256

   (d) Potential advantages
      (i) Likely to have improved accuracy in catheter tip placement and a possible greater success rate in controlling postoperative pain
      (ii) Practitioner has visual feedback (through evoked motor responses) of the location of the tip of the catheter.
   (e) Potential disadvantages
      (i) More difficult placement
      (ii) May be time consuming with increased failure rates (11)

e) **Ultrasound-guided technique**
   i) Needle in-plane, nerve in short-axis approach (10,11)
      (1) Target nerve is localized in short-axis using surface ultrasound.
      (2) The placement needle is inserted within the plane of the ultrasound beam in a trajectory perpendicular to the target nerve.
      (3) The local anesthetic solution is injected incrementally *via* the placement needle under direct visualization followed by perineural catheter insertion.
      (4) Potential advantages
         (a) Easier identification and differentiation of the nerve from surrounding structures
         (b) Needle tip location can be more easily identified relative to the target nerve.

The use of a flexible epidural-type catheter for in-plane needle/catheter guidance (target nerve in short-axis) will improve the likelihood of proper catheter tip placement.

         (c) Local anesthetic spread may be observed if the initial local anesthetic bolus is placed through the needle with adjustment of the needle tip when necessary.
         (d) Practitioners may employ a nearly identical technique for both single-injection and catheter insertion procedures.
      (5) Potential disadvantages
         (a) Catheter has the tendency to bypass the nerve when inserted past the needle tip, given the perpendicular orientation of the needle/catheter to the nerve.
         (b) Strategies to optimize catheter tip placement
            (i) Pass the catheter a minimal distance past the needle tip if using a rigid catheter design.
            (ii) Use an extremely flexible catheter in an attempt to keep the catheter tip in close proximity to the target nerve if the catheter is inserted more than a minimal distance (10,11).

ii) Needle out-of-plane, nerve in short-axis approach (20)
   (1) Target nerve is localized in short-axis using surface ultrasound.
   (2) The placement needle is inserted through the ultrasound beam in a trajectory parallel to nerve, and tissue movement surrounding the needle visible on ultrasound is used to guide needle advancement.
   (3) Potential advantages
      (a) Familiar approach to anesthesia practitioners with parallel needle-to-nerve trajectory used with traditional nerve stimulation techniques (and also vascular access)
      (b) Since the needle is nearly parallel to the target nerve, the catheter theoretically may remain in closer proximity to the nerve, especially when inserting a more rigid catheter a greater distance past the needle tip.
   (4) Potential disadvantages
      (a) Relative inability to visualize the advancing needle tip, which may increase the likelihood of unwanted contact with nerves, vessels, peritoneum, pleura
      (b) Practitioners of this technique recommend a combination of tissue movement and "hydrolocation," in which fluid is injected *via* the placement needle to infer needle tip location.
iii) Needle in-plane, nerve in long-axis approach (21)
   (1) The target nerve is visualized in long-axis using surface ultrasound.
   (2) The placement needle is advanced within the ultrasound beam with a trajectory parallel to nerve.
   (3) Potential advantages
      (a) The nerve can be viewed along with the needle shaft/tip.
      (b) The catheter may be monitored as it exits the needle parallel to the target nerve.
   (4) Potential disadvantages
      (a) Difficult to keep the needle, nerve, and catheter all in the ultrasound plane
      (b) The nerve itself must be relatively straight to be visualized in long axis; and there can be only one target nerve as opposed to multiple trunks or cords as found within the brachial plexus.
      (c) Due to disadvantages, this technique has limited applications.
f) **Hybrid technique (22)**
   i) In addition to ultrasound guidance, practitioners may elect to use nerve stimulation as a means to confirm needle tip location or to infer correct catheter tip position with a stimulating catheter.
   ii) This technique has not been compared to stimulation- or ultrasound-guided techniques in randomized fashion to date.
g) **Infusion management**
   i) Pharmacology
      (1) Majority of perineural infusion publications have involved bupivacaine (0.1% to 0.25%) or ropivacaine (0.15 to 0.4%), although levobupivacaine and shorter-acting agents have been reported (8) .
      (2) No adjuncts added to local anesthetics have been demonstrated to provide benefits during CPNB infusion (23).
   ii) Infusion regimen (24,25) (Table 35-2)
      (1) Basal infusion optimizes benefits such as analgesia and sleep quality for procedures resulting in at least moderate postoperative pain

NEURAXIAL AND REGIONAL ANESTHESIA

Table 35-2

Recommended Perineural Infusion Regimens

Catheter Location	Recommended Basal Infusion (mL/h)	Recommended Bolus
Interscalene	6–8	4 mL every 30 min
Supraclavicular/infraclavicular	6–8	4 mL every 30 min
Lumbar plexus	4–6	2–4 mL every 60 min
Femoral	4–6	2–4 mL every 60 min
Sciatic (proximal approaches)	4–6	2–4 mL every 60 min
Popliteal-sciatic	6–8	4 mL every 30 min
Paravertebral	4–6	4 mL every 30 min

    (2) Bolus capability provides patients the ability to self-administer local anesthetic doses and results in

      (a) Improved analgesia while minimizing supplemental opioids

      (b) Lower required basal infusion rate, which minimizes the risk of limb numbness and maximizes infusion duration for ambulatory patients with a finite infusion pump reservoir volume

5) **Patient education**

  a) Important for successful management of CPNB, especially in the outpatient setting

  b) Should be done preprocedure and postprocedure verbally and in written form.

    i) Patients and their caretakers need appropriate counseling on managing and troubleshooting their catheters and infusion pumps.

      (1) Provide patients with the contact number of a provider who can help them if they need assistance with managing CPNB anytime day or night.

      (2) Since patients or their caretakers will likely remove CPNB catheters in the outpatient setting, adequate instructions for removal should be provided prior to discharge.

    ii) Minimize fall risk by taking these steps

      (1) Use the minimum dose/mass of local anesthetic required for analgesia.

      (2) Provide limited-volume patient-controlled bolus doses that allow for a decreased basal dose without compromising analgesia.

      (3) Recommend non–weight-bearing status for patients with lower extremity CPNB, or consider utilizing a knee immobilizer and a walker/crutches if weight bearing is permitted.

      (4) Educate physical therapists, nurses, and surgeons of possible CPNB-induced muscle weakness and encourage fall precautions at home and on the hospital ward (e.g., signs, bed alarms, use of bedside commode).

Chapter Summary for Continuous Peripheral Nerve Block Catheters

Indications	Moderate pain Opiate intolerance Limb perfusion Physical therapy
Method of Placement	Ultrasound technique Nerve stimulation technique Hybrid technique
Complications	Catheter dislodgement Secondary block failure Nerve injury Infection Catheter knotting Postoperative fail risk
Post Placement Management	Infusion regimen Patient education Follow up Fall prevention

NEURAXIAL AND REGIONAL ANESTHESIA

References

1. Grant SA, Nielsen KC, Greengrass RA, et al. Continuous peripheral nerve block for ambulatory surgery. *Reg Anesth Pain Med* 2001;26: 209–214.
2. White PF, Issioui T, Skrivanek GD, et al. The use of a continuous popliteal sciatic nerve block after surgery involving the foot and ankle: does it improve the quality of recovery? *Anesth Analg* 2003;97:1303–1309.
3. Ilfeld BM, Morey TE, Wang RD, et al. Continuous popliteal sciatic nerve block for postoperative pain control at home: a randomized, double-blinded, placebo-controlled study. *Anesthesiology* 2002;97:959–965.
4. Loland VJ, Ilfeld BM, Abrams RA, et al. Ultrasound-guided perineural catheter and local anesthetic infusion in the perioperative management of pediatric limb salvage: a case report. *Paediatr Anaesth* 2009;19:905–907.
5. Iskandar H, Wakim N, Benard A, et al. The effects of interscalene brachial plexus block on humeral arterial blood flow: a Doppler ultrasound study. *Anesth Analg* 2005;101:279–281.
6. De Ruyter ML, Brueilly KE, Harrison BA, et al. A pilot study on continuous femoral perineural catheter for analgesia after total knee arthroplasty: the effect on physical rehabilitation and outcomes. *J Arthroplasty* 2006;21:1111–1117.
7. Tuominen M, Haasio J, Hekali R, et al. Continuous interscalene brachial plexus block: clinical efficacy, technical problems and bupivacaine plasma concentrations. *Acta Anaesthesiol Scand* 1989;33:84–88.
8. Ilfeld BM, Enneking FK. Continuous peripheral nerve blocks at home: a review. *Anesth Analg* 2005;100:1822–1833.
9. Salinas FV. Location, location, location: continuous peripheral nerve blocks and stimulating catheters. *Reg Anesth Pain Med* 2003;28:79–82.
10. Mariano ER, Cheng GS, Choy LP, et al. Electrical stimulation versus ultrasound guidance for popliteal-sciatic perineural catheter insertion: a randomized controlled trial. *Reg Anesth Pain Med* 2009;34:480–485.
11. Mariano ER, Loland VJ, Bellars RH, et al. Ultrasound guidance versus electrical stimulation for infraclavicular brachial plexus perineural catheter insertion. *J Ultrasound Med* 2009;28:1211–1218.
12. Borgeat A, Dullenkopf A, Ekatodramis G, et al. Evaluation of the lateral modified approach for continuous interscalene block after shoulder surgery. *Anesthesiology* 2003;99:436–442.
13. Borgeat A, Ekatodramis G, Kalberer F, et al. Acute and nonacute complications associated with interscalene block and shoulder surgery: a prospective study. *Anesthesiology* 2001;95:875–880.
14. Bergman BD, Hebl JR, Kent J, et al. Neurologic complications of 405 consecutive continuous axillary catheters. *Anesth Analg* 2003;96: 247–252.
15. Cuvillon P, Ripart J, Lalourcey L, et al. The continuous femoral nerve block catheter for postoperative analgesia: bacterial colonization, infectious rate and adverse effects. *Anesth Analg* 2001;93:1045–1049.
16. Capdevila X, Pirat P, Bringuier S, et al. Continuous peripheral nerve blocks in hospital wards after orthopedic surgery: a multicenter prospective analysis of the quality of postoperative analgesia and complications in 1,416 patients. *Anesthesiology* 2005;103:1035–1045.
17. Offerdahl MR, Lennon RL, Horlocker TT. Successful removal of a knotted fascia iliaca catheter: principles of patient positioning for peripheral nerve catheter extraction. *Anesth Analg* 2004;99:1550–1552.

18. Hebl JR, Neal JM. Infectious complications: a new practice advisory. *Reg Anesth Pain Med* 2006;31:289–290.

19. Salinas FV, Neal JM, Sueda LA, et al. Prospective comparison of continuous femoral nerve block with nonstimulating catheter placement versus stimulating catheter-guided perineural placement in volunteers. *Reg Anesth Pain Med* 2004;29:212–220.

20. Fredrickson MJ, Ball CM, Dalgleish AJ. A prospective randomized comparison of ultrasound guidance versus neurostimulation for interscalene catheter placement. *Reg Anesth Pain Med* 2009;34:590–594.

21. Tsui BC, Ozelsel TJ. Ultrasound-guided anterior sciatic nerve block using a longitudinal approach: "expanding the view". *Reg Anesth Pain Med* 2008;33:275–276.

22. Mariano ER, Afra R, Loland VJ, et al. Continuous interscalene brachial plexus block via an ultrasound-guided posterior approach: a randomized, triple-masked, placebo-controlled study. *Anesth Analg* 2009;108:1688–1694.

23. Ilfeld BM, Morey TE, Enneking FK. Continuous infraclavicular perineural infusion with clonidine and ropivacaine compared with ropivacaine alone: a randomized, double-blinded, controlled study. *Anesth Analg* 2003;97:706–712.

24. Ilfeld BM, Morey TE, Enneking FK. Infraclavicular perineural local anesthetic infusion: a comparison of three dosing regimens for postoperative analgesia. *Anesthesiology* 2004;100:395–402.

25. Ilfeld BM, Thannikary LJ, Morey TE, et al. Popliteal sciatic perineural local anesthetic infusion: a comparison of three dosing regimens for postoperative analgesia. *Anesthesiology* 2004;101:970–977.

36 Basic Pharmacology

Gillian Johnson, MD

A thorough understanding of the basic principles of pharmacology is paramount for the proper administration of anesthetic drugs. Due to the rapid growth of our drug armamentarium and the ever-changing clinical challenges we face, it is useful to understand the principles that influence the outcomes when drug therapies are chosen.

1) Drug administration
   a) **Intravascular**—intravenous (IV) or intra-arterial
   b) **Extravascular**—sublingual, buccal, oral, rectal, intramuscular, dermal, or pulmonary
   c) **Regional**—pleural, peritoneal, spinal, epidural, or perineural
2) Drug absorption
   a) Absorption is the process by which unchanged drug moves from the site of administration to the site of measurement within the body.
   b) Monitoring intact drug in blood or plasma is a useful method of assessing entry of drug into the systemic circulation (1) (Table 36-1).
   c) Most anesthetic drugs are given IV or are inhaled.
      i) With IV administration, the drug absorption process is eliminated, providing rapid therapeutic blood concentrations.
         (1) Toxicity or other adverse drug reactions will also be seen rapidly.
      ii) Drugs administered via **inhalation** require low molecular weight and high lipid solubility.
         (1) When combined with the high blood flow and large total surface area of the alveoli, drugs move very rapidly to the blood.
   d) **Intrathecal** administration delivers drugs directly to the site of action, allowing very low doses to be given and reduction of adverse systemic drug effects.
      i) Alternatively, **epidural or perineural** dosing requires larger doses, thereby increasing the risk of systemic effects and possible toxicity.
3) Drug distribution
   a) **Distribution** is the process of reversible transfer of a drug to and from the site of measurement, usually blood or plasma.
      i) An example is distribution between blood and muscle tissue (1).
      ii) Drugs go to **vascular areas first, for example, brain, heart, lungs, kidneys and then to muscle, skin, and finally fat**.
      iii) Equilibration of drug into all the compartments may take hours.
4) Transport across membranes
   a) Most drugs are too big to pass through aqueous membrane channels and **must cross the lipid part of the membrane**.
   b) Almost all drugs are weak acids or weak bases and are thus ionized or nonionized at physiologic pH.

Nonionized drug = lipid soluble = crosses membranes more easily

PHARMACOLOGY

275

Table 36-1

Comparison of Different Methods of Drug Administration Compared

Type of Administration	Time of Onset	First-Pass Metabolism
Transdermal	Slow	No
Oral	Slow	Yes
Sublingual/buccal	Rapid	No
Subcutaneous	Slow	No
Intramuscular	Slow	No
Intravascular	Immediate	No
Inhalational	Intermediate	No
Rectal	Slow	Small amount
Intrathecal	Immediate	No
Epidural/perineural	Rapid	No

5) **Drug elimination**
   a) **Elimination is the process of irreversible loss of drug from the site of measurement.**
   b) This can occur by two processes, either **excretion or metabolism.**

> **EXCRETION** = the irreversible loss of an unchanged drug
> **METABOLISM** = the conversion of one chemical species to another

   c) Some drugs require metabolism, as the metabolites are the active drug form; for example, codeine is metabolized to produce morphine.
   d) Occasionally, metabolites are converted back to drug (metabolic interconversion).
6) **Binding of drugs to plasma proteins**
   a) Total drug concentrations can be measured in either blood or plasma and therapeutic doses adjusted accordingly.
   b) Total drug concentration exists in two forms: that which is bound to plasma proteins and other plasma constituents and that which is free or unbound.
   c) In blood, many drugs reversibly bind plasma proteins.
   d) The degree of protein binding has important pharmacokinetic and pharmacodynamic implications, because it is the **unbound moiety that readily diffuses across biological membranes and reaches the receptor site.**
   e) The degree of plasma binding is often expressed as percentage of drug bound (2).
   f) Another term frequently used is the free fraction of drug in plasma or serum; this is equal to the free drug concentration divided by the total drug concentration.

g) Factors affecting protein binding

 i) The plasma binding of many drugs may decrease or increase due to a variety of pathophysiologic factors, for example, liver disease, burns, malabsorption syndromes.

 ii) **Because of this, measurement of total drug concentrations alone may be misleading** and cause an inappropriate increase in therapy, which might be potentially hazardous, or to the initiation of subtherapeutic dosages.

7) **Pharmacokinetic and pharmacodynamic principles**

 a) **Pharmacokinetics is the quantitative study of the absorption, distribution, metabolism, and elimination of drugs (3)** (Table 36-2).

Table 36-2
Basic Pharmacokinetic Principles

	Description	Clinical Relevance
C_{max}	Maximum concentration of a drug measured after administration.	Together with tmax, C_{max} is a surrogate marker for the rate of absorption ↑ rate of absorption may ↑ toxicity ↓ rate of absorption may lead to delayed onset of drug effect.
Steady state (C_{ss})	Concentration of a drug or a chemical in a body fluid—usually plasma—at the time a "steady state" has been achieved, and rates of drug administration and drug elimination are equal.	The effect of a drug (pharmacodynamic, toxicodynamic) can only safely be evaluated after drug concentrations reach steady state (usually after 5 terminal half-lives)
Bioavailability (F)	The percentage of dose entering the systemic circulation after administration of a given dosage form.	Oral bioavailability is usually <100%. Incomplete absorption from the gut or significant first pass metabolism in the liver decrease drug levels in the blood and hence bioavailability. In many cases, pharmacogenomics/genetics of the enzymes and transporters involved, affect oral bioavailability. Many drugs with low oral bioavailability such as immunosuppressants will require therapeutic drug monitoring. Under normal circumstances, bioavailability after IV administration is always 100%
AUC	Area under the plasma concentration vs. time curve.	The parameter that is correlated with most drug effects is systemic exposure. AUC is a surrogate marker of exposure. For many drugs, AUC can be correlated with pharmacodynamic and toxicodynamic effects and can be used to establish bioequivalence of different drug products with the same active compound.

(continued)

PHARMACOLOGY

Table 36-2

Basic Pharmacokinetic Principles (Continued)

	Description	Clinical Relevance
Volume of distribution (Vd)	The volume into which a drug appears to have been dissolved after administration.	A larger Vd will require a larger loading dose to achieve a given concentration.
Clearance (Cl)	Clearance of a drug from the body, expressed in volume/unit time	Pathological conditions such as renal disease alter the time course of clearance.
Elimination half-life ($t_{1/2}$)	The amount of time that it takes for the concentration of a drug to be reduced by half in the body.	5 terminal half-lives are required for a drug to reach steady state. Terminal half-lives determine dosing intervals (usually close to one terminal half-life to avoid accumulation) This is a critical concept when antagonizing drug effects: opioid antagonists may have shorter half-lives than opioids! This means that the opioid effects such respiratory depression may return after the antagonist is eliminated.
First-pass effect	The biotransformation and/or excretion of a drug by intestinal and hepatic, including biliary, mechanisms following absorption of the drug from the gastrointestinal tract, before drug gains access to the systemic circulation.	When dosing drugs orally, it is important to know that higher doses will be required than when given IV.
Zero-order kinetics	Mechanisms of chemical reaction in which the reaction velocity is apparently independent of the concentration of all the reactants.	Saturation of enzyme metabolism is possible. At saturation, a small ↑ in dose will result in large ↑ in plasma concentration, for example, alcohol/phenytoin.
First-order kinetics	The velocity of a chemical reaction is proportional to the concentration of the reactant.	
Elimination rate constant (k_{el})	The velocity of a chemical reaction is proportional to the product of the active masses (concentrations) of the reactants	Elimination rate determines how fast a drug is eliminated from the body and is an important component of terminal half-life. The elimination rate may be significantly altered by induction or inhibition of drug-metabolizing enzymes (induction: lower exposure, less drug effect; inhibition: higher exposure, higher risk of drug toxicity). Pharmacogenomics/genetics may play a very important role for specific drugs. There are slow and fast metabolizers. A slow metabolizer may accumulate drug quickly when treated with standard doses and result in toxicity. Fast metabolizers will eliminate the drug quickly and may have less or no drug effect. Accordingly, slow metabolizers will require much smaller doses and fast metabolizers much higher doses than "normal" metabolizers.

b) **Pharmacodynamics** describes either concentration-effect relationships or the time course of pharmacological effect after dosing (Fig. 36-1)

8) **Drug interactions**
   a) Drug–drug interactions (DDIs) are defined as "two or more drugs interacting in such a manner that the effectiveness or toxicity of one or more drugs is altered" (5).
   b) Some result in preventable medication errors (6) associated with serious adverse events and death (7,8).
   c) Alternately, some DDIs can be used to our advantage.

9) **Pharmacogenetics**
   a) Pharmacogenetic factors operate at the pharmacokinetic and the pharmacodynamic levels.
   b) Polymorphisms in drug-metabolizing enzymes, transporters, and/ or pharmacological targets of drugs may profoundly influence the dose–response relationship between individuals.
   c) Current practice of anesthesia rarely takes into account interindividual variations, and standard dosing is often applied.

As a rule of thumb, the lower the oral bioavailability of a drug, the higher the risk of substantial interpatient and intrapatient pharmacokinetic variability.

5 terminal half-lives are required for a drug to reach steady state.

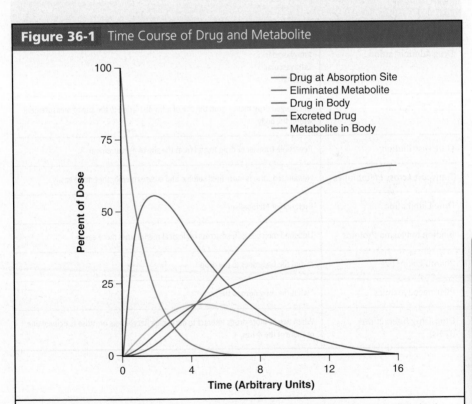

Figure 36-1 Time Course of Drug and Metabolite

— Drug at Absorption Site
— Eliminated Metabolite
— Drug in Body
— Excreted Drug
— Metabolite in Body

The amount in each compartment is expressed as a percentage of the dose administered. In this example, all the dose is absorbed. Redrawn from Rowland M, Tozer T. *Clinical Pharmacokinetics: Concepts and Applications.* 3rd ed. Philadelphia, PA: Lippincott Williams & Wilkins; 1995.

PHARMACOLOGY

d)   As more information becomes available, it is likely that pretesting pharmacogenetic variables before elective cases will increase patient safety due to a decrease in the number of adverse drug reactions.

10) **Pediatric pharmacology**

a)   Infants and children differ markedly from adult patients because their metabolism is often immature and their principal physiologic functions are different.

b)   Volumes of distribution (blood/extravascular/etc.), flows (cardiac output, cerebrospinal fluid turnover, etc.), and barriers are different from those of adult patients.

c)   For example, many cytochrome P450 isoforms are not mature until the age of 1 year, and some children are deficient until the age of 4 years (9).

d)   Due to the difficulty of studying clinical pharmacology in the pediatric population, research in this area lags behind that in adults. This leaves us to use principles defined in adult bodies when deciding on dosing regimens, which may not apply to the very young.

Chapter Summary for Basic Pharmacology

Drug Administration	Intravascular Extravascular Regional
Drug Absorption	Unchanged drug moves from the site of administration to the site of measurement within the body
Drug Distribution	Reversible transfer of drug to and from the site of measurement
Transport Across Membranes	Nonionized form is more lipid soluble and crosses membranes more easily
Drug Elimination	Excretion or Metabolism
Binding to Plasma Proteins	Unbound moieties diffuse across biological membranes more easily
Pharmacokinetics	"what the body does to the drug"
Pharmacodynamics	"what the drug does to the body"
Drug-Drug Interactions (DDIs)	When two or more drugs interact to decrease effectiveness or cause toxicity of one or more of the drugs

References

1. Rowland M, Tozer T. *Clinical Pharmacokinetics: Concepts and Applications*. 3rd ed. Philadelphia, PA: Lippincott Williams & Wilkins; 1995:17 and 18.
2. Wood M. Plasma drug binding: implications for anesthesiologists. *Anesth Analg* 1986;65(7):786–804.
3. Rescigno A. Foundations of pharmacokinetics. *Pharmacol Res* 2000;42(6):527–538.
4. Derendorf H, Lesko LJ, Chaikin P, et al. Pharmacokinetic/pharmacodynamic modeling in drug research and development. *J Clin Pharmacol* 2000 Dec;40(12 Pt 2):1399–1418.
5. Mora-Atorrasagasti O, Lertxundi-Etxebarria U, Peral-Aguirregoitia J, et al. Mechanism of clinically relevant drug-drug interactions detected by a semi-automatic method. *Eur J Hosp Pharm* 2008/5;14:32–36.
6. Peterson JF, Bates DW. Preventable medication errors: identifying and eliminating serious drug interactions. *J Am Pharm Assoc (Wash)* 2001;41(2):159–160.
7. Juurlink D, Mamdani M, Iazzetta J, et al. Avoiding drug interactions in hospitalized patients. *Healthc Q* 2004;7(2):27–28.
8. Jinks MJ, Hansten PD, Hirschman JL. Drug interaction exposures in an ambulatory Medicaid population. *Am J Hosp Pharm* 1979;36(7):923–927.
9. Mazoit JX. Pharmacokinetic/pharmacodynamic modeling of anesthetics in children: therapeutic implications. *Paediatr Drugs* 2006;8(3):139–150.

37 Local Anesthetics

Andrea J. Fuller, MD

Local anesthetics are widely used for anesthesia and analgesia. Knowledge of onset, duration, and side effects of individual agents is essential for optimal efficacy. For more information on specific local anesthetic drugs, refer to the Appendix of Drug Information, Chapter 190.

1) **Mechanism of action**
   a) Local anesthetics bind to **voltage-gated sodium channels**, preventing the influx of sodium ions necessary for nerve depolarization.

READ MORE

Appendix B Local anesthetics, Chapter 190, page 1271

2) **Structure/activity relationships**
   a) All local anesthetics are **weak bases** with pKa values above physiologic pH.
   b) The **lipophilic** (nonionized) form binds receptors.
      i) In the presence of **acidosis**, more drug is in the hydrophilic ionized form, often resulting in **poor-quality** local analgesia or anesthesia.
   c) These compounds are more stable at acidic pH, especially epinephrine-containing solutions. Only the basic, nonionized, form binds receptors.
      i) The **addition of sodium bicarbonate** can increase speed of onset by **3 to 5 minutes** and **decrease pain with subcutaneous injection** (1,2).
   d) **Differential blockade**
      i) Clinically used local anesthetics appear to affect different types of nerve fibers in different ways.
         (1) For example, **sympathetic function typically is the first affected, followed by loss of pin-prick or touch, followed by motor blockade.**
         (2) However, different agents (e.g., Ropivacaine) may affect motor function less than other agents.
      ii) The mechanism and clinical use of differential blockade are poorly understood and are an active area of research (3).
   e) **Duration of action**
      i) Amide local anesthetics bind to **alpha$_1$-gylcoprotein**.
      ii) The amount of protein binding affects duration of action and can be responsible for different clinical effects observed between individuals (3).

The amount of protein binding of local anesthetics affects duration of action and can be responsible for different clinical effects observed between individuals (3).

3) **Types of local anesthetics**
   a) All have a **lipophilic** (unsaturated aromatic ring) **moiety** and a **hydrophilic** (hydrocarbon chain) moiety connected by an **esther or amide linkage**
   b) **Esthers**
      i) Procaine, chloroprocaine, cocaine, tetracaine, benzocaine
   c) **Amides**
      i) Lidocaine, etidocaine, prilocaine, mepivacaine, bupivacaine, ropivacaine, dibucaine

Increasing the pH speeds onset of action of local anesthetics.

4) **Pharmacokinetics**
   a) Systemic absorption
      (1) Depends on the **vascularity** of the injection site
         (a) Amount of systemic absorption is as follows: **tracheal > intercostal > caudal > epidural > brachial plexus > femoral/sciatic > subcutaneous** (2)
      (2) The addition of vasoconstrictors such as epinephrine at the injection site decreases systemic absorption of local anesthetic.
         (a) This leads to **increased duration** of action and decreased **systemic toxicity.**
   b) Distribution
      i) Determined by tissue perfusion, protein binding, and tissue mass
   c) Metabolism
      i) **Amides**
         (1) Metabolized in the **liver** by microsomal enzymes
      ii) **Esthers**
         (1) Metabolized by **plasma cholinesterases**
5) **Clinical Uses**
   a) Local infiltration
   b) Topical anesthesia
   c) Peripheral nerve block
   d) Spinal, epidural, or caudal anesthesia
   e) Arrhythmia therapy
   f) Pain management
6) **Adverse effects/toxicity (Table 37-1)**
   a) **Toxic effects occur with large doses**
      i) Cardiovascular
         (1) Hypotension
         (2) Arrhythmias, including bradycardia, atrioventricular block, ventricular fibrillation

Table 37-1

Dose-Dependent Systemic Effects of Lidocaine

Plasma Concentration (µg/mL)	Effect
1–5	Analgesia
5–10	Lightheadedness Tinnitus Numbness of tongue Systemic hypotension Myocardial Depression
10–15	Seizures Unconsciousness
15–25	Coma Respiratory arrest
>25	Cardiovascular depression

Reproduced from: Stoelting RK, Hiller SC. *Local Anesthetics. In: Pharmacology & Physiology in Anesthetic Practice.* 4th ed. Philadelphia, PA: Lippincott Williams & Wilkins, 2006, with permission.

PHARMACOLOGY

Patients undergoing outpatient surgery in the lithotomy position are at increased risk of transient neurologic symptoms after lidocaine spinal anesthesia.

    ii)   Respiratory

        (1)   Depression of hypoxic drive and bronchial smooth muscle relaxation

    iii) Neurological

        (1)   Perioral numbness, tinnitus, seizures, coma

b) **Transient neurologic symptoms (3)**

    i)   **Transient** pain or sensory abnormalities in the back, buttocks, or lower extremities

    ii) Risk factors

        (1)   Lidocaine spinal anesthesia

        (2)   Lithotomy position

        (3)   Outpatient anesthesia

    iii) Not dose dependent

    iv) Symptomatic treatment with nonsteroidal anti-inflammatory drugs may improve symptoms

    v)   Symptoms are usually self-limited and resolve within 3 days (3).

Large doses of hyperbaric lidocaine delivered via small-gauge spinal catheter have been associated with cauda equina syndrome.

c) **Cauda equina syndrome**

    i)   **Diffuse injury to cauda equina nerve roots** resulting in bowel/bladder dysfunction and paraplegia

    ii) Cause is unclear but thought to be due to direct nerve damage by high concentration local anesthetics

    iii) Risk factors

        (1)   High concentration (5% or greater) hyperbaric lidocaine

        (2)   Small-gauge intrathecal catheters

           (a)   Microcatheters were removed from the market after multiple cases of cauda equina syndrome with hyperbaric lidocaine.

d) **Allergic reactions**

    i)   **Very rare with amides**

    ii) Allergic reactions to esther local anesthetics are usually due to cross-reactivity to *p*-aminobenzoic acid (PABA) because the esther linkage resembles PABA.

7) **Treatment of Toxicity**

a) Cardiovascular collapse from bupivacaine is exceptionally difficult to treat and may require **cardiopulmonary bypass.**

READ MORE

Local anesthetic toxicity, Chapter 219, page 1340

b) Recently, a **20% lipid emulsion** has been successful in treating local anesthetic toxicity.

    i)   Its use is currently limited to case reports and animal studies but has been **used to treat cardiovascular collapse** associated with local anesthetic toxicity (4–6).

    ii) Dosage of 20% lipid emulsion is **1 to 2 mL/kg IV over 1 min** while continuing chest compressions and other supportive measures.

        (1)   May be **repeated every 3 to 5 minutes to a maximum of 1 to 2 additional doses (4,6)**

    iii) Once the heart has converted to sinus rhythm, an **infusion of 0.25 to 0.5 mL/kg/min** should be given until the patient is hemodynamically stable (4,6).

Chapter Summary: Local Anesthetics

Mechanism of Action	Bind Na$^+$ channels on nerves $\rightarrow$ prevents influx of Na$^+$ ions and inhibits depolarization
Common Uses	Local and regional anesthesia, labor analgesia, treatment of arrhythmias
Adverse Effects (Cause)	Excessive plasma concentration Possible direct neurotoxicity in susceptible patients
Adverse Effects (Clinical Findings)	Seizures, arrhythmias, respiratory depression
Adverse Effects (Prevention)	Avoid inadvertent intravascular injection of large doses Consider risk factors when choosing a local anesthetic for spinal injection
Treatment of Toxicity	Symptomatic treatment with oxygenation, ventilation and cardiovascular support as needed Rapid treatment with intralipid

References

1. Carvalho B, Fuller AJ, Brummel C, et al. Local infiltration of epinephrine-containing lidocaine with bicarbonate reduces superficial bleeding and pain during labor epidrual catheter insertion: a randomized trial. *Int J Obstet Anesth* 2007;16:116–121.
2. Stoelting RK, Hiller SC. Local Anesthetics. In: *Pharmacology and Physiology in Anesthetic Practice*. 4th ed. Philadelphia, PA: Lippincott Williams & Wilkins; 2006.
3. Liu SS, Lin Y. Local anesthetics. In: Barash PG, Cullen BF, Stoelting RK, Cahalan MK, Stock MC. eds. *Clinical Anesthesia*. 6th ed. Philadelphia, PA: Lippincott Williams & Wilkins; 2009:531–548.
4. Weinberg G. Lipid rescue resuscitation from local anaesthetic cardiac toxicity. *Toxicol Rev* 2006;25:139–145.
5. Weinberg G, Ripper R, Feinstein DL, et al. Lipid emulsion infusion rescues dogs from bupivacaine-induced cardiac toxicity. *Reg Anesth Pain Med* 2003;28:198–202.
6. Rosenblatt MA, Abel M, Fischer GW, et al. Successful use of a 20% lipid emulsion to resuscitate a patient after a presumed bupivacaine-related cardiac arrest. *Anesthesiology* 2006;105:217–218.

Neuromuscular Blockade

Andrea J. Fuller, MD

Neuromuscular blocking (NMB) drugs are widely used in anesthesia and critical care. They are useful for facilitating surgery and airway management. NMB drugs can be extremely dangerous because respiratory mechanics may be impaired. Knowledge of the mechanism of action and clinical use is imperative. For more information on specific drugs, refer to the Appendix of Drug Information.

1) **Mechanism of action**
   a) Physiology of neuromuscular transmission (Fig. 38-1).
   b) Acetylcholine (ACh) is released from the motor neuron and binds to the nicotinic ACh receptor at the motor endplate on the skeletal muscle cell.
   c) A conformational change occurs in the receptor, allowing sodium ions to enter the membrane and depolarize the cell (1).
   d) NMB agents act at the ACh receptor and can be broadly classified into two categories: depolarizing and non-depolarizing.

Figure 38-1 Physiology of Neuromuscular Transmission

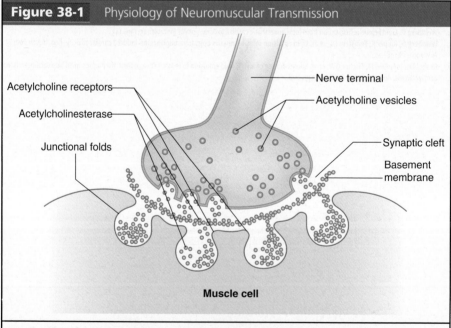

Reproduced from Donati F, Bevan DR. Neuromuscular Blocking Agents. In: Barash PG, Cullen BF, Stoelting RK, et al, eds. *Clinical Anesthesia*, 6th ed. Philadelphia: Lippincott Williams & Wilkins, 2009: 501, with permission.

- i) **Depolarizing muscle relaxants**
  - (1) **Succinylcholine** is the main depolarizing muscle relaxant in clinical use
    - (a) It is a noncompetitive agonist.
    - (b) Receptor binding induces a conformational change similar to that produced by ACh, resulting in **depolarization.**
    - (c) It remains bound to the receptor and **prevents action potentials from forming**.
  - (2) As the muscle cells depolarize, **fasiculations** are observed
    - (a) Due to uncoordinated skeletal muscle contractions
- ii) **Nondepolarizing muscle relaxants**
  - (1) **Competitive agonists**
    - (a) Compete with ACh at the receptor-binding site
    - (b) Once bound, a conformational change cannot occur, and **muscle depolarization is prevented.**

2) Monitoring neuromuscular blockade (1,3)
   a) The depth of neuromuscular blockade is best measured by a peripheral nerve stimulator.

Absence of fade with TOF stimulation does not completely exclude residual neuromuscular blockade. Clinical weakness may still occur and must always be assessed.

   - i) The ulnar nerve (stimulation of adductor pollicis) and the facial nerve (stimulation of orbicularis oculi) are the most common locations for monitor placement.
   b) **Train of four (TOF) stimulation**—occurs when the stimulator delivers four successive 200 μsec stimuli in 2 seconds (2 Hz).
   - i) The ratio of the height of the first twitch to the fourth is the TOF ratio.
   - ii) The twitches elicited from stimulation fade as neuromuscular blockade increases.
   - iii) When three of four twitches are observed, 70% to 75% of the receptors are blocked, and when one twitch is visible, 85% to 90% of receptors are blocked (1).
   c) **Tetany**
   - i) A continuous stimulus of 50 to 100 Hz is delivered to elicit tetany.
   - ii) Contraction for greater than 5 seconds without fading indicates return of neuromuscular function although TOF stimulation may be more reliable (1,2).
   - iii) **Post-tetanic potentiation**
     - (1) Occurs when the TOF is measured after tetany. The observed evoked response after tetanic stimulation is called post-tetanic potentiation.
     - (2) Due to increased ACh present at the motor endplate
     - (3) It is most helpful during profound neuromuscular blockade when TOF stimulation is undetectable (3).

3) Metabolism
   a) **Depolarizing muscle relaxants**
   - i) Diffuse away from the ACh receptor and are metabolized by plasma cholinesterase (**pseudocholinesterase**)
   - ii) **Abnormal pseudocholinesterase**
     - (1) Approximately 1:2,000 patients have a genetic mutation in the pseudocholinesterase enzyme, rendering it unable to metabolize succinylcholine (1).
     - (2) In these patients, the duration of action can be 3 to 6 hours (1,3).
     - (3) Dibucaine is a local anesthetic that inhibits normal pseudocholinesterase and has limited effect on the abnormal variant.

PHARMACOLOGY

(a) The ratio of inhibition (**dibucaine number**) indicates the amount of normal pseudocholinesterase and has historically been helpful in the diagnosis of abnormal pseudocholinesterase.

(b) Mutations in the pseudocholinesterase gene have been characterized, and newer molecular diagnostic techniques may be more informative than the dibucaine number (3,4).

   iii) **Nondepolarizing muscle relaxants**

     (1) Diffuse away from the ACh receptor and are gradually metabolized and excreted.

      (a) For more information on the metabolism and excretion of specific agents, refer to the appendix of drug information.

4) Reversal of blockade

a) **Depolarizing muscle relaxants**

READ MORE

Anticholinesterases Chapter 39, page 293

   i) **Do not have specific reversal agents**

   ii) Restoration of neuromuscular function depends on **metabolism by pseudocholinesterase**.

b) **Nondepolarizing muscle relaxants**

   i) Restoration of neuromuscular function depends on redistribution, metabolism, and excretion in addition to administration of an anticholinesterase drug.

5) Clinical uses

a) Intubation

b) Muscle relaxation to facilitate surgery (i.e., abdominal surgery)

c) Prevent movement in cases where movement could be catastrophic (i.e., intraocular or intracranial surgery)

d) Facilitate mechanical ventilation or decrease work of breathing in critically ill patients

6) Adverse effects/toxicity

a) **Awareness**

   i) Awareness is the retention of memory, pain, and consciousness while skeletal muscles are paralyzed.

   ii) NMB drugs **do not have sedative or hypnotic properties**, making **awareness** possible.

   iii) **Administration of a sedative or hypnotic agent with a comparable duration of action to the muscle relaxant is imperative when neuromuscular blockade** is employed.

When using NMB drugs, awareness is always possible. Take care to ensure that the depth of anesthesia is appropriate to prevent awareness.

b) **Depolarizing muscle relaxants**

   i) **Hyperkalemia**

     (1) Succinylcholine increases the potassium level by 0.5 to 1 mEq/L and is relatively contraindicated if the patient's serum potassium level is >5.5 mEq/L (5).

     (2) Hyperkalemia following succinylcholine administration can cause **cardiac arrest**, particularly in susceptible patients.

      (a) Risk factors

       (i) Burns, immobility, chronic infection, massive trauma, spinal cord injury, muscular dystrophy, and other neuromuscular diseases (5)

       (ii) **Increased intraocular pressure (IOP)**

        (1) Succinylcholine can increase IOP, and its avoidance with open globe injuries has been suggested due to concerns about extravasation of ocular contents.

·Drug Interactions with Neuromuscular Blocking Agents (7)

Drug	Effect on action of Depolarizing Neuromuscular Blocking Agent (Succinylcholine)	Effect on action of Nondepolarizing Neuromuscular Blocking Agent	Comments
Volatile anesthetics	↑	↑	Dose dependent
Antibiotics (except penicillins and cephalosporins)		↑	Aminoglycosides most likely to have effect
Furosemide		↑	Probably due to drug's inhibition of cAMP production
Magnesium	↑	↑	More profound with non-depolarizing agents; use extreme caution in peripartum patients treated with magnesium
Lidocaine		↑	
Quinidine	↑	↑	May interfere with prejunctional release of Ach
Lithium	↑		
Anticonvulsants (phenytoin, carbamazepine)		↓(chronic) ↑ (acute)	Chronic treatment has pharmacodynamic effect (higher plasma concentrations are required for desired effect)
Cyclosporine	↑		
Local anesthetics	↑ duration		Esther local anesthetics can prolong succinylcholine by competing for plasma cholinesterase
Corticosteroids		↑	Prolonged treatment in mechanically ventilated critically ill patients
Echothiophate	↑ duration		Inhibits both pseudocholinesterase and acetylcholinesterase; used for treatment of glaucoma

↑ refers to enhancement of blockade.
↓ refers to inhibition or decreased duration of blockade.

Medical Conditions that Affect Muscle Relaxant Function (3,5)

Medical Condition	Response to Depolarizing Agent	Response to Nondepolarizing Agent	Comments
Hypothermia		Prolonged duration	
Elderly		Prolonged duration, decreased dosage required	Due to altered pharmacodynamics and decreased elimination
Multiple sclerosis	↑ risk of hyperkalemia	Resistance	Up-regulation of ACh receptors
Amyotrophic lateral sclerosis and other motor neuron diseases	↑ risk of hyperkalemia	Resistance	Up-regulation of ACh receptors
Guillan-Barre syndrome	↑ risk of hyperkalemia	Sensitive	Loss of motor units at neuromuscular junction
Myasthenia gravis	Resistant	Extreme sensitivity	Anticholinesterases used to treat disease can make reversal difficult and prolong action of depolarizing blockade
Myotonic dystrophy	↑ risk of hyperkalemia;	Resistant	Neostigmine can cause prolonged muscle weakness
Eaton-Lambert syndrome	Sensitive	Sensitive	Neostigmine is ineffective
Muscular dystrophy	↑ risk of hyperkalemia, rhabdomyolysis, and malignant hyperthermia	Usually normal	Possible sensitivity to nondepolarizing agents in the presence of muscle weakness
Burn injury	↑ risk of hyperkalemia after the first 24 h	Resistance	Up-regulation of ACh receptors
Spinal cord injury	↑ risk of hyperkalemia after first 24 h		
Immobility and critical illness	↑ risk of hyperkalemia	Resistance	Can be associated with persistent weakness when used in critically ill patients

(2) This concern is controversial since succinylcholine has been used clinically in patients with open globe injuries, and very little clinical evidence to support its avoidance exists (6,7).

(iii) **Increased intracranial pressure**

    (1) May be related to increased $PaCO_2$ from fasiculations

    (2) When considering the increased intraocular and intracranial pressure effects of succinylcholine, it is important to remember that laryngoscopy with inadequate anesthesia and/or muscle relaxation may be far more deleterious than the small (and often controversial) effect of the drug (1,3).

    (3) **The importance of securing an airway while minimizing the risk of gastric aspiration must be considered and succinylcholine used as clinically indicated** (1,6).

(iv) **Increased intragastric pressure**

    (1) Related to fasiculations and can be prevented with a defasiculating dose of a nondepolarizing neuromuscular blocking agent (3)

    (2) Offset by increased lower esophageal sphincter tone

(v) **Myalgias**

    (1) Independent of fasiculations but can be decreased with the administration of a small dose of nondepolarizing muscle relaxant (8)

(vi) **Bradycardia**

    (1) Most common when a second dose of succinylcholine is given about 5 minutes after the first

    (2) May be prevented by atropine, thiopental, and nondepolarizing muscle relaxants (3)

(vii) **Triggers malignant hyperthermia in susceptible patients**

c) **Persistent neuromuscular blockade**

    i) Can cause postextubation respiratory failure

    ii) Prior to extubation, return of neuromuscular function must be verified via peripheral nerve stimulation (TOF monitoring or tetany) and/or clinical evidence such as sustained head lift for greater than 5 seconds.

Chapter Summary for Neuromuscular Blocking Agents

Mechanism of Action	Depolarizing: Binds receptor and facilitates muscle depolarization Nondepolarizing: Competitively binds receptor, resulting in inhibition of Ach binding
Common Uses	Facilitation of intubation and surgical conditions Patient immobility Ventilatory support for critical care
Adverse Effects	Depolarizing: Hyperkalemia, may trigger malignant hyperthermia, IOP, myalgias, bradycardia Nondepolarizing: Prolonged respiratory muscle weakness

PHARMACOLOGY

References

1. Bevan DR, Donati F. Muscle relaxants. In: Barash PG, ed. *Clinical Anesthesia*. 3 ed. Philadelphia, PA: Lippincott Williams & Wilkins; 1997:385–412.

2. Samet A, Capron F, Alla F, et al. Single acceleromyographic train-of-four, 100-Hertz tetanus or double-burst stimulation: which test performs better to detect residual paralysis? *Anesthesiology* 2005;102:51–56.

3. Naguib M, Lien CA. *Pharmacology of Muscle Relaxants and Their Antagonists*. In: Miller RD, ed. *Anesthesia*. 6th ed. Philadelphia, PA: Churchill Livingstone; 2005:481–572.

4. Cerf C. Screening patients with prolonged neuromuscular blockade after succinylcholine and mivacurium. *Anesth Analg* 2002;94:461–466.

5. Martyn JJA, Richtsfeld M, Warner DO. Succinylcholine-induced hyperkalemia in acquired pathologic states: etiologic factors and molecular mechanisms. *Anesthesiology* 2006;104:158–169.

6. Vachon CA, Warner DO, Bacon DR. Succinylcholine and the open globe. *Anesthesiology* 2003;99:220–223.

7. Stoelting RK, Hiller SC. *Neuromuscular Blocking Drugs Pharmacology and Physiology in Anesthetic Practice*. 4th ed. Philadelphia, PA: Lippincott Williams & Wilkins; 2006:208–250.

8. Schreiber JU, Lysakowski C, Fuchs-Buder T, et al. Prevention of succinylcholine-induced fasiculation and myalgia: a meta-analysis of randomized trials. *Anesthesiology* 2005;103:877–884.

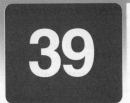

Anticholinesterases

Andrea J. Fuller, MD

39

Anticholinesterase agents reverse the effects of nondepolarizing neuromuscular blocking agents. They are also used outside of anesthetic practice to treat other neurologic and muscle diseases. For more information on specific drugs, refer to the Appendix of Drug Information, Chapter 192.

READ MORE

Neuromuscular blockade, Chapter 38, page 286

READ MORE

Myasthenia gravis Chapter 94, page 672

1) **Mechanism of action**
   a) A basic overview of neuromuscular transmission is described in Chapter 38.
   b) Anticholinesterase drugs inhibit the **acetylcholinesterase** enzyme, which increases the amount of acetylcholine (Ach) available to compete for the Ach receptor.

2) **Clinical uses and common agents**
   a) **Reversal of neuromuscular blockade**
      i) Neostigmine and edrophonium
   b) **Treatment of myasthenia gravis (1)**
      i) Pyridostigmine (most common) and neostigmine
   c) **Treatment of Alzheimer dementia**
      i) Donepezil, rivastigmine, and galantamine (2)
   d) **Treatment of central cholinergic syndrome**
      i) Physostigmine
   e) **Treatment of glaucoma**
      i) Echothiophate
         (1) Irreversible inhibitor of cholinesterase.
         (2) Also inhibits plasma cholinesterase and can increase the duration of succinylcholine (3)

3) **Pharmacology (4)**
   a) All three commonly used agents (neostigmine, edrophonium, and physostigmine) follow a two-compartment model after IV injection.
   b) All are water-soluble, ionized compounds with excretion by the kidney

4) **Reversal of neuromuscular blockade**
   a) Anticholinesterases are ineffective if such a profound neuromuscular blockade is present that all potential ACh receptors are occupied.
      i) It is advisable to wait until as much spontaneous recovery as possible has occurred prior to administering the anticholinesterase (3).
      ii) If three or four twitches are observed with train-of-four (TOF) stimulation, recovery with neostigmine will be much more effective and rapid than if one of four twitches is present (5).
   b) Evidence of effect
      i) Sustained head lift >5 seconds is a very sensitive clinical predictor of adequate reversal of blockade (4).
   c) Excessive doses of neostigmine can cause paradoxical neuromuscular relaxation.

Excessive doses of neostigmine can cause paradoxical neuromuscular relaxation.

5) Adverse Effects/Toxicity

   a) Predominantly due to the fact that **ACh is the neurotransmitter for the entire parasympathetic nervous system.**

   b) Increased ACh due to cholinesterase inhibition allows ACh to bind parasympathetic muscarinic receptors.

      i) Most adverse effects can be abated with the administration of an anticholinergic medication such as glycopyrolate or atropine.

         (1) **Bradycardia**

         (2) **Bronchospasm**

         (3) **Increased gastrointestinal peristaltic activity**

            (a) Neostigmine may cause increased nausea and vomiting.

               (i) However, this is controversial, and a recent meta-analysis did not show a difference with neostigmine use (6).

         (4) **Increased bladder tone**

         (5) **Constricted pupils**

         (6) **Diffuse CNS excitation**

            (a) **Seen only with physostigmine, an anticholinesterase that crosses that blood brain barrier**

Physostigmine crosses the blood brain barrier and can cause diffuse CNS excitation.

   c) **Cholinergic crisis**

      i) Patients present with all of the above muscarinic effects.

      ii) Seen most commonly in patients with **myasthenia gravis** undergoing treatment with anticholinesterase treatment

READ MORE

Myasthenia gravis, Chapter 94, page 672

   d) **Organophosphate poisoning (4)**

      i) Anticholinesterases are used as nerve gas agents and pesticides.

      ii) Excessive muscarinic activity as described above is observed.

      iii) Central nicotinic effects are also seen.

         (1) Can result in respiratory depression

      iv) The muscarinic effects can be reversed with large doses of atropine.

      v) Nicotinic effects require supportive care.

6) Anticholinergic medications used with anticholinesterases (4)

   a) Edrophonium has an onset of 1 to 2 minutes and is best used in conjunction with **atropine** (0.007 mg/kg).

   b) Neostigmine's peak onset is 7 to 11 minutes and is best used with **glycopyrolate** 0.007 mg/kg or atropine 0.015 mg/kg.

Chapter Summary for Anticholinesterases

Mechanism of Action	Inhibit cholinesterase → ↑ Ach available at the Ach receptor
Common Uses	Treatment of myasthenia gravis, glaucoma, central anticholinergic syndrome, Alzheimer dementia; **Reversal of neuromuscular blockade**
Adverse Effects (Cause)	Ach binding to muscarinic receptors
Adverse Effects (Clinical Findings)	Bradycardia, bronchospasm, increased peristaltic activity, miosis
Adverse Effects (Prevention)	Give with anticholinergic (atropine or glycopyrolate)

References

1. Bhatt JR, Pascuzzi RM. Neuromuscular disorders in clinical practice: case studies. *Neurol Clin* 2006;24(2):233–265.
2. Masterman D. Cholinesterase inhibitors in the treatment of Alzheimer's disease and related dementias. *Clin Geriatr Med* 2004;20(1):59–68.
3. Naguib M, Lien CA. Pharmacology of muscle relaxants and their antagonists. In: Miller RD, ed. *Anesthesia*. 6th ed. Philadelphia, PA: Churchill Livingstone; 2005:481–572.
4. Donati F, Bevan DR. Neuromuscular Blocking Agents. In: Barash PG, ed. *Clinical Anesthesia*. 6 ed. Philadelphia, PA: Lippincott Williams & Wilkins; 2009: 498–530.
5. Kirkegaard H, Heier T, Caldwell JE. Efficacy of tactile-guided reversal from cisatracurium-induced neuromuscular block. *Anesthesiology* 2002;96(1):45–50.
6. Cheng CR, Sessler DI, Apfel CC. Does neostigmine administration produce a clinically important increase in postoperative nausea and vomiting? *Anesth Analg* 2005;101(5):1349–1355.

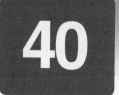

40 Benzodiazapines

Andrea J. Fuller, MD

Benzodiazapines are sedative and hypnotic drugs that can be used for anxiolysis, sedation, and induction of anesthesia.

READ MORE

Appendix of drug information, Chapter 193, page 1276

1) Overview
   a) Benzodiazapines are widely used preoperative, intraoperative, and postoperative medications.
   b) An overview of this class of drugs will be provided here. For more information on specific drugs, including dosing guidelines, refer to the Appendix of Drug Information, Chapters 193 and 205.
2) Mechanism of action (1)
   a) Benzodiazepines bind to specific receptor sites on the alpha subunits of the gamma-aminobutyric acid (GABA) receptor.
      i) Binding of benzodiazepines enhances the affinity of the receptor for GABA.
      ii) This causes increased chloride conductance and hyperpolarizes postsynaptic neurons, resulting in inhibition of synaptic transmission.
   b) Structure/activity relationships
      i) Chemical structure is a benzene ring fused to a seven-membered diazepine ring, hence the name, benzodiazepine.
         (1) Representative medications include midazolam, lorazepam, temazepam, alprazolam, diazepam, oxazepam
   c) Pharmacokinetics
      i) Absorption
         (1) Rapidly absorbed from the gastrointestinal tract with oral dose
         (2) Rapidly enter the CNS and other highly perfused organs with IV injection

Diazepam and midazolam are metabolized by hepatic microsomal enzymes and have active metabolites.

      ii) Distribution
         (1) Highly **lipid soluble**
         (2) Highly protein bound (to albumin)
            (a) Disease states that cause hypoalbuminemia (cirrhosis, malnutrition, chronic renal failure) result in increased proportion of unbound drug and lower dosage required to achieve the desired effect.
   d) Metabolism (1)
      i) Drugs with **active metabolites** include diazepam, midazolam (metabolized by hepatic microsomal enzymes)
      ii) Drugs **without active metabolites** include lorazepam, oxazepam, temazepam (metabolized by glucuronidation only)

3) **Special considerations**
   a) Benzodiazapines decrease cerebral metabolic oxygen requirements (CMRO2) and cerebral blood flow (CBF)
   b) Unlike barbiturates and propofol, **midazolam treatment does not result in an isoelectric EEG.**
   c) May cause **anterograde amnesia** (decreased ability to acquire new information)

4) **Clinical uses**
   a) Preoperative anxiolysis (especially for pediatric patients)
   b) Anticonvulsant
   c) Sedation for procedures or critical care
   d) Alcohol detoxification
   e) Skeletal muscle relaxation (spinal cord mediated)
      i) Not effective for surgical relaxation
   f) Treatment of acute insomnia

5) **Adverse effects/toxicity (1,2)**
   a) Dependence
   b) Fatigue
   c) Drowsiness
   d) Decreased ventilation (dose dependent)
      i) Most pronounced in patients with chronic pulmonary disease and in conjunction with other respiratory depressants
   e) **Potentiates the sedative effects of other medications** (especially opiates)
   f) Decreased systemic vascular resistance with large (i.e., anesthetic induction) doses
   g) May inhibit platelet aggregation (midazolam)

Benzodiazepines potentiate the sedative effects of other medications (especially opioids).

6) **Treatment of toxicity (1,2)**
   a) **Flumazenil is a specific benzodiazepine antagonist.** It reverses benzodiazepine effects, including ventilatory depression.
      i) Titrate the drug for the individual, with an initial dose of 4 to 20 µg/kg IV (0.2 mg) and additional doses of 0.1 mg given at 1 minute intervals up to 1 mg. **Typically effective doses are 0.3 to 0.6 mg.**
      ii) **Duration of action is 30 to 60 minutes. May need to be repeated** depending on the duration of action of the benzodiazepine administered. Alternatively, an **infusion of 0.1 to 0.4 mg/h** can be used.
      iii) **May precipitate withdrawal seizures in patients on antiepileptic medications**
      iv) **May increase intracranial pressure in head-injured patients**

Flumazenil is a specific benzodiazepine antagonist used to treat benzodiazepine overdose.

PHARMACOLOGY

Chapter Summary: Benzodiazepines

Definition	Benzodiazepines are sedative and hypnotic drugs with a common chemical structure of a benzene ring fused to a seven-membered diazepine ring.
Mechanism of Action	Bind to sites on the alpha subunit of the GABA receptor, increasing affinity of receptor for GABA, resulting in inhibition of synaptic transmission.
Uses	Used for sedation, anxiolysis, and induction of anesthesia.
Treatment of Toxicity	Benzodiazepine overdose can be treated with flumazenil, a specific benzodiazepine antagonist agent.

References

1. Stoelting RK, Hiller SC. *Pharmacology and Physiology in Anesthetic Practice*. Philadelphia, PA. Lippincott Williams & Wilkins; 2006: 140–154.
2. Van Hemelrijck J, White PF. Nonopoid intravenous anesthesia. In: Barash PG, Cullen BF, Stoelting RK, eds. *Clinical Anesthesia*. 3rd ed. Philadelphia, PA: Lippincott Williams & Wilkins; 1997:311–328.

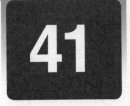

41

Opioid Analgesics and Antagonists

Andrea J. Fuller, MD

Opioids are medications that are used for pain management and adjuncts to anesthesia and critical care. Opioids are the cornerstone medication for the treatment of moderate to severe pain and are commonly used in the perioperative care of patients to provide analgesia. This chapter provides a brief overview of the mechanism of action and various routes of administration. For dosing guidelines, refer to the Appendix of Drug Information.

READ
MORE

Appendix B:
Opioids, Chapter
194, page 1278

1) **Mechanism of action (1)**
   a) Opioids bind to opioid receptors, which couple to G proteins and inhibit adenyl cyclase.
      i) Leads to inhibition of voltage-gated calcium channels and opening of potassium channels
      ii) Results in increased intracellular potassium, which leads to decreased neurotransmission
   b) **Receptor subtypes.** The physiologic function of opioid receptors is to bind endogenous opioids and provide endogenous analgesia in response to pain
      i) **Mu** receptors are in the brain, spinal cord, and periphery and are the primary receptors responsible for the analgesic and adverse effects of opioids, especially morphine.
         (1) **Mu$_1$ subtype**—analgesia
         (2) **Mu$_2$ subtype**—hypoventilation, bradycardia, and physical dependence
      ii) **Kappa** receptors inhibit neurotransmission via type N calcium channels.
         (1) Responsible for dysphoria and diuresis
      iii) **Delta** receptors modulate mu receptor activity.
         (1) **Endogenous opioids** include enkephalins, endorphins, and dynorphins.

2) **Structure/activity relationships**
   a) The term *opiate* is used to describe compounds derived from the **poppy** (Papaver somniferum).
      i) The prototype opiate is **morphine.**
   b) Opioid medications
      i) Completely synthetic or semisynthetic modifications of morphine
   c) Representative opioid medications
      i) Hydromorphone, meperidine, fentanyl, alfentanil, sufentanil, and remifentanil

3) **Administration of opioids**
   a) There are multiple routes of administration, including oral, parenteral, intramuscular, neuraxial, transdermal, and transmucosal.

b) **Parenteral administration**
   i) **Distribution**
      (1) Onset and duration of action depend on the **lipid solubility** and **ionization** of the drug.
      (2) Drugs diffuse across the blood–brain barrier and redistribute to inactive tissue sites such as skeletal muscle and fat.
      (3) High doses of lipid soluble drugs (i.e., fentanyl) lead to saturation of inactive sites and buildup of the drug in the plasma, resulting in a longer duration of action.
   ii) **Metabolism (1–3)**
      (1) Most opioids are metabolized in the liver and excreted by the kidney.
      (2) An exception is **remifentanil**, which is rapidly metabolized by **plasma esterases**.
      (3) Many opioids have **long-acting, pharmacologically active metabolites.**
         (a) **Normeperidine is the active metabolite of meperidine** and has renal elimination.
            (i) Accumulation can cause seizures and should be used with caution in patients with renal failure.
         (b) **Morphine-6-glucuronide is an active metabolite of morphine** and can accumulate in neonates and those with renal failure.

c) **Neuraxial Administration**

READ MORE

Obstetrical anesthesia Chapter 144, page 1047

   i) Neuraxial opioids act on **mu** receptors in the **substantia gelatinosa** of the spinal cord.
   ii) Epidural administration requires diffusion across the dura to bind receptors in the spinal cord.
   iii) Spinal administration requires lower doses because diffusion is not necessary.
      (1) The typical **spinal dose to produce a desired effect is five to ten times less than the epidural dose.**
   iv) Pharmacokinetics

Patients who have received neuraxial morphine should have respiratory monitoring due to the risk of delayed respiratory depression.

      (1) Lipid-soluble opioids (fentanyl) have more IV absorption and **shorter duration** of action.
      (2) Water-soluble opioids (morphine) have a longer onset but longer duration, presumably due to increased time needed to diffuse across the dura.
      (3) The duration of action depends on diffusion of the drug out of the cerebrospinal fluid (CSF) CSF and into the blood and not on metabolism.
   v) **Effects of neuraxial opioids**
      (1) **Analgesia**
      (2) **Pruritus**
      (3) **Urinary retention**
      (4) **Hypoventilation**

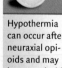

Hypothermia can occur after neuraxial opioids and may be treated with naloxone.

         (a) May be **delayed up to 12 hours**, especially after neuraxial morphine administration
      (5) **Hypothermia**
      (6) **Nausea and Vomiting**

d) **Transdermal/transmucosal administration**
   i) **Both routes avoid first-pass metabolism**
   ii) Fentanyl can be administered via either route due to its high potency and solubility in both water and lipids.

iii) The transmucosal route offers the advantage of rapid onset.

iv) The transdermal route is frequently used for treatment of chronic pain

4) **Special considerations and drug interactions**

a) The combination of **monoamine oxidase inhibitors and meperidine** can result in a severe reaction including fever, convulsions, hemodynamic instability, and coma.

5) **Clinical uses (1)**

a) Pain management

b) Sedation for procedures or critical care

c) Anesthesia for cardiac surgery (high doses)

d) Cough suppression

e) Adjuncts to anesthesia

i) The use of opioids leads to decreased MAC requirements for volatile anesthetics.

6) **Adverse effects/toxicity (1,2)**

a) **Physical dependence**

b) **Drowsiness**

c) **Decreased ventilation**

i) Opioids produce a dose-dependent change in ventilatory response to increased $PaCO_2$

d) **Potentiation of sedative effects of other medications**

e) **Analgesic tolerance**

i) May limit clinical utility

f) **Bradycardia** (dose dependent)

i) Meperidine is an exception. It has an atropine-like structure and tends to cause tachycardia.

g) **Skeletal muscle rigidity**

i) Especially seen with rapid IV administration

ii) Ventilation may be difficult and require administration of a muscle relaxant

h) **Histamine Release**

i) Most commonly associated with morphine

ii) Causes vasodilation and hypotension

i) **Miosis**

j) **Decreased gastrointestinal (GI) motility**

k) **Decreased fetal heart rate variability** when administered to pregnant patients

7) **Agonist/antagonists**

a) Representative drugs in this class: **nalbuphene, buprephenone, and butorphanol**

b) Agonist/antagonist medications have complex interactions with receptors

c) Analgesic effects when used alone but with a ceiling effect, beyond which increased doses do not produce desired results or adverse effects

i) Can result in analgesia with minimal respiratory depression

d) When combined with a full agonist acts as an antagonist

i) **Nalbuphene 2.5 to 10 mg IV is very effective in relieving pruritus induced by neuraxial opioids.**

Meperidine should be avoided in patients with renal failure, history of seizures, and those taking monoamine oxidase inhibitors.

READ MORE

Acute pain management, Chapter 149, page 1085

The opioid agonist/antagonist nalbuphene is very effective for the treatment of pruritus due to neuraxial opioids.

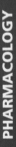
PHARMACOLOGY

8) Treatment of toxicity
   a) **Naloxone is a specific opiate receptor antagonist,** binding the receptor without causing activation.
   b) The effective dose is **1 to 4 µg/kg IV,** and the duration of action is **30 to 45 minutes.**
      i) Dose **may need to be repeated** or an **infusion** started (**5 µg/kg/h**) after administration of a long-acting opiate.
   c) **Side effects** of naloxone
      i) **Reversal of analgesia, nausea, vomiting, and increased sympathetic nervous system activity, including tachycardia, hypertension, pulmonary edema, and cardiac dysrhythmias.**

Patients who have received a long-acting opioid who require opioid antagonism may require repeat doses or an infusion of naloxone.

Chapter Summary for Opioid Analgesics and Antagonists

Mechanism of Action	Bind opioid receptors and inhibit adenyl cyclase via G protein pathway. Results in analgesia
Common Uses	Pain management, sedation, cough suppressant
Adverse Effects	Respiratory depression, pruritus, sedation, physical dependence, ↓ GI motility, miosis, potentiation of other sedative medications, skeletal muscle rigidity
Considerations with Neuraxial Opioids	Delayed respiratory depression possible (morphine), pruritus may be severe and treated with nalbuphine, spinal dose usually 5–10 times less than epidural
Treatment of Toxicity	Effects may be reversed with opioid receptor antagonist, naloxone Naloxone has a shorter half-life than most opioids and may need redosing

References

1. Stoelting RK, Hiller SC. *Pharmacology and Physiology in Anesthetic Practice*. Philadelphia, PA: Lippincott Williams & Wilkins; 2006.
2. Coda BA. Opioids. In: Barash PG, Cullen BF, Stoelting RK, Cahalan MK, Stock MC, eds. *Clinical Anesthesia*. 6th ed. Philadelphia, PA: Lippincott Williams & Wilkins; 2009:465–497.
3. Fukuda K. Intravenous opioid anesthetics. In: Miller RD, ed. *Miller's Anesthesia*. 6th ed. Philadelphia, PA: Churchill Livingstone; 2005.

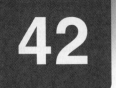

42 Nonsteroidal Anti-inflammatory Drugs and Acetaminophen

Andrea J. Fuller, MD

Nonsteroidal anti-inflammatory drugs (NSAIDs) are very commonly used medications and are widely available to patients without prescription as over-the-counter formulations. NSAIDs can be useful adjuvant drugs when given in conjunction with other anesthetic agents but have specific renal, gastrointestinal (GI), hematologic, and hepatic toxicity that can limit their use.

1) Overview
   a) NSAIDs are used for pain management and treatment of inflammatory conditions such as arthritis.
   b) An overview of this class of drugs is provided here. For more information on specific drugs, refer to the Appendix of drug information, Chapter 196.

NSAIDs inhibit COX, the enzyme responsible for converting arachidonic acid to prostaglandins.

2) Mechanism of action (1,2)
   a) **Prostaglandins** are compounds that mediate a wide variety of physiologic processes, including **platelet aggregation** and **inflammation**.
   b) NSAIDs inhibit cyclooxygenase (COX), the enzyme responsible for converting **arachidonic acid to prostaglandins**.
   c) There are two types of COX: one that is always functional, or **constitutive (COX-1)**, and one that is **inducible (COX-2)**.
3) Structure/Activity Relationships
   a) Two types of NSAIDs
      i) Nonspecific COX inhibitors (i.e., aspirin, ketorlac, ibuprofen, acetaminophen)
      ii) COX-2 inhibitors such as rofecoxib, valdecoxib, celecoxib
   b) Chemical structure
4) Pharmacokinetics
   a) All are well absorbed and have low first-pass metabolism.
   b) All are highly protein bound and have small volumes of distribution.
   c) NSAIDs are metabolized in the liver and excreted by the kidney
5) Special considerations
   a) **COX-2 inhibitors (1)**
      i) Since COX-2 is inducible mainly at inflammatory sites and not involved with platelet aggregation, COX-2 inhibitors were developed to treat inflammation and pain. **COX-2 inhibitors are as effective as conventional (nonselective) COX inhibitors at treating pain.**

      ii) Reports of **increased incidence of myocardial infarction and cerebral vascular accidents** with long-term use prompted rofecoxib to be withdrawn from the market.

      iii) Valdecoxib was also withdrawn from the market because of its association with life-threatening skin reactions and possibly increased cardiovascular events.

      iv) **Celecoxib** is still in use and does not appear to have a higher incidence of cardiovascular events compared with traditional NSAIDs (3).

Large doses of acetaminophen can cause hepatic necrosis and death.

  b) **Acetaminophen**

      i) Acetaminophen is an effective analgesic and antipyretic that **lacks anti-inflammatory properties.**

      ii) **Does not** cause gastric irritation or inhibition of platelet aggregation

      iii) May contribute to analgesic induced nephropathy

      iv) Large doses (single dose > 15 g or > 4 g/d) can cause **hepatic necrosis and death.**

        (1) Hepatotoxicity is possible at lower doses in the presence of alcohol abuse.

        (2) **N-Acetyl cystine** antagonizes the hepatotoxic effects and is an effective antidote when given within 8 hours of overdose.

6) **Clinical Uses (1-3)**

  a) Postoperative pain management

  b) Analgesia

  c) Closure of patent ductus arteriosis in neonates (indomethacin)

  d) Long-term treatment of various forms of arthritis, including osteoarthritis, rheumatoid arthritis, and ankylosing spondylitis

  e) Treatment of fever

  f) Treatment of primary dysmenorrhea

  g) Treatment of familial adenomatous polyposis (celecoxib)

7) **Adverse effects/toxicity**

  a) Renal impairment

  b) Bleeding

      i) Due to **platelet inhibition**

      ii) **Aspirin causes irreversible platelet inhibition**

  c) Gastrointestinal irritation

      i) May lead to **gastric bleeding**

  d) Asthma (in susceptible individuals)—possibly due to blocking synthesis of prostaglandin E_2

  e) Hypertension (small effect)

Chapter Summary for NSAIDS

Definition	NSAIDS are commonly used medications for the treatment of pain and inflammatory disease.
Mechanism of Action	NSAIDS inhibit COX enzyme, the enzyme responsible for converting arachidonic acid to prostaglandins.
Uses	Used for treatment of pain and inflammatory diseases. Useful adjuvant medication for the treatment of pain in conjunction with opioids and other analgesic drugs.
Adverse Effects/Toxicity	Renal impairment and bleeding can occur with NSAID use. May aggravate asthma in susceptible individuals.

References

1. Stoelting RK, Hiller SC. *Pharmacology and Physiology in Anesthetic Practice*. Philadelphia, PA: Lippincott Williams & Wilkins; 2006: 140–154.
2. Van Hemelrijck J, White PF. Nonopoid intravenous anesthesia. In: Barash PG, Cullen BF, Stoelting RK, eds. *Clinical Anesthesia*. 3rd ed. Philadelphia, PA: Lippincott Williams & Wilkins; 1997:311–328.
3. Daiani EZ, Islam K. Cardiovascular and gastrointestinal toxicity of selective COX-2 inhibitors in man. *J Physiol Pharmacol* 2008; 58 (Sup 2)117–33.

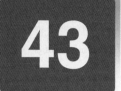

43 Intravenous Induction Agents

Jerry Ingrande, MD, MS

Intravenous (IV) induction agents are medications given at the beginning of an anesthetic to induce loss of consciousness. Each has its advantages and disadvantages. The choice of agent is determined by the procedure and the patient's coexisting diseases.

1) **Propofol**
   a) Propofol (2,6,-diisopropylphenol) is a water-insoluble IV anesthetic clinically available as a 1% emulsion containing 10% soybean oil, 2.25% glycerol, and 1.2% egg phosphatide. It is widely used, especially for ambulatory surgery, due to its fast onset and rapid recovery pharmacokinetic profile.
   b) **Mechanism of action**
      i) Selective GABA receptor agonist
   c) **Clinical use**
      i) **Induction**
         (1) Propofol is given as an IV bolus (1.5 to 2.5 mg/kg) for induction of general anesthesia (1).
         (2) Although not reported to induce histamine release, it should be used cautiously in persons with egg allergy.
            (a) Pain after injection has been reported to occur in 28% to 90% of subjects (2).
            (b) The mechanism of venous pain is unclear; however, its incidence is greater when propofol is given through small veins on the dorsum of the hand as opposed to large veins in the antecubital fossa.
      ii) **Maintenance**
         (1) Propofol is commonly used as a continuous infusion for maintenance of both general anesthesia (100 to 200 µg/kg/min) and conscious sedation (25 to 75 µg/kg/min) (1).
         (2) Supplementation with nitrous oxide can reduce maintenance requirements
   d) **Effects on major organ systems**
      i) **Central nervous system**
         (1) Decreases cerebral blood flow (CBF), cerebral metabolic activity, and intracranial pressure (ICP) (3)
         (2) Large doses may decrease cerebral perfusion pressure secondary to decreases in CBF.
      ii) **Cardiovascular system**
         (1) Causes direct myocardial depression and decreased systemic vascular resistance (SVR) that are both dose and concentration dependent (1)
            (a) **Doses should be reduced for the elderly or those who are volume-depleted.**
         (2) Attenuates the baroreflex mechanism (4)

The addition of local anesthetics (i.e., 1% to 2% lidocaine) to propofol may decrease pain upon injection.

Because propofol causes direct myocardial depression and decreases SVR, doses should be significantly reduced in the elderly or volume depleted.

iii) **Respiratory System**

 (1) Produces respiratory depression, causing apnea in approximately 25% of subjects after an induction dose.

 (2) There is a decreased ventilatory response to hypercarbia and hypoxia, which is exaggerated in the presence of opioids.

iv) **Other effects**

 (1) Propofol has antiemetic properties that popularize its use for outpatient procedures, or for maintenance of anesthesia in subjects who are prone to postoperative nausea and vomiting.

 (2) It does not trigger malignant hyperthermia and is considered the induction and maintenance agent of choice in susceptible patients (1).

e) **Pharmacokinetics**

i) Propofol's rapid recovery profile after a bolus dose is attributed to its rapid distribution from the vessel-rich group (i.e., brain), to inactive tissues (muscle and fat) (5).

 (1) Initial distribution half-life is 1 to 8 minutes with an elimination half-life of 2 to 24 hours (1).

 (2) Although propofol has a high hepatic extraction ratio, changes in hepatic blood flow have little effect on its pharmacokinetics (6).

 (3) Metabolites are cleared via the kidneys.

2) **Thiopental**

a) Thiopental [5-ethyl-5-(1-methyl-butyl)-2-thiobarbituric acid] is a highly alkaline derivative of barbituric acid with a pKa of 7.6 and pH of 9 (1).

i) Reconstitution of thiopental with acidic solutions (i.e., lactated Ringers; nondepolarizing neuromuscular blocking drugs) may result in precipitation of the compound.

b) **Mechanism of action**

i) Like propofol, the sedative-hypnotic actions of thiopental are due to its agonism of the GABA receptor.

c) **Clinical use**

i) **Induction**

 (1) The induction dose of thiopental is **3 to 5 mg/kg in adults and 5 to 6 mg/kg in children** (1).

 (2) Not commonly given in multiple doses or via infusion because of the potential for saturation of inactive tissues (muscle, fat), resulting in delayed awakening. Pain upon injection is rare.

d) **Effects on major organ systems**

i) **Central nervous system**

 (1) Thiopental reduces cerebral metabolic oxygen requirements, CBF, electroencephalogram (EEG) activity, and ICP (3).

 (2) The reduction of cerebral metabolic oxygen requirement exceeds CBF.

  (a) Thiopental is used for **neuroprotection** during periods of incomplete ischemia (carotid endarterectomy, cerebral aneurysm clipping, cardiopulmonary bypass) (7).

  (b) There is no benefit in the setting of global cerebral ischemia (8).

The incidence of pain on injection of propofol is greater when given through the small veins on the dorsum of the hand.

Because thiopental is highly basic, it can cause tissue necrosis when administered through an arterial catheter or subcutaneously (e.g., an infiltrated IV catheter).

PHARMACOLOGY

    ii) **Cardiovascular system**

        (1) Decreases cardiac output, SVR, and causes direct myocardial depression (1)

            (a) The decreased cardiac output is a function of decreased venous return secondary to peripheral vasodilatation.

            (b) Dose should be reduced in patients with hemodynamic compromise.

    iii) **Respiratory system**

        (1) Causes dose-dependent respiratory depression, with depression of central ventilatory centers (3)

        (2) Decreases the ventilatory response to hypercarbia

  e) **Pharmacokinetics**

    i) The rapid induction of anesthesia after a bolus dose of thiopental is attributed to its rapid distribution into the effect site (9).

    ii) Redistribution of drug from the central compartment into a large peripheral compartment reservoir accounts for the rapid awakening after a single induction dose (9).

    iii) Thiopental has a low hepatic extraction ratio, and hepatic clearance is dependent on the intrinsic metabolic activity of the liver (1).

3) **Etomidate**

  a) Etomidate (R-1-ethyl-1-[a-methylbenzyl] is an imidazole-containing IV induction agent that undergoes intramolecular rearrangement at physiologic pH (1).

    i) Because of its instability at physiologic pH, etomidate is formulated in a 0.2% aqueous solution containing 35% propylene glycol.

  b) **Mechanism of action**

    i) The mechanism for induction of hypnosis by etomidate is not fully understood but thought to be largely related to GABA and may be similar to the mechanism of action of propofol.

  c) **Clinical use**

    i) **Induction**

        (1) Etomidate is given as an IV bolus (0.2 to 0.4 mg/kg) for induction of general anesthesia (1).

        (2) Not commonly given in multiple doses or as a maintenance infusion secondary to adrenal suppression

  d) **Effects on major organ systems**

    i) **Central nervous system**

        (1) Reduces cerebral metabolic oxygen requirement, CBF, and ICP (3)

        (2) Cerebral perfusion pressure is maintained because of the hemodynamic stability after etomidate administration (1).

    ii) **Cardiovascular system**

        (1) Minimal changes in BP, SVR, HR, and cardiac output after administration (10)

        (2) For these reasons, etomidate is often administered to patients with cardiopulmonary compromise.

    iii) **Endocrine System**

        (1) Etomidate causes inhibition of 11-beta-hydroxylase, resulting in adrenocortical suppression after its administration (1).

            (a) Adrenal suppression occurs after administration of etomidate and may persist for 5 to 8 hours after a single bolus dose (11).

        (2) This must be taken into consideration in patients dependent on an intact stress response (i.e., septic shock or hemorrhage).

    iv) **Other effects**

        (1) Associated with a high incidence of postoperative nausea and vomiting

        (2) The propylene glycol formulation results in significant pain upon injection.

        (3) Associated with myoclonus after bolus doses, which can be attenuated with prior administration of opioids

  e) **Pharmacokinetics**

    i) Moderately lipid soluble and almost entirely unionized at physiologic pH, allowing for rapid effect site distribution and subsequent redistribution to peripheral tissues.

        (1) This accounts for the rapid induction and rapid awakening after a single IV bolus (3).

    ii) Metabolism occurs via hydrolysis of the ester side chain in the liver.

4) **Ketamine**

  a) Ketamine is a water-soluble compound with a pKa of 7.5. It is structurally related to phencyclidine.

  b) **Mechanism of action**

    i) Interacts with the NMDA receptor, in addition to opioid, and nicotinic and muscarinic acetylcholine receptors

    ii) Ketamine's analgesic, amnestic, and psychomimetic effects are thought to be due to antagonism of the NMDA receptor.

  c) **Clinical use**

    i) **Induction**

        (1) Ketamine is given as an IV bolus dose of 1 to 2 mg/kg for induction of general anesthesia.

        (2) For patients without IV access, 4 to 8 mg/kg may be given intramuscularly (1).

    ii) **Other uses**

        (1) Ketamine is also used in low doses as an adjunct to narcotics for pain relief, especially for chronic pain (1). Doses of 0.1 to 0.5 mg/kg are often given for this purpose.

  d) **Effects on major organ systems**

    i) **Central nervous system**

        (1) Produces a dissociative anesthetic state characterized by analgesia and amnesia while consciousness is maintained.

        (2) High incidence of psychomimetic reactions after awakening from ketamine.

Ketamine can increase CMRO₂, CBF, and ICP and is contraindicated in patients with intracranial pathology.

        (3) Unlike the other induction agents, ketamine *increases* cerebral metabolic oxygen requirement, CBF, and ICP (1).

           (a) It is therefore contraindicated in patients with intracranial pathology.

    ii) **Cardiovascular system**

           (a) Produces a sympathomimetic effect with an associated increase in HR, BP, and cardiac index (1)

           (b) Can cause direct myocardial depression and in the absence of autonomic control, these effects may be unmasked (12)

    iii) **Respiratory system**

        (1) Ketamine has direct bronchodilator properties.

           (a) The induction agent of choice in the setting of acute bronchospasm (1)

      (2) In contrast to the other IV induction agents, ketamine is most likely to **preserve protective airway reflexes.**

      (3) An increase in oral secretions may require concomitant use of an antisialogogue.

  e) **Pharmacokinetics**

    i) Highly lipid-soluble, which facilitates its rapid transfer into the brain (3). This, combined with the drug-induced increase in CBF, is responsible for its rapid onset of action.

    ii) Rapidly redistributed to peripheral tissues.

    iii) Duration of ketamine-induced anesthesia is approximately 10 to 20 minutes after a single bolus dose (1).

    iv) Metabolized by the cytochrome P-450 system to form norketamine, an active metabolite

    v) It has a high hepatic extraction ratio, and alterations in hepatic blood flow may affect the metabolism of ketamine.

5) **Dexmedetomidine**

  a) Dexmedetomidine is a selective alpha-2 adrenoreceptor agonist with an alpha-2 to alpha-1 ratio of 1,600:1.

  b) The anxiolytic and hypnotic responses are associated with its effects in the locus ceruleus, and are mediated by the alpha-2$_A$ receptor (13).

  c) **Clinical use**

    i) **Sedation**

      (1) Dexmedetomidine is approved for use as a continuous infusion (0.2 to 1 μg/ kg/h) for sedation of mechanically ventilated patients in the ICU (1).

      (2) Dexmedetomidine is not used for induction of general anesthesia.

      (3) It is used "off-label" for sedation during diagnostic and therapeutic procedures such as fiberoptic intubations and as an IV adjuvant during regional anesthesia.

  d) **Effects on major organ systems**

    i) **Central nervous system**

      (1) Dexmedetomidine has sedative, anxiolytic, and analgesic effects.

        (a) The level of sedation is comparable to that of midazolam (14).

      (2) The analgesic effects of dexmedetomidine reduce postsurgical opioid requirements.

    ii) **Cardiovascular system**

      (1) Increases the potential for hypotension and bradycardia because of its high alpha-2 adrenoreceptor selectivity (1).

      (2) Dexmedetomidine blunts the hemodynamic effects of direct laryngoscopy and improves hemodynamic stability when given as an anesthetic adjunct during neurosurgical procedures.

    iii) **Respiratory system**

      (1) Produces less ventilatory depression compared to other sedative-hypnotic and opioid anesthetics (15).

      (2) Bolus administration does reduce minute ventilation (16).

  e) **Pharmacokinetics**

    i) Short distribution half-life (6 minutes)

    ii) Short elimination half-life (2 hours) (13)

    iii) Metabolized in the liver and eliminated by the kidneys

      (1) Clearance is decreased with hepatic failure (13).

    iv) Age and sex do not affect pharmacokinetic parameters

Induction Doses and Physiologic Effects of IV Induction Agents

Drug	Induction Dose (mg/kg)	Physiologic Effects	Other Effects
Propofol	1.5–2.5	↓ CBF ↓ CMRO$_2$ ↓ ICP ↓ SVR	• Dose-dependent respiratory depression • Antiemetic properties • May cause pain upon injection
Thiopental	3–5	↓ CBF ↓ CMRO$_2$ ↓ ICP ↓ SVR	• Dose-dependent respiratory depression • May be used for EEG burst suppression • Concomitant administration with acidic medications may cause precipitation
Etomidate	0.2–0.3	↓ CBF ↓ CMRO$_2$ ↓ ICP ↔ SVR ↔ HR	• Myoclonus seen on injection • Adrenocortical suppression • High incidence of PONV
Ketamine	1–2	↑ CBF ↑ CMRO$_2$ ↑ ICP ↑ HR	• Preserves airway reflexes • Dissociative anesthetic • Direct bronchodilator • May increase oral secretions
Dexmedetomidine	Not used for induction Sedation dose: 1 µg/kg given over 10 min; followed by an infusion of 0.2–1 µg/kg/h	↓ HR ↓ BP ↔ MV ↔ RR	• Minimal ventilatory depression • Anxiolytic, sedative, and analgesic effects • Minimizes opioid requirements

↑ increase; ↓ decrease; ↔ no change/minimal change. CBF, cerebral blood flow; CMRO$_2$, cerebral metabolic rate for oxygen; ICP, intracranial pressure; SVR, systemic vascular resistance; HR, heart rate; MV, minute ventilation; RR, respiratory rate

Chapter Summary for IV Induction Agents

Common Uses	Induction of Anesthesia and Sedation
Mechanism of Action	Primarily through GABA (Propofol, thiopental, etomidate), NMDA (ketamine), and alpha-2 (dexmedetomidine) receptors.
Considerations	Propofol has fast onset, rapid recovery pharmacokinetics favorable for ambulatory surgery. Etomidate has minimal cardiovascular effects and may be good for patients with cardiopulmonary compromise. Ketamine has bronchodilator properties that may be good in the setting of acute bronchospasm. Dexmedetomidine is used "off label" for sedation during diagnostic and therapeutic procedures (e.g., fiberoptic intubation) and as an adjuvant during regional anesthesia.
Adverse Effects	Thiopental is highly basic and can cause tissue necrosis if administered intra-arterial or subcutaneously. Etomidate can cause adrenocortical suppression and PONV. Ketamine can have psychotomimetic effects and increases CMRO$_2$, CBF, and ICP. Dexmedetomidine can cause hypotension and bradycardia.

PHARMACOLOGY

References

1. Barash PG. *Clinical Anesthesia* . 6th ed. Philadelphia, PA: Wolters Kluwer/Lippincott Williams & Wilkins; 2009.
2. Smith I, White PF, Nathanson M, et al. Propofol. An update on its clinical use. *Anesthesiology* 1994;81:1005–1043.
3. Stoelting RK, Hillier S. *Pharmacology & Physiology in Anesthetic Practice [print]*. 4th ed. Philadelphia, PA: Lippincott Williams & Wilkins; 2006.
4. Sellgren J, Ejnell H, Elam M, et al. Sympathetic muscle nerve activity, peripheral blood flows, and baroreceptor reflexes in humans during propofol anesthesia and surgery. *Anesthesiology* 1994;80:534–544.
5. Shafer A, Doze VA, Shafer SL, et al. Pharmacokinetics and pharmacodynamics of propofol infusions during general anesthesia. *Anesthesiology* 1988;69:348–356.
6. Servin F, Desmonts JM, Haberer JP, et al. Pharmacokinetics and protein binding of propofol in patients with cirrhosis. *Anesthesiology* 1988;69:887–891.
7. Todd MM, Chadwick HS, Shapiro HM, et al. The neurologic effects of thiopental therapy following experimental cardiac arrest in cats. *Anesthesiology* 1982;57:76–86.
8. Randomized clinical study of thiopental loading in comatose survivors of cardiac arrest. Brain Resuscitation Clinical Trial I Study Group. *N Engl J Med* 1986;314:397–403.
9. Russo H, Bressolle F. Pharmacodynamics and pharmacokinetics of thiopental. *Clin Pharmacokinet* 1998;35:95–134.
10. Gooding JM, Corssen G. Effect of etomidate on the cardiovascular system. *Anesth Analg* 1977;56:717–719.
11. Wagner RL, White PF. Etomidate inhibits adrenocortical function in surgical patients. *Anesthesiology* 1984;61:647–651.
12. Schwartz DA, Horwitz LD. Effects of ketamine on left ventricular performance. *J Pharmacol Exp Ther* 1975;194:410–414.
13. Maze M, Scarfini C, Cavaliere F. New agents for sedation in the intensive care unit. *Crit Care Clin* 2001;17:881–897.
14. Alhashemi JA. Dexmedetomidine vs. midazolam for monitored anaesthesia care during cataract surgery. *Br J Anaesth* 2006;96:722–726.
15. Venn RM, Hell J, Grounds RM. Respiratory effects of dexmedetomidine in the surgical patient requiring intensive care. *Crit Care* 2000;4:302–308.
16. Bloor BC, Ward DS, Belleville JP, et al. Effects of intravenous dexmedetomidine in humans. II. Hemodynamic changes. *Anesthesiology* 1992;77:1134–1142.

Inhaled Anesthetic Agents

Ellen Choi, MD

Inhaled anesthetic agents are used to provide general anesthesia for patients. They provide analgesia, amnesia, and skeletal muscle relaxation, which allow ideal surgical conditions. The exact mechanism of action is unknown. Nitrous oxide (N_2O) and halogenated volatile anesthetic compounds are the most commonly used.

1) Pharmacokinetics
   a) The goal of inhalation anesthesia is to achieve optimal and constant partial pressure of anesthetic in the brain (P_{br}).
      i) In order to achieve this goal, the anesthetic must go from the anesthesia machine to the tissue (brain).
      ii) This creates a gradient that eventually leads to **equilibrium** between the alveolar partial pressure of the anesthetic (P_A) and the partial pressure of the anesthetic in the arterial blood (P_a).

      The goal of inhalational anesthesia

      $$P_A \Leftrightarrow P_a \Leftrightarrow P_{br}$$

      iii) **Alveolar concentration (F_A)**
         (1) Measure of anesthetic concentration and uptake
         (2) F_A quickly equilibrates with the concentrations in the blood and brain.
         (3) F_i **is the concentration of inspired anesthetic.**
         (4) The rate of rise of F_A/F_i determines the speed of inhalational induction.
            (a) If F_A/F_i increases, then speed of inhalational induction increases.
      iv) **Factors affecting delivery/input**
         (1) **Concentration of inspired gas (F_i)**
            (a) Amount of gas that is delivered
               (i) Controlled with the anesthetic vaporizer
         (2) **Fresh gas flow (FGF) rates**
            (a) Increasing the FGF rates increases the amount of anesthetic agent delivered to the patient.
         (3) **Breathing circuit**
            (a) Material of the circuit can cause absorption, decreasing the alveolar concentration of the anesthetic (F_A).
            (b) The volume of the circuit can affect the amount of gas delivered to the patient (1).
         (4) **Concentration effect**
            (a) Increasing the inspired gas concentration (F_i) will cause a more rapid rate of rise of F_A/F_i.

313

(5) **Second gas effect**

(a) A high concentration of one gas/anesthetic (usually N_2O) will accelerate the increase in the F_A of another administered gas (volatile anesthetic or O_2).

b) **Factors affecting uptake**

i) **Solubility**

(1) The solubility of an anesthetic agent can be depicted through the **blood: gas coefficient**.

(a) The blood:gas coefficient **is the ratio of concentration of an agent in blood versus the alveoli** (Table 44-1).

(b) A high blood:gas coefficient (e.g., halothane) indicates that a large amount of anesthetic agent will dissolve in blood.

(i) **The higher the blood:gas coefficient, the greater the solubility, and the slower the rise of FA/Fi.** The end result is a **slower induction**.

(c) A **low blood:gas coefficient** (e.g., N_2O) indicates **low solubility in the blood**. This results in a **faster rise of F_A/F_i and, thus, a faster induction of anesthesia.**

ii) **Alveolar ventilation**

(1) Hyperventilation—increases rate of rise of F_A/F_i.

(2) Hypoventilation—decreases rate of rise of F_A/F_i.

iii) **Cardiac output (CO)**

(1) CO determines the pulmonary blood flow available for gas exchange in the alveoli.

(2) **If CO is high, there is rapid uptake of anesthetic agent from the alveoli, slowing the rise of F_A/F_i.**

(3) **If CO is low, there is less uptake, allowing F_A to increase more rapidly. The rise of F_A/F_i is more rapid.**

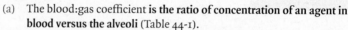

The greater the solubility of the volatile anesthetic administered, the slower the induction of anesthesia.

Table 44-1

Physiochemical Properties of Volatile Anesthetics[a]

	Halothane	Isoflurane	Sevoflurane	Desflurane	Nitrous oxide
MAC[b] (%)	0.75	1.17	1.8	6.6	104
Vapor pressure at 20°C (mm Hg)	243	238	157	669	38,770
Blood:gas partition coefficient	2.50	1.46	0.65	0.42	0.46
Brain:blood solubility	1.9	1.6	1.7	1.3	1.1
Fat:blood solubility	51.1	44.9	47.5	27.2	2.3
Muscle:blood solubility	3.4	2.9	3.1	2.0	1.2

[a]Adapted from Barash PG, Cullen BF, Stoelting RK. *Clinical Anesthesia.* 5th ed. Philadelphia, PA: Lippincott Williams & Wilkins; 2006:386.
[b]MAC value is measured in O_2, 30 to 60 yr, at 37°C P_B760

iv) **Alveolar-venous partial pressure difference (A-vD)**
  (1) A-vD gradient is determined by tissue uptake. Like the blood: gas coefficient, the tissue:blood coefficient determines solubility of anesthetic agent in the tissue.
  (2) Highly perfused tissues account for 75% of the CO. Venous partial pressure of anesthetic agent quickly rises, and thus uptake from the alveoli to the blood is slowed (1).

v) **Intracardiac shunt**
  (1) R→L shunt—slows induction (part of the CO bypasses the lung)
    (a) Clinical significance seen with less soluble agents (e.g., desflurane)
  (2) L→R shunt—speeds induction. However, decreased anesthetic delivery to peripheral tissues negates increased uptake (2).

c) **Elimination of inhaled anesthetics.**
  i) Primary mode of elimination is through **exhalation.**
  ii) Minimal metabolism and excretion
  iii) The goal is to achieve equilibrium between the alveoli, the blood, and the brain.
    (1) Factors discussed above that affect uptake and delivery (VA, CO, solubility) also play a similar role in the elimination of an anesthetic.
  iv) **Factors that affect elimination and recovery (2)**
    (1) Tissue concentrations and solubility
      (a) Tissues act as "reservoirs" for the anesthetic agent to maintain F_A as F_i is decreased to zero.
      (b) Highly soluble agents (e.g., isoflurane) will have a longer recovery time for a longer anesthetic.
      (c) Poorly soluble agents (e.g., desflurane) will have a shorter recovery time despite a prolonged anesthetic.
    (2) Lack of a concentration effect
      (a) F_i cannot be < zero; thus, one cannot "speed" the elimination such as with induction via the concentration effect (2).

2) **Minimal alveolar concentration (MAC) (Table 44-1)**
  a) **MAC is defined as the inhalational anesthetic concentration at which 50% of the population will not move to painful or noxious stimulus (e.g., surgical incision).**
    i) **Approximately 1.3 MAC will prevent movement in 95% of surgical patients.**
  b) **MAC values are an index of anesthetic potency.**
    i) For example, N_2O has a low potency at MAC of 104%. Halothane has a MAC value of 0.75% and is a highly potent anesthetic agent.
  c) **MAC values are additive**
    i) For example, 0.7 MAC of N_2O used with 0.5 MAC of halothane will give an effect of 1.2 MAC anesthetic.
  d) Other MAC values for clinical use (3)
    i) MAC-awake—the value necessary to prevent voluntary response to command.
    ii) MAC-BAR—blocks autonomic response (BAR) to surgical stimulation.
    iii) MAC-intubation—usually about 1.3 MAC; it is the MAC value that prevents response to tracheal intubation.

Table 44-2

Factors Affecting MAC[a]

Factors that Increase MAC
Increased central neurotransmitter levels (MAOIs, acute methamphetamine use, acute cocaine use, ephedrine, levodopa)
Hyperthermia
Chronic alcohol use
Hypernatremia

Factors that Decrease MAC
Anemia
Increasing age
Metabolic acidosis
Severe hypoxia
Induced hypotension (MAP < 50 mm Hg)
Decreased central neurotransmitter levels
α-2 agonists
Hypothermia
Hyponatremia
Lithium
Pregnancy
Acute alcohol ingestion
IV anesthetic agents (opioids, ketamine, barbiturates, benzodiazepines)
Lidocaine
Verapamil

[a]Adapted from Barash PG, Cullen BF, Stoelting RK. *Clinical Anesthesia*. 5th ed. Philadelphia, PA: Lippincott Williams & Wilkins; 2006:397–398.

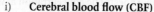

e) **Factors affecting MAC (Table 44-2)**
   i) MAC is **age-dependent**.
      (1) MAC is **greatest at infancy** (month 6 to 12) and decreases with age.
(3) **Pharmacodynamics**
   a) **Neurologic effects**
      i) **Cerebral blood flow (CBF)**

All inhaled anesthetic agents increase CBF by direct vasodilatation.

         (1) All inhaled anesthetics **increase CBF** by **direct vasodilatation** of the cerebral blood vessels.
         (2) Increase in CBF can **increase intracranial pressure**; however, this can be attenuated by hyperventilation.
      ii) **Cerebral metabolic rate of oxygen (CMRO$_2$)**
         (1) The volatile anesthetics agents **decrease CMRO$_2$**.
   b) **Cardiovascular effects (Table 44-3)**
      i) **Mean arterial pressure (MAP)**
         (1) All inhaled anesthetics cause a **decrease in MAP**.
         (2) **Halothane decreases myocardial contractility** while **isoflurane, desflurane, and sevoflurane will decrease systemic vascular resistance (SVR)**.
      ii) **Myocardial contractility**
         (1) **Halothane is direct myocardial depressant** and will decrease CO.
      iii) **Systemic vascular resistance**
         (1) Isoflurane, desflurane, and sevoflurane have a dose-dependent decrease in SVR. Halothane has minimal effects on SVR.
      iv) **Cardiac output**

Table 44-3

Cardiovascular Response to Inhalational Anesthetics

	MAP	Contractility	SVR	CO	HR
Nitrous oxide	– or ↓	↓	–	–	↑
Halothane	↓	↓	–	↓	–[a]
Isoflurane	↓	–	↓	–	↑
Sevoflurane	↓	–	↓	–	–
Desflurane	↓	–	↓	–	↑

[a]Arrhythmias seen with halothane.

    (1) Halothane decreases CO; isoflurane, desflurane, and sevoflurane have minimal effect on CO.

  v) **Heart rate (HR)**

    (1) Rapid increases in desflurane (and to a lesser extent isoflurane) can cause an increase in HR (increase sympathetic stimulation).

    (2) N$_2$O is a direct myocardial depressant; however, it also causes sympathetic stimulation, which offsets decreases in BP.

c) **Respiratory effects of inhaled anesthetics**

  i) **Tidal volume (TV)**

    (1) All inhaled anesthetics cause a **dose-dependent decrease in TV.**

d) **Respiratory rate (RR)**

  i) All inhaled anesthetics cause a **dose-dependent increase in RR.**

e) **Ventilatory response to hypoxia and hypercarbia**

  i) All inhaled anesthetics cause a **dose-dependent depression of response to hypoxia and hypercarbia.**

f) **Pulmonary vascular resistance (PVR)**

  i) N$_2$O increases PVR.

  ii) All volatile anesthetics inhibit hypoxic pulmonary vasoconstriction.

g) **Hepatic effects**

  i) All volatile anesthetics decrease hepatic blood flow.

    (1) Halothane decreases total hepatic blood flow more than other volatile anesthetics.

  ii) Halothane hepatitis has been described (see below).

h) **Renal effects**

  i) All volatile anesthetics and N$_2$O **decrease renal blood flow, glomerular filtration rate, and urinary output.**

  ii) Elevated fluoride levels (as a result of metabolism) can be seen with volatile anesthetics, particularly with sevoflurane.

  iii) **Fluoride-induced nephrotoxicity** has been described in a previously available agent, methoxyflurane, but has not been shown with sevoflurane (4).

i) **Neuromuscular effects**

N$_2$O increases PVR.

READ MORE

Malignant hyperthermia, Chapter 90, page 653, and Chapter 211, page 1328

PHARMACOLOGY

Volatile anesthetics are triggers for MH.

i) **All inhalational anesthetics (volatile agents and N2O) potentiate neuromuscular blockade.**

ii) The volatile anesthetics will cause skeletal muscle relaxation.

   (1) By contrast, N_2O does not provide significant muscle relaxation.

iii) The volatile anesthetics are triggers for **malignant hyperthermia** (MH)

   (1) N_2O is **not** a trigger and can be used safely in a MH nontriggering anesthetic.

(4) Inhaled agents in clinical use

  a) **Halothane**

    i) A halogenated alkane

    ii) **The most potent of the modern volatile anesthetics.**

    iii) It is nonpungent, making it useful for inhalational induction of anesthesia.

    iv) Not widely used in the United States due to adverse effects.

      (1) **Sensitizes the myocardium to epinephrine** and can cause **cardiac dysrhythmias**

      (2) **Halothane hepatitis** is likely due to an immune-mediated response. It occurs is 1 in 35:000

  b) **Isoflurane**

    i) Highly blood soluble, potent anesthetic

    ii) Strong coronary vasodilator and has been theorized to cause coronary steal.

  c) **Sevoflurane**

    i) Pleasant odor and low solubility

    ii) **Used for inhalational induction** in the pediatric population

    iii) Potent bronchodilator

    iv) Degraded by particular carbon dioxide absorbents (baralyme) into a vinyl ether called **Compound A**

      (1) Compound A has shown to be nephrotoxic in rats; studies in humans have had conflicting results.

      (2) The FDA recommends administering sevoflurane with FGF rates of 1 L/min if exposure is 1 hour, and 2 L/min if exposure is >1 hour. (4)

  d) **Desflurane**

    i) Ether derivative with low solubility.

    ii) Rapid onset/offset of action.

    iii) Pungent odor, thus can cause breath holding, bronchospasm, and laryngospasm

    iv) Causes carbon monoxide formation in desiccated carbon dioxide absorbents

  e) **Nitrous oxide**

    i) Inorganic gas with low solubility with quick onset and offset

    ii) With a MAC of 104%, **it cannot be used as the sole anesthetic.**

    iii) Used as an adjuvant with IV agents or other volatile anesthetics

    iv) Because N_2O is 30 times more soluble than nitrogen, **it rapidly diffuses into closed air-filled cavities.**

      (1) The use of N_2O is contraindicated in patients with pneumothorax, air embolism, middle ear surgery, and intestinal obstruction.

    v) Inhibits DNA synthesis by inactivating vitamin B_{12}-dependent enzymes

    vi) Increases PVR

    vii) **Diffusion hypoxia**

(1) Due to the low solubility of N_2O, at the elimination of an anesthetic, N_2O can diffuse out of the blood into the alveolus, displacing O_2. If room air was being administered during this time, the patient can become hypoxic.

(2) During the termination of an anesthetic with N_2O, 100% O_2 should be used to prevent diffusion hypoxia.

Chapter Summary for Inhaled Anesthetics

Definition	Inhaled anesthetics are gases that provide amnesia, analgesia, and skeletal muscle relaxation. N_2O and halogenated anesthetic compounds are most commonly used in anesthesia.
Mechanism of Action	Unknown
Pharmacokinetics and Pharmacodynamics	Higher solubility, CO, alveolar ventilation speed onset of action. All inhaled anesthetics increase CBF by direct vasodilation and decrease MAP.
Side Effects	Inhalational anesthetics can trigger MH. All inhaled anesthetics cause a dose-dependent decrease in TV, increase in RR, and potentiate neuromuscular blockade.

CO, cardiac output; CBF, cerebral blood flow; MAP, mean arterial pressure; MH, malignant hyperthermia; TV, tidal volume; RR, respiratory rate.

References

1. Stoelting RK, Miller RD. Basic pharmacologic principles. In: *Basics of Anesthesia*. 4th ed. Philadelphia, PA: Churchill Livingstone, 2000; 25–33.
2. Barash PG, Cullen BF, Stoelting RK. Inhalational anesthesia. In: *Clinical Anesthesia*. 5th ed. Philadelphia, PA: Lippincott Williams & Wilkins, 2006;384–420.
3. Eger EI II, Eisenkraft JB, Weiskopf RB. *The Pharmacology of Inhaled Anesthetics*. 1st ed. United States of America, Edmond I Eger II, M.D.; 2002.
4. Gentz BA, Malan TP Jr. Renal toxicity with Sevoflurane, a storm in a teacup? *Drugs* 2001;61(15):2155–2162.
5. Faust RJ, Cucchiara RF, Rose SH, et al. *Anesthesiology Review*. 3rd ed. Philadelphia, PA: Churchill Livingstone, 2002; 96–118.
6. Morgan Jr GE, Mikhail MS, Murray MJ. Inhalational anesthetics. In: *Clinical Anesthesiology*. 4th ed. United States: McGraw-Hill Companies, Inc.;2006, 155–178.
7. Stoelting RK, Miller RD. Effects of inhaled anesthetics on circulation and ventilation. In: *Basics of Anesthesia*. 4th ed. Philadelphia, PA:Churchill Livingstone, 2000; 46–57.

45 Adrenergic Agents

Gregory A. Wolff, MD

The autonomic nervous system (ANS) comprises two diametrically opposed forces responsible for involuntary control of cardiac muscle, smooth muscle, glandular, and visceral functions. This chapter focuses on pharmacologic manipulation of the sympathetic or the adrenergic division of the ANS responsible for reflexes consistent with the *fight or flight* response (1).

1) Sympathetic nervous system
   a) **Neurotransmission**
      i) **Preganglionic** fibers travel from thoracolumbar spine and synapse in sympathetic chain, peripheral ganglia, or adrenal medulla.
         (1) **Acetylcholine (ACh) is the neurotransmitter** (1).
      ii) **Postganglionic** fibers synapse directly at target organs.
         (1) **Norepinephrine** (NE) is the neurotransmitter in most cases.
         (2) An exception is transmission by ACh at sweat glands.
         (3) In the adrenal glands, preganglionic fibers interact directly with chromaffin cells, which release NE and Epinephrine (EPI) (1).
   b) **Adrenergic Receptors**
      i) G-protein–coupled receptors selective for NE and EPI
      ii) Subtypes have different functions and locations (1,2) (Table 45-1).
2) Mechanism of action
   a) **Adrenergic agonists/sympathomimetics**—use one or both mechanisms:
      i) **Direct-acting**—agents that directly bind a receptor, activating it
      ii) **Indirect-acting**—agents that cause the release of endogenous NE
         (1) Magnitude of response depends on patient's NE stores and adrenergic receptor density.
         (2) **Tachyphylaxis to indirect-acting sympathomimetics is common** (3).
   b) **Adrenergic antagonists/sympatholytics**
      i) **Competitively bind** receptors, preventing activation by endogenous NE or EPI (4) (Tables 45-2 and 45-3)
3) Structure/activity relationships
   a) Direct agonists are structural analogs of NE and/or EPI.
   b) Indirect agonists do not require structural similarity to NE or EPI, as they do not bind adrenergic receptors (3).
   c) Antagonists are structurally similar to NE and EPI to allow receptor binding, but sufficiently different to prevent receptor activation.

Table 45-1

Adrenergic Receptor Types (1,2)

Receptors	Sensitivity	Locations	Functions
α_1	NE > EPI	Vascular smooth muscle Heart GI smooth muscle GU smooth muscle Liver	Vasoconstriction + Inotropy Relaxation Contraction Glycogenolysis, gluconeogenesis
α_2	NE > EPI	Central nervous system Adrenergic nerve endings Vascular smooth muscle Platelets Endocrine pancreas	Sedation, decreased activity Inhibits NE release Vasoconstriction Aggregation Inhibits insulin release
β_1	EPI > NE	Heart Kidney	+ Chronotropy, + inotropy, increased AV conduction velocity Increased renin secretion
β_2	EPI > NE	Smooth muscle Liver Skeletal muscle	Relaxation Glycogenolysis, gluconeogenesis Glycogenolysis, lactate release, K^+ uptake

Esmolol is a β-blocker with a short duration of action due to its metabolism by plasma esterases.

    d) **Structural variation (agonist or antagonist) imparts receptor selectivity.**

4) **Metabolism**

    a) **Reuptake of NE and EPI at nerve endings terminates their effect.**

    b) When levels exceed reuptake capacity or reuptake inhibitors are present, metabolism becomes clinically significant.

    c) NE, EPI, and structural analogs are inactivated by monoamine oxidase (MAO) and/or catechol-O-methyltransferase, conjugated with glucuronic acid, and excreted in urine.

       i) Consequently, **MAO-inhibitors can cause an exaggerated response to sympathomimetic agents.**

    d) Ephedrine is mainly excreted unchanged in the urine.

    e) Adrenergic antagonists generally undergo liver metabolism and renal excretion. Oral administration exhibits significant first-pass metabolism.

    f) A notable exception, **esmolol, is metabolized by plasma esterases,**

       i) This results in a consistent, short duration of action regardless of dose or duration of administration (4).

5) **Adverse effects are generally dose-dependent; adverse effects tend to reflect response exceeding clinically desired magnitude.**

    a) Cardiovascular—Brady/tachycardia, hypotension/hypertension, myocardial ischemia, dysrhythmias, pulmonary hypertension, increased intrapulmonary shunting, cardiac failure

    b) Pulmonary—Increased airway resistance, pulmonary edema

PHARMACOLOGY

Table 45-2
Adrenergic Agonists (5,6)

Drug	Clinical Receptor Selectivity				CV			Airway	Notes
	α_1	α_2	β_1	β_2	HR	MAP	CO		
Albuterol				++++	+	o/–	o/+	–	Cardiovascular effects minimized by inhalational delivery.
Clonidine		++			–	–	–	o	May be used to prolong regional anesthesia. Useful adjunct in opioid withdrawal. Exhibits rebound hypertension with discontinuation.
Dexmedetomidine		++			±	±	o/–	o	MAP increases and HR decreases with loading dose. MAP decreases and HR increases after longer infusion.
Ephedrine	+	+/o	++	+	+	+	+	–	Indirect activity exceeds direct agonism. Tachyphylaxis is common.
Isoproterenol			+++	+++	+	o/–	+	–	Useful in third degree heart block until pacemaker can be placed.
Dobutamine			+++	+	+/o	o/+	+	o	Pulmonary vasodilation improves right heart function in *cor pulmonale*.
Dopamine	++	+/o	+++	+	+	+	+	o	Receptor activity varies from patient to patient. Nausea/ vomiting is common.
Norepinephrine	+++	+++	++		–	+	–	o	Extravasation can cause tissue necrosis.
Pheylephrine	+++				–	+	–/o	o	Can be used to control SVT via reflexive bradycardia. Decongestant and vasoconstrictive effects facilitate nasal intubation.
Terbutaline				++	+	o/–	o/+	–	Administered orally, subcutaneously, or by inhalation for asthma.

Table 45-3
Adrenergic Antagonists (1,4)

Drug	α_1	α_2	β_1	β_2	Elimination Half-life (h)	Notes
Esmolol			–	–	0.15	Metabolized by plasma esterases.
Labetalol	–		–	–	5–8	α:β potency is 1:7 with IV administration
Metoprolol			–		3–4	β_1 selectivity is abolished by large doses.
Phenoxybenzamine	–	–			24	Used in management of pheochromocytoma. Orthostatic hypotension is common.
Phentolamine	–	–			0.3	Used in management of phenochromocytoma. May cause cramping or diarrhea.
Propranolol			–	–	2–3	Decreases hepatic clearance of amide local anesthetics.

–, blocks receptor.

c) Neurological—Confusion, tremor, anxiety, sedation, headache, intracranial hemorrhage, cerebral vascular accident

d) Renal—Acute renal failure

e) Other—Tissue necrosis, hyperkalemia/hypokalemia

6) Clinical uses

  a) **Agonists**

    i) Increase cardiac inotropy and chronotropy

    ii) Vasopressor

    iii) Treatment of bronchospasm

    iv) Treatment of severe allergic reactions

    v) Prolong local anesthetic duration of action (peripheral and spinal)

    vi) Sedation and analgesia

  b) **Antagonists**

    i) Antihypertensive agents

    ii) Treat myocardial ischemia

    iii) Manage congestive heart failure

    iv) Prevent/treat excessive sympathetic activity

    v) Treatment of glaucoma

    vi) Treatment of benign prostatic hypertrophy

    vii) Treatment of migraine

READ MORE

Appendix of drug information, adrenergic agonists and antagonists, Chapters 199 and 200, pages 1293 and 1296

Routine use of perioperative β-blockade is recommended in patients already taking β-blockers.

Routine use of perioperative β-blockade in patients not already taking β-blockers may increase the risk of stroke and is NOT recommended.

7) **Perioperative β-blockade**
   a) Early studies showed a decrease in myocardial ischemia when patients were given β-blockers in the perioperative period.
   b) This has been a recent topic of controversy following results of POISE trial, which showed a decrease in myocardial ischemia and nonfatal myocardial infarction at the expense of **increased risk of stroke and mortality.**
      i) Evidence does not support the institution of β-blockade on the day of surgery for patients not currently on therapy.
   c) ACC/AHA Guidelines for Perioperative Evaluation were revised in 2009 (7–10).
      i) Current recommendations are to continue β-blockade in perioperative period for patients already on therapy (10).
         (1) β-Blockers should not be discontinued in the perioperative period due to increased risk of mortality.
      ii) Routine use of high dose β-blockers in the absence of titration is not recommended and may be harmful to patients not already taking β-blockers (10).

Chapter Summary for Adrenergic Agents

Mechanism of Action (Agonists)	Direct agents bind α or β receptors → activation. Indirect agents induce endogenous NE release
Mechanism of Action (Antagonists)	Competitively bind α or β receptors preventing activation.
Common Uses	Cardiovascular modulation, bronchospasm management, and anaphylaxis treatment.
Adverse Effects	Dose-dependent response exceeding clinically desired effect.
Perioperative β-Blockade	Continue in patients already on therapy; otherwise, do not routinely institute treatment.

References

1. Johnson JO, Grecu L, Lawson NW. Autonomic nervous system. In: Barash PG, Cullen BF, Stoetling RK, Cahalan MK, Stock MC, eds. *Clinical Anesthesia.* 6th ed. Philadelphia, PA: Lippincott Williams & Wilkins; 2009:326–368.
2. Williams FM, Turner TJ. Adrenergic pharmacology, In: Golan DE, Tashjian AH, Armstrong EJ, Galanter JM, Armstrong AW, Arnaout RA, Rose HS, eds. *Principles of Pharmacology: The Pathophysiologic Basis of Drug Therapy.* Baltimore, MD: Lippincott Williams & Wilkins; 2005:107–120.
3. Stoelting RK, Hiller SC. Sympathomimetics. In: *Pharmacology & Physiology in Anesthetic Practice.* 4th ed. Philadelphia: Lippincott Williams & Wilkins; 2006:292–310.
4. Stoelting RK, Hiller SC. Alpha- and beta-adrenergic receptor antagonists. In: *Pharmacology & Physiology in Anesthetic Practice.* 4th ed. Philadelphia, PA: Lippincott Williams & Wilkins; 2006:321–337.
5. Dyck JB, Maze M, Haack C, Vuorilehto L, Shafer SL. The pharmacokinetics and hemodynamic effects of intravenous and intramuscular dexmedetomidine hydrochloride in adult human volunteers. *Anesthesiology* 1993;78:813–820.
6. Westfall TC, Westfall DP. Adrenergic agonists and antagonists. In: Brunton LL, Lazo JS, Parker KL, eds. *Goodman & Gilman's The Pharmacological Basis of Therapeutics.* 11th ed. New York, NY: McGraw-Hill Medical Publishing Division; 2006.

7. POISE Study Group. Effects of extended-release metoprolol succinate in patients undergoing non-cardiac surgery (POISE trial): a randomised controlled trial. *Lancet* 2008;371:1839–1847.

8. Bangalore S, Wetterslev J, Pranesh S, et al. Perioperative β blockers in patients having non-cardiac surgery: a meta-analysis. *Lancet* 2008;372:1962–1976.

9. Fleisher LA, Beckman JA, Brown KA, et al. ACC/AHA 2007 Guidelines on Perioperative Cardiovascular Evaluation and Care for Noncardiac Surgery: A Report of the American College of Cardiology/American Heart Association Task Force on Practice Guidelines. *Circulation* 2007;116:e418–e500.

10. Fleischmann KE, Beckman JA, Buller CE, et al. ACCF/AHA Focused Update on Perioperative Beta Blockade. A Report of the American College of Cardiology Foundation/American Heart Association Task Force on Practice Guidelines. *Circulation* 2009;120:2123–2151.

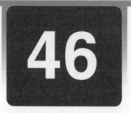

Steroids

Jeromy Cole, MD

Corticosteroids have broad applications in surgery and critical care. Since they are used to treat a wide variety of disorders, many patients encountered in the preoperative setting will be using, or will have recently used, steroids. Knowledge of different steroid preparations, their effects on the human body, and their side effects is essential. For more information on specific steroid medications, refer to the Appendix of Drug Information, Chapter 201.

1) Classification of steroids
   a) **Glucocorticoids**
      i) **Cortisol** is the endogenous form.
         (1) Produced in the zona fasciculata of the adrenal gland
      ii) Baseline secretion is 10 to 20 mg/d (1).
      iii) Peak plasma levels occur in the morning.
      iv) Varying amounts are secreted in excess of baseline in response to stress.
      v) Physiologic effects of glucocorticoids are described below.
   b) **Mineralocorticoids**
      i) **Aldosterone** is the endogenous form.
         (1) Primarily regulated by the renin-angiotensin system.
         (2) Acts at the collecting ducts in the kidney to increase reabsorption of sodium and water in exchange for potassium and hydrogen ions, which are excreted in the urine (2)
   c) **Synthetic steroids**
      i) Act primarily as glucocorticoids
      ii) Different formulations vary in their duration of action and in the amount of mineralocorticoid activity Table 46-1.
2) Mechanism of action/regulation of glucocorticoids
   i) **Mechanism of action**
      (a) Cholesterol derivatives that act upon glucocorticoid receptors at the nucleus of target cells
      (b) Bind DNA and regulate protein transcription
   ii) **Regulation**
      (a) Corticotropin-releasing factor (CRF) is released from the hypothalamus and stimulates the release of adrenocorticotropic hormone (ACTH) from the pituitary, which acts at the adrenal cortex to increase cortisol production.
      (b) Cortisol then acts to suppress both CRF and ACTH production and, through this negative feedback, helps regulate the system.
      (c) Exogenous steroids also suppress CRF and ACTH production and inhibit cortisol production (1).

Table 46-1
Glucocorticoid Preparations

Generic Name	Anti-inflammatory	Mineralocorticoid	Approximate Equivalent Dose (mg)
Short Acting			
Hydrocortisone	1.0	1.0	20.0
Cortisone	0.8	0.8	25.0
Prednisone	4.0	0.25	5.0
Prednisolone	4.0	0.25	5.0
Methylprednisolone	5.0	—	4.0
Intermediate Acting			
Triamcinolone	5.0	—	4.0
Long Acting			
Dexamethasone	30.0	—	0.75

Relative milligram comparisons with cortisol. The glucocorticoid and mineralocorticoid properties of cortisol are set as 1.0. Reproduced from Schwartz JL, Akhtar S, Rosenbaum SH. Endocrine function. In: Barash PG, Cullen BF, Stoelting RK, et al., eds. *Clinical Anesthesia*. 6th ed. Philadelphia, PA: Lippincott Williams & Wilkins; 2009:1291, with permission.

3) Physiologic effects of glucocorticoids
   a) **Metabolic**
      i) Regulate carbohydrate, protein, and fat metabolism
   b) **Endocrine**
      i) Increase serum glucose levels
      ii) Inhibit glucose uptake by muscle cells, antagonize insulin, and stimulate gluconeogenesis
         (1) Results in increased glucose availability to the brain
   c) **Hematologic**
      i) Potent **anti-inflammatory** effects
         (1) Suppress leukocyte cytokine production
         (2) Decrease histamine release by basophils and mast cells
         (3) Decrease synthesis of inflammatory mediators including prostaglandins, leukotrienes, and platelet-activating factors
      ii) **Immunosuppression**
         (1) Decrease serum levels of immunological cells including T and B cells, eosinophils, basophils, and monocytes
         (2) Disrupt the function of T cells and antigen presenting cells
   d) **Growth/fetal development**
      i) Involved in growth factor regulation
      ii) Important for fetal lung maturation, including stimulation of surfactant production (1)

PHARMACOLOGY

4) **Pharmacokinetics**
  a) **Metabolism and excretion**
    i) The majority of corticosteroids are inactivated in the liver and excreted by the kidney.
5) **Clinical uses in anesthesiology**
  a) **Transplant surgery**
    i) Used to prevent acute organ rejection and maintain immunosuppression
    ii) Steroid use may be avoided in liver recipients with hepatitis C due to concerns of disease recurrence (3).
  b) **Traumatic intubations/ENT surgery**
    i) Used to reduce airway edema/inflammation either from injury during intubation or from the surgical procedure
  c) **Neurosurgery**

READ MORE

Allergy and anaphylaxis, Chapter 67, page 484

    i) In patients with brain tumors, steroids can sometimes decrease edema surrounding the tumor and help decrease intracranial pressure (ICP).
      (1) May require hours to days of therapy before ICP decreases
      (2) Thus, steroids should be started 1 to 2 days before surgery, supplemented interoperatively, and then continued postoperatively (4).
  d) **Anaphylaxis**

READ MORE

Antiemetics, Chapter 203, page 1307

    i) Although beneficial effects can be delayed 4 to 6 hours, steroids are often administered as adjuncts in acute therapy when patients have prolonged symptoms that are refractory to other treatments.
    ii) May help attenuate late-phase reactions many hours after the acute event (5).
  e) **Antiemetic**
    i) Dexamethasone is effective alone in reducing postoperative nausea and vomiting (PONV).
    ii) PONV is further reduced when dexamethasone is combined with droperidol or ondansetron (6,7).
  f) **Chronic pain**
    i) Used extensively in both neuraxial and peripheral nerve blocks
    ii) Goal of therapy is to reduce pain by diminishing nerve root swelling, stabilizing nerve membranes, and reducing/attenuating pain signals from inflamed nerves and tissues (8).
  g) **Primary adrenal insufficiency (Addison disease)**
    i) Uncommon in the preoperative setting
    ii) Patients may require both glucocorticoid and mineralocorticoid supplementation
    iii) Hydrocortisone is commonly administered
  h) **Endocrine surgery**
    i) Adrenalectomy
    ii) Glucocorticoid and mineralocorticoid replacement is often started intraoperatively, commonly with an IV dose of 100 mg of hydrocortisone (9).
6) **Tertiary Adrenal Insufficiency (AI) or Iatrogenic AI**
  a) The most common form of AI encountered in surgical patients
  b) Secondary to exogenous steroid use causing suppression of the hypothalamic–pituitary axis and endogenous cortisol production
  c) **Steroid supplementation** or "stress dose steroids" are given to mimic the increase in cortisol that the body would normally require in response to the stress of surgery and to prevent acute AI, which is rare but can be life-threatening.

d) Risk factors for tertiary AI
       i) Can be caused by chronic use of oral, topical, or inhaled steroids
       ii) Suppression of endogenous cortisol production may persist for 6 to 12 months after treatment has been discontinued (2).

   e) **Perioperative steroid supplementation**
       i) Selecting patients who require stress dose steroids
          (1) Predicting which patients will require perioperative supplementation is difficult
             (a) Duration of adrenal suppression after steroid administration is variable.
             (b) Steroid regimens, including doses and duration of treatment, are variable.
          (2) Because the risks of single-dose therapy are low, a conservative recommendation is to give stress dose steroids to any patient who has received a steroid treatment regimen within the past year.
       ii) The optimal dose for perioperative steroid replacement is currently under debate.
          (1) The minimum dose necessary to protect the patient should be given.
          (2) For patients taking steroids at the time of surgery (Table 46-2):
             (a) Regular daily dose should be taken as prescribed.
             (b) A perioperative dose at least equal to the daily dose should be administered.
             (c) Postoperatively, the regular steroid regimen should be continued (2).
          (3) For patients who have taken steroids in the prior year but are not taking steroids at the time of surgery, steroid replacement may be necessary because recovery of the hypothalmic pituitary adrenal axis can take as long as 9–12 months (2). Two common regimens for stress dose steroid administration are listed in Table 46-2.

  7) Adverse effects/toxicity
     a) Chronic use/glucocorticoid excess
       i) Hypertension, diabetes, hyperlipidemia, weight gain, proximal muscle weakness, osteopenia, electrolyte abnormalities, impaired immunity, poor wound healing, gastrointestinal ulceration, thin skin, easy bruising, aseptic necrosis of the femoral head, and psychological effects (9)
       ii) Perioperative considerations

Table 46-2
Management Options for Steroid Replacement in the Perioperative Period
Hydrocortisone, 25 mg IV, at time of induction followed by hydrocortisone infusion, 100 mg over 24 h
Hydrocortisone, 100 mg IV before, during, and after surgery
IV, intravenous(ly). Reproduced from Schwartz JL, Akhtar S, Rosenbaum SH. Endocrine function. In: Barash PG, Cullen BF, Stoelting RK, et al., eds. *Clinical Anesthesia*. 6th ed. Philadelphia, PA: Lippincott Williams & Wilkins; 2009:1290, with permission.

PHARMACOLOGY

(1) **Hypertension**
  (a) Increased renin and volume retention result from mineralocorticoid activity, which all synthetic steroids exhibit to some degree.
  (b) Patients are often taking the aldosterone antagonist spironolactone to reduce fluid retention and hypertension.
  (c) Hypertension should be controlled perioperatively.

(2) **Positioning**
  (a) Fat distribution to the upper back can create a "buffalo hump."
    (i) Additional padding of the operating room table may be required to help the patient lie supine.
  (b) Patients must be positioned carefully due to the risks of bone fracture from severe osteopenia and easy bruising.

(3) **Electrolyte abnormalities**
  (a) Hypokalemic alkalosis and hypernatremia.
  (b) Result from mineralocorticoid activity
  (c) Patients who are taking the aldosterone antagonist spironolactone may have potassium retention.
  (d) Electrolytes should be evaluated preoperatively and abnormalities corrected accordingly.

(4) **Elevated blood glucose**
  (a) May occur due to inhibition of glucose uptake by muscle cells, antagonization of insulin, and gluconeogenesis stimulation.
  (b) Blood glucose should be checked preoperatively and hyperglycemia monitored/treated interoperatively if required.

(5) **Airway management**
  (a) Airway management for the majority of patients taking chronic steroids is routine.
  (b) Rarely, severe cushingoid features may include truncal obesity and tissue edema, with the characteristic moon facies, which may make intubation difficult.
    (i) Consider awake intubation if severe head/neck edema is present.

(6) **Preoperative muscle weakness**
  (a) Due to increased muscle wasting
  (b) Patients may be more sensitive to nondepolarizing neuromuscular blockers and require less medication for relaxation.

(7) **Increased risk of infection and poor wound healing**
  (a) Due to lympholytic and immunosuppressive effects
    (i) Suppression of wound healing may be reversible to some degree by treating with topical vitamin A (9).

b) Acute therapy
  i) Glucose may become elevated for 12 to 24 hours.
    (1) Should be used with caution in diabetics and if steroids deemed necessary glucose should be carefully monitored and controlled
  ii) There is no definitive evidence to support a clinically significant increase in infections or poor wound healing with acute therapy (2).
  iii) Rare complications include aggravation of hypertension, inducement of stress ulcers, and mental status changes (9).

8) Symptoms/treatment of acute AI (adrenal crisis)
  a) Symptoms of an acute crisis can include altered mental status; hypotension; vomiting; abdominal pain; and shock, which can be refractory to standard treatments.
  b) Treatment of acute AI is discussed in Table 46-3.

Table 46-3

Management of Acute Adrenal Insufficiency

Hydrocortisone, 100 mg IV bolus, followed by hydrocortisone, 100 mg q6h for 24 h

Fluid and electrolyte replacement as indicated by vital signs, serum electrolytes, and serum glucose

IV, intravenous(ly).
Reproduced from Schwartz JL, Akhtar S, Rosenbaum SH. Endocrine function. In: Barash PG, Cullen BF, Stoelting RK, et al., eds. *Clinical Anesthesia*. 6th ed. Philadelphia, PA: Lippincott Williams & Wilkins, 2009: 1290, with permission.

Chapter Summary for Steroids

Most Common Uses in Anesthesia	Prevent AI, airway edema, and PONV Surgical applications (i.e., transplant, ENT, neurosurgery)
Adrenal Insufficiency	Most commonly due to exogenous steroid administration (oral, topical, inhaled) within the past 6–12 months. Stress of surgery may trigger a life-threatening adrenal crisis.
Stress Dose Steroids for Patients on Current Steroid Regimen	Regular daily dose should be taken as prescribed on day of surgery. A perioperative dose at least equal to the total daily dose should be given. Preoperative regimen should be continued postoperatively.
Stress Dose Steroids for Patients not Currently Taking Steroids But Having Used a Steroid Regimen in the Past Year	Stress dose steroids may be required because recovery of the hypothalamic pituitary adrenal axis may take 9–12 months.

AI, adrenal insufficiency; PONV, postoperative nausea and vomiting; ENT, ear, nose, and throat; IV, intravenous.

References

1. Chrousos G, Margioris A. Adrenocorticosteroids & adrenocortical antagonists. In: Katzung B, ed. *Basic & Clinical Pharmacology*. 8th ed. New York, NY: McGraw-Hill Companies; 2001.
2. Schwartz J, Akhtar S, Rosenbaum S. Endocrine function. In: Barash PG, Cullen BF, Stoelting RK, Cahalan MK, Stock MC, eds. *Clinical Anesthesia*. 6th ed. Philadelphia, PA: Lippincott Williams & Wilkins, 2009:1287–1291.
3. Csete M, Glas K. Transplant anesthesia. In: Barash PG, Cullen BF, Stoelting RK, Cahalan MK, Stock MC, eds. *Clinical Anesthesia*. 6th ed. Philadelphia, PA: Lippincott Williams & Wilkins; 2009:1393–1417.
4. Kaal EC, Vecht CJ. The management of brain edema in brain tumors. *Curr Opin Oncol* 2004;16:593.
5. Levy JH. Immune function and allergic response. In Barash PG, Cullen BF, Stoelting RK, Cahalan MK, Stock MC, eds. *Clinical Anesthesia*. 6th ed. Philadelphia, PA: Lippincott Williams & Wilkins; 2009:256–270.
6. Henzi I, Walder B, Tramer M. Dexamethasone for the prevention of postoperative nausea and vomiting: a quantitative systematic review. *Anesth Analg* 2000;90:186–194.
7. Apfel C, Korttila K, Abdalla M, Kerger H, et al. A factorial trial of six interventions for the prevention of postoperative nausea and vomiting. *New Engl J Med* 2004;350:2441–2451.
8. Abram SE. Factors that influence the decision to treat pain of spinal origin with epidural steroid injections. *Reg Anesth Pain Med* 2001;26:2–4.
9. Roizen MF, Fleisher LA. Anesthetic implications of concurrent diseases. In: Miller RD, ed. *Miller's Anesthesia*. 6th ed. Philadelphia, PA: Elsevier Churchill Livingstone; 2005:1035–1042.
10. Naguib M, Lien CA. Pharmacology of muscle relaxants and their antagonists. In: Miller RD, ed. *Miller's Anesthesia*. 6th ed. Philadelphia, PA: Elsevier Churchill Livingstone; 2005:481–572.

PHARMACOLOGY

47 Antimicrobials

Andrea J. Fuller, MD

Antimicrobial agents are those used to treat or prevent infection by bacteria, fungi, or viruses. This chapter will briefly discuss concepts associated with antimicrobial administration. Classification of antimicrobials is outlined in Table 47-1. For complete information on an individual medication, please refer to the Appendix of Drug Information and/or a drug administration guide.

The emergence of drug-resistant strains of bacteria is the result of overuse of antimicrobial agents. All clinicians should be cognizant of this ever-growing problem when choosing antimicrobials.

1) Choice of antimicrobial agent
   a) **Culture**
      i) If possible, the infected tissue should be cultured to identify the organism and its antimicrobial susceptibility
   b) **Typical microorganisms**
      i) When choosing an antimicrobial for a surgical procedure or if culture is not available or impossible, the antimicrobial agent should be chosen based on typical microorganisms
   c) **Choice of narrow spectrum if possible**
      i) In order to minimize resistance, the most **narrow spectrum** agent should be chosen.
2) **Interactions with anesthetic agents**
   a) **Neuromuscular blocking agents and aminoglycosides**
      i) The most commonly cited interaction between antimicrobials and anesthetic agents is the **potentiation of neuromuscular blockade by aminoglycoside antibiotics (e.g., neomycin, gentamicin, amikacin) (1).**
         (1) This effect is resistant to reversal by neostigmine.
3) Side effects/adverse reactions
   a) **Allergic reactions/anaphylaxis**
      i) **Incidence of allergic reaction varies with the medication but is approximately 2% (2).**
      ii) It is important to obtain a thorough history of any reported drug allergy. History of rash, wheezing, or tongue swelling are suspicious for allergy. Positive skin testing is confirmatory for penicillin (PCN) allergy but is not as reliable for other antibiotics (i.e., Cephalosporins).
      iii) **Allergy to PCN**
         (1) The most commonly reported medication allergy
         (2) In fact, many patients are not allergic
            (a) **The reaction can be attributed to the underlying illness and/or IgE antibodies can be lost over time (3).**

Table 47-1

Classification of Antimicrobials

Class of Drug	Specific Drugs
Penicillinase-susceptible	Penicillin G Penicillin V
Penicillinase-resistant	Methicillin Oxacillin Nafcillin Cloxacillin Dicloxacillin
Penicillinase-susceptible with activity against Gram-negative bacilli	Ampicillin Amoxicillin Carbenicillin Mezlocillin Piperacillin Azlocillin
Penicillins with beta-lactamase inhibitors	Amoxicillin-clavulanic acid Ampicillin-sulbactam
Cephalosporins	First generation (Cefazolin) Second generation (Cefuroxime) Third generation (Cefotaxime)
Carbapenems	Imipenem
Monobactams	Aztreonam
Aminoglycosides	Streptomycin Gentamicin Tobramycin Amikacin Neomycin
Tetracyclines	Tetracycline Doxycycline
Macrolides	Erythromycin Clarithromycin Azithromycin
Lincomycins	Clindamycin
Dichloroacetic acid derivative	Chloramphenicol
Glycopeptide derivative	Vancomycin
Polymyxins	Polymyxin B
Polypeptide derivative	Bacitracin
Sulfonamides	Sulfisoxazole Sulfamethoxazole Sulfasalazine
Pyrimidine derivative	Trimethoprim

(continued)

PHARMACOLOGY

Table 47-1

Classification of Antimicrobials (*Continued*)

Class of Drug	Specific Drugs
Miscellaneous	Metronidazole
Fluoroquinolones	Norfloxacin Ciprofloxacin Ofloxacin
Urinary tract disinfectants	Nitrofurantoin Fosfomycin
Antifungal drugs	Amphotericin B Nystatin Miconazole

Source: Adapted from Stoelting RK, Hillier SC. Antimicrobials. In: *Pharmacology & Physiology in Anesthetic Practice.* 4th ed. Philadelphia, PA: Lippincott Williams & Wilkins; 2006:522, with permission.

    (3)   It is recommended that **patients with a history of adverse reaction to PCN undergo skin testing.**

        (a)   **PCN skin testing has excellent negative predictive value, making an IgE-mediated allergic reaction extremely unlikely in a patient with a negative skin test.**

        (b)   In reality, most anesthesia providers do not have this information and must rely on clinical judgment.

  iv) **Crossreactivity of PCN and cephalosporins**

    (1)   **Because cephalosporins and PCN have a common beta-lactam ring, immunologic crossreactivity has been demonstrated.**

    (2)   The exact incidence of crossreaction is debatable and confounded by many variables, including PCN contamination of early cephalosporin preparations and the phenomenon of multiple drug allergy syndrome (i.e., patients who are allergic to one medication are more likely to be allergic to another).

    (3)   Allergy to cephalosporins in a PCN allergic patient has been recently reported as high as 38% but as low as 0.17% (4,5).

        (a)   The incidence may depend on the side chain of the cephalosporin and the type of reaction (anaphylaxis vs. other) manifested by the patient.

    (4)   **It is prudent to** avoid cephalosporins in individuals with a history of anaphylaxis and/or positive skin test to PCN (3,4).

        (a)   If the allergy is questionable, one must consider the risk/benefit ratio of antibiotic administration.

        (b)   Cephalosporins have been given for surgery in this population with a very low incidence of allergic reaction (6).

  b) **Adverse reactions (Table 47-2)**

    i) Reactions associated with antimicrobials are extremely variable and range from aminoglycoside-induced ototoxicity to fluoroquinolone prolongation of the QTc interval

Table 47-2
Direct Drug Toxicity Associated with Administration of Antimicrobials

Toxicity	Antimicrobial
Allergic reactions	All antimicrobials but most often with beta-lactam derivatives
Nephrotoxicity	Aminoglycosides Polymyxins Amphotericin B
Neutropenia	Penicillins Cephalosporins Vancomycin
Inhibition of platelet aggregation	Penicillins (high doses)
Prolonged prothrombin time	Cephalosporins
Bone marrow suppression (aplastic anemia, pancytopenia)	Chloramphenicol Flucytosine
Hemolytic anemia	Chloramphenicol Sulfonamides Nitrofurantoin Primaquine
Agranulocytosis	Macrolides Trimethoprim-sulfamethoxazole
Leukopenia and thrombocytopenia (folate deficiency)	Trimethoprim
Normocytic normochromic anemia	Amphotericin B
Ototoxicity	Aminoglycosides Vancomycin (auditory neurotoxicity) Minocycline (vestibular toxicity)
Seizures	Penicillins and other beta-lactams (high doses, azotemic patients, history of epilepsy) Metronidazole
Neuromuscular blockade	Aminoglycosides
Peripheral neuropathy	Nitrofurantoin (renal failure) Isoniazid (prevent with pyridoxine) Metronidazole
Benign intracranial hypertension	Tetracyclines
Optic neuritis	Ethambutol
Hepatotoxicity	Isoniazid Rifampin Tetracyclines (high doses) Beta-lactam antimicrobials (high doses) Nitrofurantoin Erythromycin Sulfonamides

(continued)

Table 47-2

Direct Drug Toxicity Associated with Administration of Antimicrobials (*Continued*)

Toxicity	Antimicrobial
Increased plasma bilirubin concentrations	Erythromycin
Gastrointestinal irritation	Tetracyclines
Prolongation of QTc interval	Erythromycin Fluoroquinolones
Hyperkalemia	Trimethoprim-sulfamethoxazole
Tendonitis	Fluoroquinolones
Teratogenicity	Tetracyclines Metronidazole Rifampin Trimethoprim Fluoroquinolones

Source: Adapted from Stoelting RK, Hillier SC. Antimicrobials. In: *Pharmacology & Physiology in Anesthetic Practice.* 4th ed. Philadelphia, PA: Lippincott Williams & Wilkins; 2006:525, with permission.

c) **Idiosyncratic reactions**
  i) **Red-man syndrome (7)**
    (1) Manifested by an **erythematous rash on the face, neck, and torso, pruritus, hypotension, and angioedema**
    (2) **Histamine-mediated** degranulation of mast cells and basophils independent of IgE and complement
    (3) Most commonly associated with **rapid IV infusion of vancomycin** but also seen with ciprofloxicin, amphotericin B, rifampcin, and teicoplanin
      (a) To avoid this reaction, it is recommended that vancomycin 1 gram be administered over **at least 60 minutes**.
    (4) Treat with antihistamines (diphenhydramine, 50 mg) and discontinue the infusion. Vancomycin can be readministered at a slower rate.
  ii) **Stevens-Johnson syndrome (8)**
    (1) Is a serious drug reaction manifested by fever, malaise, and characteristic **mucocutaneous lesions** and can progress to multiorgan failure.
    (2) Antimicrobial drugs are among the classes of medications associated with this reaction.
    (3) Treat by discontinuing the suspected cause and prompt consultation with dermatologic and/or burn specialists

Rapid IV infusion of Vancomycin should be avoided due to its potential to cause red-man syndrome.

Always ask the surgeon about any antimicrobial prophylaxis required for the surgical procedure.

4) **Surgical site infection (SSI) prophylaxis.** Antimicrobials are commonly administered in the perioperative period to prevent SSI. The choice of agent depends on the type of surgical wound, typical microorganisms, antimicrobial resistance patterns of the institution, and consequences of SSI (1,9,10). It is important to consult with the surgeon about the antimicrobial requirements for a given procedure. If no antimicrobial is necessary, **document the reason for omission.**

Table 47-3

Cardiac Conditions Associated with the Highest Risk of Adverse Outcome from Endocarditis for Which Prophylaxis with Dental Procedures is Reasonable

Prosthetic cardiac valve or prosthetic material used for cardiac valve repair

Previous infective endocarditis

Congenital heart disease (CHD)[a]

    Unrepaired cyanotic CHD, including palliative shunts and conduits

    Completely repaired congenital heart defect with prosthetic material or device, whether placed by surgery or by catheter intervention, during the first 6 months after the procedure[b]

    Repaired CHD with residual defects at the site or adjacent to the site of a prosthetic patch or prosthetic device (which inhibit endothelialization)

Cardiac transplantation recipients who develop cardiac valvulopathy

[a]Except for the conditions listed above, antibiotic prophylaxis is no longer recommended for any other form of CHD.
[b]Prophylaxis is reasonable because endothelialization of prosthetic material occurs within 6 months after the procedure.
Source: Reused with permission from Wilson W, Taubert KA, Gewitz M, et al. Prevention of infective endocarditis: guidelines from the American Heart Association: a guideline from the American Heart Association Rheumatic Fever, Endocarditis, and Kawasaki Disease Committee, Council on Cardiovascular Disease in the Young, and the Council on Clinical Cardiology, Council on Cardiovascular Surgery and Anesthesia, and the Quality of Care and Outcomes Research Interdisciplinary Working Group. *Circulation* 2007;116:1736–1754, with permission.

a) **Clean surgical wounds** (e.g., breast surgery, joint replacement, cardiac surgery) are most commonly infected by Staphylococcal species (10).
    i) **First-generation cephalosporins** are usually recommended
b) **Clean contaminated wounds (e.g., colorectal surgery, cesarean section)** (10)
    i) Surgery in sites known to harbor bacteria such as the gastrointestinal and genitourinary tract
    ii) Choice of antibiotic depends on the type of surgery but usually requires Gram-negative coverage
c) **Contaminated wounds** (10)
    i) Known break in sterile technique, gross wound contamination by the gastrointestinal tract, a traumatic wound, or infection in biliary or urinary tract
d) **Dirty-infected wounds** (10)
    i) Infection existed prior to surgery
e) **Timing of administration**
    i) Few randomized, controlled trials exist regarding the timing of antimicrobial prophylaxis, but most evidence suggests that outcomes are optimized if antimicrobial administration occurs **within 2 hours prior to surgical incision (9,10).**

5) Infective endocarditis (IE) prophylaxis
    a) The indications for antimicrobial prophylaxis for patients who are at risk for IE and are undergoing dental, genitourinary, or gastrointestinal procedures have been recently revised (11). **Only those patients who are at highest risk for complications from IE should receive prophylaxis (Table 47-3) (11).**
    b) **Timing of administration:** A single dose of amoxicillin or cephalosporin should be given **30 to 60 minutes prior to the procedure (11).** Azithromycin or clindamycin can be substituted in allergic individuals (11).

PHARMACOLOGY

Chapter Summary for Antimicrobial Medications

Definition	Antimicrobial agents are used in medicine to treat or prevent infection by bacteria, fungi, or viruses.
Selection	Narrow-spectrum agents should be chosen, when possible, to target organisms infecting tissue and to prevent development of antibiotic resistance.
Side Effects/Adverse Reactions	Anaphylaxis Red-man syndrome (Vancomycin) Can be extremely variable (ototoxicity to QTc prolongation)
Surgical Site Infection Prophylaxis	Consult with surgeon regarding antimicrobial requirements for a given surgical procedure Consider dosing antibiotics within 2 h prior to surgical incision

References

1. Stoelting RK, Hiller SC. Antimicrobials. In: *Pharmacology and physiology in anesthetic practice*. Philadelphia, PA: Lippincott Williams & Wilkins; 2006:521–550.
2. Gomes ER, Demoly P. Epidemiology of hypersensitivity drug reactions. *Curr Opin Allergy Clin Immunol* 2005;5(4):309–316.
3. Solensky R. Drug hypersensitivity. *Med Clin North Am* 2006;90(1).
4. Miranda A, Blanca M, Vega JM, et al. Cross-reactivity between a penicillin and a cephalosporin with the same side chain. *J Allergy Clin Immunol* 1996;98(3):671–676.
5. Daulat S, Solensky R, Earl HS, et al. Safety of cephalosporin administration to patients with histories of penicillin allergy. *J Allergy Clin Immunol* 2004;113(6):1220–1222.
6. Goodman EJ, Morgan MJ, Johnson PA, et al. Cephalosporins can be given to penicillin-allergic patients who do not exhibit an anaphylactic response. *J Clin Anes* 2001;13(8):561–564.
7. Sivagnanam S, Deleu D. Red man syndrome. *Crit Care* 2003;7(2):119–120.
8. Hazin R, Ibrahimi OA, Hazin MI, et al. Stevens-Johnson syndrome: pathogenesis, diagnosis, and management. *Ann Med* 2008;40(2):129–138.
9. Classen DC, Evans RS, Pestotnik SL, et al. The timing of prophylactic administration of antibiotics and the risk of surgical-wound infection. *N Engl J Med* 1992;326(5):281–286.
10. Teplick R, Baden L, Rubin RH. Antimicrobial therapy. In: Evers AS, Maze M, eds. *Anesthetic Pharmacology: Physiologic Principles and Clinical Practice*. Philadelphia, PA: Churchill Livingstone; 2004:865–886.
11. Wilson W, Taubert KA, Gewitz M, et al. Prevention of infective endocarditis: Guidelines from the American Heart Association: a Guideline from the American Heart Association Rheumatic Fever, Endocarditis, and Kawasaki Disease Committee, Council on Cardiovascular Disease in the Young, and the Council on Clinical Cardiology, Council on Cardiovascular Surgery and Anesthesia, and the Quality of Care and Outcomes Research Interdisciplinary Working Group. *Circulation* 2007;116:1736–1754.

Antiemetics

Sunil Kumar, MD

Antiemetics are used in anesthetic practice for prevention and treatment of postoperative nausea and/or vomiting (PONV). These drugs are generally classified depending on their mechanism of action. Commonly used antiemetics are listed Table 48-1. This chapter contains a brief description of important drugs and recommendations for their use.

1) Antiemetic drugs
   a) **Serotonin (5-HT$_3$ receptor) antagonists**
      i) Effective for prevention and treatment of nausea associated with chemotherapy, radiation therapy, and PONV
      ii) Not effective for treatment of motion sickness
      iii) Most effective when given at the end of surgery
      iv) Most agents are effective orally as well as parenterally.
      v) Increasingly popular because of their **wide therapeutic index** (3)
      vi) Are **not associated with excessive sedation, or extrapyramidal side effects seen with other commonly used antiemetics**
      vii) **Can prolong QT interval**
         (1) In one study, IV boluses of 4 mg ondansetron and 0.75 mg droperidol produced similar QT prolongation (4).
      viii) Higher cost compared to other antiemetics.
      ix) **Ondansetron** is the most commonly used drug from this group.
         (1) Side effects
            (a) Generally mild and infrequent
               (i) Include headache, dizziness, constipation, and transient elevation of liver enzymes
         (2) Pharmacokinetics
            (a) Metabolized principally by liver
               (i) **Dose** should be **reduced in patients with liver dysfunction.**
            (b) Elimination half-life, 3 to 6 hours

2) **Glucocorticoids**
   a) **Dexamethasone** and other glucocorticoids are useful in the management of chemotherapy-induced emesis and PONV.
   b) Mechanism of action
      i) Animal studies suggest central antiemetic action through activation of the glucocorticoid receptors in the medulla (5).
   c) Most effective when given before induction of anesthesia
   d) Long-term use of glucocorticoids can produce side effects including wound infection and adrenal suppression. No adverse effects appear to result from single dose (1).

3) **Dopamine (D2) antagonists**
   a) **Droperidol**

Selective serotonin antagonists are most effective for PONV when given at the end of surgery.

Dexamethasone is most effective in preventing PONV when given before induction of anesthesia or at the beginning of surgery (pearl).

Glucocorticoids should be used with caution in diabetic patients as it can exacerbate hyperglycemia.

PHARMACOLOGY

i) Highly effective in prevention and treatment of PONV

ii) Side effects

  (1) Sedation, dyskinesia, restlessness, and dysphoric reactions

  (2) QTc prolongation

    (a) **"Black box" warning** was issued by the FDA in 2001, because of rare risk of **QTc prolongation**, torsades de pointes, and death.

    (b) QTc prolongation appears to be dose related and the adverse events are typically seen at doses higher than those used for PONV treatment.

    (c) FDA recommends that a 12-lead ECG should be obtained before drug administration, and ECG monitoring should be continued for 2 to 3 hours after treatment (4).

iii) **Reserve for patients not responding to other therapies**

b) **Metoclopramide**

i) Dopamine receptor antagonist

ii) **Weak antiemetic** effect in standard dose (10 mg IV). Higher dose (20 mg) may be more effective, but has higher risk of side effects.

  (1) Increases gastric and small bowel emptying, and increases lower esophageal sphincter tone. **Should be avoided in patients who may have gastrointestinal obstruction.**

  (2) Side effects

    (a) Extrapyramidal reactions, drowsiness, and restlessness

Metoclopr-amide increases gastric motility and should be avoided in patients with the potential for gastrointestinal obstruction.

c) **Perphenazine**

i) Phenothiazine derivative

ii) Best administered at the end of surgery

iii) Side effects limit the use

  (1) Sedation, postural hypotension, and extrapyramidal reactions ranging from restlessness to oculogyric crisis

4) **Anticholinergic drugs**

a) All anticholinergic drugs with central effects may have antiemetic properties.

b) **Transdermal scopolamine**, typically applied behind the ear, is effective prophylaxis for motion sickness, and has been used for PONV prophylaxis.

i) Clinical use is limited because of its **slow onset**, relatively frequent side effects and medical and age related restrictions.

ii) Onset of effect, 2 to 4 hours. The patch should be applied 4 hours prior to end of surgery, and can be worn for up to 72 hours. Generally removed after 24 hours.

iii) Side effects

  (1) Dry mouth, somnolence, dizziness, delirium, mydriasis, urinary retention

iv) **Contraindications**

  (1) **Narrow-angle glaucoma, urinary bladder neck obstruction**

  (2) **Caution** is advised **in elderly**, and patients with impaired liver and kidney function because of increased risk of CNS side effects.

  (3) Not recommended for pediatric patients

v) Care should be taken while handling the patch as contact with eyes may cause prolonged mydriasis and cycloplegia.

Hydroxyzine should always be given by intramuscular injection as it can cause thrombophlebi-tis when given intravenously.

5) **Antihistamines**

a) Particularly useful for prophylaxis and treatment of motion sickness and PONV associated with middle ear surgery

Table 48-1

Commonly Used Antiemetics for Adults, Doses, and Timing of Administration (1,2)

Drug Class/Drug	Dose	Timing
Serotonin Receptor Antagonists		
Ondansetron	4–8 mg IV	At end of surgery
Dolasetron	12.5 mg IV	At end of surgery
Granisetron	0.35–1 mg IV	At end of surgery
Tropisetron	5 mg IV	At end of surgery
Corticosteroids		
Dexamethasone	5–10 mg IV	Before induction
Dopamine Antagonists		
Droperidol	0.625–1.25 mg IV	At end of surgery
Metoclopramide	10–20 mg IV	At end of surgery
Perphenazine	5–10 mg IV	At end of surgery
Anticholinergics		
Scopolamine	Transdermal patch, 1.5 mg	Prior evening, or 4 h before end of surgery
Antihistamines		
Dimenhydrinate	1–2 mg IV	
Hydroxyzine	25–100 mg IM	
Promethazine	12.5–25 mg IV	At end of surgery
Vasopressors		
Ephedrine	0.5 mg/kg IM	

READ
MORE

Postoperative
nausea and vomiting, Chapter 7,
page 47

b) Both hydroxyzine and promethazine (a phenothiazine-derivative) are antihistamines.

c) Side effects

   i) Sedation, dizziness, and dry mouth

6) **Combination therapy**

   a) Combination of antiemetics with different mechanisms of action is **superior to monotherapy** for PONV prophylaxis, and is recommended for moderate or high-risk patients (1).

7) **General Guidelines for PONV prevention and treatment**

   a) Identify patients at higher risk of developing PONV, and reduce baseline risk factors among patients at high risk.

8) **Patients at low risk**

   a) **Routine prophylaxis** is **not recommended**

   b) If PONV occurs

   i) One drug **rescue therapy** should be provided.

   ii) A 5-HT$_3$ receptor antagonist is most common first choice in the current U.S. practice.

9) **Patients at moderate risk**

   a) **Monotherapy or combination therapy** with two or three different drugs is recommended.

   b) Combination therapy is generally recommended in children who are higher risk of PONV as compared to adults.

10) **Patients at high risk**

   a) **Combination therapy** with double or triple antiemetic combinations.

11) **PONV occurring within 6 hours after surgery**

   a) Treat with a drug different from what the patient has already received for prophylaxis.

12) **PONV after 6 hours of surgery**

   a) May be treated with any of the drugs used for prophylaxis except dexamethasone or transdermal scopolamine.

Chapter Summary for Antiemetics

Mechanism of Action	Multiple mechanisms of action that include glucocorticoids and drugs that antagonize of 5-HT$_3$, histamine, D2, and cholinergic receptors
Common Uses	Most commonly used for prophylaxis of PONV in patients at moderate-to-high risk for PONV
Adverse Effects (cause)	5-HT$_3$: QT prolongation Glucocorticoids: hyperglycemia D2 antagonists: QTc prolongation Antihistamine: sedation, dizziness Anticholinergic: dry mouth, sedation, dizziness
Treatment Guidelines	Routine prophylaxis in patients at low risk of PONV is not recommended. 5-HT$_3$ receptor antagonist is a common first-line drug choice for PONV. Consider multimodal therapy for patients at high risk or who have breakthrough PONV.

References

1. Gan TJ, Meyer TA, Apfel CC, et al. Society of Ambulatory Anesthesia Consensus Guidelines for Managing Postoperative Nausea and Vomiting. *Anesth Analg* 2007;105:1615–1628.
2. van Vlymen JM, White P. Outpatient anesthesia. In: Miller RD, ed. *Anesthesia*. 5th ed. Philadelphia, PA: Churchill Livingstone; 2000:2 213–2240.
3. Stoelting RK, Hillier SC. *Pharmacology and Physiology in Anesthetic Practice*. Philadelphia, PA. Lippincott Williams; 2006:446–448.
4. Charblt B, Albaladejo P, Funck-Brentano C, et al. Prolongation of QTc interval after postoperative nausea and vomiting treatment by droperidol and ondansetron. *Anesthesiology* 2005;102:1094–1100.
5. Ho C, Ho S, Wang J, et al. Dexamethasone has a central antiemetic mechanism in decerebrated cats. *Anesth Analg* 2004;99:734–739.

49

Hematologic Agents

Andrea J. Fuller, MD

Hematologic agents are medications that modulate blood coagulation or formation of blood cells. Surgical/anesthetic considerations are discussed in this chapter whenever possible. However, **prior to initiating regional anesthesia on any patient on anticoagulants, the American Society of Regional Anesthesia Guidelines should first be consulted (1).**

READ MORE

Regional anesthesia in the anticoagulated patient, Chapter 172, page 1171

The onset, duration, and clinical effect of heparin are highly variable between individuals and should be monitored with laboratory values.

1) **Anticoagulant medications**
 a) **Heparin**
  i) A negatively charged pentasaccharide that binds **antithrombin III**, potentiating its inhibitory effect on multiple coagulation factors, including thrombin and activated factors IX, X, XI, and XII (2)
  ii) Derived from bovine lung or porcine intestine
  iii) **Side effects**
   (1) Hemorrhage, allergic reactions, histamine release, heparin-induced thrombocytopenia
  iv) **Clinical uses**
   (1) Anticoagulation in patients undergoing coronary bypass surgery, vascular surgery, and percutaneous coronary intervention
   (2) Treatment of patients with venous thrombosis and acute myocardial infarction
  v) **Pharmacokinetics (2,3)**
   (1) **Heparin has low bioavailability due to complex protein binding.**
   (2) **Administration is intravenous (IV) or subcutaneous (SC).**
   (3) **Duration**
    (a) Approximately 4 to 6 hours (IV) and 12 hours (SC), but this is **highly variable and must be monitored.**
   (4) **Heparin does not cross the placenta, making it safe in pregnancy.**
  vi) The amount of heparin required for a given effect is **extremely variable** between individuals.
   (1) **Activated partial thromboplastin time (aPTT) and the activated clotting time (ACT)** are most commonly used to monitor heparin-induced anticoagulation.
  vii) **Considerations for surgery/anesthesia**
   (1) Elective surgery and regional anesthesia should be postponed until IV heparin has been discontinued for 4 to 6 hours or until the aPTT is normalized.

(2) If emergency surgery is required, heparin can be reversed with protamine (see below).

(3) Patients receiving low-dose SC heparin (5,000 U BID) need not have surgery and/or regional anesthesia postponed. For higher SC doses, aPTT should be checked.

b) **Low molecular weight heparin**

 i) **Derived from unfractionated heparin**

 ii) Has a uniform molecular size, resulting in **more predictable anticoagulant effects and pharmacokinetics (2)**

 iii) **Representative medications** include enoxaparin, dalteparin, fondaparinux.

 iv) **Clinical uses**

(1) Treatment of acute coronary syndrome, prevention of thrombosis, especially deep venous thrombosis and thromboembolism

 v) **Considerations for surgery/anesthesia**

(1) Timing of surgery and regional anesthesia depends on the drug and dosage but should be delayed at least 12 hours from the last dose.

 vi) Laboratory monitoring is usually not necessary, except in high-risk patient populations such as newborns, the morbidly obese, and /or those with renal failure (4).

(1) Monitoring is done using **anti-Xa** levels

(2) Therapeutic range is 0.5 to 1.1 IU/ml and should be measured 4 hours after a dose (4)

c) **Warfarin**

 i) Inhibits the production of Vitamin K–dependent coagulation proteins (2)

 ii) **Clinical uses**

(1) Prevention of venous thromboembolism, prevention of systemic embolization in patients with prosthetic heart valves or atrial fibrillation

 iii) **Pharmacokinetics (2)**

(1) **Route of administration is oral**

(2) Despite rapid absorption after oral administration the drug **does not take effect for 8 to 12 hours,** due to the elimination of clotting factors that are not affected by the drug. **Peak effects occur in 36 to 72 hours.**

(3) **Warfarin crosses the placenta and is contraindicated in pregnancy.**

 iv) **Monitoring**

(1) **Anticoagulant effects vary dramatically between individuals,** necessitating close monitoring via the **prothrombin time (PT) and INR.**

 v) **Considerations for surgery/anesthesia (2)**

(1) For elective procedures, anticoagulation should be discontinued for 1 to 5 days; the **PT/INR should be checked** and within 20% of the normal range.

(2) The exact level of anticoagulation tolerable for an elective procedure depends on the type of procedure and the patient's risk of complications from discontinuation of anticoagulation (5).

(3) **PT and INR should be checked prior to regional anesthesia.**

(4) For emergency or high-risk procedures, the anticoagulant effects can be reversed by administration of **2 to 10 mg (oral) or up to 10 mg (IV) Vitamin K (depending on the INR) or 1 to 2 units of fresh frozen plasma (6,7).**

Strongly consider obtaining the PT/INR prior to elective surgery in a patient on chronic warfarin therapy.

d) **Thrombolytic medications**

 i) Drugs that produce **thrombolysis** by facilitating the conversion of plasminogen to plasmin (2)

    ii)   **Representative medications** include streptokinase, Alteplase (recombinant tissue plasminogen activator), Anistreplase (anisolylated plasminogen streptokinase activator complex).

    iii)   **Clinical uses**

      (1)   Treatment of acute coronary syndromes, pulmonary embolism, and acute ischemic stroke

e) **Glycoprotein IIb/IIIa inhibitors**

There are no specific reversal agents for glycoprotein IIb/IIIa inhibitors.

    i)   Block fibrinogen binding at the platelet glycoprotein IIb/IIIa receptors and **inhibit the final common pathway for platelet aggregation (2)**

    ii)   **Representative medications** include abciximab, eptifibatide, and tirofiban.

    iii)   **Clinical uses**

      (1)   Treatment of patients with acute coronary syndrome and those undergoing interventional cardiology procedures such as angioplasty and stenting

    iv)   **Considerations for surgery/anesthesia**

      (1)   IIb/IIIa inhibitors should be discontinued for 24 to 72 hours prior to elective surgery.

      (2)   There are no specific reversal agents.

Patients with recent placement of a drug-eluting coronary stent are at risk of stent thrombosis and myocardial infarction if antiplatelet therapy is discontinued.

f) **Adenosine diphosphate (ADP) inhibitors**

    i)   The inhibition of ADP **prevents platelet activation, aggregation, and degranulation (2)**.

    ii)   **Representative medications** include aspirin, clopidogrel, ticlopidine, dipyridaole, and dextran.

    iii)   **Clinical uses**

      (1)   Prevention of thrombosis in patients with coronary artery disease and those who have undergone coronary artery stenting, peripheral vascular disease, and acute coronary syndromes (aspirin).

    iv)   **Considerations for surgery/anesthesia**

      (1)   Because most of these drugs are irreversible inhibitors, their effects last for the life of the platelet, which is 7 to 10 days.

Ideally, antiplatelet therapy should be discontinued 7 days prior to elective surgery or regional anesthesia.

      (2)   The decision to discontinue antiplatelet medications perioperatively depends on the indication for use.

      (3)   In patients with recent percutaneous coronary intervention and drug-eluting stent placement, discontinuation of aspirin and clopidogrel may **significantly increase the risk of stent thrombosis and acute myocardial infarction** (8,9).

        (a)   These patients may benefit from continuation of antiplatelet therapy.

        (b)   If the surgical procedure carries a high risk of bleeding, especially into a closed space such as the cranium, spine, and/or posterior chamber of the eye, discontinuation may be warranted (8).

        (c)   Consultation with the patient's cardiologist is suggested.

Platelet transfusion should be considered to treat bleeding in patients on antiplatelet therapy.

      (4)   Patients who are taking these medications for other indications should be advised to discontinue use for 7 days prior to surgery (6).

      (5)   Regional anesthesia can be performed after discontinuation of clopidogrel for 7 days.

      (6)   For aspirin therapy, regional anesthesia is not contraindicated, but special considerations should be made when the aspirin is combined with other antiplatelet medications.

      (7)   If emergency surgery is required and bleeding is encountered, platelet transfusion should be considered **(6)**.

2) Procoagulant medications
   a) **Recombinant factor VIIa**
      i) A synthetic form of **activated factor VIIa**
      ii) **Clinical uses**
         (1) FDA-approved for treatment of bleeding in patients with hemophilia A or B and inhibitors to Factors VII or XI
         (2) There is mounting evidence to support its use in **profuse and refractory bleeding in patients with massive trauma, liver dysfunction, and obstetrical bleeding (6,10,11).**
      iii) **Usual dose is 50 to 100 mcg/kg IV (10,11)**
      iv) **Side effects**
         (1) **Thrombosis**, including thrombotic stroke, acute myocardial infarction, pulmonary embolism, and clotting of indwelling devices (12)
   b) **Protamine**
      i) A specific antagonist of **heparin**
      ii) It is a positively charged protein that combines with negatively charged heparin, rendering it inactive (13).
      iii) Derived from **salmon sperm**
      iv) The dose is 1 mg of protamine for every 100 U of heparin in circulation (as calculated by the ACT).
      v) Side effects (13)
         (1) **Hypotension**
            (a) **Rapid injection is associated with histamine release and hypotension. This may be attenuated by slow injection in a peripheral rather than central injection site.**
         (2) **Pulmonary hypertension**
            (a) **Rare effect due to thromboxane and serotonin release**
            (b) **Manifested by arterial hypoxemia and pulmonary edema**
         (3) **Allergic reactions**
            (a) **Most common in patients receiving protamine-containing insulin (NPH) and those with fish allergies**
   c) Antifibrinolytics
      i) **Aminocaproic acid and tranexamic acid** are lysine analogs, which inhibit **plasminogen activator and plasmin release.**
      ii) **Inhibit fibrinolysis and decrease mediastinal bleeding in cardiopulmonary bypass (CPB) patients (6,13)**
      iii) **Aprotinin**
         (1) A nonspecific **protease inhibitor** that inhibits the intrinsic coagulation cascade, complement activation, fibrinolysis, and bradykinin formation (13).
         (2) **Decreases bleeding and transfusion requirements in CPB patients (6)**
         (3) Extracted from **beef lung**
         (4) **Potential for allergic reactions, especially with reexposure (6)**
   d) Desmopressin (DDAVP (14))
      i) A synthetic analog of **arginine vasopressin**
      ii) It **increases the amount of circulating Factor VIII available to bind to von Willebrand factor (13).**
      iii) **Clinical uses**
         (1) Treatment of bleeding or for preoperative administration in patients with **Hemophilia A or certain forms of von Willebrand's disease**
         (2) **Treatment of excessive post-CPB bleeding**

Rapid injection of protamine is associated with hypotension and should be avoided.

READ MORE
Coagulopathies, Chapter 89, page 643

PHARMACOLOGY

READ
MORE

Pituitary
disorders,
Chapter 84,
page 615

(3) **Perioperative management of diabetes insipidus (6)**

(4) 0.3 to 0.5 IV mcg/kg are given 30 minutes prior to a surgical procedure (for Hemophilia and most types of Von Willebrand's disease) (7).

Chapter Summary for Hematologic Agents

Definition	Hematologic agents are used to control the coagulation of blood and/or degradation of blood clots by modulating various aspects of the coagulation cascade.
Mechanism of Action	**Anticoagulants** interfere with proteins responsible for blood clotting or platelet aggregation such as antithrombin III (heparin) or production of vitamin K–dependent clotting factors (warfarin), glycoprotein IIb/IIIa inhibitors (abciximab), and ADP inhibitors (aspirin). **Thrombolytics** are used to dissolve formed blood clots by facilitating conversion of plasminogen to plasmin (streptokinase). **Procoagulants** such as activated factor VIIa, protamine, antifibrinolytics (aminocaproic acid), and desmopressin improve coagulation functions.
Special Considerations	Consult the ASRA guidelines prior to placement of neuraxial anesthetic blocks in patients taking anticoagulant medications.

References

1. Horlocker TT, Wedel DJ, Benzon H, et al. Regional anesthesia in the anticoagulated patient: Defining the risks (the second asra consensus conference on neuraxial anesthesia and anticoagulation). *Reg Anesth Pain Med* 2003;28(3):172–197.
2. Stoelting RK, Hiller SC. Anticoagulants. In: *Pharmacology and Physiology in Anesthetic Practice*. 4th ed. Philadelphia, PA: Lippincott Williams & Wilkins; 2006:505–520.
3. Hirsh J, Raschke R, Warkentin TE, et al. Heparin: mechanism of action, pharmacokinetics, dosing considerations, monitoring, efficacy, and safety. *Chest* 1995;108(4):258–275.
4. Laposata M, Green D, Cott EMV, et al. College of American Pathologists Conference XXXI on laboratory monitoring of anticoagulant therapy: the clinical use and laboratory monitoring of low-molecular-weight heparin, danaparoid, hirudin and related compounds, and argatroban. *Arch Pathol Lab Med* 1998;122(9):799–807.
5. Owens CD, Belkin M. Thrombosis and coagulation: operative management of the anticoagulated patient. *Surgical Clinics of North America* 2005;85(6):1179–1189.
6. Practice Guidelines for perioperative blood transfusion and adjuvant therapies: an updated report by the American Society of Anesthesiologists Task Force on perioperative blood transfusion and adjuvant therapies. *Anesthesiology* 2006;105:198–208.
7. Donnelly AJ, Baughman VL, Gonzales JP, et al. *Anesthesiology & Critical Care Drug Handbook*. 7th ed. Hudson, OH: Lexi-Comp; 2006.
8. Chassot PG, Delababys A, Spahn DR. Perioperative antiplatelet therapy: the case for continuing therapy in patients at risk of myocardial infarction. *Br J Anaesth* 2007;99(3):316–328.
9. Serruys PW, Kutryk MJB, Ong ATL. Coronary-artery stents. *New Engl J Med* 2006;354(5):483–495.
10. Martinowitz U, Kenet G, Segal E, et al. Recombinant activated factor vii for adjunctive hemorrhage control in trauma. *J Trauma* 2001;51(3):431–439.
11. Karalapillai D, Popham P. Recombinant factor viia in massive postpartum haemorrhage. *Int J Obstet Anesth* 2007;16:29–34.
12. OConnell KA, Wood JJ, Wise RP, et al. Thromboembolic adverse events after use of recombinant human coagulation factor viia. *JAMA* 2006;295(3):293–298.
13. Stoelting RK, Hiller SC. Blood components, substitutes, and hemostatic drugs. *Pharmacology and Physiology in Anesthetic Practice*. 4th ed. Philadelphia, PA: Lippincott Williams & Wilkins; 2006:623–634.
14. Drummond JC, Petrovitch CT, Lane TA. Hemostasis and transfusion medicine. In: Barash PG, Cullen BF, Stoelting RK, Cahalan MK, Stock MC, eds. *Clinical Anesthesia*. 6th ed. Philadelphia, PA: Lippincott Williams & Wilkins; 2009:369–412.

50

Challenges in Anesthesia: The Geriatric Patient Presenting for Surgery

Steven L. Shafer, MD

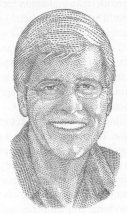

Clinical Vignette

A 76-year-old man with prostate cancer is scheduled for open radical prostatectomy. His past medical history is notable for adult-onset diabetes, coronary artery disease (CAD), and gastroesophageal reflux disease (GERD). His past surgical history included coronary artery bypass surgery (CABG) 5 years ago, and a stent placed in the past year. He smoked 1 pack per day for 50 years, but quit following his CABG. He drinks one glass of wine with dinner. His medications include metformin, simvastatin, clopidogrel, and aspirin. He had no problems with the anesthesia for his CABG surgery. His prostate biopsy was performed a one month ago, under general anesthesia, with endotracheal intubation, because his cardiologist was not comfortable stopping the clopidogrel, and the anesthesiologist was not comfortable with an laryngeal mask airway (LMA) because of the history of GERD.

Introduction

I define "old" as 20 years older than my current age. Given that I am 56, for the purposes of this chapter, the geriatric patient will be considered any patient over 76 years of age. Based on the U.S. Census projection for 2010 (www.census.gov), there are 17 million individuals in the United States who are at least 76 years old. One of them is now awaiting your preoperative assessment.

There is nothing particularly unique about the elderly patient presenting for surgery. There is no unique disease, drug sensitivity, cardiovascular risk, or anesthetic response. The primary difference in the geriatric patient is the increase in variability. Some elderly patients are very fit, have almost no systemic disease, and can be expected to respond to your anesthetic regimen as though they were young adults. However, in other elderly patients, the ravages of illness, physical trauma, poisoning (including cigarettes and alcohol), and cumulative organ injury greatly increase risk of injury from anesthesia and surgery. Indeed, since the life expectancy in 2010 is 76 years for men, and 81 years for women, half of our patient's male birth cohort have already died. The challenge in dealing with a geriatric patient is to determine where the patient is on spectrum from very fit to nearly dead.

Much of the perioperative assessment of the elderly is self-evident and routine for the experienced anesthesiologist. Citing a review by Jin and Chung (1), John and Sieber tell us that "there is increased risk for elderly

Large interindividual variability is a hallmark of caring for the geriatric patient.

349

patients with high ASA physical status (i.e., ASA III, IV, or V) who undergo emergency surgery or major vascular or prolonged surgery with large blood or fluid shifts, who have co-existing diseases: cardiac, pulmonary, renal, hepatic, diabetes; who have poor nutritional status, limited functional status (i.e., <4 METs), and who are bedridden, or not living with family" (2). This isn't news to the practicing anesthesiologist. As with any patient, the preoperative evaluation of the elderly patient requires a thorough physical examination and history, including an assessment of the status of each organ system, with our usual focus on the cardiovascular, pulmonary, and the central nervous systems.

The issues for this patient, in the order presented in the brief history, are:

1. **Adult-onset diabetes**, treated with metformin. The preoperative evaluation includes assessment of end-organ damage to the heart, kidneys, carotid arteries, peripheral vasculature, and retina, evaluation of the possibility of delayed gastric emptying, possible neurological complications (diabetic neuropathy), and assessment of the airway (which can stiffen from longstanding diabetes). There will also be an assessment of how compliant the patient is with the medical management, how well controlled the diabetes is, and the current status (morning blood sugar, did the patient take metformin?) Obviously, our patient's advancing age only increases the likelihood of finding organ damage from the diabetes.

2. **Coronary artery disease.** Not surprisingly, the next item in the patient's past medical history is coronary artery disease. Diabetes likely played a role, as did the smoking, and perhaps there is a history of hyperlipidemia or strong family history (which is less relevant in the very elderly patient). The preoperative evaluation includes a functional assessment (e.g., exercise tolerance, presence of angina), looking for evidence of advancing symptoms (e.g., is there a new Q wave on the electrocardiogram?), laboratory evaluations as indicated (e.g., cardiac catheterization), and an assessment as to whether the current medical management is optimal. If the patient says that he gets chest pain just thinking about the prostate operation, perhaps the operation can be delayed while the status of his stent is assessed. Although the primary complicating factor of

Advancing age is associated with an increased incidence of diastolic dysfunction.

the patient's age is the likelihood of cardiac disease, advancing age is specifically associated with an increased incidence of **diastolic dysfunction**. As noted in a recent review by Sanders et al. (3), the diagnosis of diastolic dysfunction is frequently missed in the elderly patient, because the symptoms (decreased exercise tolerance, weakness, fatigue, anorexia, confusion) are often ascribed to other causes, or simply dismissed as "aging."

3. **Gastroesophageal reflux disease.** Every anesthesiologist should know the right questions to evaluate GERD, regardless of the age of the patient.

4. **Previous CABG.** The questions, of course, are what was done, and is it still working? The cardiac evaluation is discussed above. It is also important to know if there were any complications related to anesthesia.

5. **A coronary stent placed in the past year.** There are voluminous reviews about the risks of stents, and the complications of managing platelet function in patients with stents. While the odds of having a stent likely increase with age, the age of the patient, per se, is not relevant. If the patient is still on clopidogrel, and it has not been stopped, then regional anesthesia is contraindicated.

6. He **smoked 1 pack per day for 50 years**, but quit following his CABG. Evaluating the damages posed by cigarettes is part of every preoperative assessment in a smoker, regardless of age. We understand how to evaluate the lungs for evidence of emphysema, COPD, and chronic bronchitis. Again, the age per se is not relevant, other than to note that the damage from cigarettes is cumulative with smoking duration.

7. He drinks one glass of wine with dinner. Provided the patient is not under-reporting his alcohol consumption (which should be considered during the interview), the modest regular alcohol intake is likely beneficial.

8. His **medications** include metformin, simvastatin, clopidogrel, and aspirin. The primary risk of metformin during anesthesia is extreme acidosis in the event of tissue hypoxia, which you don't intend to let happen. As for the clopidogrel and the aspirin, a plan should be in place, in consultation with the patient's cardiologist, for managing the patient's antiplatelet therapy in the perioperative period. For major surgery, it is likely that the clopidogrel has been stopped a week earlier, and that the patient is now on other antiplatelet therapy (e.g., aspirin, heparin).

9. His prostate biopsy was performed one month ago, under general anesthesia, with endotracheal intubation. Again, the key question is whether there was any anesthetic complication.

10. **Pain** wasn't mentioned in the clinical vignette. It's important to ask the geriatric patient about pain, even if not reported. **About 50% of patients over the age of 70 report chronic pain** (4), a much higher incidence than found in younger individuals (5,6). Understanding whether the elderly patient has pain will prompt additional questions (what are you taking for it?—Tylenol? Oops, that wasn't mentioned), as well as play an important role in determining the best plan for the patient's anesthetic and postoperative care.

Chronic pain is common in the elderly population.

The point of this clinical vignette is that the issues with the geriatric patients are usually self-evident, and based on disease, not on age per se. The key observation is that variability in physiology increases throughout life (7), so the preoperative evaluation of the geriatric patient must be especially thorough to explore just how radically his or her physiology differs from that of a healthy younger patient.

The polypharmacy required to treat multiple systemic illnesses often seen in the geriatric population places patients at risk for adverse drug reactions.

This increase in variability, and the subsequent polypharmacy to treat multiple systemic illnesses, is why elderly patients are at increased risk of adverse drug reactions (8). Elderly patients require more careful titration of drugs, particularly in the acute perioperative setting, and, if appropriate, therapeutic drug monitoring (9).

Pharmacological Implications of Aging

However, if we now turn to the question of designing an anesthetic for this patient, we must consider the impact of age, per se, on the behavior of anesthetic drugs. This is not self-evident.

Bolus injection of a drug in the elderly patient will result in higher plasma drug concentrations than in younger patients.

Table 50-1 lists the key changes in drug pharmacology with aging. **The net effect of the changes in body composition with advancing age is higher concentrations following a bolus injection of drug.** Most anesthetic drugs decrease cardiac output (10,11), particularly in elderly patients (12). This also increases the initial concentration from a bolus and explains part of the decreased drug requirement for induction of anesthesia in elderly patients. Creatinine clearance is reduced with advancing age, which is evident from the equation of Cockroft and Gault (13):

$$\text{Men: Creatinine clearance (mL/min)} = \frac{(140 - \text{age [y]}) \times \text{weight (kg)}}{72 \times \text{serum creatinine (mg\%)}}$$

Women: 85% of the above.

PHARMACOLOGY

Table 50-1

How Advanced Age Affects Dose

- There are several changes in body composition associated with age: (a) lean body mass decreases, (b) body fat increases, and (c) total body water decreases (14).
- The primary pharmacokinetic change in the elderly individual is decreased central volume of distribution. This results in higher peak concentrations following bolus injection.
- In the absence of hepatic disease, hepatic clearance is well preserved.
- GFR decreases with age, reducing the clearance of drugs excreted by renal filtration.
- The pharmacodynamic changes are usually more important than the pharmacokinetic changes. In general, the elderly are more sensitive to a given anesthetic drug concentration (about 20% more for propofol, 50% more for opioids, and >80% more sensitive for benzodiazepines).
- If the dose of anesthetics is appropriately reduced, the elderly will likely emerge from anesthesia nearly as fast as younger patients.

Figure 50-1 shows the relationship between creatinine, age, and creatinine clearance predicted by the Cockroft-Gault equation. The key observation is that *even in the presence of normal creatinine* the creatinine clearance of an 80-year-old patient will be about half that in a 20-year-old patient. This is why pancuronium is such a poor choice for muscle relaxation in the elderly patient (slow renal elimination), and also why accumulation of morphine-6-glucuronide might be a problem in the elderly patient on chronic morphine (M6G is pharmacologically active and renally eliminated) (15).

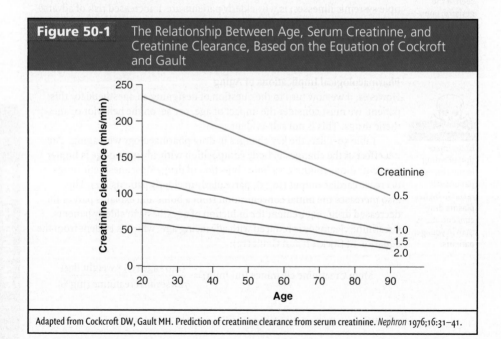

Figure 50-1   The Relationship Between Age, Serum Creatinine, and Creatinine Clearance, Based on the Equation of Cockroft and Gault

Adapted from Cockcroft DW, Gault MH. Prediction of creatinine clearance from serum creatinine. *Nephron* 1976;16:31–41.

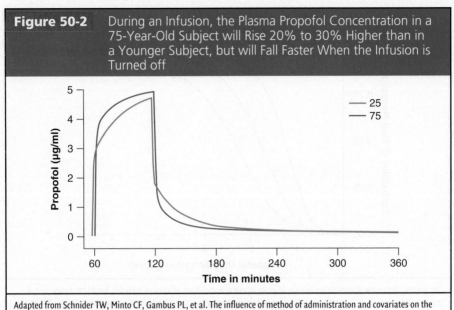

Figure 50-2 During an Infusion, the Plasma Propofol Concentration in a 75-Year-Old Subject will Rise 20% to 30% Higher than in a Younger Subject, but will Fall Faster When the Infusion is Turned off

Adapted from Schnider TW, Minto CF, Gambus PL, et al. The influence of method of administration and covariates on the pharmacokinetics of propofol in adult volunteers. *Anesthesiology* 1998;88:1170–1182.

However, the increase in sensitivity to anesthetic drugs in the elderly appears to be more driven by increased end-organ sensitivity (i.e., the brain is more sensitive) than the pharmacokinetic differences. We will explore this for 4 drugs: propofol, midazolam, fentanyl, and remifentanil.

Elderly patient's brains are more sensitive to propofol and fentanyl than younger patients.

Propofol

The induction dose for propofol in the very elderly patients is as low as 1 mg/kg in very elderly patients (16,17), well below the recommend adult dose of 2.5 mg/kg. Using pharmacokinetic/pharmacodynamic modeling, Schneider and colleagues developed a detailed model of the behavior of propofol in elderly patients (18,19). As seen in Figure 50-2, the influence of pharmacokinetic changes is modest. During a propofol infusion, the concentrations in elderly patients are about 20% to 30% higher than in younger patients. Figure 50-3 shows the influence of brain sensitivity on propofol dosing. The brain of elderly patients is about a third more sensitive to propofol than the brain of younger patients. Thus, the **reduction in propofol dose required in elderly patients is mostly, but not entirely, driven by changes in brain sensitivity.**

Midazolam

Age has a huge influence on midazolam dosing. Perhaps the most dramatic demonstration is the report by Bell on the dose of midazolam required to produce sedation in 800 patients undergoing endoscopic procedures (20), summarized in Figure 50-4. There is a 75% decrease in dose from age 20 to 90. Indeed, it appears that the 100-year-old patient is ready for colonoscopy with no midazolam at all.

PHARMACOLOGY

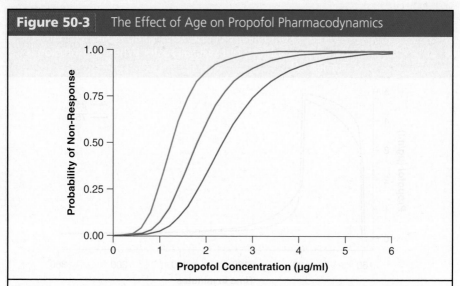

Figure 50-3   The Effect of Age on Propofol Pharmacodynamics

The logistic regression shows the probability of being asleep after a 1-hour infusion of propofol. Similar to figure 50-7, a 75-year-old subject is 30% to 50% more sensitive to propofol than a 25-year-old subject. Adapted from Schnider TW, Minto CF, Shafer SL, et al. The influence of age on propofol pharmacodynamics. *Anesthesiology* 1999;90:1502–1516.

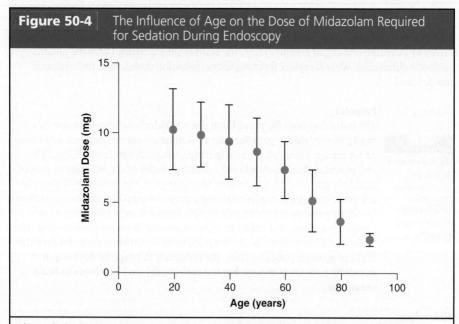

Figure 50-4   The Influence of Age on the Dose of Midazolam Required for Sedation During Endoscopy

After age 65, there is a dramatic increase in sensitivity to benzodiazepines. Adapted from Bell GD, Spickett GP, Reeve PA, et al. Intravenous midazolam for upper gastrointestinal endoscopy: A study of 800 consecutive cases relating dose to age and sex of patient. *Br J Clin Pharmacol* 1987;23:241–243.

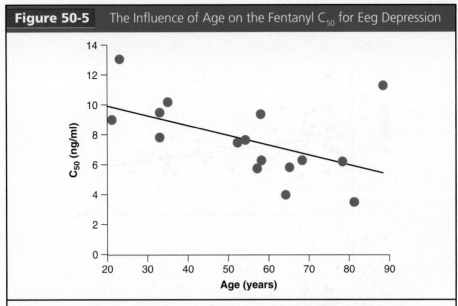

Figure 50-5 The Influence of Age on the Fentanyl C_{50} for Eeg Depression

Although there is considerable variability, there is about a 50% reduction in C_{50} from age 20 to 80, reflecting increased brain sensitivity. Adapted from Scott JC, Stanski DR. Decreased fentanyl/alfentanil dose requirement with increasing age: A pharmacodynamic basis. *J Pharmacol Exp Ther* 1987;240:159–166.

This is explained by pharmacokinetic and pharmacodynamic differences in the elderly patient. Midazolam clearance is reduced approximately 30% in 80-year-old patients, compared with 20-year-old patients (21). This accounts for about a 25% dose reduction. However, the elderly brain is far more sensitive to midazolam (22), which accounts for most of the increased sensitivity to midazolam with advancing age.

Benzodiazepines are associated with an increased risk of postoperative delirium (23). Given the increased risk of delirium in the elderly patient, I generally avoid giving benzodiazepines to elderly patients, preferring to "sedate" the patient by answering questions, providing reassurance, and developing rapport.

Fentanyl
Scott and Stanski examined the influence of age on the pharmacokinetics and the pharmacodynamics of fentanyl and alfentanil (24). These investigators did not find any effect of age on the pharmacokinetics of fentanyl or alfentanil, except for a small change in rapid intercompartmental clearance. However, they did document that the elderly brain is approximately twice as sensitive to fentanyl and alfentanil as a younger brain, as shown for fentanyl in Figure 50-5. This explains why **the dose of fentanyl should be reduced by about 50% in elderly patients compared to younger patients to achieve a given level of opioid drug effect.**

Remifentanil
The pharmacokinetics of remifentanil change with age, as shown in Figure 50-6 (25). With advancing age, the volume of the central compartment decreases about 20% and clearance decreases about 30%. Similar to fentanyl and alfentanil, the elderly brain is about twice as

PHARMACOLOGY

Figure 50-6   The Influence of Age on Remifentanil Pharmacokinetics

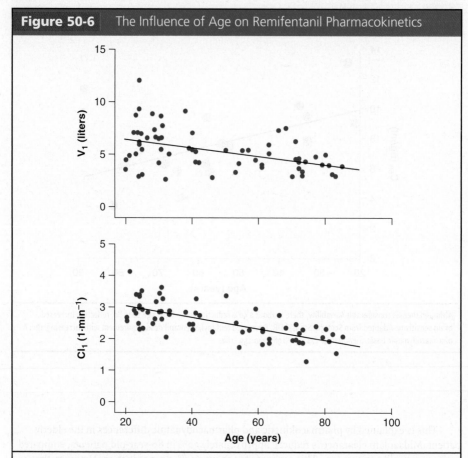

The volume of the central compartment decreases by 50% from age 20 to 80, and the clearance decreases by 66%. Adapted from Minto CF, Schnider TW, Egan T, et al. The influence of age and gender on the pharmacokinetics and pharmacodynamics of remifentanil. I. Model Development. *Anesthesiology* 1997;86:10–23.

sensitive to remifentanil as the younger brain (Fig. 50-7). Elderly patients need about half of the bolus dose of remifentanil as younger subjects to achieve the same level of drug effect (26), which is entirely due to the change in intrinsic potency as the pharmacokinetic change is offset by slower blood-brain equilibration. **Elderly subjects require only a third of the remifentanil infusion rate of a younger subject** to maintain the same level of opioid drug effect, which reflects both the change in clearance and the increased brain sensitivity.

Conclusion

There is no such thing as a typical "geriatric patient," because **the hallmark of aging is increased patient-to-patient variability.** The subject for this vignette has several common chronic conditions, no acute pathology, and is on drugs with well-understood implications for anesthesia. Preoperative evaluation begins with careful, systematic, organ-based assessment, and concludes with formulation of the anesthetic plan and anticipating age-appropriate drug dosing. Advancing age reduces anesthetic requirement, so that this subject will likely require only about half as much hypnotic and opioid as a younger subject.

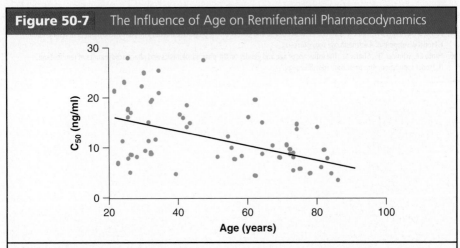

Figure 50-7   The Influence of Age on Remifentanil Pharmacodynamics

EC_{50} for Eeg depression decreases by approximately 50% from age 20 to 80, almost paralleling the influence of age on fentanyl potency. Adapted from Minto CF, Schnider TW, Egan T, et al. The influence of age and gender on the pharmacokinetics and pharmacodynamics of remifentanil. I. Model Development. *Anesthesiology* 1997;86:10–23.

References

1. Jin F, Chung F. Minimizing perioperative adverse events in the elderly. *Br J Anaesth* 2001;877:608–624.
2. John AD, Frederick E, Sieber FE. Age associated issues: geriatrics. *Anesthesiol Clin N Am* 2004;22:45–58.
3. Sanders D, Dudley M, Leanne Groban L. Cardiovascular Aging, and the Anesthesiologist. *Anesthesiol Clin* 2009;27:497–517.
4. Helme RD, Gibson SJ. Pain in older people. In: Crombie IK, Croft PR, Linton SJ, Le Resche L, Von Korff M, eds. *The Epidemiology of Pain.* 2nd ed., Seattle, WA: IASP Press; 1999:103–112.
5. Helme RD, Gibson SJ. The epidemiology of pain in elderly people. *Clin Geriatr Med* 2001;17:417–431.
6. Verhaak PF, Kerssens JJ, Dekker J, et al. Prevalence of chronic benign pain disorder among adults: a review of the literature. *Pain* 1998;77:231–239.
7. Steib H, Sargent F II. Human physiological adaptability through the life sequence. *J Gerontol* 1977;32:402–410.
8. Klein U, Klein M, Sturm H, et al. The frequency of adverse drug reactions as dependent upon age, sex and duration of hospitalization. *Int J Clin Pharmacol Biopharm* 1976;13:187–195.
9. Crooks J. Aging and drug disposition—pharmacodynamics. *J Chronic Dis* 1983;36:85–90.
10. Fairfield JE, Dritsas A, Beale RJ. Haemodynamic effects of propofol: induction with 2.5 mg kg⁻¹. *Br J Anaesth* 1991;67:618–620.
11. Brismar B, Hedenstierna G, Lundh R, et al. Oxygen uptake, plasma catecholamines and cardiac output during neurolept-nitrous oxide and halothane anaesthesias. *Acta Anaesthesiol Scand* 1982;26:541–549.
12. Tokics L, Brismar B, Hedenstierna G. Halothane-relaxant anaesthesia in elderly patients. *Acta Anaesthesiol Scand* 1985;29:303–308.
13. Cockcroft DW, Gault MH. Prediction of creatinine clearance from serum creatinine. *Nephron* 1976;16:31–41.
14. Forbes GB, Reina JC. Adult lean body mass declines with age: some longitudinal observations. *Metabolism* 1970;19:653–663.
15. Portenoy RK, Foley KM, Stulman J, et al. Plasma morphine and morphine-6-glucuronide during chronic morphine therapy for cancer pain: plasma profiles, steady-state concentrations and the consequences of renal failure. *Pain* 1991;47:13–19.
16. Maneglia R, Cousin MT. A comparison between propofol and ketamine for anaesthesia in the elderly. Haemodynamic effects during induction and maintenance. *Anaesthesia* 1988;43(suppl):109–111.
17. Steib A, Freys G, Beller JP, et al. Propofol in elderly high risk patients. A comparison of haemodynamic effects with thiopentone during induction of anaesthesia. *Anaesthesia* 1988;43(suppl):111–114.
18. Schnider TW, Minto CF, Gambus PL, et al. The influence of method of administration and covariates on the pharmacokinetics of propofol in adult volunteers. *Anesthesiology* 1998;88:1170–1182.
19. Schnider TW, Minto CF, Shafer SL, et al. The influence of age on propofol pharmacodynamics. *Anesthesiology* 1999;90:1502–1516.
20. Bell GD, Spickett GP, Reeve PA, et al. Intravenous midazolam for upper gastrointestinal endoscopy: a study of 800 consecutive cases relating dose to age and sex of patient. *Br J Clin Pharmacol* 1987;23:241–243.
21. Maitre PO, Buhrer M, Thomson D, et al. A three-step approach combining Bayesian regression and NONMEM population analysis: application to midazolam. *J Pharmacokinet Biopharm* 1991;19:377–384.
22. Buhrer M, Maitre PO, Crevoisier C, et al. Electroencephalographic effects of benzodiazepines. II. Pharmacodynamic modeling of the electroencephalographic effects of midazolam and diazepam. *Clin Pharmacol Ther* 1992;48:555–567.
23. Marcantonio ER, Juarez G, Goldman L, et al. The relationship of postoperative delirium with psychoactive medications. *JAMA* 1994;272:1518–1522.

PHARMACOLOGY

24. Scott JC, Stanski DR. Decreased fentanyl/alfentanil dose requirement with increasing age: a pharmacodynamic basis. *J Pharmacol Exp Ther* 1987;240:159–166.
25. Minto CF, Schnider TW, Egan T, et al. The influence of age and gender on the pharmacokinetics and pharmacodynamics of remifentanil. I. Model development. *Anesthesiology* 1997;86:10–23.
26. Minto CF, Schnider TW, Shafer SL. The influence of age and gender on the pharmacokinetics and pharmacodynamics of remifentanil. II. Model application. *Anesthesiology* 1997;86:24–33.

51

Part A: Cardiovascular Diseases
Ischemic Heart Disease

Bryan Ahlgren, DO

Ischemic Heart disease (IHD) is a broad term used to describe a number of closely related syndromes that share a common central pathology—an imbalance between myocardial oxygen supply and demand. Over 90% of myocardial ischemia is due to atherosclerotic obstruction of coronary artery blood flow.

1) **Epidemiology**
   a) Coronary artery disease (CAD) is the nation's leading killer of both men and women.
   b) About 1.5 million people in the United States suffer a myocardial infarction (MI) annually; one third of those will die. Both modifiable and nonmodifiable risk factors have been implicated.
      i) **Modifiable risk factors**
         (1) Include obesity, physical inactivity, high carbohydrate intake, smoking, excessive alcohol consumption, high transunsaturated fat intake, stress, hypertension, hyperlipidemia, hyperlipoproteinemia, postmenopausal estrogen deficiency, and diabetes
      ii) **Nonmodifiable risk factors**
         (1) Include advancing age, family history, and genetic abnormalities in lipid metabolism
2) **Pathophysiology**
   a) **Determinants of myocardial O₂ supply/demand**
      i) Myocardial O_2 supply is dependent on coronary artery diameter, aortic diastolic pressure, left ventricular (LV) diastolic pressure, and arterial O_2 content.
      ii) Myocardial O_2 demand is determined by ventricular wall tension, heart rate, and contractility.

Myocardial O₂ demand is dependent on ventricular wall tension, heart rate, and contractility.

         (1) **Tachycardia** increases myocardial O_2 demand through increased myocardial work. Tachycardia also shortens the diastolic filling period, thus reducing the time for optimal coronary perfusion (1).
         (2) **Hypervolemia** increases ventricular wall tension and myocardial O_2 demand. At the same time, coronary perfusion (O_2 supply) is reduced in the distended ventricle because the increased LV end diastolic pressure limits coronary flow (1).
      iii) **Anemia** can also upset both sides of the supply-and-demand equation. Decreased O_2 content reduces the O_2 supply, whereas increased heart rate and cardiac output secondary to anemia can increase demand (1).

359

b) **Atherosclerosis**

i) Atherosclerosis is the deposition of atheromatous plaques to the intimal layer of arteries.

ii) This process begins early in life and gradually narrows the lumen of coronary arteries.

iii) The risk of an individual developing detectable **IHD** depends in part on the number, distribution, and structure of atheromatous plaques, and the degree of narrowing they cause.

iv) A fixed obstructive lesion of 75% or greater generally causes symptomatic ischemia induced by exercise; with this degree of obstruction, the augmented coronary flow provided by compensatory vasodilation is no longer sufficient to meet even moderate increases in myocardial demand.

v) A 90% stenosis can lead to inadequate coronary blood flow even at rest (1).

vi) Slowly developing occlusions may stimulate collateral vessels over time, which protect against distal **myocardial ischemia** and infarction even with an eventual high grade stenosis.

(1) Common distribution patterns of stenotic lesions (1):

   (a) **Left anterior descending (LAD) 40% to 50%**

   (b) **Left circumflex (LCX) 15% to 20%**

   (c) **Right coronary artery (RCA) 30% to 40%**

(2) Clinically significant stenotic plaques may be located anywhere within these vessels but tend to predominate within the first several centimeters of the LAD and LCX and along the entire length of the RCA (1).

(3) **Atherosclerotic plaque changes**

   (a) In most patients experiencing acute coronary syndrome (unstable angina, MI, or sudden cardiac death [SCD]), a previously stable plaque has undergone one of the following acute changes followed by thrombosis:

      (i) **Rupture/fissuring**, exposing the highly thrombogenic plaque constituents.

      (ii) **Erosion/ulceration**, exposing the thrombogenic subendothelial basement membrane to blood.

      (iii) **Hemorrhage** into the atheroma, expanding its volume.

      (iv) Causes of abrupt changes in plaque configuration and superimposed thrombosis are complex and poorly understood. Influences, both intrinsic (e.g., plaque structure and composition) and extrinsic (e.g., blood pressure, platelet reactivity), are significant factors (1).

3) **Clinical syndromes of IHD**

a) **Angina pectoris**

i) Angina pectoris is a symptom complex of IHD characterized by paroxysmal and usually recurrent attacks of substernal or precordial chest discomfort (variously described as constricting, squeezing, choking, or knifelike).

ii) All angina is caused by varying combinations of increased myocardial O_2 demand and decreased myocardial perfusion, owing to disrupted plaques, fixed stenotic plaques, vasospasm, thrombosis, platelet aggregation, or embolization.

iii) Reduced blood flow causes transient (15 seconds to 15 minutes) **myocardial ischemia** that falls short of inducing the cellular necrosis that defines infarction. Three overlapping patterns of angina pectoris exist (1):

(1) **Stable or typical angina**

(2) **Prinzmetal or variant angina**

(3) **Unstable or crescendo angina**

b) **Myocardial infarction (MI)**
  i) MI, also known as "heart attack," is the **death of cardiac muscle resulting from ischemia** and is described as **transmural or subendocardial infarction**.
      (1) **Transmural**
          (a) Ischemic necrosis involves the full or nearly full thickness of the ventricular wall in the distribution of a single coronary artery.
          (b) This pattern of infarction is usually associated with coronary atherosclerosis, acute plaque change, and superimposed thrombosis.
      (2) **Subendocardial (nontransmural)**
          (a) Infarct constitutes an area of ischemic necrosis limited to the inner one third to one half of the ventricular wall. The subendocardial zone is the least well perfused region of myocardium and therefore most vulnerable to any reduction in coronary flow.
          (b) This type may extend laterally beyond the perfusion territory of a single coronary artery.
          (c) These infarcts are typically due to a plaque disruption leading to coronary thrombus which is lysed before myocardial necrosis extends across the major thickness of the wall.
          (d) Another possible mechanism is decreased perfusion due to sufficiently prolonged and severe reduction in systemic blood pressure, as in shock. In cases of global hypotension, resulting subendocardial infarcts can be global (1).

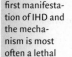

SCD may be the first manifestation of IHD and the mechanism is most often a lethal arrhythmia.

c) **Sudden Cardiac Death (SCD)**
  i) **SCD is defined as unexpected death from cardiac causes within minutes after symptom onset or without the onset of symptoms.**
  ii) Mechanism of SCD is most often a lethal arrhythmia (e.g., asystole, ventricular fibrillation).
  iii) SCD due to IHD is thought to be caused by ischemic injury impinging on the conduction system itself, or electrical irritability of myocardium that may be distant from the conduction system, induced by ischemia or other cellular abnormalities.
d) **Chronic IHD or ischemic cardiomyopathy**
  i) **Chronic heart disease is typically characterized by prior MI and often previous coronary arterial bypass graft (CABG) surgery or percutaneous interventions.**
  ii) This process usually constitutes postinfarction cardiac decompensation owing to exhaustion of the compensatory hypertrophy of viable myocardium that is in jeopardy of ischemic injury. Onset and severity of symptoms are highly variable depending on extent of disease (1).
4) **Severity or extent of MI** depends on a number of factors including
  a) Location, severity, and rate of development of coronary atherosclerotic obstructions
  b) Size of the vascular bed perfused by the obstructed vessels
  c) Duration of the occlusion
      i) Loss of contractility can occur in <2 minutes, irreversible cell injury 20 to 40 minutes, microvascular injury takes over 1 hour to develop.
  d) Metabolic needs of the myocardium at risk
  e) Extent of collateral blood vessels
  f) Presence, site, and severity of coronary arterial spasm
  g) Other **clinical factors including** alterations in blood pressure, heart rate, and cardiac rhythm.

5) **Complications secondary to MI:** Nearly three fourths of patients have one or more complications following acute MI, which include the following (1):

   a) **Contractile dysfunction**

      i) MI produces abnormalities in LV function approximately proportional to the size of infarct. This can range from mild dysfunction to cardiogenic shock.

   b) **Arrhythmias**

      i) Many patients will have MI associated arrhythmias that include sinus bradycardia, heart block (asystole), tachycardia, ventricular premature contractions or ventricular tachycardia, and ventricular fibrillation.

   c) **Myocardial rupture**

      i) Cardiac rupture syndromes result from mechanical weakening that occurs in necrotic and subsequently inflamed myocardium. These include:

         (1) Rupture of the ventricular free wall (most commonly), with hemopericardium and cardiac tamponade, usually fatal. Typically occurs 3 to 7 days postinfarction.

         (2) Rupture of the ventricular septum (less commonly), leading to a left-to-right shunt.

         (3) Papillary muscle rupture (least commonly), resulting in the acute onset of severe mitral regurgitation.

   d) **Right ventricular infarction**

      i) Rare, though may accompany septal or posterior infarct. A right ventricular infarct of either type can yield serious functional impairment.

   e) **Infarct extension**

      i) New necrosis may occur adjacent to an existing infarct.

   f) **Pericarditis**

      i) A fibrinous or fibrohemorrhagic pericarditis can develop the second or third day following a transmural infarct and usually will resolve.

   g) **Mural thrombus**

      i) Combination of a local myocardial abnormality in contractility (causing stasis) with endocardial damage (causing a thrombogenic surface) can lead to mural thrombosis and potentially to thromboembolism.

   h) **Ventricular aneurysm**

      i) True aneurysms of the ventricular wall are bounded by myocardium that has become scarred.

      ii) Aneurysms of the ventricular wall are a late complication and most commonly result from a large transmural anteroseptal infarct (often one that has undergone expansion) that heals into a large region of thin scar tissue, which paradoxically bulges during systole.

      iii) Aneurysm formation can lead to mural thrombus, arrhythmias, and heart failure, but rupture of the fibrotic wall is infrequent (unlike ventricular pseudoaneurysm).

   i) **Papillary muscle dysfunction**

      i) Rarely, early dysfunction of a papillary muscle following MI occurs due to its rupture.

      ii) More frequently, postinfarct mitral regurgitation results from early ischemic dysfunction of a papillary muscle and underlying myocardium and later from papillary muscle fibrosis and shortening or ventricular dilation.

   j) **Progressive late heart failure**

READ MORE
Congestive heart failure, Chapter 60, page 436

The most effective way to salvage ischemic myocardium threatened by infarction is to restore tissue perfusion as rapidly as possible.

6) **Treatment modalities**
a) **Reperfusion**
   i) The purpose of reperfusion therapy is to restore blood flow to the area at risk for infarction and possibly rescue the ischemic (but not yet necrotic) heart muscle.
   ii) Removal of thrombus reestablishes flow through the occluded coronary artery in most cases; early reperfusion can salvage myocardium and thereby limit infarct size, with consequent improvement in both short- and long-term function and survival.
   iii) Restoration of coronary flow *(reperfusion)* is accomplished via
      (1) **Thrombolysis**
         (a) IV administration of fibrinolytic agents, which activate plasminogen (tPA, streptokinase, alteplase, etc.)
         (b) Reserved for situations where timely access to percutaneous coronary intervention (PCI) not possible
   iv) **Percutaneous coronary intervention (PCI) with angioplasty**
      (1) **Primary PCI is preferred for acute ST elevation MI, if performed in a timely fashion by an expert operator (2).**
      (2) PCI-related delay >60 to 120 minutes appears to eliminate the survival benefit of primary PCI over fibrinolysis (2).
   v) **CABG**
      (1) Primary indications for CABG include
         (a) Two-vessel disease with proximal LAD stenosis
         (b) Single proximal left main stenosis with ischemia
         (c) Multivessel disease with ejection fraction (EF) > 50%
         (d) Failed PCI with ongoing ischemia
         (e) Significant angina despite alternative therapy.
b) **Medical therapy**
   i) **Medical therapy is critical for the postinfarct patient to optimize myocardial O₂ supply/demand, stabilize atherosclerotic plaques, and inhibit platelet function.**
   ii) In almost all instances (with the exception of anti-platelet), these medications should be continued up until the time of surgery (3) (Table 51-1).

Table 51-1

Medical Therapy Aimed at Limiting Further Cardiac Ischemic Episodes

β-adrenergic antagonists	Vasodilators: coronary or systemic
Statins	ACE inhibitors
Anti-platelet medications: (Aspirin vs. Clopidogrel)	Calcium channel blockers
	Nitrates

Table 51-2

Physical Exam in a Patient at Risk for CAD

Head and neck	Examination for evidence of jugular venous distension, or carotid bruits
Chest	Auscultation/palpation for evaluation of rales, rhonchi, wheeze, or effusions
Cardiac	Auscultation for evaluation of heaves, thrills, murmurs, rubs, arrhythmia
Abdominal	Examination for pulsatile mass, hepatomegaly, hepatojugular reflex
Extremity	Examination for the presence of cyanosis, clubbing, edema, capillary refill. Blood pressure should be checked in both arms.

7) Anesthetic considerations for the patient with CAD

   a) **Preoperative evaluation**

      i) **History**

         (1) Preoperative history should be tailored to elucidate history of symptoms that may indicate CAD.

         (2) History of known risk factors as well as of chest pain, with or without radiation to the inner aspect of the arm or neck; dyspnea on exertion, orthopnea; paroxysmal nocturnal dyspnea; nocturnal coughing; previous or current peripheral or pulmonary edema; and history of MI should all be queried.

         (3) Ability to perform moderate physical activity equal to four metabolic equivalents (walking up a flight of stairs or up a hill, walking flat at 4 mph, run a short distance) usually infers a low perioperative risk for cardiac ischemia.

      ii) **Physical exam (Table 51-2)**

      iii) **Laboratory exam**—Laboratory exam should be tailored to patient and type of surgery.

The decision to obtain further non-invasive studies in a patient with possible CAD should be instituted when suspicion is high and the outcome of these tests would alter patient care.

         (1) BUN/creatinine in any patient with known CAD

         (2) Baseline hemoglobin measurement is suggested for all patients 65 years of age or older who are undergoing major surgery, and for younger patients undergoing major surgery that is expected to result in significant blood loss.

         (3) Consider electrolyte panel based on medication regimen.

      iv) **Noninvasive studies**

         (1) Consider a pre-op ECG in vascular surgery patients or those with at least one cardiac risk factor undergoing intermediate- to high-risk surgery (4).

         (2) The predictive value of noninvasive stress imaging abnormalities for perioperative ischemic events is comparable between available techniques but the accuracy varies with the prevalence of CAD.

           (a) Dobutamine stress echocardiography may be the most cost-effective measure to identify at risk myocardium (5).

         (3) The American College of Cardiology/American Heart Association has a risk stratification algorithm in order to aid clinicians in the management of patients with CAD or significant risk factors for CAD undergoing noncardiac surgery.

READ MORE

Preanesthesia assessment, Chapter 2, page 10

b) **Intraoperative management**
   i) **Type of anesthetic**
      (1) There is no convincing evidence that either general or regional anesthesia is superior in reducing cardiac events in the perioperative period (3).
      (2) Decision on type of anesthesia should be based on type of surgery, patient preference, and skill of practitioner.
      (3) In either case, maintaining tight hemodynamic control close to patient's baseline vitals will yield the best long-term results.
   ii) **Premedication**
      (1) Premedication of the patient with CAD may alleviate sympathetic activation and its detrimental effect on myocardial O_2 demand. Careful titration is needed in order to prevent respiratory depression with respiratory acidosis, hypoxia, and hypotension.
   iii) **Monitoring**
      (1) **Intra-arterial pressure monitoring**
         (a) With few exceptions, the use of intra-arterial pressure monitoring is advisable in patients with known severe CAD or significant risk factors.
      (2) **Central venous pressure (CVP)**
         (a) CVP monitoring may be useful in prolonged procedures involving significant blood loss or fluid shifts.

↪ READ MORE

Pulmonary artery catheter, Chapter 13, page 82

      (3) **Pulmonary artery catheter (PAC) or transesophageal echocardiography (TEE)**
         (a) May provide valuable information in select patients with reduced EF (<40%), moderate or severe pulmonary hypertension, or severe valvular disease
         (b) TEE allows detection of wall motion abnormalities, and evaluation of chamber size and contractility.
      (4) Neither PAC of TEE has been shown to improve outcome in most clinical studies (3).
      (5) **Detection of ischemia**
         (a) TEE recognition of wall motion abnormalities may be the most sensitive monitor for intraoperative ischemia (5).

↪ READ MORE

Transesophageal echocardiography basic views, Chapter 162, page 1123

         (b) ECG changes may be subtle, including changes in T-wave morphology before less subtle ST segments become depressed.
         (c) Initial hemodynamic changes are commonly due to hypertension and tachycardia, with hypotension representing a later and more ominous finding.
         (d) If a Swan-Ganz catheter is in place, the pulmonary capillary wedge pressure may elevate in the presence of acute MR due to papillary muscle dysfunction or acute LV dilation.

c) **Induction and maintenance**
   i) Induction and maintenance of anesthesia are aimed at optimizing myocardial O_2 supply and demand variables. Choice of agent is not as critical as the manner delivered.
   ii) Induction goals are to maintain hemodynamic parameters as close to patients baseline as possible.
   iii) Special attention must be paid to the adrenergic stimulation caused by endotracheal intubation.
   iv) General anesthesia is typically maintained with a combination of opioid-volatile technique.

Table 51-3

Approach to the Postoperative Patient with Myocardial Ischemia

Assess and stabilize airway, breathing, and circulation

Provide oxygen; attach cardiac and oxygen saturation monitors; establish/maintain IV access

If hemodynamically unstable treat according to ACLS protocols.

Attain 12-lead EKG.

Consider giving IV β-adrenergic antagonist (metoprolol 5 mg IV) if hemodynamically stable.

Treat pain/anxiety with IV opioid medications (Morphine 2–4 mg).

Obtain blood for cardiac biomarkers (troponin preferred), electrolytes, hematocrit/hemoglobin.

Obtain emergent cardiology consultation for patients with cardiogenic shock, left heart failure, or sustained ventricular tachyarrhythmia.

Consider indications and risk/benefit ratio of giving antiplatelet medications (aspirin, Clopidogrel) to the postoperative patient.

Further intervention (PCI, anticoagulation) based on clinical scenario.

d) **Postoperative management**

Shivering can greatly increase overall oxygen consumption and should be treated once recognized (3).

  i) Emergence from anesthesia can put further stress on the myocardium.
  ii) Supplemental O_2 should be given until adequate oxygenation is confirmed.
  iii) Pain should be treated liberally in order to alleviate its sympathetic output, which will increase myocardial O_2 consumption. Control of pain with a fast-onset, short-acting opiod such as fentanyl followed by administration of a longer acting opiod such as hydromorphone is recommended.
  iv) Postoperative shivering should be treated with warming and meperidine.
  v) Hypothermia must be corrected with the use of a forced air warming blanket.

e) **Postoperative ischemia**

  i) The majority of perioperative ischemic episodes occur in the first 3 days following surgery, usually 24 to 48 hours after surgery (6,7). The use of ECG as well as laboratory tests may aid in the diagnosis (Table 51-3).

Chapter Summary for Ischemic Heart Disease

Epidemiology	Leading killer of both men and women; about 1.5 million MIs each year
Anesthetic Management	**Preoperative:** Thorough history can be invaluable. Follow current ACC/AHA guidelines for testing specific to CAD severity and surgical risk. Invasive testing should only be considered for patients with active cardiac conditions or if the outcome will significantly alter medical management. **Intraoperative:** No clear evidence of superiority between regional or general. Tight hemodynamic control critical in patients with significant CAD regardless of anesthetic choice geared to optimize myocardial oxygen supply and minimize demand **Postoperative:** Smooth emergence minimizes stress. Supplemental oxygen should be used. Avoid elevations in heart rate (pain, shivering, etc.). Pain control is critical
Monitoring	Consider arterial line for high-risk procedures. Consider central line, PAC or TEE as indicated by surgical risk and degree of CAD.

References

1. Mitchell RN, Schoen FJ. Blood vessels and the heart. In: Kumar V, Fausto N, Abbas A, eds. *Robbins and Cotran Pathologic Basis of Disease*. 7th ed. Philadelphia, PA: Elsevier Saunders; 2005.
2. Bassand JP, Danchin N, Filippatos G, et al. Implementation of reperfusion therapy in acute myocardial infarction. A policy statement from the European Society of Cardiology. *Eur Heart J* 2005;(24):2733–2741.
3. Roizen M, Fleisher L. Anesthesia implications of concurrent disease. In: Miller R, ed. Consulting editors: Fleisher L, Johns R, Savarese J, Wiener-Kronish J, Young W. *Miller's Anesthesia*. 6th ed. Philadelphia, PA: Elsevier Churchill Livingstone; 2005.
4. Fleisher, LA, Beckman, JA, Brown, KA, et al. ACC/AHA 2007 guidelines on perioperative cardiovascular evaluation and care for noncardiac surgery: a report of the American College of Cardiology/American Heart Association Task Force on Practice Guidelines (Writing Committee to Revise the 2002 Guidelines on Perioperative Cardiovascular Evaluation for Noncardiac Surgery) developed in collaboration with the American Society of Echocardiography, American Society of Nuclear Cardiology, Heart Rhythm Society, Society of Cardiovascular Anesthesiologists, Society for Cardiovascular Angiography and Interventions, Society for Vascular Medicine and Biology, and Society for Vascular Surgery. *J Am Coll Cardiol* 2007;50:e159.
5. Mantha S, Roizen MF, Barnard J, et al. Relative effectiveness of preoperative noninvasive cardiac evaluation tests on predicting adverse cardiac outcomes following vascular surgery: a meta-analysis. *Anesth Analg* 1994;79:422.
6. Battler A, Froelicher VF, Gallagher KP, et al. Dissociation between regional myocardial dysfunction and ECG changes during ischemia in the conscious dog. *Circulation* 1980;62:735–744.
7. Mangano DT, Hollenberg M, Fegert G, et al. Perioperative myocardial ischemia in patients undergoing noncardiac surgery—I: incidence and severity during the 4 day perioperative period. The Study of Perioperative Ischemia (SPI) Research Group. *J Am Coll Cardiol* 1991;17:843–850.

52

Challenges in Anesthesia: A Patient with Coronary Artery Disease for Total Hip Arthroplasty

Glenn P. Gravlee, MD

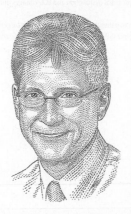

Our Patient

A 74-year-old 100-kg man (BMI 33 kg/m²) presents for a right total hip arthroplasty because of chronic degenerative arthritis. He has a history of coronary artery disease (CAD) including a lateral myocardial infarction (MI) 10 years ago, and placement of drug eluting stents in his left anterior descending (LAD) and second obtuse marginal (OM) arteries 13 months ago. His medications include atenolol, lisinopril, aspirin, and clopidogrel. His activity has been limited in the past 6 months by joint pain, but for the first several months following stent placements, he was able to walk two miles at a brisk pace and could mow his half-acre lawn using a hand-pushed power mower. A cardiac catheterization 12 months ago showed occlusion of the first OM branch of the left circumflex coronary artery, 30% narrowing of the proximal posterior descending artery, patent stents in the LAD and second OM arteries, and mild irregularities in the distal LAD artery beyond the stented segment. An echocardiogram 3 months ago showed a left ventricular ejection fraction of 0.45, akinesis of the basal-lateral and mid-lateral walls, hypokinesis of the apical lateral wall, mild mitral regurgitation, and mild diastolic dysfunction. An electrocardiogram (ECG) 1 week ago showed an old lateral MI and nonspecific ST segment changes. His preoperative vital signs are BP 134/78 mmHg, P 68 bpm, R 14/min, Temp 37°C.

Preoperative Assessment and Management

This elderly, moderately obese gentleman poses some preoperative assessment challenges. First, one must determine if he is an appropriate candidate for surgery, and if so, whether he needs additional preoperative diagnostic evaluation or therapeutic intervention. The 2007 American Heart Association (AHA) Guidelines on perioperative cardiovascular evaluation and its 2009 update (1,2) greatly aid this assessment, but common sense still serves as the best guideline. Degenerative joint disease, especially in the hips and knees, is an enemy to patients with CAD, because it restricts them from performing much-needed exercise. This provides strong motivation for joint repair or replacement. At the same time, arthritic pain-imposed limits to exercise impair bedside assessment of orthopedic patients' cardiovascular function.

In this patient, one can confidently assert that his medical condition was optimal 6 months ago. His fairly recent echocardiogram and very recent ECG do not suggest new coronary artery pathology, but neither do they definitively rule out that possibility. Since this operation falls into an intermediate risk category and there is high likelihood that his coronary artery anatomy is stable, there is no compelling need for further preoperative testing.

The patient's medications appear appropriate to his pathology, although some would argue that a resting pulse rate below 60 bpm should be attained by increasing the dose of β-blocker (3). The 2008 POISE trial argues against that approach by associating more intense β-blockade with increased mortality due to stroke and sepsis, even though myocardial events were reduced (4). A preoperative resting heart rate in the 60s is probably most appropriate for this patient. Preoperative angiotensin converting enzyme (ACE) inhibitor therapy has been linked to an increased incidence of hypotension during anesthesia (5). Although it remains somewhat controversial, a growing consensus supports withholding lisinopril on the day of surgery, but the usual dose of atenolol should be administered in the absence of bradycardia. Some evidence also suggests that perioperative administration of atorvastatin will reduce cardiovascular complications in patients such as this (6).

Drug eluting coronary artery stents have wedged anesthesiologists and surgeons between a rock and a hard place. These patients often bleed excessively if clopidogrel is continued and they have an increased risk for stent occlusion for at least the first 12 months if it is withheld. Had it been known that this patient would need a hip arthroplasty in the near future, the selection of bare metal stents might have best balanced overall risks and benefits. Unfortunately, drug-eluting stents are all-too-often placed without appropriate consideration for the likelihood that a patient may need surgery in the ensuing 12 months. Discontinuing this patient's clopidogrel for 5 to 7 days prior to surgery appears to best balance risk and benefit, since more than 12 months have elapsed since stent placement. He should continue his aspirin, which poses a much lower risk for excessive perioperative bleeding than does clopidogrel. If the patient's cardiologist should be concerned about withholding clopidogrel, the patient could be "bridged" with low molecular weight heparin until 24 hours before surgery.

Intraoperative Management
Monitoring

Although anesthesiologists worry about the choice of monitors for any given patient, there is little or no evidence basis to support any specific monitoring approach to this (or almost any) patient. Consequently, I will suggest a monitoring approach to this patient, while recognizing that other approaches may have equal merit. The ASA standard monitors, including ECG, non-invasive BP measurement, SpO_2, and temperature, constitute a baseline approach. I favor placing an arterial catheter in this patient, and since he is taking an ACE inhibitor, I would prefer to place this catheter prior to induction of anesthesia. I would not place a central venous catheter unless peripheral IV access should prove insufficient to achieve placement of one 16-gauge or two 18-gauge catheters. A pulmonary artery catheter is not needed. If the patient should experience unexplained or refractory intraoperative hypotension, I would place a transesophageal transesophageal echocardiography (TEE) probe urgently for diagnostic purposes if general anesthesia were being provided and the patient were intubated, but would try to avoid doing so if the patient were awake or lightly sedated.

V4 is the single best lead on the ECG for detecting intraoperative myocardial ischemia (7).

For intraoperative ECG monitoring, this patient would be well served by continuous monitoring of lead II and either lead V4 or V5, since the combination of those two leads misses very little myocardial ischemia (7). Landesberg et al. (7) identified V4 as the single best lead for detecting myocardial ischemia. Anesthesiology practitioners often fail to place the chest (V) lead in a position that will maximize diagnostic sensitivity myocardial ischemia. V Lead diagnostic sensitivity to myocardial ischemia falls off rapidly if the lead is placed in a position other than V4 (fifth intercostal space, mid-clavicular line) or V5 (fifth intercostal space, anterior axillary line). Erring one interspace cephalad has less impact on diagnostic sensitivity to ischemia than placing the lead too far medially or laterally. The ideal hemodynamic monitor would also provide continuous ST segment analysis in two or three leads, in which case one should select leads I, II, and V4 or V5 for this patient and place the ST segment visual analogue display on the monitor screen.

Antibiotic Prophylaxis
Anesthesiologists increasingly have been assuming responsibility for antibiotic prophylaxis. For this procedure, the use of a cephalosporin such as cefazolin 2 g prior to surgical incision is appropriate to minimize the incidence of perioperative infection.

Selection of Anesthesia
At the University of Colorado Hospital (UCH), most patients undergoing total hip replacement would preoperatively receive a single-shot lumbar plexus block using bupivacaine for early post-operative pain management. In most patients, this will block the femoral, lateral femoral cutaneous, and obturator nerves. This approach also provides considerable intraoperative analgesia but not surgical anesthesia, which is possible with the addition of a sciatic nerve block. Some centers place continuous lumbar plexus catheters to provide analgesia for 2 to 3 days, but at UCH this has most often been avoided because of concern about the potential for unrecognized epidural block and about the inability of a continuous lumbar plexus catheter infusion to sustain adequate analgesia in all three target nerve distributions. As a result of pre-emptive analgesic effects, the single shot lumbar plexus block approach may reduce postoperative pain even after the bupivacaine or ropivacaine wear off in 12 to 24 hours. In addition, regional analgesia over the first 12 to 24 hours may reduce hemodynamic stress.

↳ READ MORE

Lumbar plexus (psoas compartment) block, Chapter 180, page 1223

Debate about the relative merits of general versus regional anesthesia for patients such as this one has raged for decades without any definitive resolution. Both techniques have advantages and disadvantages, as shown in Table 52-1. For this patient, I recommend presenting the advantages and disadvantages of general and neuraxial anesthesia and letting the patient choose what he prefers. If I were in this patient's position, I would choose a spinal anesthetic because I would intuitively prefer its risk/benefit profile over that for general anesthesia. Hyperbaric bupivacaine should provide adequate blockade for a typical two-hour hip replacement procedure, and the addition of intrathecal morphine (200 to 300 µg) will provide significant analgesia through the first postoperative night. Further, I would ask to be lightly sedated because of preliminary evidence that this approach might reduce the chance for postoperative delirium. My impression is that elderly patients often are less apprehensive about being awake in the operating room than younger ones, so light sedation with midazolam alone or midazolam and fentanyl might be a good "fit" for this patient. Too often anesthesia practitioners seem compelled to administer deep sedation using a propofol infusion even when there is no obvious benefit to the patient or to the conduct of the procedure. Another attribute of spinal anesthesia is avoidance of the potential hemodynamic stress of emergence from general anesthesia.

Management of General Anesthesia
Should general anesthesia be chosen, it would be reasonable to select either a laryngeal mask airway (LMA) or an endotracheal tube. Selection of an LMA for a patient who will be undergoing surgery in the lateral position appears to make many American anesthesiology practitioners nervous. In the absence of symptomatic gastroesophageal reflux (e.g., untreated or symptomatic despite medication), there is little reason to fear the use of an LMA in this setting. Especially in the presence of a preoperative nerve block or blocks, one can maintain a lighter plane of general anesthesia with an LMA than with an endotracheal tube, and it is

Table 52-1

Advantages and Disadvantages of General or Neuraxial Anesthesia for an Elderly Total Hip Arthroplasty Patient with CAD

General anesthesia

Advantages	*Disadvantages*
Patient cooperation	Postoperative nausea and vomiting
Airway control	Sore throat/hoarseness
Likely myocardial protection	Possible "hangover" or confusion
Titratability	Increased chance of adverse drug reaction

Neuraxial anesthesia

Advantages	*Disadvantages*
Less invasive	Requires patient acceptance and cooperation
Titratability (continuous spinal or epidural)	Deep sedation may offset advantages
Possible reduced pulmonary complications	May wear off (single shot spinal)
Postoperative analgesia (especially continuous techniques)	Back pain
	Post-lumbar puncture headache
	Neuraxial complications (hematoma, abscess, retained catheter)

also easier to maintain spontaneous or lightly assisted ventilation with an LMA. The use of an endotracheal tube makes it more difficult to suppress the cough reflex without adding muscle paralysis.

For induction of anesthesia in this patient with moderately reduced left ventricular function, I favor a modest dose of fentanyl (2 to 3 μg/kg) administered 3 to 4 minutes prior to induction with propofol or etomidate. I would choose propofol 2 to 2.5 mg/kg if the systolic BP (SBP) prior to induction exceeded 125 mm Hg, and etomidate 0.2 to 0.3 mg/kg if SBP were 110 mm Hg or less. For SBPs between 110 and 125 mm Hg, either a lower dose of propofol, a combination of propofol and etomidate, or etomidate alone might be selected. If the use of an LMA is planned, I would prefer propofol for its superior airway reflex suppression, but would reduce the dose slightly. If endotracheal intubation is planned, I would be happy with succinylcholine 1 to 1.5 mg/kg or with rocuronium approximately 0.6 mg/kg. In my practice, selection of rocuronium presumes the achievement of mask ventilation prior to its administration as well as a preoperative assessment consistent with an easy intubation.

With or without an LMA, in the absence of a compelling history of perioperative nausea and vomiting I would select a volatile anesthetic agent as the primary anesthetic agent, because these agents are easily titrated and they may provide significant myocardial protection from anesthetic preconditioning. Propofol and non-synthetic opioids can also provide preconditioning effects, but protection is less well-established for those agents and it may require supraanesthetic doses. If a patient were to have an intraoperative MI, the chance of limiting the extent of the myocardial injury appears greater in the presence of a 0.5 MAC or higher dose of a volatile agent than with other techniques. For this elderly patient, I would maintain anesthesia with either sevoflurane or desflurane, but isoflurane would be equally acceptable. Some opioids will likely be needed, but if a preoperative nerve or plexus block is placed, one should keep these doses to a minimum. Failure to do this will make the resumption of spontaneous ventilation more challenging. Typically the lateral positioning used for total hip arthroplasty is compatible

The balance of myocardial oxygen supply and demand should be the primary concern when approaching the patient with CAD.

with spontaneous ventilation during the entire procedure, but occasionally the use of Trendelenberg position or the patient's body habitus (e.g., morbidly obese) renders this approach infeasible. When plausible, spontaneous or lightly assisted ventilation facilitates venous return to the heart and may reduce the incidence of hypotension. Modern anesthesia ventilators have taken the "labor" out of lightly assisted ventilation by providing a pressure support mode. Total hip arthroplasty seldom requires neuromuscular blockade in an elderly non-mesomorphic male. The absence of neuromuscular blockers somewhat eases concern about intraoperative recall, as the patient should be able to move if anesthesia becomes too "light"; and also about postoperative nausea and vomiting, as there will be no need for neostigmine.

Myocardial Oxygen Supply and Demand

When approaching a patient with CAD, the balance of myocardial oxygen (O_2) supply and demand should remain uppermost among one's concerns throughout the perioperative period. Figure 52-1 shows the traditional factors influencing this balance.

On the supply side, assuming adequate hemoglobin (Hgb) concentration, normal Hgb function, and normal arterial oxygen saturation, the principal determinant becomes diastolic arterial pressure. Assuming the absence of left ventricular volume overload, a diastolic arterial pressure of 60 mm Hg should be sufficient to maintain coronary perfusion in most patients with CAD. However, in patients with critical uncorrected stenoses (or with presumed or documented higher left ventricular diastolic pressures), it may be wise to maintain higher diastolic arterial pressures. Diastolic arterial pressures in excess of 90 mm Hg generally become counterproductive because maintaining this level will almost invariably require higher left ventricular wall tension, thereby increasing myocardial oxygen demand as well. Diastolic arterial pressures should err on the high side in patients with left ventricular hypertrophy, because coronary perfusion travels from epicardium to endocardium, hence these patients have increased susceptibility to subendocardial ischemia.

Assuming adequate oxygenation, Hgb concentration is the remaining piece of the supply side puzzle. Retrospective studies have linked Hgb concentrations below 9.0 g/dL with

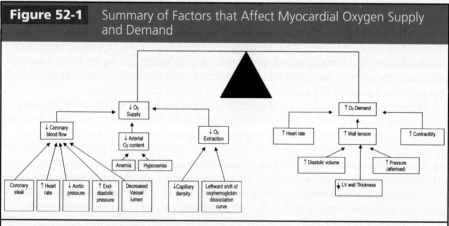

Figure 52-1 Summary of Factors that Affect Myocardial Oxygen Supply and Demand

Reprinted from Okum G, Horrow JC. Anesthetic management of myocardial revascularization. In: Hensley FA Jr, Martin DE, Gravlee GP, eds. *A Practical Approach to Cardiac Anesthesia*. 4th ed. Philadelphia, PA: Lippincott Williams & Wilkins; 2008:298, with permission.

an increased risk for myocardial ischemia, particularly in the presence of tachycardia (8). Consequently, one should probably maintain this patient's Hgb concentration above that level, but there is no compelling reason to push it higher than 10 g/dL.

On the demand side, theoretically the ideal situation is an empty left ventricle, zero intracavitary systolic pressure, absent myocardial contractility, and an aortic diastolic pressure of 60 mm Hg or higher. Since these conditions can only be achieved during cardiopulmonary bypass (or death), one must make some compromises. Pre-existing β-adrenergic blockade works well because it reduces pulse rate and myocardial contractility, although too much of it may compromise cardiac output sufficiently to compromise O_2 delivery to the other organs of the body. This probably explains the increased mortality found in the POISE trial (4). Wall tension is largely controlled by avoiding excessively high systolic pressures and left ventricular preload. Preload assessment at the bedside proves challenging, and unfortunately this task is not importantly aided by monitoring central venous pressure or pulmonary artery occlusion pressure. If preload assessment is in doubt and the patient has refractory hypotension, either a transthoracic or TEE assessment will clarify the situation.

Higher heart rates increase myocardial O_2 demand as a result of requiring more beats per minute. Myocardial O_2 consumption per beat goes up very little as heart rate increases, however, and the duration of each systolic cycle also goes down very little. Since the duration of systole diminishes only slightly, the direct inverse relationship between heart rate and R–R interval principally manifests as a reduced duration of diastole. This situation is untenable for patients with CAD, because they need maximum diastolic duration in order to replace the O_2 utilized on the preceding systolic contraction. One of my teachers, the late Dr. Myron Laver, used to say, "The heart doesn't really care how much oxygen it uses per minute. All it cares about is that the oxygen used during each systolic cycle is fully replaced during the very next diastole." Failure to replace the O_2 used during a systolic contraction results in measurable ischemia within just a few heartbeats, as reflected by new regional wall motion abnormalities seen by TEE. Consequently, avoidance of tachycardia is highly important, although only patients with critical coronary stenoses and/or severe anemia typically experience myocardial ischemia at resting pulse rates below 90 bpm. Tolerance for tachycardia can be improved by increasing diastolic BP and by keeping the left ventricle relatively empty.

Tachycardia is like double jeopardy in patients with CAD: It increases myocardial oxygen demand while also decreasing myocardial oxygen supply.

Postoperative Management

A smooth emergence from anesthesia is preferable, that is, one that lacks hypertension and tachycardia. Preoperative nerve block(s) will facilitate a smooth, pain-free emergence. Continued β-adrenergic blockade may be most important during wake-up and early recovery, especially in the absence of regional analgesia from nerve blocks or spinal anesthesia. If the patient's HR should exceed 80 bpm without an explanation such as fever or inadequate analgesia, strong consideration should be given to aggressive titration of increments of IV metoprolol sufficient to bring the HR back down into the 60s or 70s. Fever should be aggressively diagnosed and treated in order to avoid increasing myocardial O_2 demand. Continuous regional analgesia will provide excellent analgesia, but not necessarily total analgesia, so opioid-based IV patient controlled analgesic may also be required. Continuous analgesia may also assist with early mobilization as long as the local anesthetic concentration is low, for example, not higher than 0.2% ropivacaine or 0.1% bupivacaine. If the patient remains hemodynamically stable and wound drainage is low, usual preoperative medications should be resumed on the first day after surgery. Since it will take several days for clopidogrel to achieve a therapeutic effect, bridging with subcutaneous unfractionated heparin or with low molecular weight heparin is advised. This approach will also reduce the chance for deep vein thrombosis. Continuous regional analgesia can be discontinued on the second or third postoperative day, and if the postoperative course is uneventful discharge can be accomplished on postoperative day 4 or 5.

References

1. Fleisher LA, Beckman JA, Brown KA, et al. ACC/AHA 2007 Guidelines on perioperative cardiovascular evaluation and care for noncardiac surgery. *Circulation* 2007;116:e418–e500.
2. Fleisher LA, Beckman JA, Brown KA, et al. 2009 ACC/AHA focused update on perioperative beta blockade incorporated into the ACC/AHA 2007 Guidelines on Perioperative Cardiovascular Evaluation and Care for Noncardiac Surgery: a report of the American College of Cardiology Foundation/American Heart Association Task Force on Practice Guidelines. *Circulation* 2009;120:e169–e276.
3. Poldermans D, Boersma E, Bax JJ, et al. The effect of bisoprolol on perioperative mortality and myocardial infarction in high-risk patients undergoing vascular surgery: Dutch Echocardiography Study Group. *N Engl J Med* 1999;341:1789–1794.
4. Devereaux PJ, Yang H, Yusuf S, et al. Effects of extended-release metoprolol succinate in patients undergoing non-cardiac surgery (POISE trial): a randomized controlled trial. *Lancet* 2008;371:1839–1847.
5. Kheterpal S, Khodoparast O, Shanks A, et al. Chronic angiotensin converting-enzyme inhibitor or angiotensin receptor blocker therapy combined with diuretic therapy is associated with increased episodes of hypotension in noncardiac surgery. *J Cardiothorac Vasc Anesth* 2008;22:180–186.
6. Lindenauer PK, Pekow P, Wang K et al. Lipid lowering therapy and in-hospital mortality in patients undergoing major noncardiac vascular surgery. *JAMA* 2004;291:2092–2099.
7. Landesberg G, Mosseri M, Wolf Y, et al. Perioperative myocardial ischemia and infarction: identification by continuous 12-lead electrocardiogram with online ST-segment monitoring. *Anesthesiology* 2002;96:264–270.
8. Nelson AH, Fleisher LA, Rosenbaum SH. Relationship between postoperative anemia and cardiac morbidity in high-risk vascular patients in the intensive care unit. *Crit Care Med* 1993;21:860–866.

53 Valvular Heart Disease

Daryl A. Oakes, MD

Severe valvular disease is a major clinical predictor of increased perioperative risk (1). Patients with known severe, symptomatic valvular disease should be evaluated for extent of disease progression, coexisting heart disease, and need for preoperative intervention. Mild or moderate valvular disease if asymptomatic may be reasonably well tolerated perioperatively, but an understanding of these lesions can help optimize intra-operative hemodynamics. Even in the setting of severe valvular disease, intervention may not always be appropriate (e.g., age, comorbidities) or may not be possible (e.g., emergency surgery), and therefore a thorough understanding of the pathophysiology of valvular disease is important. This chapter presents on overview of pathophysiology of valvular heart disease, along with a discussion of right sided heart lesions. Aortic and mitral valve pathologies are discussed in individual chapters.

For patients with compensated valvular heart disease, anesthetic hemodynamic goals should be to maintain patients resting hemodynamic parameters.

1) General principles of caring for patients with valvular disease (2,3)

   a) **Valvular heart disease in general refers to cardiac pathology directly due to valvular abnormalities.**

   b) **In scenarios of multivalvular disease, management will generally focus on the more severe lesion in terms of hemodynamic goals.**

   c) **Maintain/optimize cardiac output (CO) (2–4)**

      i) CO = stroke volume (SV) × heart rate (HR)

      ii) CO is a measure to describe how well the heart is performing its function of delivery of oxygen, nutrients and chemicals to the cells of the body.

      iii) SV is determined by preload (venous return, left ventricular end diastolic pressure [LVEDP]), afterload (systemic vascular resistance [SVR], BP), and contractile state of myocardium.

      iv) Low HR in patients with relatively fixed SV (e.g., aortic stenosis) can severely decrease CO, even if BP is in normal range. (e.g., If HR 40 bpm and SV is normal 70 mL CO is only 2.8 L/min).

   d) **Maintain myocardial oxygen balance (2–4)**

      i) CO reflects oxygen delivery, which must increase or decrease with the demands of the body.

      ii) Myocardial O_2 balance simply reflects provision of adequate O_2 to the myocardium to prevent ischemia, particulary in settings of increased workload.

READ MORE

Ischemic heart disease, Chapter 51, page 359

      iii) Determinants of myocardial O_2 demand include HR, contractile state, wall tension (includes preload or diameter of chamber, afterload, and wall thickness), temperature, and myocardial mass.

      iv) Determinants of myocardial O_2 supply: Coronary perfusion pressure (aortic diastolic pressure – LVEDP), CO, patency of coronary vessels, oxygen content of blood = $(1.34 \times Hbg \times Sat + 0.003 \times PaO_2)$, diastolic time

e) **General principles for stenotic lesions**
  i) Maintain preload.
  ii) Maintain HR at baseline, avoid tachycardia. Significant bradycardia can compromise CO.
  iii) Maintain sinus rhythm. Prepare for cardioversion if arrhythmias are not tolerated.

f) Regurgitant lesions

READ MORE

Mitral valve disease, Chapter 55, page 394

  i) Decrease afterload by dilating subsequent vascular bed
    (1) For example, in the setting of tricuspid regurgitation (TR) or PI decrease pulmonary vascular resistance (PVR) with vasodilators and/or hyperventilation; in setting MR or AI decrease systemic vascular resistance with arterial vasodilators
  ii) Maintenance of HR normal to slightly high to compensate for decreased CO due to smaller actual ("forward") SV

2) **Pulmonary valve disease**
  a) Pulmonary regurgitation (PR)
    i) **Etiology**
      (1) Congenital PR is uncommon and is associated with idiopathic dilation of the pulmonary artery or connective tissue diseases resulting in pulmonary valve annular dilation and valve incompetence (3).
      (2) Typical Causes of PR
        (a) Secondary regurgitation in the presence of pulmonary hypertension (primary or secondary to left heart pathology)
        (b) Tetralogy of Fallot (TOF) repair with RV to PA conduit
        (c) Infective endocarditis due to IV drug abuse
        (d) Endocarditis from systemic disease (e.g., carcinoid)
    ii) **Pathophysiology (2–4)**
      (1) Regurgitation into the RV leads to RV dilation and eventually RV failure. RV enlargement can lead to tricuspid annular dilation and TR. RA enlargement and RV failure may develop if uncorrected. (Figure 53-1)
      (2) **Signs of RV failure include engorged neck veins, hepatic engorgement causing hepatic dysfunction/elevated INR, peripheral edema**
    iii) **Management considerations (5)**
      (1) For severe PR with RV dysfunction, a preinduction arterial line is recommended. CVP monitoring and TEE should be considered for intermediate to high-risk surgical procedures due to possibility of right heart failure intraoperatively.

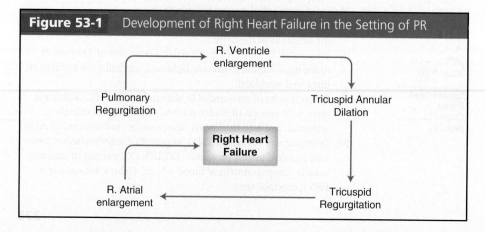

Figure 53-1 Development of Right Heart Failure in the Setting of PR

(2) A pulmonary artery catheter (PAC) may be useful depending on the degree of RV dysfunction— but may be difficult to insert due to regurgitant flow.

    (a) Mild hyperventilation will decrease pulmonary arterial pressure.

(3) Strive to maintain preload, and consider post-op intubation if RV function is severely impaired, as any increase in CO_2 due to hypoventilation will elevate PVR and further strain the right ventricle.

(4) If mild and not associated with any structural heart disease, standard anesthetic management may be appropriate.

b) **Pulmonary stenosis (3)**

  i) **Etiology**

    (1) **Congenital lesions** are the most common cause.

      (a) **Isolated PS** occurs in 8% to 12% of all congenital heart defects, with obstruction due to isolated valvular stenosis (80% to 90%), supravalvular stenosis (periperal), or subvalvular stenosis (infundibular).

      (b) **PS** as a **component of complex CHD** (e.g., TOF, single ventricle). Severe PS in neonatal life (e.g., TOF) can lead to varying degrees of pulmonary artery hypoplasia, presence of persistent intracardiac shunts (PFO) or extracardiac shunts (PDA) or coexistence of ASD, VSD to allow for adequate mixing and oxygenation of blood.

    (2) **Acquired**

      (a) Rheumatic disease, hyperplasia of RVOT tissue creating subpulmonic stenosis

    (3) **Acute causes include** pulmonary embolus, tumor, or obstruction in the pulmonary artery

  ii) **Clinical symptoms**

    (1) Children and adolescents are frequently asymptomatic even with severe PS.

    (2) Adults with longstanding PS may experience dyspnea on exertion due to an inability to increase CO.

    (3) Severe PS with severely elevated RV systolic pressures (systemic or suprasystemic) may be associated with exertional light-headedness or syncope in the setting of decreased preload, dehydration, vasodilation, and low systemic vascular resistance states such as pregnancy.

  iii) **Pathophysiology**

    (1) Longstanding resistance to flow across the pulmonic valve results in RV hypertrophy.

      (a) RV hypertrophy leads to a stiffened ventricle (diastolic dysfunction) and requires increased diastolic pressures to fill adequately.

    (2) TR may be present due to RV systolic hypertension demonstrated by a large "v wave" on the CVP tracing.

    (3) Severe TR and RV failure develops from pressure overload resulting in RV dilation.

    (4) Stretching of conduction system can lead to dysrhythmias.

    (5) High RA or RV pressures can lead to R→L shunting in presence of PFO, ASD, or VSD.

  iv) **Management considerations (3–5)**

    (1) Determine the presence of any coexisting abnormalities (e.g., PFO or other ASD, VSD). An echocardiogram may be necessary.

READ MORE

Congenital heart disease, Chapter 112, page 798

In setting of acute pulmonary stenosis (e.g., pulmonary embolus, tumor), the RV may be unable to tolerate increased workload and acutely fail, resulting in venous engorgement and cardiogenic shock.

(2) Carefully de-air IV lines, given risk of paradoxical embolism with right-to-left shunting.

(3) Monitoring considerations for severe lesions
  (a) Strongly consider a preinduction arterial line.
  (b) CVP monitoring and TEE may be necessary depending on the lesion and the procedure.

(4) Avoid large changes in preload (e.g., large boluses of propofol, nitroglycerin).

(5) Consider induction agents such as ketamine or etomidate to maintain hemodynamic stability.

(6) Avoid hypovolemia and bradycardia as CO of the RV may be decreased.

(7) Patients are at risk for dysrhythmias and the ability to perform cardioversion should be readily available.

3) Tricuspid valve disease

a) Principles and management of tricuspid disease are similar to pulmonary valve disease.

b) **Tricuspid stenosis (TS) (3–5)**
  i) **Etiology**
    (1) Congenital TS may be associated with RV hypoplasia, ASD, right-to-left shunt
    (2) Rheumatic heart disease
    (3) Mechanical due to a thrombus/mass
  ii) **Pathophysiology**
    (1) TS leads to right atrial enlargement, preload dependence, and conduction system disease (Afib/AFlutter, SVT).
    (2) Physiology resembles the restriction to venous return into the heart seen in cardiac tamponade.
  iii) **Management principles (5)**
    (1) When monitoring patients with severe TS an arterial line, central venous line, and TEE should be considered
    (2) Maintain normal preload, keep HR in the normal range, and maintain sinus rhythm.

c) **Tricuspid regurgitation**
  i) **Etiology (3–5)**
    (1) **TR with a normal valve** may be physiologic or secondary to other causes, including RV dilation and tricuspid annular dilation, or pulmonary hypertension causing RV systolic hypertension.
    (2) **TR with an abnormal valve (Table 53-1)**
  ii) **Management**
    (1) Careful history and physical exam to identify extent of disease and coexisting lesions
    (2) Management of moderate-severe or severe TR depends on the extent of RV enlargement or RV failure. Goals are to maintain adequate RV preload and decrease pulmonary valvular resistance.
    (3) For combined severe TR and RV dysfunction, PAC pressures may be helpful but TR placement of may be PAC challenging.
      (a) CO measurements by thermodilution may be unreliable.
      (b) TEE can be helpful in monitoring ventricular filling and estimating CO.

Table 53-1

Conditions which may Result in Abnormal Tricuspid Valve (3)

Common Conditions	Pathology/Etiology
Ebstein's anomaly	Inferiorly displaced septal/posterior leaflets often adherent to RV septum
Infective endocarditis	Intravenous drug abuse; indwelling catheters
Rheumatic disease	Medications (e.g., phentermine/fenfluramine "Fen-phen" pergolide, methysergide)
Trauma	Injury to leaflets or chordal elements from endocardial biopsy pacemaker wires
Systemic disease	Carcinoid, lupus
Connective-tissue disease	Ehlers-Danlos, osteogenesis imperfect, Marfan syndrome
Papillary muscle dysfunction	Ischemia, infiltration, fibrosis

4) Prosthetic valves (6)
   a) **Types of valves**
      i) **Mechanical**
         (1) Ball-in-cage (e.g., Starr-Edwards)
         (2) Disc occluder
         (3) Single tilting disc (Björk-Shiley, Medtronic-Hall, Omnicarbon)
         (4) Bileaflet (St. Jude, CarboMedics, Edwards Duromedics)
      ii) **Bioprosthetic**
         (1) Stented tissue valves (bovine pericardium, porcine valves)
         (2) Stentless tissue valves (e.g., homografts from a human cadaver, autografts such as a transplanted native valve in a Ross procedure)
   b) **Anticoagulation for prosthetic valves**
      i) **Risk of thromboembolic event**
         (1) 0.7% to 2% per year with mechanical valve despite warfarin therapy
         (2) 4% per year with mechanical valve and no anticoagulation
      ii) **High-risk patients** include those with atrial fibrillation, previous thromboembolism, hypercoagulable state, LV dysfunction, or with more than one mechanical valve.
      iii) **High-risk valves** include mitral valves, older-generation thrombogenic valves (e.g., tilting disc and Starr–Edwards cage and ball valves), mechanical tricuspid valves.
   c) **Recommended prophylactic anticoagulation (6,7)**
      i) **Aspirin alone** (or clopidogrel if aspirin not tolerated) in low-risk patients with bioprosthetic (tissue) valves
      ii) **Warfarin with a goal INR 2.0 to 3.0 plus aspirin**
         (1) Low-risk patients with Bileaflet or Medronic Hall mechanical aortic
         (2) High-risk patients with bioprosthetic aortic or mitral valves
         (3) First 3 months after bioprosthetic aortic or mitral valve in low-risk patients
      iii) **Warfarin INR 2.5 to 3.5 plus aspirin**
         (1) Any mechanical mitral valve
         (2) High-risk patients with Bileaflet or Medronic Hall mechanical aortic valve

   (3) Any disc mechanical valves (not Medronic Hall) or Starr–Edwards valves

   (4) First 3 months after mechanical aortic valve

  d) **Bridging patients with mechanical valves for invasive procedures**

   i) Low-risk patients (i.e., bileaflet valve with no risk factors)

    (1) Warfarin may be stopped 48 to 72 hours prior to procedure and restarted within 24 hours. No heparin is usually necessary.

   ii) **High-risk patients (see above)**

    (1) Warfarin is stopped and IV heparin is started when INR drops below 2.0.

    (2) Heparin is stopped 4 to 6 hours prior to procedure and restarted as soon as possible after surgery and continued until INR is again therapeutic.

   iii) Therapeutic dosing of subcutaneous heparin (15,000 units q12h) or LMWH may be used while INR is subtherapeutic.

 5) **Antibiotic prophylaxis for endocarditis (6–8)**

  a) **High-risk procedures (6)**

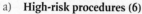

ACC/AHA 2008 guidelines on valvular heart disease recommend antibiotic prophylaxis only in patients with high-risk lesions having procedure with risk of bacteremia.

   i) Dental procedures involving manipulation of gingival tissue or periapical region of teeth or perforation of oral mucosa

   ii) Respiratory tract procedures involving incision or biopsy of the respiratory mucosa (e.g., tonsillectomy, adenoidectomy, or bronchoscopy with biopsy)

   iii) GI or GU procedures in patients with active infections of these organ systems

   iv) Procedures involving infected skin, skin structure, or musculoskeletal tissue

   v) Surgery involving placement of prosthetic heart valves, implanting of prosthetic intravascular or intracardiac materials

  b) **High-risk patients (6)**

   i) Prosthetic valve (including bioprosthetic and homografts) or prosthetic material for valve repair

   ii) Patients with history of infective endocarditis

   iii) Patients with congenital heart disease (CHD) involving (8)

    (1) Cyanotic heart lesions or lesions with palliative shunt (e.g., single ventricle, tetralogy of Fallot, transposition of great vessels)

    (2) First 6 months after complete correction CHD lesion using prosthetic materials

    (3) Partially corrected CHD with residual defects near prosthetic material

   iv) Cardiac transplant patients with valve regurgitation in a structurally abnormal valve

  c) **No prophylaxis is recommended** for the following procedures:

   i) Nondental procedures such as transesophageal echocardiogram

   ii) Invasive gastrointestinal or genitourinary procedures (e.g., procedures with mucosal disruption or biopsy such as esophagoscopy, gastroduodenoscopy, ERCP, colonoscopy, dilation of GU tract stictures, prostatectomy) in absence of active infection

  d) **No prophylaxis is recommended** for the following cardiac lesions:

   i) Bicuspid aortic valve or coarctation of aorta

   ii) Acquired aortic or mitral valve disease (including aortic stenosis or regurgitation, mitral stenosis or regurgitation)

Table 53-2
Antibiotic Therapy for Endocarditis Prophylaxis

Ampicillin 2 g p.o. (50 mg/kg in children up to 2 g)
Ampicillin 2 g IM or IV (50 mg/kg in children up to 2 g)
Cefazolin or ceftriaxone 1 g IM or IV (50 mg/kg in children up to 1 g)
If allergy to penicillin or ampicillin:
   Cephalexin 2 g p.o. (50 mg/kg in children up to 2 g)
   Clindamycin 600 mg p.o. (20 mg/kg in children up to 600 mg)
   Azithromycin or clarithromycin 500 mg p.o. (15 mg/kg in children up to 500 mg)
   Cefazolin or ceftriaxone 1 gm IM or IV (50 mg/kg in children up to 1 g)
   Clindamycin 600 mg IM or IV (20 mg/kg in children up to 600 mg)

    iii) Mitral valve prolapse with regurgitation, or history of prior valve repair
    iv) Hypertrophic cardiomyopathy with outflow obstruction
  e) **No prophylaxis is recommended** in the adolescent and young adult with congenital heart disease and native valve tissue.
  f) **No prophylaxis** is recommended in the setting of vaginal and cesarean delivery in the absence of infection with the following exceptions:
    i) In patients with the highest risk lesions (**Section 5.b.**) with established infection that could cause bacteremia (e.g., chorioamnionitis or pyelonephritis). Treatment for the underlying infection should include an IV regimen effective for infective endocarditis prophylaxis.
    ii) In select patients with the highest risk of adverse outcomes (e.g., patients with prosthetic cardiac valve, prosthetic material used for cardiac valve repair, unrepaired or palliated cyanotic heart disease, including surgically constructed palliative shunts and conduits)
  g) **Recommended therapeutic options**
    i) **Dental or respiratory tract procedures** (Table 53-2)
    ii) **For GI or GU procedures in setting of infection,** the antibiotic regimen to treat existing infection should include an agent active against enterococci, such as penicillin, ampicillin, piperacillin, or vancomycin.
    iii) **For procedures on infected skin, skin structures, musculoskeletal tissue, the** Antibiotic regimen to treat existing infection should include an agent active against staphylococci and beta-hemolytic streptococci, such as an antistaphylococcal penicillin or a cephalosporin, or, if the patient is unable to tolerate a beta-lactam or is suspected to have a methicillin-resistant strain of staphylococcus, vancomycin or clindamycin may be used.
    iv) **For Surgery to place prosthetic cardiac valves or implant intravascular or intracardiac prosthetic material.** Most commonly a first-generation cephalosporin or, in setting of high prevalence of methacillin-resistant staphylococcus, vancomycin.
    v) **Patients currently taking antibiotics for other indication at time of dental or invasive procedures.** An antibiotic of a different class should be chosen.

Chapter Summary for Anesthesia for Valvular Heart Disease

Definitions	Severity and management of valvular heart disease is defined by diagnostic findings along with degree of clinical compensation
Risks	Severe lesions are associated with markedly increased operative risk
Monitoring	Arterial line used for most procedures ± central line. PAC may be indicated, but often problematic for severe TV/PV disease. TEE as indicated by surgical risk.
Anesthetic Management Goals	Maintain/optimize CO and myocardial oxygen balance. For valvular lesions consider: **1. Insufficiency:** Gentle dilation of distal vascular bed (e.g., pulmonary vasculature with PI) to improve forward flow, HR normal to slightly elevated **2. Stenosis:** Avoids large drops in preload, avoids significant bradycardia) and significant tachycardia
Prosthetic Valves	Mechanical valves require prophylactic anticoagulation so bridging therapy should be planned prior to surgery.
Antibiotic Prophylaxis	Consider antibiotic therapy for patients with valve disease in the high risk groups based on lesion and type of procedure.

HR, heart rate; PAC, pulmonary artery catheter; PV, pulmonary valve; TEE, transesophageal echocardiography; TV, tricuspid valve.

References

1. Eagle KA, Berger PB, Calkins H, et al. ACC/AHA perioperative executive summary. *J Am Coll Cardiol* 2002;39:542–553.
2. Carabello B. Valvular Heart Disease. In Goldman L, Ausiello A eds: *Cecil Medicine*. 23rd ed. Philadelphia, PA: Saunders Elsevier; 2008: chap 75.
3. Park, M. Obstructive Lesions. *Pediatric cardiology for practitioners*. 5th ed. Philadelphia, PA: Mosby, Inc.; 2008. Chapter 13.
4. Nussmeier N. Hauser M, Sarwar M, et al. Anesthesia for Cardiac Surgical Procedures. In *Miller's Anesthesia*. 7th ed., Editor: Miller R. Contributing Editors: Eriksson L, Fleisher L, Wiener-Kronish J, Young W. Churchill Livingstone; 2009, Ch 60.
5. Bonow RO, Carabello BA, Chatterjee K, et al. 2008 Focused update incorporated into the ACC/AHA 2006 Guidelines for the Management of Patients With Valvular Heart Disease. *J Am Coll Cardiol* 2008;52:e1–e142.
6. Nishimura RA, Carabello BA, Faxon DP, et al. ACC/AHA 2008 guideline update on valvular heart disease: focused update on infective endocarditis: a report of the American College of Cardiology/American Heart Association Task Force on Practice Guidelines: endorsed by the Society of Cardiovascular Anesthesiologists, Society for Cardiovascular Angiography and Interventions, and Society of Thoracic Surgeons. *Circulation* 2008;118:887–896.
7. ACOG Committee Opinion No. 421, November 2008: antibiotic prophylaxis for infective endocarditis. *Obstet Gynecol* 2008;112:1193–1194.
8. Warnes CA, Williams RG, Bashore TM, et al. ACC/AHA 2008 Guidelines for the Management of Adults With Congenital Heart Disease: A Report of the American College of Cardiology/American Heart Association Task Force on Practice Guidelines (Writing Committee to Develop Guidelines on the Management of Adults With Congenital Heart Disease) Developed in Collaboration With the American Society of Echocardiography, Heart Rhythm Society, International Society for Adult Congenital Heart Disease, Society for Cardiovascular Angiography and Interventions, and Society of Thoracic Surgeons. *J Am Coll Cardiol* 2008;52:143–263.

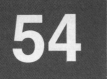
54

Aortic Valvular Disease

Judy Thai, MD

Aortic valve (AV) is a trileaflet valve located between the left ventricle (LV) and the aorta. AV disease accounts for a major portion of cardiac disease in the United States. Aortic stenosis (AS) in particular accounts for one-fourth of all chronic valvular heart diseases. In contrast, chronic aortic regurgitation (AR) may account for 5% based on the Framingham Heart Study data (1). The presence of either symptomatic AS or severe AR carries a significantly high morbidity and mortality risk compared to the general population (2,3). It is essential to understand the pathophysiology and hemodynamic consequences of aortic valvular diseases in order to anticipate problems and safely manage these patients.

1) **AS: etiology**

   a) Rheumatic heart disease is no longer the leading cause of AS. The primary etiology is idiopathic calcific degeneration of aortic valves.

   b) 1% to 2% of the general population is born with a bicuspid AV, which is prone to early stenosis; usually in their fourth to fifth decades of life (4).

   c) Senile degeneration of tricuspid aortic valves can develop with aging and their symptomatic presentations usually occur in their sixth to eighth decades of life (4).

In the setting of low cardiac output, severe AS may be present despite a "low" pressure gradient.

2) **Classification and severity grading**

   a) AS may be classified as valvular, subvalvular, or supravalvular based on the location of stenosis. The most common is valvular AS representing about 75% of the cases.

   b) AS is graded based on the severity of obstruction (**Table 54-1**)

3) **Natural history of AS**

   a) AS occurs when leaflet restriction causes outflow obstruction

   b) Generally, the rate of stenosis progression is a decrease in AV area by 0.1 cm²/y, an increase in peak pressure by 10 mm Hg/y, and an increase in mean pressure by 7 mm Hg/y (3).

   c) **Figure 54-1** shows that AS patients have a nearly normal survival rate up until symptom onset. Once symptoms develop, prognosis is dismal with a life expectancy of <5 years. The cardinal symptoms of AS are angina, syncope, and congestive heart failure (CHF).

      i) Angina is a frequent initial symptom in about two thirds of patients with critical AS (5).

      ii) With onset of CHF, the average life expectancy is 1 to 2 years (3).

   d) All AS patients are at risk of sudden death, with higher risk in symptomatic AS (3).

Table 54-1

Hemodynamic Parameters for AS

	Peak Pressure (mm Hg)	Mean Pressure (mm Hg)	AV Area (cm²)
Normal	<25	<12	2.5–3.5
Mild	25–50	12–25	1.2–1.8
Moderate	50–80	25–40	0.8–1.2
Severe	80–100	40–50	0.6–0.8
Critical	>100	>50	<0.6

Measurements assume a normal LV function.
Adapted from Bonow RO, Carabello BA, Chatterjee K, et al. ACC/AHA 2006 guidelines for the management of patients with valvular heart disease: a report of the ACC/AHA Task Force on Practice Guidelines. *Circulation* 2006;114:e124–e150.

4) Pathophysiology (5–8)

   a) **Pressure overload**

      i) The primary burden of AS is progressive pressure overload of the left ventricle.

      ii) Pressure overload directly increases myocardial wall tension in accordance with Laplace law (wall stress = pressure × radius/2 × wall thickness).

      iii) Pressure overload leads to LV concentric hypertrophy, which attempts to normalize wall tension.

Loss of sinus rhythm in patients with AS can lead to rapid clinical decline.

   b) **The cost of LV hypertrophy (LVH)**

      i) Maladaptive consequences include decrease in diastolic compliance, increase myocardial O_2 consumption, and a potential imbalance in myocardial O_2 supply and demand.

      ii) **Dependence on sinus rhythm**

         (1) Due to changes in diastolic function, atrial systole may account for up to 40% of left ventricular end-diastolic volume (LVEDV), rather than the 15% to 20% in a normal ventricle (5); loss of sinus rhythm can lead to rapid clinical deterioration.

      iii) **Diastolic dysfunction/diastolic CHF**

         (1) LVH eventually leads to poor LV compliance, which will necessitate a higher than normal LV filling pressure.

         (2) Thus with severe LVH, an elevated pulmonary wedge pressure does not indicate LV systolic dysfunction but rather LV diastolic dysfunction.

      iv) **Myocardial ischemic risks**

         (1) The major threat of LV hypertrophy is myocardial ischemia.

         (2) Myocardial O_2 consumption (demand) is elevated due to the presence of an enlarged ventricular mass and a high afterload (wall tension).

         (3) **There is a narrowing of the coronary perfusion pressure gradient due to poor ventricular compliance and an elevated LV end-diastolic pressure (LVEDP).**

Figure 54-1	Average Course of Valvular Aortic Stenosis in Adults

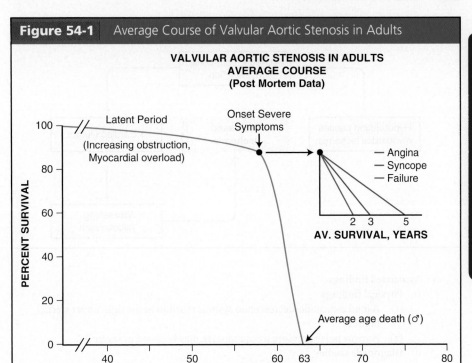

Data assembled from postmortem studies. Reproduced from Lester SJ, Heiboron B, Gin K, et al. The Natural History and Rate of Progression of Aortic Stenosis. *Chest* 1998;113:1109–1114, with permission.

Whether from vasodilation, hypovolemia, tachycardia or atrial fibrillation, all causes of hypotension need to be treated aggressively.

    (4)   Since coronary perfusion pressure is equivalent to diastolic blood pressure minus LVEDP, any systemic hypotension will also compromise an already tenuous balance of O_2 supply and demand in these patients.

    (5)   Hypertrophied hearts are much more sensitive to ischemic injury. They sustain larger infarcts and have a higher mortality rate than seen in hearts without hypertrophy (8).

  c) **"Death spiral"**

    i)   **In severe or critical AS, a precipitous drop in systemic blood pressure from any reason can lead to a vicious cycle of events (Fig. 54-2).**

    ii)   Chest compressions are often ineffective as it is difficult to generate enough mechanical force to create adequate stroke volume across the stenotic valve. Sudden death may result.

  5) **Signs and symptoms of AS**

    a) **Early stages**

      i)   During the early stages of AS, patients are asymptomatic due to adequate physiologic compensation, primarily through LV hypertrophy.

    b) **Intermediate and late stages**

      i)   AS takes years to progress to symptomatic impairment and LV failure. Ominous signs are atrial fibrillation, angina, syncope, and CHF.

      ii)   Sudden death is typically from ventricular fibrillation.

| **Figure 54-2** | Consequences of Decreased Arterial Blood Pressure in AS |

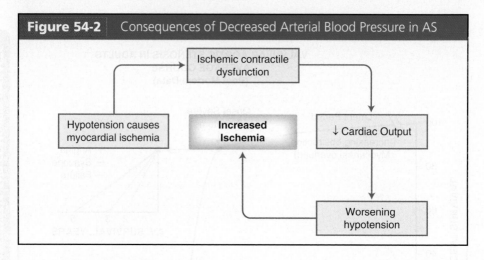

c) **Associated findings**
  i) **Physical findings**
    (1) A loud crescendo-decrescendo systolic murmur at the right upper sternal boarder
    (2) Narrow pulse pressure to <50 mm Hg may be noted in severe AS.
  ii) **Diagnostic studies**
    (1) CXR may show signs of pulmonary congestion and calcification of aortic cusp.
    (2) ECG frequently demonstrates LVH and occasionally atrial fibrillation.
    (3) Echocardiographic examination allows for a noninvasive assessment of the severity of stenosis and the adequacy of contractile function.
    (4) Coronary angiography will assess coexisting coronary artery disease.
6) **Surgical management**
  a) Except for antibiotic prophylaxis against infective endocarditis, there is no medical therapy to prevent disease progression. Treatment is surgical.
  b) **Aortic valve replacement (AVR)**
    i) AVR is the only effective treatment for symptomatic AS patients.
    ii) Averaged perioperative mortality is 3% to 4% for isolated AVR and 5.5% to 6.8% for combined AVR and coronary bypass surgery (CABG) (8).
    iii) Age alone is not a contraindication to surgery. Even in octogenarian, surgical prognosis is excellent in the absence of significant coexisting diseases (4).
  c) **Balloon valvotomy**
    i) Temporarily relieves symptoms but does not prolong survival (8).
    ii) Valvotomy is not an alternative to AVR. The rate of serious complication including death, stroke, aortic rupture, and AR exceeds 10% (4,8).
7) **Aortic regurgitation: etiology/natural history**
  a) AR results from the inability of the aortic leaflets to close tightly, which may be due to disease of the leaflets themselves and/or their supporting structures.
  b) **Acute AR**
    i) **Presentation is rare but dramatic**
    ii) Severe pulmonary congestion and hypotension refractory to medical management are the typical symptoms. Emergent valvular surgery is often required.
    iii) Causes include infective endocarditis, aortic dissection, or blunt chest trauma.
  c) **Chronic AR**

Table 54-2

General Parameters in Grading AR

Stages of AR	Mild	Moderate	Severe
Regurgitant fraction (%)	<30	30–50	>50–60
Estimated regurgitant orifice area (cm²)	<0.1	0.1–0.3	>0.3
Color Doppler jet width (as a % of LVOT)	<25	25–65	>65
Doppler vena contracta width (cm)	<0.3	0.3–0.6	>0.6

Adapted from Bonow RO, Carabello BA, Chatterjee K, et al. ACC/AHA 2006 guidelines for the management of patients with valvular heart disease: a report of the ACC/AHA Task Force on Practice Guidelines. *Circulation* 2006;114:e124–e150.

- i) Rheumatic heart disease is the leading cause of chronic AR with clinical presentation in the second or third decade of life (10). Patients tend to remain asymptomatic until late in their disease process, which may be 20+ years.
- ii) Common causes in developed countries are congenital bicuspid aortic valve, collagen vascular disease, Marfan syndrome, and idiopathic aortic root dilation, with presentation in their fourth to sixth decades of life (10).
- iii) Progression of asymptomatic AR to either symptomatic AR or LV dysfunction is on average <6%/y. Mortality is low (<0.2%/y) if asymptomatic with normal LV function (8).
- iv) I would like to put this sentence as a separate line item.
8) **Severity grading**: Doppler echocardiography is the mainstay for severity assessment in AR. General parameters for AR grading are listed on **Table 54-2**.
9) **Pathophysiology** (5–8,10,11)
   a) **Acute AR**
      - i) Sudden reflux of a large regurgitant volume back into the LV imposes a tremendous volume burden on the ventricle. LVEDP and left atrial pressure increase precipitously leading to abrupt pulmonary congestion.
      - ii) Severe systemic hypotension seen in acute AR is in distinct contrast to the systolic hypertension characteristic of chronic AR.
      - iii) Tachycardia, peripheral vasoconstriction, and increased myocardial contractility all strive to improve forward flow and are mediated through release of catecholamines.
      - iv) Myocardial ischemia and sudden death are common in acute AR.
   b) **Chronic AR**
      - i) **Volume overload**
         (1) The degree of volume overload is dependent on three factors: regurgitant orifice, pressure gradient across the AV and diastolic filling time.
         (2) Chronic volume load leads to LV dilation through eccentric hypertrophy.
         (3) A dilated LV results in high diastolic compliance thus allowing large increases in LVEDV with minimal elevation in filling pressure.
      - ii) **Pressure overload**
         (1) Ejection of a large total stroke volume creates an increased pulse pressure with systolic hypertension, which imposes an elevated pressure load on the ventricle.
         (2) According to Laplace law, LV dilation increases systolic wall tension and thus ventricular afterload (4, 8).
   c) **Decompensated AR**
      - i) Surgery is indicated prior to the development of LV dysfunction.

      ii) Progressive volume and pressure overload overcome the compensatory effect of LV hypertrophy leading to systolic dysfunction. Diastolic dysfunction is also common.

      iii) **Myocardial ischemic risks** (5,8,11)

         (1) Increased myocardial O_2 consumption occurs due to the presence of LV hypertrophy and an elevated wall tension.

         (2) Presence of low diastolic pressures results in low coronary perfusion pressure.

10) **Signs and Symptoms of AR**

  a) **Acute AR**

    i) Symptoms of severe cardiogenic shock: severe hypotension and pulmonary edema

    ii) Physical findings are minimal. Diastolic murmur, widened pulse pressure, cardiomegaly may be all missing

A widened pulse pressure is a common sign of AR, marked by high systolic and low diastolic pressures.

  b) **Chronic AR- Early Stages:**

    i) Asymptomatic

  c) **Chronic AR- Intermediate & Late Stages:**

    i) Symptoms generally appears when regurgitant volume is >60% of stroke volume

    ii) Fatigue, dyspnea on exertion, orthopnea and paroxysmal nocturnal dyspnea are common.

    iii) Angina portends a mortality >10%/y and CHF >20%/y (8).

11) **Findings (of chronic AR)**

  a) Classic decrescendo early diastolic murmur at upper left sternal boarder

  b) Bounding carotid pulse, head bobbing, and pulsation of the uvula

  c) With significant LV enlargement, S3 is present and the apical impulse may be displaced to the left.

12) **Diagnostic studies**

  a) CXR may show pulmonary congestion and cardiomegaly.

  b) Echocardiography is useful for classifying AR severity, assessing LV function and evaluating the mechanism for AR.

Table 54-3

New York Heart Association Classification of Cardiovascular Disease

- Class I
  - ➤ Patients with cardiac disease but no limitation to their physical activity No symptoms of cardiac decompensation (angina, palpitations, dyspnea, fatigue) occurs with activity.
- Class II
  - ➤ Patients who have mild limitations in physical activity due to cardiac disease. Patients are comfortable at rest but develop symptoms with mild to moderate exertion.
- Class III
  - ➤ Patients with marked impairment in physical activity due to cardiac disease. Typically asymptomatic at rest, but minimal exertion will result in symptoms of cardiac decompensation.
- Class IV
  - ➤ Patients with severe functional limitation with minimal exertion due to cardiac disease. These patients may also be symptomatic at rest.

NYHA Criteria: Adapted from: The Criteria Committee of the New York Heart Association. *Nomenclature and Criteria for Diagnosis of Diseases of the Heart and Great Vessels.* 9th ed. Boston, MA: Little Brown & Co., 1994:253–256.

    c) Cardiac catheterization may confirm echocardiography findings or diagnose coexisting coronary artery disease.

13) **Medical management versus surgical management**

    a) **Medical management**

        i) **Acute AR**

            (1) Nitroprusside and IV hydralazine have been shown to ↓ regurgitant volume, ↓ LVEDV, and improve ventricular function (8).

            (2) Inotropes such as dopamine, dobutamine, or milrinone may also be helpful in temporarily managing these acutely ill patients prior to valve surgery (8).

        ii) **Chronic AR**

            (1) Medical therapy is not an alternative to surgery.

            (2) Since patients remain clinically compensated for years, they can be safely followed for symptom onset, LV dilation, or LV dysfunction (8,11).

            (3) Long-term use of oral hydralazine and nifedipine in asymptomatic severe AR patients with normal LV function can potentially delay the need for surgery by several months to 2 years (4,8,11).

    b) **Surgical management**

        i) **Surgery** should not be delayed until symptom appearance.

        ii) **Indications for surgery**

            (1) **Symptomatic AR: Patients with severe symptoms (NYHA class III or IV) are at especially high risk with about 25%/y mortality rate without surgery. Even mild symptoms (class II) have a 6.3%/y mortality rate (10). (Table 54-3)**

            (2) **LV dysfunction: defined as EF < 55%**

            (3) **Marked LV enlargement: defined as end-systolic diameter >55 mm**

14) **Anesthetic implications (5-7)**

    a) **General hemodynamic goals for AS and AR are listed in Table 54-4.**

        i) **AS**

Use of venodilators such as nitroglycerin may seriously drop cardiac output in patients with AS.

            (1) **Heart rate/rhythm**

                (a) **Extremes of heart rate are not well tolerated.**

                (b) Goal is to maintain a low normal heart rate, giving time for adequate systolic ejection.

                (c) Maintaining sinus rhythm is crucial. Any dysrhythmia should be treated aggressively.

            (2) **Preload**

                (a) Poor ventricular compliance necessitates preload augmentation.

                (b) Serial cardiac output measurements during fluid augmentation can help find patient's optimal loading condition.

Table 54-4
Hemodynamic Management Goals in AV Disease

	Heart Rate	Preload	Afterload (SVR)	Contractility
AS Management	Sinus Low normal HR	↑	Normal to slightly elevated	Maintain
AR Management	↑	↑	↓	Maintain

"Fast, full and forward" is a useful phrase that summarizes the pertinent hemodynamic goals for AR.

(3) **Afterload**

(a) Preserving systemic vascular resistance (SVR) and adequate diastolic pressure are critical for coronary perfusion.

(b) A relatively fixed stroke volume exists in severe AS so severe changes in SVR are not tolerated. **Medications causing arterial dilation should be used cautiously.**

(c) Hypotension from any cause should be avoided

ii) **AR**

(1) **Heart rate/rhythm**

(a) Elevated heart rate (HR), (~80 to 90 bpm), improves forward flow by decreasing diastolic duration → ↓regurgitant volume, and ↑EF.

(b) Improved coronary perfusion is also seen with an elevated HR due to a higher mean diastolic pressure and a lower LVEDP (6,7).

(2) **Preload**

(a) Adequate preload is necessary to maintain forward flow. Often a fluid bolus of 250 to 500 mL of crystalloid or albumin is effective.

(3) **Afterload**

(a) Afterload reduction through peripheral arteriolar dilation improves forward flow by reducing ventricular stroke work. When initiating vasodilator therapy, additional preload is usually needed.

(4) **Contractility:** If ventricular systolic dysfunction is present, **consider** "inodilators" such as dobutamine or milrinone.

b) **Preoperative management**

i) Obtain a thorough history of symptoms and associated comorbidities.

ii) Recent studies evaluating AS/AR severity, adequacy of LV function and LV chamber size should be done prior to any surgery (cardiac or noncardiac).

iii) Symptomatic severe AS/AR are active cardiac conditions—all elective noncardiac surgeries should be deferred until valve replacement completed.

iv) In patients without heart failure, light premedication with a benzodiazepine is beneficial to blunt anxiety-induced tachycardia and its potential ischemic risk.

v) Prophylactic antibiotic against infective endocarditis should be given.

c) **Monitoring**

i) A 5-lead ECG will monitor for ischemia and arrhythmias.

READ MORE
Pulmonary artery catheter, Chapter 13, page 82

ii) **Intra arterial blood pressure monitoring, often placed prior to induction, is strongly recommended for moderate to severe lesions.**

iii) Pulmonary artery catheter (**PAC**) and/or transesophageal **echocardiography** use depends on the type of surgery and aortic valvular disease severity.

iv) Central venous pressure (CVP) and wedge pressure can both underestimate true LVEDP via different mechanisms (6).

(1) Severe AR may result in elevated LV diastolic filling, leading to mitral valve closure before end diastole → underestimation of LVEDP

(2) AS results in a thickened, stiff LV and resultant diastolic dysfunction. This decreased LV compliance is the most common cause of LVEDP underestimation by the PAC.

v) A risk of PAC insertion is arrhythmia-induced hypotension.

d) **Induction**
   i) **Table 54-4 outlines hemodynamic goals**
   ii) **Aortic stenosis**
      (1) A defibrillator should be readily available for immediate cardioversion if necessary.
      (2) **Regional anesthesia**
         (a) Neuraxial anesthesia is relatively contraindicated in severe AS due to concerns of sympathectomy-induced vasodilation.
         (b) If a neuraxial method is chosen, consider a more gradual onset of sympathetic blockade offered through an epidural rather than a spinal.
      (3) **General anesthesia**
         (a) Many clinicians prefer a heavier narcotic and benzodiazepine-based technique.
         (b) Volatile anesthetics are usually tolerated in moderate amounts.
   iii) **Aortic regurgitation**
      (1) **Regional anesthesia**
         (a) **Has a theoretical advantage in decreasing SVR and thus afterload**
         (b) Neuraxial anesthesia may also increase venous capacitance, which can severely decrease preload and cardiac output.
         (c) If a high block occurs due to local anesthetic blockade of cardiac accelerator fibers, bradycardia and reduced forward flow may result.
      (2) **General anesthesia**
         (a) Ketamine and pancuronium may be useful due to increased heart rate.

e) **Maintenance**
   i) Often accomplished via a combination of volatiles and narcotics
   ii) Blood loss must be promptly replaced in order to maintain adequate intravascular volume.
   iii) Atropine or glycopyrolate may be considered for the treatment of significant bradycardia or junctional rhythm, but used with extreme caution in AS because the goal HR is 70 to 80.
   iv) Hemodynamically significant arrhythmias should be treated with electrical cardioversion.
   v) **AS**
      (1) Treat intraoperative hypotension with α-adrenergic agonists such as phenylephrine.
      (2) Sinus tachycardia needs to be swiftly rate-controlled. Short-acting β-adrenergic antagonists such as esmolol may be administered with caution since it may adversely affect inotrope and stroke volume.
      (3) Lidocaine or amiodarone may be used to stabilize ventricular ectopy prior to its degeneration into ventricular fibrillation.
   vi) **AR**
      (1) Phenylephrine should be used cautiously, as this can elevate the regurgitant fraction. A mixed agonist such as ephedrine may be a better choice.
      (2) Intra-aortic balloon pump is contraindicated in AR patients since diastolic augmentation will worsen the regurgitant volume.

f) **Emergence**
   i) At the conclusion of surgery the decision to extubate will be dependent on the patient's baseline condition, intraoperative course, and type of surgery.
   ii) If extubation is deemed appropriate, preparation needs to be made to control the sympathetic activation that is inevitable with emergence.

Chapter Summary for Aortic Valvular Disease

	Aortic Stenosis	Aortic Regurgitation
General Considerations	Long latent period without symptoms/complications Onset of symptoms results in large increase in mortality—surgery is the only effective therapy.	Acute AR may present with severe hemodynamic instability. Emergent cardiac surgery is usually necessary Chronic AR imposes both components of pressure and volume overload on the left ventricle.
Indications for Surgery	Symptomatic severe AS Asymptomatic severe AS + reduced systolic function Moderate AS + CAD requiring heart surgery	Symptomatic AR LV dysfunction (EF<55%) Severe LV enlargement (end-systolic diameter >5.5 cm)
Anesthetic Management		
Preoperative	Complete cardiac history focusing on cardiac evaluative studies, current exercise tolerance, along with comorbid conditions. For noncardiac surgery—evidence of above indications should be sought and considered before elective procedures.	
Intraoperative (Hemodynamic Goals)	Aortic Stenosis	Aortic Regurgitation
	Maintain sinus rhythm and low normal heart rate Maintain normal intravascular volume Expect a higher than normal CVP/wedge Avoid hypotension Maintain adequate ventricular contractility	Maintain an elevated heart rate Preload augmentation Low-normal SVR Maintain contractility
Postoperative	For cardiac surgery—plan transport to ICU with goal to control blood pressure in normal range as patient emerges (reduce bleeding). For noncardiac surgery, emergence needs to focus on hemodynamic goals listed above.	
Monitoring	Arterial line, Central line ± PAC, +/- TEE	

CAD, coronary artery disease; CVP, central venous pressure; LV, left ventricle; PAC, pulmonary artery catheter; SVR, systemic vascular resistance; TEE, transesophageal echocardiography.

References

1. Singh, JP, Evans JC, Levy D, et al. Prevalence and clinical determinants of mitral, tricuspid, aortic regurgitation. *Am J Cardiol* 1999;83: 897–902.
2. Dujardin KS, Enriquez-Sarano M, Schaff HV, et al. Mortality and morbidity of aortic regurgitation in clinical practice: a long-term follow-up study. *Circulation* 1999;99:1851–1857.
3. Lester SJ, Heilbron B, Gin K, et al. The natural history and rate of progression of aortic stenosis. *Chest* 1998;113:1109–1114.
4. Carabello, BA, Crawford FA. Valvular heart disease. *N Engl J Med* 1997;337:32–41.
5. Cook DJ, Housmans, PR, Rehfeldt KH. Valvular heart disease: replacement and repair. In: Kaplan JA, Reich DL, Lake CL, eds. *Kaplan's Cardiac Anesthesia*. 5th ed. Elsevier Saunders; 2006:645–666.
6. Skubas N, Lichtman AD, Sharma A. et al, Anesthesia for cardiac surgery. In: Barash P, Cullen BF, Stoeling RK, eds. *Clinical Anesthesia*. 5th ed. Philadelphia, PA: Lippincott Williams & Wilkins; 2006:898–902.

7. Moore RA, Martin DE. Anesthetic Management for the treatment of Valvular Heart Disease. In: Hensley FA Jr, Martin DE, Gravlee GP, eds. *A Practical Approach to Cardiac Anesthesia*. 3rd ed. Philadelphia, PA: Lippincott Williams & Wilkins; 2003:302–309.
8. Bonow RO, Carabello BA Chatterjee K, et al. ACC/AHA 2006 Guidelines for the management of patients with valvular heart disease: a report of the ACC/AHA Task Force on Practice Guidelines. *Circulation* 2006;114:e84–e111.
9. Sidebotham D, Merry A, Legget M. Practical Perioperative Transoesophageal Echocardiography. *Butterworth-Heinemann*. Elsevier Limited,2003:131–170.
10. Enriquez-Sarano M, Tajik AJ. Aortic regurgitation. *N Engl J Med* 2004;351:1539–1545.
11. Bekeredjian R, Grayburn PA. Valvular heart disease-aortic regurgitation. *Circulation* 2005;112:125–134.
12. The Criteria Committee of the New York Heart Association. *Nomenclature and Criteria for Diagnosis of Diseases of the Heart and Great Vessels*. 9th ed. Boston, MA: Little, Brown & Co., Lippincott Williams & Wilkins; 1994:253–256.

ANESTHESIA AND COMORBID DISEASES

55

Mitral Valve Disease

Judy Thai, MD

Mitral valve (MV) is a bicuspid valve located between the left atrium and left ventricle. Mitral stenosis (MS), typically from rheumatic disease, is highly prevalent in developing countries and remains a substantial cause of morbidity worldwide. In the United States, chronic moderate to severe mitral regurgitation (MR) continues to be one of the most common valve lesions despite reduction in rheumatic fever (1). Both MS and MR are discussed sequentially in this chapter.

1) **Mitral stenosis**
   a) **Etiology**
      i) MS is typically rheumatic in origin, affecting women twice as often as men (1,2).
      ii) Isolated MS occurs in only 40% of all rheumatic heart disease. More often MS exists in combination with mitral or aortic regurgitation (2).
      iii) MS may occur as a result of severe annular calcification or complication after MV repair.

READ MORE

TEE evaluation of the mitral valve, Chapter 164, page 1136

   b) **Severity grading (Table 55-1).** Echocardiography is the primary diagnostic tool for grading MS. General parameters are listed in Table 55-1.

2) **Natural history**
   a) Rheumatic fever may cause chronic inflammatory valve injury.
   b) The progressive process of fibrosis, calcification, and fusion of the leaflets/subvalvular apparatus occur gradually over decades (2,3). Valve area narrows on average by 0.1 to 0.3 cm²/y (2,4).
   c) Symptoms rarely appear until the valve area decreases to <2.5 cm².

Table 55-1

Hemodynamic Parameters for MS

	Mean Pressure (mm Hg)	MV Area (cm²)	PHT (ms)
Normal	Negligible	4–6	
Mild	<5	1.5–2.5	<150
Moderate	5–10	1.0–1.5	150–220
Severe	>10	<1.0	>220

PHT, pressure half-time, which measures the rate of pressure decline across MV (an echocardiography parameter).
Adapted from Bonow RO, Carabello BA, Chatterjee K, et al. ACC/AHA 2006 guidelines for the management of patients with valvular heart disease: a report of the ACC/AHA task force on practice guidelines. *Circulation* 2006;114:e124–e150.

    i)   Valve area >1.5 cm², symptoms may occur with provocation such as with atrial fibrillation, or conditions that increase blood flow (pregnancy, exercise, infection) (3).

    ii)   Valve area <1.5 cm², symptoms may occur at rest or with minimal exertion (4).

  d) Survival correlates with symptom severity (2,3) (Table 54-3).

    i)   NYHA classes I and II have a 10-year survival of about 80%, with 60% of these patients demonstrating no progression in symptoms.

    ii)   NYHA classes III and IV have a 10-year survival as low as 15%.

    iii)   Presence of severe pulmonary hypertension (HTN), mean survival drops to <3 years.

3) **Pathophysiology**

  a) **Left atrial pressure (LAP) overload**

    i)   Progressive narrowing of the mitral orifice eventually causes an increase in LAP, LAP overload, and LA enlargement (2,3).

READ MORE
Pulmonary hypertension, Chapter 62, page 447

    ii)   ↑LAP transmitted to the lung can lead to pulmonary edema (3). If the increase in pulmonary venous pressure is gradual, compensatory increase in lymphatic drainage can enable patients to remain minimally symptomatic for a period of time (4).

    iii)   Pulmonary arterioles may react to chronic elevation in pulmonary venous pressure with vasoconstriction and hypertrophy (2,3). The resultant pulmonary arterial hypertension can translate to right ventricular (RV) pressure overload.

  b) **Right and left ventricular consequences**

    i)   RV is ultimately responsible for driving blood through the stenotic MV. Compensatory RV hypertrophy develops.

    ii)   The RV may dilate and fail in later stages of MS resulting in signs of peripheral congestion (i.e., ascites, peripheral edema) (5).

    iii)   LV is protected from volume and pressure overload because it is chronically underfilled.

    iv)   Poor LV filling leads to poor cardiac output. The combination of pulmonary congestion and limited LV output mimics LV systolic failure despite normal LV contractile function (1–3).

    v)   Although still controversial, it appears that about one third of MS patients have load-independent LV contractile dysfunction (1,3–6)

  c) **Special circumstances**

    i)   Severity of pressure gradient across a valve is dependent on both the valve orifice and its transvalvular blood flow.

    ii)   Any conditions that increase cardiac demand can significantly increase transvalvular gradient and worsen symptoms (2,3). Examples of such conditions are atrial fibrillation, pregnancy, fever, infection, and anemia (1–4).

4) **Signs and symptoms**

  a) Initial presentations are typically that of "LV failure" (dyspnea on exertion, orthopnea, paroxysmal nocturnal dyspnea). Occasionally, an embolic event is the first presenting symptom, which is often related to atrial fibrillation (4).

  b) Rarely, hemoptysis occurs as a result of high pulmonary venous pressure. Hoarse voice may appear secondary to an enlarged LA impinging on the recurrent laryngeal nerve (6).

  c) At the terminal stage, RV failure results in ascites and peripheral edema (7).

  d) **Physical findings**

     i) There is classically an opening snap followed by a rumbling diastolic murmur.

     ii) Narrowed pulse pressure is present when stroke volume is reduced (6).

     iii) RV hypertrophy may be palpated as a heave at the left sternal border. With RV dysfunction, JVD, ascites, hepatomegaly, and peripheral edema may be present.

     iv) ECG commonly shows LA enlargement, atrial fibrillation, and RV hypertrophy.

     v) CXR may reveal pulmonary congestion and enlarged left atrium.

5) Medical management versus surgical management

  a) **Medical management**

     i) All patients with MS require appropriate antibiotic prophylaxis against recurrent rheumatic fever and infective endocarditis (6).

     ii) Anticoagulation in patients with MS and atrial fibrillation is paramount (6).

     iii) **Once significant symptoms develop, the only effective treatment is surgical relief of the mechanical obstruction caused by MS (2).**

  b) **Percutaneous balloon valvotomy (PBV)**

     i) Unlike aortic stenosis, most MS cases can be successfully treated with PBV. This technique is as effective as surgical valvotomy in patients with favorable valve anatomy (2).

     ii) Favorable mitral anatomy includes noncalcified pliable valves, no calcium in the commissures and mild subvalvular pathology (2,6).

     iii) Contraindications to PBV are significant MR, LA thrombus, and clinically significant tricuspid regurgitation (2,6).

     iv) Immediate postvalvotomy hemodynamic improvement is predictive of long-term clinical outcome. Generally, immediate results include doubling of the MV area and a 50% reduction in transmitral gradient (2).

  c) **Surgical management**

     i) Patients presenting for surgical correction are those who are poor PBV candidates.

     ii) Operative risk for mitral valve replacement (MVR) may be 3% to 8% in the absence of pulmonary HTN and other comorbidities (2,6). In older patients with severe symptoms, perioperative mortality may be as high as 10% to 20% (2).

6) **Anesthetic implications**

  a) **General hemodynamic goals for MS** (Table 55-2)

     i) **Heart rate/rhythm**

       (1) Primary goal should be the prevention and treatment of tachycardia. A rapid heart rate shortens diastolic filling time and worsens transvalvular gradient (3).

       (2) The most detrimental component of atrial fibrillation is the presence of an elevated ventricular rate rather than the loss of atrial kick (3). Thus, rate control is the primary concern.

       (3) Excessive bradycardia is also undesirable as MS creates a relatively fixed stroke volume (5).

     ii) **Preload**

Table 55-2

Hemodynamic Goals for MV Lesions

	Heart Rate	Preload	Afterload (SVR)	RV and LV Contractility	PVR
MS management	↓	↑	↑	Maintain	↓
MR management	↑	↑	↓	Maintain	↓

Prevention and treatment of tachycardia is the primary goal in anesthetic management of patients with MS.

Hypoxia, hypercapnia, acidosis, hypothermia, pain (sympathetic activation) increase PVR and should be avoided in both MS and MR.

(1) Another important goal is to maintain adequate preload without exacerbating pulmonary edema, pulmonary HTN, or precipitating RV failure.

(2) Pulmonary artery catheter (PAC) can aid fluid management. Pulmonary capillary wedge pressure and pulmonary artery (PA) diastolic pressures will both overestimate LV filling. Thus, it is more important to monitor PAC trends and responses to interventions (3).

iii) **Afterload (SVR)**

(1) As a result of limited cardiac output, preserving an elevated SVR is necessary to avoid hypotension.

iv) **Contractility**

(1) Adequate cardiac output is dependent on both adequate RV and LV contractility. Inotropic support may be necessary.

v) **Pulmonary vascular resistance (PVR)**

(1) Pulmonary HTN is frequently present in MS patients. The RV may be quite sensitive to increases in PA pressure; diligent avoidance of factors that increase PVR is necessary (2).

b) **Preoperative management**

i) Obtain a thorough history of symptoms, associated comorbidities, valve lesion severity, and adequacy of LV/RV function.

ii) Mild premedication to prevent anxiety-induced tachycardia may be necessary. Caution must be taken not to cause excessive sedation, which may result in hypoxia or hypercapnia with worsening pulmonary HTN.

iii) Supplemental O_2 should be given with any premedication.

iv) Prophylactic antibiotic against infective endocarditis should be given.

v) Maintain patient's antiarrthymics and nodal blockers up to the day of surgery.

c) **Monitoring**

i) **Invasive monitoring, including arterial line, PAC,** and/or **transesophageal echocardiography** are invaluable in assessing volume status, LV filling, and biventricular function.

d) **Induction**

i) General anesthesia is preferred over regional approaches as MS patients cannot tolerate sudden decreases in SVR.

ii) Choose an induction agent that maintains hemodynamic goals listed on Table 55-2.

iii) Tachycardia must be treated aggressively with medication or cardioversion (for tachydysrhythmias).

e) **Maintenance**

i) Meticulous attention to CO_2 and pH management should be taken to avoid aggravating preexisting pulmonary HTN.

ii) Blood loss must be diligently replaced to maintain volume status and cardiac output.

iii) Maintain an adequate level of anesthesia. Light anesthesia can trigger sympathetic activation with a resultant ↑SVR, ↑PVR and worsen cardiac output.

f) **Postoperative management**

i) See section 13e of this chapter for general postoperative considerations.

Table 55-3

General Parameters in Grading MR

	Mild	Moderate	Severe
Regurgitant fraction (%)	<30	30–50	>50
Estimated regurgitant orifice area (cm²)	<0.2	0.2–0.4	>0.4
Doppler vena contracta width (cm)	<0.3	0.3–0.6	>0.6
Associated findings			LAE, LVE

LAE, left atrial enlargement; LVE, left ventricular enlargement.
Adapted from Bonow RO, Carabello BA, Chatterjee K, et al. ACC/AHA 2006 guidelines for the management of patients with valvular heart disease: a report of the ACC/AHA task force on practice guidelines. *Circulation* 2006;114:e124–e150.

7) **Mitral regurgitation**
   a) **Etiology**
      i) MR may result from any process that distorts the mitral leaflets, chordae tendineae, papillary muscles, valve annulus, or LV geometry.
      ii) MR maybe classified as organic or functional.
      iii) The most common cause of organic MR is MV prolapse. Others include rheumatic heart disease, mitral annular calcification, endocarditis, and connective tissue disorders (i.e., Marfan or Ehlers-Danlos) (2,3).
      iv) Functional MR
         (1) Refers to MR, which occurs despite normal mitral leaflets and chordal structures.
         (2) Often occurs from ischemic heart disease or dilated cardiomyopathy where distortion in LV geometry or mitral annulus prevents adequate mitral leaflets coaptation. Rarely, functional MR is secondary to papillary muscle rupture (2,3).
   b) **Severity grading (Table 55-3)**
      i) Echocardiography is the primary tool for assessing MR severity.

8) **Natural history**
   a) **Acute MR**
      i) Acute severe MR may occur rarely as a result of rupture papillary muscle, rupture major chordae tendineae, or endocarditis.
      ii) Cardiogenic shock may develop rapidly, necessitating emergent cardiac surgery.
   b) **Chronic MR**
      i) MR tends to be a progressive process.
      ii) Regurgitant volume over time causes atrial and ventricular enlargement and annular dilatation, which in turn increases the regurgitant orifice and thus worsens MR.
      iii) MR progression has a variable time course (3).
         (1) **Predictors of increased mortality are the presence of severe MR, NYHA III-IV symptoms, or reduced LV function (defined as EF < 60% or LVEDV > 40 mm) (2,7).**
      iv) Once severe symptomatic MR develops, the average mortality rate is ~5%/y (7).
      v) Prognosis for functional/ischemic MR is quite different from that of organic MR. In general, functional MR has a worse outcome even when MR severity is only mild. This is due to its underlying pathology of ischemic cardiomyopathy (2,8).

9) **Pathophysiology**
   a) **Acute MR**

LV ejection fraction <60% implies overt LV dysfunction in patients with MR.

i) Sudden large volume overload into an uncompensated LA and LV can cause severe pressure increase in both chambers with resultant florid pulmonary edema.

ii) Volume overload increases LV preload and thus allows for a modest increase in LV stroke volume via the Frank-Starling mechanism. However, this is inadequate to maintain normal forward flow in the presence of significant regurgitation and the absence of LV dilation (2,7).

iii) Clinical presentation is that of left-sided heart failure (HF) despite myocardial function being normal or even hyperdynamic due to sympathetic activation.

b) **Chronic MR**

  i) **Volume overload**

    (1) MR results in both ventricular and atrial volume overload.

    (2) Compensatory LA and LV enlargement via **eccentric hypertrophy** permits accommodation of regurgitant volume without significant increases in filling pressures.

    (3) Promoted by LA enlargement, as many as 75% of MR patients develop chronic atrial fibrillation (5).

  ii) **LV and RV consequences**

    (1) The left ventricular volume in MR favors LV ejection as preload is increased while afterload remains normal to low. Thus a "supra-normal" ejection fraction is expected with normal myocardial function (2,7).

    (2) Prolonged volume overload eventually leads to LV dysfunction (2).

    (3) LV ejection fraction (EF) <60% implies overt LV dysfunction (2).

    (4) Development of LV dysfunction often initiates a vicious cycle of decline (8) (Fig. 55-1)

    (5) With declining LV function, forward stroke volume decreases and filling pressures rise. Elevated pressures transmitted to the pulmonary and right-sided system can eventually result in pulmonary edema, pulmonary HTN, and RV failure.

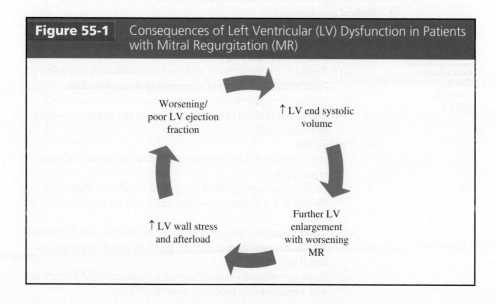

Figure 55-1 Consequences of Left Ventricular (LV) Dysfunction in Patients with Mitral Regurgitation (MR)

Worsening/ poor LV ejection fraction

↑ LV end systolic volume

Further LV enlargement with worsening MR

↑ LV wall stress and afterload

10) **Signs and symptoms**

   a) **Acute MR**

READ MORE

Heart failure, Chapter 60, page 436

      i)   Patients with acute severe MR are almost always severely symptomatic with significant HF symptoms

      ii) Physical findings may be minimal. Diastolic murmur may be short and soft or even absent because of rapid equalization of pressures between LA and LV. A third heard sound (S$_3$) may be the only physical finding (2).

   b) **Chronic MR**

      i)   **Early Stages**

         (1) Slow onset of MR allows compensatory mechanisms to develop, which enables patients to remain asymptomatic with minimal activity limitation.

      ii) **Intermediate and Late Stages**

         (1) Initial symptoms may be that of easy fatigability (5).

         (2) Regurgitant fraction <60% generally causes HF symptoms (5).

         (3) Presence of pulmonary HTN and RV dysfunction indicate advanced disease with poor prognosis (2). Patients with severe MR can progress into a decompensated stage of irreversible LV dysfunction without symptoms (2).

      iii) **Physical findings**

         (1) Classical findings are apical holosystolic murmur that radiates to the axilla, a third heart sound, and a displaced apical pulse.

      iv) **Studies**

         (1) ECG may show left atrial enlargement and atrial fibrillation.

         (2) CXR: cardiomegaly, prominent pulmonary vessels, pulmonary edema

         (3) Echocardiography allows accurate assessment of MR severity and mechanism.

         (4) Cardiac catheterization is indicated if there is inconsistency between clinical and echocardiographic findings or if coronary artery disease is a concern.

11) **Medical management versus surgical management**

   a) **Medical management**

      i)   **Acute MR**

READ MORE

Aortic valvular disease, Chapter 54, page 383

         (1) Medical therapy may help stabilize hemodynamics prior to emergent cardiac surgery.

         (2) If patient is normotensive, infusion of vasodilators may help improve forward flow while decreasing regurgitant flow.

         (3) Patients are typically hypotensive, so use of an intraaortic balloon pump (IABP) can decrease afterload and support coronary perfusion (2,8).

      ii) **Chronic MR**

         (1) Medical therapy does not change the disease course of chronic organic MR (2).

         (2) Unlike aortic regurgitation, long-term vasodilator therapy in chronic MR is ineffective as afterload is already normal to low (2,8).

         (3) Vasodilators may improve symptoms in patients with functional MR where preload reduction can promote better coaptation of mitral leaflets.

         (4) Yearly surveillance echocardiogram is recommended for patients with asymptomatic moderate to severe MR (2).

b) Surgical Management is the only approach with noted clinical success (7).

    i) Surgical options for MR are MV repair versus MV replacement.

    ii) Compared to replacement, MV repair yields improved hemodynamics and ventricular function, avoids the risks of prosthesis, and avoids long-term anticoagulation (2,7,8).

    iii) Reoperation rate is similar for both MV repair and replacement (7% to 10% at 10 years).

    iv) General indications for MV surgery are symptomatic severe MR, LV dysfunction (EF < 60%), or LV dilation (LVESV > 40 mm) (2,7).

    v) Well-timed surgical correction can restore MR patients' life expectancy back to that of the general population. If surgery is delayed and patient develops significant CHF symptoms NYHA III-IV or EF < 50%. Surgical correction at this point may not be able to reverse the LV dysfunction, but it should prevent further deterioration (2,8).

Anesthetic management for patients with MR should optimize forward flow.

12) Anesthetic implications

a) **General hemodynamic goals for MR (Table 55-2)**

    i) **Heart rate/rhythm**

        (1) Bradycardia should be avoided.

        (2) Increased diastolic filling time may cause LV distention and worsen MR

Slow heart rate increases diastolic time and increased LV filling, which may cause LV distention and worsen MR.

    ii) **Preload**

        (1) Maintaining adequate preload is essential for adequate forward flow.

        (2) However, excessive fluid administration may dilate both LV and mitral annulus and worsen MR and pulmonary congestion.

        (3) Preload optimization should be guided by a PA catheter ± echocardiography.

    iii) **Afterload**

        (1) Decreasing SVR should facilitate forward flow.

        (2) Avoid sudden increases in SVR, which can worsen MR and cause LV decompensation.

    iv) **Contractility**

        (1) Maintain biventricular contractility for adequate cardiac output.

        (2) In MR patients, a "supranormal" EF is expected.

        (3) If EF declines to a "low normal" level (i.e., EF < 60%), recognize this already represents LV dysfunction and inotropic support may need to be implemented.

    v) **Pulmonary vascular resistance**

        (1) Most patients with long-standing severe MR will have some degree of pulmonary HTN.

        (2) **Factors to avoid include hypoxia, hypercapnia, acidosis, hypothermia, pain (sympathetic activation) (7).**

13) Anesthetic considerations

a) **Preoperative considerations**

    i) Premedication with benzodiazapines may be helpful in preventing anxiety-induced elevation in SVR and PVR.

    ii) Premedication should be given carefully as oversedation can worsen pulmonary HTN.

    iii) Prophylactic antibiotic against infective endocarditis is recommended.

b) **Monitoring**

    i) Standard ASA monitors, 5-lead ECG, **arterial line**, **PAC**, and transesophageal **echocardiography** are useful intraoperative monitors especially in patients with severe MR and LV dysfunction.

c) **Induction**

    i) Regional anesthesia may have a theoretical advantage due to reduction in afterload, thus promoting forward flow, but its abrupt onset and its potential compromise on preload detract from its use.

    ii) For general anesthesia, any induction agent may be used if it maintains the overall hemodynamic goals listed in **Table 55-2**.

        (1) Ketamine and pancuronium may be beneficial agents due to their ability to increase heart rate.

d) **Maintenance**

    i) As adequate preload is vital, diligent maintenance of intravascular volume is necessary. Thus, replace blood loss promptly.

    ii) Correlate end-tidal CO_2 with arterial blood gas to maintain near normal $PaCO_2$ to prevent aggravating pulmonary HTN.

    iii) If LV and/or RV dysfunction is present, consider inotropic support from agents such as milrinone or dobutamine.

    iv) If an inodilator cannot be tolerated, consider dopamine or even epinephrine. Caution with excessive use of α-constrictor, which can cause LV decompensation.

    v) If patient remains unstable despite maximal medical therapy, consider IABP

e) **Postoperative management**

    i) Cardiac surgery

        (1) Most patients will be admitted to the intensive care unit (ICU) on the ventilator with anticipation of emergence and extubation over the next few hours.

        (2) Vital signs may be variable depending on patient's baseline function, intraoperative course and the degree of inotropic support needed.

        (3) Blood pressure should be kept to a safe minimum to reduce postoperative bleeding with consideration given to any preexisting hypertension.

        (4) Ensure adequate reversal of protamine and normalization of coagulation parameters

        (5) Ensure ABG is in normal range and the hemoglobin levels are adequate (>8 g/dL)

        (6) TEE can be invaluable in assessing adequacy of mitral repair/replacement, cardiac function and further tailoring intropic requirements.

    ii) Noncardiac surgery

        (1) Management should be based on degree of preoperative disease.

        (2) All of the above hemodynamic considerations should be applied to emergence and the postoperative period.

ANESTHESIA AND COMORBID DISEASES

Chapter Summary for MV Disease

	Mitral Stenosis	Mitral Regurgitation
General Considerations	Primarily the result of rheumatic heart disease. Slow progressive disease taking decades for symptom onset. Survival correlates with symptom severity. Can be effectively treated with balloon valvuloplasty in certain cases	Acute MR is poorly tolerated and usually results in cardiogenic shock. Chronic severe MR may progress into irreversible LV dysfunction without symptoms. Mitral repair preferable to replacement
Indications for Surgery	Severe MS (valve area < 1.0 cm²) Moderate MS (valve area <1.5 cm²) + HF symptoms Poor balloon valvuloplasty candidate	Symptomatic severe MR LV dysfunction (EF < 60%) LV dilation (LVEDV > 40mm) **Only surgical correction has any documented survival benefit.**

Anesthetic Management

Preoperative	Complete cardiac history focusing on cardiac evaluative studies, current exercise tolerance, along with comorbid conditions. For noncardiac surgery—evidence of above indications should be sought and considered before elective procedures.	
Intraoperative (Hemodynamic Goals)	Control heart rate. Aggressively prevent tachycardia Maintain adequate preload. Avoid factors that may aggravate pulmonary HTN Maintain an elevated SVR Maintain contractility	Maintain an elevated heart rate Preload augmentation Avoid factors that elevate PVR Lower SVR/avoid sudden increase in SVR Maintain contractility
Postoperative	For cardiac surgery—plan transport to ICU with goal to control blood pressure in normal range as patient emerges (reduce bleeding). For noncardiac surgery, emergence needs to focus on hemodynamic goals listed above.	
Monitoring	Arterial line, central line ± PAC, +/− TEE	

LV, left ventricle; SVR, systemic vascular resistance; EF, ejection fraction; PAC, pulmonary artery catheter; TEE, transesophageal echocardiography.

References

1. Carabello BA, Crawford FA. Valvular heart disease. *N Engl J Med* 1997;337:32–41.
2. Bonow RO, Carabello BA, Chatterjee K, et al. ACC/AHA 2006 Guidelines for the management of patients with valvular heart disease: a report of the ACC/AHA Task Force on Practice Guidelines. *Circulation* 2006;114:e124–e150.
3. Cook DJ, Housmans, PR, Rehfeldt KH. Valvular heart disease: replacement and repair. In: Kaplan JA, Reich DL, Lake CL, eds. Kaplan's Cardiac Anesthesia. 5th ed. Elsevier Saunders; 2006:670–678.
4. Chandrashekhar Y, Westaby S, Narula J. Mitral stenosis. *Lancet* 2009;374:1271–1283.
5. Hensley FA Jr, Martin DE, Gravlee GP. A practical approach to cardiac anesthesia. In: Moore RA, Martin DE, eds. *Anesthetic Management for the Treatment of Valvular Heart Disease*. 3rd ed. Philadelphia, PA: Lippincott Williams & Wilkins; 2003:313–323.
6. Carabello BA. Modern management of mitral stenosis. *Circulation* 2005;112:432–437.
7. Enriquez-Sarano M, Akins CW, Vahanian A. Mitral regurgitation. *Lancet* 2009;373:1382–1394.
8. Carabello, BA. Progress in mitral and aortic regurgitation. *Prog Cardiovasc Dis* 2001;43:457–475.
9. Sidebotham D, Merry A, Legget M. *Practical Perioperative Transoesophageal Echocardiography*. Butterworth-Heinemann. Elsevier Limited, 2003:131–170.

56 Ventricular Assist Devices

Benjamin Kratzert, MD • Charles Hill, MD

Ventricular assist devices (VADs) are pumps that can partially or fully take over the function of the ventricles of the heart. Mechanical ventricular support has become an increasingly employed adjunct in the medical treatment of acute cardiogenic shock, as well as short- and long-term support of the patient awaiting orthotopic heart transplantation. Devices exist for left, right, and biventricular support. With rapidly improving technology and an increasing number of long-term VADs in use, the need to provide care to the stable VAD patient undergoing elective or semielective surgery will continue to grow. This chapter focuses on the anatomy, physiology, and perioperative management of short- and long-term VADs.

1) VAD indications

a) **Short-term support** (1)

   i) Short-term VADs are being used as a bridge-to-recovery in patients with conditions expected to improve over time, such as acute viral myocarditis, acute cardiogenic shock, postcardiotomy cardiogenic shock, and left ventricular assist device (LVAD)-associated right ventricular (RV) failure.

   ii) These devices are extracorporeal (pump is located outside the body), less technically difficult to implant, and less operator-dependent.

   iii) Cumbersome external control and power components and require the patient to be hospitalized.

   iv) Short-term devices may be placed percutaneously or via thoracotomy with direct cannulation of the heart.

   v) If the ventricle does not recover, these devices become the bridge-to-bridge and need to be replaced by a long-term device.

2) **Long term support** (1)

   a) VAD therapy as a bridge-to-heart transplantation has marked survival benefits and improvement in quality of life in end-stage heart failure.

   b) Additionally, improvements in size, durability, and mobility are leading to an increase in the use of the VAD as destination therapy.

   c) Most of these devices are intracorporeal (pump implanted in pre-peritoneal cavity). The only extracorporeal component is the subcutaneously tunneled driveline that connects to a control device and a wearable battery (Table 56-1).

3) **VAD anatomy.** The mechanical principles of all devices are similar and consist of the following parts.

   a) **Cannulas**

   i) The inflow and outflow cannulas, most commonly placed in the LV apex and the ascending aorta, respectively, bring blood from the heart into the pumping chamber of the device and back into the systemic circulation.

Table 56-1
Commonly Used VADs

Location		Device	Type	SV/rpm	Maximum Flow	Anti-Coagulation
Short term	External	ABIOMED BVS	Pulsatile	80 mL	6 l/min	Yes
		THORATEC PVAD	Pulsatile	65 mL	7 l/min	Yes
	Internal	THORATEC CENTRIMAG	Continuous	1,500–5,500 rpm	10 l/min	Yes
		IMPELLA	Continuous	10,000–50,000 rpm	2.5/5 l/min	No
Long term	Internal	THORATEC IVAD	Pulsatile	65 mL	7 l/min	Yes
		HEARTMATE I	Pulsatile	85 mL	10 l/min	No
		NOVACOR LVAS	Pulsatile	65 mL	12 l/min	Yes
		ABIOMED AB5000	Pulsatile	80 mL	6 l/min	Yes
		DEBAKEY VAD	Continuous	7,000–12,000 rpm	5.5 l/min	Yes
		JARVIK 2000	Continuous	8,000–12,000 rpm	5.5 l/min	Yes
		HEARTMATE II	Continuous	6,000–15,000	10 l/min	Yes

rpm, revolutions per minute; SV, stroke volume.

It is important to differentiate between pulsatile and nonpulsatile flow devices.

RV failure can be catastrophic as there is not adequate filling pressure for the LVAD pump.

b) **Flow generating chamber**

    i) Consists of either pusher plates or a diaphragm to create pulsatile flow; in an axial flow device, a rotating impeller provides continuous nonpulsatile blood flow.

c) **External parts**

    i) The pumping chamber connects via a driveline to external controls/power source.

4) VAD histology (2)

    a) A VAD is a mechanical pump, which depends on adequate filling. A left VAD therefore relies on the native right ventricle to pump venous blood through the lungs and into the left heart circulation.

    b) Most second- and third-generation VADs are now nonpulsatile continuous flow devices with the advantage of higher durability, smaller size, decreased disruption of RV function, and increased long-term hemodynamic stability.

    c) **Pulsatile devices**

        i) Pulsatile devices function similarly to the native ventricle by filling the pumping chamber and emptying it sequentially

ii) This action is independent of the native cardiac rate and rhythm.

iii) In most pulsatile devices, the pump chamber will fill with gravity, which makes adequate left ventricular preload of paramount importance.

iv) Two modes of operation exist for these pulsatile pumps.

    (1) **"Fill-to-empty"** (automatic) mode

        (a) Most commonly used.

        (b) Ejection occurs each time the control unit senses the blood chamber being nearly full.

        (c) While providing a constant device stroke volume, the cycling time of the device (i.e. the device "heart rate") changes with fluctuating VAD preload.

    (2) **"Asynchronous"** (fixed) mode

        (a) Used mainly when initiating VAD support and during states of fluctuating preload

        (b) Filling-emptying cycle remains constant resulting in variable device stroke volume.

        (c) Only very high increases in afterload impair emptying of the device, therefore cardiac output (CO) is mainly dependent on VAD preload.

v) Devices are either pneumatically or electronically powered.

    (1) In case of control unit or power source failure, all devices capable of pneumatic powering can be manually powered using a handheld pneumatic pump.

d) **Continuous (axial) flow devices**

i) Continuous flow devices function by axial or centrifugal flow.

ii) Driven by a centrally rotating propeller, blood is accelerated through the device into the systemic circulation.

iii) Nonpulsatile flow may be adjusted by changing the device rotation speed given in revolutions per minute (rpm). As flow rates are increased, so is the amount of support.

iv) Ventricular function is indicated by the pulsatility seen on the arterial line tracing, as well as the pulsatility index in some devices.

v) Axial flow devices will cycle off 8 to 10 seconds per minute to allow ejection through the aortic valve and movement of blood antegrade through the aortic root.

vi) **Continuous flow devices are dependent on preload as well as afterload.** While the LV cavity does not need to be as filled as in pulsatile devices, hypovolemia and cannula malposition will cause decrease in device output.

vii) Increased afterload has a slowing effect on forward flow and can impair output.

5) **Perioperative approach to the patient with a VAD (3)**

a) **Preoperative evaluation** should be a systematic evaluation for any major organ system dysfunction.

i) **Neurologic**

    (1) With increased risk of thromboembolic events and hypoperfusion, a comprehensive baseline neurologic exam should be obtained.

ii) **Pulmonary**

    (1) Signs of pulmonary congestion on preoperative exam can indicate possible device malfunction with suboptimal drainage of the left cardiac chamber by the LVAD.

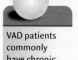

VAD patients commonly have chronic systemic disease secondary to long standing heart failure.

iii) **Cardiovascular**
  (1) Evaluate for symptoms and signs of LV and RV failure.
  (2) Backward failure with pulmonary edema, elevated JVD, hepatosplenomegaly, and pedal edema, or forward failure, with hypoperfusion and worsening end-organ function, could be signs of suboptimal device function.
  (3) The presence of intracardiac or device-associated thrombi should be assessed as these patients are at significant risk for intraoperative cerebrovascular accidents, ischemic bowel, and vasoocclusive damage to the peripheral vasculature.
  (4) Assessment of RV contractility and volume status is critically important, as this represents the ability to fill the left VAD in cases of left ventricular support.

iv) **Hematologic**
  (1) Patients are at increased risk of perioperative bleeding.
  (2) Mechanical destruction of cells leads to anemia and thrombocytopenia.
  (3) Hepatic and splenic congestion, chronic renal dysfunction, and poor nutritional status all lead to impairment of the coagulation cascade.
  (4) Systemic anticoagulation is required with the use of VADs to prevent thrombus formation.
    (a) Anticoagulation with warfarin should be held with a transition to heparin infusion.

v) **Endocrine**
  (1) In patients with chronic illness, on preoperative steroids, or exhibiting insensitivity to vasopressor agents, stress dose steroids should be considered.

vi) **Gastrointestinal**
  (1) VAD patients should be considered a "full stomach," secondary to the intraperitoneal or preperitoneal placement of the assist device.

vii) **Hepatic**
  (1) Chronic heart failure can cause hepatic congestion with impaired synthetic function, most commonly exhibited by mild coagulopathy and hypoalbuminemia.
  (2) Patients are at high risk for intraoperative and postoperative hepatic dysfunction.

viii) **Renal**
  (1) Chronic low cardiac output states lead to chronic kidney disease with electrolyte imbalances, platelet dysfunction, and hypervolemia.

6) **Anesthetic management (4) (Table 56-2)**
  a) **VAD coordination**
    i) Preoperative coordination with the LVAD team is imperative.

In a patient with a VAD, careful transportation and positioning is crucial to avoid kinking of cannulas, hemodynamic instability, and interruption of power supply.

      (1) The cardiothoracic surgery team, perfusionists and cardiac anesthesiologist, should all be aware of the case and available in the event of an emergency.
      (2) LVAD-trained nursing personnel should be available at all times.
      (3) Careful transport and positioning is imperative.
      (4) Adequate device battery life and power supply in the OR must be guaranteed.
      (5) Anticoagulation with warfarin should be held prior to surgery, with a transition to heparin infusion to maintain therapeutic levels of anticoagulation.
      (6) Availability of blood products should be assured prior to incision.
      (7) With the risk of VAD infection, care should be taken to minimize contamination.

Table 56-2
Preoperative Checklist

✓ VAD team notified and emergency contact available
✓ VAD-trained nursing personnel available
✓ Anticoagulation management discussed
✓ Plan for transport discussed with OR personnel
✓ Adequate perioperative power supply assured
✓ Defibrillator in the OR
✓ Emergency drugs available
✓ Blood products available
✓ Adequate vascular access and monitoring
✓ Place electric cautery away from device
✓ VAD in "asynchronous" mode

b) **Device management**
   i) Optimization of device function is important for hemodynamic stability.
   ii) Electromagnetic interference should be avoided.
   iii) The device should be set to "asynchronous" mode to simplify the variables affecting hemodynamic management during the case.
   iv) Bipolar cautery should be used and the grounding pad placed away from the VAD.
   v) The VAD device console should be clearly visible and in close proximity.

c) **Monitoring**
   i) Type and extent of surgery determine the need for invasive intraoperative monitoring.
   ii) In patients with continuous flow VADs, an arterial line is needed to adequately assess blood pressure.
   iii) Central venous access to monitor CVP and/or pulmonary artery catheter monitoring depends upon the type of surgery, comorbidities, risk of blood loss, and possibility of fluid shifts.
   iv) Pulse rate as measured by pulse oximetry or the arterial catheter reflects the VAD ejection rate and may differ from the native heart rate measured by the ECG.

d) **Anesthetic plan**
   i) Rapid sequence induction recommended due to increased aspiration risk.
   ii) Induction goal should be maximal hemodynamic stability maintaining mean arterial pressures between 60 and 90 mm Hg.
   iii) Rapid alterations in afterload during induction and maintenance of anesthesia should be avoided.
   iv) Careful preoperative and intraoperative positioning should be done to avoid changes in VAD preload or compromise of inflow and outflow cannulas. Patients with pulsatile devices should receive a fluid bolus prior to induction of general anesthesia (Table 56-3).
   v) Criteria for postoperative extubation are similar to patients without VADs.
   vi) The patient should be then closely monitored in the post-anesthesia care unit (PACU) or the intensive care unit (ICU) by LVAD-trained personnel.

e) **Intraoperative complications (5) (see Table 56-3)**
   i) **Hemodynamic instability**
      (1) Hemodynamic instability manifested by hypotension and low or fluctuating device flows is a frequently encountered intraoperative complication.
      (2) Gradual decreases in systemic blood pressure associated with decreasing VAD output are most often the result of reduced VAD preload.

Table 56-3

Intraoperative Complications

Problem		Etiology		Treatment
Low device flow	Normotensive/ hypertensive	↑ SVR	→	↓ SVR (deepen anesthesia, vasodilators)
	Hypotensive	Arrhythmias Hypovolemia RV failure	→ → →	ACLS protocol Give volume Increase RV function
Arrhythmias	Stable	Supraventricular	→	Rate control + pharmacologic Conversion
	Instable	Ventricular	→	Cardioversion
Hypoxemia		Volume overload Inadequate LV Unloading Intracardiac shunt	→ → →	↑ FiO_2 + diuresis + ↑ peep ↑ FiO_2 + ↓SVR + ↑ peep ↑ FiO_2 + ↑ RV function + ↑ device flow
Device failure		Power supply	→	Battery backup Pneumatic hand pump
		Pump failure	→	Optimize native heart function
Bleeding			→	Blood products DDAVP

SVR, systemic vascular resistance; ACLS, advanced cardiac life support; DDAVP, (1-deamino-8-D-arginine vasopressin).

(a) Clinically presents as fluctuating device output. In patients with extracorporeal devices, pulsation of inflow and outflow lines, called "chattering," is often observed as a first sign of hypovolemia.

(b) Hypotension as a result of hypovolemia should resolve with volume resuscitation.

(3) If RV failure is the cause of instability, treatment becomes a challenging task.

(a) Pulmonary vascular resistance (PVR) lowering maneuvers, such as hyperoxia, hyperventilation, correction of acidosis should be considered.

(b) Attempts to optimize RV systolic function with phosphodiesterase inhibitors and β-adrenergic agonists as inodilators

(c) Vasopressors may be needed for maintenance of systemic blood pressure.

(d) Inhaled nitric oxide (iNO) is a potent pulmonary vasodilator and may be useful in cases of elevated PVR.

(e) Assessment of RV function by TEE is very helpful.

(4) Less commonly encountered causes, such as inflow cannula obstruction, outflow graft kinking, or cardiac tamponade should always be ruled out. These mechanical causes usually require surgical intervention.

(5) With continuous flow devices, significant increases in mean arterial pressure secondary to sympathetic stimulation or iatrogenic drug administration can lead to decreased device output with subsequent end-organ malperfusion and intracardiac or device thrombus formation.

f) **Arrhythmias (6)**

   i) VAD patients are at high risk to develop supraventricular and ventricular arrhythmias.

   ii) Preoperative consultation with the LVAD team should address mode selection, treatment algorithms, and potential pitfalls.

   iii) In an unstable patient with a new arrhythmia, the "asynchronous" mode should be ensured.

      (1) Once VAD flows and BP are stable and acceptable, treatment of the arrhythmia should proceed.

   iv) Ventricular arrhythmias should be treated by pharmacological or electrical termination.

   v) Notification of primary teams and support staff should occur as soon as possible.

   vi) Electrical defibrillation and synchronized cardioversion may cause fluctuating device flows or resetting of the device into a fixed mode.

g) **Hypoxemia**

   i) VADs pose a unique risk for hypoxemia due to disruption of the natural cardiovascular anatomy and physiology.

   ii) Pulmonary edema may result from hypervolemia or inadequate unloading of the left side of the heart.

   iii) Admixture of oxygenated and deoxygenated blood secondary to a newly formed or previously unrecognized intracardiac right to left shunt may also lead to hypoxemia.

   iv) Hypervolemia should be treated with medical interventions such as diuresis or dialysis if needed.

      (1) Inadequate ventricular unloading often does not respond to device output adjustments and treatment usually requires involvement of a cardiac anesthesiologist and cardiac surgeon.

   v) Diagnosis of intracardiac shunts usually requires TEE for confirmation and often warrants cessation of any nonurgent or emergent surgery and notification of the primary cardiac surgical team.

      (1) Immediate interventions include decreasing right to left pressure differences by decreasing RV preload and decreasing RV afterload (PVR) to improve forward flow.

      (2) For certain devices VAD-trained personnel can decrease the suction pressure applied to the left atrium by the VAD.

h) **Bleeding**

   i) Hemodynamically significant bleeding should be treated as in the non-VAD patient.

   ii) Recombinant factor VIIa/pharmacologic clotting adjuncts should be avoided unless discussed with the VAD team, due to thrombosis risk.

i) **ACLS**

   i) Standard pharmacologic ACLS protocols measurements need to account for the unique VAD physiology; defibrillation is acceptable in most devices in case of emergencies.

j) **Device failure**

   i) Failure can occur in any of the device components; however, the most common cause is lack of power supply.

   ii) Pulsatile devices can be pneumatically driven by hand pump.

   iii) Newer continuous flow devices lack this backup option, and the patient will be dependent on their native heart function until the failure can be fixed.

Chest compression should be strictly avoided due to the risk of cannula dislodgement or disruption.

  iv) In any case of device failure, prompt contact of the LVAD team is warranted to mini-mize the time without mechanical support.

7) **Postoperative considerations**

  a) Early complications are quite similar to the above-described intraoperative problems, and may appear in the immediate perioperative period in the PACU or ICU.

  b) Late complications include thromboembolic events, infection, and multiorgan system failure.

Chapter Summary for VAD

Definitions	Mechanical circulatory support device assuming the role of the left, right, or both ventricles
Assessment	Thorough history can be invaluable. Assess volume status, current device function/settings, and existing RV function.
Risks	Patients are high risk surgical candidates. Bleeding risk may be elevated due to VAD alteration in coagulation/platelet function. Do not do chest compressions if VAD is in place.
Monitoring	Assure adequate VAD function and power supply preoperatively. Pulse oximetry will not work in presence of axial flow devices—arterial line monitoring may be necessary. VAD monitor provides pump flows/output.
Anesthetic Management	Maintain preload and avoid large changes in SVR. Reduced pump flows/hypotension often responds to fluid bolus. Maintaining RV function is essential—avoid hypoxia, hypercarbia, and acidosis.

References

1. Cohn LH, ed. Aggarwal S, Cheema F, Oz MC, et al. Long-term mechanical circulatory support. In: *Cardiac Surgery in the Adult*. New York, NY: McGraw-Hill; 2008:1609–1628.

2. Mudge GH, Fang JC, et al. The physiologic basis for the management of ventricular assist devices. *Clin Cardiol*. 2006;29:285–289.

3. Nicolosi AC, Pagel PS. Perioperative considerations in the patient with a left ventricular assist device. *Anesthesiology* 2003;98:565–570.

4. Stone ME, Soong W, Krol M, et al. The anesthetic consideration in patients with ventricular assist devices presenting for non-cardiac surgery: a review of eight cases. *Anesth Analg* 2002;95:42–49.

5. Goldstein DJ, Oz MC, Rose EA. Implantable left ventricular assist devices. *N Engl J Med* 1998;339:1522–1533.

6. Goldstein DJ, Mullis SL, Delphin ES, et al. Non-cardiac surgery in long-term implantable left-ventricular assist device recipients. *Ann Surg* 1995;222: 203–207.

Cardiac Arrhythmias and Pacemakers

Matt Koehler, MD

Monitoring and treatment of cardiac rhythm and rhythm disturbances are of paramount importance to the practicing anesthesiologist. Knowledge of the most common rhythm disturbances encountered in the OR will help with perioperative decision making. In addition to this, more and more patients are coming to the OR with some electronic rhythm management device—pacemaker, automated implantable cardioverter-defibrillator (AICD), or both. It is important to keep up to date with the current recommendations on management of these devices in the perioperative period. This chapter reviews these topics and presents the current accepted guidelines.

1) Cardiac arrhythmias: (1).
   a) **Normal EKG (Fig. 57-1)**
      i) Normal intervals
         (1) PR interval < 0.12 seconds
         (2) QRS interval < 0.40 seconds
         (3) QT interval (corrected) < 0.42 seconds
      ii) Arrhythmias are most notable in lead II, as one gets the best view of the P wave.
   b) **Abnormal rhythms**
   Note: All pharmacologic doses listed are for adults only (pediatric doses may vary).
   c) **AV block**
      i) **First-degree AV block (Fig. 57-2)**
         (1) PR interval > 0.20 seconds
         (2) Clinically insignificant
      ii) **Second-degree AV block (Fig. 57-3)**
         (1) Mobitz Type I (Wenckebach)
            (a) Gradual lengthening of PR interval until a beat is "dropped"
            (b) Commonly insignificant, but can be seen with drug toxicity

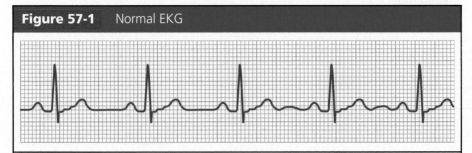

Figure 57-1   Normal EKG

Adapted from Barash P, Cullen B, Stoelting R, et al., eds. *Clinical Anesthesia.* 6th ed. Philadelphia, PA: Lippincott Williams & Wilkins; 2009.

(2) Mobitz Type II **(Fig. 57-4)**
   (a) Intermittent "dropped" beats
   (b) Infranodal block
   (c) Can progress to third-degree AV block
   (d) Treatment: Atropine (0.2 to 1 mg), isoproterenol (20 to 60 µg), or pacing (1,2)

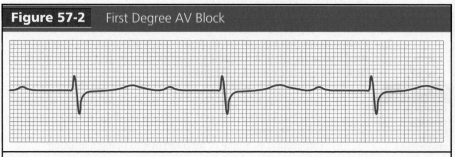

Figure 57-2   First Degree AV Block

Adapted from Zaidan JR, Barash PG. Appendix: Electrocardiography. In: Barash P, Cullen B, Stoelting R, et al., eds. *Clinical Anesthesia*. 6th ed. Philadelphia, PA: Lippincott Williams & Wilkins; 2009:1580.

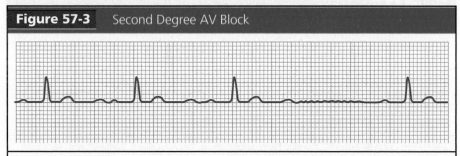

Figure 57-3   Second Degree AV Block

Adapted from Zaidan JR, Barash PG. Appendix: Electrocardiography. In: Barash P, Cullen B, Stoelting R, et al., eds. *Clinical Anesthesia*. 6th ed. Philadelphia, PA: Lippincott Williams & Wilkins; 2009:1580.

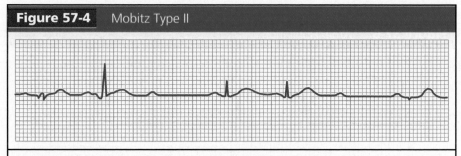

Figure 57-4   Mobitz Type II

Adapted from Zaidan JR, Barash PG. Appendix: Electrocardiography. In: Barash P, Cullen B, Stoelting R, et al., eds. *Clinical Anesthesia*. 6th ed. Philadelphia, PA: Lippincott Williams & Wilkins; 2009:1581.

iii) **Third-degree AV block (Fig. 57-5)**
   (1)   No interaction between atrial and ventricular conduction
   (2)   Ventricular beat morphology may be variable
   (3)   Treatment: Atropine (0.2 to 1 mg), isoproterenol (20 to 60 μg), and likely pacing (transcutaneous or transvenous pacing if unstable in OR)
d) **Supraventricular dysrhythmias**
   i) **Atrial fibrillation (Fig. 57-6)**
      (1)   Variable HR (typically 100 to 200 bpm)
      (2)   No discernible P wave
      (3)   Variable R-R cycle
      (4)   Treatment is either rate control or cardioversion depending on length of time atrial fibrillation present (Chronic atrial fibrillation tends to be difficult to cardiovert—so rate control is the goal) (1,2).

Rule out atrial thrombus before cardioversion.

         (a)   Rate control with β-adrenergic antagonists or calcium channel blockade:
             (i)   Esmolol 500 μg/kg load over 1 to 2 minutes, followed by 50 μg/kg/min. May increase rate every 5 minutes titrating to effect (max dose 300 μg/kg/min)
             (ii)   Diltiazem 0.25 mg/kg IV followed by 5 to 15 mg/h infusion

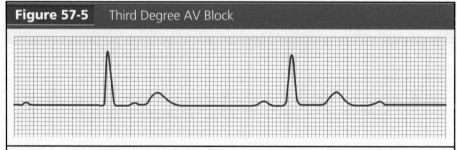

Figure 57-5   Third Degree AV Block

Adapted from Zaidan JR, Barash PG. Appendix: Electrocardiography. In: Barash P, Cullen B, Stoelting R, et al., eds. *Clinical Anesthesia*. 6th ed. Philadelphia, PA: Lippincott Williams & Wilkins; 2009:1581.

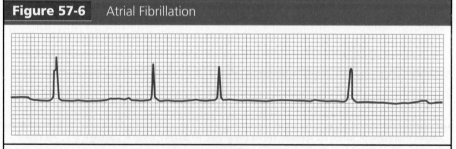

Figure 57-6   Atrial Fibrillation

Adapted from Zaidan JR, Barash PG. Appendix: Electrocardiography. In: Barash P, Cullen B, Stoelting R, et al., eds. *Clinical Anesthesia*. 6th ed. Philadelphia, PA: Lippincott Williams & Wilkins; 2009:1580.

    (b)   Pharmacologic cardioversion with calcium channel blockers (Diltiazem or Verapamil—bolus and infusion rates usually guided with the assistance of a cardiologist).

    (c)   May require immediate electrical cardioversion⋆ if hemodynamically unstable

ii) **Atrial flutter (Fig. 57-7)**

    (1)   Rapid, regular HR (atrial rate typically 250 to 300 bpm)

    (2)   Typically set ratio of ventricular conduction (i.e., 1:1, 2:1, 3:1, etc.)

    (3)   Flutter waves may display a "sawtooth" pattern

    (4)   Treatment is the same as atrial fibrillation

iii) **Supraventricular tachycardia (SVT) (Fig. 57-8)**

    (1)   Rapid, regular HR (typically 150 to 250 bpm)

    (2)   P wave location and orientation are variable, but will be 1:1 with QRS

    (3)   Treatment (1,2)

        (a)   Vagal maneuvers or adenosine (6 or 12 mg)

            (i)   Vagal maneuvers include Valsalva (e.g., coughing, "bearing down," or blowing through straw) and carotid sinus massage (look for history of carotid disease prior to this).

        (b)   β-adrenergic antagonists (Esmolol 30 to 50 mg), calcium channel blockers (Verapamil 2.5 to 5 mg), amiodarone (150 mg), or procainamide (500 mg over 30 min)

        (c)   If hemodynamically unstable, electrical cardioversion⋆

iv) **Junctional rhythm (Fig. 57-9)**

    (1)   Common under general anesthesia secondary to halogenated agents slowing SA and AV nodes (1)

    (2)   May occur due to increased junctional automaticity or in response to decreased sinus node firing

    (3)   Regular, narrow QRS

    (4)   May have decreased cardiac output due to loss of atrial contribution

    (5)   Treatment (1,2)

        (a)   Usually, no treatment required

        (b)   Atropine (0.2 to 1 mg), isoproterenol (30 to 60 μg), or ephedrine (5 to 20 mg) if in response to nodal bradycardia (i.e., junctional beats occur as an escape rhythm to decreased firing from the SA node)

        (c)   Amiodarone (150 mg) if junctional tachycardia (i.e., junctional beats occur faster than SA nodal depolarization)

Figure 57-7   Atrial Flutter

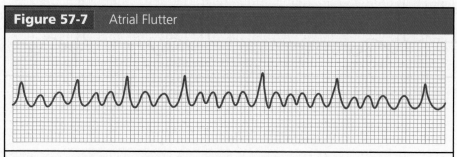

*Cardioversion and defibrillation at 360J in a single shock—see ACLS guidelines for complete ALCS protocols.
Adapted from Zaidan JR, Barash PG. Appendix: Electrocardiography. In: Barash P, Cullen B, Stoelting R, et al., eds. *Clinical Anesthesia*. 6th ed. Philadelphia, PA: Lippincott Williams & Wilkins; 2009:1580.

Figure 57-8 | Supraventricular Tachycardia

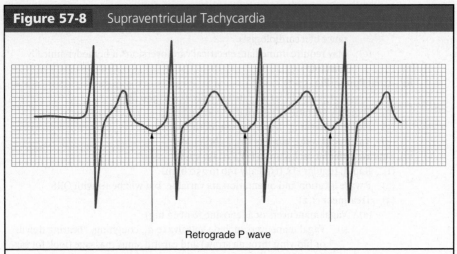

Retrograde P wave

PR interval may be difficult to distinguish because of tachycardia obscuring the P wave. P wave may be precede, be included in, or follow the QRS complex. Adapted from Zaidan JR, Barash PG. Appendix: Electrocardiography. In: Barash P, Cullen B, Stoelting R, et al., eds. *Clinical Anesthesia*. 6th ed. Philadelphia, PA: Lippincott Williams & Wilkins; 2009: 1583.

---

e) **Ventricular dysrhythmias**
  i) **Premature ventricular contraction (Fig. 57-10)**
     (1) Irregular, typically slower HR (<100 bpm) with wide QRS
     (2) Can occur every other beat (bigeminy) or every third beat (trigeminy)
     (3) If frequent, may be indicative of myocardial stress (i.e., ischemia, electrolyte abnormality, "light" anesthesia)
     (4) "R on T" phenomenon can result in ventricular tachycardia (VT) or fibrillation
         (i) "R on T" occurs when a ventricular depolarization ("R wave") occurs during the repolarization phase of a preceding beat (on the "T wave").

Figure 57-9 | Junctional Rhythm

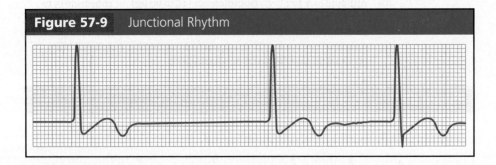

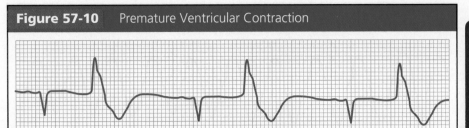

Figure 57-10   Premature Ventricular Contraction

Adapted from Zaidan JR, Barash PG. Appendix: Electrocardiography. In: Barash P, Cullen B, Stoelting R, et al., eds. *Clinical Anesthesia*. 6th ed. Philadelphia, PA: Lippincott Williams & Wilkins; 2009:1584.

   (5) Treatment (1,2)
     (a) Relieve stressor
     (b) First-line treatment is lidocaine (1 to 1.5 mg/kg).
     (c) Second-line treatments include β-adrenergic antagonists and calcium channel blockers.
  ii) **Torsades de pointes (Fig. 57-11)**
     (1) Rapid, irregular ventricular rhythm (150 to 250 bpm)
     (2) Wide QRS with "twisting" phases of variation
     (3) Most commonly seen in severe electrolyte derangements (low K^+, Ca^{2+}, Mg^{2+}) and long QT syndrome
     (4) Treatment (1,2)
       (a) Correct underlying abnormality
       (b) Magnesium sulfate (1 to 2 g)
       (c) Amiodarone (300 mg) or isoproterenol (30 to 60 μg)
       (d) Overdrive pacing
  iii) **Ventricular tachycardia (Fig. 57-12)**
     (1) Rapid, ventricular rhythm (100 to 250 bpm) can be regular or irregular.
     (2) May be confused with SVT with aberrant conduction (requires 12-lead EKG), but SVT often shows AV association and S–R in V1.
     (3) Treatment (1,2)
       (a) Electrical cardioversion if hemodynamically unstable.
       (b) If stable, amiodarone (300 mg) for pharmacologic conversion

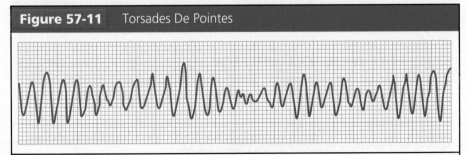

Figure 57-11   Torsades De Pointes

Adapted from Zaidan JR, Barash PG. Appendix: Electrocardiography. In: Barash P, Cullen B, Stoelting R, et al., eds. *Clinical Anesthesia*. 6th ed. Philadelphia, PA: Lippincott Williams & Wilkins; 2009: 1584.

Figure 57-12 Ventricular Tachycardia

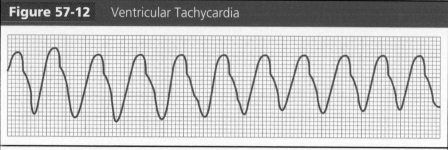

Adapted from Zaidan JR, Barash PG. Appendix: Electrocardiography. In: Barash P, Cullen B, Stoelting R, et al., eds. *Clinical Anesthesia*. 6th ed. Philadelphia, PA: Lippincott Williams & Wilkins; 2009:1585.

    iv) **Ventricular fibrillation (VF) (Fig. 57-13)**
        (1) Vacillating, irregular baseline without discernible P, QRS, or T
        (2) Treatment: immediate CPR with defibrillation (1,2)
2) **Electronic rhythm control devices.** Pacemakers and AICD placement are becoming more frequent as the population ages and technology improves. New therapeutic options include biventricular pacing for heart failure patients along with antitachycardia devices.
    a) **Major indications for pacemaker/AICD implantation** (For full literature review, see the ACC/AHA/HRS 2008 Guidelines for Device-Based Therapy of Cardiac Rhythm Abnormalities)
      i) **Pacemaker indications**
        (1) Sinus node dysfunction (SND)
          (a) SND with symptomatic bradycardia, including frequent pauses
          (b) Syncope with history of SND
        (2) AV node dysfunction
          (a) Third-degree heart block
          (b) Mobitz Type II heart block
        (3) Chronic bifascicular block
          (a) Alternating bundle-branch block
          (b) Prolonged bundle of His conduction time (>100 ms)
        (4) Residual problems after myocardial infarction such as persistent Mobitz II, third-degree or alternating bundle branch block, or prior ST segment elevation myocardial infarction

Figure 57-13 Ventricular Fibrillation

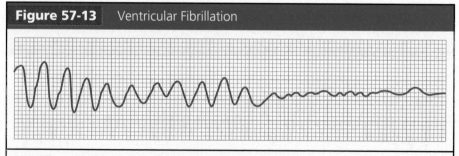

Adapted from Zaidan JR, Barash PG. Appendix: Electrocardiography. In: Barash P, Cullen B, Stoelting R, et al., eds. *Clinical Anesthesia*. 6th ed. Philadelphia, PA: Lippincott Williams & Wilkins; 2009:1585.

(5) Hypersensitive carotid sinus syndrome and neurocardiogenic syncope

(a) Syncope caused by spontaneously occurring carotid sinus stimulation that induces asystole for >3 seconds

(b) Syncope without clear, provocative events and with a hypersensitive cardioinhibitory response of 3 seconds or longer

(6) Arrhythmia avoidance

(a) Recurrent SVT proven to be prevented with pacing

(b) Pause-dependent VT (i.e., long-QT syndrome)

ii) **AICD indications**

(1) VT or VF (especially with syncope or structural heart disease)

(2) Low ejection fraction (<35%)

(3) May be indicated in dilated cardiomyopathy, hypertrophic cardiomyopathy, and long QT syndrome

Electroconvulsive therapy has *not* been shown to affect cardiac rhythm management device (CRMD) function, but the device should be interrogated and ICD function should be disabled prior to procedure.

b) **Sources of electromagnetic interference**—potential causes of AICD/pacer discharge/malfunction

i) Unipolar electrocautery (i.e., "the bovie")

ii) Radiofrequency ablation

iii) Lithotripsy

iv) Magnetic resonance imaging

v) Radiation therapy

c) **Magnet functions**

ALWAYS know what the magnet function does prior to using a magnet.

i) Pt should carry an ID card documenting the type and number of device.

ii) CXR will reveal devices ID number and can be referenced.

iii) Almost all pacemakers are supplied by either Medtronic or Boston Scientific (formerly Guidant) as of the printing of this text.

iv) **With a magnet, the pacer will typically convert to VOO (HR 80 to 100) and ICD will be disabled when magnet is applied**

d) **Pacemaker/AICD nomenclature system** (Revised NASPE/BPEG code, 2002) (Tables 57-1 to 57-3 printed with permission from the ASA's "Practice advisory for the perioperative management of patients with cardiac rhythm management devices: Appendix 2").

e) **Examples (further simplification)**

i) DDD—Paces atrium and/or ventricle if no depolarization sensed; Senses both atrium and ventricle; If depolarization sensed, can inhibit or trigger (used only during pacemaker interrogation) atrium or ventricle, respectively.

ii) AAI—Paces atrium only; senses atrium only; inhibits pacemaker if atrial depolarization sensed (good for sick sinus syndrome and hypersensitive cardioinhibitory responses)

iii) VVI—Paces ventricle when no depolarization sensed; senses ventricle only; inhibits pacer when depolarization sensed.

iv) DOO—Asynchronous pacing of both atrium and ventricle without regard to underlying rhythm.

f) Stepwise Approach to the Perioperative Treatment of the Patient with a CRMD (printed with permission from the ASA's "Practice advisory for the perioperative management of patients with cardiac rhythm management devices: Appendix 2") (Tables 57-3)

Table 57-1

Generic Pacemaker Code (NBG*): NASPE/BPEG Revised (2002)

Position I, Pacing Chamber(s)	Position II, Sensing Chamber(s)	Position III, Response(s) to Sensing	Position IV, Programmability	Position V, Multisite Pacing
O = none A = atrium V = ventricle D = dual (A + V)	O = none A = atrium V = ventricle D = dual (A + V)	O = none I = inhibited T = triggered D = dual (T + I)	O = none R = rate modulation	O = none A = atrium V = Ventricle D = dual (A + V)

Examples:

AAI = Atrial-only antibradycardia pacing. In the AAI mode: any failure of the atrium to produce an intrinsic event within the appropriate time window (determined by the lower rate limit) results in an atrial pacing pulse emission. There is no ventricular sensing; thus, a premature ventricular event will not likely reset the pacing timer.

AOO = Asynchronous atrial-only pacing. In this mode, the pacing device emits a pacing pulse regardless of the underlying cardiac rhythm.

DDD = Dual-chamber antibradycardia pacing function in which every atrial event within programmed limits, is followed by a ventricular event. The DDD mode implies dual-chamber pacing with atrial tracking. In the absence of intrinsic activity in the atrium, it will be paced, and. after any sensed or paced atrial event, an intrinsic ventricular event must occur before the expiration of the atrioventricular timer or the ventricle will be paced.

DDI = Dual-chamber behavior in which the atrial activity is tracked into the ventricle only when the atrial event is created by the antibradycardia pacing function of the generator In the DDI mode, the ventricle is paced only when no intrinsic ventricular activity is present.

DOO = Asynchronous atrioventricular sequential pacing without regard to the underlying cardiac rhythm.

VOO = Asynchronous ventricular-only pacing without regard to the underlying cardiac rhythm.

VVI = Ventricular-only antibradycardia pacing. In the VVI mode, any failure of the ventricle to produce an intrinsic event within the appropriate time window (determined by the lower rate limit) results in a ventricular pacing pulse emission. There is no atrial sensing; thus, there can be no atrioventricular synchrony in a patient with a VVI pacemaker and any intrinsic atrial activity.

* NBG: N refers to NASPE. B refers to BPEG, and G refers to generic.

Table 57-2

Generic Defibrillator Code (NBD): NASPE/BPEG

Position I, Shock Chamber(s)	Position II, Antitachycardia Pacing Chamber(s)	Position III, Tachycardia Detection	Position IV, * Antibradycardia Pacing Chamber(s)
o = none A = atrium V = ventricle D = dual (A + V)	o = none A = atrium V = ventricle D = dual (A + V)	E = electrogram H = hemodynamic	O = none A = atrium V = ventricle D = dual (A + V)

* For robust identification, position IV is expanded into its complete NBG code, For example, a biventricular pacing-defibrillator with ventricular shock and antitachycardia pacing functionality would be identified as VVE-DDDRV, assuming that the pacing section was programmed DDDRV. Currently, no hemodynamic sensors have been approved for tachycardia detection (position III).

Table 57-3

Stepwise Approach to the Patient with a CRMD

Perioperative Period	Patient/CRMD Condition	Intervention
Preoperative Evaluation	Patient has CRMD	Focused history and physical examination
	Determine CRMD type	Manufacturer's CRMD identification card Chest x-ray studies if no data available Consider other resources such as manufacturer Web site, cardiology consultation, etc.
	Determine whether patient is CRMD-dependent for pacing function	Verbal history Bradyarrhythmia symptoms Atrioventricular node ablation No spontaneous ventricular activity
	Determine CRMD function	Comprehensive CRMD evaluation by electrophysiology service Determine if pacing pulses are present and create paced beats
Preoperative Preparation	EMI unlikely during procedure	Special precautions are not needed
	EMI likely; CRMD is pacemaker	Reprogram to asynchronous mode when indicated Suspend rate-adaptive functions
	EMI likely; CRMD is ICD	Suspend antitachyarrhythmia functions If patient is dependent on pacing function, alter pacing functions as above
	EMI likely; all CRMD	Use bipolar cautery; ultrasonic scalpel Temporary pacing and external cardioversion-defibrillation should be available
	Intraoperative physiologic changes likely (e.g., bradycardia, ischemia)	Plan for possible adverse CRMD-patient interaction
Intraoperative Management	Monitoring	ECG per ASA standard Peripheral pulse monitoring
	Electrocautery interference	CT/CRP—no current through PG/leads Avoid proximity of CT to PG/leads Short bursts of lowest possible energy Use bipolar cautery; ultrasonic scalpel
	MRI	Generally contraindicated If required, consult ordering physician, cardiologist, radiologist, and manufacturer
	ECT	If required, consult ordering physician, cardiologist, radiologist, and manufacturer

(continued)

Table 57-3

Stepwise Approach to the Patient with a CRMD *(Continued)*

Perioperative Period	Patient/CRMD Condition	Intervention
Emergency defibrillation-cardioversion	ICD; magnet disabled	Terminate all EMI sources Remove magnet to reenable therapies Observe for appropriate therapies
	ICD; programming disabled	Programming to reenable therapies or proceed directly with external cardioversion/defibrillation
	ICD; either of above	Minimize current flow through PG/leads PP as far as possible from PG PP perpendicular to major axis PG/leads To extent possible, PP in anterior-posterior location
	Regardless of CMD type	Use clinically appropriate cardioversion/defibrillation energy
Postoperative Management	Immediate postoperative period	Monitor cardiac rate and rhythm continuously Backup pacing and cardioversion/defibrillation capability
	Postoperative interrogation and restoration of CRMD function	Interrogation to assess function and appropriate settings Restore antitachycardia therapies if ICD Use cardiology/pacemaker-ICD service if needed

CRP, current return pad; CRT, cardiac resynchronization therapy; CT, cautery tool; ECT, electroconvulsive therapy; EMI, electromagnetic interference; ICD, internal cardioverter-defibrillator; MRI, magnetic resonance imaging; PG, pulse generator; PP, external cardioversion-defibrillation pads or paddles.

Chapter Summary for Cardiac Arrhythmias

Arrhythmias	Abnormal cardiac rhythms are common in the perioperative period. Key disturbances are significant heart block (second and third degree), atrial flutter or fibrillation with hemodynamic disturbance, and ventricular disturbances with hemodynamic compromise.
Pacemakers and AICDs	**Pacemakers:** Always find the underlying rhythm and reason for pacemaker. If the patient is pacemaker-dependent and significant EMI is anticipated, the device should be set to a VOO mode to avoid electrical interference. A magnet will typically convert the device to VOO/DOO for newer devices, but needs to be interrogated following magnet placement (see Table 57-1 for explanation of terms "DOO" and "VOO"). **AICD:** Antitachyarrhythmia function should be disabled prior to surgery. Once disabled, some method of cardioversion should be available (external pads) and monitoring needs to be employed. **Magnet:** Most new devices respond by disabling the AICD portion and setting the pacing function to VOO. This needs to be verified prior to placing the magnet.

References

1. Barash P, Cullen B, Stoelting R, et al., eds. *Clinical Anesthesia.* 6th ed. Philadelphia, PA: Lippincott Williams & Wilkins; 2009.
2. Miller. In: Consulting editors: Fleisher L, Johns R, Savarese J, Wiener-Kronish J, Young W. *Miller's Anesthesia.* 6th ed. Elsevier Churchill Livingstone; 2005.
3. Practice advisory for the perioperative management of patients with cardiac rhythm management devices: pacemakers and implantable cardioverter-defibrillators: a report by the American Society of Anesthesiologists Task Force on Perioperative Management of Patients with Cardiac Rhythm Management Devices. *Anesthesiology* 2005;103:186–198.
4. Epstein AE, Dimarco JP, Ellenbogen KA, et al. ACC/AHA/HRS 2008 guidelines for Device-Based Therapy of Cardiac Rhythm Abnormalities: executive summary. *Circulation* 2008;117:e350–408.

58 Essential Hypertension and Anesthetic Considerations

Hien Nicole Tran, MD • Marek Brzezinski, MD, PhD

Essential hypertension (HTN) is a common problem with 66 million Americans suffering from elevated blood pressure (BP), defined as systolic BP ≥ 140 mm Hg or diastolic BP ≥ 90 mm Hg (1). Of these, 63% are aware of their HTN, 45% are receiving treatment, and only 34% are under control using a threshold of 140/90 mm Hg. Proper periopera-tive management is essential in anesthetic practice.

1) **General principles**
   a) **Definition**
      i) Essential HTN
         (1) No secondary cause for HTN can be identified such as pheo-chromocytoma, hyperaldosteronism, Cushing syndrome, renovascular HTN, aortic coarctation.
         (2) Essential HTN comprises 95% of all cases of HTN
   b) **Classification (1,2) (Table 58-1)**
   c) **Risk Factors (1,3,4) (Table 58-2).**
2) **Complications**
   a) **Uncontrolled HTN (5,6)**
      i) Defined as systolic BP > 180 mm Hg and/or diastolic BP > 110 mm Hg

Table 58-1
Classification of HTN

BP Classification	Systolic BP (mm Hg)	Diastolic BP (mm Hg)
Normal	<120	<80
Pre-HTN	120–139	80–89
Stage 1 HTN	140–159	90–99
Stage 2 HTN	160–179	100–109
Stage 3 HTN	180–209	110–119
Stage 4 HTN	≥210	≥120

Table 58-2	
Risk Factors for Essential HTN	
Increased Age	Excessive Dietary Sodium Intake
African american race	Alcohol consumption of ≥2 drinks per day (4)
Genetic/family history	Tobacco use
Obesity	Stress

b) **Perioperative considerations for uncontrolled HTN**
   i) Delay elective surgery in case of uncontrolled HTN or existing target organ damage that can be improved or should be evaluated further (see Section 4.a).
   ii) Increase or modify antihypertensive therapy, consider adding β-adrenergic antagonist.
   iii) For emergency surgery consider invasive monitoring of perioperative hemodynamics (arterial line, central line).
c) **End-organ damage**
   i) Cardiovascular
      (1) Coronary artery disease
      (2) Cerebral vascular disease
         (a) Transient ischemic attacks, ischemic stroke
      (3) Peripheral vascular disease (PVD)
      (4) Left ventricular hypertrophy (LVH), congestive heart failure (CHF)
      (5) Retinopathy
   ii) Kidney failure
   iii) Neurologic
      (1) hemorrhagic stroke, hypertensive encephalopathy
d) **Perioperative considerations for patients with end-organ damage**
   i) Detailed preoperative assessment with a focus on end-organ damage should be performed in any patient with essential HTN
   ii) Appropriate referrals should be made and the patient's medical condition optimized prior to elective surgery
3) **Treatment and management**
a) **Lifestyle changes (5-7)**
   i) Weight loss, moderate alcohol consumption, smoking cessation, reduced sodium intake
b) **Pharmacology (5)**
   i) ACE inhibitors, β-adrenergic antagonists, thiazide diuretics, calcium channel blockers, angiotensin receptor blockers
4) **Anesthetic management of the patient with HTN**
a) **Preoperative evaluation (5,6)**
   i) Assess the patient's baseline BP and self-management at home to identify possible shift in cerebral autoregulation (see below).
   ii) Patients with untreated severe HTN have a higher incidence of stroke, myocardial ischemia, and kidney failure because of chronic changes in the autoregulation of end-organ perfusion (8,9).

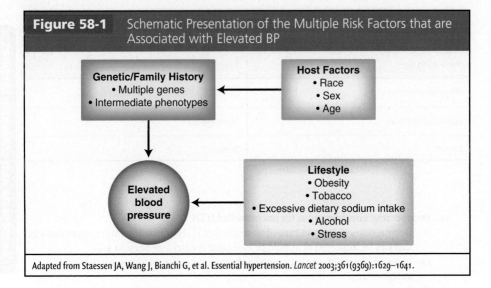

Figure 58-1 Schematic Presentation of the Multiple Risk Factors that are Associated with Elevated BP

Adapted from Staessen JA, Wang J, Bianchi G, et al. Essential hypertension. *Lancet* 2003;361(9369):1629–1641.

iii) No clear consensus exists regarding the timing of elective surgery in patients with uncontrolled HTN. However, recommendations according to HTN stage are as follows (10):
- (1) Stage 1 and 2 HTN: Proceed with anesthesia and surgery.
- (2) Stage 3 HTN: Consider postponing anesthesia and surgery, especially in patients with other cardiovascular risk factors (end organ damage).
- (3) Stage 4 HTN: Defer anesthesia and surgery whenever possible, begin appropriate antihypertensive therapy, and arrange for follow-up or inpatient BP control.

Patients who have taken ACE inhibitors or angiotensin II receptor antagonists the day of surgery are at high risk for intraoperative hypotension.

iv) Evaluate for end-organ damage
- (1) Including angina pectoris, LVH, CHF, cerebrovascular disease, stroke, PVD, renal insufficiency
- (2) Laboratory studies
  - (a) Complete blood count
  - (b) Coagulation studies
  - (c) Basic Metabolic Panel to determine the extent of renal disease and electrolyte status

v) **Presume ischemic heart disease in patients with essential HTN until proven otherwise (6).**
- (1) Assess patient's exercise tolerance with the focus on dyspnea or angina.
- (2) Check ECG for abnormal conduction or ischemia and consider stress test.
- (3) If cardiac exam suggests valvular disease or myocardial dysfunction, consider echocardiography.

vi) Continue current antihypertensive regimen prior to surgery.

vii) Review antihypertensive medication for pharmacology and potential side effects.
- (1) ACE inhibitors and angiotensin receptor blockers can be associated with severe hypotension during general anesthesia.
- (2) Complications due to cessation of antihypertensive medications

        (a)   β-Adrenergic antagonists → myocardial ischemia

        (b)   Clonidine → hypertensive crisis

b)   **Intraoperative management**

    i)   **Induction (5,6)**

      (1)   Direct laryngoscopy and tracheal intubation can cause significant HTN, tachycardia, and myocardial ischemia.

      (2)   The use of IV drugs cannot definitely suppress the cardiovascular responses to tracheal intubation.

      (3)   Management

        (a)   In patients at high risk for myocardial ischemia, consider deep inhalation anesthesia or injection of opioid, lidocaine, β-adrenergic antagonists, or vasodilator to suppress tracheal reflexes and reduce autonomic responses to laryngoscopy.

    ii)   **Intraoperative hemodynamic management (6)**

      (1)   Patients with essential HTN have an increased incidence of perioperative HTN.

        (a)   Volatile anesthetics can attenuate pressor responses of sympathetic nervous system resulting in dose-dependent decrease in BP, systemic vascular resistance, and myocardial depression.

      (2)   Intraoperative hypotension may occur, when ACE-inhibitors and angiotensin II antagonists were not discontinued 24 hours before surgery (11).

Patients with preoperative uncontrolled HTN are at high risk of hemodynamic lability intraoperatively.

        (a)   Vasoconstrictor treatment may be required such as low-dose vasopressin (12).

      (3)   No volatile agents or muscle relaxants appear to be more preferable in this patient population.

        (a)   Pancuronium has dose-related sympathomimetic and vagolytic effects and one should consider avoiding this drug (13).

      (4)   **Cerebral autoregulation (14)**

        (a)   Typically maintained between mean BP between 50 and 150 mm Hg.

        (b)   In chronic HTN, the lower BP limit of autoregulation of cerebral blood flow is shifted toward a higher BP.

        (c)   The clinical consequence of this shift is an impaired tolerance to lower BP

        (d)   Long-term antihypertensive treatment can help readapt to normal autoregulation of cerebral blood flow illustrating the importance of the preoperative baseline evaluation (15).

Due to changes in cerebral autoregulation with chronic HTN, rapid BP drops to normotensive levels can result in decreased cerebral blood flow and possibly cause ischemic brain damage.

   iii)   **Monitoring**

      (1)   ECG, preferably 5-lead, to recognize myocardial ischemia during periods of intense painful stimulation such as laryngoscopy and tracheal intubation.

      (2)   Invasive monitoring (arterial or central line, pulmonary artery catheter) are useful for extensive surgery or in case of left ventricular dysfunction or other significant end-organ damage.

      (3)   Transesophageal echocardiography to monitor left ventricular function and intravascular volume replacement in major surgical cases or critical condition of the patient

5) **Postoperative management** (5,6)
   a) Postoperative HTN is common in patients with essential HTN
      i) Close monitoring of BP with prompt assessment and treatment is required to decrease risk of myocardial ischemia, arrhythmias, CHF, cerebrovascular ischemia, and maintain surgical wound hemostasis.
      ii) Adequate management of postoperative pain
         (1) Pain is an important contributor to postoperative HTN.
         (2) Useful approaches to pain management may include epidural analgesia (16).
      iii) Temporary IV administration of antihypertensive agents may be necessary.
         (1) Medications should be chosen based on the patient's vital signs and coexisting diseases.
         (2) One approach is to use labetalol IV intermittently 20 mg over 2 min, then double at 10 minute intervals until desired response, a single maximal dose of 80 mg, toxicity or a cumulative dose of 300 mg/d, or infusion of 2 mg/min initially, then titrate in 2 mg increments every 10 minutes until response, toxicity, or a cumulative dose of 300 mg/24 h (17).
         (3) In the presence of a low heart rate and/or contraindications to β-adrenergic antagonists, hydralazine is an alternative agent.

Chapter Summary for Essential HTN and Anesthetic Considerations

Definition	Essential HTN—No secondary cause for HTN can be identified such as pheochromocytoma, hyperaldosteronism, Cushing syndrome, renovascular HTN, aortic coarctation. Essential HTN comprises 95% of all cases of HTN		
Classification		Systolic BP (mm Hg)	Diastolic BP (mm Hg)
	Normal	<120	<80
	Pre-HTN	120–139	80–89
	Stage 1 HTN	140–159	90–99
	Stage 2 HTN	160–179	100–109
	Stage 3 HTN	180–209	110–119
	Stage 4 HTN	≥210	≥120
Preoperative Considerations	Review medications, assess baseline and end-organ damage In Stage 3 and 4 HTN and Stage 2 HTN with end-organ damage, consider deferring surgery for patient optimization		
Intraoperative Considerations	Increased risk of perioperative HTN and BP lability Cerebral autoregulation may altered		
Postoperative Considerations	Close monitoring and management of BP to avoid myocardial ischemia and maintain surgical wound hemostasis Adequate pain management essential		

BP, blood pressure; HTN, hypertension.

References

1. Mc Phee SJ, Papadakis MA, Tierney LM. *Current Medical Diagnosis and Treatment*. 4th ed. McGraw-Hill Medical; 2008.
2. The Joint National Committee on detection, evaluation, and treatment of high blood pressure. *Arch Intern Med* 1993;153:154–183.
3. Lloyd-Jones DM, Evans JC, Levy D. Hypertension in adults across the age spectrum: current outcomes and control in the community. *JAMA* 2005;294(4):466–472.
4. Stranges S, Wu T, Dorn JM, et al. Relationship of alcohol drinking pattern to risk of hypertension. *Hypertension* 2004;44:813–819.
5. Pardo M, Sonner JM. *Manual of Anesthesia Practice*. 2nd ed. New York, NY: Cambridge University Press; 2007.
6. Hines, RL, Marshall KE. *Stoelting Anesthesia and Co-disease*. 5th ed. Churchill Livingstone, Elsevier; 2008.
7. Staessen JA, Wang J, Bianchi G, et al. Essential hypertension. *Lancet* 2003;361(9369):1629–1641. Review.
8. Cheung AT. Exploring an optimum intra/postoperative management strategy for acute hypertension in the cardiac surgery patient. *J Card Surg* 2006;21(Suppl 1):S8–S14.
9. Immink RV, van den Born BJ, van Montfrans GA, et al. Impaired cerebral autoregulation in patients with malignant hypertension. *Circulation* 2004;110:2241–2245.
10. Dix P, Howell S. Survey of cancellation rate of hypertensive patients undergoing anaesthesia and elective surgery. *Br J Anaesth* 2001;86(6):789–793.
11. Bertrand M, Godet G, Meersschaert K, et al. Should angiotensin II antagonists be discontinued before surgery? *Anesth Analg* 2001;92:26–30.
12. Eyrau D, Brabant S, Nathali D, et al. Treatment of intraoperative refractory hypotension with terlipressin in patients chronically treated with an antagonist of the renin angiotensin system. *Anesth Analg* 1999;88:980–984.
13. Paulissian R, Mahdi M, Joseph NJ, et al. Hemodynamic responses to pancuronium and vecuronium during high-dose fentanyl anesthesia for coronary artery bypass grafting. *J Cardiothorac Vasc Anesth* 1991;5(2):120–125.
14. Strandgaard S. Autoregulation of cerebral blood flow in hypertensive patients. *Circulation* 1976;53:720–727.
15. Vorstrup S, Barry DI, Jarden JO, et al. Chronic antihypertensive treatment in the rat reverses hypertension- induced changes in cerebral blood flow autoregulation. *Stroke* 1984;15:312–8. 98–1.
16. Laslett L. Hypertension-Preoperative assessment and perioperative management. *West J Med* 1995;162:215–219.
17. Varon J, Marik PE. Perioperative hypertension management. *Vasc Health Risk Manag* 2008;4(3):615–627.

ANESTHESIA AND COMORBID DISEASES

Anterior Mediastinal Mass

Haley G. Hutting, MD

The patient with an anterior mediastinal mass provides an anesthetic challenge. Anterior mediastinal masses can cause compression of the airways and great vessels within the mediastinum and the administration of general anesthesia can be associated with a host of intraoperative complications. Careful preoperative planning is essential to providing safe perioperative care.

The causes of anterior mediastinal mass can be remembered as the four "T"s: Thymus, Teratoma, Thyroid, Terrible lymphoma.

Patients with anterior mediastinal mass are at high risk for airway obstruction or cardiovascular collapse under general anesthesia.

1) **Introduction**
   a) **Anatomy**
      i) The anterior mediastinum normally contains the thymus, lymph nodes, ascending aorta, pulmonary artery (PA), phrenic nerves, thyroid, and fat
   b) **Causes of anterior mediastinal mass**
      i) Tumors
         (1) Children—most common is lymphoma.
         (2) Adults—most common is thymoma.
      ii) Others include teratoma, germ cell tumors, goiter, parathyroid adenoma, lipoma, carcinoma, aortic aneurysm (Table 59-1)
   c) **Presenting symptoms**
      i) Shortness of breath, cough, hemoptysis, hoarseness, Horner syndrome, superior vena cava (SVC) syndrome
         (1) SVC syndrome is due to obstruction of SVC and presents with dyspnea, facial swelling, cough, orthopnea, headache.
   d) Surgical interventions
      i) Biopsy via mediastinoscopy or video-assisted thoracoscopic surgery
      ii) Definitive resection via sternotomy or thoracotomy
2) **Perioperative physiology**
   a) **Effects of the supine position**
      i) Decreased transverse diameter of thorax
      ii) Cephalad displacement of diaphragm
      iii) Central blood volume increases, causing vascular tumors to enlarge
      iv) The result is decreased thoracic airway cross-sectional area and increased external compression pressure on airways (1).
      v) If airways or great vessels in the mediastinum are already compromised from the effect of the mass, the supine position may be problematic.
   b) **Effects of general anesthesia**
      i) **Decreased transverse diameter of thorax** due to decreased intercostal muscle tone
      ii) **Decreased inspiratory and abdominal muscle tone**
      iii) **Cephalad displacement of abdominal contents decreases thoracic volume** by 500 to 1,000 mL (1,2).
      iv) **Relaxation of bronchial smooth muscles** worsens large airway compressibility.

ANESTHESIA AND COMORBID DISEASES

Table 59-1

Decision Making in Airway Management of Patients with Anterior Mediastinal Mass

Safe Airway	Unsafe	Uncertain
Asymptomatic adult	Severely symptomatic adult or child	Mild/moderate symptomatic child with tracheobronchial diameter >50% of normal
Minimum tracheobronchial diameter >50% normal	Children with tracheobronchial diameter <50% of normal, regardless of symptoms	Mild/moderate symptomatic adult with tracheobronchial diameter <50% of normal Adult or child unable to give history

Infants and small children have more compressible airways, making them more susceptible than adults to extrinsic airway obstruction.

    v)   If neuromuscular blockade is used, loss of craniocaudal movement of the diaphragm decreases transpleural gradient, worsening airway compression.

        (1)   The normal transpleural pressure gradient dilates the airways during inspiration, minimizing the effects of extrinsic intrathoracic airway compression.

    vi)   Controlled ventilation preferentially ventilates anterior lung segments causing dorsal atelectasis, leading to **V/Q mismatch and shunt (1)**

c) **Hemodynamic physiology**

    i)   Patients are at risk for hemodynamic decompensation if the heart or major vessels are surrounded by tumor.

    ii)   SVC is most susceptible to external compression.

        (1)   Decreased venous drainage from upper half of body → decreased RV filling → decreased cardiac output (CO)

    iii)   The pulmonary artery (PA) is more resistant to compression, but decreased PA flow can lead to hypoxemia, acute RV failure, cardiac arrest.

    iv)   Large tumors can directly compress the heart leading to arrhythmias and low CO (tamponade physiology).

3) **Preoperative considerations**

a) History should include questions about the following symptoms:

    i)   Supine dyspnea or cough suggests possibility of airway compression on induction of anesthesia.

    ii)   Supine syncope suggests vascular compression.

    iii)   Identify patient positions that exacerbate and ameliorate symptoms, bearing in mind that it may be more difficult to ascertain symptoms in pediatric or elderly patients.

b) **Evaluation (Table 59-1)**

    i)   Chest x-ray

    ii)   Most important pre-op test is CT chest/trachea.

        (1)   **A cross-sectional tracheal area <50% of normal predicts frequent perioperative respiratory complications with general anesthesia (2,3).**

    iii)   Fiberoptic bronchoscopy may be helpful to assess the airways and potential dynamic compressibility (4).

    iv)   Pulmonary function tests (PFTs)

        (1)   May be helpful in determining the degree of airway compression

        (2)   Determine flow-volume curves in the recumbent and sitting positions

(3) A decrease in flow or plateau during expiratory phase suggests intrathoracic obstruction.

(4) MEF_{50}/MIF_{50} is one of the most useful parameters of the PFTs (1).

   (a) MEF_{50} is the maximum expiratory flow (MEF) at 50% vital capacity

   (b) MIF_{50} is the maximum inspiratory flow (MIF) at 50% vital capacity

   (c) **$MEF_{50}/MIF_{50} < 1$ is concerning for intrathoracic obstruction.**

v) Echocardiogram

   (1) If CT or clinical exam suggests hemodynamic compromise, transthoracic or transesophageal echocardiography is indicated and should be performed in the recumbent and lateral positions to assess for compression and changes in filling.

vi) Consider preoperative irradiation or chemotherapy to decrease the tumor mass and decrease perioperative complications (4).

vii) Labs to consider

   (1) CBC should be obtained to estimate allowable blood loss and evaluate for associated thrombocytopenia.

   (2) Type and cross

   (3) ABG if respiratory symptoms

4) **Intraoperative management**

   a) **Preduction**

   i) Adequate personnel should be available **prior to induction**, including surgeons (prepared for immediate rigid bronchoscopy), a second anesthesiologist, and nurses.

   ii) Perfusionist should be present for high-risk patients.

   iii) Minimize preoperative sedation, which may produce respiratory depression or muscle relaxation.

   iv) **Ensure adequate IV access**

      (1) In patients with SVC syndrome, large-bore lower extremity access will likely be most effective.

   v) Pulse oximeter or arterial line should be placed on the **right upper extremity** to monitor for perfusion of brachiocephalic trunk.

   vi) In patients classified as uncertain or unsafe, central venous access and arterial line should be placed prior to induction.

   vii) Consider airway backup plans, including

      (1) Various tube sizes

      (2) Reinforced tubes

      (3) Flexible fiberoptic scope

      (4) Rigid bronchoscope

      (5) For "unsafe" patients, primed bypass circuit and perfusionist (1)

   b) **Induction (Fig 59-1)**

   i) **Optimal positioning**

      (1) Consider tumor location (based on imaging) and document patient's positions of comfort. Induction should be performed in the position of greatest comfort.

      (2) Transport to and from the operating room should be done in patient's position of comfort.

      (3) Patients with evidence of SVC syndrome should be transported with the upper body elevated (semi-Fowler position).

      (4) Induction should be performed in a stepwise manner with continuous respiratory and hemodynamic monitoring and maintenance of spontaneous ventilation

Prior to anesthetizing a high-risk patient with anterior mediastinal mass, personnel including the surgeon, a second anesthesiologist, nurses, and possibly a perfusionist should be present in the OR.

Patients with anterior mediastinal mass should have anesthesia induced and be transported in their position of greatest comfort.

Avoid muscle relaxants in patients with anterior mediastinal mass due to the risk of airway compression.

ii) **Short-acting medications are preferable.**
   (1) Sevoflurane is preferred for inhalational induction
   (2) Etomidate is ideal for IV induction due to short duration of action, mainte-
       nance of muscle tone, maintenance of spontaneous breathing, and minimal
       effect on hemodynamics (1).
   (3) Remifentanil is a good opiate choice due to its very short half-life (1).
iii) **Avoid use of muscle relaxants due to risk of worsening airway compression**
   (1) If the procedure necessitates muscle relaxation, attempt a trial of mask venti-
       lation first.

Figure 59-1 Preoperative Decision Making in Patients with Anterior Mediastinal Mass

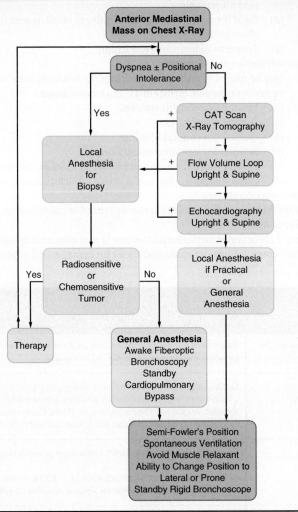

Reused from Neustein SM, Eisenkraft JB, Cohen E. Anesthesia for thoracic surgery. In: Barash P, Cullen B, Stoelting R, et al., eds. *Clinical Anesthesia.*, 6th ed. Philadelphia, PA: Lippincott Williams & Wilkins; 2009:1059, with permission.

(2) As anesthetic depth is slowly increased, begin to assist the patient with respirations incrementally. Small doses of succinylcholine injected slowly may be considered during this trial (1).

(3) If airway pressures are not significantly changed, you can cautiously proceed with muscle relaxation and mechanical ventilation (2).

c) **Potential intraoperative complications**

  i) **Problems with oxygenation**

   (1) May be due to **airway compression.** Maneuvers to relieve the compression include:

     (a) Reposition the patient, recalling positions of comfort from preoperative evaluation.

     (b) Confirm ETT position with fiberoptic bronchoscope.

     (c) Advance ETT past any obstruction under visualization with bronchoscope if possible.

     (d) Rigid bronchoscopy may be effective to ventilate past the point of obstruction.

     (e) Return to spontaneous ventilation.

  ii) **Hemodynamic complications**

   (1) May be related to mass compression of the heart and great vessels and include severe hypotension, arrhythmias, and cardiac arrest

   (2) Consider the following treatments:

     (a) Volume resuscitation

     (b) Evaluate for surgical bleeding

     (c) Evaluate for tension pneumothorax

     (d) Prompt surgical decompression via sternotomy for severe cases

     (e) Cardiopulmonary bypass for severe refractory hemodynamic instability

5) **Postoperative considerations**

  a) Tracheal obstruction after extubation may be related to postoperative edema or surgical complications

  b) Continued reduction in ventrodorsal movement may worsened by oversedation and poor pain control. Consider epidural catheter for management of postoperative pain

Chapter Summary for Anterior Mediastinal Mass

General Considerations	Patients with anterior mediastinal masses are at risk for airway and cardiovascular compromise with general anesthesia
Preoperative Considerations	Careful preoperative evaluation including history, physical, and imaging. Consider whether general anesthesia is absolutely necessary at this time. Can this procedure be done under local or regional anesthesia? Can an alternate node be biopsied? Can the patient proceed to radiation prior to operative intervention?
Intraoperative Considerations	Potential for cardiovascular collapse on induction of general anesthesia. Avoid muscle relaxants. NPIC induction (noli pontes ignii consumere, i.e., "don't burn your bridges")—maintain spontaneous ventilation until either the airway is secured or the procedure is complete
Postoperative Considerations	Continue to monitor patients closely during the postoperative period for signs of airway or cardiovascular compromise.

References

1. Erdos E, Tzanova I. Perioperative anaesthetic management of mediastinal mass in adults. *Eur Soc Anaesthesiol* 2009;26:627–632.
2. Miller RD. *Anesthesia*. 7th ed. Philadelphia, PA: Churchill Livingstone; 2009.
3. Barash PG. *Clinical Anesthesia*. 5th ed. Philadelphia, PA: Lippincott Williams & Wilkins; 2009.
4. Stoelting RK, SF Dierdorf. *Anesthesia and Co-Existing Disease*. 4th ed. New York, NY: Churchill Livingstone; 2008.

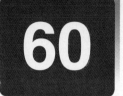

60

Heart Failure

Steven B. Edelstein, MD • Scott W. Byram, MD

In this chapter, we will investigate the anesthetic implications of heart failure (HF). As the population continues to age, the overall incidence of HF is projected to rise. Not only does this have implications for the medical management of these patients but also for costs to the entire healthcare system.

1) Incidence, risk factors, and evaluation
   a) **Incidence**
      i) The history of HF is a preoperative diagnosis commonly encountered, especially in patients presenting for elective noncardiac procedures.
      ii) In the most recent report of the Heart Disease and Stroke Statistics (1), it is estimated that the incidence of HF approaches 10 per 1,000 after the age of 65 years; 75% of these patients have a prior history of hypertension (HTN).
      iii) At age 40 the lifetime risk for development of HF is approximately 1 in 5 and the lifetime risk for people with HTN (BP > 160/90 mm Hg) is twice that of those with normal or high normal BP (<140/90 mm Hg).

2) **Risk factors.** The Framingham Heart Study reported the risk factors associated with HF (2) .
   a) HTN is the most common risk factor, followed by antecedent myocardial infarction (MI)
   b) Diabetes mellitus was the strongest risk factor for HF in postmenopausal women with established coronary artery disease, especially in combination with elevated body mass index or reduced creatinine clearance
   c) Other risk factors include increased circulating concentrations of resistin and inflammatory markers (3)

3) **Definition of HF.**
   a) HF is generally defined as inability of the heart to supply sufficient blood flow to meet the body's needs. The American Heart Association has defined HF in four stages (4) (Table 60-1).

4) **Symptoms**
   a) **Nonspecific** symptoms include dyspnea at rest or on exertion, easy fatigability, and peripheral edema.
   b) **More specific** signs (but not necessarily specific) include orthopnea, paroxysmal nocturnal dyspnea, jugular venous distention, cardiac enlargement, and a third heart sound (5).

Table 60-1
Stages of Heart Failure

Stage A	Patient at high risk but with no symptoms or signs of HF (e.g., patient with a history of HTN, atherosclerotic disease, or metabolic syndrome)
Stage B	Patient with structural heart disease strongly associated with HF, but without signs and symptoms (e.g., prior MI, asymptomatic valvular disease)
Stage C	Symptomatic HF with structural heart disease
Stage D	Advanced disease with symptoms at rest despite maximal medical therapy

Reproduced from Jessup M, Abraham WT, Casey DE, et al. 2009 Focused update: ACCF/AHA guidelines for diagnosis and management of heart failure in adults. *J Am Coll Cardiol* 2009;53:1343–1382, with permission.

5) Evaluation

    a) Defining whether the patient has preserved or reduced left ventricular function (as determined by ejection fraction) has significant implications with two entities being important to differentiate: **heart failure with reduced ejection fraction (HFREF) and heart failure with normal ejection fraction (HFNEF).**

    b) **Diagnostics.** Consider the following tests in patients with suspected HF:

        i) Routine electrocardiography

        ii) Chest x-ray with a focus on pulmonary edema or possible cardiomegaly

        iii) Plasma concentrations of natriuretic peptides

            (1) Natriuretic peptides (e.g., b-type or brain natriuretic peptides—BNP and NT-proBNP—N-terminal fragment of prohormone of BNP) are elevated in the presence of left ventricular failure.

            (2) Sensitivity may be impaired in the presence of obesity (6)

            (3) Other causes of increased BNP include ventricular hypertrophy, volume expansion, decreased renal clearance, hypoxia, tachycardia, and female gender (7).

        iv) Transthoracic echocardiography—two-dimensional echocardiography with Doppler to assess left ventricular ejection fraction, left ventricular size, wall thickness, and valve function (4)

Elective surgery in the setting of new onset HF or worsening symptoms should be delayed for further evaluation.

    c) Based on the 2007 American College of Cardiology/American Heart Association Guidelines (8), it is clear that one must answer the following question prior to proceeding to the operating room. **"Are the symptoms of heart failure new?"**

        i) If so, elective surgical procedures should be postponed until optimization has occurred.

        ii) The patient who has a known history of HF but worsening symptoms (i.e., decompensation) should also have elective surgery delayed.

6) HF with reduced ejection fraction. **The perioperative management of patients with HFREF can be quite complex. There are several important implications for the anesthetic care.**

    a) Medical management of the patient with HFREF

        i) Diuretic therapy

        ii) β-adrenergic antagonists used judiciously

        iii) Angiotensin converting enzyme (ACE) inhibitors, or angiotensin II receptor blockers (ARBs), in patients who are ACE inhibitor intolerant

iv) For African Americans, guidelines suggest the addition of hydrala-zine and nitrates for refractory symptoms (4)

v) Hospitalized patients with HFREF may be on more powerful vasodilators or inotropic medications such as:

(1) Vasodilators: nitroglycerin, nitroprusside, or nesiritide with the goal of decreasing left ventricular filling pressures (LVFP) (9)

(2) Inotropes: dobutamine and milrinone have the benefit of not only lowering the LVFP but also increasing cardiac output.

vi) Avoid calcium channel blockers due to their negative inotropic qualities.

vii) Avoid nonsteroidal anti-inflammatory agents due to their potential to aggravate the cardiorenal syndrome commonly seen in this patient population.

b) Implantable cardioverter-defibrillator (ICD) is indicated for all patients with: (4)

i) Nonischemic dilated cardiomyopathy

ii) Ischemic heart disease at least 40 days post MI

iii) LVEF ≤35%

iv) History of cardiac arrest/ventricular fibrillation/ventricular tachycardia

v) Life expectancy of >1 year

c) Cardiac resynchronization therapy (CRT)

i) Playing a growing role in the management of HFREF.

ii) CRT addresses dyssynchronous contraction commonly found in HFREF by activating the right and left ventricular chambers via a biventricular pacemaker and is at times combined with ICD therapy.

d) **Anesthetic implications in patient with HFREF (Table 60-2)**

i) **Invasive monitoring**

(1) Arterial BP or central pressure monitoring may be indicated

(2) Surgical risk should guide the choice of monitors selected. For low risk procedures (e.g., ambulatory-based such as hernia repairs, cystoscopies, and cataract surgery), requires no inva-sive devices; intermediate- to high-risk surgery requires more intensive monitoring

(3) Pulmonary artery catheters are not routinely recommended for all HFREF patients presenting for noncardiac surgery (11).

ii) **Inhalational anesthetics**

(1) Cause a dose-dependent decrease in cardiac output and cardiac contractility

(2) Nitrous oxide, though having the benefit of allowing lower concentrations of inhaled agents to be administered, is also associated with myocardial depression in the presence of HF, especially when administered with opioids.

(3) Nitrous oxide may have a deleterious effect on the pulmonary vascular resistance, causing an increase in right atrial pressures secondary to sympathetic stimulation (12).

7) **HF with normal ejection fraction. Approximately 50% of HF patients have poor systolic function (13), the rest of the patients presenting with HF will have what is known as HFNEF. These patients are likely to be older women with HTN.**

a) **Symptoms and signs**

i) Clinical signs consistent with HF as mentioned previously, notably shortness of breath

ii) Preserved ejection fraction on echocardiographic exam

iii) Increased filling pressures and impaired left ventricle (LV) filling

READ MORE

Cardiac arrhythmias and pacemakers, Chapter 57, page 412

Electrosurgical units are known to interfere with the function of pacemakers and ICDs and a thorough investigation of the patient's device is war-ranted (10).

READ MORE

Pulmonary artery catheter, Chapter 13, page 82

b) **Pathophysiology of HFNEF**

i) Patients with HFNEF have a normal ejection fraction, but have diastolic dysfunction (DD), a hallmark of HFNEF

ii) DD is a result of both impaired relaxation and increased LV passive stiffness, and may be part of the normal aging process (14).

iii) Impaired relaxation is likely due to ineffective calcium removal from the cytosol resulting in a slow LV isovolemic relaxation phase, which is worsened by myocardial ischemia.

iv) The net result of the impaired relaxation and increased stiffness is an elevated left ventricular end diastolic pressure, which can translate to an increase in left atrial pressure as well as pulmonary capillary pressure.

v) In HFNEF, an increase in blood volume coupled with tachycardia-induced decreased diastolic filling time can cause dyspnea on exertion and pulmonary edema (seen in response to exercise).

vi) Noncompliant LV is unable to accept more preload and thus is unable to use the Frank-Starling mechanism to augment stroke volume (15).

Atrial kick becomes increasingly important with atrial fibrillation decreasing cardiac output by 30% or more in patients with HFNEF, similar to what is seen in patients with aortic stenosis.

c) **Medical management of HFNEF.** In contrast to HFREF, evidence is lacking for any specific therapy to reduce mortality in patients with HFNEF (16–19). The 2005 ACC/AHA guidelines do offer some recommendations for treatment of HFNEF (20). Main therapeutic goals include:

i) Avoid tachycardia

ii) Avoid ischemia

iii) Avoid HTN

READ MORE

Quantitative echocardiography, Chapter 165, page 1143

Challenges in anesthesia: the geriatric patient presenting for surgery, Chapter 50, page 349

d) **Medication recommendations**

i) β-Adrenergic antagonists and/or calcium channel blockers have value in that they both help reduce heart rate, improve diastolic filling time, decrease BP, and decrease myocardial ischemia.

ii) ACE inhibitors/ARBs in addition to decreasing afterload may help in the regression of myocardial fibrosis (21).

e) **Anesthetic implications of HFNEF Table 60-2**

i) **Preoperatively**

(1) Up to 61.5% of geriatric surgical patients exhibit evidence of abnormal diastolic filling, DD and HFNEF (22).

(2) Patient must be medically optimized by addressing uncontrolled HTN, atrial fibrillation, HF, or myocardial ischemia.

(3) Patients should continue their cardiac medications the day of surgery to avoid HF exacerbations.

In HFNEF, pulmonary capillary wedge pressure and central venous pressure may be elevated at baseline, so estimation of volume status requires following the trends rather than the raw numbers.

ii) **Intraoperative**

(1) Standard ASA monitors are usually all that is required for the patient with HFNEF.

(2) The decision for invasive monitoring should be individualized and take into account the anticipated surgical stress, anticipated volume shifts, and comorbidities.

(3) **IV and inhalational anesthetic agents**

(a) Both can adversely affect cardiac diastolic function (23)

(b) Maintaining hemodynamic parameters seems to be more important than avoiding certain anesthetic agents

(c) In fact, diastolic function may actually improve after induction of general anesthesia (24).

(4) Avoid tachycardia since it shortens diastolic filling time

Fluid management is critical under general anesthesia, as too much fluid predisposes to pulmonary edema and atrial fibrillation on emergence.

(5) Blood pressure should be maintained within 10% of baseline since HTN can impede ejection, exacerbate ischemia, and increase LV volume, whereas hypotension, especially diastolic hypotension, can cause a decrease in coronary perfusion pressure resulting in ischemia

(6) Avoid hypercarbia and hypoxia, both of which may exacerbate any preexisting pulmonary HTN

(7) Close management of volume status is mandatory since patients are very sensitive to alterations in preload

(8) **Key point. General or regional anesthetic induced venodilation may decrease venous return and preload. Caution is advised, however, in indiscriminately administering fluid because upon emergence, venous return is restored and this may precipitate pulmonary edema or atrial fibrillation.**

iii) **Postoperative**

(1) Patients with HFNEF should be observed closely in the early postoperative period.

(2) Volume overload may occur not only in the postanesthesia care unit, but around postoperative day 3 as any third spaced fluid is reabsorbed.

(3) Pain control is important to limit tachycardia and HTN.

Chapter Summary for Key Anesthetic Considerations for HFREF and HFNEF

Preoperative	Optimization of HTN, ischemia, HF, arrhythmias Continue home medications Understand the clinical effects of concomitantly administered diuretic, vasodilator, or inotrope and the interaction with anesthetic agents Be aware of any pacemaker/defibrillator and plan accordingly
Intraoperative	Consider invasive monitors if clinically indicated Hemodynamic goals are more important than choice of anesthetic technique Avoid tachycardia (HFNEF) Avoid hypertension or excessive hypotension Avoid hypoxia and hypercarbia, which may adversely affect pulmonary vascular resistance
Postoperative	Observe for volume overload and provide adequate pain control

HF, heart failure; HFNEF, heart failure with normal ejection fraction; HTN, hypertension.

References

1. Lloyd-Jones D, Adams RJ, Brown TM, et al. Heart disease and stroke statistics 2010 update. A Report From the American Heart Association. *Circulation* 2010;121:e46–e215.

2. Levy D, Larson MG, Vasan RS, et al. The progression from hypertension to congestive heart failure. *JAMA* 1996;275:1557–1562.

3. Frankel DS, Vasan R, D'Agostino RB Sr, et al. Resistin, adiponectin, and risk of heart failure the Framingham offspring study. *J Am Coll Cardiol* 2009;53:754–762.

4. Jessup M, Abraham WT, Casey DE, et al. 2009 Focused update: ACCF/AHA Guidelines for Diagnosis and Management of Heart Failure in Adults. *J Am Coll Cardiol* 2009;53:1343–1382.

5. Mant J, Doust J, Roalfe A, et al. Systematic review and individual patient data meta-analysis of diagnosis of heart failure, with modeling of implications of different diagnostic strategies in primary care. *Health Technol Assess* 2009;13:1–207.

6. Maisel A, Mueller C, Adams K Jr, et al. State of the art: using natriuretic peptide levels in clinical practice. *Eur J Heart Fail* 2008;10:824–839.

7. Omland T. Advances in congestive heart failure management in the intensive care unit: B-type natriuretic peptides in evaluation of acute heart failure. *Crit Care Med* 2008;36(1 suppl):S17–S27.

8. Fleisher LA, Beckman JA, Brown KA, et al. ACC/AHA 2007 Guidelines on Perioperative Cardiovascular Evaluation and Care for Noncardiac Surgery: Executive Summary. *Circulation* 2007;116:1971–1996.

9. Gheorghiade M, Pang PS. Acute heart failure syndromes. *J Am Coll Cardiol* 2009;53:557–573.

10. Zaidan JR, Atlee JL, Belott P, et al. Practice advisory for the perioperative management of patients with cardiac rhythm management devices: pacemakers and implantable cardioverter-defibrillators. *Anesthesiology* 2005;103:186–198.

11. Vincent JL, Pinsky MR, Sprung CL, et al. The pulmonary artery catheter: *In medio virtus Crit Care Med* 2008;36:3093–3096.

12. Stoelting RK, Hillier S. *Chapter 2: Inhaled Anesthetics. Pharmacology & Physiology in Anesthetic Practice*. 4th ed. Philadelphia, PA: Lippincott Williams & Wilkins; 2006:42–86.

13. Owan TE, Hodge DO, Herges RM, et al. Trends in prevalence and outcome of heart failure with preserved ejection fraction. *N Engl J Med* 2006;355:251–259.

14. Zile MR, Baicu CR, Gaash WH. Diastolic heart failure-abnormalities in active relaxation and passive stiffness of the left ventricle. *N Engl J Med* 2004;350:1953–1959.

15. Kitzman DW, Higginbotham MB, Cobb FR, et al. Exercise intolerance in patients with heart failure and preserved left ventricular systolic function: failure of the Frank–Starling mechanism. *J Am Coll Cardiol* 1991;17:1065–1072.

16. Yusuf S, Pfeffer MA, Swedberg K, et al. Effects of candesartan in patients with chronic heart failure and preserved left-ventricular ejection fraction: the CHARM-Preserved Trial. *Lancet* 2003;362:777–781.

17. Ahmed A, Rich MW, Fleg JL, et al. Effects of digoxin on morbidity and mortality in diastolic heart failure: the ancillary digitalis investigation group trial. *Circulation* 2006;114:397–403.

18. Cleland JG, Tendera M, Adamus J, et al. The perindopril in elderly people with chronic heart failure (PEP-CHF) study. *Eur Heart J*. 2006;27:2338–2345.

19. Massie BM, Carson PE, McMurray JJ, et al. Irbesartan in patients with heart failure and preserved ejection fraction. *N Engl J Med* 2008;359:2456–2467.

20. Hunt SA, Abraham WT, Chin MH, et al. ACC/AHA 2005 Guideline Update for the diagnosis and management of chronic heart failure in the adult: a report of the American College of Cardiology/American Heart Association task force on practice guidelines (writing committee to update the 2001 guidelines for the evaluation and management of heart failure): developed in collaboration with the American College of Chest Physicians and the International Society of Heart and Lung Transplantation: endorsed by the Heart Rhythm Society. *Circulation* 2005;112:e154–e235.

21. Diez J, Querejeta R, Lopez B, et al. Losartan-dependent regression of myocardial fibrosis is associated with reduction of left ventricular chamber stiffness in hypertensive patients. *Circulation* 2002;105:2512–2517.

22. Phillip B, Pastor D, Bellows W, et al. The prevalence of preoperative diastolic filling abnormalities in geriatric surgical patients. *Anesth Analg* 2003;97:1214–1221.

23. Pagel PS, Grossman W, Haering JM, et al. Left ventricular diastolic function in the normal and diseased heart. *Anesthesiology* 1993;79:1104–1120.

24. Couture P, Denault AY, Shi Y, et al. Effects of anesthetic induction in patients with diastolic dysfunction. *Can J Anesth*. 2009;56:357–365.

61

Cardiomyopathy

Gurdev Rai, MD

Cardiomyopathies represent a broad class of structural heart diseases that are of major concern to the anesthesiologist. The American Heart Association defines cardiomyopathies as "a heterogeneous group of diseases of myocardium associated with mechanical or electrical dysfunction that usually exhibit inappropriate ventricular hypertrophy or dilation and are due to a variety of causes (1)." Classically, cardiomyopathies were defined by emphasizing the clinical implications of these diseases (2). Therefore this chapter focuses on the familiar approach of classifying the cardiomyopathies into hypertrophic, dilated, restrictive, or arrythmogenic right ventricular. This approach allows the anesthesiologist to focus on the clinical implications on anesthetic care of each of these disorders.

1) **Epidemiology and pathophysiology**
   a) **Hypertrophic cardiomyopathy (HCM)** occurs at a rate of 1:500 in the adult population of the United States and is characterized by a large, nondilated left ventricle (LV) (1). This characteristic must exist in the absence of any other known causes of LV hypertrophy. The causes of HCM are both genetic and nongenetic.
      i) The nongenetic form is usually seen in athletes and is a milder hypertrophy.
      ii) The genetic form is due to mutations in one of up to 11 genes and thus, results in large amounts of clinical variability (3).
      iii) Pathophysiology
         (1) The hypertrophic LV becomes harder to fill passively, resulting in diastolic dysfunction.
         (2) The hypertrophic muscle requires more oxygen to function, making it prone to ischemia (3).
         (3) In cases involving hypertrophy of the interventricular septum, dynamic left ventricular outflow tract obstruction can pose a unique challenge to the anesthesiologist.
   b) **Dilated cardiomyopathy (DCM)** has a prevalence of 1:20,000 in the middle-aged population and is characterized by ventricular dilation secondary to toxic, metabolic, or infectious causes leading to myocyte damage (1).
      i) Etiologies include viral or alcohol-related myocyte degeneration with a pattern of irregular myocyte hypertrophy and atrophy. Histologically, one also sees perivascular and interstitial fibrosis.
         (1) Viral DCM is most common in young, previously healthy individuals subjected to coxsackie B or echovirus.
         (2) Alcohol-related DCM results from chronic ingestion and is most often reversible.

c) **Restrictive cardiomyopathy (RCM)** is the least common and defined by impaired ventricular filling of normal sized ventricles. This is usually due to a fibrosed or scarred endomyocardium. Causes include:

   i) Deposition of abnormal substances like amyloid, iron, glycogen, or tumor.

   ii) Scarring related to anthracycline toxicity, radiation, or endomyocardial diseases such as hypereosinophilic syndrome.

   iii) Recently, scientists are describing a genetic component to RCM as well (1).

d) **Arrythmogenic right ventricular cardiomyopathy (ARVD)** is defined by a segmental loss of right ventricular myocytes. This is noticeable as segmental wall motion abnormalities of the right ventricle on echocardiography.

   i) Death in ARVD occurs secondary to arrhythmia related sudden death or eventual right heart failure. Its prevalence in this country is 1:10,000 (4).

   ii) Histologically, one sees the displacement of normal cardiac tissue with adipocytes or fibrous tissue.

   iii) Genetic disease with autosomal dominant inheritance and variable penetrance.

2) **Signs and symptoms**

a) The normal heart can be described as a pump consisting of four chambers with an intrinsic electrical system.

b) There are two systems of interest in a normally functioning heart, the mechanical and the electrical.

   i) These systems are dependent on each other to provide baseline functioning of the heart.

   ii) In times of stress, the two systems must have adequate reserves to meet the body's demands.

   iii) **Cardiomyopathies result from a defect in the mechanical system associated with decreased cardiac performance.**

c) **Systolic failure**

   i) As remodeling of the ventricular structure progresses, the associated changes in the mechanics of the heart eventually start impacting the heart's functional reserve.

   ii) Systolic failure occurs more often in DCM.

   iii) Increased end-diastolic volume and decreased ejection fraction result in signs of decreased O_2 delivery. The body tries to compensate by increasing heart rate and increasing vascular tone.

   iv) **Thus, with DCM the classical signs of systolic heart failure including cyanosis, cold extremities, and decreased exercise tolerance are observed.**

d) **Diastolic dysfunction**

   i) With HCM and RCM a combination of systolic and diastolic dysfunction is observed.

   ii) The decreased compliance of the LV results in increased filling pressures, increased left ventricular end diastolic pressure, and decreased end-diastolic volume.

   iii) The left atrium may hypertrophy and eventually dilate, increasing the risk of atrial fibrillation or flutter; further decreasing the end-diastolic volume in a very preload dependent ventricle.

Cardiomyopathies may be asymptomatic during the early phases with symptoms becoming evident as the disease progresses.

READ MORE

Heart failure, Chapter 60, page 436

       iv) Clinically, the body compensates with tachycardia and increased systemic vascular resistance.

       v) **Symptoms include dyspnea upon exertion, pulmonary edema, atrial fibrillation, and vascular congestion/edema.**

  e) **Arrhythmias**

       i) A dilated or hypertrophic heart may have impaired conduction of electrical impulses.

       ii) Commonly, patients exhibit bundle branch blocks, first-degree heart blocks, and an increased incidence of tachyarrythmias (5).

       iii) Sudden death is a constant threat to all patients with cardiomyopathy (2).

  f) **Left Ventricular Outflow Tract Obstruction.** With HCM, one must pay special attention to left ventricular outflow tract obstruction.

       i) **Symptoms/signs include**

           (1) Fainting spells and angina during stressful situations or conditions, which increase preload.

       ii) A dynamic holosystolic murmur is typically heard on ascultation.

       iii) **Echocardiographic** imaging usually shows a large interventricular septum.

           (1) As flow increases, the septum and mitral valve leaflet get pulled together based on the Bernoulli Effect. This causes an obstruction of the outflow tract during systole.

       iv) During anesthesia, any stimulus, which increases contractility or preload, can cause hypotension and heart failure in these patients.

3) **Treatment options** depend primarily on the cardiomyopathy classification

  a) **Lifestyle modifications** such as weight control, abstinence from tobacco, and moderation of alcohol intake.

  b) **Pharmacotherapy**

       i) Emphasis is on ACE-inhibitors, potassium sparing diuretics, vasodilators, and digitalis, all of which prevent further remodeling of the heart.

       ii) In addition, the antiarrhythmogenic therapy is employed.

       iii) In patients with severe dysfunction, warfarin is utilized to decrease the viscosity of blood and encourage flow. It also prevents the formation of clot in a low flow state.

       iv) The definitive treatment is cardiac transplantation. In patients who are not candidates for transplantation or those on the waiting list, ventricular assist devices can be used.

4) **Anesthetic implications**

  a) **Preoperative considerations**

       i) One must define the type of cardiomyopathy present and the patient's functional status.

       ii) The physical exam includes a thorough heart and lung exam.

       iii) If the patient has signs of heart failure, the surgery should be delayed until further workup including chest films, ECG, and echocardiogram can be obtained (6).

       iv) In emergent situations, the goal is to maintain normal hemodynamics with the aid of invasive monitors.

       v) An arterial line and a central venous pressure line are the minimum to provide a safe anesthetic in a patient with an unknown cardiomyopathy

       vi) Preparedness for arrhythmias, cardiac arrest, and potentially death is absolutely relevant to the perioperative care of these patients. This must be discussed with the patients as well as the care team.

b) **Intraoperative**

   i) **Hypertrophic Cardiomyopathy (HCM)**

READ MORE

Cardiac arrhythmias and pacemakers, Chapter 57, page 412

   (1) Typically, these patients are on β-adrenergic antagonists or amio-darone and may even have an implanted defibrillator. One must ensure that the patient has had all scheduled medications. The defibrillator must be turned off if interference from surgical devices like unipolar electrocautery is expected and external defibrillating equipment must at hand.

Outflow obstruction in patients with HCM can lead to sudden death—recognize warning signs early and treat aggressively with IV fluid, phenylephrine, and b-adrenergic blockade.

   (2) The main goals to help prevent obstructive physiology are: maintain preload and afterload, maintain a relatively slow sinus rhythm, and recognize undiagnosed obstruction (6).

   (3) Afterload and preload are maintained with heart rate control and maintenance of systemic vascular resistance during induction, maintenance, and emergence from anesthesia.

   (4) Junctional rhythms are not tolerated well due to the dependence of the left ventricular end diastolic volume on atrial kick. Early detection and treatment of a junctional rhythm is imperative.

   (5) **Sudden hypotension and a dynamic systolic murmur should raise the suspicion of undiagnosed LV outflow obstruction.** In these cases, drugs that increase heart rate or contractility should be avoided. Emphasis should be on filling the ventricles and slowing the heart rate. This can be accomplished with fluid boluses, phenylepherine, and beta-blockade.

   ii) **Restrictive Cardiomyopathy (RCM)**

   (1) Initially, try to determine the levels of venous congestion by looking for jugular venous distension, hepatojugular reflex, or peripheral edema.

   (2) In patients with evidence of congestion, diuretics are the preferred treatment.

   (3) One must also be wary of arrhythmias. Antiarrhythmogenic treatment with beta-blockers or amiodarone is the mainstay.

   (4) Preoperative echocardiographic studies are essential to define the level of diastolic dysfunction.

   (5) Restrictive hearts are rate-dependent for cardiac output. Thus, rate control and maintenance of sinus rhythm are keys to a safe anesthetic (6).

   iii) **Dilated Cardiomyopathy (DCM)**

   (1) Hemodynamic goals of maintaining preload and sinus rhythm should be accomplished by avoiding myocardial depression and preventing large increases in afterload.

   (2) Careful induction using a technique that preserves myocardial contractility, preload, and rhythm (6).

   (3) Moderately elevated heart rates are better tolerated since they prevent large increases in end-diastolic volume. Therefore, drugs like ephedrine, epinephrine, and dopamine become the treatments of choice for hypotension.

   iv) **Arrythmogenic right ventricular cardiomyopathy (ARVD)**

   (1) The main goal in patients with ARVD is to promote forward flow out of the right side of the heart. This depends on balancing adequate preload with the myocardium's ability to contract.

   (2) **A pulmonary artery catheter (PAC), or transesophogeal echocardiography,** is indicated in intermediate- to high-risk procedures. However, one must be ready to handle any potential malignant arrhythmia associated with PAC placement or anesthesia administration.

   (3) Familiarity with AICDs and antiarrhythmia medications is essential.

(4) Afterload reduction by maintaining low pulmonary vascular resistance and left ventricular function are also imperative. **The emphasis must be on maintaining normocapnea, preventing hypoxia or acidosis to minimize changes in pulmonary vascular resistance (4).**

c) **Postoperative care** depends on the operation.

   i) For minor procedures, it may be adequate to monitor in a telemetry or stepdown unit. For moderate- to high-risk surgery, intensive care settings are the safest.

   ii) Restarting the patient's preoperative medications in a timely fashion is critical.

   iii) For patients with AICDs that were turned off, trained personnel must be available to reprogram the device after surgery. If not, one must keep a defibrillator at hand and monitor the patient closely for malignant arrhythmias (5).

5) **Follow-up**

   a) Cardiologists should be alerted to, if not involved with, these patients prior to the operative day and informed of any perioperative events.

   b) The patient should be evaluated to ensure that their medications have been restarted and that their AICD is functional.

   c) If any clinical signs of decompensation are evident, an evaluation of cardiac function involving an echocardiogram must be pursued, with any changes worked up as potential myocardial infarction or a need to further optimize medications.

Chapter Summary for Cardiomyopathies

Epidemiology	Prevalence varies with classification. Most adult patients arrive with their diagnosis in hand prior to surgery. HCM and DCM are the most common.
Preoperative Considerations	Input from cardiologists is imperative during a very thorough preoperative workup of these patients. Once the type of cardiomyopathy is determined, one must plan an anesthetic that preserves the compensatory mechanisms in place to overcome the pathology. This entails a complete understanding of medications and monitors.
Intraoperative Considerations	HCM—Dynamic outflow tract obstruction is major concern. Maintain preload/afterload, relatively slow sinus rhythm. Avoid tachycardia DCM—Avoid myocardial depression and large increases in afterload
Monitoring	Low-risk procedures may be safely performed with standard monitors. For intermediate- and high-risk procedures, invasive arterial monitoring should be employed ± central venous monitoring or TEE.

HCM, hypertrophic cardiomyopathy; DCM, dilated cardiomyopathy.

References

1. Maron BJ, Towbin JA, Thiene G, et al. Contemporary Definitions and Classifications of the Cardiomyopathies: An American Heart Association Scientific Statement from the Council on Clinical Cardiology, Heart Failure, and Transplantation Committee; Quality of Care and Outcomes Research and Functional Genomics and Translational Biology Interdisciplinary Working Groups; and Council on Epidemiology and Prevention. *Circulation* 2006;113:1807.

2. Elliot P, Anderson B, Arbustini E, et al. Classification of the Cardiomyopathies: a position statement from the European Society of Cardiology Working Group on Myocardial and Pericardial Disease. *Eur Heart J* 2008;29:270.

3. Neubauer S. The failing heart-an engine out of fuel. *N Engl J Med.* 2007;356:1140–1151.

4. Alexoudis AK. Anaesthetic implications of arrhythmogenic right ventricular dysplasia cardiomyopathy. *Anaesthesia* 2009;64:73–78.

5. Practice advisory for the perioperative management of patients with cardiac rhythm management devices: pacemakers and implantable cardioverters-defibrillators; a report by the American Society of Anesthesiologists Task Force on Perioperative Management of Patients with Cardiac Rhythm Management Devices. *Anesthesiology* 2005;103:186–198.

6. Stoelting R, Dierdorf S. *Anesthesia and Coexisting Disease.* 4th ed. Philadelphia, PA: Churchill Livingstone; 2002.

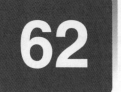

Pulmonary Hypertension

Nathaen Weitzel, MD

Pulmonary Hypertension (PH) represents a clinical challenge to the practicing anesthesiologist because it places patients presenting for surgery in a high risk category. This risk, coupled with relatively limited therapeutic options for PH, complicates the perioperative care. This chapter outlines the pathophysiology of PH and anesthetic considerations when caring for these patients.

⌐ READ
▶ MORE
Challenges in anesthesia: laparoscopic cholecystectomy in the patient with pulmonary hypertension, Chapter 66, page 476

1) Definitions and etiology

   a) PH is defined as a syndrome with elevated pulmonary artery pressures (mean PAP > 25 mm Hg at rest) (1–3).

   b) PH is associated with reduced nitric oxide (NO) and prostacyclin synthesis as well as with increased thromboxane production (4).

      i) Histologic features include medial thickening and intimal fibrosis (5).

   c) Classically, PH was described as primary or secondary PH. In 1998, the World Health Organization adopted a new classification system describing five categories of PH:

      i) **Isolated pulmonary arterial hypertension** (PAH)

         (1) Includes primary PH, systemic to pulmonary shunts and collagen vascular disease

         (2) PAH is defined as exclusion of secondary causes, elevated mean PAP (>25 mmHg), and elevated PVR of >3 Woods units

      ii) **PAH associated with diseases of the respiratory system and/or hypoxia**

         (1) Includes chronic obstructive pulmonary disease, obstructive sleep apnea

      iii) **Pulmonary venous hypertension**

         (1) Includes mitral valve disease, chronic left ventricle [LV] dysfunction

      iv) **PH associated with chronic embolic/thrombotic disease**

      v) **PH attributed to direct obstruction of the pulmonary vasculature** (inflammatory pulmonary capillary hemangiomatosis) (1)

2) Pathophysiology

   a) **Acute changes**

      i) The normal pulmonary vascular resistance (PVR) is <90% of the systemic vascular resistance (SVR).

      ii) Because the right ventricle (RV) is designed for a low pressure system, an acute increase in pulmonary pressure often results in rapid right ventricular failure (i.e., acute pulmonary embolus, acute severe MR) (1,5).

   b) **Chronic PH**

      i) PH tends to develop over time, allowing the RV to compensate for the increased work via hypertrophic changes.

        ii)   Unfortunately, the RV has limited ability to compensate in this manner and will eventually dilate and fail. RV failure leads to a variety of events including (1,5)

           (1)   Reduced RV stroke volume, decreased preload to the LV, and resultant hypotension

           (2)   Intraventricular septum of the dilated RV shifts toward the LV, further decreasing LV output.

           (3)   Reduced RV coronary blood flow secondary to disruption of the normal systolic and diastolic coronary blood flow pattern

        iii)   Right-to-left shunt may develop in patients with a patent foramen ovale (~30% of adults) resulting in hypoxia.

3) **Surgical and anesthetic risks**

    a)   PH patients are high-risk surgical candidates.

        i)   Published series demonstrate a range of surgical mortalities from a low 4% to high of 24% depending on disease severity and surgical procedure (1).

        ii)   Surgical and anesthetic risk should be clearly stated to the patient, especially for an elective case.

    b)   **Hemodynamic spiral**

"Death spiral" secondary to RV failure is always a possibility in PH patients.

        i)   Acute deterioration is possible as RV failure causes reduced pulmonary blood flow, leading to hypoxia, which subsequently increases the PVR.

        ii)   The elevated PVR ultimately leads to increased strain on the RV.

        iii)   This initiates a **catastrophic hemodynamic chain of events** where the decreased RV stroke volume decreases LV output and coronary blood flow decreases to both the LV and RV.

        iv)   The already failing RV may not be able to recover from this, resulting in cardiac arrest. This "death spiral" is always a potential in PH patients; the anesthesia provider should be aware of it and take steps to prevent it.

4) **Preoperative evaluation**

    a)   Patients with PH are high-risk patients who should be evaluated by a PH specialist before surgery and should be started on appropriate medication as indicated.

    b)   The goal of the pre-op evaluation is to determine if the patient suffers from PH, RV failure, or a combination of these, as this knowledge affects management (5).

Symptoms of low cardiac output and metabolic acidosis along with hypoxia, syncope, and evidence of RV failure indicate severe disease state (1).

    c)   **Clinical findings**

        i)   The signs of PH are often vague, but the most common sign is dyspnea with exertion.

        ii)   This symptom can progress to dyspnea at rest, chest pain, fatigue, and syncope. A history of syncope is an extremely poor prognostic sign (1).

    d)   The **etiology** of the PH should be determined if possible, and a cardiac echocardiographic exam should be obtained (1,5).

        i)   Valvular structures, size and function of both RV and LV, and the presence of any intracardiac shunts should be evaluated.

        ii)   Echocardiography can measure mean PAP; however, this is often underestimated; therefore, cardiac catheterization is the gold standard of measure.

    e)   Pulmonary vascular reactivity can also be determined at catheterization to test responsiveness to vasodilators.

    f)   **Medications**

        i)   Common medications for the treatment of PH include calcium channel blockers, digoxin, diuretics, prostaglandin infusion, and sildenafil.

ii) Patients with PH are often taking warfarin, and they should be transitioned to low molecular weight heparin prior to their surgery.

g) **PH medications should be continued and doses should not be missed on the day of surgery.**

h) A complete blood count, metabolic panel, and coagulation panel should be evaluated. Consider preoperative blood gas analysis.

i) An ECG should be performed to evaluate signs of ischemia or right-sided ventricular strain.

5) **Anesthetic management**

a) **Type of anesthetic**

i) Regional anesthesia is likely the best approach for PH patients if possible (peripheral nerve block or epidural but not spinal anesthesia), although data is limited and retrospective in nature.

ii) Martin et al. showed that operative mortality in patients with Eisenmenger syndrome was 18% with general anesthesia versus 5% with regional anesthesia (6).

iii) Conversely, Weiss et al. conducted a review of obstetric outcomes over 18 years, demonstrating similar outcomes using either general or regional anesthesia (7).

iv) For moderate to severe PH, spinal anesthesia is contraindicated due to chance for abrupt alterations in SVR and preload.

b) Maintain preoperative medications and continue the prostaglandin infusion, as even brief infusion interruptions can cause rapid deterioration and death.

i) For patients taking sildenafil, avoid nitroglycerin and nitroprusside, which can cause severe hypotension.

ii) Outpatient therapy is typically titrated slowly and carefully, so it is critical that this is not disrupted for elective surgery.

c) **Monitoring**

i) **Arterial lines** are indicated for all but the lowest risk surgeries.

ii) **Central venous access**

(1) Caution should be taken during placement to avoid inducing arrhythmias.

(2) If atrial arrhythmias develop, cardioversion will avoid the rapid cardiovascular collapse that can occur.

iii) **Pulmonary artery catheters** (PAC)

(1) The information gained by this monitor may provide critical information for ventilatory and inotropic management, making it recommended for most intermediate and all high-risk procedures.

(2) Caution must be used when inserting a PAC, which may be more difficult to place in a PH patient.

Management of either regional or general anesthesia requires utmost vigilance in patients with PH.

READ MORE

Pulmonary artery catheter, Chapter 13, page 82

Table 62-1

Anesthetic and Hemodynamic Goals for patients with PH

1. **Avoid elevations in PVR:** Prevent hypoxemia, acidosis, hypercarbia, and pain. Provide supplemental oxygen at all times.
2. **Maintain SVR:** Decreased SVR dramatically reduces CO due to "fixed" PVR.
3. **Avoid myocardial depressants and maintain myocardial contractility.**
4. **Maintain preload.**
5. **Maintain sinus rhythm.**

(3) **PAC should not be placed in patients with Eisenmenger physiology (4).**

iv) **TEE** should be considered if available.

d) **General anesthesia**

   i) **Sedation**

   (1) Supplemental oxygen should be used and preoperative sedation minimized to avoid hypoxia and hypercarbia.

   ii) **Induction**

   (1) Anesthetic induction can be challenging due to the high resting sympathetic tone and resultant deficiency of catecholamine levels (5).

   (2) This can result in exaggerated hemodynamic compromise following induction and as such, induction should be titrated slowly to effect.

   (3) Induction are be carried out using a slow titration of narcotics, followed by an induction agent such as etomidate (0.2 to 0.4 mg/kg) to limit hemodynamic changes. Lidocaine (1 mg/kg) may also help blunt response to intubation and should be considered.

Intraoperative hypotension in a patient with PH may be caused by RV failure or inadequate preload.

   iii) **Maintenance of anesthesia**

   (1) Combinations of inhaled agents along with IV narcotics/benzodiazepines should be titrated to effect.

   iv) **Fluid management**

   (1) Attempt to maintain euvolemia as close to baseline as possible.

   (2) TEE/PAC measurements should guide fluid management with care taken not to overwhelm the RV function.

e) **Hemodynamic management**

   i) If hypotension is observed, determine if it is due to RV failure or inadequate preload.

   ii) Assuming euvolemia, inotropic therapy must be considered. **(Table 62-2)**

   iii) Consider dobutamine (β_1 agonist) or milrinone (PDE III inhibitor) as IV inotropic therapy.

   (1) Both agents are considered "inodilators" and may result in systemic vasodilation and hypotension, which can usually be treated with phenylephrine or norepinephrine.

Table 62-2

Therapeutic Options for Hemodynamic Support in PH

Direct acting Pulmonary Vasodilators (requires modifying circuit, consult respiratory therapy for assistance)

- Inhaled NO 20–40 ppm blended into inspiratory arm of circuit
- Inhaled prostacyclin nebulized 50 ng/kg/min or 50 μg over 15 min q1h

Pulmonary and Systemic Vasodilators Plus Increased Cardiac Contractility

- Dobutamine infusion 2–20 μg/kg/min
- Milrinone infusion 0.5–0.75 μg/kg/min
- Dipyridamole bolus 0.2–0.6 mg/kg over 15 min q12h
  - Consider for cases of PH refractory to NO therapy.

Systemic Vasoconstrictors

- Phenylephrine infusion 10–200 μg/min
- Norepinephrine infusion 0.2–3.3 μg/kg/min

Adapted from Blaise G, Langleben D, Hubert B. Pulmonary arterial hypertension: pathophysiology and anesthetic approach. *Anesthesiology* 2003;99:1415–1432.

iv) **Inhaled NO**
  (1) A potent pulmonary vasodilator (starting dose 20 to 40 ppm), which has minimal effect on systemic circulation (8).
  (2) NO requires special equipment to administer inline in the anesthesia circuit, and not all hospitals have NO available.
  (3) NO must be weaned slowly, so once started the patient will need to remain intubated as NO is weaned in the ICU.
  (4) Inhaled prostacyclin has also been used intraoperatively either as continuous inhalational therapy (50 ng/kg/min) (9) or as an hourly inhaled bolus (50 µg over 15 minutes) (10).
  v) Vasoconstrictors such as phenylephrine, norepinephrine, and vasopressin may have variable responses on PVR, but may be needed in the setting of persistent systemic hypotension.
f) **Ventilator management**
  i) Avoidance of hypoxia and hypercarbia is critical, but must be balanced by avoidance of lung hyperinflation.
  ii) Large alterations in lung volumes by positive pressure ventilation, along with either excessive or inadequate PEEP, can dramatically alter PVR in PH patients (5).
  iii) Low Tidal Volume Ventilation with low PEEP levels may be the ideal strategy, adjusting respiratory rate to prevent hypercarbia. Hypercarbia dramatically elevates PVR, and is a risk with this ventilation strategy and must be monitored carefully.
6) **Postoperative management**
  a) The postoperative period is a high risk time for PH patients.
  b) PH patients should be monitored in an intensive care setting in the first few days following surgery as there is high risk for sudden death.
  c) Patients may benefit from epidural anesthesia for postoperative analgesia.
  d) Finally, the patients should be transitioned back to their usual oral anticoagulation postoperatively.

Chapter Summary for PH

Definitions	Mean PAP > 25 mm Hg. Can be either primary or secondary PH.
Assessment	Thorough history can be invaluable. Evaluation by specialist in PH before elective surgery is recommended. TEE or right heart catheterization is key in evaluation of etiology, current RV function, and response to vasodilators. Consider preoperative ABG.
Risks	Patients are high-risk surgical candidates. Elevations in PAP can result in RV failure leading to hemodynamic collapse.
Monitoring	Arterial line for most procedures. Consider central line, PAC, or TEE as indicated by surgical risk.
Anesthetic Management	Regional anesthesia probably is first choice. Tailor anesthetic to minimize alterations in preload/afterload. Avoid hypercarbia, acidosis, and hypoxia. Consider inhaled NO for severe PH patients. Maintain all outpatient PH medications throughout perioperative period.

References
1. Blaise G, Langleben D, Hubert B. Pulmonary arterial hypertension: pathophysiology and anesthetic approach. *Anesthesiology* 2003;99: 1415–1432.
2. Weitzel N, Gravlee G. Cardiac disease in the obstetric patient. In: Bucklin B, Gambling D, Wlody D, eds. *A Practical Approach to Obstetric Anesthesia*. 1st ed. Philidelphia, PA: Lippincott Williams & Wilkins; 2009:403–434.

3. McLaughlin VV, Archer SL, Badesch DB, et al. ACCF/AHA 2009 expert consensus document on pulmonary hypertension: a report of the American College of Cardiology Foundation Task Force on Expert Consensus Documents and the American Heart Association: developed in collaboration with the American College of Chest Physicians, American Thoracic Society, Inc., and the Pulmonary Hypertension Association. *Circulation* 2009;119:2250–2294.

4. Ray P, Murphy G, Shutt L. Recognition and management of maternal cardiac disease in pregnancy. *Br J Anaesth* 2004;93:428–439.

5. Huffmyer J, Rich G. Managing the patient with pulmonary hypertension who requires cardiac surgery. In: Cohen N ed. *Medically Challenging Patients Undergoing Cardiothoracic Surgery*. Philadelphia, PA: Lippincott Williams & Wilkins; 2009:185–214.

6. Martin JT, Tautz TJ, Antognini JF. Safety of regional anesthesia in Eisenmenger's syndrome. *Reg Anesth Pain Med* 2002;27:509–513.

7. Weiss BM, Zemp L, Seifert B, et al. Outcome of pulmonary vascular disease in pregnancy: a systematic overview from 1978 through 1996. *J Am Coll Cardiol* 1998;31:1650–1657.

8. Sitbon O, Brenot F, Denjean A, et al. Inhaled nitric oxide as a screening vasodilator agent in primary pulmonary hypertension. A dose-response study and comparison with prostacyclin. *Am J Respir Crit Care Med* 1995;151:384–389.

9. Fiser SM, Cope JT, Kron IL, et al. Aerosolized prostacyclin (epoprostenol) as an alternative to inhaled nitric oxide for patients with reperfusion injury after lung transplantation. *J Thorac Cardiovasc Surg* 2001;121:981–982.

10. Hoeper MM, Schwarze M, Ehlerding S, et al. Long-term treatment of primary pulmonary hypertension with aerosolized iloprost, a prostacyclin analogue. *N Engl J Med* 2000;342:1866–1870.

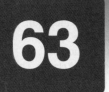

63 Anesthesia for Aortic Surgery

James Sederberg, MD • Nathaen Weitzel, MD

Surgical repair of aneurysms have represented a challenge for physicians from the time of the first attempted aneurysm repair by Antyllus in the 4th century AD. Abdominal and thoracic aneurysms remain one of the more challenging anesthetic cases in major vascular surgery, and place patients at elevated risk. A thorough knowledge of the pathophysiology of both the disease and operation is critical to managing these patients.

1) Epidemiology and incidence of thoracic and abdominal aortic disease
   a) **Definition and etiology**
      i) An aneurysm is a permanent focal dilation of an artery to 1.5 times its normal size.
      ii) Aneurysms develop from the degradation of extracellular matrix proteins—elastin and collagen.
      iii) Smoking and infection may also play an important part by creating inflammation in the vessel wall (1).
   b) **Surgical intervention** is recommended based on overall aneurysm size, rate of expansion, patient age, and comorbidities. The annual risk of rupture is 3% in aneurysms 5 to 5.9 cm (2).
      i) **Ascending thoracic aneurysm**
         1) Surgery recommended for diameter **>5.5 cm**, or **>6 cm** in patients with increased operative risk. If patients are at increased risk of rupture or dissection, then repair is recommended at **>5 cm** (2).
      ii) **Descending thoracic and abdominal aortic aneurysms (AAA)**
         (1) Intervention is recommended if aneurysm is **>6 cm** or growth rate >1 cm per year (3–5).
   c) **Typical surgical and anesthetic complications**
      i) **Elective AAA repair has a mortality of < 2%, whereas rupture carries a mortality of up to 70% to 80% with 1% mortality per hour for the first 48 hours.**
      ii) Complication rates are influenced by comorbid disease (Table 63-1) (6).

Table 63-1
Complications Associated with AAA Repair

Myocardial infarction
Respiratory failure
Renal failure (depending on cross-clamp time and location of aneurysm)
Bleeding
Spinal cord injury (depending on ischemia duration and surgical technique)
Stroke

2) Physiology of aortic cross clamping
   a) Thoracic/supraceliac (Table 63-2)
      Hemodynamic changes associated with proximal aortic occlusion include (10):
      i) **Increased afterload,** with an increase in proximal aortic pressure
      ii) **Elevated LV wall tension** with increased myocardial O_2 consumption
      iii) **Increased preload** due to decreased venous capacitance below the clamp. This results in volume redistribution from the splanchnic and nonsplanchnic beds toward the heart.
      iv) **Severe hypertension (HTN) during aortic occlusion**
         (1) Often associated with clamping along with a reflexively decreased heart rate
         (2) Increase in cardiac contractility secondary to cathecholamine release
         (3) Treatment of HTN is often difficult while still maintaining spinal cord and distal perfusion pressures.
            (a) Nitroglycerin, sodium nitroprusside, esmolol, epidural infusions, high-dose narcotics, and increased anesthetic depth may be used to treat HTN during aortic occlusion.
   b) **Abdominal/infraceliac (Table 63-2)**
      i) The same effects on afterload and contractility occur when the abdominal aorta is cross-clamped; however, effects on preload are inconsistent (8).
      ii) Preload has been observed to increase, likely secondary to the same mechanism as in a supraceliac clamp.
   c) **Unclamping** (Table 63-3)—As the cross-clamp is released, the opposite physiologic effects are seen with a marked decrease in systemic vascular resistance (SVR), central hypovolemia, and hypotension.
      i) This is caused by blood pooling in reperfused tissues, hypoxia-mediated vasodilation, and accumulation of myocardial depressant and vasodilatory metabolites such as lactate.
      ii) Left ventricular end-diastolic pressure decreases and myocardial blood flow increases (7,8).
      iii) The celiac and/or superior mesenteric arteries are often involved with suprarenal cross-clamp placement. This can produce visceral ischemia and profound lactic acidosis, therefore sodium bicarbonate, along with slow release of the cross clamp, is beneficial.
      iv) If severe unclamping shock occurs, replacement of the clamp will restore BP until further volume resuscitation can be accomplished.

Table 63-2

Physiologic Changes Associated with Aortic Cross-Clamping (7,8)

Supra-Celiac Clamping

↑ Afterload
↑ Preload→ due to redistribution of venous capacitance below clamp
HTN (potentially severe)
↓ Heart rate
↑ or ↓ cardiac output
Catecholamine release → increase contractility
↑ Myocardial oxygen demand can lead to ischemia

Infraceliac Clamping

Same as above except preload may ↑ or ↓ and is inconsistent

Table 63-3

Physiologic Changes Associated with Aortic Cross-Clamp Release (7,8)

↓ SVR
Central hypovolemia
Blood pooling in reperfused tissues
Vasodilatation
Myocardial depression from metabolites like lactate
↓ LVEDP
↑ Myocardial blood flow
Lactic acidosis from ischemic tissue, which can be severe

When the aortic cross-clamp is released, be prepared for decreased SVR, hypovolemia, and hypotension.

Anesthetic management for repair of thoracic aortic aneurysms is one of the greatest challenges to the anesthesiologist (3).

3) **Thoracic aortic aneurysms (TAAA)**
   a) Descending thoracic aneurysms begin distal to the left subclavian artery and are classified using the Crawford classification (**Fig. 63-1**)
      i) Type I aneurysms originate below the left subclavian artery and extend to the celiac axis
      ii) Type II originate as Type I, but extend to the infrarenal aorta.
      iii) Any aneurysm involving the ascending aorta or arch is also considered a Type II aneurysm.
      iv) Type III begins in the distal thoracic aorta and involves the remainder of the abdominal aorta.
      v) Type IV begins at the diaphragm and involves the entire abdominal aorta.
   b) **Anesthetic considerations**
      i) **Preoperative considerations**
         (1) Preanesthesia evaluation
            (a) Many patients are smokers with cardiac and/or pulmonary disease including HTN, coronary artery disease, Chronic Obstructive Pulmonary Disease (COPD), or bronchitis.
            (b) A thorough preoperative multisystem workup must be carried out with special focus on the cardiac and pulmonary systems.
               (i) Pulmonary Function Testing, chest radiograph, and cardiac stress testing are often indicated. Basic labs should also be obtained.
      ii) **Intraoperative considerations**
         (1) Monitoring choices and considerations.
         (2) Standard ASA monitors plus an arterial line is typically used.
         (3) A right radial arterial line is preferred in case the cross clamp is applied proximal to the subclavian artery. An additional femoral arterial line may be useful depending on the surgical clamping strategy.
         (4) Large bore peripheral IV and central venous access are essential.

Figure 63-1   Crawford Classification of Thoracoabdominal Aneurysms

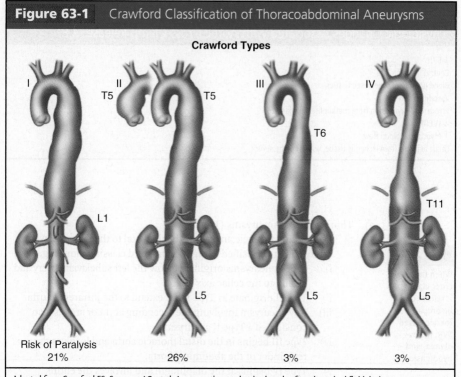

Crawford Types

Risk of Paralysis
21%   26%   3%   3%

Adapted from Crawford ES, Svensson LG, et al. A prospective randomized study of cerebrospinal fluid drainage to prevent paraplegia after high-risk surgery on the thoracoabdominal aorta. *J Vasc Surg* 1991;13:36–45.

Consider a right radial arterial line for thoracic aortic aneurysm repair in case the cross-clamp is applied proximal to the subclavian artery.

(5) A pulmonary artery catheter (PAC) or transesophageal echocardiography (TEE) can give vital information about hemodynamic changes and volume status, and is indicated in patients with known cardiac disease (9).

(6) The patient should have a type and cross for four units of packed red blood cells.

(7) Vasoactive infusions and heparin should be readily available.

iii) For **induction**, the choice of agent is not as critical as is the manner delivered.

(1) Induction should be achieved with careful and slow titration of narcotics, hypnotics, and muscle relaxants.

(2) The goal is to maintain hemodynamic stability while preventing overt HTN, and to blunt the sympathetic response to endotracheal intubation.

iv) **Airway management**

(1) Lung isolation is usually necessary for Crawford type I, II, and some type III aneurysm repairs (3).

(2) Double lumen endotracheal tube is preferred over endobronchial blockers because of the increased ability to clear secretions and the ability to provide Positive End Expiratory Pressure (PEEP) to the dependent lung and/or Continuous Positive Airway Pressure (CPAP) to the nondependent lung.

v) **Surgical considerations**

   (1) A left-sided thoracotomy is the preferred approach with patients typically placed in a modified right lateral decubitus position. The exact location of the incision depends on the extent of aortic pathology.

c) **Specific perfusion scenarios**

   i) **Circulatory arrest**

      (1) The goals of deep hypothermic circulatory arrest (DHCA) are to protect the vital organs by reducing metabolic rate and to protect the brain and heart from re-warming.

      (2) Temperatures are typically reduced to 10°C to 18°C, which allows a safe duration of approximately 40 minutes.

      (3) Cooling and re-warming should be gradual, and a differential temperature gradient (esophageal-blood) of more than 10°C should be avoided.

      (4) During DHCA, the head should be packed in ice (with care taken to avoid the eyes), which typically achieves isoelectricity on an electroencephalogram (EEG) or processed EEG monitor before arrest.

      (5) Use of steroids, propofol, or barbiturates may be also helpful.

   ii) **Anterograde cerebral perfusion (ACP)**

      (1) The goal is to maintain the brain temperature at selected levels, meet the demands of metabolism, and remove the cerebral metabolic waste during ischemia.

READ
MORE

Coagulopathies,
Chapter 89,
page 643

      (2) The subclavian or innominate artery can be cannulated for this purpose, or to provide bihemispheric protection, the left common carotid artery as well.

      (3) This is a low flow scenario using approximately 10 mL/kg/min flow rates (to achieve pressures near 40 mm Hg), coupled with hypothermia for protection. Studies demonstrate conflicting data regarding absolute length of time ACP can be safely carried out (9,10).

   iii) **Partial bypass or left heart bypass (11)** may be required during more extensive aortic repairs. Oxygenation can be through the lungs or an oxygenator.

d) Anti-coagulation considerations

   i) **Coagulopathy**

      (1) Platelet dysfunction and coagulopathy are often seen following prolonged cardiopulmonary bypass and DHCA.

      (2) Coagulation studies can help guide transfusion decisions, and thromboelastography can be invaluable.

e) **Spinal cord protection/neurologic protection**

   i) Neurological injury is a devastating consequence of aneurysm repair, especially thoracic aorta aneurysm repair.

   ii) **Risks include** emergency surgery, dissection, extensive disease, prolonged cross clamp time, rupture, level of clamp, age, and history of renal dysfunction.

Cross-clamping
of the aorta
increases CSF
pressure and
increases the
risk for spinal
cord ischemia.

   iii) **Cerebrospinal fluid (CSF) drain**

      (1) Aortic cross-clamping causes elevation of CSF pressure.

      (2) The spinal cord perfusion pressure (SCCP) is the difference between spinal arterial pressure and CSF pressure. ↓CSF pressure → improved SCCP.

      (3) Goals are to keep spinal drain pressure around 10 mm Hg, and drainage should be limited to a maximum of 20 mL/h.

The anterior artery of Adamkiewicz supplies the upper thoracic spinal cord and is at risk for ischemia during aortic surgery.

READ MORE

Neurophysiologic monitoring and anesthetic management, Chapter 16, page 100

iv) **Spinal cord blood flow**

(1) The spinal cord is perfused by two posterior arteries, which supply approximately 25% of the spinal cord and one anterior artery that supplies 75% of the spinal cord.

(2) The most important radicular artery is the **artery of Adamkiewicz,** which arises from T9 to T12 in 60% of people, and supplies the anterior spinal artery of the upper thoracic spinal cord. If this artery comes from the aneurysm wall or below the cross-clamp, then spinal cord ischemia and anterior spinal artery syndrome are possible.

v) **Electrophysiologic monitoring of spinal cord**

(1) Monitoring of evoked potentials provides the surgeon with opportunity to promptly intervene if the monitoring shows potential neurological compromise. A decrease in amplitude or an increase in latency can be indicative of pathway interruption.

(2) Somatosensory evoked potentials (SSEPs) monitor the integrity of the posterior sensory pathway, the posterior and lateral column of the spinal cord.

(3) Motor evoked potentials (MEPs) stimulate the motor cortex and record at the level of the spinal cord, peripheral nerves, or muscles and monitor the vulnerable anterior portion of the spinal cord.

(4) Monitoring SSEPs and MEPs are often used in conjunction in TAAA surgery (7).

f) **Renal protection and fluid management**

i) Renal failure is a common occurrence in aortic surgery and carries a high risk of mortality. There have been multiple techniques used to protect the kidneys including

ii) **Low-dose dopamine**

(1) Dopamine has α, β, and DA2 as well as DA1 receptor effects (which may actually limit renal blood flow, GFR, and sodium excretion and thus contributing to renal injury). Current evidence indicates no benefit associated with the use of dopamine for renal protection (12).

iii) **Fenoldopam**

(1) DA-1 specific agonist with systemic vasodilator properties has been used to help protect the kidneys.

(2) Used at low doses (0.05 to 1.0 µg/kg/min), it has been shown to increase urine output and decrease renal replacement therapy and all cause mortality (13).

(3) Should be continued into the perioperative period for at least 48 hours.

iv) **Mannitol**

(1) Often given as well to help improve renal blood flow and protect the kidneys.

v) **Fluid therapy**

(1) Replace fluid and blood loss aggressively to maintain renal perfusion.

(2) The goal is to keep renal perfusion adequate and to maintain a urine output of ≥0.5 mL/kg/h (13,14).

4) Abdominal aortic aneurysms

a) **Anesthetic considerations**

i) **Preanesthesia evaluation**

(1) Patients who present with AAA often have coronary artery disease, HTN, lung disease, diabetes, and renal disease.

(2) Cardiac studies including ECG, along with stress testing when indicated, pulmonary function tests, and basic labs including a complete blood count, complete metabolic profile, and coagulation studies should be examined.

ii) **Monitors**

(1) Standard ASA monitors and an arterial line.

(2) A central line to measure CVP and determine volume status is important.

(3) As stated (Section 3.b), a PAC and TEE may be useful to help manage hemodynamics and volume status in certain patients, but are not routinely indicated.

iii) **Induction/maintenance of anesthesia (Section 3.b)**

iv) **Renal protection and fluid management (Section 3.f)**

b) **Regional anesthesia**

i) A mid-thoracic epidural catheter may be placed to provide postoperative analgesia or to help provide anesthesia during the operation. The placement can be problematic in the face of the necessary anticoagulation, and the risk of postoperative epidural hematoma, which may be confused with spinal cord ischemia from the operation.

ii) If the patient has normal coagulation parameters during placement and anticoagulation is maintained with unfractionated heparin, as opposed to low molecular weight heparin, epidural catheters can be placed safely.

5) **Surgical approaches**

a) **Open abdominal**

i) The open abdominal approach, or transabdominal approach to a AAA repair, is indicated for history of previous left retroperitoneal surgery and the need to perform either mesenteric or right renal artery revascularization.

ii) Involves supine positioning and a large abdominal incision (15). This was the original approach described, and is preferred by many surgeons despite its association with greater pain and complications

b) **Retroperitoneal approach to AAA repair**

i) Usually performed with the patient in the lateral decubitus position, although midline incisions have been described.

ii) Associated with fewer postoperative complications (especially reduced ileus), less fluid shifts, shorter hospital and intensive care unit stays, and lower cost in one study. May potentially be associated with increased pain (15).

iii) Indications for the retroperitoneal approach include, severe COPD, history of abdominal surgeries, presence of horseshoe kidney, inflammatory aneurysm, and abdominal wall stomas

6) **Endovascular repairs**

a) **Endovascular repair of an aortic aneurysm**

i) Interventional percutaneous alternative to the open procedure where an endograft is placed in the aorta usually via the femoral artery.

ii) Benefits include minimal invasiveness, reduced hemodynamic stress, earlier patient ambulation with less pain, and shorter hospital stays.

iii) Often used for patients with severe comorbidities where an open procedure would be contraindicated.

iv) More patients are requesting endovascular repair of AAA, due to its decreased hospital stay and morbidity (16).

b) **Anesthetic considerations**

i) **Monitors**

(1) Standard ASA monitors + invasive arterial monitoring.

(2) A CVP monitor and TEE are rarely needed for abdominal grafts. TEE can help visualize the graft depending on where it is to be placed (often used for thoracic stents, but not abdominal).

(3) It is necessary to monitor urine output as well during these procedures because intravenous contrast dye can be nephrotoxic.

TEE is often used for thoracic but not abdominal endovascular grafts.

ii) **Anesthetic technique**

(1) A balanced general anesthetic technique is common.

(2) As the stent is deployed, the aorta is momentarily occluded, and this can cause a rapid increase in BP, which can cause the stent to migrate.

(a) Control hemodynamics with short-acting IV medications like esmolol, nitroprusside, or nitroglycerin.

(3) Most patients will achieve extubation so dose narcotics/muscle relaxants accordingly.

iii) **Complications**

(1) Include hemorrhage, vessel damage, endovascular leak, aortic rupture necessitating emergent surgery, migration of grafts, distal embolization, and paraplegia (17).

7) **Emergency aortic surgery**

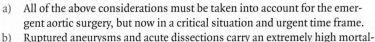

a) All of the above considerations must be taken into account for the emergent aortic surgery, but now in a critical situation and urgent time frame.

b) Ruptured aneurysms and acute dissections carry an extremely high mortality, with time to aortic cross-clamping being the most important factor.

Ruptured aortic aneurysms have an extremely high mortality rate. Patients may acutely decompensate on anesthetic induction.

c) The patient should be prepped and draped, with adequate IV access in place prior to induction.

d) Consider interventional/surgical placement of femoral arterial access with use of intraaortic balloon catheter to occlude the aorta above the aneurysm prior to induction.

i) Agents with minimal hemodynamic changes on induction such as etomidate should be considered.

Chapter Summary for Anesthesia for Aortic Surgery

Definitions	Crawford classification system commonly used.
Risks	Patients are considered high-risk surgical candidates. Comorbid conditions must be assessed carefully
Monitoring	Arterial line utilized for most procedures. Consider central line, PAC, or TEE as indicated by surgical risk.

Anesthetic Management Goals	Induction:
	    Goals are hemodynamic stability avoiding HTN and risk of aneurysm rupture.
	Maintenance:
	    Avoid HTN from cross-clamp with vasodilators/anesthetic depth.
	    Fluid management critical to reduce unclamping shock.
	    Renal protection should be considered for suprarenal clamp applications.

Thoracic Aneurysm	Represents challenging anesthetic and surgical case. Variations of cardiopulmonary bypass, including circulatory arrest, often required.

References

1. Upchurch GR Jr, Schaub TA. Abdominal aortic aneurysm. *Am Fam Pract* 2006;73:1198–1204.
2. Isselbacher EM. Thoracic and abdominal aortic aneurysms. *Circulation* 2005;111:816–828.
3. Levine WC, Lee JJ, Cambria RP, et al. Thoracoabdominal Aneurysm Repair: Anesthetic Management. *Int Anesthesiol Clin* 2005;43:39–60.
4. The United Kingdom Small Aneurysm Trial Participants. Final 12-year follow-up of surgery versus surveillance in UK small aneurysm trial. *Br J Surg* 2007;94:702–708.
5. Lederle FA, Wilson SE, Johnson GR, et al. Immediate repair compared with surveillance of small abdominal aortic aneurysm. *N Engl J Med* 2002;346:1437–1444.
6. Rubin LA. Abdominal aortic aneurysm repair. In: Yao FSF, Fontes ML, Malhotra V, eds. *Yao and Artusio's Anesthesiology: Problem Oriented Patient Management.* 6th ed. Philadelphia, PA: Lippincott Williams & Wilkins; 2008:271–295.
7. Kahn RA, Stone ME, Moskowitz DM. Anesthestic considerations for descending thoracic aortic aneurysm repair. *Semin Cardiothorac Vasc Anesth* 2007;11:205–223.
8. Gelman S. The pathophysiology of aortic cross-clamping and unclamping. *Anesthesiology* 1995;82:1026–1057.
9. Levine WC, Lee JJ, Black JH, et al. Thoracoabdominal aortic aneurysm repair: anesthetic management. *Int Anesth Clin* 2005;43:39–60.
10. Apostolakis E, Akinosoglou K. The methedologies of hypothermic circulatory arrest and of anterograde and retrograde cerebral perfusion for aortic arch surgery. *Ann Thorac Cardiovasc Surg* 2008;14:138–146.
11. Pantin EJ, Cheung AT. Thoracic aortic disease. In: Kaplan JA, Reich DL, Lake LL, Konstadt SN, eds. *Kaplans Cardiac Anesthesia.* 5th ed. Philidelphia, PA: Saunders Elsevier; 2006:723–764.
12. Zacharias M, Conlon NP, Herbison GP, et al. Interventions for protecting renal function in the perioperative period. *Cochrane Database Syst Rev* 2008:CD003590.
13. Landoni G, Biondi-Zoccai GL, Marino G, et al. Fenoldopam reduces the need for renal replacement theapy and in-hospital death in cardiovascular surgery: a meta-analysis. *J Cardiothorac Vasc Anesth* 2008;22:27–33.
14. Oliver WC, Nuttall GA, Cherry KJ, et al. A comparison of fenoldopam with dopamine and sodium nitroprusside in patients undergoing cross-clamping of the abdominal aorta. *Anesth Analg* 2006:103;833–840.
15. Sicard GA, Reilly JM, Rubin BG, et al. Transabdominal versus retroperitoneal incision for abdominal aortic surgery: report of a prospective randomized trial. *J Vasc Surg* 1995;21:174–183.
16. Eliason, JL, Clouse WD. Current management of infrarenal abdominal aortic aneurysms. *Surg Clin North Am* 2007;87:1017–1033.
17. Jaffe RA, Samuels SI, eds. *Anesthesiologists Manual of Surgical Procedures.* 3rd ed. Philadelphia, PA: Lippincott Williams & Wilkins; 2004.
18. Crawford ES, Svensson LG, Hess KR, et al. A prospective randomized study of cerebrospinal fluid drainage to prevent paraplegia after high-risk surgery on the thoracoabdominal aorta. *J Vasc Surg* 1991;13:36–45.

64

Peripheral Vascular Disease

Gurdev Rai, MD

Peripheral vascular disease (PVD) refers to any pathologic, chronic process causing obstruction to blood flow in the arteries (not including coronary and cerebral vessels). In the United States, the prevalence of PVD is increasing as the population ages. In the Baltimore Longitudinal Study of Aging (BLSA), a high incidence of increased pulse pressure and pulsed wave velocities in even asymptomatic, otherwise healthy persons over the age of 55 years was demonstrated (1). This indicates that the hardening of vessels with age occurs even in the absence of atherosclerosis or hypertension. As the disease progresses, this can lead to cerebral vascular ischemia, critical limb ischemia (CLI)/loss, and in some cases hemorrhage from large vessel rupture. Anesthesiologists need to be familiar with the pathophysiology of PVD and its anesthetic implications.

1) **Pathophysiology**
   a) The molecular mechanism leading to PVD is related to certain risk factors resulting in deposition of calcium and the "hardening" of vessels. These risk factors include:
      i) Hypertension
      ii) Diabetes
      iii) Smoking
      iv) Hyperlipidemia
      v) The BLSA indicates that aging in itself might be a risk factor.

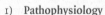

In patients with symptomatic PVD, mortality rates can be as high as 25% to 30% over 5 years (2).

2) **Epidemiology**
   a) The National Health and Nutrition Examination Survey found that the prevalence of PVD, as measured by ankle brachial index (ABI) <90%, is estimated at 14.5% in the population over the age of 70 years (3).
   b) The **ABI** is defined as the ratio of the blood pressure in the lower legs compared to the blood pressure in the arms.

3) **Signs and symptoms**
   a) **Neurologic system**
      i) Stroke, transient ischemic attacks, or reversible ischemic neurologic deficits.
      ii) With primary carotid disease, the number of strokes increases and vascular dementia can set in. Due to these catastrophic endpoints, early detection and intervention is critical.

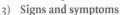

PVD leads to symptoms of ischemia in the area supplied by the diseased vessel.

   b) **Peripheral extremities**
      iii) The initial symptom is pain or **claudication.**
      iv) With peripheral disease, increasing pain from claudication and infection can lead to eventual limb loss or systemic shock.
      v) Involvement of larger vessels leads to aneurysms with potential rupture.
      vi) Patients can present with no symptoms, intermittent claudication, or CLI.

(1) Intermittent claudication

    (a) Associated with functional disability due to pain.

    (b) This disability is measured as the maximal walking time and overall walking ability before the onset of symptoms.

    (c) Fortunately, most patients do not progress beyond this point due to the formation of collateral circulation, which alleviates some of the disability.

(2) **Critical Limb Ischemia (CLI)**

    (a) CLI is defined by intractable pain at rest or limb ulceration of sufficient severity to warrant hospitalization (4).

    (b) The risk of limb loss and death associated with stroke or coronary events is much higher in this patient population.

The best predictors of progression to more serious disease in patients with intermittent claudication tend to be an ABI <50%, diabetes, and smoking.

d) Associated findings

    i) Many patients with PVD have comorbid conditions such as: hypertension, diabetes, smoking history, and hyperlipidemia, which increase the risk of coronary artery disease (CAD) and myocardial ischemia.

4) Medical therapy

The goal of care of patients with PVD is to minimize disability and provide either improvement or stability in disease progression. Fortunately, these interventions have an added benefit of decreasing the risk of stroke and MI (2–4).

  a) **Smoking cessation**

    i) Smoking is not only a risk factor for developing PVD; it also increases the rate of disease progression and the incidence of CLI and limb loss. **Therefore, smoking cessation is the most important single modifiable risk factor.**

    ii) Smoking cessation decreases the severity of claudication and the risk of stroke or MI in this population (2–4).

  b) **Exercise**

    i) Walking until the point of maximal pain three times a week for 6 months improves disability associated with claudication and is more effective than antiplatelet therapy or angioplasty (4).

  c) **Statins**

    i) Statin therapy increases maximal walking time in patients with intermittent claudication and decreases the incidence of new claudication in patients otherwise at risk of developing vascular disease.

  d) **Blood pressure control**

    i) Angiotensin converting enzyme (ACE) inhibitors appear to be the best at decreasing BP and improving the risk of cardiovascular events in this population.

    ii) β-Adrenergic antagonists may lower the risk of perioperative cardiac events when used long term.

  e) **Glucose control**

    i) Patients with diabetes have a higher risk of disease progression.

    ii) As the levels of glycosylated hemoglobin rises, so does the risk of PVD.

    iii) Aggressive management of diabetes is highly desirable.

  f) **Antiplatelet therapy**

    i) May delay disease progression and improve symptoms.

    ii) Decreases the risk of stroke, MI, and cardiovascular death in this population

    iii) Aspirin is the mainstay of treatment. Ticlodopine is the other most often used and studied.

- iv) Clopidogrel has become popular due to its effectiveness in decreasing the risk of cardiovascular events and strokes more so than aspirin.
- v) TASC II recommends that all patients with PVD with evidence of atherosclerosis should be on an antiplatelet agent.
- vi) Perioperative planning must address the use, preoperative discontinuation, and postoperative reinstatement of antiplatelet therapy.

g) **Phosphodiesterase inhibitors**
- i) Mechanism of action is suppression of platelet aggregation and direct arterial vasodilation.
- ii) Cilastozol is the only agent in this class approved for treatment of claudication.
- iii) Reserved for patients with moderate to severe disease due to associated side effects.

h) **Other**
- i) Homeopathic treatment with ginko biloba, use of chelation therapy, prostaglandins, and other numerous treatment methods are also employed in the medical management of these patients.
- ii) Anesthesia caregivers must be thorough in their review of patient medication lists and histories to avoid any perioperative issues that may arise secondary to these interventions.

5) **Interventional/surgical treatment**
- a) When disease progression can be predicted or medical therapy has failed, percutaneous or surgical revascularization becomes an option.
- b) Revascularization is the only option in patients with threatened limb loss.
- c) The ACC/AHA Guidelines indicate that percutaneous interventions should be attempted first if access is available to the diseased vessel (5).

All major vascular surgery falls into the high-risk surgical procedure category.

d) **Surgical intervention**
- i) Surgery is reserved for otherwise healthy patients with limited disease and a predicted improvement in quality of life.
- ii) Type of surgery depends on the location of the lesion, the patient's comorbidities, and ease of access.
- iii) **Inflow disease (aortoiliac)** usually requires the most extensive access and exposure.
  - (1) The procedure could require aortoiliac, aortofemoral, or iliofemoral bypass in conjuction with femoral-femoral bypass
  - (2) This is a very high-risk surgical procedures with similar risks to abdominal aortic surgery

READ MORE

Anesthesia for aortic surgery, Chapter 63, page 453

- iv) **Outflow disease**
  - (1) Outflow disease affects vessels below the inguinal ligament.
  - (2) Surgical access and exposure are limited.
  - (3) For distal lower-extremity revascularization procedures the perioperative mortality is very low (5).
- v) **Salvage operations**
  - (1) Despite aggressive medical and surgical interventions, some patients continue to have progressive disease and may require limb debridement or amputation procedures.
  - (2) These patients have either had failed interventions or were never candidates for surgical revascularization due to comorbidities.
  - (3) The biggest surgical risk is blood loss, which is typically controlled with tourniquets.

Figure 64-1	Exercise Capacity

Expressed in metabolic equivalents (METS)
- POOR: eat, dress, use toilet (1 MET)
- MODERATE: one flight of stairs (4 METS)
- GOOD: Heavy house work (4-10 METS)
- Excellent: Strenuous sports (>10 METS)

– 1 MET = 3.5 mL O2 uptake/kg per minute
- Resting O2 uptake while sitting
– <4 METS = higher risk

6) **Anesthetic implications**

a) Preoperative considerations

READ
MORE

Challenges in
anesthesia: the
geriatric patient
presenting for
surgery,
Chapter 50,
page 349

i) PVD is associated with risk factors that are associated with increased perioperative morbidity and mortality. It is imperative to look for these risk factors preoperatively.

ii) **Age** is a significant risk factor for PVD; the prevalence of PVD increases disproportionately in the elderly population.

(1) Functional reserve might be the single most important indicator of perioperative morbidity in the elderly population.

(2) If one cannot exert at least four metabolic equivalents of activity (Fig. 64-1), he/she is at increased risk of perioperative complications.

(3) In these patients, further evaluation of reserve capacity in the form of frailty indices and eventually cardiac stress tests are suggested (5).

iii) **Coronary disease**

(1) Evaluation of cardiac risk is imperative in patients with PVD.

(2) The anesthesiologist must be familiar with the various risk indices and interventions available to minimize the risk of adverse cardiovascular events.

(3) Some patients may benefit from further studies and interventions prior to surgery.

(4) **Risk indices** predict which patients will have increased cardiac morbidity or mortality during noncardiac surgery.

READ
MORE

Ischemic heart
disease,
Chapter 51,
page 359

(5) The Modified Cardiac Risk Index has been recently adopted into the ACC/AHA guidelines for the evaluation of perioperative risk for patients having noncardiac surgery, often these patients fall in the intermediate to high-risk groups.

iv) **β-Adrenergic antagonists**

(1) Should be continued perioperatively in patients with a history of coronary artery disease undergoing major vascular surgery.

(2) There is a possible benefit to start β-adrenergic antagonists in patients, not on them previously, prior to major vascular surgery. Ideally, these should be started weeks in advance and titrated to a heart rate >60 and <80 bpm.

(3) Starting β-adrenergic antagonists in the immediate pre-operative period may be detrimental and remains debatable (5).

v) **Stress tests**

READ MORE

Ischemic heart disease
Chapter 51, page 359

(1) In many cases, the patients are so handicapped by their disease that an accurate indication of exercise tolerance cannot be obtained from history alone.

(2) In these patients, with the presence of other cardiac risk factors, a cardiac stress test might be the only way to predict potential problems or diagnose unrecognized CAD.

b) Cardiac intervention

i) If during risk assessment, it is found that the patient has high probability or CAD the patient may require intervention prior to any elective noncardiac surgery.

ii) **The CARP trial and DECREASE trials state that in the absence of active angina or other indications for immediate intervention, these patients should be medically managed through the perioperative period (6,7).**

c) **Elective intervention**

i) Indicated in the presence of left main disease, greater than three vessel disease, and unstable angina despite medical optimization.

ii) The anesthesiologist and surgeon should be involved in the decision of which type of intervention occurs because if percutaneous intervention is planned, the need for platelet inhibitors afterwards should not be overlooked.

iii) **Plain angioplasty** requires 1 month of antiplatelet medication while the coronary endothelium heals.

iv) **Stenting**

(1) When stents are placed, the length for antiplatelet therapy increases.

(2) With bare metal stents, medication needs to be continued for at least 4 to 6 weeks.

(3) Drug eluting stents require up to a year of antiplatelet therapy.

(4) If these guidelines are not followed, the risk of rethrombosis during the perioperative period increases (5). Therefore, potential need for surgery should be evaluated prior to the intervention.

d) **Intraoperative considerations**

i) Depend on the type of surgical intervention planned

(1) For inflow disease, where the aorta is entered surgically, one must be ready for the fluid shifts associated with laparotomy, hemodynamic changes associated with clamp placement and eventual revascularization of an ischemic limb, plus the usual issues involving high risk surgery.

(2) For outflow procedures, the hemodynamic insult is far less but still clinically relevant.

READ MORE

Invasive arterial blood pressure monitoring
Chapter 11, page 70 and
Central venous monitoring,
Chapter 12, page 75

ii) **Fluid management**

(1) One can anticipate the normal insensible loss associated with abdominal surgery.

(2) The risk of blood loss must be addressed with these procedures, with strong consideration for blood product availability.

(3) Appropriate monitors, potentially including central venous pressure and arterial blood pressure monitoring, should be utilized to help predict and monitor fluid replacement.

    iii) **Temperature control**

        (1) In order to achieve surgical access, the patient can sometimes be exposed from the xyphoid to the toes.

        (2) Beyond measuring core temperature, one must be ready to actively warm these patients.

            (a) Potential techniques include increasing ambient room temperature, fluid warmers, warming pads, and forced air blankets.

        (3) Failure to maintain reasonable core body temperature increases the patients' risk of coagulopathies, infection, delayed emergence, and cardiac dysrhythmias.

    iv) **Aortic arteriotomy**

READ MORE

Anesthesia for aortic surgery, Chapter 63, page 453

        (1) Hemodynamic changes depend on the placement of the aortic clamp.

        (2) If the only viable place for anastomosis is on the proximal aorta, one must be ready for the hemodynamic changes associated with AAA repair surgery.

        (3) Fortunately, a partial aortic clamp is usually adequate and the physiologic derangements are minimized.

    v) **Revascularization**

        (1) Once circulation is restored to the limb, the products of anaerobic metabolism are washed into systemic circulation. Consequences of this at the time of reperfusion are:

            (a) **Drop in temperature**

            (b) **Lactic acidosis**

            (c) **Hyperkalemia**

            (d) **Hypercarbia**

            (e) **Decreased preload**

        (2) For healthy patients, these effects can be managed with minimal intervention.

        (3) For unhealthy patients, one must be ready for the cardiac and pulmonary implications of this washout.

            (a) Cardiac manifestations can include hypotension and arrhythmias.

            (b) The hypercarbia and acidosis can increase pulmonary vascular resistance and lead to hypoxia, further stressing a compromised heart.

    4) Reperfusing the limb in stages may ameliorate some of these problems.

    5) Prophylactic treatment may include increasing intravascular volume, hyperventilation, and active warming.

    6) Often, more aggressive intervention including the use of sodium bicarbonate, calcium, and pressors is required.

7) **Anesthesia techniques**

  a) **The goal of any anesthesiologist is to prescribe or administer the safest possible plan in this fragile patient population.**

  b) **Monitored anesthesia care**

    i) Most procedures associated with PVD are not conducive to monitored anesthesia care.

    ii) Procedures involving minor débridement or amputation of nonviable tissue lacking sensation could be performed with minimal anesthesia.

  c) **Regional techniques**

READ MORE

Atlas of regional anesthesia, Chapter 172, page 1171

    i) Many studies imply better outcomes and patient satisfaction associated with regional anesthesia. Anesthesia staff should be familiar with lower extremity regional anesthesia.

ii) Most débridements or amputations of lower extremities may be performed with a peripheral nerve block, depending on the location of the surgery.

iii) For procedures involving the foot, **an ankle block** can be invaluable.

iv) In procedures involving the lower limb near the ankle, a **popliteal and saphenous** nerve block is typically adequate for surgical anesthesia.

v) For below knee amputations, a **femoral and sciatic nerve block** can be used.

vi) Above the knee, one must consider the lateral femoral cutaneous nerve and weigh the costs and benefits of lumbar plexus blocks versus neuraxial blockade.

d) **Neuraxial anesthesia/analgesia**

i) May be used as a primary anesthetic technique or as an adjunct to general anesthesia.

ii) Neuraxial techniques reduce morbidity and increase graft patency in surgeries involving arteries of the lower extremities (8).

iii) For patients scheduled for elective open aortic or femoral artery procedures, an epidural is a standard approach to perioperative anesthetic management. **One must take special notice of the ASRA guidelines here due to the use of anticoagulants during the perioperative period (9).**

e) **General anesthesia**

i) General anesthesia remains the most reliable anesthetic in this patient population.

ii) It can be safely administered as long as an adequate preoperative workup has been performed.

iii) Techniques involving total intravenous, high opiate, volatile anesthetics have equal results provided hemodynamic stability is maintained.

iv) One must be familiar with the placement and interpretation of invasive monitoring including arterial lines, central venous lines, pulmonary artery catheters, and basic transesophageal echocardiography. Interpretation infers that the anesthesiologist recognizes the importance of intraoperative hemodynamic stability in these patients.

f) **Postoperative care**

i) An adequate preoperative assessment and a well-managed anesthetic are essential to an uncomplicated postoperative course.

ii) Postoperative pain management is critical to ensure a rapid recovery. Options include neuroaxial, regional, or intravenous/oral medications. Refer to the above discussions.

iii) Control of heart rate and blood pressure is still relevant. Patients' preoperative medications should be restarted as soon as tolerated.

iv) Monitoring for potential postoperative cardiac events should continue into the immediate postoperative period. For patients with multiple comorbidities having major vascular surgery, intensive care settings are justified for recovery.

v) Deep vein thrombosis prophylaxis should be addressed until the patient has gained adequate mobility or is discharged from the hospital.

Chapter Summary for PVD

Epidemiology	PVD is increasing in prevalence as the population of the United States ages.
Risk factors	The main risk factors associated with PVD include advanced age, hypertension, smoking, diabetes, and hyperlipidemia.
Anesthetic Concerns	Cardiac events are very common in this population, making perioperative cardiac risk stratification and management the primary goal of the preoperative evaluation. Vascular surgery is classified as a high-risk procedure. Therefore, one must be familiar with the medical treatment of PVD and the implications of these interventions on anesthesia care.
Anesthetic Management	Intraoperative events can pose a challenge to anesthesiologists. One must be aware of the type of procedure planned in order to anticipate some of the associated physiologic aberrations. Although multiple anesthesia techniques can be used successfully in this patient population, the thoroughness of the preoperative evaluation is not minimized by less invasive anesthesia.

References

1. Lakatta EG, Levy D. Arterial and cardiac aging: major shareholders in cardiovascular disease enterprises: part 1: aging arteries: a "Set Up" for vascular disease. *Circulation* 2003;107:139–146.
2. Hirsch AT, Haskal ZJ, Hertzer NR, et al. ACC/AHA 2005 Practice Guidelines for the management of patients with peripheral arterial disease (lower extremity, renal, mesenteric, and abdominal aortic): a collaborative report from the American Association for Vascular Surgery/ Society for Vascular Surgery, Society for Cardiovascular Angiography and Interventions, Society for Vascular Medicine and Biology, Society of Interventional Radiology, and the ACC/AHA Task Force on Practice Guidelines (Writing Committee to Develop Guidelines for the Management of Patients With Peripheral Arterial Disease): endorsed by the American Association of Cardiovascular and Pulmonary Rehabilitation; National Heart, Lung, and Blood Institute; Society for Vascular Nursing; TransAtlantic Inter-Society Consensus; and Vascular Disease Foundation. *Circulation* 2006;113:e463.
3. Norgren L, Hiatt WR, Dormandy JA, et al. Inter-society consensus for the management of peripheral arterial disease (TASC II). *J Vasc Surg.* 2007;45(suppl S):S5–S67.
4. Hankey GJ, Norman PE, Eikelboom JW. Medical treatment of peripheral arterial disease. *JAMA* 2006;295:547–553.
5. Fleisher LA, Beckman JA, Brown KA, et al. ACC/AHA 2007 guidelines on perioperative cardiovascular evaluation and care for noncardiac surgery: a report of the American College of Cardiology/American Heart Association Task Force on Practice Guidelines. *J Am Coll Cardiol* 2007;50:e159.
6. McFalls EO, Ward HB, Moritz TE, et al. Coronary-artery revascularization before elective major vascular surgery. *N Engl J Med* 2004;351:2795–2804.
7. Poldermans D, Schouten O, et al. A clinical randomized trial to evaluate the safety of a noninvasive approach in high-risk patients undergoing major vascular surgery. The DECREASE-V Pilot Study. *J Am Coll Cardiol* 2007;49:1763–1769.
8. Grass J. The role of epidural anesthesia and analgesia in postoperative outcome. *Anesthesiol Clin North Am* 2000;18:407–428.
9. Neal JM, Bernards CM, Hadzic A, et al. ASRA practice advisory on neurologic complications in regional anesthesia and pain medicine. *Reg Anesth Pain Med* 2008;33:404–415.

65 Deep Vein Thrombosis and Pulmonary Embolism

Cosmin Guta, MD • Xiang Qian, MD, PhD

Deep-vein thrombosis (DVT) and pulmonary embolism (PE) are major causes of significant morbidity and mortality, which are frequently, but not exclusively, associated with surgery, injury and other reasons for hospitalization. DVT of the lower extremity is subdivided into either distal (calf vein) or proximal (popliteal, femoral, or iliac vein) thrombosis. Proximal vein thrombosis is of greater importance clinically, since it is more commonly associated with PE.

Up to 200,000 deaths in the United States are either caused or related to PE each year.

1) Prevalence
   a) The estimated annual incidence of venous thromboembolism (VTE) from a 25-year population-based study is about 117 per 100,000, and up to 900 per 100,000 by the age of 85 years (1).
   b) Approximately 30% of these patients (around 600,000 cases per year) develop symptomatic PE.
   c) Up to 200,000 deaths annually in the United States are either caused or related to PE.
2) Risk factors (Tables 65-1 and 65-2)
3) Pathophysiology
   a) An embolic occlusion in the pulmonary circulation increases the total dead space.
   b) A theoretical increase of $PaCO_2$ is expected but often not clinically observed, due to compensation from increased minute ventilation, triggered by medullary chemoreceptors sensing of the rise of $PaCO_2$.

Table 65-1
Risk Factors for DVT and PE

Risk factors for DVT	Alterations of blood flow (stasis)
	Injury to vascular endothelium
	Abnormal blood coagulation, also known as *Virchow triad* (hypercoagulopathy, hemodynamic changes, and endothelial injury/dysfunction), which is often present in the perioperative period
Risk factors for PE	Malignancy
	Trauma
	Inflammatory bowel disease
	Immobilization
	Surgery (especially orthopedic)
	Presence of a central venous catheter
	Oral contraceptives
	Pregnancy
	Sickle cell anemia
	Hormone replacement therapy

Table 65-2	
Causes of Venous Thrombosis	
Inherited disorders	Protein S deficiency
	Protein C deficiency
	Antithrombin deficiency
Acquired disorders	Malignancy
	Trauma
	Inflammatory bowel disease
	Immobilization
	Surgery (especially orthopedic)
	Presence of a central venous catheter
	Oral contraceptives
	Pregnancy
	Sickle cell anemia
	Hormone replacement therapy

     c)   When hypercapnia becomes evident, massive PE should be suspected.

     d)   Hypoxemia is more often seen during a PE.

         i)   V/Q mismatch in which there is "dead space" ventilation in some parts of the lung and overperfusion in others

         ii) Atelectasis caused by loss of surfactant within hours after PE

         iii) Right-to-left intrapulmonary shunting when overperfusion and decreased vascular resistance occur in nonembolic parts of the lung

         iv) Intracardiac shunting may occur due to increased pulmonary artery (PA) pressure and enlarged opening of preexisting patent foramen ovale.

     e)   A pulmonary embolus reduces the cross-sectional area of the pulmonary vasculature, resulting in increased pulmonary vascular resistance.

         i)   In addition, intrapulmonary reflexes stimulate the release of humoral substances that lead to vasoconstriction throughout the lungs and thus further increases pulmonary vascular resistance.

            (1) As a result, high PA pressure could acutely develop, especially in patients with preexisting cardiopulmonary diseases, and potentially precipitate or lead to acute right ventricular failure (RVF).

  4)   **Diagnosis**

     a)   Deep vein thrombosis

         i)   **Clinical presentation**

             (1) Often nonspecific

             (2) Low predictive value (~15%) (2)

             (3) **Symptoms**

                 (a) Local swelling

                 (b) Discoloration of the legs

                 (c) Increased warmth over the skin

                 (d) More visible surface veins

                 (e) Calf or leg pain or tenderness

                 (f) Classical Homan sign (pain when dorsiflexion of the affected foot), which is often difficult to distinguish from simple muscle strain, injury, or skin infection.

         ii) **Lab studies**

             (1) A positive D-dimer test has limited clinical value.

Contrast venography is the gold standard test to diagnose deep venous thrombosis.

iii) **Doppler ultrasonography**

    (1) Most commonly used test, but a normal result cannot rule out DVT.

iv) **Contrast venography**

    (1) Considered as the gold standard test to diagnose DVT.

v) **Other**

    (1) Spiral computed tomography (CT)

    (2) Impedance plethysmography

    (3) Magnetic resonance imaging (MRI)

b) **Pulmonary embolism**

  i) **Clinical presentation**

    (1) Clinical features are mild and nonspecific.

    (2) Diagnosis is difficult to establish on clinical presentations alone.

    (3) **Preoperative and postoperative presentation of pulmonary embolism**

      (a) Most consistent

        (i) Acute dyspnea (75%)

        (ii) Tachypenea (70%)

      (b) Observable with PE near pleural surface

        (i) Pleuritic or chest pain (60%)

        (ii) Rales (50%)

        (iii) Cough (40%)

      (c) Others

        (i) Possible wheezing on auscultation

        (ii) Wide S2 splitting

        (iii) Tachycardia (3).

Intraoperative signs of PE include sudden onset of hypoxemia, low EtCO$_2$, bronchospasm or high airway pressures.

    (4) **Intraoperative presentation of pulmonary embolism**

      (a) Often transient and nonspecific.

        (i) Includes the sudden onset of the following symptoms

          1. Hypoxemia

          2. Low EtCO$_2$

          3. Bronchospasm

          4. High airway pressure

  ii) **Lab Studies**

    (1) Normal D-dimer test has a high negative predictive value of up to 99.6% (4)

    (2) ECGs could be abnormal but the findings listed are not specific or sensitive.

      (a) ST-T wave change

      (b) Peaked P wave

      (c) RV strain

      (d) Right bundle branch block (RBBB)

      (e) An S-wave in lead I and a Q-wave and T-wave inversion in lead III (S1Q3T3), in up to 70% of patients with PE and no preexisting cardiovascular disease.

    (3) Chest x-ray is often normal.

    (4) An arterial blood gas (ABG) may show respiratory alkalosis, hypoxemia, and increased A-a gradient.

  iii) **V/Q scan**

    (1) Used to be the first-line study but has been associated with high false-positive results up to 50%.

    (2) A negative scan is of high value and can essentially rule out PE. Currently, the test is reserved for patients with major renal impairment, anaphylaxis to intravenous contrast, or pregnancy.

iv) **High resolution CT-scan**
- (1) Currently the standard diagnostic imaging test to evaluate a suspected PE
- (2) Sensitivity and specificity nearly 90% for main and lobar emboli
- (3) Negative predictive values up to 99.1% (5)

v) **Pulmonary angiography**
- (1) Gold standard test to diagnose PE.
- (2) Used when other imaging modalities are nondiagnostic or contradicted, and a high clinical suspicion for PE persists with homodynamic instability.

vi) **Transesophageal echocardiography**
- (1) May show acute dilation of right atrium (RA) and right ventricle (RV).

5) Treatment

a) **The primary objectives of treatment of VTE are to prevent and/or treat the following complications:**
- i) Prevent further clot extension
- ii) Prevention of acute PE
- iii) Reducing the risk of recurrent thrombosis
- iv) Treatment of massive iliofemoral thrombosis with acute lower limb ischemia and/or venous gangrene
- v) Limiting the development of late complications, such as the postthrombotic syndrome, chronic venous insufficiency, and chronic thromboembolic pulmonary hypertension (6)

b) **Deep vein thrombosis**
- i) **Supportive care**
  - (1) Limb elevation, local warming blanket, graded elastic compression stockings, with minimal activity for at least several days.
- ii) **Anticoagulation**
  - (1) Heparin followed by warfarin at least 6 to 12 weeks (7).

c) **Pulmonary embolism**
- i) **Anticoagulation**

Intracranial hemorrhage risk may be as high as 3% with tPA.

  - (1) Intravenous **unfractionated heparin** (IUH) (bolus followed by continuous infusion, to titrate the prothrombin time to two to three times the upper limit (around 60 to 80 seconds) **is the mainstream therapy.**
  - (2) Patients with stable vital signs, normal BP, and no evidence of RV dysfunction generally responded well with anticoagulation and other supportive measures, such as supplemental oxygen.
  - (3) **LMWHs such as enoxaparin can also be used** and are as safe and effective as IUH.
- ii) **Fibrinolysis with tissue plasminogen activator (tPA)** (100 mg as continuous infusion over 2 hours)
  - (1) Reserved for massive PE with acute RVF and hemodynamic instability
  - (2) Intracranial hemorrhage risk may be as high as 3.0%.
  - (3) In one study, fibrinolytics did not reduce mortality or recurrent PE at 90 days (8).
- iii) **Pulmonary embolectomy**
  - (1) Reserved for massive PE in whom fibrinolysis is contraindicated or has failed or for patients with homodynamic or respiratory compromises requiring cardiopulmonary resuscitation
- iv) **Inferior vena cava (IVC) Filter**

    (1) Filters are reserved for patients who have contradictions for anticoagulation, are having recurrent PE despite adequate anticoagulation, and those undergoing pulmonary embolectomy.

    (2) A recent analysis showed a significant reduction in 90-day mortality associated with IVC filters (8).

6) Prophylaxis

  a) **The best treatment for VTE is prevention.**

  b) Proper prophylaxis may decrease perioperative VTE risk more than 10-fold (9).

  c) The methods of thromboprophylaxis proven to be clinically effective and relevant are low-dose anticoagulants and mechanical devices.

  d) All patients should be well hydrated and early mobilization after surgery is mandatory.

    i) **Non-pharmacological strategies**

      (1) Early ambulation should be encouraged.

      (2) Mechanical compression devices should be initiated prior to induction of the anesthesia and continued intraoperatively and then into the postoperative period, and have to be worn at least 18 to 20 hours a day to be effective.

      (3) IVC filter may be offered to patients who have contradictions to pharmacological prophylaxis.

    ii) **Pharmacological strategies (Table 65-3)**

      (1) Based on the 2008 ACCP guidelines, prophylaxis is recommended by both level of procedural thromboembolic risk and individual patient risk factors.

      (2) In general, prophylaxis should be initiated 8 to 24 hours postoperatively, with either unfractionated heparin or low molecular weight heparins (LMWHs).

        (a) Low-dose unfractionated heparin administered at a dose of 5,000 units subcutaneously, every 8 or 12 hours, reduces the risk of developing a DVT by approximately 60% with a similar reduction in PE-associated mortality.

          (i) There is, however, a marginal increase in the risk of hemorrhage, particularly in patients undergoing surgery.

        (b) Low-dose LMWHs are as effective, if not slightly more effective when compared with low-dose unfractionated heparin with fewer side effects and usually require only daily dosing.

        (c) Up to 28 days of VTE prophylaxis is recommended in selected high-risk general or gynecological surgical patients, and extended prophylaxis is indicated after major orthopedic procedures.

        (d) LMWH is preferable to warfarin, and aspirin alone is not recommended in any patient population (10).

Table 65-3	
Thromboprophylactic Recommendations (11)	
Low risk	No thromboprophylaxis is recommended.
Moderate risk	An effective form of thromboprophylaxis is recommended. This should be either in the form of an effective low-dose anticoagulant or an effective mechanical method. The thromboprophylaxis should ideally be started before the risk commences and should continue as long as the risk persists.
High risk	An effective form of thromboprophylaxis is mandatory and consideration should be given to using a combination of low-dose anticoagulants and mechanical devices. Continuation of thromboprophylaxis beyond the period of hospitalization should be considered.

Chapter Summary for Deep Venous Thrombosis

Prevalence	The estimated annual incidence of VTE is about 117 per 100,000, and up to 900 per 100,000 by the age of 85 y (1).
Risk Factors	Surgical patients, especially elderly, and patients undergoing orthopedic procedures are at high risk of VTE.
Causes	Causes of venous thrombosis can be classified as inherited or acquired disorders
Pathophysiology	When hypercapnia becomes evident, massive PE should be suspected. Hypoxia is more often seen in PE
Diagnosis	For DVT, Doppler ultrasonography is most commonly used, while contrast venography is considered the gold standard test. For PE, CT scan and pulmonary angiography are the gold standard tests to evaluate suspected PE and diagnose PE, respectively.
Treatments	Treatment for DVT should include supportive care and anticoagulation. Treatment for PE should include anticoagulation, fibrinolysis, pulmonary embolectomy, and IVC filters.
Prophylaxis	The best treatment for VTE is prevention. The methods of thromboprophylaxis proven to be clinically effective and relevant are low-dose anticoagulants and mechanical devices.

VTE, venous thromboembolism; PE, pulmonary embolism; DVT, deep venous thrombosis; IVC, inferior vena cava.

References

1. Silverstein MD, Heit JA, Mohr DN, et al. Trends in the incidence of deep vein thrombosis and pulmonary embolism: a 25-year population-based study. *Arch Intern Med* 1998;158(6):585–593.
2. Wells PS, Anderson DR, Bormanis J, et al. Value of assessment of pretest probability of deep-vein thrombosis in clinical management. *Lancet* 1997;350:1795–1798.
3. Stein PD, Terrin ML, Hales CA, et al. Clinical, laboratory, roentgenographic, and electrocardiographic findings in patients with acute pulmonary embolism and no pre-existing cardiac or pulmonary disease. *Chest* 1991;100(3):598–603.
4. Dunn KL, Wolf JP, Dorfman DM, et al. Normal D-dimer levels in emergency department patients suspected of acute pulmonary embolism. *J Am Coll Cardiol* 2002;40:1475–1478.
5. Quiroz R, Kucher N, Zou KH, et al. Clinical validity of a negative computed tomography scan in patients with suspected pulmonary embolism: a systematic review. *JAMA* 2005;293:2012–2017.
6. Landaw S, Bauer,K. Approach to the diagnosis and therapy of deep vein thrombosis, In: UpToDate, Leung LL (Ed), UpToDate, Waltham, MA, 2010.
7. Hyers TM, Agnelli G, Hull RD, et al. Antithrombotic therapy for venous thromboembolic disease. *Chest* 2001;119(1 suppl):176S–193S.
8. Kucher N, Rossi E, De Rosa M, et al. Massive pulmonary embolism. *Circulation* 2006;113:577–582.
9. Michota FA. Prevention of venous thromboembolism after surgery. *Cleve Clin J Med* 2009;76(suppl 4):S45–S52.
10. Geerts WH, Bergqvist D, Pineo GF, et al. Prevention of venous thromboembolism: American College of Chest Physicians Evidence-Based Clinical Practice Guidelines (8th Edition). *Chest* 2008;133(6 suppl):381S–453S.
11. Nicolaides AN, Fareed J, Kakkar AK, et al. Prevention and treatment of venous thromboembolism. International consensus statement (Guidelines according to scientific evidence). *Int Angiol* 2006;25:101–161.

66 Challenges in Anesthesia: Laparoscopic Cholecystectomy in the Patient with Pulmonary Hypertension

Ronald G. Pearl, MD, PhD

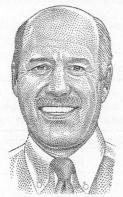

Clinical Vignette

A 45-year-old female patient is scheduled for laparoscopic cholecystectomy. One week ago she had acute cholecystitis that required admission to the intensive care unit for hypotension. She had a similar episode 2 months ago. Her medical history is significant for pulmonary hypertension (PH). What is the approach to perioperative management?

In 1973, when the World Health Organization organized the first international conference on PH, there were no effective therapies, and median survival for patients with primary PH (now termed idiopathic pulmonary arterial hypertension [IPAH]) was under 3 years. Today, there are multiple therapies and survival has more than doubled. As a result, more patients with PH undergo anesthesia and surgery. PH markedly increases morbidity and mortality among patients undergoing surgery (1–3). Successful management involves five steps: (1) diagnosing PH and its etiology, (2) assessing the severity of the disease, (3) assessing the risks and benefits of anesthesia and surgery, (4) developing an anesthetic plan, and (5) managing the perioperative complications of systemic hypotension and right heart failure (4–7) (Table 66-1).

Diagnosis and Evaluation of Pulmonary Hypertension

Understanding the pathophysiology of PH allows accurate risk assessment, optimization prior to surgery, and rational intraoperative and postoperative treatment (4,7–13). The pulmonary circulation is normally a low pressure, low resistance circulation. In patients with PH, altered vascular endothelial and smooth muscle function lead to vasoconstriction, localized thrombosis, and vascular growth and remodeling. These processes increase pulmonary vascular resistance (PVR). The normal thin-walled right ventricle (RV) decreases stroke volume in response to increased afterload, so PH can result in RV failure, systemic hypotension, and death.

The pulmonary circulation is normally a low pressure, low resistance circulation.

Table 66-1

Approach to Perioperative Management of PH

Diagnosis and evaluation of PH
Assessment of the severity of PH
Assessment of the risks and benefits of anesthesia and surgery
Development of an anesthetic plan
    Choice of general vs. regional anesthesia
    Monitoring
    Induction of anesthesia
    Maintenance of anesthesia
    Emergence issues
    Postoperative management
Plan for treatment of systemic hypotension

PH is defined as a mean pulmonary artery pressure (PAP) ≥25 mm Hg at rest.

The diagnosis of PH is usually suspected either from symptoms or from associated diseases that increase risk. Patients with PH have three major symptoms: (1) exertional dyspnea, (2) chest pain, and (3) syncope. Suspicion of PH should prompt evaluation with electrocardiogram (for RVH and RV strain) and echocardiogram (RV hypertrophy, enlargement and decreased systolic function with elevated RV pressures by Doppler). PH is confirmed by right heart catheterization.

In 2008, the 4th World Symposium on Pulmonary Hypertension reviewed classification, diagnosis, evaluation, and therapy of PH (14). PH is defined as a mean PAP ≥ 25 mm Hg at rest.

An approach to understanding PH is derived from the equation for PVR:

$$PVR = (PAP - LAP) \times 80/CO$$

Rearranging this equation for PAP demonstrates that

$$PAP = LAP + (CO \times PVR)/80.$$

Choice of perioperative therapy for PH requires assessment of LAP, CO and PVR.

Thus, the three factors that increase PAP are (1) left atrial pressure (LAP), (2) cardiac output (CO), and (3) PVR. Perioperative therapy requires assessing the quantitative contribution of each component. For example, pulmonary vasodilator therapy will only be appropriate when PH is associated with increased PVR. In patients with PH, analyzing whether CO remains normal or is markedly decreased has prognostic value in assessing perioperative risk.

The current classification of PH involves five major categories: (1) pulmonary arterial hypertension, (2) pulmonary venous hypertension, (3) PH associated with disorders of the respiratory system and/or hypoxemia, (4) chronic thrombotic and/or embolic disease, and (5) PH due to disorders directly affecting the pulmonary vasculature. The above equation for PAP can be used to classify the common etiologies.

Increased LAP includes LV failure and valvular heart disease (particularly mitral stenosis). Increased CO includes patients with congenital heart disease with cardiac shunts. The major categories of chronically increased PVR are pulmonary disease (parenchymal or airway), hypoxia without pulmonary disease (hypoventilation syndromes, high altitude), pulmonary arterial obstruction (thromboembolism), and idiopathic (primary) pulmonary arterial hypertension.

In addition to these etiologies of chronic PH, acute increases in PVR may result from hypoxia, hypercarbia, acidosis, increased sympathetic tone, and endogenous or exogenous pulmonary vasoconstrictors such as catecholamines, serotonin, thromboxane, and endothelin. Most perioperative patients with decompensated PH have a combination of chronic PH with an acute increase in PVR; in general, therapy is directed at reversing this acute increase in PVR.

Evaluation of the patient with PH should investigate the underlying etiology and severity of the disease.

Evaluation of the patient with PH should determine the underlying etiology and the severity of the disease. In patients without an identified etiology, ventilation-perfusion lung scan should be performed to exclude chronic thromboembolic PH, since patients with this disorder should be considered for surgical thromboendarterectomy. Echocardiography with Doppler measurements can determine RV function and RV systolic pressure (15).

Pulmonary artery catheterization will demonstrate pulmonary hemodynamics and whether the pulmonary circulation is reactive to vasodilators. Measurement of vasodilator responsiveness should be performed with a short-acting vasodilator such as inhaled nitric oxide, inhaled prostacyclin, intravenous prostacyclin, or intravenous adenosine. Measurement of PAP, cardiac index, and right atrial pressure can be used to predict survival. Other major prognostic factors include the etiology of PH, functional status, mixed venous oxygen saturation, and evidence of right heart failure. The 6-minute walk test evaluates functional impairment, prognosis, and response to chronic therapy.

In this patient, IPAH was diagnosed 2 years ago when she developed severe dyspnea on exertion and an episode of syncope. Evaluation for cardiac and pulmonary etiologies was negative, and chronic thromboembolic PH was excluded by a normal ventilation-perfusion scan. She is currently on continuous intravenous prostacyclin (epoprostenol; Flolan) and oral sildenafil (Revatio) with class III heart failure (dyspnea with minimal exertion). What additional evaluation is necessary prior to surgery?

Assessing the Risks and Benefits of Surgery

In the face of increased impedance to RV ejection, the compensatory reserves of the RV are limited. Reductions in RV stroke volume and CO occur, eventually resulting in ventricular interdependence with decreased LV filling. Anesthesia and surgery may produce additional increases in PVR and decreases in RV function, resulting in progressive hemodynamic deterioration and death. Patients with PH have markedly increased morbidity and mortality with anesthesia and surgery (1–3). Mortality is as high as 70% in patients with Eisenmenger syndrome undergoing cesarean section. Patients undergoing liver transplantation have mortality rates as high as 80% when the mean PAP exceeds 45 mm Hg. The risks associated with idiopathic (primary) PH appear to be even higher than those related to secondary PH.

Patients with PH have markedly increased morbidity and mortality with anesthesia, as high as 70% in patients with Eisenmenger syndrome undergoing cesarean section.

Survival in patients with PH correlates with the ability of the RV to compensate for the increased PVR as assessed by CO, right atrial pressure, and functional status. These factors also are major predictors of perioperative risk in the surgical patient. Perioperative risk is also related to the surgical procedure (2).

Procedures with rapid blood loss may result in fatal hypotension since adequate RV filling is required to compensate for increased RV afterload. Major procedures, which result in a systemic inflammatory response syndrome, may exacerbate PH. Finally, some procedures may pose special risks for the patient with PH, such as pulmonary embolization of air, bone marrow, and cement during joint replacement surgery. Risk assessment requires balancing the functional reserves of the patient against the anticipated increased demands of the surgical procedure.

In patients who pose an unacceptably high risk, consideration should be given to lung or heart-lung transplantation or to chronic treatment to decrease PH to acceptable levels before surgery. In general, oral calcium channel blockers are used for patients with a positive acute vasoreactivity test, and prostanoids (epoprostenol or treprostinil), endothelin antagonists (bosentan), and PDE5 inhibitors (sildenafil) are used in patients who either do not have acute vasoreactivity or fail calcium channel blocker therapy (14).

The patient initially had class IV heart failure from her PH. Three months after treatment with continuous intravenous prostacyclin (Flolan) and oral sildenafil, she had significant improvement to class III heart failure and has remained stable since. Her improved functional status was confirmed by a 6-minute walk test of 304 m. Her PAPs were 95/60 prior to starting therapy and 78/42 on therapy. Her echocardiogram 1 month ago demonstrated moderate RV enlargement and moderate RV systolic dysfunction with an estimated RV systolic pressure of 80 mm Hg.

She was therefore considered to be at markedly increased perioperative risk, including the effects of pneumoperitoneum and associated carbon dioxide absorption intraoperatively and diaphragmatic dysfunction postoperatively. However, based on her two recent episodes of acute cholecystitis and her inability to increase CO in response to sepsis-induced vasodilation, the decision was that surgery was inevitable and that her risk with emergency surgery far outweighed the risk of an elective procedure.

Preparation of the Patient for Anesthesia and Surgery

Prior to anesthesia and surgery, patients with PH should have an electrocardiogram, chest x-ray, arterial blood gas, and echocardiogram. Evidence of significant RV dysfunction should prompt reevaluation of the need for surgery. Patients receiving chronic therapy for PH should continue on such therapy throughout the perioperative period. Patients on chronic prostacyclin or treprostinil infusions should have the infusion continued throughout the perioperative period, and patients on chronic inhaled iloprost should receive a treatment prior to surgery.

The patient's prostacyclin infusion was switched to a hospital infusion system by an experienced nurse. She received her morning dose of sildenafil in the preoperative area.

Anesthetic management

The anesthetic management of patients with PH undergoing noncardiac surgery is controversial (4,6–8,10,11,16,17). Most authors agree that the way a specific anesthetic technique is managed is as important as the choice of the technique. In the absence of evidence-based recommendations, anesthesiologists focus on hemodynamic principles.

The anesthetic management of patients with PH undergoing noncardiac surgery is controversial and anesthesiologists should focus on hemodynamic principles.

Physiologic Considerations and Goals

The major patholophysiology in PH is due to the elevated PVR, which increases RV afterload, thereby increasing RV work and decreasing RV (and thus LV) output (4,9,12). Based on the underlying pathophysiology, the major anesthetic considerations include:

1. **Preload:** Maintenance of preload (intravascular volume) at normal or increased levels is required to maintain CO with increased RV afterload.
2. **Systemic vascular resistance (SVR):** In normal hemodynamic states, SVR is a major determinant of LV afterload (and, therefore, CO). In PH, CO is limited by RV function and is therefore independent of SVR. In order to avoid systemic hypotension, SVR must be maintained in the normal-to-high range.
3. **Contractility:** Maintenance of normal-to-high contractility is essential to maintain CO in the face of increased RV afterload.
4. **Heart rate and rhythm:** Sinus rhythm is important for adequate filling of a hypertrophied RV. Stroke volume is limited by ventricular afterload, so bradycardia should be avoided. Patients with PH commonly have excess vagal activity.
5. **Avoidance of myocardial ischemia:** RV subendocardial ischemia due to myocardial oxygen supply-demand imbalance is common in PH. Systemic hypotension and excessive increases in preload, contractility, and heart rate must be avoided.

Table 66-2

Hemodynamic Goals in Management of PH

Maintain preload (normal to high)
Maintain SVR (normal to high)
Maintain contractility (normal to high)
Maintain heart rate and sinus rhythm
Avoid myocardial ischemia
Avoid increases in PVR
Avoid systemic hypotension

6. **PVR:** In PH, PVR is the major factor governing RV afterload and CO. Therefore, increases in PVR must be avoided and therapy to decrease PVR may be required.
7. **Avoidance of hypotension:** Systemic hypotension precipitates RV failure by decreasing coronary perfusion of the RV and by decreasing the contribution of the interventricular septum to RV ejection (Table 66-2).

Perioperative Monitoring

Monitoring during anesthesia must detect the causes and complications of increased PVR. Arterial catheterization is almost always indicated since hypotension may be precipitous and require rapid intervention. Intraoperative transesophageal echocardiography (TEE) allows continuous assessment of the filling and function of both ventricles (15). Pulmonary artery catheterization can guide therapy of systemic hypotension (see below), but the risks and benefits of pulmonary artery catheterization must be assessed for each patient.

After a small dose of midazolam, a radial arterial catheter was inserted. Pulmonary artery catheterization (performed after induction of general anesthesia) demonstrated PAP 65/38 with a mean pressure of 48 mm Hg and systemic mean arterial pressure of 65 mm Hg. CO was 2.8 L/min.

Choice of Anesthetic Technique

Many anesthetic techniques have been successfully used in individual patients with PH. Since general anesthesia in patients with PH has significant risks, peripheral nerve blocks should be considered when appropriate. The use of

Nitrous oxide increases PVR and should be avoided in patients with PH.

neuraxial techniques (spinal or epidural) may decrease SVR and thereby produce systemic hypotension when CO is limited due to PH. Epidural anesthesia is preferable to spinal anesthesia since it allows a slower onset so that adverse hemodynamic effects may be recognized in early stages and corrected. Intrathecal and epidural narcotics may provide excellent pain relief postoperatively or during labor without producing sympathetic blockade.

General anesthesia is usually required for major surgery. Isoflurane, sevoflurane, and desflurane may produce beneficial pulmonary vasodilation, but decreased contractility and

SVR can result in systemic hypotension. In general, patients with PH with adequate functional reserve will tolerate volatile agents. Nitrous oxide increases PVR and should be avoided. In poorly compensated patients, a high-dose narcotic-oxygen technique maintains preload, SVR, and

Etomidate is the drug of choice for inducing anesthesia in patients with PH.

contractility without increasing PVR; the use of 100% oxygen may produce pulmonary vasodilation.

Anesthetic induction is an unstable period during which patients with PH are prone to develop systemic hypotension and cardiovascular collapse. Propofol decreases SVR. Ketamine as an induction agent in adults may increase

PVR and decrease contractility. Etomidate, which maintains systemic hemodynamics without affecting PVR, is the drug of choice.

Ventilatory management may affect PVR. Hypercarbia is a potent pulmonary vasoconstrictor, and hypocarbia is a pulmonary vasodilator. PVR is dependent upon functional residual capacity (FRC), such that PVR is increased whenever FRC is increased or decreased from its normal value. FRC is decreased during general anesthesia; this decrease in FRC can be reversed with positive end-expiratory pressure (PEEP). However, excessive PEEP will increase FRC above optimal values and increase PVR. The effect of tidal volume on PVR may similarly be bimodal. At low tidal volumes, alveolar hypoxia and hypercarbia may occur and increase PVR. At high tidal volumes, excess lung volume results in compression of intra-alveolar vessels and increased PVR. Ventilation of the patient with PH should use high concentrations of oxygen, moderate tidal volumes, rates sufficient to achieve mild hypocarbia, and low levels of PEEP.

Ventilatory goals in patients with PH should be to use high concentrations of oxygen, moderate tidal volumes, rates sufficient to achieve mild hypocarbia and low levels of PEEP.

> Induction of anesthesia was achieved with 250 mcg fentanyl, 14 mg etomidate, and 40 mg rocuronium. Anesthesia was maintained with 1% isoflurane in oxygen and incremental doses of fentanyl. Initial ventilator settings were TV 400 mL, PEEP 5 cm, and rate 14 with a goal of maintaining an end-tidal CO_2 of 30 mm Hg.
>
> The start of surgery with creation of the pneumoperitoneum (thereby restricting lung expansion) and surgical stimulation (producing pulmonary vasoconstriction) was a time of potential instability. The surgeon agreed to use low insufflation pressures.

> Since laparoscopic cholecystectomy is performed in reverse Trendelenberg position (vs. pelvic procedures), tidal volumes were maintained with only a small increase in airway pressures. PAPs were monitored with a plan for discontinuing the pneumoperitoneum and proceeding to an open procedure if there was evidence of decompensation.
>
> The ratio of pulmonary to systemic artery pressure was monitored as an index of stability. Surgical stimulation increased PAP but did not change the ratio, allowing deepening of the anesthetic with additional fentanyl. CO measurements confirmed stability. During the case, the ventilator rate was progressively increased to 24 in response to CO_2 absorption from the pneumoperitoneum. Volume status was monitored by TEE (focusing on both the right and left ventricles) and by CVP, in addition to estimated blood loss.

Management of emergence from anesthesia is often the most challenging problem. Hemodynamic stability depends on the ratio of pulmonary to systemic vascular tone. Extubation in a light plane of anesthesia can produce pulmonary vasoconstriction, but extubation in a deep plane of anesthesia can produce inadequate ventilation.

> Pulmonary hemodynamics were monitored during emergence following optimization of narcotic administration and a lidocaine bolus. If the patient had developed increased PH and systemic hypotension, the plan was for high dose narcotics with transfer to the ICU for slow weaning. Although PAP increased during emergence, systemic blood pressure also increased with no change in the ratio of pulmonary to systemic pressures, so nitroglycerin was used for transient treatment of hypertension.

Treatment of Perioperative Hypotension

Hemodynamic management in PH should maintain blood pressure and CO and minimize PVR. When CO is low, inovasodilator agents such as dobutamine and milrinone can increase CO and decrease PVR. Systemic hypotension should be aggressively treated since it decreases RV myocardial perfusion (producing ischemia) and decreases the contribution of the interventricular septum to RV CO. Systemic hypotension may result from four etiologies, each with a specific hemodynamic pattern that can be diagnosed by pulmonary artery catheterization (Table 66-3).

Decreased preload is the only etiology with decreased CVP. Volume therapy is indicated, but must be monitored since excess volume in a patient with a failing RV may result in further

Table 66-3

Etiologies of Systemic Hypotension in Patients with PH

Etiology	CVP	PAP	Pulmonary Artery Occlusion Pressure (PAOP)	CO
Decreased preload	↓↓	↓	↓	↓
Decreased contractility	↑	↓	↑	↓
Decreased SVR	↔	↔	↔ or ↓	↑ or ↔
Increased PVR	↑	↑	↓	↓

distention and dysfunction. Decreased contractility increases CVP but not PAP; inotropic therapy is indicated. When decreased systemic blood pressure occurs without a decrease in PAP, the ratio of PVR to SVR has increased. The initial approach should be to reverse correctable causes of increased PVR such as hypoxia, hypercarbia, and acidosis. In patients with hypotension but maintained CO, decreased SVR can be treated by systemic vasoconstriction with phenylephrine or vasopressin. A combined inotropic-vasopressor agent such as epinephrine or norepinephrine may also be useful.

When exacerbation of PH results in systemic hypotension and decreased CO, inhaled pulmonary vasodilators such as inhaled nitric oxide or inhaled prostacyclin may produce selective pulmonary vasodilation (4,12,18–21). A trial of 20 ppm inhaled NO is sufficient to determine if the patient will have a beneficial response. Inhibition of cyclic guanosine monophosphate (GMP) phosphodiesterase with sildenafil can increase the response to inhaled NO but may itself produce systemic hypotension. Although drugs with combined inotropic and pulmonary vasodilator effects such as dobutamine and milrinone can increase CO in patients with PH, their systemic vasodilator effects frequently contraindicate their use in patients with PH-induced systemic hypotension.

This patient never developed hypotension, but inhaled NO was available if needed in the operating room and the ICU.

Postoperative Management

Although intraoperative management of PH is challenging, most patients who die in the perioperative period do so several days after surgery. Causes of death include progressive increases in PVR, progressive decreases in cardiac function, and sudden death. Patients should be monitored at least overnight in the ICU. The use of epidural narcotics and local anesthetics, continuous regional anesthesia, and non-narcotic analgesic adjuvants should be considered.

The patient was monitored in the ICU overnight after surgery with continuation of her prostacyclin infusion and oral sildenafil. She was discharged home 2 days later and has subsequently done well.

References

1. Price LC, Montani D, Jaïs X, et al. Non-cardiothoracic non-obstetric surgery in mild-moderate pulmonary hypertension: perioperative management of 28 consecutive individual cases. *Eur Respir J* 2010;35:1294–1302.
2. Ramakrishna G, Sprung J, Ravi BS, et al. Impact of pulmonary hypertension on the outcomes of noncardiac surgery: predictors of perioperative morbidity and mortality. *J Am Coll Cardiol* 2005;45:1691–1699.
3. Carmosino MJ, Friesen RH, Doran A, et al. Perioperative complications in children with pulmonary hypertension undergoing noncardiac surgery or cardiac catheterization. *Anesth Analg* 2007;104:521–527.
4. Pritts CD, Pearl RG. Anesthesia for patients with pulmonary hypertension. *Curr Opin Anaesthesiol* 2010;23:411–416.

5. Hill NS, Roberts KR, Preston IR. Postoperative pulmonary hypertension: etiology and treatment of a dangerous complication. *Respir Care* 2009;54:958–968.
6. Subramaniam K, Yared JP. Management of pulmonary hypertension in the operating room. Semin Cardiothorac Vasc Anesth 2007;11:119–136.
7. Blaise G, Langleben D, Hubert B. Pulmonary arterial hypertension: pathophysiology and anesthetic approach. *Anesthesiology* 2003;99:1415–1432.
8. Gordon C, Collard CD, Pan W. Intraoperative management of pulmonary hypertension and associated right heart failure. *Curr Opin Anaesthesiol* 2009;23:49–56.
9. Afifi S, Shayan S, Al-Qamari A. Pulmonary hypertension and right ventricular function: interdependence in pathophysiology and management. *Int Anesthesiol Clin* 2009;47:97–120.
10. Fischer LG, Van Aken H, Burkle H. Management of pulmonary hypertension: physiological and pharmacological considerations for anesthesiologists. *Anesth Analg* 2003;96:1603–1616.
11. Fox C, Kalarickal PL, Yarborough MJ, et al. Perioperative management including new pharmacological vistas for patients with pulmonary hypertension for noncardiac surgery. *Curr Opin Anaesthesiol* 2008;21:467–472.
12. Zamanian RT, Haddad F, Doyle RL, et al. Management strategies for patients with pulmonary hypertension in the intensive care unit. *Crit Care Med* 2007; 35:2037–2050.
13. Forrest P. Anaesthesia and right ventricular failure. *Anaesth Intensive Care* 2009;37:370–385.
14. Humbert M, McLaughlin VV. The 4th World Symposium on Pulmonary Hypertension. *J Am Coll Cardiol* 2009;54:S1–S2.
15. Pedoto A, Amar D. Right heart function in thoracic surgery: role of echocardiography. *Curr Opin Anaesthesiol* 2009;22:44–49.
16. Friesen RH, Williams GD. Anesthetic management of children with pulmonary arterial hypertension. *Paediatr Anaesth* 2008;18:208–216.
17. MacKnight B, Martinez EA, Simon BA. Anesthetic management of patients with pulmonary hypertension. *Semin Cardiothorac Vasc Anesth* 2008;12:91–96.
18. Haj RM, Cinco JE, Mazer CD. Treatment of pulmonary hypertension with selective pulmonary vasodilators. *Curr Opin Anaesthesiol* 2006; 19:88–95.
19. Creagh-Brown BC, Griffiths MJ, Evans TW. Bench-to-bedside review: Inhaled nitric oxide therapy in adults. *Crit Care* 2009; 13:221.
20. Lowson SM. Inhaled alternatives to nitric oxide. *Crit Care Med* 2005;33:S188–S195.
21. Winterhalter M, Simon A, Fischer S, et al. Comparison of inhaled iloprost and nitric oxide in patients with pulmonary hypertension during weaning from cardiopulmonary bypass in cardiac surgery: a prospective randomized trial. *J Cardiothorac Vasc Anesth* 2008;22:406–413.

ANESTHESIA AND COMORBID DISEASES

67

Part B: Immunology and Infectious Diseases
Allergy and Anaphylaxis

T. Kyle Harrison, MD • Andrea J. Fuller, MD

In everyday anesthetic practice, patients with a history of immune-mediated reactions are encountered. While there are many different types of immune-mediated reactions, anaphylaxis is a potentially fatal allergic reaction that can occur during anesthesia or in daily life and will be the focus of this chapter. Potentially, any drug or substance can cause anaphylaxis; the most commonly associated agents during anesthesia are the neuromuscular blocking drugs (NMBDs).

1) Pathophysiology
   a) Immune-mediated reactions
      i) **Type I hypersensitivity reactions**
         (1) Exposure to causative agent (antigen) results in production of IgE antibodies
         (2) When the individual is later re-exposed to the same antigen, the IgE antibodies promote release of histamine and other vasoactive substances from mast cells and basophils.
         (3) Examples include anaphylaxis, asthma, allergic rhinitis.
         (4) **Anaphylaxis is the most severe Type I hypersensitivity reaction**
            (a) The severity of anaphylaxis is dose-independent.
            (b) The incidence of anaphylaxis is estimated to be between 1:10,000 and 1:20,000, with the mortality rate approaching 5% (1,2).
            (c) Women are at greater risk than men of developing anaphylaxis (3).
      ii) **Type II hypersensitivity reactions**
         (1) Also known as antibody-dependent cell-mediated cytotoxic reactions
         (2) Mediated by IgG or IgM antibodies
         (3) Antigens are on the surface of foreign cells.
         (4) Examples include ABO-incompatible transfusion reactions and heparin-induced thrombocytopenia.
      iii) **Type III hypersensitivity reactions**
         (1) Also known as immune complex reactions
         (2) Antigens and antibodies bind in the bloodstream to form complexes.
         (3) Complexes deposit in the vasculature, which may result in injury.
      iv) **Type IV (delayed) hypersensitivity reactions**
         (1) Peak 2 to 4 days after exposure to antigen
         (2) Sensitized lymphocytes react with antigens.

(3) Mediated by cytotoxic T cells

(4) Examples include tissue rejection and graft-versus-host reactions.

b) **Anaphylactoid (nonimmunologic) reactions**

  i) Clinically indistinguishable from anaphylaxis

  ii) Causative agent directly stimulates the release of the vasoactive substances, **without IgE mediation.**

  iii) Severity of an anaphylactoid reaction is dose-dependent.

  iv) Treatment is the same as for anaphylaxis (Table 67-1).

2) **Causative agents for Type I hypersensitivity section Table 67-1**

a) Almost 70% of anaphylaxis events during anesthesia are caused by NMBDs.

  i) The order of frequency is: rocuronium, succinylcholine and vecuronium.

  ii) All NMBDs can cause anaphylaxis, and they can be cross-reactive with one another.

b) Other causes of anaphylaxis in order of their frequency

  i) Latex exposure, antibiotics, colloids, opioids, and hypnotics.

c) **Allergic reactions to local anesthetics**

  i) Extremely rare

  ii) Ester-based local anesthetics are more likely than amides to cause a reaction.

  iii) Some patients react to the preservatives used in the preparation.

d) **Latex allergy**

Table 67-1

Anesthetic Agents Implicated in Allergic Reactions

Anesthetic Agents

Induction agents (cremophor-solubilized drugs, barbiturates, etomidate, propofol)

Local anesthetics (paraaminobenzoic ester agents)

Muscle relaxants (succinylcholine, gallamine, pancuronium, d-tubocurarine, metocurine, atracurium, vecuronium, mivacurium, doxacurium)

Opioids (meperidine, morphine, fentanyl)

Other Agents

Antibiotics (cephalosporins, penicillin, sulfonamides, vancomycin)

Aprotinin

Blood products (whole blood, packed cells, fresh-frozen plasma, platelets, cryoprecipitate, fibrin glue, γ-globulin)

Bone cement

Chymopapain

Corticosteroids

Cyclosporin

Drug additives (preservatives)

Furosemide

Insulin

Mannitol

Methylmethacrylate

Nonsteroidal anti-inflammatory drugs

Protamine

Radiocontrast dye

Latex (natural rubber)

Streptokinase

Vascular graft material

Vitamin K

Colloid volume expanders (dextrans, protein fractions, albumin, hydroxyethyl starch)

Reprinted with permission from Levy JH. *Anaphylactic Reactions in Anesthesia and Intensive Care.* 2nd ed. Boston, MA: Butterworth-Heinemann; 1992.

Full-blown
anaphylaxis may
present with
hypoxia, cardio-
vascular collapse,
and death.

Anesthesia
providers and
other health
care workers
are at risk for
developing
latex allergy.

When a patient
with a latex allergy
has surgery, it
is important to
check all equip-
ment for the pres-
ence of latex.

READ
MORE

Crisis man-
agement:
anaphylaxis,
Chapter 212,
page 1330

i) Incidence of latex allergy and anaphylaxis associated with latex products has been increasing.

ii) Populations at increased risk include children who have had numerous surgeries, patients with spina bifida, and health care workers.

iii) **Management of latex allergy**

    (1) A patient with known hypersensitivity to latex should be scheduled as the first case of the day in a latex-free environment, with special latex-free equipment and carts.

    (2) Whereas anaphylaxis from drugs often occurs during induction, latex anaphylaxis often occurs during the maintenance phase of the anesthetic.

3) **Clinical manifestations**

  a) Type I hypersensitivity reactions can present with a mild rash or hive.

    i) Full-blown anaphylaxis may present with hypoxia, cardiovascular collapse, and death.

    ii) The signs and symptoms often present suddenly, following administration of the causative agent, which causes mast cell degranulation and release of vasoactive substances such as histamine and tryptase.

    iii) The most common feature is a rash or hives followed by cardiovascular collapse (hypotension and tachycardia or bradycardia), bronchospasm, and angioedema.

    iv) The patient may present with only a single manifestation of anaphylaxis or with multiple associated findings.

4) Treatment of anaphylaxis (Table 67-2)

  a) The treatment is supportive with the goal of providing adequate oxygenation and maintaining adequate hemodynamic stability.

  b) If you suspect a patient of having an anaphylaxis event, eliminate further exposure to the suspected agent.

    i) Airway and ventilation

      (1) Place the patient on 100% oxygen.

      (2) If the patient is not already intubated, consider early airway intervention, to avoid the development of angioedema.

      (3) Treat bronchospasm with low-dose epinephrine in moderate to severe cases.

        (a) Albuterol or other inhaled β2 agonists can be used in milder cases.

    ii) Circulatory support

      (1) Administer epinephrine IV (in moderate to severe cases) to treat hypotension.

      (2) Epinephrine also decreases mast-cell degranulation, thus decreasing the amount of histamine circulating in the blood.

      (3) Give an initial dose of 5 to 10 μg, increasing it (usually doubling) every 2 minutes, until you observe clinical improvement.

        (a) If clinical improvement is observed, an epinephrine infusion should be considered at the rate of 4 to 8 μg/min and titrated to effect.

        (b) Patients on β-blockade therapy may require large doses.

Table 67-2

Management of Anaphylaxis During General Anesthesia

Initial Therapy

Stop administration of antigen.

Maintain airway and administer 100% O_2.

Discontinue all anesthetic agents.

Start intravascular volume expansion (2–4 L of crystalloid/colloid with hypotension).

Give epinephrine (5–10 μg IV bolus with hypotension, titrate as needed; 0.1–1.0 mg IV with cardiovascular collapse).

Secondary Treatment

Antihistamines (0.5–1 mg/kg diphenhydramine)

Catecholamine infusions (starting doses: epinephrine, 4–8 μg/min; norepinephrine, 4–8 μg/min; or isoproterenol, 0.5–1 μg/min as an infusion; titrated to desired effects)

Bronchodilators: inhaled albuterol, terbutaline, and/or anticholinergic agents with persistent bronchospasm)

Corticosteroids (0.25–1 g hydrocortisone; alternatively, 1–2 g methylprednisolone)[a]

Sodium bicarbonate (0.5–1 mEq/kg with persistent hypotension or acidosis)

Airway evaluation (before extubation)

Vasopressin for refractory shock

---

[a]Methylprednisolone may be the drug of choice if the reaction is suspected to be mediated by complement.

IV, intravenous(ly).

Reprinted with permission from Levy JH. *Anaphylactic Reactions in Anesthesia and Intensive Care.* 2nd ed. Boston, MA: Butterworth-Heinemann; 1992:162.

When treating a patient for anaphylaxis, epinephrine is the drug of choice.

Doses of epinephrine should initially be small (5 to 10 μg) and increased incrementally to avoid the possibility of severe hypertension and tachycardia.

Patients treated for anaphylaxis are at risk of relapsing several hours after the initial event.

(4) Vasodilation must also be treated with IV fluid.
    (a) Large volumes (2 to 4 L) are sometimes required.
    (b) Consider central venous access to guide therapy.
(5) Consider administering vasopressin if the patient continues to be hypotensive following treatment with epinephrine (4).
(6) H_1 antagonists such as diphenhydramine (0.5 to 1 mg/kg) should be administered.

iii) Although no data exists to support using H2 blockers or corticosteroids in the acute-phase treatment of anaphylaxis, these agents might decrease the incidence of rebound or the return of symptoms that can occur after successful treatment.

iv) Consider obtaining a serum mast cell tryptase level.
    (1) Marker for anaphylaxis and can be used as part of the differential diagnosis
    (2) Can be measured from 1 to 6 hours after the event
    (3) May take several days for results

5) Postevent follow-up
a) If successfully treated, most anaphylaxis events will resolve within one hour.
    i) Depending on the severity of the reaction, the patient may require continuing treatment.
b) Monitor patients with moderate to severe anaphylaxis in an intensive care setting.
    i) Continued intubation is usually warranted.
c) Update the patient's chart to reflect the most likely cause of anaphylaxis.

  d) Inform the patient of his/her allergy status.
  e) Perform postoperative allergy testing for all medications used prior to the event.
    i) If allergy to NMBD is suspected, recommend that the patient be tested for reactions to all NMBDs, and note which one(s) does not cause a reaction, for future reference when anesthetics will be used.
      (1) However, it is important to bear in mind that if the patient has an allergy to a particular NMBD there is still a risk of cross-reaction; hence, avoiding all neuromuscular drugs if possible is the best action.

Chapter Summary for Allergic Reactions and Anaphylaxis

Pathophysiology	IgE mediated histamine release in response to antigen exposure. Anaphylactoid reactions are not IgE mediated, but signs and symptoms are clinically indistinguishable from anaphylaxis.
Cause	Many drugs and environmental exposures
Symptoms	Rash, bronchospasm, airway edema, hypotension, tachycardia, leading to circulatory collapse
Treatment	Supportive care focusing on oxygenation, IV fluid management, and treatment of symptoms with epinephrine

References

1. Fisher MM, Baldo BA. The incidence and clinical features of anaphylactic reactions during anesthesia in Australia. *Ann Fr Anesth Reanim* 1993;12:97–104.
2. Mitsuhata H, Hasegawa J, Matsumoto S, et al. The epidemiology and clinical features of anaphylactic and anaphylactoid reactions in the perioperative period in Japan: a survey with a questionnaire of 529 hospitals approved by Japan Society of Anesthesiology. *Masui* 1992;41: 1825–1831.
3. Mertes PM, Laxenaire MC. Allergic reactions occurring during anaesthesia. *Eur J Anaesthesiol* 2002;19:240–262.
4. Kill C, Wranze E, Wulf H. Successful treatment of severe anaphylactic shock with vasopressin. Two case reports. *Int Arch Allerg Immunol* 2004;134:260–261.

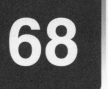

Human Immune Deficiency Virus

Andrea J. Fuller, MD

Human immune deficiency virus (HIV) is a virus whose infection is responsible for acquired immune deficiency syndrome (AIDS). In parts of sub-Saharan Africa, HIV infection is reaching epidemic proportions. In 2004, the number of people in the United States infected with HIV approached 1 million, with as many as 20% unaware of their illness. Approximately, 20% to 25% of HIV-positive patients will require surgery throughout the course of their lifetime (1).

1) **Pathophysiology**
   a) **HIV-1** is the most commonly encountered strain which causes AIDS.
   b) **Transmission**
      i) Through blood, saliva, sexual contact, and vertically (mother to infant)
         (1) **Vertical transmission** is substantially reduced by cesarean delivery and antiretroviral therapy.
   c) HIV-1 is a **single-strand RNA** virus. Upon entering a cell, it produces double strand DNA via an enzyme called **reverse transcriptase.**
   d) **CD4 T lymphocytes** are predominantly infected.
   e) HIV-2 predominates in western Africa.
2) **Diagnosis**
   a) **Testing for HIV**
      i) Recommended in patients with a high-risk lifestyle (injection drug use, unprotected sexual intercourse), pregnant women, health care workers with occupational exposure, and routinely for patients in hospital settings where the prevalence in the population is >1% (2).
      ii) **ELISA testing for** anti-HIV antibody is the most common means of testing.
         (1) Because of the high sensitivity with ELISA testing, a second test with high specificity is usually performed after a positive result (3).
   b) **Acquired immune deficiency syndrome**
      i) **Defined as a CD4 count <200 cells/uL** (1,3)
      ii) **High risk of opportunistic infections and malignancy (index conditions)** such as Kaposi sarcoma, *Pneumocystis carinii* pneumonia, coccidioidomycosis, or recurrent bacterial infections
   c) **HIV RNA viral load** is a measurement of viral activity.
      i) **Patients with a high viral load are at increased risk for disease progression (3).**
3) **Clinical manifestations**
   a) **Neurologic**
      i) Occur early in the disease and throughout its course
         (1) **Early:** Myelopathy, peripheral neuropathy, Guillian-Barré syndrome

489

(2) **Latent:** Autoimmune demyelinating neuropathies resembling Guillian-Barre syndrome

(3) **Late:** Opportunistic meningitis (cryptococcal most common), CNS lymphoma, AIDS dementia complex (cognitive, motor, and behavioral changes)

b) **Pulmonary**

i) Opportunistic infections predominate. Thorough evaluation for residual pulmonary impairment is essential prior to formulating an anesthetic plan.

(1) **P. carinii, tuberculosis, aspergillosis,** and other bacterial organisms are frequent pathogens.

c) **Cardiovascular**

HIV positive patients on long-term antiretroviral therapy are at high risk for coronary artery disease.

i) **Coronary artery disease** appears to be increasing with antiretroviral therapy. **Protease inhibitors** appear to be associated with **dyslipidemias** (1).

ii) The incidence of **cardiomyopathy, pulmonary hypertension, myocarditis, pericardial effusions** is higher in untreated HIV-positive patients compared to the general population (1).

d) **Hematologic**

i) **Mild thrombocytopenia, bone marrow suppression from AZT**

4) Treatment

a) Drugs involved in the treatment of HIV can be divided into four major classes. Common side effects and interactions are reported in Table 68-1.

i) **Nucleoside analog reverse transcriptase inhibitors.**

ii) **Nonnucleoside analog reverse transcriptase inhibitors.**

iii) **Protease inhibitors**

(1) **Ritonavir (1)**

(a) **Potent inhibitor of** cytochrome P-450 3A and 2D6

(b) Increases effectiveness of other HIV treatment regimens

(c) **Can affect fentanyl metabolism**

(2) **Other protease inhibitors induce cytochrome P-450.**

iv) **Fusion inhibitors** bind to HIV and prevent fusion with target cell membranes.

v) **Prophylactic agents** are usually antimicrobials given to prevent or treat opportunistic infections.

5) **Anesthetic implications**

a) **Preoperative**

i) **History should include a review of medications and side effects.**

(1) A consultation with the primary care physician and/or HIV specialist may be warranted if the medications are unfamiliar.

(2) Include questions about the patient's general health including exercise tolerance, presence of pulmonary disease, and neurologic history.

ii) **Physical exam**

(1) A general physical with a thorough evaluation of the patients cardiac, pulmonary, and neurologic systems is necessary.

iii) **Labs and tests**

(1) Should include CBC, liver enzymes, CD4 count, and a review of viral load. Some patients will require EKG, CXR, cardiac echo, PFTs, and ABGs depending on their overall health status.

ANESTHESIA AND COMORBID DISEASES

Table 68-1

Medications Used to Treat HIV-1 Infection

Drug Class	Mechanism of Action	Example	Side Effects	Special Concerns
Nucleoside/ nucleotide analogs	Inhibits reverse transcriptase by preventing DNA elongation	Zidovudine (AZT, Retrovir) Didanosine	Bone marrow suppression, anemia, GI disturbances Pancreatitis, peripheral neuropathy	Few drug interactions
Protease inhibitors	Prevent HIV protease from making functional proteins	Ritonavir (Norvir) Nelfinavir mesylate (Viracept)	Potent inhibitor of cytochrome P-450, increased triglycerides, increased transaminases GI effects (nausea, vomiting, diarrhea), induces cytochrome P-450	May alter metabolism of sedative hypnotics, antiarrhythmics May decrease serum levels of some drugs
Nonnucleoside reverse transcriptase inhibitors	Inhibit proper function of reverse transcriptase	Nevirapine (Viramune) Delavirdine (Rescriptor)	Severe skin rash, induces cytochrome P-450 Inhibits cytochrome P-450	May decrease serum levels of some drugs May increase serum concentrations of warfarin, calcium-channel blockers, and antiarrhythmic drugs
Fusion inhibitors	Binds to HIV and prevents viral fusion with target cell membranes	Enfuvirtide (Fuzeon)	Injection site reactions	

Adapted from Hughes SC. HIV and anesthesia. *Anesth Clin North America* 2004;22:379–404.

b) **Intraoperative**
  i) **All HIV positive patients should be considered immunosuppressed.**
  ii) **General anesthesia**
    (1) There are no specific concerns with GA except those pertaining to the patient's underlying illness and drug interactions.
  iii) **Regional anesthesia**
    (1) Epidural and spinal anesthesia are generally considered safe.
    (2) Viral infection of the CNS occurs early in the disease so **it is unlikely that neuraxial anesthesia will spread HIV infection to the CNS** (1).
  iv) **Epidural blood patch is safe** in this population and is reasonable to attempt when conservative measures fail to treat a post-dural puncture headache (1).
c) Postoperative
  i) Postoperative considerations are related to the underlying disease processes.

Epidural and spinal anesthesia are considered safe in HIV-positive patients.

Chapter Summary for HIV

Definition	HIV is a retrovirus that infects the immune system and causes AIDS	
Laboratory Assessment	CD4 count is a measure of the immune system's strength	
	CD4 <200 cells/uL indicates patient is at high risk for opportunistic infections	
Anesthetic Considerations	Preoperative	Thorough history and physical
		Review labs
		Review medications
	Intraoperative	Regional anesthesia NOT contraindicated
	Postoperative	Patients on antiretroviral therapy may be at increased risk of CAD

AIDS, acquired immune deficiency syndrome; CAD, coronary artery disease; HIV, human immunodeficiency virus.

References

1. Hughes SC. HIV and anesthesia. *Anesth Clin North Am* 2004;22:379–404.
2. www.cdc.gov/mmwr/preview/mmwrhtml/rr5514a1.htm. Center for Disease Control. Accessed February 20, 2009.
3. Hull MW, Harris M, Montaner JSG. Principles of management of HIV in the developed world. In: Cohen J, Opal SM, Powderly WG, eds. *Infectious Disease*, 3rd ed. Philadelphia: Elsevier, 2010.

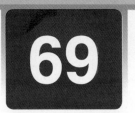

Needlestick Injury

Andrea J. Fuller, MD

Anesthesia providers are at high risk for needlestick injury, with an estimated incidence of 1:2600 anesthetics (1). Approximately, 30% of sharps injuries in the operating room (OR) are high risk for disease transmission (1). All operating room personnel are at risk for injury and in one multicenter study, anesthesia residents had the highest incidence of injury of all anesthesia providers (1).

1) Mechanisms of injury
   a) The most common needlestick injuries in anesthesia personnel are from **intravascular catheter insertion, injection of intradermal local anesthesia, and suturing intravascular catheters** (1).
   b) **Large, hollow bore needles that have been used to enter a blood vessel are most likely to cause** seroconversion.
   c) Other modes of transmission include contact of infected blood or body fluid (semen, vaginal secretions, etc.) with mucous membranes or nonintact skin.

2) Pathophysiology
   a) Diseases transmitted by needlestick injury
      i) The hepatitis B virus (**HBV**), hepatitis C virus (**HCV**), and human immune deficiency virus (**HIV**) are the most thoroughly studied organisms transmitted by needlestick injury.
      ii) Other transmissible diseases include bacteria, fungi, protozoa, and tumors.
   b) Seroconversion
      i) Incidence depends on
         (1) Type of injury
         (2) Incidence of disease in the patient population
         (3) Infectivity of the virus
      ii) Average incidence of seroconversion
         (1) **HBV**
            (a) 1% to 30% risk of developing clinical hepatitis from a percutaneous injury, depending on the infection status of the patient
   c) **HCV**
      i) 1.8% from hollow-bore needle stick injury (2)
      ii) Transmission across mucus membranes or nonintact skin is low.
   d) **HIV**
      i) 0.3% for percutaneous and 0.09% for mucous membrane exposure (2)

3) Treatment and management
   a) **Immediate treatment** (3)
      i) **Wash sites** of potential contamination with soap and water.

Blood contaminated with HBV can still be infectious on environmental surfaces for 1 week (2).

When a needlestick injury occurs, it is important to report the injury to the appropriate authorities as soon as possible.

493

       ii) **Irrigate exposed mucous membranes** with water or sterile saline solutions.
- b) **Determine risk associated with exposure**
  - i) **Type of fluid** (blood is highest risk)
  - ii) **High-risk exposure**
    - (1) **Large, hollow-bore needle**
    - (2) **Deep penetration**
    - (3) **Visible blood contamination**
    - (4) **Needle used to enter a blood vessel**
    - (5) **Mucous membrane exposure with large volume blood splash (2)**
- c) **Report the injury**
  - i) It is estimated that only **50% or less** of sharps injuries in health care workers are reported to the appropriate authorities (1,4).
  - ii) Every health care facility is required to comply with federal regulations by the Occupational Safety and Health Administration (OSHA) and will have an Employee Health Department or other agent responsible for handling reported occupational exposures.
- d) **Test patient or source of exposure** as soon as possible so the injured worker can begin drug therapy if necessary (3).
  - i) **Testing discarded needles or syringes is not recommended (2).**
  - ii) In cases of a **known source (usually a patient)**, State and federal laws for patient confidentiality must be followed.
    - (1) **Informed consent** is usually required. The medical record should be examined for any information about disease status.
  - iii) In cases of an **unknown source**, risk is based on prevalence of disease in the patient population.
- e) **Begin therapy if necessary**
  - i) **HBV**
    - (1) **Hepatitis B immunoglobulin** and **vaccination** are given for individuals who are unvaccinated or incompletely vaccinated.
    - (2) **There is no therapy for vaccinated individuals** with acceptable levels of anti-HBs antibody.
  - ii) **HCV**
    - (1) **No postexposure prophylaxis is currently available (2).**
    - (2) If the source of exposure is anti-HCV positive, perform baseline testing for **anti-HCV and liver function tests (ALT).**
      - (a) Follow-up testing for anti-HCV and ALT should be done at 4 to 6 months.
      - (b) If earlier detection is desired, HCV RNA can be done at 4 to 6 weeks (2).
    - (3) Some evidence supports that early treatment of acute infection with interferon or an antiviral agent decreases the risk of chronic infection (2).
    - (4) It is important for workers exposed to HCV to follow up with the appropriate agents (employee health department, primary care or specialist physician) to receive up-to-date information and treatment.
  - iii) **HIV**
    - (1) HIV antibody test is performed at **baseline** and for at least **6 months postexposure.**
    - (2) Antiretroviral therapy
      - (a) The decision to begin antiretroviral therapy and which drugs to use depends on
        - (i) The **HIV status of the source** (including viral load and the presence of AIDS)
        - (ii) The **severity of exposure**

The source and type of exposure are important factors in determining a preventative regimen after HIV exposure.

The CDC recommends that all health care workers and trainees without immunity be vaccinated for HBV (2).

    (b)   Most antiretroviral therapy prophylaxis regimens consist of **at least** two drugs and last 4 weeks.

    (c)   Side effects vary depending on the drug, but are quite significant and can include

        (i)   Myalgia

        (ii) Fatigue

        (iii) Nausea

        (iv) Peripheral neuropathy

        (v) Neutropenia

        (vi) Pancreatitis

    (d)   Up-to-date recommendations from the CDC should be consulted and an appropriate regimen determined for the prescribing agent.

    (e)   Regardless of the regimen used, **antiretroviral therapy is most effective when started as soon as possible, preferably within hours of exposure** (2).

  (3) **Secondary transmission should be prevented,** especially while the exposed person is taking drug prophylaxis. Measures taken should include

    (a)   Sexual abstinence or use of condoms

    (b)   Refraining from blood or tissue donation

    (c)   Discontinuation of breast-feeding.

  4) Prevention

    a) Vaccination

      i)   The vaccine for HBV is the only one currently available.

    b) Universal precautions

      i)   This term is based on the 1985 CDC recommendation that the **blood of all persons should be regarded as infectious.**

      ii) **Use barrier devices** such as gloves, masks, protective eyewear, and possibly gowns or other protective garments whenever there is a possibility of exposure to blood or bodily fluids (4).

The blood of all persons should be regarded as infectious. Universal precautions should be followed.

Sharps injuries are more common when practitioners are rushing, distracted, or angry, or when multiple attempts are required to complete a procedure.

    c) **Appropriate management of sharps**

      i)   All needles and sharp objects should be disposed of in puncture-resistant containers.

      ii) Avoid recapping needles and touching needles or other sharps.

      iii) Sharps passed between personnel should be done via a "neutral zone" such as an emesis basin or Mayo stand to avoid touching the sharp (4).

      iv) When performing procedures, place needles in areas provided for sharps. Attempt to do the procedure the same way every time in order to know where sharps are located.

    d) **Communication**

      i)   Communication among personnel regarding the location of sharps is paramount.

      ii) A recent study showed that sharps injuries were more common when practitioners were rushing, distracted, angry, or required multiple attempts to complete a procedure (5).

    e) **Safety devices**

      i)   Multiple safety devices are available that decrease sharps injuries (6,7).

      ii) It is advisable to become familiar with the use of such devices and use them whenever possible (6,8)

Chapter Summary for Needlestick Injury

Most Common Infectious Agents	HBV, HCV, HIV
Highest Risk Injuries	Occur from hollow bore needles used to enter a blood vessel.
What to do when an Injury Occurs?	Report to authorities and follow their recommendations. Wash and irrigate the wound. Test source of contamination.

HBV, hepatitis B virus; HCV, hepatitis C virus; HIV, human immune deficiency virus.

References

1. Greene ES, Barry AJ, Hagger J, et al. Multicenter study of contaminated percutaneous injuries in anesthesia personnel. *Anesthesiology* 1998;89(6):1362–1372.
2. Centers for disease control and prevention. Updated US Public Health Service guidelines for the management of occupational exposures to HBV, HCV, and HIV and recommendations for postexposure prophylaxis. *Morb Mortal Wkly Rep* 2001;50(No. RR-11):1–52.
3. Berry AJ. Needle stick and other safety issues. *Anesthesiol Clin North Am* 2004;22(3):493–508.
4. Berguer R, Heller PJ. Strategies for preventing sharps injuries in the operating room. *Surg Clin North Am* 2005;85(6):1299–1305.
5. Fisman DN, Harris AD, Mittleman MA. Sharps-related injuries in health care workers: A case crossover study. *Am J Med* 2003;114(8):688–694.
6. Cullen BL, Genasi F, Symington I, et al. Potential for reported needlestick injury prevention among healthcare workers through safety device usage and improvement of guideline adherence: Expert panel assessment. *J Hosp Infect* 2007;63(4):445–451.
7. Rouges AM, Verdun-Esquer C, Buisson-Valles I, et al. Impact of safety devices for preventing percutaneous injuries related to phlebotomy procedures in health care workers. *Am J Infect Control* 2004;32(8):441–444.
8. Joint commission for accreditaion of health care organizations. Sentinel alert: Preventing needle stick and sharps injuries. August 2001. Http://www.Jointcommission.Org/sentinelevents/sentineleventalert/sea_22.Htm accessed 5/29/2010.

70

Challenges in Anesthesia: The Septic Patient Requiring Urgent Surgery

Myer Rosenthal, MD

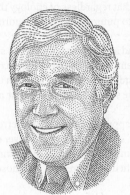

Clinical Vignette

A 68-year-old, 5'2", 80 kg female is scheduled for an urgent exploratory laparotomy for a ruptured diverticulum complicated by peritonitis and hemodynamic insufficiency. She was admitted 36 hours ago with abdominal pain accompanied by diffuse tenderness and rebound. She relates a history of diverticulitis.

There was delay in proceeding with diagnostic testing and treatment and finally an abdominal CT done 3 hours ago revealed a fluid collection and obvious perforation in the region of her sigmoid colon.

Over the past several hours she has become progressively more hypotensive and oliguric. Antibiotics have been instituted, a nasogastric tube and Foley catheter placed, and she has received 1,500 mL of normal saline over the past 3 hours. Her current vital signs are blood pressure 80/30 mm Hg, pulse (P) 110 per minute and full, respirations (R) 22 per minute and temperature 38.4°C. She is experiencing some shortness of breath although her lungs sound clear to auscultation. Her heart sounds are normal and her abdominal exam is as described above. Her airway also appears normal.

Her past medical history is significant for a myocardial infarction 3 years ago at which time she was in mild congestive heart failure. Angiography was performed at that time which revealed a 100% left anterior descending coronary artery (LAD) lesion with <50% lesions in her right main and circumflex coronary arteries. An angioplasty of the LAD was performed without stent placement. Since that time she has been asymptomatic. She is very active without any limitations.

Her medications have included atenolol 50 mg twice daily, which has not been administered since her admission, and furosemide 20 mg once daily with potassium supplementation. Available laboratory studies performed 24 hours ago showed a hemoglobin of 11 gm/dL, white blood count of 16,000 with a left shift and normal appearing platelets. Her electrolytes were sodium 145 mEq/L, potassium 4.2 mEq/L, chloride 104 mEq/L, and CO_2 18 mEq/L. Additional findings were a BUN of 25 mg/dL, creatinine 1.4 mg/dL, and glucose 98 mg/dL. Her chest x-ray on admission was normal without any evidence of infiltrates or failure and her EKG showed a sinus rhythm at 72 per minute with evidence of an old inferior myocardial infarction, but no signs of acute ischemia.

Preoperative Evaluation and Preparation

Although in acute distress with signs consistent of septic induced shock, necessitating a surgical procedure for drainage of a likely abscess with bowel resection and diversion, the urgent, not emergent, nature of this procedure should allow for some stabilization prior to induction of anesthesia. Such must be discussed with the surgeon along with the offer to provide whatever assistance is necessary for this preoperative management. As antibiotic therapy has been instituted along with gastrointestinal drainage and urinary catheterization, the therapy now should be directed at stabilization of her hemodynamic dysfunction with the goal of improved tissue perfusion.

A definition of shock indicates that regardless of etiology this state is a manifestation of failure of the heart to pump blood into the aorta in sufficient quantity and under sufficient pressure to maintain the pressure-flow relationship for adequate tissue perfusion and aerobic metabolism. As such the clinician must first be aware of normal hemodynamic physiology, have the ability to assess existing pathophysiology and the therapeutic acumen to correct the abnormalities minimizing the adverse sequelae of both disease and therapy induced major organ dysfunction.

Controversy may exist as to the best monitoring approaches and the preferred pharmacologic manipulations to optimize tissue perfusion in shock, however, whatever options are taken should focus on the physiologic principles outlined by awareness of the models created by Starling with the ventricular function curves identified in Figure 70-1 and those of Otto Frank with the pressure volume loop diagram in Figure 70-2.

A full physiologic discussion is both beyond the scope of this presentation and is also assumed to be well understood by clinicians involved in the perioperative care of critically ill patients.

The most important assessment is to develop an initial hypothesis based on an understanding of the underlying disease and the information gained from selected laboratory and monitoring data. In the patient under consideration here, it is recognized that the

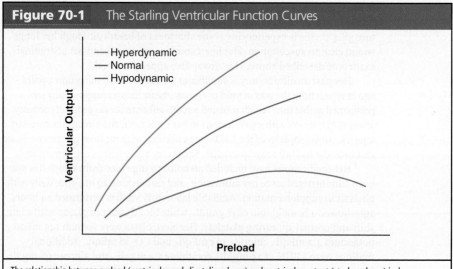

Figure 70-1 The Starling Ventricular Function Curves

The relationship between preload (ventricular end-diastolic volume) and ventricular output (stroke volume) is demonstrated. Altered states of contractility are depicted as hyperdynamic and hypodynamic as compared to normal.

Figure 70-2   The Pressure-Volume Loop Diagram for Ventricular Function

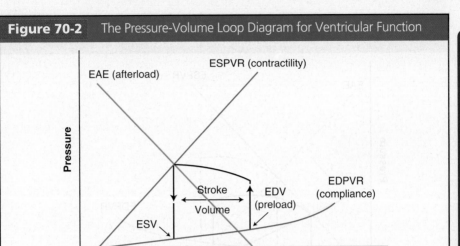

The loop shown in black begins at the EDV with a period of isovolumic contraction, followed by opening of the ventricular outflow valve with ventricular ejection. Following ejection of the stoke volume the valve closes and a period of isovolumic relaxation ensues. Lastly, at ESV, the atrio-ventricular valve opens and the ventricle fills along the EDPVR. The loop is determined by (A) the EDPVR influenced by ventricular compliance and diastolic function, (B) the slop of the ESPVR depicting the inotropic/contractility, systolic function of the ventricle, and (C) the slope of the EAE that depicts vascular resistance, a major determinant of afterload. ESPVR, end systolic pressure volume relationship; EDPVR, end diastolic pulmonary vascular relationship; EDV, end diastolic volume; ESV, end systolic volume; EAE, effective arterial elastance.

principle etiology of her hemodynamic compromise is septic (likely gram-negative bacteremic) induced, but one must also be cognizant of the potential complicating role of her underlying ischemic cardiac disease.

As shown in Figure 70-3 using the pressure volume loop diagram, the patient's initiating pathophysiology would be a dramatic fall in vascular resistance as a result of likely endotoxin and other cytokine-induced vasodilation. Accompanying this drop in resistance as shown by the decreasing slope of the effective arterial elastance (EAE) will be a profound decrease in preload—ventricular end-diastolic volume (EDV)—both as a result of vascular dilation but also an increase in endothelial permeability resulting in a loss of intravascular volume to the adjacent interstitium.

An experienced echocardiographer can gain useful information in evaluating the volume status of the left ventricle.

Central venous or pulmonary artery pressure measurement can minimize the risk of pulmonary edema from excessive fluid administration.

Options that exist for the assessment of her intravascular volume include central venous pressure (CVP), pulmonary artery occlusive pressure (PAOP) and echocardiography. Each clinician will have her/his preference based on experience, concerns over complications of the invasive procedure and awareness of the evidence in peer reviewed scientific literature.

Where the experienced echocardiographer can gain useful information in evaluating the volume status of the left ventricle, it should be recognized that the assessment of central venous or pulmonary arterial pressure provides the added benefit of minimizing the risk of development of hydrostatic pressure induced pulmonary edema from over aggressive fluid administration.

In recent years, there has been increasing reluctance to place the flow-directed pulmonary artery (PA) catheter based on concerns for complications and lack of scientific data in support of its

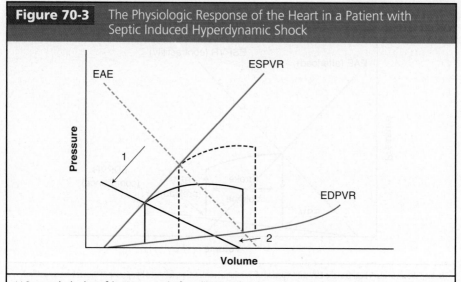

Figure 70-3 The Physiologic Response of the Heart in a Patient with Septic Induced Hyperdynamic Shock

(1) Decrease in the slope of the EAE as a result of vasodilation and (2) decrease in preload. No change in myocardial contractility (ESPVR) is evident, however, there is an increase in stroke volume as the ejection fraction increases.

ESPVR, end systolic pressure volume relationship; EDPVR, end diastolic pulmonary vascular relationship; EDV, end diastolic volume; ESV, end systolic volume; EAE, effective arterial elastance.

benefits. As a result, increasing reliance on the central venous pressure (CVP) attained from catheters placed in the superior vena cava has developed. It must be recognized, however, that reliance on right-sided filling pressures may provide insufficient information regarding the optimization of left ventricular preload particularly in a patient such as the one presented here with underlying cardiac disease.

Measurement of mixed venous or central venous oxygen saturation ($S_{cvp}O_2$) can help assess the efficacy of tissue oxygen delivery.

The availability of both end-diastolic related pressure assessment of the left ventricle measuring the pulmonary artery occlusive or wedge pressure (PAOP) and direct measurement of thermal dilution cardiac output (CO) and, thus calculation of stroke volume (SV) and systemic vascular resistance (SVR) are advantages of the PA catheter. The absence of some means to accurately assess the adequacy of CO is a limitation of the use of most commonly placed CVP catheters.

More recently the addition of oximetry to both PA and CVP catheters permits the clinician to assess mixed venous (S_vO_2) or central venous ($S_{cvp}O_2$) oxygen saturation as a means to evaluate the effectiveness of treatment to improve tissue oxygen delivery. If CVP measurement is to be the choice to assess the adequacy of preload in a patient such as the one here, the availability of direct measurement of central venous oxygen saturation ($S_{cvp}O_2$) either using a CVP catheter with oximetry or repeated measurement of central venous blood samples for oxygen saturation must be considered.

Assessment of the patient presented here shows her to be hypotensive, tachycardic, tachypneic, and oliguric. These findings along with her history and presentation indicate that she is suffering from septic shock likely with insufficient tissue perfusion. Steps to be considered at this time would be added oxygen by face mask and placement of an arterial catheter for blood pressure assessment and withdrawal of blood for evaluation of arterial blood gases (ABG) and other laboratory studies.

While awaiting the results of her ABG, central venous cannulation should be done using ultrasound guidance. For the purposes of this discussion, initial placement of a CVP catheter with oximetry will be used. Once accomplished, the following results are attained—mean arterial pressure (MAP) 50 mm Hg, P 110, CVP

3 mm Hg, and $S_{cvp}O_2$ 58%. An ABG reveals a PaO_2 95 mm Hg (receiving 4 lpm oxygen), $PaCO_2$ 32 mm Hg, and pH 7.29. She remains anuric.

The results of the initial assessment following scheduling of her surgery demonstrate her to have insufficient perfusion as evidenced by her anuria, metabolic acidosis, and low central venous oxygen saturation (normal = 70%). Given her low CVP, further volume administration remains the principal means for resuscitation.

At this point one may consider temporizing with a vasoconstrictor—phenylephrine or norepinephrine; however, reliance on such a pharmacologic approach in the presence of insufficient preload would only aggravate her tissue hypoperfusion. Pending assessment of her hemoglobin, fluid therapy using either crystalloid or colloid would be acceptable. Should crystalloid be chosen, lactated ringer may be preferable to normal saline to avoid aggravating her acidosis by making her hyperchloremic.

Although her pH is low, the hazards of bicarbonate administration, including left shift of the oxyhemoglobin dissociation curve and decreased ionized calcium, should cause hesitation while observing to see if correction of her tissue hypoperfusion improves her apparent lactic acidosis. A reasonable goal for fluid administration would either be a return of reasonable blood pressure (MAP > 65 mm Hg) in the absence of vasopressor agents, or a CVP of 12 mm Hg whichever comes first. Once either goal is reached the $S_{cvp}O_2$ should be reassessed.

As one proceeds with treatment there should be anticipation for moving to the operating room (OR) as surgery will obviously be required to remove the offending etiology. The goal of preoperative stabilization should be to enhance the ability of the patient to withstand anesthesia induction and surgery and to allow the anesthesiologist to become more aware of the patient's pathophysiology and ability to withstand the anesthesia and surgery.

After about 1 hour of therapy with fluid and vasopressor administration the patient remains hypotensive (MAP = 55 mm Hg) and anuric. At this point having received 2.5 liters of lactated ringer solution and a current infusion of phenyleprine at 120 μg/min, her CVP is 12 mm Hg and her $S_{cvp}O_2$ is 65%. Her arterial oxygen saturation is 95% and she is not showing signs of worsening respiratory function although she remains tachypneic and her ABG shows a $PaCO_2$ of 33 mm Hg and a pH of 7.26.

With her CVP having reached a reasonable level and her blood pressure remaining below acceptable levels the clinician must determine if the patient's CO is inadequate requiring inotropic support or if further increase in SVR is necessary. This is the most common dilemma faced by clinicians in evaluating patients in septic shock, particularly in the older population with decreased cardiac reserve.

The questions to be answered are (1) Does the patient have sufficient CO to provide satisfactory perfusion or will the vasopressor while normalizing blood pressure further decrease perfusion through profound vasoconstriction? (2) Is mixed venous oxygen saturation a reliable indicator of satisfactory vital organ perfusion and oxygen delivery in a state of septic shock known to be accompanied by peripheral shunting?

Finally, to complicate matters further, caution must be exercised in evaluating the response to various vasoconstrictor and inotropic agents in the presence of reduced adrenergic receptor responsiveness known to be present in patients with bacteremic septic shock. Figure 70-4 demonstrates an algorithm that might be considered in treating patients with hemodynamic instability regardless of etiology. In reviewing this approach the author has indicated examples of data to be considered; however, the clinician must individualize each patient as to the values to assign for the parameters described. The influences of preexisting hypertension, coexisting cardiac disease, influence of current processes on mixed venous oxygen saturation and adverse responses to therapy must all be considered.

Accompanying any decision to institute pharmacologic support in the form of vasoconstrictors agents to increase SVR or inotropes to increase CO, the clinician must consider both

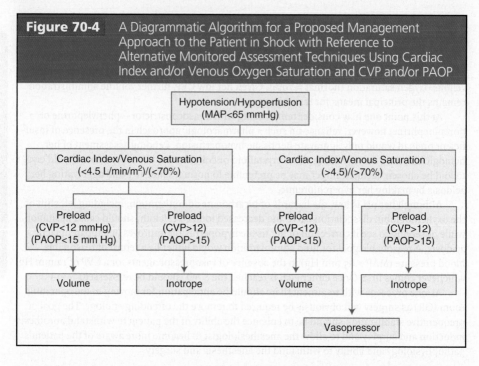

Figure 70-4   A Diagrammatic Algorithm for a Proposed Management Approach to the Patient in Shock with Reference to Alternative Monitored Assessment Techniques Using Cardiac Index and/or Venous Oxygen Saturation and CVP and/or PAOP

the side effects of these agents and their mechanisms of action. Table 70-1 outlines expected responses to these agents and groups them by their mechanisms of action. The importance of the mechanism relates to reduced responsiveness of the adrenergic receptors—alpha and beta—with resultant decrease in adenyl cyclase production and thus decrease in cyclic-AMP. It is the cyclic-AMP that increases the availability of ionized calcium facilitating muscle contractility. Should responsiveness to adenyl cyclase stimulation be impeded, agents with alternative mechanisms should be considered.

Further consideration in evaluating the response to these agents must include the ionized calcium level as all agents ultimately cause their desired effect by increasing intracellular ionized calcium to facilitate the bond between the actin and myosin protein units for increasing muscular contractility be it the myocardium or the smooth muscle of the media layer of arteries. A decision to directly treat the patient's acidosis may be influenced by the failure of responsiveness to adrenergic agents in an acidotic environment.

In the patient considered here, a decision is made to place a flow-directed PA catheter using the existing CVP site. With placement it is found that the patient's PAOP is 14 mm Hg and CO is 3.6 lpm. As a result an infusion of epinephrine is selected to provide inotropic support while attempting to decrease the phenylephrine and maintaining the PAOP and CVP at current levels. Over the next 20 minutes with epinephrine now at 80 ng/kg/min and phenylephrine at 30 μg/min, the patient has attained a MAP of 72 mm Hg, P 92, PAOP 13 mm Hg, and CO of 6.2 lpm. The patient appears stable with satisfactory arterial oxygen saturation and she is brought to the OR for her procedure.

Figure 70-5 demonstrates the pathophysiology indicated by the data attained from the PA catheter demonstrating normalized EDP with persistent vasodilation and decreased myocardial contractility.

Although a favorable result has been described with this choice of therapy, it must be recognized that alternative choices regarding both the vasopressor and inotropic agents could have been made. Norepinephrine and vasopressin have been demonstrated to provide satisfactory

Table 70-1

A Summary of Available Inotropes and Vasopressors Grouped by their Mechanisms of Action also Showing the Expected Hemodynamic Responses

Inotropes and Vasopressors for Treatment of the Septic Patient	
Adenyl cyclase stimulants	
Isoproterenol	Inotrope/vasodilator
Dobutamine	Inotrope/vasodilator
Dopamine	Inotrope/vasoconstrictor
Epinephrine	Inotrope/vasoconstrictor
Norepinephrine	Vasoconstrictor/inotrope
Phenylephrine	Vasoconstrictor
Glucagon	Inotrope
Phosphodiesterase inhibitor	
Milrinone	Inotrope/vasodilator
Na-K ATPase inhibitor	
Digoxin	Inotrope/splanchnic constrictor
Endothelin stimulation	
Vasopressin	Vasoconstrictor

increases in SVR. Dobutamine has been recommended as the preferable inotrope although one has to recognize that it is a far weaker beta-adrenergic stimulant when compared to epinephrine and has associated vasodilator effects that may be undesirable in this patient.

As one proceeds, careful attention to acid-base balance, lactic acid levels, urine output and clinical assessment of capillary filling must be continually evaluated as indicative of adequate tissue perfusion. The added benefit of echocardiography in assessing EDV as well as observing for any indications of myocardial ischemia should also be considered. Reliance on end-diastolic pressure as indicative of adequate EDV can be misleading in patients with cardiac disease manifested by diastolic dysfunction and altered ventricular compliance. Certainly, once under anesthesia should trans-esophageal echocardiography be available, it should be considered.

Finally, prior to anesthetic induction a repeat hemoglobin measurement should be attained as administration of crystalloid may have induced hemodilution and transfusion may be indicated. A hemoglobin level of at least 10 g/dL should be considered to minimize cardiac work and provide tissue oxygenation in the face of increased tissue demands in this hypermetabolic state. Blood availability and that of coagulation products should be assured prior to anesthetic induction and surgery.

| **Figure 70-5** | The Physiologic Response of the Heart in a Patient with Septic-Induced Hyperdynamic Shock After Treatment |

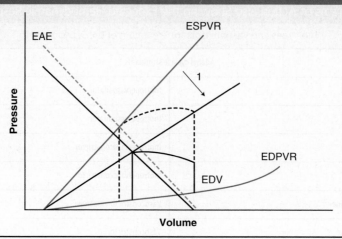

In comparison to Figure 70-3, there has been vasoconstriction with increased slope of the EAE, yet still with some vasodilation when compared to normal (dashed EAE line). Also the EDV has returned to normal as a result of fluid administration. A major change depicted has been (1) the recognition of a reduction in contractility as shown by the decrease in the slope of the ESPVR with a reduction in stroke volume.

ESPVR, end systolic pressure volume relationship; EDPVR, end diastolic pulmonary vascular relationship; EDV, end diastolic volume; ESV, end systolic volume; EAE, effective arterial elastance.

Intraoperative Management

As the patient is brought to the OR the anesthesia caregiver must determine how best to induce anesthesia. The hemodynamic instability of this patient and the likelihood of coagulopathy would make a regional technique a poor choice. Thus, induction of general anesthesia must be considered.

With all of the monitoring in place and therapy satisfactorily applied the choice of induction agents is not as critical as the method of administration. Slow careful titration should be considered regardless of the agents selected. Gastric evacuation with the nasogastric tube should have decreased the risk of aspiration and made a rapid sequence induction (RSI) less necessary. If a RSI is planned than choice of induction agent may be more crucial with avoidance of propofol or thiopental, as a bolus of either could lead to profound hypotension and instability. In such a situation etomidate or even ketamine may be desirable.

Propofol or thiopental for induction of the septic patient should be avoided because they can lead to profound hypotension and instability.

The patient is transported to the OR with full monitoring and oxygen administration while continuing to administer the hemodynamic agents selected. Upon arrival in the OR the patient is moved to the operating table and monitors transferred. Availability of CO and venous saturation monitoring in addition to all pressures should be present upon arrival.

After re-establishment of the monitors and insuring continued stability the anesthesiology care proceeds with induction of general anesthesia. After preoxygenation, the choice is made to slowly titrate doses of intravenous midazolam and fentanyl until loss of lid reflex followed by intravenous administration of rocuronium. During induction the patient's MAP decreases to 58 mm Hg and 100 μg of phenylephrine is administered. Following satisfactory muscle relaxation the patient is intubated and placed on mechanical ventilatory support. Anesthetic maintenance commences with titration of further intravenous opioid and inhalation of sevoflurane as tolerated. The surgical procedure then commences.

Acute respiratory distress syndrome, renal and hepatic ischemia and failure, cardiac ischemia and infarction and coagulopathy must all be anticipated.

Although an example of anesthetic management is provided it must be acknowledged that multiple possibilities exist. Rather than focusing on the choices of anesthetic agents for induction and maintenance it is of far more importance to emphasize the continued monitored physiologic approach to therapy instituted in the preoperative period.

Now complicated by the application of surgical and anesthetic procedures and the stress accompanying those interventions, the anesthesia clinician must remain attentive to the existing monitors, assessing blood samples for acid base balance, hemoglobin levels, electrolytes, ionized calcium and coagulation factors, and responding to changes that can be expected to occur aggravated by the surgical manipulations including fluid shifts and hemorrhage. During the surgical procedure attention must also be focused on expected sequelae of the hemodynamic compromise and resuscitation that has taken place.

The development of respiratory insufficiency in the form of acute respiratory distress syndrome (ARDS), renal and hepatic ischemia and failure, cardiac ischemia and infarction, or coagulopathy must all be anticipated. Dependent on the magnitude of the surgery and its duration, one cannot underestimate the implications of intraoperative management on the postoperative course and eventual outcome. The role of the anesthesia caregiver in this patient goes far beyond that of providing insensibility to pain, lack of awareness and muscle relaxation. Barring a surgical catastrophe and a reasonable intraoperative time the patient should be expected to tolerate the procedure with minimal further disruption of hemodynamics.

Postoperative Management

The surgical procedure has taken about 90 minutes during which time incision and drainage of an abscess cavity, resection of the sigmoid colon and a descending colostomy has been performed with minimal blood loss. The patient has remained stable and trans-esophageal echocardiography (TEE) used during the procedure has not indicated any evidence of myocardial ischemia and has verified adequacy of ventricular EDV.

The agents used for hemodynamic support have been epinephrine now at 70 nanog/kg/min and phenylephrine at 50 μg/min. A recent ABG while receiving 50% oxygen showed a PaO_2 105 mm Hg, $PaCO_2$ 37 mm Hg and a pH of 7.31. Ionized calcium was 0.98 and 1,000 mg of $CaCl_2$ was administered. During the surgery a hemoglobin of 8.8 gm/dL was noted and she received 2 units of packed cells. Her coagulation profile was acceptable and there was not excessive bleeding. She also received 2,200 mL of crystalloid keeping her CVP and PAOP at presurgical levels. Her urine output during the procedure remained scant. The decision is made to leave her intubated and sedated and to transport to the ICU with full monitoring and manual ventilation with oxygen.

The decision to leave the patient intubated and sedated for the early postoperative period provides the opportunity to maintain stability during the transport and reestablishment of intensive care while transitioning to a new nursing and medical team. This is not the time to add the potential development of respiratory insufficiency and effects of pain and anxiety while attempting to maintain a stable environment dealing with hemodynamic, renal, cardiac, and other system dysfunction.

In most clinical environments the anesthesia caregiver will provide a full and complete report to both the accepting nursing and medical teams who will be assuming further management. However, the knowledge gained and the experience with this patient over that last 3 to 5 hours provides a substantial amount of accumulated information that is invaluable to the physicians and nurses assuming care.

The postoperative period will present tremendous challenges in continuing to provide proper hemodynamic support with the hoped for restitution of vital organ function most

ANESTHESIA AND COMORBID DISEASES

notably splanchnic and renal. What has been demonstrated in this patient thus far is that proper management resulting in provision of satisfactory central hemodynamic function as evidenced by SVR, CO, indices of preload, mixed venous oxygen saturations and acid base status do not insure that those most sensitive tissues to ischemia—splanchnic and renal—will be preserved. Current monitoring technology is limited in provided evidence of perfusion and tissue oxygenation of these vascular compartments. Thus, continued management to avoid further insults is critical.

It must also be recognized that although the primary insult has been addressed and proper antibiotics will be provided based on results of microbial culture assessment, the progress of the septic process with its concurrent systemic inflammatory response syndrome will likely continue. Should decreasing responsiveness to inotropic and vasopressor agents be noted, in addition to consideration for agents with alternative mechanisms of action as described above, the possibility for adrenal suppression should be addressed with either the assessment of baseline cortisol levels or a corticotropin stimulation test. Should adrenal suppression be identified replacement therapy should ensue with recommended dosing of 125 mg of hydrocortisone IV every 8 hours.

Once the patient is stabilized with satisfactory hemodynamics, weaning from ventilatory support and extubation should be considered. This assumes that no evidence of ARDS has appeared and the patient has satisfactory oxygenation and acid-base equilibrium is evident.

Suggested Reading

1. Dellinger RP, Carlet GM, Masur H, et al. Surviving sepsis campaign guidelines for management of severe sepsis and septic shock. *Crit Care Med* 2004;32:858–873.
2. Doyle CA, Rosenthal MH. Hypotension and shock states. In: Gravenstein N, Kirby R, Lobato E, eds. *Complications in Anesthesiology*. Philadelphia, PA: Lippincott-Raven; 2007.
3. Gilbert EM, Hershberger RE, Weichmann RJ, et al. Pharmacologic and hemodynamic effects of combined beta-agonist stimulation and phosphodiesterase inhibition in the failing heart. *Chest* 1995;108:1524–1532.
4. Moran JL, O'Fathartaigh MS, Peisach AR, et al. Epinephrine as an inotropic agent in septic shock: a dose-profile analysis. *Crit Care Med* 1993;21:70–77.
5. Rivers E, Nguyen B, Havsted S, et al. Early goal-directed therapy in the treatment of severe sepsis and septic shock. *N Engl J Med* 2001;345:1368–1377.
6. Rozenfeld V, Cheng JW. The role of vasopressin in the treatment of vasodilation in shock states. *Ann Pharmacotherap* 2000;34:250–254.
7. Silverman HJ, Penaranda R, Orens JB, et al. Impaired beta-adrenergic stimulation of cyclic adenosine monophosphate in human septic shock: associated with myocardial hyporesponsiveness to catecholamines. *Crit Care Med* 1993;21:31–39.

71

Part C: Respiratory Diseases
Chronic Obstructive Pulmonary Disease

Binbin Wang, MD • Linda L. Liu, MD

Chronic obstructive pulmonary disease (COPD) is characterized by an obstructive pattern on pulmonary function testing, progressive airway limitation that is not fully reversible and an abnormal inflammatory response to noxious particles or gases. COPD can include chronic obstructive bronchitis and/or emphysema, and is distinguishable from asthma by the irreversibility of the obstructive pattern.

COPD is the fourth leading cause of chronic morbidity and mortality in the United States.

"Pink puffers" have emphysematous lung disease, "Blue bloaters" more often meet criteria for chronic bronchitis.

1) **Epidemiology**
   a) COPD is the fourth leading cause of chronic morbidity and mortality in the United States (1).
   b) Prevalence can be as high as 5% to 10% in the age-matched general surgery population, and up to 40% of thoracic surgery patients (2).

2) **Pathophysiology**
   a) Pathological changes consist of chronic inflammation seen in the proximal and peripheral airways, lung parenchyma, and pulmonary vasculature.
      i) The gas exchange abnormalities of severe COPD depends on whether the inflammation leads to emphysema with alveolar wall and pulmonary capillary destruction or chronic bronchitis with airway obstruction and cough/sputum production.
   b) "Pink puffers" have emphysematous lung destruction and they tend to have $PaO_2 > 65$ mm Hg, with a normal to slightly decreased $PaCO_2$.
   c) "Blue bloaters" more often meet criteria for chronic bronchitis and have:
      i) Hypoxia from V/Q mismatch and
      ii) Hypercapnia from **increased dead space ventilation,** and **impairment of ventilatory muscles** (3).

3) **Risk factors**
   a) **Tobacco smoke is the primary cause**
   b) However, indoor and outdoor air pollution and genetic predisposition also factor prominently

4) **Clinical features**
   a) Patients often present with a history of smoking, presence of chronic cough, sputum production and dyspnea on exertion (1).

5) **Physical examination**
   a) Depending on severity of disease, patients can have
      i) Decreased breath sounds, wheezes, prolonged expiratory phase
      ii) Increased A–P diameter of the chest

507

iii) Evidence of hyperinflation on CXR

iv) Use of accessory muscles for respiration

6) Pulmonary function tests (PFTs)

a) Narrowing **of the small airways and decreased lung elastic recoil** lead to the airflow limitations in COPD. This translates into

i) **Reduced FEV_1 and FEV_1/FVC,** and

ii) Increased residual volume, functional residual capacity, and total lung volume

7) Prognosis

a) 14% of medical patients admitted for COPD exacerbation will die within 3 months of admission.

b) In patients with COPD, the incidence of respiratory failure and pneumonia after non-cardiac surgery has been shown to be 1% to 3% and 1% to 5%, respectively (2), representing a large socioeconomic burden.

8) Preoperative considerations

a) **Identification of high risk patients is essential to improving their postoperative course** (Table 71-1).

i) The odds ratio for postoperative pulmonary complications (PPC) is increased in patients with COPD **(OR 1.79),** with an unadjusted **PPC rate of 18.2%** (5).

ii) The incidence of **PPCs often increases with increasing severity** of disease, especially in the severe to very severe range (**Grade III–IV**) or if patients have concomitant abnormal clinical findings (wheezes, ronchi, prolonged expiration, decreased breath sounds) (2,6).

(1) Individual disease stratification can be done according to the GOLD criteria, a frequently updated evidence based consensus report assembled by an expert panel on obstructive lung diseases (2).

Table 71-1
COPD Disease Grade

GOLD COPD Disease Grade (1)	Symptoms (4)	Characteristic Therapy
0: At risk—$FEV_1 \geq 80\%$ predicted	None	Recommend smoking cessation PRN
I: Mild—$FEV_1/FVC < 0.7$, $FEV_1 \geq 80\%$ predicted	± chronic cough, sputum	Short acting bronchodilator PRN
II: Moderate—$FEV_1/FVC < 0.7$, FEV_1 50%–79% predicted	+ DOE ± chronic cough, sputum	Short acting bronchodilator PRN, ± scheduled long acting bronchodilator
III: Severe—$FEV_1/FVC < 0.7$, FEV_1 30%–49% predicted	SOB, fatigue, reduced exercise capacity, repeated exacerbations	Above, ± inhaled glucocorticoids
IV: Very severe—$FEV_1/FVC < 0.7$, $FEV_1 < 30\%$ or $FEV_1 < 50\%$ with chronic respiratory failure	Above, ± respiratory failure, cor pulmonale	Above, ± chronic oxygen therapy

Respiratory failure = $PaO_2 < 60$ mm Hg or $PaCO_2 > 50$ mm Hg on room air at sea level.
DOE, dyspnea on exertion; SOB, shortness of breath.

iii) **PFTs are usually not necessary** for preoperative screening as clinicians can diagnose and assess COPD severity with high accuracy based on history and physical examination alone (1,2,6). Other **patient related risk factors** include
  (1) Current smoking
  (2) Acute COPD exacerbation
  (3) Advanced age, and
  (4) Poor general health

b) **Procedure related risk factors** should also be kept in mind, with increased risk associated with
  i) Operative site (incision closer to diaphragm)
  ii) Surgery >3 hours, and
  iii) Disruption of normal respiratory muscle function from anesthesia drugs, neuromuscular blocking drugs, and surgical trauma

c) Preoperative risk factor reduction strategies can include
  i) **Smoking cessation (preferably >2 months prior to surgery)**
  ii) **Treatment of underlying COPD exacerbation (bronchodilators, glucocorticoids)**
  iii) Antibiotics for infections, if present, and
  iv) Preoperative teaching and institution of lung expansion exercises (6)

9) **Intraoperative considerations**

a) Care consists mainly of optimal airway and ventilator management, and the realization that these patients are susceptible to PPCs.

b) **Preoperative anxiolytics** such as benzodiazepines can be used in COPD patients. However, because of their dose-dependent depressant effects on minute ventilation, they **should be used with caution** or avoided in patients with severe COPD (7).

Benzodiazepines can be used in COPD patients, but should be used cautiously or avoid in those with severe COPD due to repiratory depressant effects.

Anesthetic Concerns for Patient with COPD

Airway Management	•Face mask, LMA, tracheal intubation can all be appropriate: •If tracheal intubation - ensure **adequate anesthetic depth,** strongly consider inhaled beta-agonists,inhaled anticholingeric agents, inhaled or IV steroids, and IV lidocaine (2)
Ventilator Management	•Warm and humidfy freash gas, especially in long surgeries •Reduce autoPEEP: low RR and increase I:E ratio - if suspect, autoPEEP, disconnect circuit, suction, and increase E time(2) •Avoid post-hypercapnic alkalosis by avoiding hyperventilation •All volatile anesthetics are equipotent bronchilators except desflurane which can cause airway hyperreactivity •**Ensure full neuromuscular blockade reversal prior to extubation (2-5)**
Regional Anesthesia	•Lack of consensus if intraop neuraxial aneshetic vs GA lowers risk of PPC (2-5) •Unclear if intrathecal opioids lower PPC as compared to systemic opioids (2-5) •**Postoperative maintenace of epidural local analgesia reduces PPC compared to systemic opioids and is recommended when appropriate(4)**

c) Multidisciplinary team approach works best in the care of COPD patients. Consideration should be given to use of minimally invasive surgery (laparoscopy) when possible. PPCs are less after laparoscopic cholecystectomy than after open cholecystectomy (8).

d) Volatile anesthetics except for desflurane are good bronchodilators.

e) Ensure full reversal of neuromuscular blocking agents prior to extubation.

f) Consider regional anesthesia, although the idea that regional anesthesia has less risk of PPC compared to general anesthesia has not been supported fully by evidence based medicine. Thoracic epidurals seem to reduce risk of PPC in high-risk surgeries such as abdominal aortic surgery (9).

10) **Postoperative considerations**

a) Whether in the ICU, PACU, or on the ward, it is important to minimize the incidence and severity of PPC.

b) **Analgesia** is important to maintain respiratory function, and minimize splinting, which may permit early tracheal extubation or prevent reintubation.

c) Epidural local analgesia preserves diaphragmatic function, increases tidal volume and vital capacity (3).

d) PCA analgesia reduces PPC as compared to nurse administered analgesia (6).

e) **Lung expansion** techniques help to prevent/reopen atelectatic regions and to prevent postoperative fall in lung volumes.

f) Incentive spirometry and deep breathing exercises each can reduce the incidence of PPC, but the combination of these techniques fails to confer additional benefits.

g) Noninvasive positive pressure ventilation (NIPPV), continuous positive airway pressure (CPAP), or inspiratory positive airway pressure (IPAP) are equally effective, but less cost-efficient and require sophisticated devices and the availability of trained personnel.

h) **Respiratory rehabilitation and frequent pulmonary toileting** improves secretion handling.

i) Head up position is an effective way to decrease pulmonary aspiration.

Chapter Summary for COPD

Definition	COPD is characterized by chronic inflammation of the airways and lung parenchyma and pulmonary vasculature. Patients exhibit obstructive respiratory physiology on pulmonary function testing.
Preoperative Issues	Identify those at risk: Severe COPD, acute exacerbation, active smoking, poor general health, advanced age, high risk surgery PFT not usually needed Antibiotic, bronchodilator, glucocorticoid therapy as needed
Intraoperative Issues	Laparoscopic approach better if feasible Consider regional anesthesia and epidural analgesia Ensure adequate anesthetic depth if general anesthesia Avoid desflurane if possible

Postoperative Issues	Maximize analgesia:
	Epidural or PCA preferred
	Lung expansion techniques are crucial and include:
	    Incentive spirometry
	    Deep breathing exercises
	    Non-invasive ventilation as needed
	    Frequent pulmonary toileting
	    Keep head up position

References

1. The GOLD Committee. Global Strategy for the Diagnosis, Management, and Prevention of Chronic Obstructive Pulmonary Disease. Global Initiative for Chronic Obstructive Lung Disease. 2008 Update.
2. Licker M, Schweizer A, Ellenberger C, et al. Perioperative medical management of patients with COPD. *Int J Chron Obstruct Pulmon Dis* 2007;2:493–515.
3. Qaseem A, Snow V, Fitterman N, et al. Risk assessment for and strategies to reduce perioperative pulmonary complications for patients undergoing noncardiothoracic surgery: a guideline from the American College of Physicians. *Ann Intern Med* 2006;144:575–580.
4. Sutherland ER, Cherniack RM. Management of chronic obstructive pulmonary disease. *NEJM* 2004; 350:2689–2697.
5. Smetana GW, Lawrence VA, Cornell JE. Preoperative pulmonary risk stratification for noncardiothoracic surgery: systematic review for the American College of Physicians. *Ann Intern Med* 2006:144;581–595.
6. Smetana G. A 68 year old man with COPD contemplating colon cancer surgery. *JAMA* 2007;297:2121–2130.
7. Yamakage M, Iwasaki S, Namiki A. Guideline-oriented perioperative management of patients with bronchial asthma and chronic obstructive pulmonary disease. *J Anesth* 2008;22:412–428.
8. Karayiannakis AJ, Makri GG, Mantzioka A, et al. Postoperative pulmonary function after laparoscopic and open cholecystectomy. *Br J Anaesth* 1996;77:448–452.
9. Liu SS, Wu CL. Effect of postoperative analgesia on major postoperative complications: a systematic update of the evidence. *Anesth Analg* 2007;104:689–702.

ANESTHESIA AND COMORBID DISEASES

72 Asthma and Reactive Airway Disease

Lisa Gramlich, MD

Asthma is a chronic inflammatory disease of the airways and is the most common chronic disease of childhood in the United States. As the leading cause of absenteeism from school and the most prevalent cause of hospital admission, asthma wields a major impact on education and health care dollars. In 2002, the total cost of asthma care was $14 billion (1).

1) Incidence
   a) More than 20 million people are affected and 6 million of those are children. One in four children have wheezing which persists into adulthood or relapses in later life (1). From 1980 to 1996, the prevalence was noted to increase by 4.3% per year (2). A higher incidence is seen in:
      i) Ex-premature infants in the preadolescent period (3)
      ii) Two thirds have a familial predisposition (1)
      iii) Afrrican-Americans and Puerto Ricans (1)
      iv) Prepubertal males (1)
      v) Those with problem allergies, especially when associated with atopy
      vi) Infants and children who develop lower respiratory tract viral infections, especially respiratory syncytial virus (RSV) (4)
2) Pathophysiology
   a) Eosinophils and mast cells are triggered in the airways and release cytokines, leukotrienes, and histamine. Airway obstruction ensues due to these mediators via:
      i) Smooth muscle spasm
      ii) Airway mucosal edema
      iii) Hypersecretion
      iv) Mucous plugging
3) Precipitating factors
   a) Lower respiratory viral infections, especially RSV, provoke hyperreactivity even in nonasthmatics for up to 6 weeks (5).
   b) Gastroesophageal reflux disease (GERD)
      i) GERD is part of the triad of the Sandifer syndrome, which is GERD, asthma, and opisthotonos.
      ii) Treatment of GERD with H_2 receptor antagonists and prokinetics decrease morbidity and the need for asthma medications (6).
   c) Emotional stress
   d) Inhaled allergens such as dust mites, animal dander, mold, and dust
   e) Inhaled irritants (cigarette smoke, caustic cleansers, inhaled anesthetics)

If possible, intubation should be avoided in patients with reactive airways as it is associated with an increase in pulmonary complications (10).

Patients at risk for imminent respiratory arrest have the following symptoms: Drowsy, confused, no wheezing (little air movement), peak flow rate (PEF) < 25% (though probably unlikely to perform test), bradycardia, absence of pulsus paradoxus (due to muscle fatigue). These patients should be intubated urgently.

    i) All inhaled anesthetics are bronchodilators, but initially act as an irritant (7).

    ii) This effect can be primarily ablated by use of β_2-adrenergic agonists immediately preoperatively (8).

    iii) Secondhand smoke increases severity and frequency of symptoms, but an increased incidence is not consistently shown in studies (9).

  f) Inhaled dry and/or cold air

  g) Mechanical irritation such as intubation

4) **Symptoms**

  a) Can follow circadian rhythms and worsen at night, especially around 04:00 (1)

  b) Dyspnea and tachypnea may lead to difficulty speaking.

  c) Chest tightness and tachycardia

  d) Wheezing, except when severe bronchospasm limits air movement.

  e) Coughing

  f) Pulsus paradoxus (a fall in BP > 10 mm Hg during spontaneous inspiration when BP should stay the same or slightly increase)

  g) Visible use of accessory muscles and pursed lip breathing

  h) Prolonged expiration with I:E (inspiratory to expiratory time) ratio > 1:3

  i) Altered consciousness, especially when SpO_2 < 90% and $PaCO_2$ > 45 mm Hg

5) **Severity scoring (Table 72-1)**

  a) Included in Table 72-1 are guidelines to aid the clinician in assessing asthma severity and control.

6) **Differential diagnosis of wheezing**

  a) Asthma—wheezing is polyphonic and extends into the periphery, frequently accompanied by dry cough.

  b) Foreign body—wheezing is usually fixed and central.

  c) Secretions—moist cough with rhonchi frequently associated.

  d) Mainstem intubations or endotracheal tube (ETT) cuff herniations (over the end of the ETT) partially blocking the opening.

  e) Anaphylaxis—will be associated with other symptoms, namely flushing, urticaria, angioedema and hemodynamic instability.

  f) Pneumothorax—unilateral wheezing is noted verses bilateral wheezing in asthma.

  g) Congestive heart failure—associated with cardiovascular symptoms and rales

  h) Acute tracheobronchiolitis

  i) Tracheomalacia—onset is usually at birth.

  j) Tuberculosis or other granulomatous disease

  k) Mechanical obstruction—vascular rings or mediastinal masses would be extrinsic causes and laryngeal webs or bronchial stenosis intrinsic causes.

7) **Treatments (Table 72-2)**

  a) **β_2 adrenergic agonists**

    i) The mainstay of asthma treatment

    ii) Mechanism of action is an increase in cAMP resulting in smooth muscle relaxation and bronchiole dilation.

    iii) Greatest effect on medium and small airways (11)

  b) **Anticholinergics**

    i) Ipratropium bromide nebulized or via metered-dose inhaler (MDI)

    ii) Slower onset but longer duration of action than β_2-adrenergic agonists

    iii) Slightly more effective on the larger conducting airways (11)

Table 72-1

Severity Assessment for Asthma

Symptoms	Classification		
	Well Controlled (Mild)	Not Well Controlled (Moderate)	Poorly Controlled (Severe)
Frequency of symptoms	≤2 d/wk	> 2 d/wk	Throughout the week
Nighttime awakening	≤2 times/mo	1–3 times/wk	≥4 times/wk
Interference with activity	None	Some limitations	Extreme
Breathlessness	Occurs while walking or with excercise	At rest (infant with softer cry and difficulty feeding)	At rest (infant stops feeding)
Position when breathless	Is able to lie down	Prefers sitting	Sits upright
Speaks in	Sentences	Phrases	Words
Alertness	May be agitated	Usually agitated	Usually agitated
Use of accessory muscles	Usually not	Common	Usually
Wheezing	Moderate, usually end expiratory	Loud throughout exhalation	Usually loud in both inspiration and expiration

HR
   <1 y
   1–2 y
   2–8 y
	
	 <160
	 <120
	 <110
		
		 160
		 120
		 >110
			
			 160
			 120
			 >110

Pulsus paradoxus	Absent; 0–9 mm Hg	Occasional; 10–20 mm Hg	Often; >20 mm Hg
*FEV_1, or PEF *[PEF (L/M) = (5 × height in cm) – 400]	≥75%	50%–75%	<50%
No. of asthma meds	0	1–2	≥3
Use of rescue inhaler	≤2 d/wk	>2 d/wk	Several times/day
Exacerbation requiring PO steroids	0–1/y	≥2/y	≥2/y

c) **Leukotriene-modifying drugs**
   i) Two major categories
      (1) Leukotriene receptor antagonists (zafirlukast and montelukast = Singulair)
      (2) Leukotriene synthesis inhibitors (zileuton)
   ii) Leukotrienes are 1,000 times more potent bronchial constrictors than histamine so for moderate to severe asthma these have become a mainstay of treatment (12).

Table 72-2
Drugs for Asthma Treatment

	Maintenance	Emergency Treatment
β₂-adrenergic agonists		
(SABA= short acting) Albuterol (Proventil, Ventolin)	MDI, 2 puffs q4-6hrs Nebulizer, 01–0.15 mg/kg	Up to 10 puffs (1 mg) q20min 2.5–5.0 mg q20min or continuous nebulization of 10 mg/h (requires special nebulizer)
Terbutaline		IV bolus: 15 µg/kg over 20 min followed by infusion 1–5 µg/k/min
(LABA = long acting) Salmeterol (Serevent)	MDI, 1–2 puffs bid	Not indicated
Anti-Inflammatory		
Beclomethasone (Vanceril) Budesonide (Pulmicort) Flunisolide (AeroBid) Fluticasone propionate (Flovent)	MDI, 2–4 puffs bid MDI, 1–2 inhalations bid MDI, 1–2 puffs bid MDI, 1 inhalation bid	Methylprednisolone 2 mg/kg IV *Will not give immediate relief, but should be given Effect not usually seen for an hour. IV: 4 mg/kg hydrocortisone
Prednisone or prednisolone (Prelone, Pediapred)	0.25–2 mg/kg qod Preop 1 mg/kg/day × 3 days	Oral: 1–2 mg/kg prednisolone
Anticholinergics		
Ipratropium bromide (Atrovent)	MDI, 1–2 puffs qid	5–10 mg/kg nebulized q6h
Leukotriene Modifiers		
Montelukast (Singulair)	≥15 y/o, 10 mg qd 6–14 y /o, 5 mg qd 1–5 y/o, 4 mg qd	Peak plasma concentration achieved in 3–4 h; single preoperative dose may be beneficial
Nedocromil (Tilade)	2–4 puffs bid	Little added utility in acute setting.
Methylxanthines		
Theophylline (therapeutic level 5–15 µg/mL)	5 mg/kg/d up to 200 mg	5 mg/kg over 10 min followed by 1 mg/kg/h
Magnesium		50 mg/kg over 10 min
Anesthetics		
Ketamine		1–2 mg/kg bolus followed by 15–45 µg/kg/min
Inhalational		0.5–1.5 MAC

d) **Corticosteroids**
  i) Inhaled corticosteroids limit negative systemic effects while still providing potent anti-inflammatory effects on the airways.
  ii) Routine use reduces airway reactivity and inflammation which results in improved symptom control and lung function (13).
  iii) Oral or parenteral steroids are reserved for acute exacerbations of asthma unresponsive to maximal bronchodilator therapy (14).

e) **Methylxanthines**
  i) Inhibit adenosine-induced bronchoconstriction.
  ii) Fell out of favor because narrow therapeutic window requires routine blood level monitoring.
  iii) These drugs can still be helpful adjunct, especially with nighttime wheezing.

f) **Cromolyn sodium and nedocromil sodium**
  i) Prophylactic only not useful in acute period
  ii) Stabilizes mast cells to reduce IgE mediated release of histamine and leukotrienes

g) **Immunomodulators**
  i) Namely omalizumab, are anti-IgE antibodies reserved for severely allergic asthmatics with elevated IgE levels.
  ii) May decrease steroid requirements, but has been associated with anaphylaxis.
  iii) Administered subcutaneously every 2 to 4 weeks.

h) **Magnesium**
  i) 50 mg/kg to treat acute presentation of moderate to severe asthma
  ii) Has not been shown to be helpful in mild asthma or used as a prophylactic agent

8) **Preoperative management**
  a) Pulmonary function tests, namely peak expiratory flow rates are commonly used to monitor asthmatics but are rarely required perioperatively.
    i) FEV$_1$ (forced expiratory volume)
      (1) >75% predicted = good prognostic indicator
      (2) 50% to 75% predicted = fair to poor prognostic indicator
      (3) <50% predicted = very poor prognostic indicator

In an asthmatic who has had a recent URI, strongly consider postponing elective surgery for 6 weeks (10).

  b) Patients should be queried about triggers, effective treatments, side effects to medications, and general respiratory well-being over past month.
  c) If the **need for rescue medication has escalated** or symptoms worsened and the surgery is elective, patients should be referred to their primary care physician to optimize their pulmonary status.
  d) A **recent URI** (upper respiratory infection) should prompt postponing elective surgery for 6 weeks (10).
    i) In some patients, URIs are so frequent that a window of opportunity to operate becomes so narrow as to become impractical.
    ii) Proven RSV infections should elicit heightened concern due to their strong association with worsening bronchospasm.

READ MORE

Corticosteroids, Chapter 201, page 1300

  e) **Ascertain the need for steroid therapy**
    i) Symptomatic asthmatics on maximal therapy may benefit from 3 days of oral steroids prior to surgery (prednisone 1 mg/kg up to 60 mg).
    ii) Stress dose steroids

(1) Short courses of prednisolone can affect hypothalamic-pituitary-adrenal (HPA) function for up to 10 days (15).

(2) High doses, treatment with steroids for >3 weeks, evening and daily dosing verses every other day dosing all increase likelihood and duration of HPA suppression, which may lasts up to a year (16).

(3) Inhaled steroids are usually not an indication for stress dose steroids perioperatively (17), but high doses (>440 µg/d) of fluticasone (Flovent) may reduce cortisol levels and lead to symptomatic adrenal suppression in children (18).

Inhaled steroids are usually not an indication for stress dose steroids perioperatively.

9) **Intraoperative management**

a) **Maximizing a patient's preoperative status** is crucial, but patient compliance and the urgency of the case may make this difficult.

b) **Prophylactic use of a MDI or nebulizer prior to going to the operating room** is helpful at decreasing bronchospastic response to airway manipulation.

A calm patient is important especially in patients with exercise-induced asthma to avoid triggering an attack.

i) Most commonly a β_2-adrenergic agonist is used, but combination with an anticholinergic agent should be considered (see discussion of each drug above).

ii) During severe attacks, medications nebulized with a helium and oxygen mixture, verses oxygen have been shown to demonstrate a better response.

c) **Warm and humidify gases to avoid tracheal irritation**

i) HME (heat and moisture exchanger) with low flows on the vent

ii) Heated humidifiers attached inline to the anesthesia circuit

d) Induction

i) If inhalation induction is indicated, a mask induction with nitrous, oxygen and sevoflurane is a suitable choice.

e) **IV induction**

i) Propofol may be the best choice because it provides bronchiole dilation (19).

ii) As long as hemodynamically tolerated, fairly large doses of an induction agent with the quick addition of an inhalational agent so the peak effect of the IV agent does not dissipate, is important.

iii) Ketamine is a consideration due to its bronchodilatory effects. A ketamine infusion may also be used then for maintenance. Alternatively, inhalationals may be used for maintenance. There are no comparative trials to argue for the choice of one agent (ketamine or inhalational anesthetics) over the other.

f) Lidocaine may also blunt airway hyperresponsiveness. Consider giving 1 mg/kg, up to 100 mg, just prior to induction in anyone with active wheezing or on multimodal therapy.

g) **Avoid drugs that may cause histamine release**, that is, morphine and atracurium.

h) Volatile technique may be superior to a heavier narcotic technique due to the benefits of bronchiole dilatation.

i) Avoidance of an ETT whenever applicable is desirable to prevent triggering bronchospasm.

j) Deep extubation may be of great value in patients with hyperreactive airways.

k) Consider avoidance of NSAIDs (nonsteroidal anti-inflammatory drugs) in the rhinitis prone patient who previously has not used non-steroidals.

   i) Consider acetaminophen in asthmatics who have taken acetaminophen previously without sequelae.

   ii) NSAIDs have been shown to cause a sudden exacerbation of asthma symptoms (20,21).

   iii) COX-2 (cyclooxygenase-2) inhibitors may be safely used. These anti-inflammatory drugs also do not cause significant anti-platelet effects (22).

10) **Ventilatory management for asthma**

a) Choose tidal volumes (TV) of 6 to 10 mL/kg.

   i) In the presence of bronchospasm, high peak pressures are not transmitted to the alveoli. If plateau pressures are >35 cm H_2O, then reduction in TV is prudent to prevent risk of pneumothorax.

b) Breath stacking occurs when obstruction to air flow does not allow full expiration before another breath is given.

   i) In order to avoid breath stacking, which leads to air-trapping and auto-PEEP, I:E ratios are changed from the usual 1:2 to 1:3 to 5.

   ii) Flow rates may need to be increased to assure adequate volume delivery with shortened inspiratory times and the respiratory rate may need to be slightly decreased.

c) Permissive hypercapnea (up to $PaCO_2$ 80 mm Hg) keeping the pH > 7.2 is frequently adopted to minimize barotrauma during periods of sustained severe bronchospasm (status asthmaticus).

d) Intubation criteria:

   i) Cardiac arrest

   ii) Respiratory arrest or profound bradypnea

   iii) Physical exhaustion

   iv) Altered sensorium, such as lethargy or agitation

   v) $PaCO_2$ > 80 mm Hg

   vi) PaO_2 < 60 mm Hg on >60% FiO_2

   vii) pH < 7.2

   viii) Worsening symptoms despite escalating treatment should prompt preparation for intubation.

11) **Postoperative management**

a) **Extubation criteria/considerations**

   i) There are no well-defined postoperative extubation criteria and decisions must be made based on the severity of reactive airway disease (RAD), the surgical procedure, and the potential for difficult airway management.

   ii) **Preparation for extubation**

     (1) Intraoperative events should be reviewed

      (a) When anesthesia is lightened, signs of bronchospasm may be witnessed:

        (i) Increased airway pressures

        (ii) Upsloping CO_2 curves

        (iii) Desaturation

When preparing the patient for extubation, be aware that surgical interventions may impair respiratory status.

(2) If any perioperative wheezing has occurred, preparations should be made to immediately administer nebulized β_2-adrenergic agonist and possibly an anticholinergic should bronchospasm occur post-extubation.

(3) Consideration for a deep extubation should be made if signs of bronchospasm are seen, which were readily relieved by a deepening of the anesthetic.

(4) A deep extubation means the patient is without spontaneous reflexes, i.e. gag, blink. A patient may be deeply extubated on inhalational agents or lightened and given a small dose (0.5 to 1 mg/kg) of propofol immediately before extubation.

   (a) Patients should not be transported until they can support their own airway and have a return of spontaneous reflexes.

(5) Shortly before extubation, consider administering the same agents to decrease airway reactivity that may have been given at induction such as β_2-adrenergic agonists and/or IV lidocaine.

(6) At least an hour before extubation, consider administration of methylprednisolone 2 mg/kg or hydrocortisone 4 mg/kg for patients who have active wheezing/bronchospasm preoperatively or intraoperatively.

(7) If a patient was or is considered to be a difficult mask ventilation or reintubation, then a deep extubation should not be considered.

(8) Postoperative pain control should be considered

   (a) Regional anesthesia may help to minimize opioids and crying/agitation, which is a known asthmatic trigger.

READ MORE
Atlas of peripheral nerve block procedures, Section 13, page 1171

   (b) Care must be taken to spare blocking the diaphragm (phrenic paralysis) which has demonstrated a 25% reduction in FEV_1.

      (i) Interscalene block carries a 100% risk of phrenic nerve paralysis

      (ii) Infraclavicular and axillary blocks have a <1% risk of phrenic nerve paralysis

   (c) Low-dose ketamine infusions (5 to 15 µg/kg/m) may decrease opioid usage while also providing bronchodilation. Ketamine is less likely to depress respiratory drive.

iii) Drug management postoperatively is the same as preoperatively.

iv) CPAP or BiPAP open up bronchioles to prevent alveolar air trapping, improving symptoms more than air exchange. These modalities also improve delivery of nebulized drugs.

v) VapoTherm (high flow warmed, humidified O_2) with oxygen flows of 6 to 40 L/m have been shown to improve oxygenation and symptoms and also improves delivery of nebulized drugs.

12) **Status asthmaticus and the use of isoflurane in the ICUs**

a) Isoflurane may be indicated for refractory status asthmaticus in the intubated patient already on multidrug therapy.

b) Stringent criterias for instituting and weaning need to be established for the institution.

Chapter Summary for Asthma and RAD

Preoperative Considerations	All routine medications should be administered the day of surgery
	Albuterol (β_2-adrenergic agonist) $\pm$ ipratropium bromide (anticholinergic) inhaler/ nebulizer within an hour of induction
	Administer inhaled steroids and consider IV steroids
Intraoperative Considerations	Ensure a deep level of anesthesia before instrumenting airway
	Consider lidocaine 1 mg/kg up to 100 mg maximum prior to instrumenting airway and before extubation
	Favor volatiles to opioids
	Repeat nebulizer treatments every 2 h if any signs of bronchospasm
	Avoid traditional NSAIDs. Acetaminophen and COX-2 inhibitors are generally tolerated
	Warm anesthesia gases
	For ventilation, TV of 6–10 mL/kg and I:E with greater than normal expiratory time
	Consider deep extubation if bronchospasm has occurred with lightening of anesthesia
Postoperative Considerations	Consider leaving intubated and sedated (possibly with a ketamine infusion) if bronchospasm refractory to intraoperative measures
	Utilize BiPAP or VapoTherm when indicated postextubation
	Repeat nebulizers and steroids when indicated

References

1. "Asthma: Merck Manual Professional". *Merck & Co., Inc. – We Believe the Most Important Condition Is the Human One* http://www.merck.com/mmpe/seco5/cho48/cho48a.html. 21 May 2010.
2. Akinbami LJ, Schoendorf KC. Trends in childhood asthma: prevalence, healthcare utilization, and mortality. *Pediatrics* 2002;110(2 Pt 1): 315–322.
3. von Mutius E, Nicolai T, Martinez FD. Prematurity as a risk factor for asthma in preadolescent children. *J Pediatr* 1993;123(2):223–229.
4. Rooney JC, Williams HE. The relationship between proved viral bronchiolitis and subsequent wheezing. *J Pediatr* 1971;79(5):744–747.
5. Empey DW, Laitinen LA, Jacobs L, et al. Mechanisms of bronchial hyperreactivity in normal subjects after upper respiratory tract infection. *Am Rev Respir Dis* 1976;113(2):131–139.
6. Sheikh S, Stephen TC, Sisson B. Prevalence of gastroesophageal reflux in infants with recurrent brief apneic episodes. *Can Respir J* 1999 Sep–Oct;6(5):401–404.
7. Bishop MJ, Rooke GA. Sevoflurane for patients with asthma. *Anesth Analg* 2000;91:245–246.
8. Scalfaro P, Sly PD, Sims C. Salbutamol prevents the increase in respiratory resistance caused by tracheal intubation during Sevoflurane anesthesia in asthmatic children. *Anesth Analg* 2001;93:898–902.
9. Soussan D, Liard R, Zureik M, et al. Treatment compliance, passive smoking, and asthma control: a three year cohort study. *Arch Dis Child* 200388(3):229–333.
10. CoteC, Lerman J, Todres ID. *A Practice of Anesthesia for Infants and Children*. 4th ed. Saunders, Philadelphia, PA. 2009.
11. Labiris NR, Dolovich MB. Pulmonary drug delivery. Part I: Physiological factors affecting therapeutic effectiveness of aerosolized medications. *Br J Clin Pharmacol* 2003;56(6): 588–99.
12. Hardman JG, Linnbird LE, Ed. *Goodman & Gilmans: Pharmacological Basis of Therapeutics*. 10th ed. McGraw Hill New York; 2001.
13. Juniper EF, Guyatt GH, Ferrie PJ, et al. Measuring quality of life in asthma. *Am Rev Respir Dis* 1993;147:832–838.
14. Chapman KR, Verbeek PR, White JG, et al. Effect of a short course of prednisone in the prevention of early relapse after the emergency room treatment of acute asthma. *N Engl J Med* 1991;324(12):788–94.
15. Zora JA, Zimmerman D, Carey TL. Hypothalamic-pituitary-adrenal axis suppression after short-term, high-dose glucocorticoid therapy in children with asthma. *J Allergy Clin Immunol* 1986;77:9–13.
16. Dolan LM, Kesarwala HH, Holroyde JC. Short-term, high-dose glucocorticoid therapy in children with asthma: the effect on the hypothalamic-pituitary-adrenal axis. *J Allergy Clin Immunol* 1987;80:81–7.
17. Barnes PJ, Pedersen S. Efficacy and safety of inhaled corticosteroids in asthma. *Am Rev Respir Dis* 1993;148:S1.
18. Drake AJ, Howells RJ, Shield JP. Symptomatic adrenal insufficiency presenting with hypoglycaemia in children with asthma receiving high-dose fluticasone proprionate. *BMJ* 2002;324:1081.
19. Hirota K, Sato T, Hashimoto Y. Relaxant effect of propofol on the airway in dogs. *Br J Anaesth* 1999;83:292–295.
20. Jenkins C, Costello J, Hodge L. Systemic review of prevalence of aspirin induced asthma and its implications for clinical practice. *BMJ* 2004;328: 434–440.
21. Lesko SM. The safety of ibuprofen suspension in children. *Int J Clin Pract Suppl* 2003;50–53.
22. West PM. Safety of COX-2 inhibitors in asthma patients with asthma hypersensitivity. *Ann Pharmacother* 2003;37(10):1497–1501.

73 Restrictive Lung Disease

Daniel Zaghi, MD

Restrictive lung diseases are a varied group of disorders characterized by reduced lung compliance and lung volumes. They are defined and distinguished from the more common obstructive lung diseases through pulmonary function tests (PFTs).

1) Definition
   a) **The classical definition of restrictive lung disease is a decrease in vital capacity in the presence of a normal forced expiratory volume (FEV$_1$) (2).**
   b) Characterized by reduced lung compliance and lung volumes
   c) Diagnosis
      i) **Reduced FEV$_1$**
      ii) Reduced forced vital capacity (FVC)
      iii) Normal ratio of FEV$_1$/FVC (1)
      iv) Vital capacity of < 15 mL/kg (normal 70 mL/kg) (4) and a total lung capacity < 50% of the predicted value are indicators of severe disease.

2) Pathophysiology
   a) **Can be acute or chronic and vary in etiology**
   b) Underlying pathophysiology is **reduced compliance of the lung, pleura, diaphragm, or chest wall**
      i) Increases the work of breathing, resulting in a characteristic rapid but shallow breathing (3)
      ii) This hyperventilation keeps the PaCO$_2$ at normal or depressed levels until the restrictive disorder is very severe (2).
   c) Gas exchange is usually maintained until the disease process is advanced.

Patients with restrictive lung disease tend to hyperventilate and will likely have a normal PaCO$_2$.

3) **Causes of restrictive lung disease (4)**
   a) Can often be delineated by history, exam, PFTs, and radiographs (3)
   b) **Intrinsic**
      i) Inflammation or scarring of the lung parenchyma
         (1) Examples include pulmonary fibrosis, cardiogenic and non-cardiogenic pulmonary edema, ARDS, pneumonia, and aspiration pneumonitis
   c) **Extrinsic**
      i) Disorders of the pleura, diaphragm, or chest wall that limit lung expansion
         (1) Examples include morbid obesity, massive pleural effusion, kyphoscoliosis, ascites, and pregnancy
   d) **Neuromuscular**
      i) Any pathology of the chest wall muscles or nerves that limits the ability of respiratory muscles to inflate the lung.
         (1) Examples include respiratory muscle myositis or myopathy of any cause, myasthenia gravis, quadriplegia, and phrenic neuropathy

521

4) **Anesthetic considerations**
   a) Preoperative
      i) Associated BP disturbances and respiratory infections should be aggressively treated (4).
      ii) **Pulmonary function testing**

Ensuring optimal pulmonary function in the pre-op assessment is a major step in reducing post-op complications.

      (1) Routine PFTs for all patients with restrictive lung disease are unnecessary as the results are often unlikely to change the anesthetic plan (5).
      (2) PFTs may be useful in patients with moderate to advanced restrictive lung disease undergoing major abdominal or thoracic procedures.
         (a) In these patients, PFTs can be used to compare the patient's pre-op pulmonary function to baseline, to determine surgical risk, and to gauge the potential for postoperative complications.
      iii) **Preoperative smoking cessation**
      (1) Prolonged tobacco use results in chronic obstructive lung disease.
      (2) Cessation just 12 to 18 hours before surgery may reduce carboxyhemoglobin levels, normalize the oxyhemoglobin dissociation curve and lessen sympathetic tone (5).
      (3) The ASA has sponsored a Smoking Cessation Initiative to help surgical patients quit smoking, by having anesthesiologists advise tobacco users to quit and refer them to other resources for materials, support and follow-up such as a telephone helpline like 1–800-NO-BUTTS for California residents.
      iv) Elective surgery should be delayed in patients experiencing an episode of acute restrictive lung disease.
5) **Intraoperative considerations**
   a) Perioperative management varies with the etiology of the restriction.
   b) A lowered FRC means reduced ability for pre-oxygenation and decreased time until hypoxia occurs when the patient is apneic.
   c) Neuraxial blocks may provide some benefit versus general anesthesia (5).
   d) Restrictive lung diseases do not influence the drug choice for induction or maintenance of general anesthesia (4).

Patients with restrictive lung disease are at high risk for barotrauma with positive pressure ventilation.

   e) A high inspired FiO_2 and PEEP may be required to oxygenate in the setting of a poorly compliant lung or chest wall (4).
      i) Poor lung compliance translates into high peak inspiratory pressures during positive pressure ventilation.
      (1) Patients are at higher risk for barotrauma and volutrauma
      (2) Consider lowering the TV to 4 to 8 mL/kg, increasing the RR to 14 to 18 breaths/min, and allowing higher end-tidal CO_2 levels (permissive hypercapnia) (4)
      (3) Although higher peak inspiratory pressures are to be expected, it is advisable to keep airway pressures below 30 cm H_2O (4)
   f) Longer acting opioid use intraoperatively needs to be evaluated in this patient population due to risk of postoperative sedation.
6) **Postoperative considerations** (Table 73-1, Table 73-2)
   a) Patients with respiratory muscle weakness may require prolonged postoperative respiratory support to overcome normal decreases in respiratory function after surgery and anesthesia (5).
   b) Common occurrences in the PACU can add their own restrictive effect to a patient with baseline restrictive lung pathology.

Table 73-1

Six Risk Factors for Postoperative Pulmonary Complications in Patients with Restrictive Lung Disease

Risk Factors	Pre-existing pulmonary disease
	Thoracic or upper abdominal surgery
	Smoking
	Obesity
	Age > 60 y
	Prolonged general anesthesia >3 h

Table 73-2

Postoperative Factors that Exacerbate Restrictive Lung Disease

Post-op factors	Pain
	Restrictive dressings
	Sedation from opioids
	Recumbent position further reducing FRC
	Residual anesthetic and neuro-muscular blocking drug effects
	Operations near the diaphragm causing diaphragmatic dysfunction

Chapter Summary for Restrictive Lung Disease

Definition	Decrease in VC with normal FEV_1
Pathophysiology	Acute or chronic reduction in pulmonary compliance from multiple etiologies
Causes	Intrinsic Extrinsic Neuromuscular
Preoperative Considerations	Optimize pulmonary function Aggressively treat respiratory infections Encourage smoking cessation PFTs usually not necessary
Intraoperative Considerations	Consider neuraxial anesthesia/analgesia Higher PEEP and FiO_2 may be required Recommend maintaining airway pressures < 30 cm H_2O
Postoperative Considerations	Multiple patient, surgical, and PACU risk factors may exacerbate preexisting disease

FEV_1, forced expiratory volume; FiO_2, fractional inspired oxygen concentration; PEEP, positive end-expiratory pressure; VC, vital capacity.

References

1. Miller RD, ed. *Anesthesia.* 6th ed. Philadelphia, PA: Elsevier/Churchill Livingstone; 2005:Section III, chap. 26.
2. Stoelting RK, Miller RD. *Basics of Anesthesia.* 4th ed. Philadelphia, PA: Churchill Livingstone; 2000:271–281.
3. Mason RJ, Murray JF, Broaddus CV, eds. *Murray and Nadel's Textbook of Respiratory Medicine.* 4th ed. St. Loius, MO: Saunders Company; 2005:chap. 83.
4. Morgan GE, Mikhail MS, Murray MJ, eds. *Clinical Anesthesiology.* 4th ed. New York, NY: Lange medical Books/McGraw-Hill Medical Publishing Division; 2006:571–584.
5. Faust FJ, Cucchiara RF, Rose SH, eds. *Anesthesiology Review.* 3rd ed. Philadelphia, PA: Churchill Livingstone; 2002:87–88.

74 Obstructive Sleep Apnea

Danielle B. Ludwin, MD

Obstructive sleep apnea (OSA), a common and often undiagnosed medical condition, is caused by airway obstruction leading to pauses in breathing during sleep. OSA has significant perioperative implications including an increased risk of difficult ventilation and intubation, postoperative hypoxemia and cardiopulmonary arrest (1,2). Thus, several screening tools have been developed to assess for undiagnosed sleep apnea including the ASA guidelines, Berlin questionnaire and the STOP-BANG and a number of perioperative strategies have been suggested to minimize these complications.

1) Prevalence

The majority of OSA patients are undiagnosed.

a) The incidence of OSA is 2% of middle-aged females and 4% of middle-aged males.
   i) It is estimated that four times as many middle-aged adults are undiagnosed (3,4)
      (1) **The majority of OSA patients are undiagnosed.**

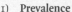

2) Diagnosis
   a) The gold standard for diagnosis is polysomnography (sleep study).
   b) An **apnea-hypopnea index (AHI)** is measured detailing the number of events per hour.
      i) Typically, apnea is defined as no breathing for $\geq$ 10 seconds.
      ii) Hypopnea is a decrease in oxygen saturation $\geq$ 4% or a decrease in airflow of 25% to 50%.
      iii) There are no universally accepted cutoffs but a general guide is AHI <5 is normal, 5 to 15 is mild OSA, 16 to 30 is moderate OSA and >30 is severe OSA (5).

The cycle of OSA is: an episode of apnea/hypopnea causing hypoxemia, hypercarbia, and acidosis, which is followed by CNS arousal and commencement of ventilation.

3) Pathophysiology
   a) Obesity leads to increased adipose tissue in the pharynx **reducing pharyngeal diameter.**
   b) **Decreased muscle tone** leads to collapse of the pharyngeal tissues.
      i) During wakefulness the pharyngeal muscle tone is adequate to maintain an airway, but during sleep, especially REM when muscle relaxation is most pronounced, obstruction occurs until sleep is interrupted and tone is restored.
   c) The cycle of OSA is an episode of apnea/hypopnea causing hypoxemia, hypercarbia and acidosis, which is followed by CNS arousal and commencement of ventilation.
      i) This leads to poor sleep hygiene, daytime sleepiness, hypertension, right heart failure, pulmonary hypertension, left heart failure, and arrhythmias (5)

4) Preoperative management for OSA patients
   a) Since OSA is commonly undiagnosed, screening patients for OSA is important.

b)   There are a number of screening tools including the ASA guidelines (Table 74-1), the Berlin questionnaire, and the STOP-BANG (6–8).

  i)   The ASA guidelines for OSA include physical characteristics that suggest OSA and the second category is a history of apparent airway obstruction during sleep.

   (1)   If a patient meets criteria by physical characteristics and has a history of obstruction, then there is a significant probability that the patient has OSA.

   (2)   A grading scale is done with points awarded for the **severity of OSA**, the **invasiveness of surgery and anesthesia,** and the **likely postoperative opioid requirement** (8).

   (3)   It is controversial whether or not OSA patients can be safely treated in an ambulatory surgery setting.

    (a)   Considerations include the severity of the OSA, the type of procedure, the likeliness of opioid requirement postoperatively, and the ability to transfer the patient to the inpatient setting as needed (8).

    (b)   If OSA patients are candidates for ambulatory surgery, they ideally should be scheduled as the first case of the day.

  ii)   The Berlin questionnaire asks patients to quantify their snoring history including the loudness, quantity, if other people complain about their snoring and presence of apnea.

   (1)   There are questions about tiredness and fatigue after sleep, falling asleep while driving, and the presence of high blood pressure (7).

  iii)   The STOP-BANG screening tool (Table 74-2) stands for S, Snoring; T, Tiredness/fatigue during the day; O, Observed apnea; P, high blood Pressure; B, BMI > 35 kg/m²; A, age > 50; N, neck circumference > 40 cm and G, Male gender.

   (1)   Patients are considered high-risk for OSA if they answer yes to three or more of the above (6).

c)   For patients with diagnosed OSA, weight loss and avoidance of alcohol and sedatives can improve symptoms.

d)   Patients on continuous positive airway pressure (CPAP) should bring their devices with them to the hospital.

  i)   Since patients with OSA are prone to co-morbidities, a thorough cardiopulmonary assessment should be done.

Table 74-1

Adapted from ASA Guidelines

Physical Characteristics	History of Airway Obstruction
BMI > 45 kg/m²	Snoring
Neck circumference > 17 in (men), > 16 in (women)	Observed pauses in breathing during sleep
Craniofacial abnormalities	Awakening with a feeling of choking
Anatomical nasal obstruction	Frequent arousals from sleep
Tonsils that touch/nearly touch	

Table 74-2			
STOP-BANG Screening Tool			
S	Snoring	B	BMI > 35 kg/m²
T	Tiredness/fatigue during the day	A	Age > 50
O	Observed apnea	N	Neck circumference > 40 cm
P	High blood Pressure	G	male Gender

Chung F, Yesneswaran B, Liao P, et al. STOP questionnaire: a tool to screen patients for OSA. *Anesthesiology* 2008; 108:812–821.

5) **Intraoperative management**
    a) The ASA guidelines recommend:
        i) Local anesthetics and/or peripheral nerve blocks are preferred over general anesthesia for peripheral surgery.
        ii) A spinal or epidural technique is preferred over general anesthesia for peripheral surgery.
        iii) For intra-abdominal surgery the recommendations are equivocal over whether a general or regional technique is superior (8).
    b) A **semiupright or lateral position** decreases airway obstruction compared to the supine position.
    c) For patients receiving general anesthesia, they should be extubated when **fully awake** and **reversed** if neuromuscular blockade has been given.
    d) For patients receiving monitored anesthetic care, EtCO₂ should be monitored to help assess adequate ventilation.
    e) Consider using CPAP/biPAP/oral appliances intraoperatively.
    f) Medications that **do not cause respiratory depression** are preferable including ketamine, dexmedetomodine, NSAIDS, and other adjuvants (9).
    g) Minimize/avoid opioids if possible.

6) **Postoperative management**
    a) There is a risk of rebound rapid eye movement sleep postoperatively so OSA patients may be at increased risk of apnea for 1 week postoperatively (10).
        i) Epidural opioids are linked to respiratory depression in this patient population (11).
    b) CPAP/biPAP should be instituted in the recovery room for patients using these devices preoperatively.
        i) Patients with undiagnosed OSA who meet criteria and exhibit signs of OSA in the operating room should be considered for a respiratory consult postoperatively for use of CPAP.
    c) Avoid recovery in the supine position when possible.
    d) Supplemental O₂ should be given until the patient can maintain baseline SpO₂ on room air (8).
    e) For patients with moderate-severe OSA, a monitored setting with continuous pulse oximetry is recommended with possible ICU admission (12).

READ MORE

Outpatient anesthesia, Chapter 130, page 909

7) Discharge criteria a panel of expert consultants convened by the ASA taskforce on perioperative management of patients with OSA developed monitoring indications. The following are based on the ASA Guidelines:
   a) Patients should meet standard outpatient discharge criteria.
   b) Be able to maintain their baseline SpO_2 on room air.
   c) No hypoxemia or airway obstruction when left alone.
   d) The group as a whole indicated that patients with OSA should be monitored for a median of 3 hours longer than non-OSA patients and for a median of 7 hours after a hypoxic or airway obstruction event (8).
   e) It is controversial if OSA patients with upper airway surgery should be admitted or discharged. The consultants disagree that these procedures can be done safely on an outpatient basis for patients at increased risk of OSA.
   f) Additional factors to consider when assessing discharge readiness include severity of OSA, type of surgery, need for postoperative opioids, use of CPAP, and recovery room status (stable vs. episodes of desaturation) (8).

Chapter Summary for OSA

General Considerations	OSA is a common and often undiagnosed disease.
Preoperative Considerations	Several screening tools are available to assess patients for undiagnosed OSA
Intraoperative Considerations	Increased risk of difficult ventilation and intubation When appropriate use regional/local anesthesia, NSAIDS, and other adjuvants that do not cause respiratory depression If general anesthesia is given, patients should be fully awake and reversed prior to extubation
Postoperative Considerations	Increased risk of postoperative hypoxemia and cardiopulmonary arrest Avoid the supine position if possible. A lateral or head-up position is preferable

References

1. Kheterpal S, Martin L, Shanks AM, et al. Prediction and outcomes of impossible mask ventilation. *Anesthesia* 2009;110:891–897.
2. Liao P, Yegneswaran B, Vairavanathan S, et al. Postoperative complications in patients with obstructive sleep apnea: a retrospective matched cohort study. *Can J Anesth* 2009;56:819–828.
3. Young T, Palta M, Dempsey J, et al. The occurrence of sleep-disordered breathing among middle-aged adults. *N Engl J Med* 1993;328: 1230–1235.
4. Young T, Evans L, Finn L, et al. Estimation of the clinically diagnosed proportion of sleep apnea syndrome in middle-aged men and women. *Sleep* 1997;20(9):705–706.
5. Benumof JL. Obstructive sleep apnea in the adult obese patient: implications for airway management. *Anesth Clin North Am* 2002;20: 789–811.
6. Chung F, Yesneswaran B, Liao P, et al. STOP questionnaire: a tool to screen patients for OSA. *Anesthesia* 2008;108:812–821.
7. Chung F, Yesneswaran B, Liao P, et al. Validation of the Berlin Questionnaire and American Society of Anesthesiologists Checklist as Screening Tools for Obstructive Sleep Apnea in Surgical Patients. *Anesthesia* 2008;108:822–830.
8. American Society of Anesthesiologists Task Force on Perioperative Management of Patients with Obstructive Sleep Apnea. Practice guidelines for the perioperative management of patients with obstructive sleep apnea. *Anesthesia* 2006;104:1081–1093.
9. Chung SA, Yuan H, Chung F. A systemic review of obstructive sleep apnea and its implications for anesthesiologists. *Anesth Analg* 2008;107:1543–1563.
10. Kaw R, Michota F, Jaffer A, et al. Unrecognized sleep apnea in the surgical patient implications for the perioperative setting. *Chest* 2006;129(1):198–205.
11. Ostermeier AM, Roizen MF, Hautkappe M, et al. Three sudden postoperative respiratory arrests associated with epidural opioids in patients with sleep apnea. *Anesth Analg* 1997;85:452–460.
12. Isono S. Obstructive sleep apnea of obese adults. *Anesthesia* 2009;110:908–921.

Intracranial Pressure

Leslie C. Andes, MD

Intracranial pressure (ICP) is the pressure exerted throughout the cranium by the tissues and fluids inside the skull. It is normally tightly regulated but can become elevated in many pathological conditions. Increased ICP, also called intracranial hypertension (ICH), can require emergency treatment if severe, due to potential compressive effects on tissue and restriction of cerebral blood flow (CBF).

1) **General principles**
   a) Intracranial constituents
      i) Brain parenchyma
      ii) Cerebrospinal fluid (CSF)
      iii) Blood
   b) Intracranial volume
      i) Considered to be fixed and incompressible (the "Monro–Kellie Doctrine").
      ii) If the volume of one constituent increases, the volume of at least one other must decrease for ICP to remain normal.
         (1) Adjustable components of ICP
            (a) CSF production and drainage
            (b) Blood flow in the brain and spinal cord
         (2) Normal ICP is 5 to 15 mm Hg in healthy supine adults and 3 to 7 mm Hg in children.

Due to the high turnover of CSF, obstruction of CSF flow may cause ICH within a few hours, necessitating emergency treatment.

2) **Cerebrospinal fluid (CSF)**
   a) Nourishes and cushions the brain in the cranial vault
   b) Redistribution provides a compensatory mechanism for increased ICP
   c) Primarily produced by the choroid plexus (CP) in the ventricles
   d) Circulates from the ventricles through the subarachnoid space of the brain and spinal cord, and is passively absorbed into the venous circulation primarily via the arachnoid granulations
   e) Total CSF volume is 75 to 150 mL in adults with normal production rate 450 to 750 mL/day.

3) **ICP and ICH**
   a) When growth of an intracranial lesion is slow, ICP will remain stable for a while because of shunting of CSF into spinal reservoirs and blood into the central vascular system.
   b) When an increase in volume can no longer be accommodated, ICP will increase rapidly with any small change in volume of any of the three components (Fig. 75-1).
   c) ICP above 20 mm Hg will reduce cerebral perfusion pressure (CPP) (CPP = MAP – ICP), and thus needs to be treated.
      i) When local tissue pressure exceeds perfusion pressure of the arterioles, the resultant ischemia can cause endothelial injury and increased transudation across capillary membranes, leading to cerebral edema.

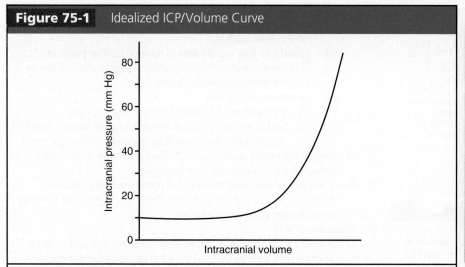

Figure 75-1   Idealized ICP/Volume Curve

From Kass IS. Physiology and metabolism of the brain and spinal cord. In: Newfield P, Cottrell JE, eds. *Handbook of Neuroanesthesia*. 4th ed. Philadelphia, PA: Lippincott Williams & Wilkins; 2007:21.

    ii) If ICH remains untreated, CBF will be low due to maximal arterial constriction, and death will quickly ensue due to limited CBF and/or herniation.

    iii) ICH is associated with poor outcome after traumatic brain injury (TBI), and uncontrolled rise in ICP is the most common cause of death in these patients (1).

  d) Conditions in which ICH may occur:

    i) Parenchymal volume increase due to hemorrhage, tumor, TBI, edema following ischemic events, encephalopathies, and idiopathic ICH (IIH, also called pseudotumor cerebri).

    ii) Hydrocephalus due to absolute or relative excess of CSF. Causes include:

      (1) Increased CSF production (meningeal disease, CP tumor, or cyst)

      (2) Obstruction to CSF flow (Arnold–Chiari malformation, mass effect from tumors, blood in the ventricles from subarachnoid hemorrhage)

      (3) Normal pressure hydrocephalus

        (a) Characterized by near-normal ICP that slowly increases due to gradually worsening obstruction of flow

        (b) Patients are typically older than 60, and develop a triad of dementia, gait problems, and incontinence; etiology is unknown.

    iii) Increased cerebral blood volume

      (1) Cerebral arterial dilation (hypoxemia, arterial hypertension, volatile anesthetic administration, hypoventilation with resultant hypercapnia)

      (2) Increased venous pressure (venous sinus thrombosis, right sided heart failure, or obstruction of jugular or great thoracic veins)

4) **CSF leak**

  a) May occur from several sites, including the nose (rhinorrhea), external auditory canal (otorrhea), or traumatic or operative defects in the skull or spine

  b) Causes

    i) CSF rhinorrhea may follow trauma and skull base surgery (e.g., transsphenoidal resection of pituitary tumor, translabyrinthine acoustic neuroma resection, mastoid surgery).

ii) Otorrhea can be seen in perforated tympanic membrane with fracture of the petrous or temporal bone, and mastoid or trans-labyrinthine surgery.

READ
MORE

Postdural
puncture
headache and
epidural blood
patch,
Chapter 32,
page 247

iii) Spinal CSF leak may be seen in trauma, lumbar puncture (LP), inadvertent "wet tap" during epidural placement, Valsalva or nose-blowing, or postoperatively.

iv) Spontaneous CSF leak
   (1) Rare and may be difficult to diagnose and treat
   (2) Recent research indicates that 90% of these patients have ICH, and often the best closure success is with endoscopic repair.

c) Depending on the cause, epidural blood patch may be used as in therapy for post-dural puncture headache.

d) If unplanned durotomy is suspected intraoperatively, one may differentiate between CSF and other fluids by using a urine test strip to test for the presence of glucose.

Signs and symptoms of increased ICP are diminished consciousness, nausea/vomiting, visual problems, and headache.

5) **Diagnosis of ICH**

a) Symptoms may be subtle, depending on the etiology and anatomy involved, and include decreased level of consciousness, breathing irregularities, visual problems, headache, nausea and vomiting, irritability and personality changes, memory loss, ataxia, and weakness.

b) Signs include papilledema, neurologic deficit, and unstable vital signs (hyper- or hypotension, arrhythmias)

c) Diagnostic imaging
   i) May be normal or show enlarged ventricles and/or lateral shift.
   ii) Evaluate scan for CVA, mass effect from tumor or hemorrhage, as well as signs of impending herniation.

d) If patient is pregnant, preeclampsia should be ruled out.

Lumbar puncture, used to diagnose various neurologic conditions, may induce herniation and should not be performed if ICH is suspected.

6) **Monitoring**

a) Monitoring of ICP assists in determining optimal therapy and may prevent herniation.

b) Direct ICP monitoring is performed via ventriculostomy and manometry.
   i) An external ventricular drain (EVD) or lumbar drain can be placed pre- or intraoperatively when anticipated that brain relaxation could be needed during the case, or if potential for postoperative CSF leak exists (see above).
   ii) Removal of 3 to 5 mL can be quickly accomplished and may be sufficient to treat acute ICH.

c) Measurement of ICP
   i) ICP is measured relative to a reference level, above which positive ICPs will result in CSF flow if the system is open.

An extraventricular drain should be zeroed at the level of the external auditory meatus.

   ii) Zero the catheter at the level of the external auditory meatus, then raise the top of the reservoir to a height above the ear that equals the acceptable ICP; CSF will flow into the reservoir bag once the ICP exceeds this level.
      (1) Care must be used in determining the height at which to hang the reservoir bag as it is possible to over-drain CSF, with potential complications such as SDH, intracranial hypotension, rupture or re-bleed of an aneurysm, or even herniation (2).
      (2) Volume-limited (20 to 30 mL) CSF drainage systems have been recently introduced.

Dextrose-containing fluids should not be administered to patients with ICH because once the dextrose is metabolized, free water remains which can worsen brain edema.

d) Other types of ICP monitors (subarachnoid bolt, epidural sensor, fiberoptic direct tissue monitor (intraparenchymal) with a pressure transducer) are used primarily in the ICU.

e) Patients in whom ICP therapy is ongoing may need CVP and arterial line to optimize volume status and CPP.

7) **Medical treatment of ICH**

a) Elevation of the patient's head up to 30 degrees is rapidly effective.

b) Ensure there is no obstruction to venous drainage from the head.

c) Hyperventilate patient to $ETCO_2$ of 25 to 30.

    i) $ETCO_2$ will return to normal via bicarbonate buffering after 4 to 8 hours of hyperventilation.

    ii) Over-ventilation to $ETCO_2 < 25$ may cause ischemia secondary to severe vasoconstriction.

d) Control BP to maintain systolic BP 110 > MAP > 70

e) Treat hypoxia

f) IV fluids should be isotonic or hypertonic to avoid further increase in brain water

g) Osmotic or loop diuretics

    i) Mannitol is currently the first line agent at a dose of 0.25 to 1 g/kg.

    ii) Hypertonic saline (HS) may be more effective than mannitol (3–5) with fewer side effects.

        (1) There are few studies of intraoperative HS use (6,7), and none show a difference in effectiveness between HS and mannitol.

        (2) HS expands plasma volume and may increase CPP, unlike mannitol which can decrease intravascular volume (4,8–10).

        (3) A reasonable starting dose would be 30 mL of 23.4% HS via central venous catheter over 15 to 20 minutes, after which 3% HS may be infused at 30 to 50 mL/h to keep serum Na+ at 140 to 145 (checked with osmolality at least every 4 hours) (9).

Patients with ICH should get little or no preoperative sedation.

h) Prevent shivering, muscle movements, pain, and seizures with narcotics, paralytics, anti-epileptics, sedatives or barbiturates as necessary, once appropriate ventilation is assured.

8) **Surgical treatment of ICH**

a) **Preoperative planning**

Extreme care should be taken when intubating a patient with ICH as hypertension on laryngoscopy can cause uncal herniation.

    i) Patients with ICH who are awake and responsive should get little or no preoperative sedation because hypoventilation can further increase ICP, possibly causing herniation.

    ii) ABG after induction may be helpful in determining the best ventilatory parameters in patients where significant end-tidal to arterial CO_2 gradient may exist.

b) **Intraoperative technique**

    i) Voluntary hyperventilation while awake followed by early mask hyperventilation during anesthetic induction may assist in minimizing changes in ICP or CPP during induction and intubation.

    ii) Assurance of anesthetic depth before intubation is important.

    iii) Anesthetic agents

        (1) Propofol, thiopental, and etomidate decrease ICP.

        (2) Ketamine recently shown to be safe in patients with ICH under certain conditions, although its use is still controversial (11).

(3)   Volatile anesthetic agents may cause a small increase in ICP via cerebral vasodilation, but this effect may be overcome by mild hyperventilation.

(4)   The effects of N₂O on ICP vary with concentration.

    (a)   Increase in ICP has been shown in humans but is largely attenuated with prior hyperventilation or administration of induction agents which cause decreased ICP.

    (b)   N₂O should not be used when there is a chance of intracranial air and some anesthesiologists do not use it at all for intracranial procedures.

(5)   Narcotics have no direct effect on ICP but may cause hypoventilation leading to ICH.

(6)   Barbiturates are occasionally administered to prevent brain herniation upon dural opening if the dura looks "tight" upon turning the bone flap.

  c)   **Surgical procedures**

   i)   **Shunt procedures**

(1)   For urgent but non-emergent increases in ICP due to obstruction of CSF flow (patient symptomatic but herniation not imminent)

(2)   Shunts are silastic catheters used to drain CSF from an area of high pressure (ventricles or cistern) to one of lower pressure

VP Shunts have a fairly high failure rate over time and are frequently revised, or may be removed and subsequently replaced if infection develops.

(3)   The proximal end is most often placed in the right lateral (intracranial) ventricle

(4)   The distal end is tunneled under the skin to one of several locations (the right atrium via the internal jugular vein, pleural cavity, peritoneal cavity, gall bladder)

    (a)   Venous placement of the distal end is most often used if the patient is obese, has peritonitis or previous abdominal surgery.

    (b)   The hypertensive response frequently seen with skin tunneling of the catheter should be forestalled by increasing anesthetic depth (narcotics, propofol, sevoflurane) or β adrenergic antagonists.

(5)   If there is free communication between intracranial and spinal CSF, an LP shunt may be used instead (from lumbar subarachnoid space into peritoneum).

(6)   For shunt removal due to infection, hold antibiotics until cultures are taken.

(7)   No special intraoperative monitoring is necessary for a shunt procedure.

   ii)   **Minimally invasive neuroendoscopic surgery for treatment of CSF obstruction**

(1)   Used effectively to treat many types of obstructive hydrocephalus, and may be lower risk than craniotomy or shunt procedures (12).

(2)   Infection rate of endoscopic third ventriculostomy for resection of colloid cyst is lower than with transcallosal craniotomy (13).

(3)   Aqueductoplasty and aqueductal stenting are examples of other therapeutic options afforded with the endoscope.

(4)   Long-term patency rates are as yet unknown and require follow up studies.

   iii)   **Emergency craniotomy for refractory ICH**

(1)   Decompressive craniectomy solely for ICH is still somewhat controversial.

(2)   Rarely, surgical resection of brain tissue may be necessary.

(3)   If ICP remains elevated at the end of a craniotomy (surgeon unable to put on bone flap without compressing brain tissue), the bone may be frozen and replaced at a later date.

9) **Postoperative care**
   a) Maintain slight head up position.
   b) If an ICP monitor or EVD is in place, watch the level of the bag and ICP as the patient is moved and transported.
   c) Carry sedative agent, vasoconstrictors, and vasodilators with you during transport in case needed urgently to keep patient sedated or manipulate BP.

Chapter Summary for the Patient with Increased ICP

Definition	ICP is defined as the pressure exerted throughout the cranium by the tissues and fluids inside the skull.
General Considerations	The cranium is a fixed compartment consisting of brain, blood, and CSF. CPP = MAP−ICP Increases in any of these may result in severe decrease in CPP and potentially herniation of the brain through the foramen magnum, which is life threatening.
Preoperative	Do not over-sedate patients with ICH.
Intraoperative	Hyperventilate to ETCO$_2$ 25–30 mm Hg until ICH resolved. Other treatments for acutely increased ICP are head up position, placement of CSF drain, osmotic diuretics.
Postoperative	Watch patient for signs of increased ICP.

ICP, intracranial pressure; CPP, cerebral perfusion pressure; CSF, cerebrospinal fluid; MAP, mean arterial pressure; ICH, intracranial hypertension; ETCO$_2$, end-tidal carbon dioxide.

References

1. Grande PO, Bentzer P. Hypertonic saline: a marker for discrimination between a disrupted and intact blood-brain barrier? *Crit Care Med* 2006;34(12):3057–3058.
2. Muraskin SI, Roy RC, Petrozza PH. Overdrainage of cerebrospinal fluid during central venous catheter exchange in a patient with an external ventricular drain. *Anesth Analg* 2007;105(5):1519–1520.
3. Qureshi AI, Wilson DA, Traystman RJ. Treatment of elevated intracranial pressure in experimental intracerebral hemorrhage: comparison between mannitol and hypertonic saline. *Neurosurgery* 1999;44(5):1055–1063; discussion 1063–1064.
4. Levine JM. Hypertonic saline for the treatment of intracranial hypertension: worth its salt. *Crit Care Med* 2006;34(12):3037–3039.
5. Battison C, Andrews PJ, Graham C, et al. Randomized, controlled trial on the effect of a 20% mannitol solution and a 7.5% saline/6% dextran solution on increased intracranial pressure after brain injury. *Crit Care Med* 2005;33(1):196–202; discussion 257–258.
6. Gemma M, et al. 7.5% hypertonic saline versus 20% mannitol during elective neurosurgical supratentorial procedures. *J Neurosurg Anesthesiol* 1997;9(4):329–334.
7. Rozet I, et al. Effect of equiosmolar solutions of mannitol versus hypertonic saline on intraoperative brain relaxation and electrolyte balance. *Anesthesiology* 2007;107(5):697–704.
8. Bentsen G, Breivik H, Lundar T, et al. Hypertonic saline (7.2%) in 6% hydroxyethyl starch reduces intracranial pressure and improves hemodynamics in a placebo-controlled study involving stable patients with subarachnoid hemorrhage. *Crit Care Med* 2006;34(12):2912–7.
9. Qureshi AI, Suarez JI. Use of hypertonic saline solutions in treatment of cerebral edema and intracranial hypertension. *Crit Care Med* 2000;28(9):3301–3313.
10. Schwarz S, Georgiadis D, Aschoff A, et al. Effects of hypertonic (10%) saline in patients with raised intracranial pressure after stroke. *Stroke* 2002;33(1):136–140.
11. Himmelseher S, Durieux ME. Revising a dogma: ketamine for patients with neurological injury? *Anesth Analg* 2005;101(2):524–534.
12. Schroeder HW, Oertel J, Gaab MR. Endoscopic treatment of cerebrospinal fluid pathway obstructions. *Neurosurgery* 2007;60(2 Suppl 1): ONS44–ONS51; discussion ONS51–ONS52.
13. Horn EM, Feiz-Erfan I, Bristol R, et al. Treatment options for third ventricular colloid cysts: comparison of open microsurgical versus endoscopic resection. *Neurosurgery* 2007;60(4):613–618; discussion 618–620.

76 Anesthesia and Diseases of the Nervous System

Divya Chander, MD, PhD

Assessment of underlying neurological disease in the patient undergoing anesthesia is critical. The nervous system exerts control over all physiological systems affected by anesthesia, including the respiratory and cardiac systems. The autonomic branch controls compensatory mechanisms to anesthetic perturbations, and all three branches contribute to maintenance of intact reflex systems, most notably, airway reflexes. Certain motor system diseases share susceptibility to malignant hyperthermia triggers. Anatomically, the nervous system is vulnerable to injury with delivery of anesthetics, especially when regional or neuraxial techniques are used. Finally, the nervous system itself is the target of anesthetics; cerebral vasoregulation, cerebral excitatory and inhibitory balance, traffic along peripheral nerves, and proper function of the neuromuscular junction are altered. Anesthesia also modulates the global arousal system and may therefore have long-lasting cognitive effects in select, vulerable patient populations. Therefore, knowledge of how to manage patients with neurological derangements contributes to the safety of anesthetic delivery.

1) **Motor System Diseases**

READ MORE

Muscular dystrophy, Chapter 114, page 820 and Malignant hyperthermia, Chapter 90, page 653

When performing a history and physical in any patient with neurologic disease, rigorous documentation of pre-existing deficits, and a full risk-benefit discussion of anesthetic technique with patients is mandatory.

a) Motor system dominated diseases include myopathies and muscular dystrophies, motor end-plate denervation, motor neuron degeneration, spinal motor tract disorders, and disuse atrophy. Motor system disease involving other branches of the nervous system includes peripheral nerve disease, polyneuropathies, and spinal cord injury.

b) **Amyotrophic lateral sclerosis (ALS)**
   i) Progressive loss of both upper and lower motor neurons leading to fasciculations, flaccid paralysis, hyperreflexia, and spasticity.
   ii) Treatment
      (1) There are no effective therapies at this time.
      (2) Patients may be on a number of experimental treatments that rarely have anesthetic interactions (e.g. high dose antioxidants, or riluzole, an anti-glutamatergic drug).

c) Duchenne muscular dystrophy (DMD)
   i) X-linked disorder of the dystrophin gene leading to muscle wasting and weakness, dilated cardiomyopathy (in 50% of patients by age 15), ultimately resulting in early death (1).
   ii) Administration of malignant hyperthermia (MH) triggers can lead to perioperative, hypermetabolic complications reminiscent of MH (1–3).

d) Central core disease (muscle channelopathy)/King Denborough syndrome (myopathy)
   i) A group of rare muscle disorders directly linked to MH (3).

e) **Anesthetic management**
   i) Preoperative considerations
      (1) Risk of aspiration and requirement for postoperative ventilatory support should be rigorously assessed.

(2) Regional anesthesia is not contraindicated, though nervous system deficits should be meticulously documented and risks explained thoroughly to patients so pre-existing deficits are not confused with nerve injury.

(3) Prepare an anesthesia machine free of MH-triggering agents for those disorders that are MH-susceptible (3,4).

ii) Induction

(1) **Succinylcholine should be avoided** secondary to muscle denervation and up-regulation of extrajunctional receptors **in all motor neuron diseases.** Severe hyperkalemia my lead to intractable bradycardia and/or cardiac arrest.

(2) Patients may be more sensitive to non-depolarizing muscle relaxants.

(3) In the **dystrophies and myopathies** such as central core disease and King Denborough syndrome, **both succinylcholine and potent volatile anesthetics should be avoided because they may lead to rhabdomyolysis or hypermetabolic states reminiscent of MH** (1,3).

Neurologic diseases resulting in muscle denervation secondary to disuse atrophy or lower motor neuron denervation (e.g. ALS, post-polio syndrome, tetanus, MS, or GBS with motor involvement) can cause a proliferation of extrajunctional receptors and an exaggerated release of extra-cellular potassium in response to sub-paralytic doses of succinylcholine.

iii) Maintenance and emergence

(1) A total intravenous anesthetic (TIVA) technique and a "clean" machine are recommended for the dystrophies and myopathies (2,3).

(2) In all motor system diseases, monitoring of muscle twitch with a nerve stimulator should be on an unaffected limb, if one is available.

(3) Autonomic nervous system (ANS) is typically not impaired in pure motor diseases, and hemodynamic responses will be more stable.

(4) In peripheral nerve disease, polyneuropathies (see below) and spinal cord injury, the ANS may show variable impairment and could alter hemodynamics significantly.

iv) Postoperative considerations

(1) Preparation for postoperative ventilatory support should be undertaken in select populations.

(2) Suspicion of hypermetabolic syndromes or rhabdomyolysis should be monitored appropriately in the PACU (e.g. serial serum potassium and creatine kinase levels, urine myoglobin).

2) **Peripheral Demyelinating Diseases: Guillian-Barré syndrome (GBS)**

a) Demyelinating diseases typically have motor and sensory nervous system involvement; sometimes autonomic nervous system involvement is also present.

Demyelinating diseases can affect both peripheral and central nervous system, and involve all three branches – motor, sensory and autonomic. When *multiple peripheral nerves* are involved the disease is considered a *polyneuropathy.*

b) **Guillain–Barré syndrome (GBS): Acute inflammatory demyelinating polyneuropathy (AIDP)**

i) GBS is an infrequent, autoimmune response against peripheral nerves, triggered 60–70% of the time by an acute viral respiratory or gastrointestinal infection.

ii) Sequelae occur days to weeks after exposure to infection.

iii) GBS is characterized by an ascending paralysis, affecting limbs before trunk, and loss of deep tendon reflexes.

(1) Cranial nerves are involved 50% of the time.

iv) Treatment for acute episodes is via IV-IG or plasmapheresis exchange. Steroids are not considered useful.

c) **Anesthetic management**

i) Preoperative considerations

(1)   A focused understanding of involved systems is imperative to managing the patient safely – a thorough chart review and patient history must be taken. Targets with important anesthetic implications include:

(a)   Autonomic/cardiac system

(i)   BP lability in the absence of compensatory cardiovascular reflexes, requiring vasoactive treatment at various intraoperative time points

(ii)   Dysrhythmias and possibly cardiac arrest

(b)   Brainstem

(i)   Compromised pharyngeal reflexes which may contribute to reflux or inability to protect the airway, necessitating unplanned intubation or tracheostomy

(ii)   Disordered swallowing

(iii) Vocal cord paralysis

(c)   Respiratory system

(i)   Increased risk of pulmonary embolus

(ii)   Diaphragmatic paralysis necessitating intubation or tracheostomy

(d)   Secondary skeletal muscle denervation or atrophy

(2)   Regional and neuraxial anesthesia are not contraindicated; there are several case reports of safe neuraxial anesthesia undertaken in GBS patients (5–9).

(a)   There is an increased risk of complications due to exaggerated hemodynamic responses in patients with autonomic involvement (10).

(b)   There is the potential for exaggerated receptor responses to local anesthetics.

(c)   Use of regional techniques should be balanced against the other risks and benefits of such approaches in these patients.

(d)   These techniques may have increased benefit in the GBS parturient, but increased risk in the patient with lung disease.

(e)   A detailed discussion of these risks should be undertaken with the patient and all pre-existing neurological deficits should be meticulously documented so pre-existing deficits are not confused with nerve injury.

(f)   The choice must be made on a case-by-case basis.

ii) Induction

(1)   Stress-dose steroids are only required in patients on long-term steroids, which is unusual in this population.

(2)   Autonomic involvement will lead to exaggerated responses to:

(a)   Induction agents (hypotension, brady- or tachycardia)

(i)   Anticipate and consider pre-treatment with vasoactive agents as necessary

(b)   Direct laryngoscopy (hypertension, tachycardia)

(i)   Consider pre-medication (e.g. 3–5 mcg/kg fentanyl) prior to laryngoscopy to blunt autonomic responses

(3)   Bulbar involvement may increase risk of aspiration – anticipate and use a modified rapid sequence technique with cricoid pressure if deemed necessary.

(4)   Skeletal muscle denervation, even subclinical, can lead to an upregulation of extrajunctional receptors. Avoid succinylcholine because of the risk for hyperkalemic bradycardia or cardiac arrest.

(5)   There are no known contraindications to use of non-depolarizing muscle relaxants, though there is the potential for increased sensitivity and delayed recovery.

Patients with GBS are at high risk for autonomic instability and respiratory failure.

      iii) Maintenance/Emergence

         (1) Autonomic instability will lead to exaggerated responses to:

           (a) addition of PEEP (hypotension)

           (b) surgical stimulation (hypertension)

           (c) blood loss (hypotension)

           (d) changes in posture (hypo- and hypertension)

         (2) Invasive arterial monitoring can assist management in patients with autonomic instability.

         (3) Indirect-acting vasopressors may elicit exaggerated responses secondary to up-regulation of postsynaptic receptors.

         (4) Myocardial irritants or sensitizers should be avoided (e.g. halothane).

         (5) Wildly fluctuating blood pressure responses during emergence should be anticipated and pre-treated if possible (e.g. β-adrenergic antagonists).

         (6) If there is motor involvement, monitoring of muscle twitch with a nerve stimulator should typically be on an unaffected limb.

         (7) Careful attention to extubation criteria must be followed:

           (a) Appropriate respiratory mechanics (11)

           (b) Return of airway reflexes

           (c) Full recovery of neuromuscular tone

           (d) A warmed patient

           (e) Recovery of mental status

           (f) Normalized blood gases

           (g) Minimal intraoperative hemodynamic shifts

           (h) Normal electrolytes

      iv) Postoperative

         (1) Depending on severity of disease and involvement of the respiratory system, the GBS patient may require post-surgical ventilatory support.

READ MORE

Post-op ventilation of the surgical patient, Chapter 148, page 1079

  3) Central demyelinating diseases: Multiple sclerosis

    a) **Multiple sclerosis (MS)**

      i) Autoimmune disorder against CNS myelin.

      ii) Has a relapsing and remitting course, with variable periods of latency in-between.

      iii) Disease severity and expression is based on the burden and distribution of CNS lesions.

      iv) Sensory, motor, and autonomic nervous system involvement is possible.

    b) Treatment includes:

      i) Chronic immunosuppressive therapies (e.g. cyclophosphamide, azathioprine).

      ii) Steroid treatment during acute flares.

      iii) Intravenous ACTH if afflicted with optic neuritis.

      iv) Antispasmodics if suffering severe spasticity or bladder involvement.

    c) **Anesthetic management**

      i) Preoperative considerations

         (1) As with GBS, a focused but thorough chart review and patient history must be taken. Central white matter loss may affect critical targets with anesthetic implications:

- (a) Autonomic/cardiac system resulting in blood pressure lability with poor compensatory reflexes
- (b) Brainstem nuclei affecting respiration, pharyngeal reflexes, swallowing or vocal cord function
- (c) Secondary skeletal muscle denervation or atrophy
- (2) Regional and neuraxial anesthesia are not contraindicated though controversial. Retrospective studies have not found an increase in MS exacerbations or documented neurotoxicity with neuraxial anesthesia or nerve blocks (12).
  - (a) There is a theoretical risk of increased sensitivity of nerve conduction to either single or repeated doses of local anesthetics, particularly with intrathecal administration (13), or concern for secondary crush injury to already compromised nerves (14–15).
  - (b) There is the potential for exaggerated receptor responses to local anesthetics.
  - (c) Use of regional techniques should be balanced against the other risks and benefits of such approaches in these patients. The benefits may be more strongly seen in the MS parturient; increased caution should be exercised in the patient with documented spinal cord lesions. The decision to use regional techniques should be made on a case-by-case basis.
  - (d) A detailed discussion of these risks should be undertaken with the patient, and all pre-existing neurological deficits should be meticulously documented so pre-existing deficits are not confused with nerve injury.
  - (e) If utilized, one should consider use of lower local anesthetic doses, supplemented with opioids.
- ii) Induction
  - (1) Stress-dose steroids are only required in patients on long-term steroids, which is unusual in this population.
  - (2) Autonomic involvement will lead to exaggerated responses to:
    - (a) Induction agents (hypotension, brady- or tachycardia)
      - (i) Anticipate and consider pre-treatment with vasoactive agents as necessary
    - (b) Direct laryngoscopy (hypertension, tachycardia)
      - (i) Consider premedication (e.g. 3–5 mcg/kg fentanyl) prior to laryngoscopy to blunt autonomic responses
  - (3) Bulbar involvement may increase risk of aspiration – anticipate and use a modified rapid sequence technique with cricoid pressure if deemed necessary.
  - (4) Skeletal muscle denervation, even subclinical, can lead to an up-regulation of extrajunctional receptors. Avoid succinylcholine because of the risk for hyperkalemic bradycardia or cardiac arrest.
  - (5) There are no known contraindications to use of non-depolarizing muscle relaxants, though there is the potential for increased sensitivity and delayed recovery.
- iii) Maintenance/Emergence
  - (1) Autonomic instability will lead to exaggerated responses to:
    - (a) Addition of PEEP (hypotension)
    - (b) Surgical stimulation (hypertension)
    - (c) Blood loss (hypotension)
    - (d) Changes in posture (hypo- and hypertension)

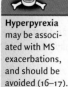

Hyperpyrexia may be associated with MS exacerbations, and should be avoided (16–17).

Neuraxial and other regional techniques are generally safe in patients with peripheral nervous or neuromuscular involvement. However, the decision to perform these techniques should be made on a case-by-case basis with thorough discussion of risks and benefits with the patient.

(2) Invasive arterial monitoring can assist management in patients with autonomic instability

(3) Indirect-acting vasopressors may elicit exaggerated responses secondary to up-regulation of postsynaptic receptors.

(4) Wildly fluctuating blood pressure responses during emergence should be anticipated and pre-treated if possible (e.g. β-adrenergic antagonists).

(5) If there is motor involvement, monitoring of muscle twitch with a nerve stimulator should typically be on an unaffected limb.

(6) Careful attention to extubation criteria must be followed:

    (a) Appropriate respiratory mechanics

    (b) Return of airway reflexes

    (c) Full recovery of neuromuscular tone

    (d) A warmed patient

    (e) Recovery of mental status

    (f) Normalized blood gases

    (g) Minimal intraoperative hemodynamic shifts

    (h) Normal electrolytes

iv) Postoperative

    (1) Depending on severity of disease and involvement of the respiratory system, the MS patient may require post-surgical ventilatory support.

4) **Inflammatory neurologic disease**

  a) **Lyme disease**

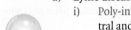

Up to 10% of cases of Lyme disease have significant cardiac involvement.

    i) Poly-inflammation of multiple organ systems (joints, heart, muscle, central and peripheral nervous system) is the hallmark of the disease.

    ii) Early manifestations include erythema migrans and influenza-like symptoms.

    iii) Later systemic manifestations can masquerade as many other diseases.

    iv) As many as 10% of cases can have significant cardiac involvement (18), complicating anesthetic management.

        (1) Most common problem is atrioventricular block; other dysrhythmias/conduction abnormalities are possible.

        (2) Rarer cardiac manifestations include pericarditis, myocarditis, cardiomyopathy and degenerative valvular disease.

        (3) Unstable patients may require temporary pacing (18).

  b) Neurologic Lyme disease (*neuroborreliosis*)

    i) Occurs 1 to 4 weeks after initial infection in 10% to 15% of cases.

    ii) Causes inflammation of the peripheral nerves, meningeal lining, or brain parenchyma.

    iii) Manifestations include meningitis, meningoradiculitis, cranial neuritis, encephalopathy, peripheral neuropathy, encephalitis, and encephalomyelitis (19).

  c) Treatment

    i) Nervous system infection responds well to parenteral high-dose penicillin, ceftriaxone, and cefotaxime in both adults and children.

    ii) Oral doxycycline is often used in adults with meningitis, cranial neuritis, and radiculitis (14).

  d) **Anesthetic Management**

    i) Preoperative considerations

        (1) Anesthetic risk depends on the portion of the nervous system involved. As with GBS and MS, an extremely thorough preoperative evaluation is needed to identify these affected systems to develop an anesthetic plan. Any system can be involved in Lyme Disease.

(a) Cardiac involvement most prominently leads to dysrhythmias, and can result in arrest.

(b) Myelitis can result in weakness, sensory loss, and dysautonomia, leading to autonomic lability. Denervation can affect the neuromuscular junction and respiratory muscles.

(c) Cranial neuritis may affect airway reflexes, cause vocal cord paralysis, and impact the ability to protect the airway.

(d) Management of peripheral neuritis depends on severity and distribution of lesions. It has maximal impact if autonomic fibers or muscles of respiration are affected.

(e) In rare cases, vasculitic involvement can lead to stroke (see Ischemic Vascular Disease/CVA).

(f) Parenchymal involvement can infrequently lead to seizures (see Epilepsy/ Seizure Disorder).

(2) Similar considerations (ALS, GBS, MS patients) for the use of neuraxial anesthesia in *neuroborreliosis* with peripheral neuritis hold. A strict risk-benefit analysis and meticulous documentation of pre-existing deficits should be performed.

ii) Induction

(1) Cardiac and autonomic involvement may lead to dysrhythmias or exaggerated responses to:

(a) Induction agents (hypotension, brady- or tachycardia)

(i) Anticipate and consider pre-treatment with vasoactive agents as necessary

(b) Direct laryngoscopy (hypertension, tachycardia)

(i) Consider pre-medication (e.g. 3–5 mcg/kg fentanyl) prior to laryngoscopy to blunt autonomic responses.

(2) Cranial neuritis and/or bulbar involvement may increase risk of aspiration – anticipate and consider using a modified rapid sequence technique with cricoid pressure.

(3) Myelitis leading to muscle denervation carries high risk of hyperkalemia-induced bradycardia or arrest. Motor compromise may be impossible to document, so it is safer to avoid succinylcholine.

(4) There are no contraindications to non-depolarizing muscle relaxants, though sensitivity to them may be slightly increased.

iii) Maintenance/Emergence

(1) Autonomic instability will lead to exaggerated responses to:

(a) Addition of PEEP (hypotension)

(b) Surgical stimulation (hypertension)

(c) Blood loss (hypotension)

(d) Changes in posture (hypo- and hypertension)

(2) Invasive arterial monitoring can assist management in patients with autonomic instability.

(3) Indirect-acting vasopressors may elicit exaggerated responses secondary to up-regulation of postsynaptic receptors.

(4) Myocardial irritants or sensitizers should be avoided (e.g. halothane).

(5) Wildly fluctuating blood pressure responses during emergence should be anticipated and pre-treated if possible (e.g. β-adrenergic antagonists).

(6) If there is motor involvement, monitoring of muscle twitch with a nerve stimulator should typically be on an unaffected limb.

(7) Careful attention to extubation criteria must be followed (see ALS, GBS, MS).

iv) Postoperative considerations

(1) If myelitis or cranial neuritis affects the respiratory system or ability to protect the airway, the patient with Lyme Disease may require post-surgical ventilatory support.

5) Cerebral disease: Epilepsy
   a) **Epilepsy/seizure disorder**
      i) *Seizures* are paroxysmal, transient disturbances of brain function characterized by excessive or hypersynchronous discharge of neurons.
      ii) The electrical signature of seizures can be measured by surface scalp electrodes (EEG).

READ MORE
Anesthesia for intracranial and neurovascular procedures, Chapter 139, page 979

      iii) The clinical manifestations can be sensory, motor, or psychic, and be accompanied by loss of consciousness.
      iv) The hypermetabolic activity of brains undergoing seizure discharge necessitates supportive function, especially if seizure activity is not self-limited (*status epilepticus*).
      v) *Epilepsy* is a chronic disorder characterized by recurrent seizures.
   b) Pro- and anti-convulsant effects of anesthetic drugs

Patients with seizure foci in a speech or other eloquent sensory center may require awake craniotomy for resection of seizure focus.

      i) Many anesthetic agents have dose-dependent paradoxical pro- and anticonvulsant effects (21).
         (1) Lower doses are more likely to be proconvulsant.
         (2) Higher doses or infusions (propofol, ketamine, thiopental) are more likely to be anticonvulsant.
      ii) The opposing effects may be related to dose-dependent effects on differential recruitment of GABAergic circuits.
      iii) Narcotics may show the reverse effect (22–23).
   c) **Anesthetic management of the patient for intracranial resection of seizure focus.**
      i) Preoperative considerations
         (1) May require an awake craniotomy if the seizure focus overlaps with speech (motor or receptive), sensory, or motor ("eloquent") centers.
            (a) Only motor centers can be tested with the patient asleep.

For awake craniotomies requiring adjunct sedation, have a carefully thought out back-up plan in case of loss of airway, especially since the patient's head may be far from the anesthesiologist, fixed (i.e., pins), and difficult to access; discuss plan with the surgeon if necessary, especially if the patient has predictable airway difficulties (e.g., craniofacial compromise, obesity).

         (2) Benzodiazepines are usually avoided as pre-medication in both awake and asleep craniotomies
            (a) They raise the seizure threshold
            (b) They may interfere with intraoperative assessment during awake craniotomies
         (3) IV access is obtained on the side of the patient not involved with (motor) seizures.
      ii) Induction
         (1) Choose a method of sedation that:
            (a) Provides patient comfort
            (b) Is rapidly titratable/reversible
            (c) Does not interfere with the seizure threshold
            (d) Does not induce profound apnea
               (i) Adjuncts often include propofol, remifentanil, and dexmetetomidine
         (2) Have a carefully thought out back-up plan in case of loss of airway, especially since the patient's head may be far from the anesthesiologist, fixed (i.e. pins), and difficult to access.
            (a) Discuss this airway plan with the surgeon if necessary, especially in high-risk patients (e.g. craniofacial compromise, obesity)
      iii) Maintenance
         (1) Intraoperative brain mapping is common

      (a) May be done with electrocorticography (ECoG), electrodes placed directly on the cortical surface overlying the focus, or with intracranial depth electrodes in the region of interest

      (b) The neurosurgeon may ask for pharmacological adjuncts for stimulation of the epileptogenic focus.

        (i) Methohexital: 10 to 50 mg IV

        (ii) Propofol: 10 to 20 mg IV

        (iii) Thiopental 25 to 50 mg IV

        (iv) Etomidate 2 to 8 mg IV

d) Anesthetic management of the epileptic patient undergoing non-epilepsy surgery.

  i) Preoperative evaluation

Patients on antiseizure medication may require increased dose and frequency of medications.

    (1) Thoroughly assess co-morbidities, including psychiatric illnesses, head trauma, or associated syndromes, some more common in childhood.

      (a) West syndrome, Lennox–Gastaut syndrome, mitochondrial syndromes such as MERRF and MELAS, neurofibromatosis, tuberous sclerosis, multiple endocrine adenomatosis.

    (2) Knowledge of the patient's anticonvulsant therapy and associated complications is imperative.

      (a) Phenytoin: gum disease/poor dentition, airway management issues.

      (b) Valproate: altered platelet function, thrombocytopenia.

      (c) Carbamazepine: bone marrow suppression, cardiac toxicity.

  ii) Maintenance

In any setting where a seizure takes place, the first goal is to ensure a patent airway, administer supplemental O2, and maintain adequate perfusion (ABCs).

    (1) Avoid anesthetic agents that potentiate the seizure threshold such as etomidate and methohexital.

    (2) Avoid hypocapnia (through hyperventilation and control of minute ventilation)

      (a) Potentiates the seizure threshold and decreases cerebral blood flow through vasoconstriction.

    (3) For long intraoperative procedures, ongoing anticonvulsant therapy may need to be administered. Consult with the surgical team to determine the patient's dosing schedule.

    (4) Most anticonvulsants (especially phenytoin and phenobarbital) undergo hepatic transformation and up-regulate the P450 enzyme system.

      (a) This usually necessitates an **increased amount or frequency of dosing** of many anesthetic drugs, especially the muscle relaxants.

e) Anesthetic management of the epileptic patient in status epilepticus.

  i) Status epilepticus is ongoing, intractable seizure activity, either convulsive or non-convulsive.

    (1) **Status epilepticus is a neurological emergency**

  ii) Treatment

Hypoglycemia should always be considered and treated in a patient who is seizing.

    (1) Primary goal is prevention of brain damage.

    (2) Secondary goal is prevention of injury due to involuntary convulsions.

    (3) Brain damage prevention includes:

      (a) ABC: Secure the airway, provide supplemental O_2, maintain adequate perfusion/circulation.

      (b) Decrease or silence neuronal activity.

ANESTHESIA AND COMORBID DISEASES

Anesthesia for intracranial and neurovascular procedures, Chapter 139, page 979

(i) Decreases neuronal metabolism and secondary glutamate excitotoxicity.

(c) If hypoglycemia has not been ruled out and cannot be ruled out quickly, supplement with D50 as a slow IV push.

    (i) Dextrose 50% = 25 g D-glucose in 50 mL water.

(d) Commonly used medications to decrease convulsive activity include:

    (i) Benzodiazepines

    (ii) Barbiturates

    (iii) Propofol

    (iv) Phenytoin

(e) Most intravenous anesthetics have anticonvulsant properties when used at adequate dosages as infusions.

    (i) Anticonvulsant therapy can be titrated to a simultaneously monitored EEG.

6) **Cerebral disease: Ischemia**

  a) **Ischemic vascular disease/cerebrovascular accident CVA**

    i) Rupture or obstruction of a blood vessel feeding the brain parenchyma that results in sudden impairment of consciousness, sensory, or motor function.

  b) Treatment

    i) Medical

      (1) Multifactorial treatment

        (a) Anticoagulation (if ischemic disease)

        (b) Decrease the risk of the associated comorbidities

          (i) Hypertension, dyslipidemia, tobacco use, diabetes

    ii) Surgical

      (1) Open or endovascular carotid endarterectomy (CEA).

        (a) Performed to correct stenosis of the carotid artery in ischemic disease.

      (2) Open clipping or endovascular coiling treatment of aneurysm or AVMs is performed for hemorrhagic strokes.

  c) Anesthetic implications

    i) **Anesthetic management of the patient with ischemic vascular disease undergoing non-CEA surgery.**

      (1) Preoperative considerations

        (a) Meticulous attention should be paid to multiple comorbidities. These patients are generally pan-vasculopaths with small and large vessel atherosclerosis. They present with associated pro-inflammatory conditions including:

          (i) Hypertension

          (ii) Diabetes

          (iii) Coronary artery disease

          (iv) Obesity

          (v) Obstructive lung disease

        (b) History should emphasize exercise tolerance, use of home O_2, symptoms of chest pain, orthopnea, dyspnea on exertion, and those consistent with obstructive sleep apnea.

          (i) Pre-existing neurological deficits should be documented.

        (c) Medications, electrolyte abnormalities (especially glucose, potassium, bicarbonate), coagulopathies, and anemia should be noted.

          (i) The ECG should be examined, and compared to prior ECGs if available.

Ischemic heart disease, Chapter 51, page 359

      (d) Physical exam should focus on thorough airway and cardiopulmonary evaluation, including carotid auscultation.

   (2) Intraoperative management

      (a) Induction

         (i) Minimize significant hemodynamic swings during induction and direct laryngoscopy.

            1. β-adrenergic antagonists, opioids or lidocaine may blunt tachycardia associated with direct laryngoscopy.

        (ii) A slow, controlled induction is preferred (with or without etomidate) supplemented by pressor support (e.g. phenylephrine) as necessary.

      (iii) If significant cardiac comorbidities or autonomic instability exist, pre-induction invasive arterial monitoring may be necessary to ensure rapid responses to hemodynamic shifts.

      (b) Heart rate is the most significant driver of myocardial O_2 consumption.

         (i) Therefore strict control of heart rate (<80 bpm) is important to preventing transient myocardial ischemia by balancing O_2 supply and demand.

      (c) Blood pressure (BP) should be kept within 20% of baseline mean arterial pressure (MAP) or systolic pressure to prevent further cerebral ischemia.

         (i) The cerebral autoregulation curve is generally shifted to the right; higher MAPs are required to maintain cerebral perfusion.

        (ii) Choice of pressor is based on baseline heart rate and other co-morbid conditions.

      (iii) Note: If these patients have associated elevations in intracranial pressure (ICP), elevated MAPs are required to maintain cerebral perfusion (CPP).

            1. $CPP = MAP - ICP$

      (d) Hypocapnia/hyperventilation should be avoided except to acutely decrease brain swelling.

         (i) May cause cerebral vasculature constriction and contribute to cerebral ischemia.

        (ii) $PaCO_2$ should be kept within 5 mm Hg of the patient's baseline.

            1. This can be determined by comparing the $ETCO_2$ with a $PaCO_2$ from an arterial blood gas.

            2. The $PaCO_2$ gradient will allow the anesthesiologist to optimize ventilation to maintain cerebral perfusion.

READ MORE
Intracranial pressure, Chapter 75, page 528

   (3) Emergence/postoperative management:

      (a) Avoid sympathetic surges (hypertension, tachycardia) associated with emergence by having β-adrenergic antagonists readily available.

      (b) This elevated sympathetic drive may continue into the postoperative period in recovery, and up to 24 hours following the procedure. The perioperative risk for myocardial events and elevated ICP also continues well into this period.

      (c) IV or tracheal lidocaine can be used to blunt the response to extubation.

      (d) Adequate pain control is imperative to blunt sympathetic overdrive.

7) **Cerebellar and basal ganglia diseases: Dementia and cognitive decline**

   a) Dementia and cognitive decline refer to a mixed group of disorders that represent a global decline in cognitive processing, and may result from a global cerebral insult or neurodegenerative process.

      i) Well-known neurodegenerative dementias include Parkinson's and Alzheimer's Disease.

    ii)   Global ischemic or hypoglycemic insults may occur during development (e.g. cerebral palsy) or in adulthood (e.g. following a seizure or secondary to traumatic brain injury).

  b) **Anesthetic management**

    i)   Preoperative

        (1) Document pre-existing neurological and cognitive defects.

        (2) A large subset of these patients are older; a thorough preoperative evaluation to assess for co-morbidities is imperative.

        (3) Familiarize yourself with the patient's targeted medication list; many of the drugs alter cholinergic (e.g. donepezil, a reversible acetylcholinesterase inhibitor) and dopaminergic (L-DOPA) balance.

           (a) Side effects should be anticipated.

           (b) Interactions with anesthetic medications (e.g. neostigmine, metoclopramide) should be considered.

        (4) Regional anesthesia may be preferred in this population (where appropriate) to decrease exposure to general anesthesia (24).

Diphenhydramine and other anticholinergics can be used for decrease of tremor in awake patients with PD, and may ease IV placement if given as preoperative medication.

    ii)   Induction

        (1) Hemodynamic swings to induction and laryngoscopy should be anticipated and managed appropriately (see Cerebral disease: Ischemia).

    iii)   Maintenance/Emergence

        (1) There is increasing evidence that pre-existing cognitive decline may predispose to delayed emergence and postoperative cognitive worsening. This postoperative decline may be irreversible (24).

        (2) One approach is to minimize depth of anesthesia and length of procedure/anesthetic exposure time; the evidence for this approach is suggestive but not conclusive (24).

           (a) The patient should be kept just beyond a level of MAC aware.

           (b) Autonomic responses and pain should be appropriately blunted by pharmacological intervention, judicious use of regional anesthesia, etc.

Patients on L-dopa for PD are at increased risk of catecholamine-induced tachyarrhythmias.

    iv)   Postoperative

        (1) Cognitive engagement/enrichment during this period may hasten recovery and increase the likelihood that the patient will return to their preoperative baseline.

        (2) Restart any critical medications that enhance cognitive performance.

8) **Cerebellar & basal ganglia diseases: Parkinson's Disease**

  a) **Parkinson's Disease (PD)**

    i)   Neurodegenerative disease that causes a relative deficiency of dopamine relative to acetylcholine (ACh) in the basal ganglia. In addition to bradykinetic manifestations, it may also result in dementia (see Cerebral disease: demntial and cognitive decline).

    ii)   Treatment

        (1) Patients are usually on medications that increase dopamine (DA) delivery or prevent its degradation.

        (2) Chronic increase in DA delivery can result in myocardial irritability, decreased intravascular volume, orthostatic hypotension, or nausea and vomiting.

        (3) Anticholinergic therapy may be added to decrease dyskinesias from dopaminergic therapy.

  b) **Anesthetic management**

    i)   Preoperative considerations

(1) Therapeutic agents should be continued through the morning of surgery.

(2) IV access may be more difficult secondary to tremor.

(3) Note baseline neurological defects and any concomitant dementia (see Cerebral disease: dementia and cognitive decline).

ii) Induction

   (1) Hypotension may occur secondary to relative hypovolemia

      (a) Consider fluid-loading prior to giving an induction agent

      (b) Treat with direct-acting pressors (phenylephrine rather than ephedrine).

   (2) Succinylcholine and nondepolarizing neuromuscular blockers are generally considered acceptable.

      (a) If muscle denervation secondary to disuse atrophy is suspected, succinylcholine should be avoided because of the potential for hyperkalemic bradycardia and arrest.

iii) Maintenance/Emergence

   (1) Maintain euvolemia to prevent hypotension.

   (2) Avoid medications that can precipitate extra-pyramidal symptoms:

      (a) Phenothiazines

         (i) chlorpromazine, promethazine

      (b) Butryophenones

         (i) droperidol, haloperiodol

      (c) Benzamides

         (i) Metoclopramide

   (3) There is an increased potential for catecholamine-induced tachyarrhythmias with L-DOPA.

      (a) Use epinephrine with extreme caution in these patients.

      (b) Avoid myocardial irritants or sensitizers (e.g. halothane).

   (4) Although these medications are generally used safely in PD, there are isolated case reports suggesting:

      (a) exaggerated hypertensive responses to ketamine

      (b) increased rigidity to fentanyl and inhaled anesthetics

      (c) increased predisposition toward dyskinesias with high dose morphine).

iv) Postoperative considerations

   (1) Propofol may block PD tremors in the immediate post-operative period.

   (2) Resume the patient's therapeutic medications as soon as possible.

9) Brain death (25–26)

  a) Brian death is defined as the absence of cerebral function (unresponsiveness/coma), absence of brainstem function, and loss of respiratory drive (apnea). Absence of cerebral function (unresponsiveness/coma).

  b) Diagnosis

   i) Two independent exams must be conducted by two physicians at least six hours apart.

   ii) Absence of cerebral function can only be diagnosed when the cause of coma is identified and conditions that mimic brain death have been ruled out.

     (1) Brain death mimicking conditions

       (a) Drug overdose

          (i) Includes drugs of abuse, anesthetic agents, neuromuscular blockers

       (b) Hypothermia

       (c) Locked-in syndrome

       (d) Stroke variants that may prevent a patient from responding

       (e) Shock/hypotension

      (f)   Guillain–Barré syndrome

      (g)   Encephalitis/encephalopathy

  iii) Brainstem reflexes (sequential cranial nerve testing) (Table 76-1)

  iv) Apnea test

     (1) Absence of respiratory drive with a $PaCO_2 \geq 60$ mm Hg or 20 mm Hg above normal baseline (25).

     (2) Connect pulse oximeter.

     (3) Disconnect the patient from the ventilator.

     (4) Deliver apneic oxygenation (6 L/min flow) into trachea.

       (a) Can be done via catheter through the endotracheal tube to the level of the carina.

     (5) Observe for spontaneous ventilation (abdominal, chest excursions).

     (6) A $PaCO_2$ rise of 3 mm Hg/min of apnea is expected.

       (a) Therefore, 8 to 10 minutes is usually sufficient for assessment of the return of respiratory drive.

       (b) Reconnect the patient to the ventilator after obtaining arterial blood gas for assessment of $PaCO_2$, PaO_2, and pH.

  v) Ancillary testing for diagnosing brain death (if complete brainstem evaluation not possible)

     (1) Isoelectric EEG for at least 30 minutes.

     (2) Absence of cerebral perfusion as demonstrated by angiography, T-99 scan, or transcranial Doppler ultrasound (usually of the middle cerebral artery).

     (3) Absence of somatosensory and brainstem auditory evoked potentials.

e) Organ donation (27)

  i) If designated for organ donation, the brain dead patient must be optimally cared for to preserve remaining organ function.

Table 76-1

Criteria for Diagnosis of Brain Death in Adults and Children

Diagnosis	Absence of cerebral function	• Cause for coma must be sought • Conditions mimicking brain death must be ruled-out
	Absence of brainstem reflexes	• Pupillary light response • Corneal, jaw reflex • Oculocephalic reflex (doll's eyes) • Oculovestibular reflex (cold water calorics) • Gag, cough reflex • Sucking, rooting reflex (infants)
	Absence of respiratory drive	• Apnea test: no attempt to breathe at $PaCO_2 \geq 60$ or 20 mm Hg above baseline
Evaluation Interval by Patient Age	• Adult (>18 y) • Child, 1–18 y • Toddler, 2 mo–1 y • Infant, term–2 mo	• 2 exams, usually 6 h apart • 2 exams, 12 h apart • 2 exams, 24 h apart • 2 exams, 48 h apart
Confirmatory Tests	• EEG • Cerebral perfusion testing • Cerebral somatosensory evoked responses • Brainstem auditory evoked responses	• Optional in adults • Required in children

    ii) Brain death is often accompanied by dysautonomia.

       (1) Loss of systemic sympathetic tone and relative or absolute hypovolemia.

       (2) Causes fast deterioration of donor organ viability.

    iii) Perioperative monitoring

       (1) Standard ASA monitors

       (2) Temperature

       (3) Urine output

       (4) Invasive arterial pressure

       (5) Central venous/pulmonary artery pressure

    iv) Physiological goals are geared toward maintaining normal parameters.

       (1) Oxygen saturation 97% to 100%

       (2) HR 60 to 100 beats per minute, sinus rhythm

       (3) MAP 60 to 80 mm Hg

       (4) CVP 8 to 12 mm Hg

       (5) Pulmonary artery wedge 10 to 15 mm Hg

       (6) CI > 2.1 L/min/m²

       (7) Urine output 1 to 2 mL/kg/h

       (8) Volume replacement approximately 50 mL/h > urine output

10) **Summary Considerations**

  a) A systematic approach can assist the anesthesiologist in management of patients with neurological diseases, and can simplify the understanding of how to care for the patient with uncommon nervous system disorders as well.

    i) Which branches of the nervous system are involved: sensory, motor or autonomic? (Table 76-2)

    ii) What treatment or drug therapy is the patient on that can interact with anesthetic management and anesthetic drugs?

    iii) How can baseline nervous system function be preserved?

    iv) How can baseline organ function be preserved?

  b) Disuse atrophy is often overlooked in bed-ridden (e.g. ICU), wheelchair bound, or young, healthy, but casted patients who have been unable to use limbs for longer than 3 days. These conditions predispose toward succinylcholine-induced hyperkalemia and cardiac arrest.

  c) Rigorous documentation of pre-existing deficits and attention to the full risk-benefit discussion with patients must be undertaken.

    i) The decision to use epidural, spinal or nerve block anesthetics should be made on a case-by-case basis.

Table 76-2
Anesthetic Risk Associated with Disorders of the Nervous System

Nervous System Division	Associated Disorders	Anesthetic Risk
Sensory	Includes peripheral nerve disease, myelin disorders, polyneuropathies, cord insult: • Guillain–Barré syndrome (GBS) • Multiple sclerosis (MS) • Lyme disease • Spinal cord injury • Burn injury	• Nerve injury with regional techniques • Increased sensitivity to local anesthetics • Impaired airway reflexes, sensory arc (e.g. gag)

(continued)

Table 76-2
Anesthetic Risk Associated with Disorders of the Nervous System (*Continued*)

Nervous System Division	Associated Disorders	Anesthetic Risk
Motor	Includes myopathies, motor end-plate denervation, motor neuron disorders, spinal motor tract disorders, peripheral nerve disease, polyneuropathies, cord injury: • Amyotrophic lateral sclerosis (ALS) • Spinal muscular atrophy (SMA) • Spinal cord injury • Guillain–Barré syndrome (GBS) • Multiple sclerosis (MS) • Lyme disease • Parkinson disease (PD) • Duchenne muscular dystrophy (DMD) • Trauma • Burn injury • Disuse atrophy	• Aspiration • Respiratory muscle weakness necessitating perioperative ventilatory support • Muscle denervation increasing the risk of hyperkalemic arrest with succinylcholine administration • Impaired airway reflexes, motor arc (e.g. cough)
Autonomic	Includes peripheral nerve disease, myelin disorders, polyneuropathies, cord injury: • Guillain–Barré syndrome (GBS) • Multiple sclerosis (MS) • Lyme disease • Parkinson disease (PD) • Familial dysautonomia • Spinal cord injury (upper thoracic, cervical) • Diabetes • Alcoholism • Burn injury	• Baseline hypotension • Blood pressure lability with absence of appropriate compensatory reflexes • Lack of response to indirect-acting pressors • Increased catecholamine sensitivity • Increased myocardial irritability • Exaggerated responses to fluid shifts (e.g. blood loss) • Exaggerated responses to sympathetic stimulation (e.g. laryngoscopy, surgical stimulation) • Exaggerated responses to changes in intrathoracic pressure (e.g. PEEP, CO_2 insufflation, Trendelenburg position)

Chapter Summary for Anesthesia and Diseases of the Nervous System

General Principles	Neurologic diseases are extremely variable in their presentation and clinical severity
Preoperative	Assess and document degree of neurologic dysfunction Anesthetic plan, including possibility of regional anesthesia, made on a case-by-case basis depending on degree of bulbar involvement, autonomic dysfunction, and sensory/motor deficits
Intraoperative	Succinylcholine usually contraindicated May have hemodynamic instability due to autonomic dysfunction Medications may alter anesthetic drug metabolism Extubation may not be easily achieved if high degree of respiratory muscle involvement
Postoperative	Pain management may be difficult due to co-existing pain issues Neurologic assessment should be performed May require ICU care

References

1. Hayes J, Veyckemans F, Bissonnette B. Duchenne muscular dystrophy: an old anesthesia problem revisited. *Ped Anes* 2008; 18:100–106.
2. Bellinger AM, Reiken S, Carlson C, et al. Hypernitrosylated ryanodine receptor calcium release channels are leaky in dystrophic muscle. *Nat Med* 2009;15(3):325–329.
3. Malignant Hyperthermia Association of the United States, http://www.mhaus.org/index.cfm/fuseaction/Content.Display/PagePK/MedicalFAQs.cfm
4. Gunter, JB, Ball J, Than-Win S. Preparation of the Dräger Fabius Machine for the Malignant Hyperthermia Susceptible Patient. *Anesth Analg* 2008;107(6):1936–1945.
5. Brooks H, Christian AS, May AE. Pregnancy, anaesthesia and Guillain-Barré syndrome. *Anaesthesia* 2000;55(9):894–898.
6. Vassiliev DV, Nystrom EU, Leicht CH. Combined spinal and epidural anesthesia for labor and cesarean delivery in a patient with Guillain-Barré syndrome. *Reg Anesth Pain Med* 2001;26(2):174–176.
7. Alici HA, Cesur M, Erdem AF, et al. Repeated use of epidural anaesthesia for caesarean delivery in a patient with Guillain-Barré syndrome. *Int J Obstet Anesth* 2005;14(3):269–270.
8. Kuczkowski KM. Labor analgesia for the parturient with neurological disease: what does an obstetrician need to know? *Arch Gynecol Obstet* 2006;274(1):41–46.
9. Kocabas S, Karaman S, Firat V, et al. Anesthetic management of Guillain-Barré syndrome in pregnancy. *J Clin Anesth* 2007;19(4):299–302.
10. Dalos NP, Borel C, Hanley DF. Cardiovascular autonomic dysfunction in Guillain-Barré syndrome. Therapeutic implications of Swan-Ganz monitoring. *Arch Neurol* 1988;45(1): 115–117.
11. Tobin M. Advances in Mechanical Ventilation. *NEJM* 2001;344(26):1986–1996.
12. Argyriou AA, Makris N. Multiple Sclerosis and Reproductive Risks in Women. *Reprod Sci* 2008;15(8):755–764.
13. Bader AM, Hunt CO, Datta S, et al. Anesthesia for obstetric patients with multiple sclerosis. *J Clin Anesth* 1988;1:21–24.
14. Blumenthal S, Borgeat A, Maurer K, et al. Preexisting subclinical neuropathy as a risk factor for nerve injury after continuous ropivacaine administration through a femoral nerve catheter. *Anesthesiology* 2006;105:1053–1056.
15. Koff MD, Cohen JA, McIntyre JJ, et al. Severe brachial plexopathy after an ultrasound-guided single-injection nerve block for total shoulder arthroplasty in a patient with multiple sclerosis. *Anesthesiology* 2008;108(2):325–328.
16. Steinman L. Nuanced roles of cytokines in three major human brain disorders. *J Clin Invest* 2008;118(11):3557–3563.
17. Baranov D, Kelton T, McClung H, et al. Neurological Diseases. In: Fleisher LA, ed. Anesthesia and Uncommon Diseases, 5th ed. Saunders Elsevier, Philadelphia 2006: 261–302.
18. Lelovas P, Dontas I, Bassiakou E, et al. Cardiac implications of Lyme disease, diagnosis and therapeutic approach. *Int J Cardiol* 2008;129(1):15–21.
19. Fallon BA, Levin ES, Schweitzer PJ, et al. Inflammation and central nervous system Lyme disease. *Neurobiol Dis* 2010;37:534–541.
20. Halperin JJ, Shapiro ED, Logigian E, et al. Quality Standards Subcommittee of the American Academy of Neurology. Practice parameter: treatment of nervous system Lyme disease (an evidence-based review): report of the Quality Standards Subcommittee of the American Academy of Neurology. *Neurology.* 2007;69(1):91–102.
21. Modica PA, Tempelhoff R, White PF. Pro- and anticonvulsant effects of anesthetics (Part II). *Anesth Analg.* 1990 Apr;70(4):303–444.
22. Tempelhoff R, Modica PA, Bernardo KL, et al. Fentanyl-induced electrocorticographic seizures in patients with complex partial epilepsy. *J Neurosurg* 1992;77(2):201–208.
23. Wang B, Bai, Q, Jiao, X, et al. Effect of sedative and hypnotic doses of propofol on the EEG activity of patients with or without a history of seizure disorders. *J Neurosurg Anesthesiol* 1997;9(4):335–340.
24. Mason SE, Noel-Storr A, Ritchie CW. The impact of general and regional anesthesia on the incidence of post-operative cognitive dysfunction and post-operative delirium: a systematic review with meta-analysis. *J Alzheimers Dis* 2010; 22 Suppl 3: 67–79.
25. Goila AK, Pawar M. The diagnosis of brain death. *Indian J Crit Care Med* 2009;13:7–11.
26. Wijdicks EF. The diagnosis of brain death. *NEJM* 2001; 344(16):1215–1221.
27. Mascia L, Mastromauro I, Viberti S, Vincenzi M, Zanello M. Management to optimize organ procurement in brain dead donors. *Minerva Anestesiol* 2009;75(3):125–133.

Suggested Readings

Gupta AK, Gelb AW, eds. *Essentials of Neuroanesthesia and Neurointensive Care*. Elsevier Saunders; 2008.
Newfield P, Cottrell JE, eds. *Handbook of Neuroanesthesia*. 4th ed. Lippincott Williams & Wilkins; 2006.
Pasternak JJ, Lanier WJ. Diseases affecting the brain. In: Hines RL, Marschall KE, eds. *Stoelting's Anesthesia and Co-Existing Disease*. 5th ed. Churchill Livingstone; 2008:199–238.

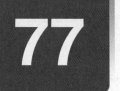

77

Diseases of the Liver and Biliary Tract

Matthew J. Fiegel, MD

Although comprising only 2% of adult body weight, the liver serves many vital functions. Its synthetic and metabolic activities allow for physiologic homeostasis and any disruption results in numerous physiologic derangements. These derangements can be acute or chronic and are best categorized as parenchymal liver disease (including the hepatidides and cirrhosis) and cholestatic disease.

Mortality in cirrhotic patients undergoing non-hepatic surgery can be as high as 80% (1).

1) Functional hepatic anatomy and circulation
  a) **Macroscopic anatomy**
    i) The liver is divided into four anatomic lobes (left, right, caudate, and quadrate).
    ii) The falciform ligament divides the left and right lobes.
    iii) Physiologically, the liver can be divided into eight segments (I to VIII) and each segment is classified according to its blood flow and biliary drainage (2).
  b) **Microscopic anatomy**
    i) Liver acinus is a functional anatomic unit representing the distance of a hepatocyte to a portal triad (hepatic arteriole, portal venule, and bile ductule).
      (1) The acinus possesses three zones.
        (a) Hepatocytes in zone 1 are located closest to the portal triad and receive more blood flow and nutrients.
        (b) Hepatocytes in zone 3 receive less blood flow and are prone to ischemic injury (3).
  c) **Circulation**
    i) The liver receives approximately **20% to 25% of the cardiac output** and possesses 10% to 15% of total blood volume.
      (1) The **proper hepatic artery**, a branch of the celiac axis, provides **25% to 30%** of the liver's blood flow and **50% of its O$_2$ requirements**.
        (a) Hepatic artery flow is regulated by
          (i) α_1, α_2, and β_2 sympathetic nervous system receptors
            1. α_1 Stimulation vasoconstricts the hepatic artery whereas β_2 stimulation vasodilates it (4).
          (ii) Local metabolic factors (adenosine and nitric oxide).
      (2) The **portal vein** (draining the intestines, spleen, pancreas, and stomach) provides **70% to 75%** of the liver's blood flow and **50% of its O$_2$ requirements**.
      (3) Hepatic blood is returned to the inferior vena cava via hepatic veins (4).

2) **Hepatic function**

a) **Protein synthesis and degradation**

i) Hepatocytes synthesize almost all plasma proteins (excluding hemoglobin and gamma globulins).

ii) Through transamination and oxidative deamination, the liver contributes to protein metabolism.

(1) Amino acids are degraded to ammonia, which is eliminated as urea (5).

iii) **Albumin** accounts for 15% of the protein made by the liver and 50% of all circulating proteins.

(1) Albumin binds to drugs, hormones, and bile and dictates plasma oncotic pressure.

iv) α_1-**Acid Glycoprotein** binds amide-type local anesthetics, opioids and propranolol.

v) **Butyrylcholinesterase, or pseudocholinesterase,** is an enzyme which metabolizes succinylcholine and ester-type local anesthetics.

vi) With the exception of factors III (tissue thromboplastin), IV (calcium), and the factor VIII–Von Willebrand complex, all **coagulation factors are synthesized by the liver.**

vii) Fibrinolytic factors such as plasminogen activator inhibitor, protein C, protein S, and antithrombin III are also produced in the liver

(1) **Vitamin K dependent factors include II, VII, IX, X, and proteins C and S (6).**

b) **Carbohydrate metabolism**

i) In the fed state, the liver converts glucose to glycogen.

ii) During starvation, the liver stimulates gluconeogenesis from lactate and amino acid substrates.

iii) **Hepatic glycogen stores can provide glucose for a starvation period of 12 to 24 hours (8).**

c) **Lipid metabolism**

i) When glycogen stores are full, **hepatocytes convert proteins and carbohydrates to fats.**

ii) Other hepatic sources of lipids include plasma lipoproteins, exogenous fatty acids, and cytoplasmic triglycerides.

(a) The acetyl-CoA portion of these lipids produce **ATP, the body's main source of fuel.**

iii) **Cholesterol is formed and metabolized in the liver.**

(1) **Steroid hormones** are a byproduct of cholesterol.

(2) In the presence of hepatic disease, diminished breakdown of **aldosterone** results in sodium retention, hypokalemia, and volume overload.

d) **Bile metabolism**

i) The liver synthesizes 600 to 800 mL of bile per day (9).

ii) Bile salts, the primary component of bile, are chiefly composed of cholesterol and bilirubin.

iii) Bile is stored in the gallbladder and its release is governed by the enzyme cholecystokinin.

iv) Bile carries waste to the intestine and promotes fat micelle formation, which is needed for intestinal uptake of fats (i.e., vitamins A, D, E, and K).

e) **Erythopoesis**

i) **The liver is responsible for 20% of heme production (10).**

Administration of vitamin K to a patient with cirrhosis **does not** improve coagulation (7).

Spider angiomata, testicular atrophy, and gynecomastia are sequelae of chronic liver disease which result from estrogen excess.

Acute intermittent porphyria, is the most common porphyria and presents as abdominal pain and neurologic dysfunction (11).

Thiopental and etomidate are two anesthetic drugs which can porphyria in susceptible individuals.

The liver serves as the main organ of drug metabolism.

  ii) Accumulation of heme substrates from abnormal heme synthesis results in **porphyria.**

  iii) **Hepatocytes convert heme to biliverdin and bilirubin.**

    (1) Albumin binds bilirubin in the plasma.

    (2) The liver extracts bilirubin from the blood and conjugates it with glucuronic acid. It is then secreted as bile into the intestines and excreted in the urine or feces.

3) Endocrine functions of the liver

 a) **Degradation of approximately half of the insulin produced by the pancreas** before it reaches the systemic circulation (12).

 b) **Conversion of thyroxine (T_4) to triiodothryonine (T_3).**

 c) Production of hormones such as angiotensinogen and insulin-like growth factor (6).

 d) Degradation of aldosterone, estrogens, and anti-diuretic hormone.

4) Immune function

 a) **Kupfer cells** filter splanchnic venous blood. These cells scavenge and phagocytize bacteria, protecting the body from systemic bacterial exposure and infection (13).

5) Drug metabolism

 a) **Drug elimination is governed by hepatic blood flow, hepatic clearance, and protein binding.**

  i) The **extraction ratio** measures the liver's ability to eliminate a drug (ER = hepatic clearance/hepatic blood flow).

    (1) Drugs such as propofol, morphine, and metoprolol have a high extraction ratio. They are rapidly metabolized and their elimination is blood flow dependent (14).

  ii) **Conversely, hepatic clearance is the product of hepatic blood flow and extraction ratio.**

    (1) Drugs with a low extraction ratio, such as ethanol, acetaminophen, and anticonvulsants, **are more dependent on hepatic clearance and have a slow metabolism (14).**

 b) Only drugs that are **unbound** to a carrier protein ("free" drug fraction) are clinically active and **undergo metabolism.**

 c) **Drug Metabolism is governed by three hepatic reactions**

  i) **Phase 1 reactions**

    (1) **Utilize the cytochrome P450 family of proteins**

    (2) Consist of oxidation, reduction or hydrolysis

    (3) Resulting metabolites may be clinically active

    (4) Because of the newly acquired polar moiety, these metabolites are more hydrophilic and easily excreted in the urine or bile.

 d) **Phase 2 reactions**

  i) **Drugs undergo conjugation with substances such as glucuronic acid and amino acids.**

  ii) Metabolites are more hydrophilic and readily excreted in the urine or bile.

 e) **Phase 3 reactions**

  i) **Involve elimination reactions**

  ii) Endogenous hepatic proteins utilize ATP to excrete various substances (15).

6) Hepatic pathophysiology

 a) **Acute parenchymal liver disease**

  i) **Most commonly secondary to viral infection but can also be caused by drugs and toxins.**

    (1) **Viral Hepatitis is usually due to Hepatitis A, B, C, D, and E.**

      (a) Traditionally, hepatitis B (HBV) was the most common cause of acute viral hepatitis.

DILI causing an elevation in bilirubin of more than twice the upper limit carries a 10% mortality rate (17).

      (b) With the advent of the HBV vaccine, Hepatitis A and C are accounting for a larger percent of cases worldwide.

    (2) **Cytomegalovirus** and **Epstein-Barr virus** can also cause acute hepatitis (16).

  ii) **Drug-induced liver injury (DILI)** clinically resembles acute viral hepatitis. It is typically idiosyncratic but can be toxic or cholestatic in etiology.

    (1) **The most common causes of DILI are alcohol, antibiotics, and NSAIDs.**

    (2) Other causes include analgesics, volatile anesthetics, antihypertensives, anticonvulsants, statins, and antiretroviral therapy.

    (3) Of note, acetaminophen can cause hepatic dysfunction ranging from acute hepatitis to massive hepatic necrosis and failure

  iii) Symptoms

    (1) Dark urine, fatigue, anorexia, and nausea.

    (2) In some instances, acute hepatitis can progress to hepatic failure requiring transplant.

 b) **Chronic parenchymal liver disease**

  i) **Chronic hepatitis** is defined as elevated liver chemistries and hepatocyte inflammation, for **>6 months**.

  ii) Signs and symptoms

    (1) Fatigue, malaise, jaundice and abdominal pain.

  iii) The most common causes are **HBV and HCV.**

    (1) Chronic hepatitis is seen in approximately 2% to 10% of patients with acute HBV cases and 50% to 85% of HCV cases.

    (2) Other causes include drugs, Wilson Disease, Hemochromatosis, Nonalcoholic steatohepatitis, and α_1-antitrypsin deficiency (16).

 c) **Hepatic cirrhosis**

  i) The most serious sequelae of chronic hepatitis and represents end stage liver disease.

    (1) Histologically characterized by liver fibrosis and parenchymal nodular regeneration.

    (2) HBV, HCV, and alcohol are the most common of cirrhosis causes worldwide (18).

 d) **Cholestatic liver disease**

  i) Signs and symptoms

    (1) Pruritus, hyperbilirubinemia (with jaundice), and right upper quadrant pain.

    (2) A rise in alkaline phosphatase and gamma-glutamyl-transpeptidase are common.

  ii) Although often benign, cholestatic liver disease can progress to liver failure and/or cirrhosis (19).

  iii) **Intrahepatic**

    (1) Causes include drugs, alcoholism, pregnancy, sepsis, primary biliary cirrhosis, and primary sclerosing cholangitis.

  iv) **Extrahepatic**

    (1) Most common cause is cholelithiasis. Other causes include chronic bile duct stricture or bile duct/pancreatic tumor.

7) Perioperative risk assessment in patients with cirrhosis

 a) **Child–Turcotte–Pugh (CTP) score** (Table 77-1)

  i) Places patients in three different classes: A (low risk), B (medium risk), and C (high risk).

Table 77-1
Modified Child-Turcotte-Pugh Score (20)

Presentation	Points		
	1	2	3
Albumin (g/dL)	>3.5	2.8–3.5	<2.8
INR	<1.7	1.7–2.3	>2.3
Bilirubin(mg/dL)	<2	2–3	>3
Ascites	Absent	Moderate	Tense
Encephalopathy	None	Grade I–II	Grade III–IV

Class A, 5 to 6 points; Class B, 7 to 9 points; Class C, 10 to15 points.

Independent risk factors such as emergent surgery, open abdominal procedures, ascites, azotemia, and perioperative infection increase mortality in cirrhotics undergoing surgery (23).

    ii)   Studies have shown one month mortality ranges of 5% to 10%, 14% to 30%, and 51% to 80% for patients undergoing surgery in each respective class.

        (1)   **Non-cardiac elective surgery is not recommended for patients with Class C cirrhosis (21).**

    b)   **The model for end-stage liver disease (MELD) (Table 77-2)**

        i)   Created as a **more objective system** for assessing perioperative risk in cirrhotic patients.

        ii)   The MELD formula is **comprised of INR, total bilirubin, and serum creatinine.**

            (1)   MELD scores of <10, 10 to 14, and >14 correlate well with CTP classes A, B, and C (22).

        iii)   **The MELD score is a superior predictor of surgical risk in patients with cirrhosis.**

    8)   Physiologic derangements of cirrhosis (Table 77-3)

        a)   **Central nervous system (CNS)**

        i)   **Hepatic encephalopathy represents CNS dysfunction**

            (1)   Presentation ranges from confusion to coma and may be secondary to increased dietary protein consumption or GI bleeding.

            (2)   Increased ammonia levels do not correlate **with the degree of encephalopathy.**

            (3)   Treatment is lactulose, rifaximin, or neomycin.

        ii)   Acute liver failure may present with cerebral edema and increased intracranial pressure (23).

Table 77-2
Model for End Stage Liver Disease (21)

MELD score = (0.957 * Ln(Serum Cr) + 0.378 * Ln(Serum Bilirubin) + 1.120 * Ln(INR) + 0.643) * 10

Ln, natural logarithm; INR, international normalized ratio; Cr, creatinine.

Table 77-3

Physiologic Derangements in Patients with Cirrhosis

Organ System	Physiologic Derangement
Central nervous system	Encephalopathy, confusion, coma
Pulmonary	Hypoxemia resulting from atelectasis or HPS; Portopulmonary hypertension
Cardiovascular	Hyperdynamic state/increased cardiac output, decreased SVR, decreased arterial blood volume, decreased response to vasoconstrictors
Gastrointestinal	Portal hypertension with resulting esophagogastric varices, splanchnic hypervolemia
Renal	Renal Hypoperfusion with resulting AKI/acute tubular necrosis, hepatorenal syndrome
Hematologic	Anemia, thrombocytopenia, coagulopathy

HPS, hepatopulmonary syndrome; SVR, systemic vascular resistance; AKI, acute kidney injury.

The **response to vasopressors is decreased** with cirrhosis (26).

Cardiomyo-pathy should always be considered in patients with a history of alcoholic cirrhosis.

b) **Pulmonary**

    i)   Patients may have hypoxemia secondary to atelectasis from ascites/ hydrothorax or **hepatopulmonary syndrome (HPS).**

        (1) HPS is caused by intrapulmonary arteriovenous shunting of blood.

        (2) Clinical features include orthodeoxia and platypnea (24).

    ii) **Portopulmonary hypertension**

        (1) Defined as mean pulmonary artery pressure >25 mm Hg, is seen in 2% to 4% of patients with cirrhosis.

        (2) Severe portopulmonary **hypertension is a contraindication to liver transplantation (25).**

c) **Cardiovascular**

    i)   Patients with cirrhosis may have a hyperdynamic state consisting of **increased cardiac output** and **decreased systemic vascular resistance (SVR).**

    ii) It is postulated that numerous systemic arteriovenous shunts, as well as an increase in endogenous vasodilators, result in the decreased SVR. Cardiac output increases to compensate.

    iii) Patients typically have a low-normal BP.

    iv) Hypoalbuminemia results in decreased plasma oncotic pressure and **decreased effective arterial blood volume** (with increased total body volume).

    v)   Development of portal hypertension leads to splanchnic hypervolemia.

d) **Gastrointestinal**

    i)   Complications result from **portal hypertension (>10 mm Hg)**

        (1) Leads to the development of porto-systemic venous collaterals, including esophagogastric varices.

        (2) Ruptured varices with hemorrhage account for **one third of the mortality** in patients with cirrhosis (27).

         (3)   Treatment of bleeding varices consists of sclerotherapy, endoscopic ligation, β blockade, vasopressin, somatostatin, and transjugular intrahepatic portosystemic shunt (TIPS)

         (4)   Portal hypertension also leads to the development of ascites, splenomegaly, and hemorrhoids.

e) **Renal dysfunction**

    i)   Common in advanced liver disease and is almost always secondary to hypoperfusion.

    ii)   It manifests as either acute kidney injury or hepatorenal syndrome (HRS)

    iii) **Acute kidney injury (AKI)**

         (1)   Due to decreased blood flow to the kidneys

         (2)   May be caused by hemorrhage (ruptured varices), splanchnic sequestration of blood, ascites formation, or dehydration.

         (3)   Restoring intravascular volume typically corrects AKI but it can progress to acute tubular necrosis.

    iv) **Hepatorenal syndrome (HRS)** is seen with cirrhosis and portal hypertension.

         (1)   Although unknown, the etiology is thought to be renal hypoperfusion from a decrease in vasodilating prostaglandins or profound splanchnic sequestration of blood.

         (2)   HRS is defined as a **plasma creatinine >1.5 mg/dL in the absence of other causes of renal disease.**

         (3)   Type I HRS progresses rapidly and **requires hemodialysis and liver transplantation.**

         (4)   Type II HRS is more stable and responsive to conservative treatments, including terlipressin, midodrine, and TIPS procedure (22).

f) **Hematologic dysfunction**

    i)   **Anemia**

         (1)   May be secondary to bleeding, malnutrition, or bone marrow suppression.

    ii)   **Thrombocytopenia**

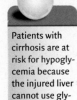

Patients with cirrhosis are at risk for hypoglycemia because the injured liver cannot use glycogen stores to create glucose.

         (1)   Caused by splenic sequestration, bone marrow depression, and immune-mediated destruction.

    iii) Coagulopathy

         (1)   Due to decreased synthesis of vitamin K dependent clotting factors and accelerated fibrinolysis.

         (2)   Cirrhotics often present with chronic disseminated intravascular coagulation.

g) **Metabolic abnormalities**

    i)   Include susceptibility to hypoglycemia and hyponatremia.

    ii)   Hyponatremia is typically dilutional and is treated with volume restriction.

9) Anesthetic implications of liver disease

a) **Preoperative considerations**

    i)   Due to the high perioperative morbidity and mortality associated with liver disease, a thorough preoperative evaluation is necessary.

    ii)   Assessment of the type of liver disease and preoperative fluid and coagulation optimization may improve postoperative outcome.

    iii) **Identification of risk factors**

         (1)   History of blood transfusions, IV drug abuse, sexual promiscuity, alcoholism, and a family history of liver disease should increase your suspicion for liver disease.

         (2)   **History** of jaundice, pruritis, and anorexia may indicate liver dysfunction.

iv) **Physical exam** may yield stigmata of chronic liver disease including ascites, hepatosplenomegaly, caput medusae, spider angiomata, and gynecomastia.

b) **Determine the type and severity of liver disease**

 i) Patients with acute hepatitis or Child type C (MELD > 15) cirrhosis **should have elective surgeries cancelled** due to increased mortality (26).

 ii) **Child's class A (MELD < 10) cirrhotics can safely undergo elective surgery.**

 iii) Patients requiring emergency surgery should be warned of their high perioperative risk of morbidity and mortality.

c) **Organ system review** should be performed specifically looking for encephalopathy, ascites, portal hypertension, and renal insufficiency.

d) **A complete laboratory evaluation** should be performed.

Intraoperative hypoxemia, hemorrhage, and hypotension in a patient with liver disease may further reduce hepatic blood flow.

 i) Elevation of aminotransferases (AST and ALT) **reflects hepatocellular injury.**

 ii) Increased serum bilirubin indicates decreased hepatic excretory function, increased hemolysis, or hepatocellular injury.

 iii) Elevated INR or decreased serum albumin reflects **decreased hepatic synthetic capacity.**

e) **Correct coagulopathy, volume status, and electrolyte imbalances** prior to surgery if possible

 i) Fresh frozen plasma and platelet concentrates may be required.

 ii) For major surgery, an INR of <1.5, a platelet count of >100×10^9, and fibrinogen >100 mg/dL is preferred (26).

 iii) A thromboelastogram may help to guide component therapy.

 iv) Hyponatremia should be corrected **slowly** with an increase of **no more than 8 meq in 24 hours.**

f) **Operating room preparations**

 i) Include transducers for invasive monitoring, a fluid warming/rapid infusion device, and increased room temperature.

10) **Intraoperative considerations**

a) Management goals include preserving hepatic blood flow and existing hepatic function.

b) Regional anesthesia is a good option if coagulopathy is not present.

c) Drug selection and dosing

Cisatracurium and atracurium are the neuromuscular blockers of choice for patients with liver disease due to their organ-independent elimination.

 i) **IV induction agents**

 (1) Have a modest effect on hepatic blood flow.

 (2) Thiopental and etomidate decrease hepatic blood flow

 (3) Propofol and ketamine increase blood hepatic blood flow.

 (4) Awakening from short acting induction agents is not prolonged by liver disease, likely due to redistribution and a larger volume of distribution.

 (5) **Hypoalbuminemia can cause an exaggerated induction response with both etomidate and thiopental.**

 (6) Propofol, etomidate, and ketamine possess a high hepatic extraction ratio, and their pharmacokinetic profile is relatively unchanged in mild to moderate cirrhosis.

 ii) **Neuromuscular blocking agents (NMBs)**

 (1) Should be titrated and monitored appropriately.

 (2) Although pseudocholinesterase levels may be decreased, **clinical prolongation of succinylcholine is not significant.**

All benzodiazepines should be dosed cautiously in patients with liver disease due to the potential for worsening pre-existing encephalopathy.

(3) Succinylcholine is the neuromuscular blocking induction agent of choice as patients are at risk for aspiration and rapid sequence induction is indicated.

(4) Intermediate acting non-depolarizing agents, such as rocuronium and vecuronium, **have a prolonged effect in the presence of liver disease**, which is accentuated with repeated dosing.

(5) Benzyl isoquinoline neuromuscular blockers, such as atracurium and cisatracurium, undergo organ-independent elimination via ester hydrolysis and Hoffman degradation.

iii) Volatile anesthetics

(1) **The newer volatile anesthetics do not significantly alter hepatic blood flow or oxygenation.**

(2) At levels below 1 MAC, limited human data suggests that sevoflurane, desflurane, and isoflurane minimally decrease hepatic blood flow and undergo minimal hepatic metabolism (<2%) with no significant clinical sequelae.

iv) Other commonly used medications

(1) **Benzodiazepines**

(a) Midazolam and Diazepam are metabolized by phase I oxidative reactions and have a prolonged duration of action.

(b) Lorazepam is cleared by phase II reactions via glucuronidation and undergoes normal metabolism.

Fentanyl and remifentanil are the opioids of choice in patients with liver disease.

(2) **Opioids**

(a) Metabolism is decreased in liver disease.

(b) Morphine and meperidine have a prolonged half-life and can precipitate hepatic encephalopathy.

(c) Fentanyl, although completely metabolized by the liver, does not show a prolonged effect in cirrhosis.

(d) Remifentanil, metabolized solely by blood esterases, is not affected by liver disease.

(e) All opioid agonists can increase sphincter of oddi pressure

(i) Agonist/antagonists (nalbuphine, tramadol) seem to have less of an effect.

(3) **Intravascular volume status**

(a) Can be very difficult to assess in patients with liver disease as they are usually "arterially underfilled" and clinically hypovolemic.

(b) Arterial blood volume should be monitored via arterial pH, urine output, and central venous pressure.

(c) A transesophageal echocardiogram may also be useful, but one must be cautious with varices.

d) **Postoperative considerations**

i) **Postoperative liver dysfunction** is common in patients with liver disease.

(1) With mild disease, the dysfunction may be limited to elevation of transaminases or postoperative jaundice.

(2) In patients with class C (MELD >14) cirrhosis, 1 month mortality ranges from 60% to 100%.

(3) The most common postoperative complications **include new onset ascites, volume overload, worsening hepatic encephalopathy, upper gastrointestinal hemorrhage, sepsis, renal failure, and decreased liver function with coagulopathy.**

(4) Poor outcomes are common in emergency or major surgery especially with coexisting renal failure.

(5) **Preoperative jaundice** is a risk factor for postoperative renal failure.

ii) **Manifestations of alcohol withdrawal should be monitored for 48 to 72 hours in patients with suspected alcohol abuse**

iii) All postoperative patients with preexisting liver disease should be monitored closely for 24 hours in a step down or ICU setting as morbidity and mortality is extremely high.

Chapter Summary for the Patient with Liver Disease

Preoperative Evaluation	Assessment and optimization of coagulation, electrolyte, and intravascular volume status, correct INR to <1.5 and platelet count to >100 × 10⁹, warm room and fluids, warn patient of high perioperative risk
Induction of Anesthesia	RSI with succinylcholine for presumed full stomach, expect exaggerated desaturation due to decreased FRC from ascites, minimize preoperative benzodiazepines, use short acting induction agents (propofol)
Maintenance of Anesthesia	Maintain hepatic/renal blood flow, atracurium, and cisatracurium are the NMBs of choice, volatile anesthetics at <1 MAC, use short acting opioids (fentanyl and remifentanil), invasive monitoring may be used to assess/restore intravascular volume, acid/base, and electrolyte status
Postoperative Concerns	Monitor closely in a stepdown/ICU setting for signs of volume overload, worsening renal/liver dysfunction, sepsis, encephalopathy

FRC, functional residual capacity; ICU, intensive care unit; INR, international normalized ratio; MAC, minimum alveolar concentration; NMB, neuromuscular blocking drugs; RSI, rapid sequence induction.

References

1. Mansour A. Watson W. Shayani V, et al. Abdominal operations in patients with cirrhosis: Still a major surgical challenge. *Surgery* 1997;22: 730–736.
2. Gazelle GS, Lee MJ, Muelle PR. Cholangiographic segmental anatomy of the liver. *Radiographics* 1994;14(5):1005–1013.
3. Jones AL. Anatomy of the normal liver. In: Zakim D, Boyer T, eds. *Hepatology: A Textbook of Liver Disease.* 3rd ed. Philadelphia, PA: WB Saunders; 1996:3–32.
4. Mushlin P, Gelman S. Hepatic physiology and pathophysiology. In: Miller R, ed. *Miller's Anesthesia.* 6th ed. Philadelphia, PA: Elsevier; 2005:743–775.
5. Jalan R, Hayes PC. Hepatic encephalopathy and ascites. *Lancet* 1997;350(9087):1309–1315.
6. Fitz JG. Hepatic encephalopathy, hepatopulmonary syndromes, hepatorenal syndrome, coagulopathy, and endocrine complications of liver disease. In; Feldman M, Friedman LS, Sleisenger MH, eds. *Sleisenger and Fordtran's Gastrointestinal and Liver Disease: Pathophysiology/ Diagnosis/ Management.* 7th ed. St. Louis, MO: WB Saunders; 2002:1543–1567.
7. Otero Fernández MA, Romero-Gómez M, Martínez Delgado C, et al. Usefulness of vitamin K in cirrhosis. *Aten Primaria* 1999;24:242–243.
8. Zakim D. Metabolism of glucose and fatty acids by the liver. In: Zakim D, Boyer TD, eds. *Hepatology: A Textbook of Liver Disease.* 3rd ed. Philadelphia, PA: WB Saunders; 1996:58–92.
9. Fitz JG. Cellular mechanisms of bile secretion. In: Zakim D, Boyer TD, eds, *Hepatology: A Textbook of Liver Disease.* 3rd ed. Philadelphia, PA: WB Saunders; 1996:362–376.
10. Fujita H. Molecular mechanism of heme biosynthesis. *Tohoku J Exp Med* 1997;183(2):83–99.
11. Stoelting R. Dierdorf S. *Anesthesia and Coexisting Disease.* 4th ed. Philadelphia, PA: Churchill Livingstone; 2002:456.
12. Rojdmark S, Bloom G. Hepatic extraction of exogenous insulin and glucagon in the dog. *Endocrinology* 1978;102(3):806–813.
13. Laskin DL. Nonparenchymal cells and hepatotoxicity. *Semin Liver Dis* 1990;10(4):293–304.
14. Adedoyin A. Branch RA. Pharmacokinetics. In: Zakim D, Boyer T, eds. *Hepatology: A Textbook of Liver Disease.* 3rd ed. Philadelphia, PA: WB Saunders; 1996:3–32.
15. Estabrook R. An introduction to the cytochrome P450. *Mol Aspects Med* 1999;20(1–2):5–137.
16. Stoelting R, Dierdorf S. *Anesthesia and Coexisting Disease.* 4th ed. Philadelphia, PA: Churchill Livingstone; 2002:299–323.

17. Hussaini SH. Farrington EA. Idiosyncratic drug-induced liver injury: an overview. *Expert Opin Drug Saf* 2007;6(6):673–684.
18. Quinn P. Johnston D. Detection of chronic liver disease: costs and benefits. *Gastroenterologist* 1997;5(1):58–77.
19. Elferink RO. Cholestasis. *Gut* 2003;52(2):ii42–ii48.
20. Barash P, Cullen B, Stoelting R. *Clinical Anesthesia.* 5th ed. Philadelphia, PA: Lippincott Williams & Wilkins; 2006:1103.
21. Befeler A. Palmer D. The safety of intra-abdominal surgery in patients with cirrhosis. *Arch Surg* 2005;140(7):650–654.
22. Farnsworth B. Fagan S. Child-Turcotte-Pugh versus MELD score as a predictor of outcome after elective and emergent surgery in cirrhotic patients. American Journal of Surgery 2004; 188(5): 580–583.
23. Millwala F, Nguyen GC. Outcomes of patients with cirrhosis undergoing non-hepatic surgery: risk assessment and management. *World J Gastroenterol* 2007;13(30):4056–4063.
24. Rakela J, Krowka MJ. Cardiovascular and pulmonary complications of liver disease. In: Zakim D, Boyer TD, eds. *Hepatology: A Textbook of Liver Disease.* 3rd ed. Philadelphia, PA: WB Saunders; 1996:58–92.
25. Castro M. Krowka MJ. Frequency and clinical implications of increased pulmonary artery pressures in liver transplant patients. *Mayo Clin Proc* 1996;71(6):543–551.
26. Ziser A. Plevak D. Morbidity and mortality in cirrhotic patients undergoing anesthesia and surgery. *Curr Opin Anaesthesiol* 2001;14(6):707–711.
27. de Franchis R. Primignani M. Natural history of portal hypertension in patients with cirrhosis. *Clin Liver Dis* 2001;5(3):645–663.

The gastrointestinal (GI) tract's main function is to absorb water, electrolytes, and nutrients. Derangement can adversely affect many other organ systems. It is the responsibility of the anesthesiologist to ensure preoperative optimization of fluids, electrolytes, and nutrition. One must also search for other organ involvement (e.g., anemia from B12 deficiency) and treat these systems accordingly. Intraoperatively, manipulation of the GI tract can lead to bacteremia and sepsis. This should always be anticipated and treated as necessary with volume, antibiotics, and vasopressive agents.

I) **Esophageal diseases**

  a) **Gastroesophageal reflux disease (GERD)**

    i) **Pathophysiology**

      (1) Risk factors for GERD and/or delayed gastric emptying include:

        (a) Obesity

        (b) Diabetes

        (c) Obstructive sleep apnea

        (d) Collagen vascular diseases

      (2) Patients with GERD are at risk for aspiration of gastric contents upon induction of anesthesia.

        (a) May result in a life-threatening aspiration pneumonitis.

    ii) GERD is one of the more common problems anesthesiologists encounter.

      (1) Increasing in frequency due to the rise in obesity.

    iii) Signs and Symptoms

      (1) Dysphagia

      (2) Retrosternal pain

      (3) Acidic taste

    iv) **Pharmacologic treatment**

      (1) Of the protective medications, proton pump inhibitors (PPIs) appear to raise gastric pH the most (1).

        (a) Allow 45 to 60 minutes for full onset of action.

      (2) Metoclopromide, H_2 blockers, and oral antacids may also be implemented.

    v) **Perioperative considerations**

      (1) Preoperative considerations

        (a) Because no good evidence-based therapy exists, treatment and prophylaxis should be according to the judgment of the clinician.

        (b) **Measures which lessen the likelihood of significant aspiration include:**

          (i) Removal of gastric contents

Approximately 25 mL of a gastric aspirate with a pH of 2.5 or 50 mL of a gastric aspirate with a pH of 3.5 is necessary to cause clinically significant chemical pneumonitis.

        (ii) Cricoid pressure

        (iii) Proper starvation status

        (iv) Head-up position

    (c) The ASA **does not recommend** preoperative treatment with an antireflux medication as the evidence is equivocal (1).

    (d) Patients on chronic antireflux therapy should take their medication the day of surgery.

  (2) Intraoperative considerations

    (a) No clear cut recommendations exist on which patient population should undergo rapid sequence induction (RSI).

        (i) Each clinician should use his/her best judgment.

    (b) Patients at high risk for pulmonary aspiration include:

        (i) **Full stomach by nil per os (NPO) guidelines**

        (ii) **Bowel obstruction**

        (iii) **Multiple risk factors for delayed gastric emptying listed above**

        (iv) Patients at high risk for aspiration should always be considered for RSI with succinylcholine or high dose rocuronium.

        (v) **Succinylcholine is not contraindicated.** It increases **both** intragastric and lower esophageal sphincter pressure (2).

  (3) Postoperative considerations

    (a) Patients at risk for aspiration on induction are still at risk for aspiration with emergence and should be treated with caution.

    (b) Awake extubation with intact airway reflexes is recommended.

2) **Diffuse esophageal spasm**

  a) Esophageal spasm does not present many anesthetic-related concerns.

  b) It can mimic angina and must therefore be considered in a patient with chest pain in the perioperative setting.

3) **Esophageal bleeding**

  a) **Causes**

    i) Esophageal varices

    ii) Mallory–Weiss tears

    iii) Erosive esophagitis

  b) Esophageal varices

    i) Result from portal hypertension

    ii) Varices may be treated medically

        (1) Vasopressin or octreotide are common medications for treatment of varices

        (2) Sclerotherapy

        (3) Transjugular intrahepatic portosystemic shunt procedure.

        (4) Surgical treatment includes banding

  c) **Perioperative considerations**

    i) If a patient is presenting for control of active bleeding, resuscitation should be anticipated.

    ii) The airway will need to be secured with endotracheal intubation.

    iii) Adequate IV access should be obtained and blood products should be available.

    iv) If varices are chronic and stable, manipulation of the esophagus should be kept to a minimum.

        (1) Placement of an oro/nasogastric tube as well as a transesophageal echocardiogram should be done with caution.

4) **Peptic ulcer disease (PUD)**

  a) Pathophysiology

    i) PUD is seen in approximately 10% of men and 4% of women (3).

      ii) Represented by focal ulceration in the esophagus, stomach, or duodenum.

      iii) Causes of ulcers include:

          (1) Helicobacter pylori (H. pylori)

          (2) Non-steroidal anti-inflammatory drugs (NSAIDs)

          (3) Stress

          (4) Excessive gastrin secretion (Zollinger–Ellison disease)

      iv) Smoking and steroid use are also implicated in the development of PUD.

  b) **Chronic ulcer disease**

    i) **Does not warrant any major anesthetic alterations**

    ii) Treatment includes:

        (1) Eradication of H. Pylori

        (2) PPIs

        (3) H_2 receptor antagonists

        (4) Cessation of offending agents

  c) **Acute bleeding ulcers**

    i) As with esophageal variceal bleeding, resuscitation must be anticipated.

        (1) Adequate IV access should be obtained.

        (2) Volume should be replaced in the form of crystalloid, colloid, or blood.

    ii) Intraoperative considerations

        (1) Airway management

           (a) If the patient is unable to maintain his/her airway, a RSI and intubation should be performed.

        (2) After assessment of volume status and airway stability, endoscopy should be performed to treat the bleeding.

        (3) Consider a PPI infusion as it may decreases the risk of recurrent bleeding.

  d) Perforated ulcers

    i) **Typically secondary** to NSAID use or cancer

    ii) Signs and symptoms

        (1) **Present as fever, abdominal pain, and free air on imaging.**

        (2) Patients can deteriorate quickly.

    iii) 30-day mortality is approximately 10%

        (1) However, **it can be as high as 38% in patients with advanced age, multi-organ failure, and prolonged, diffuse peritonitis (4).**

    iv) Perioperative considerations

        (1) Electrolyte and volume status should be corrected prior to surgery.

        (2) Vasopressive agents may be necessary if peritonitis and sepsis are present.

        (3) Broad spectrum antibiotics should be initiated.

5) **Zollinger-Ellison (ZE) syndrome**

  a) **Causes and pathophysiology**

    i) Patients have duodenal ulcers resulting from a gastrinoma.

        (1) Usually treated with PPIs and H_2 blockers.

    ii) Although not usually an acute process, ZE syndrome sometimes necessitates surgery.

  b) **Perioperative considerations**

    i) Preoperative liver function tests and electrolytes should be obtained.

    ii) Malabsorption may be present

        (1) Results from secretion of large volumes of gastric fluid.

        (2) Can influence clotting factors and electrolytes (5).

    iii) Preoperative nasogastric tube is often necessary to remove these large gastric volumes.

    iv) All patients should undergo a RSI

6) **Inflammatory Bowel disease (IBD)**
   a) The IBDs, Crohn's disease and ulcerative colitis (UC), are the second most common inflammatory disease in the body.
   b) Both are autoimmune mediated and therefore may affect many different organ systems.
   c) **Crohn's disease**
      i) Can affect the entire GI tract but is typically confined to the ileum and colon.
      ii) Chronic disease results in rectal fissures, fistulas, and abscesses.
      iii) Anemia, with accompanying malnutrition, is often present.
      iv) Immunosuppressive treatments
         (1) Includes steroids and anti tumor necrosis factor antibodies.
      v) Patients often require total parenteral nutrition and bowel rest to treat the fistulas.
         (1) If drug therapy fails, then surgery is required (6).
   d) **Ulcerative colitis**
      i) Signs and symptoms
         (1) Presents as intermittent diarrhea and is confined to the colon.
         (2) Can progress to toxic megacolon, bowel stricture/perforation and colon cancer.
         (3) Extraintestinal manifestations
            (a) **Iritis**
            (b) **Ankylosing arthritis**
            (c) **Primary sclerosing cholangitis (PSC)**
         (4) If PSC is present, patients typically develop cirrhosis of the liver.
      ii) Treatment
         (1) Initial treatment consists of sulfasalazine and mesalamine.
         (2) If these are ineffective, more potent immunomodulating agents may be necessary.
            (a) Steroids, anti tumor necrosis factor antibodies, and cyclosporine.
         (3) Patients require surveillance colonoscopies and often a colectomy for prevention/treatment of colon cancer (6).
   e) **Anesthetic management of patients with IBD**
      i) **Preoperative considerations**
         (1) Assess **volume and electrolyte status**
         (2) Determine the **extent of the extraintestinal manifestations**
         (3) If cirrhosis is present from PSC/UC, blood products and adequate IV access should be made available.
      ii) **Intraoperative considerations**
         (1) RSI should be considered in anyone with obstruction from the IBD.
         (2) The choice of muscle relaxant may be influenced by the presence of liver disease.
         (3) If ankylosing spondylitis is present, a fiberoptic intubation may be necessary.
         (4) Stress dose steroids may be required in patients with long term use.
         (5) Avoidance of nitrous oxide is prudent as it may distend an already scarred bowel lumen.
7) **Carcinoid tumors**
   a) **Pathophysiology**
      i) Carcinoid tumors arise from enterochromaffin cells and reside in the GI tract 75% of the time.

READ MORE

Arthritis, Chapter 92, page 663

Diseases of the liver and biliary tract, Chapter 77, page 551

      (1)   The most common location for benign tumors is the appendix.

      (2)   The ileum and cecum are the most common sites for malignant tumors.

  ii) Cells of these tumors secrete a variety of vasoactive hormones including:

      (1)   **Serotonin**

      (2)   **Histamine**

      (3)   **Bradykinin**

      (4)   **Prostaglandins (7)**

b) **Carcinoid syndrome**

  i) Results from metastasis of the tumor to the liver.

  ii) The affected liver cannot metabolize the secreted hormones and carcinoid syndrome ensues.

      (1)   Although most tumors secrete hormones, only about 7% to 18% of people with these tumors develop carcinoid syndrome.

  iii) Signs and symptoms

      (1)   **Cutaneous flushing**

      (2)   **Diarrhea**

      (3)   **Right sided cardiac symptoms**

         (a)   Tricuspid and pulmonic valve dysfunction

      (4)   **Bronchoconstriction and hypotension** may also be present (7).

  iv) Treatment

      (1)   The mainstay treatment of carcinoid disease is the somatostatin analogue **octreotide** (sandostatin) (5,7).

         (a)   Inhibits release of the vasoactive hormones from the tumor.

         (b)   Dosing ranges from 50 to 100 µg two to three times daily.

         (c)   A long acting depot formulation also exists.

c) **Perioperative considerations**

  i) **Preoperative considerations**

      (1)   **Extraintestinal manifestations should be evaluated.**

      (2)   A preoperative echocardiogram may diagnose right sided heart disease (8).

      (3)   Patients should be on octreotide before surgery.

  ii) **Intraoperative considerations**

      (1)   Octreotide should be available for potential intraoperative release of hormones.

      (2)   If refractory hypotension ensues, vasopressin should be used.

      (3)   Steroids and H_2 blockers have both been studied in carcinoid disease.

         (a)   However, neither has been shown to be effective in decreasing any of the carcinoid symptoms (7).

8) **Pancreatic disease**

a) **Acute pancreatitis**

  i) Defined as inflammation of the pancreas

  ii) **Pathophysiology**

      (1)   Gallstones obstructing the ampulla of Vater or alcohol consumption (70% of cases) (9).

      (2)   May also be secondary to trauma, hypercalcemia, or an endoscopic retrograde cholangiopancreatography (10).

  iii) Signs and symptoms

      (1)   Patients present with nausea, vomiting, fever, and abdominal pain.

      (2)   Can progress to systemic inflammatory response syndrome/shock, acute respiratory distress disease (ARDS), acute kidney injury (AKI), and pancreatic infection.

Patients with acute pancreatitis may become critically ill very quickly and require ICU care.

iv) Treatment

    (1) In the acute form of the disease, cessation of the offending agent will allow the pancreas to return to its normal function.

    (2) Supportive care includes NPO status, IV hydration, occasional antibiotics, cessation of alcohol, and/or removal of gallstones.

    (3) Surgery is only required if infection is confirmed.

v) **Perioperative considerations**

    (1) When surgery is required, the anesthesiologist must **assess the degree of organ dysfunction and treat accordingly.**

        (a) Vasopressive medications and fluids may be necessary for septic shock.

        (b) Lung protective ventilation strategies and/or an ICU ventilator may be necessary for ARDS.

        (c) Meticulous volume management and/or hemodialysis may be necessary for AKI.

        (d) Coagulation status should be assessed as pancreatitis can progress to disseminated intravascular coagulation.

b) **Chronic pancreatitis**

i) Defined as repeated injury to the pancreas resulting in loss of normal function.

ii) Chronic pancreatitis is almost always secondary to alcohol use (10)

iii) Signs and symptoms

    (1) Loss of exocrine function leads to lack of digestive enzymes and chronic malabsorption.

    (2) Loss of endocrine function can lead to diabetes.

    (3) Chronic pain is often present.

iv) **Perioperative considerations**

    (1) If a patient with chronic pancreatitis presents for surgery, **volume, coagulation, metabolic, and electrolyte status should be evaluated.**

    (2) A perioperative, **multimodal plan for pain control** should be instituted as these patients are often taking large amounts of opioids.

9) **Diverticular and appendiceal disease**

a) **Diverticulosis**

i) Causes

    (1) Diverticulosis results from herniations through the colonic muscular layer.

    (2) Patients who consume low-fiber diets are at highest risk.

ii) Signs and symptoms

    (1) Are infrequent but can include abdominal pain and lower GI bleeding.

iii) Perioperative considerations

    (1) If surgery is required to control bleeding, preoperative volume status should be assessed.

    (2) Adequate IV access is necessary and blood should be available.

b) **Diverticulitis**

i) Approximately 10% to 25% of patients with diverticulosis progress to diverticulitis (11).

ii) Signs and symptoms

    (1) Patients present with fever, nausea, vomiting, and right-sided abdominal pain.

Approximately 10% to 20% of the population older than 50 years of age are known to be affected by diverticular disease (11).

Duodenal ulcers are responsible for the majority of upper GI bleeding, diverticuli are responsible for the majority of lower GI blood loss.

(2) Abscess and fistula formation may necessitate surgical intervention.

iii) Perioperative considerations

(1) RSI should be considered.

(2) Patients are at high risk for sepsis so invasive hemodynamic monitoring and vasopressor therapy should be considered.

c) **Appendicitis**

i) Often mimicking diverticulitis, inflammation of the appendix occurs in 7% to 9% of the population during their lifetime (11).

ii) Signs and symptoms

(1) Patients present with anorexia, fever, and periumbilical/right lower quadrant pain.

(2) If the patient is febrile, appendiceal rupture with peritonitis should be suspected.

(3) Surgical removal is often necessary.

iii) **Perioperative considerations**

(1) RSI should be considered.

(2) Vital signs should be monitored for signs of sepsis or hemodynamic instability.

Chapter Summary for Diseases of the GI System

Definition	Diseases of the GI tract are varied and include esophageal, stomach, pancreatic, intestinal, and appendiceal processes.	
GI Diseases	Esophageal	GERD, Esophageal spasm, and esophageal bleeding
	Stomach	Bleeding/perforated peptic ulcers and Zollinger–Ellison syndrome
	Pancreatic	Acute and chronic pancreatitis
	Intestinal	IBD, diverticular disease, and carcinoid Syndrome
	Appendix	Acute appendicitis
Anesthetic Implications	The anesthetic implications of almost every GI process include assessment of the nutrition, volume, electrolyte, and hemodynamic status	

GERD, gastroesophageal reflux disease; GI, gastrointestinal; IBD, inflammatory bowel disease.

References

1. Practice Guidelines for preoperative fasting and the use of pharmacologic agents to reduce the risk of pulmonary aspiration: Application to healthy patients undergoing elective procedures. A report by the American Society of Anesthesiologists Task Force of Preoperative Fasting. *Anesthesiology* 1999;90:896.
2. Stoelting R, Dierdorf S. *Anesthesia and Coexisting Disease*. 4th ed. Philadelphia, PA: Churchill Livingstone; 2002:326.
3. Feldman M. Peptic ulcer diseases. *Sci Am Med* 2000;5:1–13.
4. Lohsiriwat V, Prapasrivorakul S. Perforated peptic ulcer: clinical presentation, surgical outcomes, and the accuracy of the boey scoring system in predicting postoperative morbidity and mortality. *World J Surg* 2009;33(1):80–85.
5. Holdcroft A. Hormones and the gut. *Br J Anaesth* 2000;85:58–68.
6. Hanauer SB. Inflammatory bowel disease. *N Engl J Med* 1996; 334: 841–848.
7. Kulke MH. Mayer RJ. Carcinoid tumors. *N Engl J Med* 1999;340:858–868.
8. Botero M, Fuchs R. Carcinoid heart disease: A case report and literature review. *J Clin Anesth* 2002;14:57–63.
9. Steinberg W, Tenner S. Acute pancreatitis. *N Engl J Med* 1994;330:1198–1210.
10. Young HS. Diseases of the pancreas. *Sci Am Med* 1997;7:1–16.
11. Harford WV. Diverticulosis, diverticulitis, and appendicitis. *Sci Am Med* 1998;2:1–8.

79 Kidney Disease

John Sang Lee, MD • Binbin Wang, MD

The kidneys perform the major functions of **volume regulation, electrolyte homeostasis, and toxin excretion**, along with the production of hormones involved in blood pressure regulation (renin) and red blood cell production (erythropoietin). Despite being 0.5% of the body weight, the kidneys normally receive 20% to 25% of the cardiac output. Renal blood flow is normally **autoregulated between mean arterial pressures of 60 to 150 mm Hg (1)**.

The nomenclature to describe kidney diseases has recently been updated.

Diabetes is the leading cause of CKD in the United States.

1) Nomenclature update
   a) Suggested by international panel of nephrologists and intensivists.
   b) Acute renal failure => Acute kidney injury **(AKI)**
   c) Chronic renal failure => Chronic kidney disease **(CKD)**
   d) The nomenclature has been modified to ensure more accurate definition of kidney injury, better predictive measures of mortality, and recognition of early kidney injury before onset of failure (2).
   e) The nomenclature AKI and CKD will be used in this chapter.

2) Epidemiology
   a) Perioperative acute kidney failure (AKF) accounts for one-half of cases of acute hemodialysis (HD) in the United States (3).
   b) Kidney disease is the ninth leading cause of death in the United States.

3) Pathophysiology
   a) Renal dysfunction can be categorized by the glomerular filtration rate (GFR) and the rapidity of onset.
   b) GFR is the volume of fluid filtered from the renal glomerular capillaries per unit time.
      i) Varies with age, sex, and body size, and declines with age.
      ii) GFR ≥ 40% of normal is usually asymptomatic.
      iii) **GFR between 10% to 40% of normal.**
         (1) May not require HD, but are **more likely to sustain nephrotoxic insults (4)**.
      iv) **GFR < 10% of normal is associated with end-stage renal disease (ESRD).**
         (1) Uremic toxins accumulate and **HD is usually required.**
   c) **AKI versus CKD**
      i) Acute kidney injury
         (1) Rapid progressive loss of kidney function, characterized by:
            (a) **Oliguria** of less than 400 mL/day in adults.
            (b) **Retention of waste products,** such as **hydrogen ions, potassium, and nitrogenous compounds.**
      ii) Chronic kidney injury
         (1) Slow progression of disease resulting in **irreversible AKI or chronic worsening of underlying disease.**
      iii) Acute on chronic is AKI that presents in a patient with pre-existing CKD.

569

4) **Acute kidney failure**
   a) Clinical symptoms and signs
      i) Nausea/vomiting, anorexia, pruritis, fatigue, **altered mental status**, decreased urine output.
      ii) **Volume overload** causing peripheral and **pulmonary edema.**
      iii) Pericarditis, **hyperkalemia, metabolic acidosis, coagulopathy** from platelet dysfunction.
   b) Etiologies of AKF
      i) **At risk patient population**
         (1) CKD, hypertension, cardiac disease, peripheral vascular disease, diabetes mellitus, liver disease, and age > 60.
      ii) **Pre-renal**
         (1) Hypoperfusion from decreased intravascular volume, decreased cardiac output, or intrarenal vasoconstriction.
         (2) Integrity of renal tissue is preserved.
         (3) NSAIDS can provoke acute pre-renal failure in patients with other risk factors for developing AKI.
      iii) **Intra-renal**
         (1) Acute tubular necrosis (ATN) secondary to ischemia (hypoperfusion > 30 to 60 minutes) most common, sepsis, acute contrast nephropathy, nephrotoxic drugs, and trauma.
         (2) Postoperative ATN accounts for 20% to 25% of all hospital acquired AKF (5).
         (3) Other risk factors include cardiopulmonary bypass.
      iv) **Post-renal**
         (1) **Obstruction to urine flow from the kidneys.**
         (2) Causes include prostatic hypertrophy, abdominal or pelvic mass impinging on ureters.
   c) Diagnosis of AKF (Table 79-1) (6). Differentiation between the different causes of AKF can be aided by
      i) Measuring urine and serum indices.
      ii) Calculating **Fractional Excretion of Na (FENa)** = (Urine Na/Plasma Na)/(Urine Cr/Plasma Cr).
   d) Classification and prognosis
      i) **RIFLE (Risk, Injury, Failure, Loss, End-stage) classification (Table 79-2)(7,8).**
         (1) A system recently devised by an international panel of experts.
         (2) Used to provide a standardized definition of AKI severity and aid in prognosis in the acute phase of injury.

Table 79-1

Indices for Diagnosis of AKF (6)

Diagnostic Test	Prerenal	Intrarenal (ATN)	Postrenal
Urine Na	<10 mEq/L	>20 mEq/L	>20 mEq/L
FENa	<1%	>2%	>2%
Urine Osmolarity	>500	<350	<350
Serum BUN/Cr	>20	=10	=10

Table 79-2

RIFLE Categories and Associated Mortality in ICU Patients (7,8)

RIFLE Category	Serum Creatinine	Urine Output	Associated Mortality (%)
Risk	Increased by 1.5× (or Cr increased ≥ 0.3 mg/dL)	<0.5 mL/kg/h × 6 h	8.8–20
Injury	Increased 2×	< 0.5 mL/kg/h × 12 h	11.4–45.6
Failure	Increased 3× or Cr ≥ 4 mg/dL (acute rise ≥ 0.5 mg/dL)	< 0.4 mL/kg/h × 24 h OR anuric × 12 h	26.3–56.8
Loss	complete loss of renal function >4 wk		
ESRD	End-stage renal disease		

5) **Chronic kidney disease**
  a) Definition
    i) GFR < 60 mL/min/1.73 m^2 for 3 or more months.
    ii) Kidney damage leading to decreased GFR present for 3 months or more, irrespective of the cause (3).
  b) **Multiple organ systems are affected**
    i) **Hematologic**

CKD affects multiple organ systems.

      (1) **Anemia**—decreased production of erythropoietin.
      (2) **Coagulopathy**
        (a) Normal PT/INR, PTT and platelet count.
        (b) **Poor platelet adhesion** from defective interaction of the von Willebrand Factor and platelet glycoprotein IIb/IIIa receptors.
      (3) Hypercoagulation
        (a) Despite platelet dysfunction, thromboelastographic indices show tendency towards clotting
    ii) **Electrolyte disturbances (Table 79-3)**
    iii) **Cardiovascular**
      (1) Hypertension
        (a) Present in 80% of patients.
        (b) May be primary cause or as a result of kidney disease.
      (2) **Left ventricular hypertrophy** due to volume and pressure overload.
      (3) **Accelerated atherosclerosis** due to dyslipidemia and inflammation.
      (4) **Vascular and valvular** disease due to abnormal calcium deposition.
      (5) **Predisposition to arrhythmias** due to conduction system abnormalities.
      (6) **Pericarditis** due to uremia.
    iv) Neurologic
      (1) Autonomic neuropathy
        (a) Present in 38% to 87.5% of patients with CKD on HD (3).
        (b) **Characterized by reduced baroreceptor sensitivity, sympathetic overactivity, and parasympathetic dysfunction.**
      (2) Peripheral sensory neuropathy correlates with cardiovascular autonomic neuropathy.

Table 79-3

Common Electrolyte Disturbances in Renal Failure

Electrolyte Abnormality	Pathophysiology	Signs/Symptoms	Treatment
Hyperkalemia	Poor excretion, transcellular shifts due to **acidemia** and insulin deficiency	Weakness, paresthesias **Peaked T waves, ST depression, prolonged PR, QRS widening, sine wave, ventricular fibrillation**	**IV calcium stabilizes myocardium** sodium bicarbonate, insulin/dextrose, hyperventilation shifts K intracellularly, HD
Hypocalcemia	Elevated parathyroid hormone	Usually well tolerated, can cause tetany, seizures if severe or sudden	Vitamin D, calcium supplements
Hypermagnesemia	Poor excretion	Usually well tolerated, can cause hypoventilation, altered mental status, prolongation of neuromuscular blocking drugs if severe	Avoid magnesium containing medications, HD
Metabolic acidosis	Inadequate hydrogen ion excretion	Respiratory distress, hypotension, **cardiac arrythmias,** hyperkalemia	**Hyperventilation, sodium bicarbonate,** HD

A large number of patients with CKD on HD have autonomic neuropathy.

Preoperative evaluation of the patient on HD includes HD history, assessment of volume status, and evaluation of electrolytes.

  v) Gastrointestinal
   (1) **Delayed gastric emptying** seen in up to 69% of patients
  vi) Immunologic
   (1) Patients are immunocompromised and have a higher prevalence of systemic and superficial infections.
6) **Anesthetic considerations**
 a) **Preoperative considerations**
  i) If patient is not on HD
   (1) Assess level of current renal function using creatinine and urine output.
   (2) Assess whether renal function is stable, worsening, or improving by trending creatinine and urine output.
  ii) If patient is on HD
   (1) **Assess volume status using current vital signs and weight as compared to dry weight.**
   (2) **Review when patient last received HD and HD record if available.**
  iii) Consider invasive monitoring or echocardiogram to aid in volume assessment.
  iv) **Careful review of electrolytes, especially serum potassium, is mandatory.**
  v) **Evaluation of pH status is helpful**
 b) **Intraoperative Considerations**
  i) Induction of anesthesia
   (1) Oral non-particulate antacid should be used if appropriate.

  (2) **Rapid sequence induction (RSI)** should be considered as delayed gastric emptying is seen in the majority of patients.

 ii) Medication dosing

  (1) Patients will have decreased excretion of drugs cleared by the kidneys.

  (2) Sensitivity to drugs that suppress the central nervous system is increased.

 iii) Muscle relaxation

  (1) **Succinylcholine can be an acceptable choice** for muscle relaxation **if there is no pre-existing hyperkalemia**, as the associated potassium release is not increased in AKI/CKD or ESRD as compared to usual (0.5 to 1 mEq/L).

  (2) **Vecuronium and rocuronium** have **prolonged duration of action** especially with repeated dosing.

  (3) **Cisatracurium is the muscle relaxant of choice** as its duration of action is unaffected by renal disease (it is degraded by Hoffman degradation).

  (4) **Neostigmine** has prolonged duration of action, therefore re-curarization is unlikely.

 iv) Maintenance of anesthesia

  (1) Volatile anesthetics can be used.

   (a) Sevoflurane in the setting of low flows and dry CO_2 absorbant may result in accumulation of the nephrotoxic agent, compound A.

 v) Pain medication

  (1) Morphine

   (a) Leads to accumulation of active and toxic metabolites.

   (b) Lowers seizure threshold.

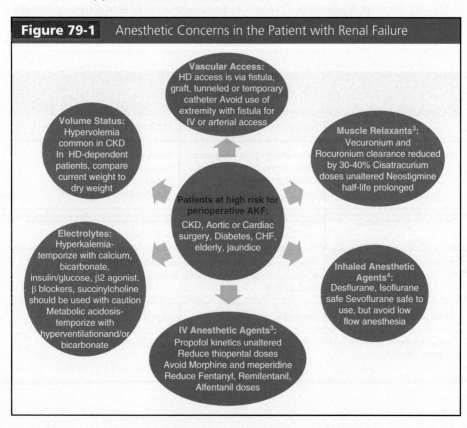

Figure 79-1 Anesthetic Concerns in the Patient with Renal Failure

(c) May cause delayed respiratory depression.

(d) **Doses should be reduced.**

(2) Meperidine

(a) **Metabolite normeperidine accumulates**

(i) Associated with **seizures, myoclonus and altered mental status.**

(3) Fentanyl

(a) Has no active metabolites, but clearance is reduced.

vi) Intraoperative **low urine output (< 0.5 mL/kg/h**, if not oliguric at baseline):

(1) **Rule out new post-renal cause**

(a) **Check foley patency,** flush if necessary.

(b) Maintain suspicion for surgical ureteral obstruction in gynecologic and pelvic procedures, communicate with the surgeons.

(2) **Rule out pre-renal cause**

(a) **Ensure adequate intravascular volume.**

(b) **Maintain renal perfusion** by optimizing cardiac output.

(c) **Laparoscopic surgery** often causes transient low urine output due to renal hypoperfusion and ureteral compression.

(3) **Consider intra-renal cause**

(a) Pre-existing CKD

(b) Recent use of nephrotoxic agents such as IV contrast

c) **Postoperative considerations**

i) Hypertension is common.

(1) If volume overload is suspected, urgent HD should be considered

ii) Fentanyl, remifentanil, alfentanil, hydromorphone can be used at reduced dosages for pain management (Fig. 79-1)

Chapter Summary for Kidney Disease

	Non-HD Dependent	HD Dependent
Preoperative Evaluation	Assess volume status, urine output Initiate preoperative HD if needed Check K+, pH, BUN/Cr, CO_2	**Assess volume status** Check timing of last HD Check K+, pH, BUN/Cr Check location of AVF if present
Induction of Anesthesia	Assume full stomach, use RSI if appropriate, avoid hypoventilation, succinylcholine only if preoperative K+ normal, reduce dose of induction agents and opioids	
Maintenance of Anesthesia	Inhaled agents safe, cisatracurium neuromuscular blockade of choice, reduce dose of opioids, monitor for signs of cardiac ischemia, if AVF present—palpate intermittently for thrill	
Postoperative Concerns	May need to initiate HD	May need urgent HD

AVF, arteriovenous fistula; BUN, blood urea nitrogen; Cr, creatinine, HD, hemodialysis; K+, potassium; RSI, rapid sequence induction.

References

1. Morgan G, Mikhail, M. *Clinical Anesthesiology*. San Mateo, CA: Appleton & Lange; 1992.
2. Warnock DG. Towards a definition and classification of kidney injury. *J Am Soc Nephrol* 2005;16:3149–3150.
3. Craig RG, Hunter JM. Recent developments in the perioperative management of adult patients with chronic kidney disease. *J Anaesth* 2008;101(3):296–310.
4. Stoelting R, Dierdorf S. *Anesthesia and Co-existing Disease*. 3rd ed. New York, NY: Churchill Livingstone; 1993.
5. Lameie N, Biesen WV, Vanholder R. Acute renal failure. *Lancet* 2005;365:417–430.
6. Saperstein A. Specific considerations with renal disease. In: Hurford WE, ed. *Clinical Anesthesia Procedures of the Massachusetts General Hospital*. 6th ed. Philadelphia, PA: Lippincott Williams & Wilkins; 2002.
7. Osterman M, Chang R. Acute kidney injury in the intensive care unit according to RIFLE. *Crit Care Med* 2007;35:1837–1843.
8. Srisawat N, Hoste EA, Kellum JA. Modern classification of acute kidney injury. *Blood Purif* 2010;29:300–307.

80 Water, Electrolyte, and Acid/Base Disturbances

Ludwig Lin, MD • Bassam Kadry, MD

Water, electrolyte, and acid/base disturbances are commonly encountered in chronic illness and hospitalized patients presenting for surgery. These derangements in the cellular milieu can lead to multisystemic pathophysiology, including arrhythmias, hemodynamic changes, and neuromuscular dysfunctions. Proper diagnosis and treatment may be essential to decrease the likelihood of complications in the perioperative anesthetic course.

1) Overview of water, electrolyte, and acid/base disturbances
   a) **Incidence/prevalence**
      i) Electrolyte disturbances in the hospitalized patient population is fairly common.
         (1) Acid–base disturbances are documented with an incidence of as high as 56% (1).
         (2) Hypernatremia is present in >1%, with hyponatremia at an incidence of 1% to 2% among hospitalized patients (2).
            (a) They are more common in patients with multiple diseases, and are associated with disorders of the older patient population, such as congestive heart failure (CHF) and dementia.
   b) **Clinical implications**
      i) Because water, electrolyte, and acid/base disturbances affect the overall cellular milieu, they can have major influences on normal physiologic function when left untreated.
      ii) **Arrhythmias**
         (1) Electrolyte and pH abnormalities lead to cardiac conduction abnormalities and eventually, conduction abnormalities that can lead to lethal hemodynamic collapse.
         (2) Intravascular volume abnormalities can contribute toward those electrolyte and pH abnormalities.
            (a) It is also the primary cause in arrhythmogenesis by distension of the atrial wall.
      iii) **Hemodynamic changes**
         (1) Electrolyte disturbances by themselves do not affect the hemodynamics, but they can result in hemodynamic consequences, such as hypotension.
         (2) A pH <7.2 leads to ineffective adrenergic receptor activity, and results in a suboptimal environment for catecholamine action (3).
      iv) **Impact on enzymatic function**
         (1) Most enzymes require a physiologic pH environment for optimal functional activity.

Hypocalcemia, hyper- and hypokalemia, and hypophosphatemia can lead to respiratory muscle weakness and paralysis.

(a) pH changes affect the oxygen–hemoglobin dissociation curve (Bohr effect)

(i) Creates decreased peripheral dissociation and availability of oxygen in extreme alkalosis.

v) **Impact on work of breathing**

(1) Hypocalcemia, hyper- and hypokalemia, and hypophosphatemia can lead to respiratory muscle weakness and paralysis.

(2) Pulmonary edema from fluid overload can lead to increased V/Q shunt and hypoxemia, as well as increased work of breathing leading to eventual respiratory failure due to fatigue.

2) **Water disturbances**

a) Total body water (TBW)

   i) 70% to 75% of the total body mass of an infant.

   ii) 65% to 70% of a toddler.

   iii) 55% to 60% of an adult.

   iv) TBW is compartmentalized into intracellular water and extracellular water.

   v) The amount that is relevant to a patient's hemodynamic profile is the intravascular portion of the extracellular water

   (1) Intravascular water + interstitial water = extracellular water.

b) When discussing "hyper-" and "hypovolemia," we most frequently are referring to the intravascular component of water.

c) The intravascular volume and the TBW do not demonstrate a consistent relationship.

   i) Some disease states, such as cirrhosis and anasarca (e.g., a result of persistent capillary leak during sepsis), may result in an increase in the TBW.

   (1) Due to continued renal water resorption in an attempt to maintain a depleted intravascular volume.

d) **Hypervolemia**

   i) **Hypervolemia with increased intravascular volume**

   (1) **Causes**

       (a) CHF

       (b) Cirrhosis

       (c) Renal failure

       (d) Primary hyperaldosteronism

   ii) **"Hypervolemia" with decreased intravascular volume**

   (1) Capillary leak

       (a) Sepsis, anaphylaxis, burn injury

   (2) Hypoalbuminemia

       (a) Decreased production

           (i) Malnutrition, cirrhosis

       (b) Increased loss

           (i) Nephrotic syndrome, enteropathy, exudative ascites

   iii) **Mechanisms**

   (1) Activation of carotid baroreceptors releases anti-diuretic hormone (ADH), and results in increased tubular resorption of water.

     (2) Activation of juguloglomerular apparatus to activate the renin–angiotensin system to increase water/sodium resorption as well as increased vasomotor tone.

   iv) **Symptoms**
     (1) Peripheral edema
     (2) Pulmonary edema
      (a) Increased V/Q mismatch and hypoxia.
     (3) Congestive hepatopathy
      (a) Increased liver enzymes (LFTs), coagulopathy.
     (4) Hypertension
   v) **Treatment**
     (1) Treat the etiology of the water retention.
     (2) Intravascular hypervolemia
      (a) Diuretics
      (b) Preload reduction
     (3) Intravascular hypovolemia
      (a) Increase intravascular oncotic pressure.

 e) **Hypovolemia**
   i) Can be associated with both hyper- and hyponatremia.
   ii) **Causes**
     (1) Diarrhea
     (2) Vomiting
     (3) Renal losses
     (4) Hemorrhage
     (5) Insensible water losses
     (6) Other fluid losses
      (a) Thoracentesis
      (b) Paracentesis
      (c) Drainage output
   iii) If the volume loss (from water loss alone or water combined with sodium loss) is not replaced, then hypernatremia is the result.
     (1) If there is access to continued water ingestion, then stimulation of ADH release leads to water retention and results in hyponatremia.
   iv) **Preoperative assessment**
     (1) Dry mucosa
     (2) Delayed capillary refill
     (3) Increased sympathetic activity to increase cardiac output—tachycardia and increased cardiac contractility, and increased systemic vascular resistance (SVR)
     (4) Hypotension
      (a) May be a late sign
      (b) If patient is not able to compensate for the decreased preload.
     (5) Sodium derangements
   v) **Treatment**
     (1) Preoperative optimization as well as intra-operative management.
     (2) Hydration with iso-osmolar fluids.
      (a) With sodium, which most likely was lost in addition to water.

 3) **Electrolyte disturbances**
  a) **Sodium**
   i) **Hypernatremia (2)**
     (1) **Iatrogenesis**

Consider preoperative optimization of the hypovolemic patient with hydration using iso-osmolar fluids.

  (a) Hypertonic NaCl administration

  (b) Water loss

   (i) Increased insensible losses, diabetes insipidus.

   (ii) Unable to replenish due to decreased mental status or water restriction.

 (2) **Treatment**

  (a) Hydration

   (i) Need to decide on the osmolarity as well as the route of hydration.

  (b) If the patient has lost water—but has normal sodium stores—then free H_2O replacement via PO or feeding tube route should be sufficient.

  (c) The free water deficit can be calculated.

   (i) Free water deficit (in L) = 0.6 × weight (kg) × ([current Na/140] − 1)

  (d) If the patient has lost both water and solutes (e.g., sodium), then intravenous (IV) or PO administration of an isotonic solution is the best plan.

 ii) **Hyponatremia**

  (1) **Iatrogenesis**

   (a) Hypo-osmolar intravenous fluid administration

   (b) Psychogenic polydipsia

   (c) Syndrome of inappropriate antidiuretic hormone hypersecretion (SIADH)

   (d) Hypovolemia leading to increased ADH secretion and water retention

   (e) Thiazides

   (f) Pseudohyponatremia

    (i) High protein (multiple myeloma) or high lipid states decrease the percentage of water and electrolytes occupying the intravascular volume.

     1. Leads to a decreased sodium reading

   (g) Hyperosmolarity

    (i) Mannitol administration hyperglycemia lead to movement of H_2O into intravascular space.

     1. Effectively diluting the sodium and therefore to a decreased reading.

  (2) **Treatment**

   (a) Syndrome of inappropriate antidiuretic hormone hypersecretion (SIADH) and polydipsia

    (i) Water restriction

   (b) Hypovolemia

    (i) Isotonic fluid replacement

     1. Treating the cause of the hypovolemia.

b) **Potassium**

 i) **Hyperkalemia**

  (1) **Causes (4)**

   (a) Normal total body potassium, but extracellular movement of potassium cations

   (b) Sudden depolarization at neuromuscular junctions via administration of succinylcholine

   (c) Hyperkalemia results in patients with abnormal proliferation of neuromuscular junctions following denervation injuries

   (d) Spinal cord injuries

   (e) Cerebral vascular accidents

   (f) Burn injuries

   (g) Prolonged state of immobilization (e.g., ICU stay)

   (h) Even in patients without such injuries, succinylcholine administration can elevate plasma potassium by 0.5 mEq/L

(i)   So, in certain patients with elevated plasma potassium levels (such as patients with renal insufficiency, or recent red blood cell transfusions with acute hyperkalemia) such an increase can lead to dangerously high potassium concentrations.

(i)   Acidosis

    (i)   Diabetic ketoacidosis

(j)   Increased tissue breakdown

    (i)   Rhabdomyolysis

    (ii) Hemolysis

(k)   Increased total body potassium

    (i)   Impaired renal excretion

        1.   Estimate the transtubular potassium concentration gradient (TTKG)

            a.   TTKG = [urine K/(urine osmolality/serum osmolality)]/ serum K

            b.   TTKG should be above 10 with normal renal function

            c.   If <5 to 7, then it is highly suggestive of hypoaldosteronism.

        2.   Hypoaldosteronism

        3.   Adrenal insufficiency

        4.   Renal failure

        5.   Severe hypovolemia leading to increased renal resorption.

        6.   Drug effect

        7.   ACE-inhibitors

        8.   NSAIDs

        9.   Spironolactone

(2) Signs/symptoms

(a)   Very few signs or symptoms until plasma potassium is >7.0 mEq/L, unless rise has been rapid.

(b)   Muscle weakness leading to flaccid paralysis.

    (i)   Including respiratory muscles.

(c)   ECG conduction abnormalities

    (i)   Peaked T waves and shortened QT interval, with lengthening of PR and QRS intervals.

    (ii) Eventual loss of P waves and QRS widening, leading to "sine wave."

    (iii) Ventricular arrhythmias

(3) Treatment

(a)   Above 7.0 mEq/L

    (i)   Life-threatening, and needs immediate treatment.

    (ii) IV calcium chloride or calcium gluconate (calcium chloride has more elemental calcium) 1,000 mg.

A serum potassium above 7.0 mEq/L is life-threatening and requires immediate treatment.

    (iii) Sodium bicarbonate (45 mEq bolus over 5 minutes).

    (iv) Insulin (10 units and accompanied D50 50 mL push, followed by D10 infusion).

    (v)   Beta-agonists

        1.   The goal is to drive potassium into intracellular space.

(b)   Emergent hemodialysis is also an option.

(c)   Between 6 and 7 mEq/L

    (i)   Use an oral cation exchange resin.

        1.   Sodium polystyrene sulfonate—kayexalate.

    (ii) May be harmful in patients with ileus or decreased gut motility, because its contact with gut mucosa can lead to intestinal necrosis.

(d) Below 7 mEq/L
- (i) Encourage excretion by use of loop or thiazide diuretics and low-potassium diet.

ii) **Hypokalemia**
- (1) **Causes**
  - (a) Decreased total body stores of potassium through GI or renal losses.
    - (i) GI
      1. Emesis
      2. Gastric tube drainage
      3. Diarrhea
      4. Laxatives
      5. VIPoma
    - (ii) Renal loss
  - (b) Decreased renal tubular absorption from metabolic alkalosis.
    - (i) Loss of both bicarbonate and associated potassium absorption.
  - (c) Hyperaldosteronism
  - (d) Hypomagnesemia is associated with increased potassium excretion.
  - (e) Amphotericin B
  - (f) Various nephropathies
- (2) **Signs/symptoms**
  - (a) Muscle weakness
  - (b) Skeletal muscle
    - (i) Respiratory muscle weakness and resulting respiratory failure.
  - (c) Cramps, paresthesias, tetany
    - (i) Plasma potassium <2.5 mEq/L can cause rhabdomyolysis.
  - (d) Smooth muscle
    - (i) Ileus
  - (e) Arrthythmias and ECG abnormalities
    - (i) Premature atrial complex (PAC)s, premature ventricular complex (PVC)s, sinus bradycardia, paroxysmal atrial, or junctional tachycardias
    - (ii) A–V block
    - (iii) Ventricular tachycardia or ventricular fibrillation
    - (iv) "U" waves on ECG
    - (v) Combination of hypomagnesemia and hypokalemia leads to increased risk for prolonging the QT interval and development of torsade de pointes

Intravenous potassium administration can irritate veins and cause lethal arrhythmias. Administer through a central line no faster than 20 mEq/h.

- (3) **Treatment**
  - (a) Potassium replacement
    - (i) 10 mEq replacement leads to approximately an increase in plasma potassium of 0.1 mEq/L
    - (ii) PO and IV formulations
      1. IV potassium is irritating to veins, and boluses can lead to lethal arrhythmias; therefore the maximal IV replacement rate is 20 mEq/h through a central line.

c) **Phosphate**
- i) **Hyperphosphatemia (5)**
  - (1) **Causes**
    - (a) Any massive tissue necrosis leads to loss of intracellular phosphate to the intravascular plasma.
      - (i) Tumorlysis syndrome

(ii) Rhabdomyolysis

(iii) Massive hemolysis

(b) Extracellular shift of phosphate from lactic acidosis, diabetic ketoacidosis (DKA), and insulin deficiency.

(c) Decreased excretion of phosphate from renal failure.

(d) Increased exogenous administration of phosphate.

(i) Laxatives

(e) Increased renal tubular absorption of phosphate.

(i) Hypoparathyroidism

(ii) Acromegaly

(iii) Bisphosphonates

(iv) Vitamin D toxicity

(v) Familial tumoral calcinosis

(2) **Sequelae**

(a) Phosphate binds calcium, and causes acute hypocalcemia, which is life-threatening.

(3) **Treatment**

(a) Brisk intravenous fluid administration can increase renal secretion of phosphate; hemodialysis; oral phosphate binding agents.

ii) **Hypophosphatemia**

(1) **Causes**

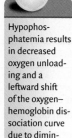

Hypophosphatemia results in decreased oxygen unloading and a leftward shift of the oxygen–hemoglobin dissociation curve due to diminished intracellular levels of 2,3-DPG.

(a) Intracellular shift

(i) Increased insulin secretion

(ii) Acute respiratory alkalosis

(iii) Hungry bone syndrome

(b) Decreased intestinal absorption

(i) Decreased phosphate intake

(ii) Ingestion of aluminum or magnesium containing antacids

(iii) Steatorrhea and chronic diarrhea

(c) Increased urinary secretion

(i) Phosphate wasting

(ii) Fanconi syndrome

(iii) Vitamin D deficiency/resistance

(iv) Hyperparathyroidism (1 and 2 degrees)

(2) **Sequelae**

(a) Decreased oxygen release from hemoglobin because of decreased intracellular levels of 2,3-diphosphoglycerate (DPG) and a shift of the oxygen–hemoglobin dissociation curve to the left.

(b) Decreased availability of ATP.

(c) Results

(i) Encephalopathy

(ii) Respiratory and skeletal muscle weakness

(iii) Smooth muscle weakness manifesting in ileus.

(iv) Hypercalciuria

(v) Red blood cell hemolysis

(vi) Decreased WBC phagocytic activity

(vii) Abnormal platelet function

(3) **Diagnosis and treatment**

(a) Calculate the urinary fractional excretion of phosphate.

(i) If higher than 5% in setting of hypophosphatemia, then renal wasting is the cause, and replacement is needed.

2. Intravenous replacement (2.5 mg [0.08 mmol]/kg of body weight over 6 hours) is dangerous.
   a. Can precipitate with calcium and cause lethal hypocalcemia.
   b. Can be done if patient is symptomatic.
3. Nonsymptomatic patients should be corrected with oral phosphate replacement (2.5 to 3.5 g, or 80 to 110 mmol/d)

(b) If fractional excretion of phosphate is <5%, then other causes of hypophosphatemia are present, and correction of the cause should be sufficient.

(c) Vitamin D replacement if due to vitamin D deficiency.

d) **Calcium**
  i) **Hypocalcemia (6)**
    (1) **Definition**
      (a) Serum calcium <8 mg/dL, or ionized calcium <1 mmol/L
    (2) **Causes**
      (a) Acute hypocalcemia
        (i) Transfusions
          1. Sequelae of chelation by citrate in banked blood products.
        (ii) Critical illness
          1. Associated with sepsis, burns, acute renal failure (ARF), pancreatitis.
        (iii) Hypoalbuminemia
          1. Decreased binding to albumin reduces total calcium concentration (but normal *ionized* calcium concentration)
        (iv) Metabolic alkalosis
          1. Increases calcium's binding to protein, so will decrease ionized calcium concentration.
        (v) Postop s/p parathyroidectomy or thyroidectomy
          1. **Causes**
            a. Chronic hypocalcemia due to parathyroid hormone (PTH) abnormalities
        (vi) Hypoparathyroidism
          1. Congenital
          2. Hypomagnesemia
          3. Surgical removal of parathyroids
        (vii) Ineffective PTH
          1. Pseudohypoparathyroidism
          2. Vitamin D deficiency
        (viii) Overwhelmed PTH
          1. Hyperphosphatemia from tumor lysis or rhabdomyolysis.
    (3) **Treatment**
      (a) Hypoparathyroidism
        (i) Vitamin D or calcitriol
        (ii) Calcium supplement
      (b) Hypomagnesemia
        (i) IV magnesium administration
    (4) **Preop**
      (a) Evaluation
      (b) Systemic effects of hypocalcemia
        (i) CNS
          1. Numbness and circumoral paresthesia, confusion, seizures

(ii) Hypotension

1. Increased left ventricular filling pressures

(iii) Prolonged QT interval

(iv) Weakness and fatigue, skeletal muscle spasm, laryngospasm

1. Chvostek and Trousseau signs indicate neuromuscular irritability.

2. Chvostek sign: tapping on facial nerve anterior to ear results in ipsilateral facial muscle twitching.

3. Trousseau sign: inflating blood pressure cuff above systolic pressure for several minutes results in muscular contraction of the hand.

(c) Management

(i) Confirm hypocalcemia with an ionized calcium measurement (to exclude the contribution of the albumin level to the total calcium level).

(ii) Obtain ECG to look for QT prolongation

1. Rarely ST segment prolongation and depression/elevation can manifest, mimicking an acute myocardial infarction.

2. Extremely rarely, arrythmias such as torsade des pointes can result (7).

(5) **Intraop**

(a) Administer 500 mg to 1 g calcium chloride or calcium gluconate IV, check ionized calcium, and repeat IV calcium administration as needed to correct hypocalcemia.

(b) Avoid hyperventilation, as respiratory alkalosis can increase calcium binding to serum proteins.

(c) Consider checking phosphate and magnesium levels.

(6) **Postop**

(a) Continue to follow serum and ionized calcium levels

(b) Continue replacement as necessary

ii) **Hypercalcemia**

(1) **Causes**

(a) Parathyroid related

(i) Primary, lithium therapy, familial.

(b) Malignancy-related

(c) Vitamin D-related

(i) Vitamin D intoxication, sarcoidosis, idiopathic hypercalcemia of infancy

(d) Increased bone turnover

(i) Hyperthyroidism, immobilization, thiazides, vitamin A intoxication

(e) Renal failure

(f) Secondary hyperparathyroidism, aluminum intoxication, milk–alkali syndrome

(2) Diagnosis

(a) Measurement of calcium, albumin, PTH, or ionized calcium

(3) Usual Rx

(a) Depends on specific cause, but general measures include hydration with saline, with or without diuresis with loop diuretics (furosemide or ethacrynic acid).

(4) Other treatments

Chvostek sign is ipsilateral facial twitching by tapping on facial nerve anterior to the ear.

Trousseau sign is muscular contraction of the hand after inflating blood pressure cuff above systolic pressure for several minutes.

Avoid hyperventilation in the setting of hypocalcemia as respiratory alkalosis can increase calcium binding to serum proteins.

- (a) Biphosphonates
  - (i) Etidronate and pamidronate
- (b) Calcitonin
- (c) Glucocorticoids, in dosages of 40 to 100 mg QD in four divided doses
  - (i) Increase urinary calcium excretion and decrease intestinal calcium absorption.
  - (ii) Effective antitumor agent in certain malignancies.
- (d) Dialysis
- (e) Gallium nitrate
  - (i) Inhibits bone resorption
  - (ii) Nephrotoxin
- (f) Mithramycin
  - (i) Inhibits bone resorption
  - (ii) Can lead to thrombocytopenia and hepatocellular necrosis
- (g) PO and IV phosphates
  - (i) Can lead to ectopic calcification
- (h) Parathyroid surgery for primary hyperparathyroidism
- (5) **Preop**
  - (a) **Issues/evaluation**
    - (i) For severe symptomatic hypercalcemia, consider postponing elective surgery to determine cause and appropriate therapy.
    - (ii) Although most patients have only mild symptoms, hypercalcemia can cause multisystem abnormalities
      1. Neuromuscular
         a. Generalized weakness, fatigue, mild depression, proximal muscle weakness, confusion
      2. **Renal**
         a. Renal stones with renal colic, polyuria, dehydration, renal insufficiency
      3. **Cardiovascular**
         a. Shortened QT interval, increased sensitivity to digoxin
      4. **GI**
         a. Anorexia, constipation, nausea, and vomiting
      5. **Other**
         a. Bone demineralization, arthralgias, bone pain, pruritus
    - (iii) Get ECG to assess for prolonged PR or shortened QT intervals and cardiac arrhythmias.
    - (iv) Serum calcium >13 mg/dL
      1. Leads to calcification in tissue and renal insufficiency.
    - (v) Serum calcium >15 mg/dL
      1. Medical emergency because of the risk of coma and cardiac arrest.
- (6) **Management**
  - (a) IV hydration with normal saline (2.5 to 4 L/d)
  - (b) Consider IV furosemide diuresis once hydration is adequate.
    - (i) Follow other electrolytes closely during this process
- (7) **Intraop**
  - (a) Maintain normocarbia.
    - (i) Hyperventilation may be deleterious by decreasing plasma potassium, which can counterbalance the effects of calcium.
    - (ii) However, it may be beneficial because it decreases the ionized calcium fraction.
  - (b) Preop muscle weakness should be considered when dosing muscle relaxants.

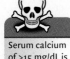

Serum calcium of >15 mg/dL is a medical emergency due to the risk of coma and cardiac arrest.

Avoid thiazide diuretics in the setting of hypercalcemia: they enhance renal tubular resorption.

(8) **Management**
- (a) Avoid thiazide diuretics
  - (i) They enhance renal tubular resorption of calcium
- (b) Avoid prolonged immobilization
  - (ii) Calcium release from resorbed bone increases.

(9) Postop
- (a) Treatment options such as calcitonin and mithramycin take hours for onset and hence are not helpful intraop
- (b) May be beneficial postop.
  - (i) Magnesium

4) Acid–Base Disturbances

a) **Arterial Blood Gas can be used to assess:**
   - i) Acid-Base disturbances and causes
   - ii) Adequacy of Ventilation
   - iii) Adequacy of Oxygenation

b) **Assessing Acid-Base Disturbances (See Fig. 80-1)**
   - i) **Step 1: Assess pH**
     - (1) Normal 7.35-7.45
     - (2) Acidemic Less than 7.35
     - (3) Alkalemic Greater than 7.45
   - ii) **Step 2: Assess $PaCO_2$**
     - (1) Normal 35-45 mmHg
     - (2) Primary Respiratory Acidosis greater than 45 mmHg
     - (3) Primary Respiratory Alkalosis less than 35 mmHg
   - iii) **Step 3: Assess HCO_3**
     - (1) Normal 22-26 mmol/L
     - (2) Primary Metabolic Alkalosis greater than 26 mmol/L
     - (3) Primary Metabolic Acidosis less than 22 mmol/L
   - iv) **Step 4: Calculate Serum Anion Gap (SAG) to help determine cause**
     - (1) $SAG=(Na^+-(Cl^- + HCO_3)$
     - (2) High Anion Gap Acidosis > 12 mEq/L (See Table 80-1)
     - (3) Normal Anion Gap Acidosis (See Table 80-1)
   - v) **Step 5: Identify type of compensation if present (See Fig. 80-1 & Table 80-2)**
   - vi) **Step 6: Identify a Mixed Acid-Base condition if present (See Table 80-3)**

c) **Assessing Adequacy of Ventilation**
   - i) Bohr Dead Space Equation to assess adequacy of ventilation
     - (1) $(P_ACO_2 - ETCO_2)/P_ACO_2$
       - (a) Normal < 0.3
       - (b) Elevated > 0.3

Causes of gap acidosis are "CUTE DIMPLES" and non-gap acidosis is "FUSED CARS."

   - (2) Differential Diagnosis due to decreased perfusion
     - (a) Hypotension
     - (b) Low Cardiac Output
     - (c) Pulmonary Embolus
     - (d) PEEP
     - (e) Blebs or Cysts

d) **Assessing Adequacy of Oxygenation**
   - i) P/F Ratio
     - (1) Ratio of PaO_2 mmHg : F_iO_2
     - (2) The lower the ratio the worse the oxygenation
       - (a) Acute Lung Injury < 300
       - (b) Acute Respiratory Distress Syndrome < 200

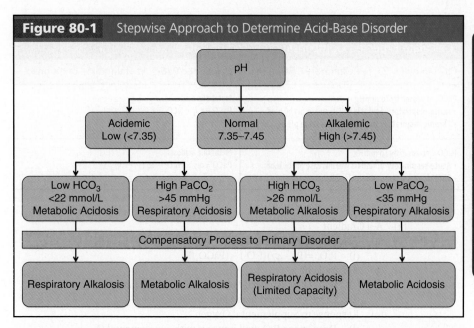

Figure 80-1 Stepwise Approach to Determine Acid-Base Disorder

Table 80-1
Metabolic Acidosis Differential Diagnosis

High Anion Gap Acidosis > 12 mEq/L (CUTE DIMPLES)	NormalAnion Gap Acidosis 8-12 mEq/L (FUSED CARS)
Cyanide	Fistula-pancreatic
Uremia	Uretogastric conduits
Toluene	Saline administration
Ethylene glycol	Endocrine disorders-*hyperparthyroidism*
Diabetic ketoacidosis	Diarrhea
Isoniazid	Carbonic anhydrase inhibitors-*acetazoloamide*
Methanol	Ammonium chloride
Paraldehyde/Propylene glycol	Renal tubular acidosis
Lactic acidosis	Spironolactone
Salicylates	

Table 80-2

Calculate Expected Compensation Based on $PaCO_2$

Calculated $PaCO_2$ in Respiratory Conditions	Calculated $PaCO_2$ in Metabolic Conditions
$PaCO_2$ *increased* by 10 mmHg • **Acute respiratory acidosis** will decrease pH by 0.08 • **Chronic respiratory acidosis** will decrease pH by 0.03	Metabolic acidosis $PaCO_2 = 1.5 \times HCO_3 + 8 \ (+/-2)$
$PaCO_2$ *Decreased* by 10 mmHg • **Acute respiratory alkalosis** will increase pH by 0.08 • **Chronic respiratory alkalosis** will increase pH by 0.03	Metabolic acidosis $PaCO_2 = 0.7 \times HCO_3 + 20 \ (+/-1.5)$

(3) A-a Gradient
    (a) Calculating P_AO_2 (Alveolar)
        (i) $P_AO_2 = (P_B - 47)(F_iO_2) - (PaCO_2/R)$
    (b) A-a gradient
        (i) $P_AO_2 - P_aO_2$ (Arterial Measured from blood gas)
        (ii) Large gradient due to Shunt or Dead Space
    (c) Response to Supplemental Oxygen
        (i) Dead space-P_aO_2 will improve with supplemental O_2
        (ii) Shunt-P_aO_2 will NOT improve with supplemental O_2
           1. Atelectasis
           2. Pulmonary Edema
           3. Endobronchial Intubation
           4. Aspiration
           5. Airway obstruction
e) **Metabolic alkalosis**
  i) **Causes**
    (1) Emesis
      (a) Loss of HCl
    (2) Contraction alkalosis
    (3) Posthyperventilation

Table 80-3

Determine If Mixed Acid-Base Disorder is Present

Identify if a Mixed Acid-Base Condition is Present

Step 1: Calculate delta gap:
• Measured Serum Anion Gap (SAG) – Normal SAG

Step 2: Calculate delta-delta:
• Add the Delta Gap to the measured bicarbonate from the basic metabolic panel taken at the same time the arterial blood gas was analyzed

Step 3: Compare delta-delta to normal HCO_3
• If Delta-Delta < 22 there is a non-anion gap metabolic acidosis
• If Delta-Delta > 26 there is an additional metabolic alkalosis

f) **Metabolic acidosis**
  i) **Decide if there is an anion-gap present**
    (1) Anion gap = [sodium] − [chloride] − [bicarbonate].
    (2) If >12, then gap acidosis is present.
      (a) Adjust for hypoalbuminemia
        (i) Add 2 to the calculated gap for every decrease in plasma albumin level of 1 g/dL below normal.
        (ii) Albumin behaves as an unmeasured anion.

5) **Gap Acidosis**
  a) **Causes**
    i) **"CUTE DIMPLES"**
      (1) C = cyanide
      (2) U = uremia
      (3) T = toluene
      (4) E = ethylene glycol
      (5) D = diabetic ketoacidosis
      (6) I = isoniazid
      (7) M = methanol
      (8) P = propylene glycol
        (a) Traditionally used to denote paraldehyde, but that is now archaic
      (9) L = lactic acidosis
      (10) S = salicylates

6) **Non-gap acidosis**
  a) **Causes**
    i) **"FUSED CARS"**
      (1) F = fistula-pancreatic
      (2) U = uretogastric conduits
      (3) S = saline administration
      (4) E = endocrine disorders-*hyperparthyroidism*
      (5) D = diarrhea
      (6) C = carbonic anhydrase inhibitors − *acetazoloamide*
      (7) A = ammonium chloride
      (8) R = renal tubular acidosis
      (9) S = spironolactone
      (10) **Other causes**
        (a) Hyperalimentation (e.g. TPN)
        (b) Hyperaldosteronism
        (c) Hyperchloremic acidosis from liberal administration of intravenous 0.9%sodium chloride administration.
  b) Treatment
    i) Respiratory acidosis and lactic acidosis
      (1) Treat the cause
    ii) If the pH is <7.2, then rapid correction may be necessary to avoid impending hemodynamic collapse.
    iii) Traditionally, sodium bicarbonate has been utilized.
      (1) 2 mmol/kg of IV sodium bicarbonate, administered over 15 minutes, can increase the pH by 0.14 (8).
      (2) However, clinical studies demonstrate no improvement in outcome from such a strategy (9).
      (3) In fact, multiple studies demonstrate *worsened* intracellular acidosis in situations of lactic acidosis from hypoperfusion, because of the lack of removal of the resulting bicarbonic acid if the patient is not ventilated adequately.

iv) In many ways, a better choice for acidosis treatment is **THAM**.

THAM may be better than sodium bicarbonate for the treatment of metabolic acidosis.

   (1) THAM
      (a) Tris–hydroxymethyl aminomethane
      (b) Buffer compound that chelates protons and is then cleared via renal secretion
   (2) The amount of THAM (a 0.3 M solution) needed to correct acidosis, in mL units, can be calculated:
      (a) Multiply the patient's body weight (kg) by the base deficit (mmol/L) (10).
   (3) No benefit to utilizing sodium bicarbonate in treatment of respiratory acidosis.
      (a) Hypoventilation
         (i) The cause of respiratory acidosis
      (b) The inability to clear carbon dioxide, which is the way to clear bicarbonic acid (the resulting compound when sodium bicarbonate combines with H+ ions) from the circulation
         (i) Leads to lactic acidosis
v) Renal etiology acidosis
   (1) Consider treatment with sodium bicarbonate infusion.

Chapter Summary for Water, Electrolytes, and Acid/Base Disorders

Water Disturbances	**TBW** is 55%–60% of an adult total body mass **Hypervolemia** can occur in the setting of increased or decreased intravascular volume. Treat the cause of the water retention. **Hypovolemia** is associated with both hyper- and hyponatremia. Hydrate with iso-osmolar fluids.

Electrolyte Disturbances

Disturbance	Diagnostic Information	Physiologic Effects	Anesthetic Implications and Concerns	Treatment
↑ Na⁺	>145 mEq	Mental status Δ's	Mental status Δ's	Replace free H_2O deficit
↓ Na⁺	<135	Mental status Δ's	Mental status Δ's	IV NS or ½ NS
↑ K⁺	>5.5	Myocardial depolarization changes	Arrhythmias	Kayexalate or dialysis
↓ K⁺	<3.5	Myocardial depolarization changes	QT-prolongation and torsades des pointes	IV or PO potassium
↑ PO₄	>4.5 mg/dL	Hypocalcemia	Hemodynamic collapse	IV hydration; PO binding agents; dialysis
↓ PO₄	<2.5 mg/dL	Muscle weakness; encephalopathy	Respiratory failure	PO phosphate

Acid/Base Disorders	Obtain arterial blood gas sample to evaluate. a) pH > 7.4, then alkalosis b) pH < 7.4, then acidosis **Respiratory acidosis:** PCO_2 of 10 mm Hg decreases pH by 0.08. **Metabolic acidosis:** If base deficit is a negative number, there is a component of metabolic acidosis. Gap acidosis: "CUTE DIMPLES" Non-gap acidosis "FUSED CARS"

References

1. Palange P, Carlone S, Galassetti P, et al. Incidence of acid–base and electrolyte disturbances in a general hospital: a study of 110 consecutive admissions. *Recenti Prog Med* 1990;81(12):788–791.
2. Bagshaw SM, Townsend DR, McDermid RC. Disorders of sodium and water balance in hospitalized patients. *Can J Anaesth* 2009;56(2): 151–167.
3. Modest VE, Butterworth JF. Effect of pH and lidocaine on beta-adrenergic receptor binding. Interaction during resuscitation? *Chest* 1995;108(5):1373–1379.
4. Nyirenda MJ, Tang JI, Padfield PL, et al. Hyperkalaemia. *BMJ* 2009;339:b4114.
5. Kuhlmann MK. Management of hyperphosphatemia. *Hemodial Int* 2006t;10(4):338–345.
6. Kraft MD, Btaiche IF, Sacks GS, et al. Treatment of electrolyte disorders in adult patients in the intensive care unit. *Am J Health Syst Pharm* 2005;62(16):1663–1682.
7. RuDusky BM. ECG abnormalities associated with hypocalcemia. *Chest* 2001;119(2):668–669.
8. Forsythe SM, Schmidt GA. Sodium bicarbonate for the treatment of lactic acidosis. *Chest* 2000;117(1):260–267.
9. Aschner JL, Poland RL. Sodium bicarbonate: basically useless therapy. *Pediatrics* 2008;122(4):831–835.
10. Nahas GG, Sutin KM, Fermon C, et al. Guidelines for the treatment of acidaemia with THAM. *Drugs* 1998;55(2):191–224.

81

Part D: Endocrine Diseases
Diabetes Mellitus

Christopher Lace, MD

Diabetes Mellitus (diabetes) is a prevalent metabolic disorder of glucose regulation, with the long term potential for serious organ damage and the possibility of acute metabolic derangements. Anesthesia providers must understand the treatment and complications of this disease to provide adequate perioperative care.

1) Overview
   a) **Epidemiology (1)**
      i) The overall incidence in the United States in 2007 was 23.6 million (7.8% of the population).
      ii) Diabetes is the seventh leading cause of death in the United States.
2) **Classification**
   a) **Insulin-dependent diabetes mellitus (IDDM)**
      i) Characterized by a total deficiency in insulin production.
      ii) Patients must receive exogenous insulin in order to live.
      iii) Occurs most frequently in those <20 years of age, but has been reported in persons in their 50s.
      iv) Patients are at risk for **diabetic ketoacidosis (DKA)** and may rarely present with hyperosmolar, hyperglycemic nonketotic coma (HHNC).
   b) **Non–insulin-dependent diabetes mellitus (NIDDM)**
      i) Characterized by resistance to insulin.
      ii) Most common form of diabetes in the United States, with a prevalence of 23% in those over age 60 (1).
      iii) Extremely uncommon in those <10 years of age, but prevalence is increasing.
      iv) More common in those who are overweight and sedentary.
      v) Patients are at risk for hyperosmolar, hyperglycemic nonketotic coma (HHNC), but very rarely present with DKA.

Patients with IDDM are at much higher risk for DKA than those with NIDDM.

3) **Long term complications from poorly controlled diabetes**
   a) Patients are at higher risk for heart disease, peripheral vascular disease, stroke, kidney disease, peripheral neuropathy, vision impairment, delayed gastric emptying, and autonomic dysfunction.
   b) **Heart disease**
      i) Patients with diabetes have two to three times the risk for coronary artery disease than the general population.
      ii) Due to the neuropathy from diabetes, these patients are at high risk for silent myocardial ischemia.
   c) **Autonomic dysfunction**
      i) Results in abnormal vascular tone responses.

Diabetic patients have a two to threefold higher risk of coronary artery disease than the general population.

Patients with autonomic dysfunction due to diabetic neuropathy may have blunted responses to β-blockers and atropine.

Patients with DKA may have severe intravascular volume depletion and may require 5 to 8 L of intravenous fluid.

ii) Patients are at risk for hypotension and hypothermia, and may have blunted responses to changes in heart rate seen with β-adrenergic antagonists and atropine (2).

d) **Delayed gastric emptying**
   i) Patients have impaired motility and delayed gastric emptying.
   ii) May be at higher risk for aspiration events.

4) **Diabetic ketoacidosis**
   a) A serious, potentially fatal, complication of diabetes.
   b) Most common in insulin dependent diabetics, but has been reported in noninsulin dependent diabetics.
   c) It is characterized by ketone formation (from a lack of insulin), an anion gap acidosis, profound dehydration (5 to 8 L), and electrolyte abnormalities (especially hypokalemia) (Table 81-1).

5) **Treatment of DKA (3)**
   a) If severe CNS depression is present, intubate the trachea to protect the airway.
   b) **Administer regular insulin IV to facilitate glucose-based cellular metabolism.**
      i) Start with a 10-unit bolus, followed by an infusion at 5 to 10 units/hour.
   c) Restore intravascular volume.
   d) If patient needs to go emergently to OR, consider 20 mL/kg bolus(es) of normal saline to restore intravascular volume prior to induction.
   e) **Once hemodynamically stable, or if time permits, replace volume with normal saline 5 to 10 mL/kg/hour.**
      i) Add 5% glucose when serum glucose level is <250 mg/dL.
      ii) Consider placement of a central venous catheter to guide volume replacement.
   f) Restore total body potassium deficit (0.3 to 0.5 mEq/kg/hour)
   g) **Closely monitor blood glucose, serum potassium, and pH**

Table 81-1

Signs and Symptoms of DKA (3)

Clinical Signs and Symptoms	Laboratory Abnormalities
Nausea and vomiting	Hyperglycemia
Dehydration	Metabolic Acidosis
Hypotension	Arterial pH <7.3
Tachycardia	Bicarbonate <15 mEq/L
Kussmaul respirations	Ketones present in urine and blood
Abdominal pain	Hyperosmolarity
Ileus	Hypokalemia
Somnolence or coma	Increased BUN and/or creatinine

h) **Patients with DKA have large total body potassium deficits.**

    i) Yet, they often have normal or elevated serum potassium levels due to insulin deficiency and hyperosmolarity.

        (1) When insulin is administered the potassium is pumped back into cells, resulting in a precipitous fall in the serum potassium level.

            (a) Potassium repletion should begin once the serum level is below approximately 5.3 mEq/L.

6) **Hyperosmolar, hyperglycemic nonketotic coma (HHNC) (3)**

    a) **A serious complication of diabetes with mortality rates approaching 50%.**

        i) Characterized by severe hyperglycemia (>600 mg/dL).

        ii) Profound dehydration

        iii) Hyperosmolarity (>350 mOsm/kg)

        iv) Electrolyte abnormalities (especially hypokalemia)

        v) **A normal pH.**

            (1) Most prevalent in elderly noninsulin dependent diabetics.

    b) **Signs and symptoms**

        i) **Similar to DKA**

            (1) However, there is a lack of metabolic acidosis and ketone formation.

            (2) CNS symptoms tend to predominate.

            (3) Unlike DKA where symptoms arise rapidly, in HHNC, symptoms tend to be gradual in onset.

    c) **Treatment**

        i) Administer hypotonic saline to correct severe hyperosmolarity and restore intravascular volume

        ii) Insulin infusions are useful to help lower the blood glucose below 300 mg/dL

        iii) Potassium replacement is often needed to replace losses from the osmotic diuresis.

        iv) As with DKA, frequent laboratory monitoring is indicated.

Perioperative glucose control is extremely important because hyperglycemia and hypoglycemia are associated with poor outcomes.

7) **Perioperative insulin management**

    a) There is no clear consensus on the best regimen for perioperative glucose control in the diabetic patient.

    b) **The optimal range for blood glucose in the perioperative period is controversial.**

        i) However, both hyperglycemia and hypoglycemia in the perioperative period are associated with negative outcomes.

    c) **The guiding principle should be to maintain the patient as close to normal as possible, while avoiding certain conditions.**

        i) Hypoglycemia

        ii) Hyperglycemia

        iii) Ketoacidosis

        iv) Dlectrolyte abnormalities

Perioperative patients who have taken their diabetes medications are at high risk for hypoglycemia and should be monitored carefully.

    d) **This may be accomplished through multiple different routes.**

        i) The easiest is via a continuous IV insulin infusion (Table 81-2).

8) **Perioperative approach to the diabetic patient**

    a) **Preoperative considerations**

        i) Determine what type of diabetes the patient has, how long they have had the disease, and how well it is controlled.

Table 81-2

Continuous IV Insulin Infusion Protocol for Use with Continuous Pump Delivery Systems (3,4)

1. Mix regular insulin to a concentration of 1 unit/mL (250 units/250 mL).
2. Initiate infusion at 0.5 to 1 unit/h.
3. Measure blood glucose concentrations as necessary (every 1–2 h) and adjust infusion rate accordingly.
4. Provide sufficient glucose 5 to 10 g/h and potassium (2–4 mEq/h).

Blood Glucose Value	Action to be Taken
<80 mg/dL	Turn infusion off for 30 min Administer 25 mL of 50% Glucose Measure blood glucose in 30 min
80–120 mg/dL	Decrease infusion by 0.3 units/h
120–180 mg/dL	No change in infusion
180–220 mg/dL	Increase infusion by 0.3 units/h
>220 mg/dL	Increase infusion by 0.5 units/h

Table 81-3

Pharmacologic Properties of Commonly Available Insulin

Name	Type	Onset*	Peak*	Duration
Humalog (Lispro)	Rapid	5–15 min	30–75 min	2–3 h
Apidra (Glulisine)	Rapid	5–15 min	30–75 min	2–4 h
Novolog (Aspart)	Rapid	10–20 min	Hours	3–5 h
Regular (R)	Short-acting	Minutes	Hours	5–8 h
NPH (N)	Intermediate	1–3 h	6–12 h	16–24 h
Lente (L)	Intermediate	Hours	6–12 h	16–24 h
Ultralente (U)	Long-acting	Hours	8–14 h	18 h
Glargine (Lantus)	Very long-acting	1 h	Evenly for 24 h	24–28 h
NPH and regular mixed in either 50/50 mix, or 70/30 mix	Premixed	30–60 min	2–12 h	Up to 18 h

Note: All times are approximate. Individual patient factors may alter these times.
Reproduced from www.isletsofhope.com, with permission.

Table 81-4

Common Oral Diabetes Medications

Drug Class	Mechanism of Action	Brand and Generic Names	Half-life	Perioperative Considerations
Sulfonylurea	Stimulates pancreatic islet beta cell insulin secretion	Amaryl (glimepiride) DiaBeta (glyburide) Micronase (glyburide) Glynase (glyburide) Glucotrol (glipizide)	9–10 h	Risk of hypoglycemia
Meglitinides	Stimulates pancreatic islet beta cell insulin secretion	Prandin (repaglinide)	1 h	Risk of hypoglycemia
Phenlalanine derivatives	Stimulates pancreatic islet beta cell insulin secretion	Starlix (nategilnide)	1.5 h	Risk of hypoglycemia
Biguanides	Decreases hepatic glucose production; increases insulin sensitivity	Glucophage (metformin)	6 h	Black box warning: risk of lactic acidosis
Alpha-Glucosidase Inhibitors	Delays glucose absorption from the intestines	Precose (acrabose) Glyset (miglitol)	2 h	Risk of ileus
Thiazolidinediones	Increases insulin sensitivity	Avandia (rosiglitazone) ACTOS (pioglitazone)	3–7 h	Black box warning: may cause or exacerbate CHF
DPP-4 inhibitors	Slows incretin metabolism, increases insulin release, decreases glucagon levels	JANUVIA (sitagliptin)	12 h	Risk of angioedema and pancreatitis

ii) **Determine what medications they have taken on the morning of surgery.**
  (1) Be wary of the risk of hypoglycemia in NPO patients who have taken either insulin or oral drugs that stimulate insulin secretion (Tables 81-3 to 81-4).
iii) **Obtain a blood glucose value in the preoperative area.**
  (1) If it is significantly elevated, consider starting an insulin infusion before going to the OR.
iv) **Be very alert to the possibility of DKA in the following cases.**
  (1) The patient is an insulin dependent diabetic who is acutely ill.
  (2) The patient has not been taking their insulin.
v) **Attempt to ascertain the extent of end-organ damage that has occurred.**
  (1) Keep in mind that not only are patients with diabetes at higher risk of cardiovascular disease, but the neuropathy from diabetes can lead to silent myocardial ischemia.
    (a) A good cardiac risk evaluation is essential.
vi) **For patients who have significant peripheral neuropathy.**
  (1) Weigh the risks and benefits of peripheral nerve blocks, as there is the possibility of increased neurotoxicity.

ANESTHESIA AND COMORBID DISEASES

b) **Intraoperative considerations**

  i) In diabetic patients, especially those with neuropathy, gastric emptying may be significantly delayed.

  ii) **The autonomic dysfunction in diabetes leads to abnormal vascular tone responses.**

    (1) This leads to increased risk of hypotension and hypothermia.

  iii) For patients who are felt to be at high risk for myocardial ischemia.

    (1) Precordial V-lead EKG monitoring should be a strong consideration.

  iv) Monitor blood glucose at regular intervals during the case.

    (1) Consider starting an insulin infusion early if levels are consistently elevated.

In any patient with postoperative confusion, delayed emergence, or seizures, RULE OUT HYPOGLYCEMIA.

c) **Postoperative considerations**

  i) For patients with delayed emergence or who are confused in the recovery area, always rule out hypoglycemia as a cause.

  ii) If the patient required an insulin infusion in the operating room, consider continuing it in the recovery area.

  iii) Patients with diabetes are at risk for many postoperative complications.

    (1) Poor wound healing

    (2) Infection

    (3) Pressure ulcers

Chapter Summary for Diabetes Mellitus

Diabetes	Prevalent disease that is the seventh leading cause of death in the United States.
Long-Term Complications	Heart disease, peripheral vascular disease, stroke, kidney disease, peripheral neuropathy, vision impairment, delayed gastric emptying, and autonomic dysfunction
Insulin Dependent Diabetes	Characterized by lack of endogenous insulin. Patients are at risk for DKA, which can be life-threatening.
Noninsulin Dependent Diabetes	Characterized by resistance to insulin. Most common form of diabetes in the United States. DKA is rare.
Diabetic Ketoacidosis (DKA)	Potentially deadly complication characterized by ketone formation, an anion gap acidosis, profound dehydration (5–8 L), and electrolyte abnormalities (especially hypokalemia).
Intraoperative Care	Maintain the blood glucose as close to normal as possible, while avoiding hypoglycemia, hyperglycemia, ketoacidosis, and electrolyte abnormalities.

References

1. National Diabetes Information Clearinghouse. www.diabetes.niddk.nih.gov/index.htm
2. Tsueda K, Huang KC, Diamond SW, et al. Cardiac sympathetic tone in anaesthetized diabetics. *Can J Anaesth* 1991;38:20–23.
3. Stoelting RK. *Anesthesia and Co-Existing Disease*. 4th ed. Philadelphia, PA: Churchill Livingston; 2002.
4. Hirsch IB, McGill JB, Cryer PE, et al. Perioperative management of surgical patients with diabetes mellitus. *Anesthesiology* 1991;74(2): 346–359.

82 Thyroid Disease

Athina Kakavouli, MD

The thyroid is one of the largest endocrine glands in the body and produces hormones that regulate cellular metabolism, growth, and rate of function of other body systems and regulation of calcium levels. This chapter will discuss the implications of diseases of the thyroid on anesthetic management.

I) Overview

   a) The thyroid gland consists of two lobes connected by the isthmus. It is located anteriorly in the neck below the cricoid cartilage.

   b) The functional unit of the thyroid is the colloid filled follicle consisting mostly of thyroglobulin. Two-thirds of iodine that is absorbed from the follicle binds to thyroglobulin to become the thyroid hormones thyroxine (T_4) and triiodothyronine (T_3).

      i) T_3:T_4 hormones are secreted in a ratio of 1:10. 80% of plasma T_3 comes from deiodination of T_4 by peripheral tissues.

      ii) T_3 is three to four times more potent than T_4. Elimination half time for T_4 and T_3 is 7 and 1.5 days respectively.

      iii) T_3 and T_4 are mostly inactive and bound to thyroxine binding globulin (80%), albumin (5% to 10%) and prealbumin (10% to 15%). Biological active free-T_4 (fT_4) represents 0.03% of total T_4 plasma levels while free-T_3 (fT_3) represents 0.3% of total T_3.

   a) T_3 and T_4:

      i) Promote gene transcription and basal cell metabolism, body growth, bone maturation and formation.

      ii) Increase gut reabsorption and cell utilization of glucose, enhance cell glycolysis and gluconeogenesis.

      iii) Increase lipid utilization from the adipose tissue with increase in plasma free fatty acids and decrease of plasma cholesterol, phospholipids and triglycerides.

      iv) Increase the number of β-adrenergic receptors and the sensitivity of those receptors to catecholamines thus increasing myocardial contractility, reducing systemic vascular resistance, and increasing intravascular volume via direct vasodilation (sympathetic stimulation).

      v) Promote brain development in the intrauterine and neonatal periods. T_3/T_4 deficiency may lead to depression, psychosis, and delayed peripheral reflexes.

   b) Thyroid function is regulated through thyrotropin (TSH), thyrotropin-releasing hormone (TRH) T_3, T_4, and iodine plasma levels.

      i) TSH, is an anterior pituitary gland hormone, that enhances iodine uptake, T_3/T_4 production and secretion by the thyroid gland.

Thyroid hormones increase the number of beta-adrenergic receptors and the sensitivity of those receptors to catecholamines, thus increasing myocardial contractility.

Hyperthyroidism is a state of thyroid gland hyperfunction which may present with signs of hypermetabolism and sympathetic overstimulation.

ii) TRH, is a hormone produced by the hypothalamus, that promotes TSH secretion.

iii) High (or low) plasma levels of T3/T4 down (or up)-regulate the secretion of both TRH and TSH through down (or up) regulation of T3/T4 receptors in the hypothalamus and anterior pituitary gland.

iv) High plasma iodine levels down regulate T3/T4 production through down regulation of iodine transport and sensitivity to TSH. The opposite occurs with low plasma iodine levels.

c) Scattered between the follicles are parafollicular cells which secrete calcitonin as a response to increased calcium plasma levels. Calcitonin decreases the levels of calcium and phosphorus by osteoblast inhibition and by renal inhibition of calcium and phosphorus reabsorption.

2) **Hyperthyroidism**

a) **Etiology**

i) Hyperthyroidism is a state of thyroid gland hyperfunction (goiter) with excessive secretion of thyroid hormones. Thyroid hyperfunction causes suppression of TSH levels.

b) **Causes**

i) Graves disease

(1) Multinodular diffuse autoimmune disease affecting females between 20 and 40 years due to circulating stimulating IgG antibodies to the TSH thyroid receptor.

ii) Thyroid single adenoma or multi-nodular goiter

(1) Autonomic functioning thyroid tissue that is not down regulated by increased thyroid hormone levels.

iii) Endemic goiter due to iodine deficiency

iv) Subacute (de Quervain) thyroiditis

(1) Inflammation of the thyroid with flu-like symptoms and thyroid pain that develops usually after an upper respiratory infection and is treated with anti-inflammatory medications.

v) Ectopic thyroid tissue/neoplasm

vi) Exogenous, usually iatrogenic, administration of thyroid hormone or iodine/iodine rich medications (e.g., amiodarone) in patients with chronically low iodine intake or nodular goiters (1,2).

c) **Prevalence**

i) More common in females.

ii) 60% to 80% of patients have Graves disease (3–5).

All patients with thyroid abnormalities undergoing elective procedures should be euthyroid (normal thyroid function tests). This is usually clinically represented by a heart rate <85 bpm and no hand tremor before the procedure.

d) **Signs and Symptoms** (Table 82-1)

i) **Hypermetabolism** and **sympathetic overstimulation**

e) **Associated findings**

i) Graves disease is associated with myasthenia gravis and exophthalmos opthalmopathy (2,3,5,6).

f) **Treatment** (2,5,7) Can be pharmacologic with β-adrenergic antagonists, antithyroid agents, glucocorticoids or with radioactive iodine or with surgical intervention.

i) **Pharmacologic.** This is recommended for children and pregnant/breast-feeding women.

(1) **β-adrenergic antagonists** (propanolol, metoprolol, esmolol). Control of adrenergic manifestations. Propanolol additionally reduces peripheral conversion of T4 to T3.

(2) **Antithyroid agents.** Decrease thyroid hormone production, and circulation.

Table 82-1	
Hyperthyroidism Signs	
Symptoms	Tachycardia
	Palpitations/ectopic heart beats
	Atrial fibrillation
	Heat intolerance
	Emotional lability
	Exophthalmos ophthalmopathy:
	Upper lid retraction,
	Increased intraocular pressure,
	Proptosis and ocular muscle weakness due to
	Retro-orbital tissue inflammation and edema.
	Fine hand tremor
Signs	Patients may have sympathetic overstimulation:
	↑HR
	↑Systemic blood pressure (SPB)
	↑Ejection fraction
	↑Left ventricular contractility
	Atrial fibrillation, ectopic heart beats
	Thrombocytopenia
	Anemia
	Hypercalcemia
	Weight loss
	Diarrhea
	Skeletal muscle weakness
	Heat intolerance
	Anxiety

(a) **Thionamides** (propylthiouracil [PTU] or methimazole). Block the production of T3, T4. PTU additionally prevents peripheral conversion of T4 to T3.

(b) **Non-radioactive iodines** (Lugol iodine, potassium iodine, sodium iodine). Reduce thyroid gland vascularity and block release of T3, T4. They are iodine substrates and should be given 2 to 3 hours after administration of thionamides to avoid a thyrotoxic crisis in a hyperthyroid patient.

(c) **Glucocorticoids** (dexamethasone, hydrocortisone). Inhibit peripheral conversion of T4 to T3 and correct subsequent adrenal suppression.

ii) **Radioactive iodine.** Reduces thyroid hormone production through thyroid gland destruction. It is not used for pregnant/ breastfeeding women or patients with Graves ophthalmopathy (may deteriorate ophthalmopathy). A thionamide should be administered prior to radioactive iodine to avoid thyrotoxic crisis.

iii) **Surgical thyroidectomy.** In patients refractory to medication treatment, retrosternal or large goiter, thyroid cancer or lymphoma, and obstructive symptoms.

g) **Preoperative anesthesia evaluation**

i) All patients undergoing **elective procedures** should be **euthyroid** (normal thyroid function tests). This is usually clinically represented by a **heart rate <85 bpm and no hand tremor** before the procedure.

ii) Usually takes 1 to 8 weeks of treatment to become euthyroid (5,6).

iii) Patients undergoing **emergency surgery**

Patients undergoing emergency surgery should be given a β-blocker (usually propanolol), thionamide and a stress dose of glucocorticoid.

Be sure to evaluate for signs of tracheal compression in patients with a thyroid mass.

READ MORE

Anterior mediastinal mass, Chapter 59, page 430

Consider awake FOB or inhalational induction for patients with signs of tracheal compression.

(1) β-adrenergic antagonist (usually propanolol), thionamide and a stress dose of glucocorticoid should be given.

(2) Inorganic iodine should be given 2 to 3 hours after the thionamide (5).

iv) **Labs**

  (1) Thyroid function tests (TSH and free T4 and T3), CBC, comprehensive metabolic panel and urinalysis.

  (2) An ECG to evaluate for ischemia, left ventricular hypertrophy, tachycardia, atrial fibrillation.

  (3) Chest xray (CXR) to evaluate for tracheal compression/deviation and for retrosternal thyroid extension should be ordered in large goiters.

    (a) A CT or MRI should be done to further evaluate the airway if there is >50% narrowing of the trachea, a retrosternal thyroid mass, or any signs/symptoms of airway compression.

  (4) An ENT consult or fiberoptic evaluation may be needed to document for vocal cord dysfunction or paralysis due to laryngeal nerve damage and pharyngeal displacement in patients with neoplasms or previous neck surgeries.

    (a) Fiberoptic evaluation should be considered in patients with a difficult airway or airway obstruction (2,6).

v) **Preoperative medications (1,5,6)**

  (1) Goals are to reduce thyroid hyperfunction, sympathetic stimulation, anxiety, and pain.

  (2) All anti-thyroid and β-adrenergic antagonists medications should be continued through the morning of surgery.

    (a) Consider an esmolol IV infusion perioperatively to control tachycardia to <90 bpm.

    (b) Benzodiazepines can be useful as anxiolytics.

  (3) Regional anesthesia with a superficial and deep cervical block may be used for intraoperative sympathetic blockade and for postoperative analgesia.

  (4) Consider omitting epinephrine to avoid stimulation of an up-regulated sympathetic system.

  (5) If a patient has signs of tracheal compression, an awake fiberoptic bronchoscopy (FOB) or an inhalational induction may be indicated.

h) **Intraoperative treatment (1,4,6,8)**

i) Maintain adequate anesthesia and pain control.

ii) Complications to be prepared for include:

  (1) Difficult ventilation/intubation

  (2) Cardiac arrhythmias

  (3) Sympathetic hyperactivity

  (4) Hyperthermia requiring active cooling and excessive airway pressures during surgical manipulations

iii) Patient's head and neck should be positioned in a slight head-up tilt position.

  (1) Careful eye padding in exophthalmos patients

iv) **Medications**

(1) **Avoid adrenergic stimulation or parasympathetic blockade** to avoid exacerbated responses from an up regulated sympathetic system. Medications that cause hypertension or tachycardia are best avoided and when needed smaller doses should be used to avoid exacerbated elevations of blood pressure and heart rate.

    (a) Avoid ketamine, halothane, pancuronium, anticholinergics, indirect acting vasopressors (e.g., ephedrine), and epinephrine.

    (b) For hypotension, a decreased dose of a direct acting vasopressor (e.g., phenylephrine) can be used.

    (c) Esmolol and lidocaine can be used for tachycardia or supraventricular arrhythmias.

    (d) If β-adrenergic antagonist intolerance consider diltiazem for heart rate reduction.

(2) Patients are often hypovolemic and vasodilated.

    (a) Give all IV medications slowly and titrate to effect.

(3) Minimal alveolar concentration (MAC) of volatile anesthetics is increased in hyperthermic patients (5% MAC increase for every degree above 37°C).

(4) Muscle relaxants: Initial and maintenance doses of muscle relaxants should be reduced since subclinical myopathy may be present and reversal with an anticholinergic medication may be unwanted.

(5) Avoid salicylates, NSAIDs or furosemide which can increase levels of thyroid hormones by increasing fT3 and fT4.

    (a) Consider ethacrinic acid for diuretic.

  v) **Postoperative treatment**

    (1) Supplemental O$_2$

    (2) Monitor patient's vital signs including temperature

    (3) Provide adequate pain control

j) **Thyroid storm (TS).** A life threatening condition that develops rapidly in patients with poorly treated hyperthyroidism.

  i) TS is due to marked hypersensitivity to increased catecholamine secretion.

  ii) Due to acute emotional or physical stress from conditions such as:

    (1) Emergent surgery

    (2) Surgical manipulations of an overactive thyroid gland

    (3) Cardiovascular stress

    (4) Trauma

    (5) Infection

    (6) Diabetic ketoacidosis

    (7) Pregnancy-induced hypertension

  iii) **Symptoms that may present**

    (1) Anxiety

    (2) Agitation

    (3) Delirium

    (4) Hyperthermia

    (5) Hypertension

    (6) Tachycardia

    (7) Arrhythmias

    (8) Nausea/vomiting

    (9) Diffuse abdominal pain/obstruction

    (10) Myocardial ischemia

    (11) Congestive heart failure (CHF)

  iv) TS most commonly presents 6 to 18 hours postoperatively.

v) Mortality rates can be up to 10% to 75%.

    (1) Immediate diagnosis of TS is critical (2,5,6,8).

vi) **Treatment and resuscitation**

    (1) Treatment should focus on ventilation and cardiovascular support.

        (a) Supplemental O_2 to maximize oxygen delivery.

        (b) Maintaining a HR < 100 bpm.

        (c) Decreasing temperature.

        (d) Treating the precipitating factor.

    (2) Since drug metabolism is slowed, consider reducing drug dosages.

    (3) The following should be given promptly:

        (a) β-adrenergic antagonist (esmolol infusion or propranolol 10 to 40 mg po q4–6h)

        (b) Corticosteroids (hydrocortisone 100 to 200 mg IV q6h) to reduce peripheral T4 to T3 conversion and because relative adrenal deficiency may be present.

        (c) Antithyroid medications (PTU 200 to 400 mg po/NGT q8h)

        (d) Give iodine (Lugol iodine or potassium iodine) 3 to 4 hours after PTU

    (4) Invasive monitoring including arterial, central venous and potentially a pulmonary artery catheter and continuous temperature monitoring should be established.

    (5) Consider ice packs or hypothermic blankets for cooling. Give acetaminophen for temperature control (8,9).

    (6) Correct fluid deficits and metabolic abnormalities. Dehydrate with IV saline and glucose.

    (7) Avoid salicylates or furosemide which can increase levels of thyroid hormone.

    (8) Thyroid levels return to normal after 24 to 48 hours and recovery occurs after 1 week.

    (9) If conventional therapy is not successful, consider direct removal of circulating thyroid hormones with cholestyramine, plasmapheresis and peritoneal dialysis.

3) **Hypothyroidism**

  a) **Etiology**

    i) Hypothyroidism is a state of thyroid gland hypofunction with decreased production of thyroid hormones.

  b) **Primary hypothyroidism**

    i) TSH is increased above the upper limit of normal.

    ii) The most common causes are iatrogenic.

       (1) Surgical resection

       (2) Iodine or amiodarone treatment

         (a) High iodine content causes a reduction in thyroid hormone synthesis and release.

       (3) Lithium use

         (a) Lithium blocks thyroid hormone synthesis and release.

       (4) Hashimoto disease

         (a) Autoimmune disease with lymphocytic infiltration of the thyroid gland

       (5) Other causes are thyroiditis (e.g., de Quervain thyroiditis that initially can cause hyperthyroidism)

  c) **Secondary hypothyroidism (pituitary)**

    i) Thyroid hormone and TSH levels are decreased due to decreased TRH

    ii) Due to any pituitary abnormality

       (1) Postpartum pituitary necrosis (Sheehan syndrome)

       (2) Expansive pituitary mass

        (3)   Surgical resection

        (4)   Intracranial radiation

d) **Secondary hypothyroidism (hypothalamic)**

    i)   Thyroid hormone and TSH levels are decreased due to decreased TRH.

    ii)   Due to neoplasms and surgical resection (7,10)

e) **Prevalence**

    i)   Hypothyroidism is seen in 1% to 2% of patients.

    ii)   More common in females and older patients (10).

f) **Signs and symptoms**

    i)   Often insidious in onset

    ii)   Decreased metabolism

    iii) Lethargy

    iv) Depressed cardiac and respiratory function

        (1)   Bradycardia

        (2)   ↓CO

        (3)   ↓ventilatory response to hypoxia and hypercapnia

    v)   Cold intolerance (4,5,11)

g) **Associated findings in untreated hypothyroidism**

    i)   Obesity

    ii)   Obstructive sleep apnea

    iii) Hyperlipidemia

    iv) Hypothermia

    v)   Delayed gastric emptying

    vi) Cardiomegaly

    vii) CHF

    viii)Pericardial/pleural effusions

    ix) Peripheral edema

    x)   Anemia

    xi) Adrenal insufficiency

    xii) Hyponatremia

    xiii)Hashimoto disease

        (1)   Associated with other autoimmune diseases including primary adrenal insufficiency and diabetes mellitus (2,4,5,7,10).

h) **Treatment**

    i)   **Pharmacologic**

        (1)   **Thyroid replacement**

            (a)   Levothyroxine is most commonly used at doses of 1.6 µg/kg/day.

            (b)   6 to 8 weeks after initiation of treatment, T4 and TSH levels should be checked and doses modified accordingly. (7,10).

        (2)   **Drug interactions** are common.

            (a)   Levothyroxine can increase warfarin levels.

            (b)   Iron sulfate, sucralfate and aluminum hydroxide interfere with levothyroxine absorption.

            (c)   Phenytoin, rifampin, and carbamazepine decrease levothyroxine levels (7).

i) **Preoperative anesthesia evaluation**

    i)   For patients with mild-moderate hypothyroidism elective surgery is probably safe.

    ii)   For patients with severe hypothyroidism or pregnant, a euthyroid state (HR > 60) should be established prior to elective surgery (5,6,8).

    iii) Hypothyroid patients with coronary artery disease (CAD) are at increased risk of myocardial ischemia during establishment of a euthyroid state due to a sudden increase in metabolic O_2 demands.

For patients with hypothyroidism, the goals are to protect from respiratory depression, hypovolemia, hypoglycemia, hyponatremia, and hypothermia.

      (1) Should be assessed for β-adrenergic antagonist therapy or emergency coronary revascularization (2,4,6,9).

iv) For patients undergoing emergency surgery with severe hypothyroidism, aggressiveness of therapy should be based on the patient's clinical status (4).

v) **Labs.** The same labs should be obtained as for patients with hyperthyroidism.

vi) **Preoperative medications**

      (1) Treatment goals are to protect from respiratory depression, hypovolemia, hypoglycemia, hyponatremia and hypothermia (5,6,9).

      (2) Levothyroxine has a $t_{1/2}$ of 5 to 7 days but ideally should be continued perioperatively.

      (3) Thyroid hormone medications are associated with wrong dose safety issues with conversions from μg to mg and adjusting IV to PO dosing.

         (a) Oral dosing has 50% bioavailability versus IV dosing with 100% bioavailability (2).

      (4) Patients may have heightened sensitivity to respiratory depression from sedatives.

      (5) Since patients may have delayed gastric emptying and occult adrenal insufficiency, consider histamine H_2 antagonists, metoclopramide, rapid sequence induction, non-particulate antacid and corticosteroids (1,10).

Myxedema coma is a life threatening condition of severe hypothyroidism which can be precipitated by sepsis, omission of thyroid replacement therapy, trauma or surgery.

j) **Intraoperative treatment** (1,4,5,6).

i) Anticipate the potential for difficult intubation (generalized edema, tracheal compression/deviation) in patients with goiter and complications:

      (1) Exaggerated effects of cardiodepressant drugs

      (2) Prolonged muscle relaxation with neuromuscular blockade

      (3) Hypocarbia

      (4) Hyponatremia

      (5) Hypoglycemia

      (6) CHF

ii) For patients with refractory hypotension, consider adrenal insufficiency.

iii) For patients with severe hypothyroidism, consider invasive monitoring.

iv) Preventing hypothermia

      (1) Increase ambient OR temperature.

      (2) Warm IV fluids

      (3) Use forced air warming devices

k) **Postoperative treatment**

i) Anesthesia recovery may be delayed.

ii) Ensure patients have adequate muscle strength and are normothermic prior to extubation.

iii) Non-opioid analgesics like ketorolac and peripheral and or central neuraxial blockade are preferable for postoperative pain management (1,5,7,9).

4) **Myxedema coma (MXC)** (2,5,8–10)

a) A life threatening condition of severe hypothyroidism.

b) Sepsis, omission of thyroid replacement therapy, trauma, or surgery can precipitate MXC in hypothyroid patients.

c) Mortality can be as high as 15% to 60%.

d) Strong mortality predictors include:

i) Low mean arterial pressure (MAP)
ii) Need for mechanical ventilation
iii) Sepsis

e) The diagnosis can be made by very low blood levels of free T4, T3 with or without TSH elevation.

f) **Signs and Symptoms**
   i) Impaired mental status
   ii) Seizures
   iii) Loss of deep tendon reflexes
   iv) Hypoventilation
   v) Hypothermia
   vi) Hyponatremia
      (1) Due to inappropriate antidiuretic hormone (ADH) secretion.
   vii) Hypoglycemia
      (1) Due to concomitant adrenal insufficiency.
   viii) Ileus
   ix) Effusions
   x) ECG abnormalities
      (1) Sinus bradycardia
      (2) Low-voltage
      (3) Non-specific ST and T wave changes
   xi) CHF
      (1) Dilated cardiomyopathy
      (2) Pericardial effusion

g) **Treatment and Resuscitation**
   i) Patients should be in an ICU setting.
      (1) Mechanical ventilation
      (2) Cardiovascular support
      (3) IV thyroid hormone
      (4) Steroids
      (5) Saline

Complications after thyroid surgery include superior laryngeal nerve damage, recurrent laryngeal nerve damage, tracheal compression and hypoparathyroidism.

      (6) Glucose for gradual correction of hyponatremia and hypoglycemia.
   ii) A loading dose of levothyroxine 200 to 500 μg is given until the patient regains consciousness.
      (1) Followed by a maintenance dose of 50 to 200 μg daily.
   iii) Continuous ECG monitoring should be done.
   iv) Steroid replacement with hydrocortisone 100 mg every 8 hours should be given to prevent adrenal insufficiency.
   v) Patients become euthyroid after 3 to 5 days.
   vi) External warming for correction of hypothermia should be done gradually to avoid cardiovascular collapse due to sudden peripheral vasodilatation of a hypovolemic patient.

5) Complications after thyroid surgery (5,8)
  a) **Superior laryngeal nerve damage**
    i) Hoarseness.
    ii) Loss of sensation above the vocals cords which can place the patient at risk for aspiration.
  b) **Recurrent laryngeal nerve damage**
    i) Unilateral can present with hoarseness.
    ii) Bilateral can present with airway obstruction and aphonia.
    iii) To assess vocal cord function postoperatively, ask the patient to say "e."

c) **Tracheal compression**
   i) Can be secondary to hematoma or tracheomalacia.
   ii) May require surgical intervention and/or reintubation.
d) **Hypoparathyroidism**
   i) Due to inadvertent removal of the parathyroid glands.
   ii) Typically presents with hypocalcemia 24 to 96 hours postoperatively.
   iii) Patients may present with laryngospasm.
   iv) Treatment is with calcium carbonate/gluconate.
      (1) Magnesium levels should also be followed.

Chapter Summary for Thyroid Disease

Hyperthyroidism Perioperative Considerations	Defined as $\uparrow T_4$ and $\uparrow T_3$, $\downarrow$TSH Presents with signs and symptoms of hypermetabolism and increased sympathetic activity. Treat with medications (β-blockers, thionamides, glucocorticoids, iodine) or surgical treatment. Patients should be euthyroid (HR < 85) prior to elective surgery. TS (severe hyperthyroidism) can be life threatening.
Hypothyroidism Perioperative Considerations	Defined as $\downarrow T4$ and $\downarrow T3$, $\uparrow$TSH. Presents with signs and symptoms of decreased metabolism and lethargy. Treat with thyroid replacement. Severe hypothyroidism should be corrected prior to elective surgery. MXC (severe hypothyroidism) can be life threatening.
Thyroid Surgery Perioperative Considerations	Be concerned for tracheal compression and vocal cord dysfunction Postoperatively patients can have superior laryngeal nerve damage (hoarseness, aspiration risk), recurrent laryngeal nerve damage (hoarseness, risk of complete obstruction), tracheal compression (hematoma), and hypoparathyroidism (low calcium).

References

1. McQuillan PM, Allman KG, Wilson IH. Endocrine and metabolic disease, endocrine surgery. In: *Oxford American Handbook of Anesthesiology.* Oxford 1st ed. New York, NY: Oxford; 2008:155–192, 575–586.
2. Breivik H. Perianaesthetic management of patients with endocrine disease. *Acta Anaesthesiol Scand* 1996;40:1004–1015.
3. Little JW. Thyroid disorders. Part I: Hyperthyroidism. *Oral Surg Oral Med Oral Path Oral Radiol Endod* 2006;101(3):276–284.
4. Connery LE, Coursin DB. Assessment and therapy of selective endocrine disorders. *Anesth Clin N Am* 2004;22:93–123.
5. Wall, RT. Endocrine disease. In: Hines RL, Marschall KE, eds. *Stoelting's Anesthesia and Co-Existing Disease.* 5th ed. Philadelphia, PA: Churchill Livingstone; 2008:378–393.
6. Roizen MF, Fleisher LA. Anesthetic implications of concurrent diseases. In: Miller RD, ed. *Miller's Anesthesia.* 7th ed. Philadelphia, PA: Churchill Livingstone; 2009:1067–1089.
7. Arora N, Dhar P, Fahey TJ, et al. Seminars: local and regional anesthesia for thyroid surgery. *J Surg Oncol* 2006;94:708–713.
8. Schwartz JJ, Shamsuddin A, Rosenbaum SH. Endocrine function. In: Barash, PG, Cullen BF, Stoelting RK, et al., eds. *Clinical Anesthesia.* 6th ed. Philadelphia, PA: Lippincott Williams & Wilkins; 2009:1279–1286.
9. Vedig AE. Thyroid emergencies. In: Bersten AD, Soni N, Oh TE, eds. *Oh's Intensive Care Manual.* 5th ed. Edinburgh, UK: Butterworth Heinemann; 2003:559–566.
10. Little JW. Thyroid disorders. Part II: Hypothyroidism and thyroiditis. *Oral Surg Oral Med Oral Path Oral Radiol Endod* 2006;102(2):148–153.
11. Farling PA. Thyroid disease. *Br J Anaesth* 2000;85(1):15–28.

Adrenal Disorders

83

Jessica Spellman, MD

The adrenal gland is responsible for catecholamine, mineralocorticoid, glucocorticoid, and androgen production and secretion. Excess catecholamines from pheochromocytomas, excess aldosterone, or derangements in cortisol secretion can result in physiologically significant disease with impact on perioperative management.

1) Overview
   a) **The adrenal glands** are small (4 to 5 g) triangular shaped endocrine glands that sit on top of the kidneys
      i) Synthesize and store essential hormones
      ii) Release hormones in conjunction with stress
      iii) Divisions of the adrenal glands
         (1) **Adrenal cortex** produces and stores three hormones
            (a) **Mineralocorticoids (aldosterone)** responsible for regulation of extracellular volume via urinary sodium and potassium exchange in the Renin–Angiotensin–Aldosterone system
            (b) **Glucocorticoids (cortisol)** responsible for gluconeogenesis, elevation of blood glucose, promotion of glycogen storage, protein, lipid and carbohydrate metabolism, anti-inflammatory actions, and blood pressure maintenance
            (c) **Androgens**
         (2) **Adrenal medulla** produces catecholamines that function as hormones throughout the body
            (a) **Epinephrine and norepinephrine**
            (b) Embryologically derived from neuroectodermal cells
   b) **Disorders of the adrenal gland** can be described in four main categories
      i) Disorders which cause increased output
         (1) Increased catecholamine production
            (a) **Pheochromocytoma**
            (b) **Paragangliomas**
         (2) Increased aldosterone production
            (a) Primary (**Conn syndrome**)
            (b) Secondary from increased renin production
         (3) Increased cortisol
            (a) **Cushing syndrome**
            (b) **Exogenous administration**
      ii) Disorders which cause decreased output
         (1) Decreased cortisol
            (a) **Addison disease**
            (b) **Secondary to decreased ACTH production**
            (c) **Tertiary (iatrogenic)**

2) Disorders of increased output
   a) **Pheochromocytoma**
      i) Rare but significant disease
         (1) Incidence is <0.2% of patients with hypertension
         (2) Sometimes associated with familial syndromes such as multiple endocrine neoplasia (MEN), von Hippel–Lindau, Neurofibromatosis-1, and familial paragangliomas (1)
         (3) High perioperative mortality
             (a) Without preoperative treatment mortality can be as high as 45%
             (b) With appropriate preoperative treatment mortality is <3%
         (4) Surgical excision of the tumor is curative in >90% of patients (1)

"Classic" signs of pheochromocytoma: headache, palpitations, sweating, hypertension.

      ii) **Pathophysiology**
         (1) Pheochromocytomas are tumors that arise from chromaffin cells of the adrenal medulla
         (2) **Secrete epinephrine and norepinephrine** which leads to clinical manifestations
         (3) **Paragangliomas** are pheochromocytomas that grow outside of the adrenal glands
      iii) **Signs and symptoms result from catecholamine release**
         (1) Hypertension, headache, palpitations, tremor, sweating, anxiety, hyperglycemia, and catecholamine induced cardiomyopathy (2)
         (2) Signs and symptoms may be **sustained or paroxysmal** as a result of episodic increased secretion of catecholamines
         (3) **Paroxysmal catecholamine release may be precipitated by:**
             (a) **Stimulation,** including: laryngoscopy, displacement of abdominal contents, pneumoperitoneum, tumor manipulation
             (b) Tyramine containing **foods**
             (c) Certain **drugs** such as TCAs and metoclopromide
             (d) Micturition, in the case of urinary bladder tumors (1)
      iv) **Diagnosis**
         (1) **Excess catecholamines or metabolites** (metanephrine, normetanephrine, or VMA) found in **urine or plasma** testing
             (a) Plasma-free metanephrines or urinary-fractionated metanephrines are the most sensitive tests for diagnosis and exclusion of pheochromocytoma (1)
             (b) False positive elevated catecholamine levels may occur with physiologic stimuli
             (c) True positive elevated catecholamines can be distinguished by the magnitude of elevation often two to three times the upper reference limit (1,4)
         (2) Imaging allows localization of the tumor (1)
             (a) CT imaging with and without contrast
                 (i) Contrast may have an effect on plasma catecholamines
                 (ii) Patients should be protected from catecholamine release by alpha and beta blockade (see below) prior to contrast administration
             (b) MRI is preferred for extra-adrenal tumors or tumors found in pregnant patients, children, or patients allergic to CT contrast
             (c) MIBG scanning allows for functional and anatomic coupling which may be required for metastatic or multifocal tumors

α-blockade is continued for 10 to 14 days before surgery along with intravascular volume expansion to avoid excessive orthostatic hypotension.

      v) **Perioperative management**

(1) **Preoperative goals** are to prevent the effects of tumor released catecholamines

    (a) *α*-**Blockade**

        (i) Prevents the hypertensive effects of catecholamines (4).

        (ii) *α*-**Blockade is continued for 10 to 14 days before surgery along with intravascular volume expansion to avoid excessive orthostatic hypotension.**

        (iii) α-Blockers

           1. Long acting α-blockers (irreversible, noncompetitive)

              a. Phenoxybenzamine 10 mg BID, increasing every 2 to 3 days by 10 to 20 mg to maximum dose of 1 mg/kg

           2. Short acting α-blockers (competitive)

               b. Doxazosin increasing from 1 to 16 mg/day

               c. Prazosin 2 to 5 mg two to three times a day

               d. Terazosin 2 to 5 mg/day

β-blockade should only be added after several days of α-blockade to avoid the possibility of unopposed α-constriction resulting in severe hypertension, ischemia, and heart failure as well as other hypertension related end-organ dysfunction.

    (b) *β*-**Blockade**

        (i) Patients with **dysrhythmias or persistent tachycardia** require β-blockade

        (ii) *β*-**blockade should only be added after several days of α-blockade** to avoid the possibility of unopposed α-constriction resulting in severe hypertension, ischemia, and heart failure as well as other hypertension related end-organ dysfunction (1)

        (iii) β-Blockers

           1. Propranolol 20 to 80 mg one to three times a day

           2. Atenolol 12.5 to 25 mg two to three times a day

           3. Metoprolol 25 to 50 mg three to four times a day (4)

    (c) Other agents

        (i) **Labetalol** is a nonselective α and β blocker with predominant effects at β-receptors

        (ii) **Calcium channel blockers** do not completely prevent hemodynamic instability

        (iii) *α*-**methyl-paratyrosine or metirosine** can be used to block catecholamine synthesis

    (d) Preoperative treatment endpoints

        (i) Blood pressure control of <160/90 for more than 24 hours

        (ii) Presence of orthostatic hypotension (not <80/45 standing)

        (iii) Less than one premature ventricular contraction every 5 minutes

        (iv) Absence of ST segment changes and T wave inversions on ECG for 1 week (1)

        (v) Hematocrit decrease of 5% to suggest the adequacy of intravascular volume expansion and satisfactory α-blockade (3)

vi) **Intraoperative considerations**

    (1) Arterial blood pressure monitoring should be initiated prior to induction and intubation.

    (2) Large bore IV access and/or central venous access should be established for administration of fluids and vasoactive infusions.

    (3) Adequate monitoring for ischemia from catecholamine induced acute, severe hypertension should be used.

        (a) ECG

        (b) Transesophageal echocardiography (TEE) in patients with cardiomyopathy or uninterpretable ECG

    (4) Adequate depth of anesthesia should be achieved prior to laryngoscopy to minimize catecholamine responses

Pheochromocytoma patients should be watched for hypotension and hypoglycemia postoperatively.

(5) Acute increases in blood pressure can be treated with short acting agents such as: sodium nitroprusside, phentolamine, nicardipine, or magnesium infusions.

(6) Tachycardia can be treated with esmolol

(7) Short acting agents are preferred as hypotension may ensue following ligation of the venous drainage of the tumor

(8) **If hypotension occurs, IV fluids and phenylephrine or norepinephrine infusions are the initial treatment.**

vii) **Postoperative considerations**

    (1) **Hypotension** may result from an abrupt fall in circulating catecholamine levels combined with the residual effects of preoperative α blockade.

    (2) **Hypoglycemia** may ensue from a rebound hyperinsulinemia effect due to insulin release after tumor excision (1)

    (3) Following surgery patients should remain in a close watch unit for 24 hours for monitoring of blood pressure and glucose.

b) **Adrenal pathology with increased aldosterone production (2)**

  i) Two types

    (1) Primary increased adrenal cortex production (**Conn syndrome**)

    (2) Secondary to increased renin production

  ii) Pathophysiology

    (1) **Increased aldosterone** causes increased urinary sodium and potassium exchange that leads to **sodium and water retention, potassium loss**

  iii) Signs/symptoms of increased aldosterone

    (1) Hypertension, extracellular volume expansion, weakness

  iv) Perioperative management

    (1) Normalization of intravascular fluid volume and electrolytes

    (2) Preoperative sodium restriction

    (3) Aldosterone antagonists (spironolactone)

    (4) Potassium repletion

c) **Adrenal pathology with increased cortisol production (Cushing syndrome) (2)**

  i) Cortisol production is regulated by the hypothalamic-pituitary-adrenal (HPA) axis

    (1) Hypothalamic corticotrophin-releasing factor (CRF) stimulates anterior pituitary adrenocorticotropic hormone (ACTH) release, which stimulates the adrenal cortex to release cortisol.

    (2) Normal daily production of cortisol is 20 mg, with up to 300 mg produced in times of stress.

  ii) Excess cortisol production caused by adrenocortical overproduction (pituitary microadenoma or neuroendocrine tumors producing excess ACTH, adrenal neoplasm), or exogenous administration of cortisol

  iii) Signs/symptoms

    (1) Truncal obesity, hypertension, hyperglycemia, increased intravascular fluid volume, hypokalemia, osteoporosis, and muscle weakness

  iv) **Perioperative management**

    (1) Management of hypertension

    (2) Management of blood glucose

    (3) Normalization of intravascular fluid volume and electrolytes

    (4) When adrenalectomy is performed on these patients, glucocorticoid replacement must be initiated (see below)

3) **Adrenal Disorders with decreased output**

a) **Adrenal pathology with decreased cortisol production**

  i) **Adrenal Insufficiency (AI) (5)**

(1) Three types

(a) Primary adrenal insufficiency

(i) Loss of adrenal tissue

(ii) Results from autoimmune destruction (Addison's), infection (tuberculosis, advanced HIV, sepsis), malignancy, or hemorrhage

(iii) Patients are deficient in both mineralocorticoids and glucocorticoids

(b) Secondary adrenal insufficiency

(i) Decreased pituitary ACTH production

(ii) Patients usually have intact mineralocorticoid function via the renin–angiotensin system

(c) **Tertiary or iatrogenic HPA axis suppression**

(i) **Most common form of AI**

(ii) Results from chronic exogenous corticosteroid therapy

(iii) Patients usually have intact mineralocorticoid function via the rennin–angiotensin system

(2) AI may be seen in critically ill patients.

(3) Signs/Symptoms

(a) **AI is characterized by fatigue, weakness, anorexia, weight loss, hypotension, and hyperkalemia**

(b) **Acute AI may result in refractory distributive shock**

(4) Treatment of AI

(a) Mineralocorticoid and glucocorticoid administration

(i) **Patients suspected of acute AI should receive immediate steroid replacement with hydrocortisone** (100 mg IV every 6 hours continued for 24 hours), doses may be reduced following stabilization

(ii) electrolyte correction

(5) **Perioperative management (5)**

(a) **All patients with AI who undergo a procedure should receive their normal daily corticosteroid dose orally or intravenously.**

(b) Patients with primary or secondary AI are often unable to increase endogenous cortisol production during stress and should receive supplemental corticosteroid therapy.

(c) Patients on hydrocortisone doses >50 mg/day do not require additional mineralocorticoid supplementation (see Table 83-1 for steroid equivalencies among different glucocorticoid preparations)

(d) **Patients with tertiary AI who receive prednisone ≤5 mg/day (or equivalent) may have adequate HPA response to stress and usually do not require additional supplementation other than their normal daily dose.**

(e) Patients with tertiary AI on higher doses should receive supplemental corticosteroid therapy.

(f) Preoperative testing of adrenal function in patients with tertiary AI is not required as it does not predict clinical outcome or development of adrenal crisis (5,6)

(g) **Supplemental corticosteroid dosing**

(i) Corticosteroid doses should be administered based on the degree of surgical stress:

1. **Minor procedures** (hernia repair): hydrocortisone 25 mg or methylprednisolone 5 mg IV on the day of surgery only

2. **Moderate procedures** (open cholecystectomy): hydrocortisone 50 to 75 mg or methylprednisolone 10 to 15 mg IV on the day of surgery tapered quickly over 1 to 2 days to normal daily dose.

Adrenal insufficiency may be seen in critically ill patients.

Adrenal insufficiency usually presents with fatigue, weakness, anorexia, weight loss, hypotension and/or hyperkalemia.

Table 83-1

Equivalent Doses of Glucocorticoid Preparations

Generic Name	Anti-Inflammatory	Mineralocorticoid	Approximate Equivalent Dose (mg)
Short Acting			
Hydrocortisone	1.0	1.0	20.0
Cortisone	0.8	0.8	25.0
Prednisone	4.0	0.25	5.0
Prednisolone	4.0	0.25	5.0
Methylprednisolone	5.0	—	4.0
Intermediate Acting			
Triamcinolone	5.0	—	4.0
Long Acting			
Dexamethasone	30.0	—	0.75

Relative milligram comparisons with cortisol. The glucocorticoid and mineralocorticoid properties of cortisol are set as 1.0. Reproduced from Schwartz JJ, Akhitar S, Rosenbaum SH. Endocrine Function. In: Barash PG, Cullen BF, Sotelting RK, et al. Clinical Anesthesia. 6th ed. Philadelphia, PA: Lippincott, Williams & Wilkins, 2009:1291, with permission.

3. **Major procedures**: hydrocortisone 100 to 150 mg or methylprednisolone 20 to 30 mg IV on the day of procedure with rapid taper over 1 to 2 days to normal daily doses.

(ii) **Excessive doses (>200 to 300 mg) or prolonged duration of glucocorticoids are of no benefit** and deleterious effects may include: hyperglycemia, immunosuppression, accelerated protein catabolism, altered wound healing, volume overload, and acute psychosis (5).

Chapter Summary for Adrenal Disorders

Adrenal Gland Functions	Synthesis and secretion of hormones including aldosterone, cortisol, androgens, and catecholamines
Adrenal Gland Disorders	May involve increased hormone production (pheochromocytoma, hyperaldosteronism, Cushing syndrome), or decreased hormone production (AI)
Pheochromocytoma	Marked catecholamine release with resulting severe hypertensive disease. Careful preoperative preparation, intraoperative monitoring and treatment, and postoperative monitoring of blood pressure and glucose are required.
Adrenal Insufficiency (AI)	Most commonly results from exogenous steroid administration and suppression of the HPA axis. Perioperatively, patients may require additional cortisol supplementation.

References

1. Lenders JW, Eisenhofer G, Mannelli M, et al. Phaeochromocytoma. *Lancet* 2005;366:665–675.
2. Schwartz JJ, Akhtar S, Rosenbaum SH. Endocrine function. In: Barash PG, Cullen BF, Stoelting RK, et al., eds. *Clinical Anesthesia*. 6th ed. Philadelphia, PA: Lippincott Williams & Wilkins; 2009:1287–1295.
3. Stoelting RK, Dierdorf SF. Endocrine diseases. In: *Anesthesia and Co-Existing Disease*. 4th ed. Philadelphia, PA: Churchill Livingstone; 2002:424–434.
4. Pacak K. Preoperative management of the pheochromocytoma patient. *J Clin Endocrinol Metab* 2007;92(11):4069–4079.
5. Coursin DB, Wood KE. Corticosteroid supplementation for adrenal insufficiency. *JAMA* 2002;287(2):236–240.
6. Marik PE, Varon J. Requirement of perioperative stress doses of corticosteroids: a systematic review of the literature. *Arch Surg* 2008;143(12):1222–1226.

84 Pituitary Disorders

Andrea J. Fuller, MD

The pituitary gland is responsible for the secretion of many different endocrine hormones. Disorders may be due to under or over secretion of one or more hormones, each with its characteristic clinical signs and symptoms. Pituitary surgery is most commonly performed for a pituitary adenoma and the anesthesiologist must be aware of the intraoperative management of patients with specific pituitary disorders such as acromegaly.

1) **Anatomy**
   a) The pituitary gland is located in the **sella turcica** at the base of the brain.
   b) The lateral border of the sella turcica is the **cavernous sinus,** which contains **the internal carotid artery, cranial nerves III, VI, V (maxillary and ophthalmic divisons), and VI.**
   c) Anterior to the pituitary is the **optic chiasm.**

2) **Physiology:** The pituitary gland is under the control of the hypothalamus and secretes many different hormones (1).
   a) **Anterior pituitary**
      i) **Thyroid stimulating hormone (TSH)**
         (1) Stimulates the thyroid gland to release thyroid hormone
      ii) **Follicle stimulating hormone (FSH)**
         (1) Stimulates estradiol production in females
      iii) **Adrenocorticotropic hormone (ACTH)**
         (1) Stimulates the secretion of cortisol and androgens
      iv) **Prolactin**
         (1) Stimulates lactation
      v) **Growth hormone**
         (1) Acts throughout the body and has a variety of metabolic and endocrine functions.
         (2) Exerts much of its effects via insulin-like growth factors.
      vi) **Luteinizing hormone**
         (1) Stimulates progesterone production and ovulation in females.
         (2) In males it results in testosterone production and spermatogenesis.
   b) **Posterior pituitary:** The hormones released by the posterior pituitary are synthesized in the hypothalamus and released by the posterior pituitary.
      i) **Vasopressin (ADH or antidiuretic hormone) (2)**
         (1) Controls water retention in the kidney
         (2) Causes **systemic vasoconstriction** in higher doses
         (3) Increases the level of plasma von Willebrand factor and factor VIII.
         (4) Synthetic analog is desmopressin (DDAVP)
      ii) **Oxytocin**
         (1) **Contracts the uterus** during parturition and aids in **expressing milk** during lactation.

615

3) **Pituitary disorders** (2)

a) **Hyposecretory**
   i) Involves **decreased hormone secretion.**
   ii) Causes include postpartum necrosis (Sheehan syndrome), trauma, radiation therapy, and compression from adjacent tumor.
   iii) Treatment is hormone replacement therapy, including cortisol, thyroid hormone, and possibly DDAVP

Endocrine abnormalities caused by a pituitary adenoma should be normalized prior to surgery whenever possible.

b) **Hypersecretory**
   i) Involve **excess hormone secretion**, most commonly caused by a pituitary adenoma (see below for specific hypersecretory disorders).
   ii) **Treatment is surgical excision**

4) **Hypersecretory disorders of concern for anesthesiologists** (2,3):
   a) **Signs/symptoms**
      i) Visual field disturbances (bitemporal hemianopsia), headaches, papilledema, nausea, vomiting, and physiologic changes due to hormone hypersecretion.
      ii) **Laboratory evaluation should include ECG, electrolytes, and blood glucose.**
   b) **Prolactinoma**
      i) Causes galactorrhea and amenorrhea but has few other physiologic implications.
   c) **Cushings disease**
      i) Excess cortisol secretion by the adrenal gland due to excess secretion of ACTH by the pituitary (2).
      ii) **Signs/symptoms**
         (1) Weight gain accompanied by thickened facial fat (moon faces), hyperglycemia, hypertension, skeletal muscle wasting, hypokalemia
   d) **Acromegaly**
      i) Results from excess secretion of growth hormone (2,3)
      ii) **Signs/symptoms**
         (1) Distorted facial anatomy including mandibular expansion and enlarged tongue

Patients with acromegaly are at high risk for difficult airway.

         (2) Airway changes such as enlarged epiglottis, overgrowth of cricoarytenoid joints, vocal cord dysfunction, enlargement of nasal turbinates
            (a) **Airway management can be difficult in patients with acromegaly and appropriate precautions should be taken.**
               (i) Signs concerning for difficult airway include a history of **stridor, hoarseness, and dyspnea**
               (ii) Patients are at risk for postoperative respiratory failure or airway obstruction
         (3) Patients often have glucose intolerance so blood glucose should be monitored
         (4) Abnormal collateral blood flow in the ulnar artery (3)
         (5) Systemic hypertension
         (6) Ischemic heart disease
         (7) Skeletal muscle weakness

5) Pituitary surgery and anesthetic considerations
   a) The most common surgical approach is transphenoidal but a transcranial approach can be used (3,4).
   b) **Preoperative considerations**
      i) A thorough history and physical should be performed, concentrating on possible signs/symptoms of hypersecretion.
      ii) Laboratory tests should be reviewed, including serum glucose, electrolyte panels and hormone levels. A type and cross should be performed.
      iii) Imaging studies should be performed and reviewed with the radiologist or surgeon to determine the extent of tumor invasion.
      iv) **Cardiac considerations**
         (1) ECG should be reviewed, looking for signs of left ventricular hypertrophy and arrythmias (especially in the presence of acromegaly).
         (2) If the hormone imbalance has been longstanding and/or the patient has symptoms of cardiac dysfunction an echocardiogram may be helpful in determining possible ventricular dysfunction and/or valvular anomalies.
         (3) Cardiac function should be optimized prior to surgery.
   c) **Intraoperative considerations**
      i) **Invasive monitoring**
         (1) An arterial line is usually necessary for monitoring BP and laboratory values.
         (2) A central venous catheter may be required if significant hemodynamic changes will require vasoactive infusions.
      ii) A lumbar drain may be placed by the surgeon. Saline may be injected to aid in visualization of the pituitary gland during surgery.
      iii) Difficult airway equipment should be available in all acromegalic patients and any whose exam is concerning for difficult intubation or ventilation.

Consider cortisol deficiency when faced with refractory intraoperative hypotension during pituitary surgery.

      iv) **Intraoperative hypotension**
         (1) May be due to inadequate cortisol production, especially in patients with Cushing Disease or impaired cortisol production.
         (2) **Cortisol should be replaced with hydrocortisone 50 to 100 mg IV** in this situation (5).
      v) **Blood loss**
         (1) Usually minimal although there is the potential for massive blood loss if the cavernous sinus is entered inadvertently.
      vi) **Venous air embolism** is possible but very uncommon due to the semi-seated position required for the procedure.
   d) **Postoperative**
      i) **Diabetes insipidus (DI)**
         (1) Characterized by excessive urine production and high plasma osmolality.
         (2) May occur intra or postoperatively
         (3) Usually due to reversible trauma to the posterior pituitary resulting in insufficient ADH production.
         (4) If DI is suspected, the diagnosis can be made by measuring serum electrolytes, plasma osmolality, and urine osmolality (2)
            (a) Patients will have a low urine osmolality, high plasma osmolality, and hypernatremia
         (5) Treatment
            (a) Monitor urine output and electrolytes
         (b) Ensure adequate fluid replacement.
         (c) ADH can be replaced with intranasal or intravascular DDAVP (2).

Chapter Summary for Pituitary Surgery

Pituitary Gland Function	Responsible for initiating secretion of many hormones
Pituitary Surgery	Typically transsphenoidal approach
Preoperative Considerations	Evaluate for visual field defects, cardiac disease, glucose intolerance and difficult airway (especially in acromegaly)
Intraoperative Considerations	Blood loss usually not high, closely monitor glucose, consider cortisol deficiency with refractory hypotension
Postoperative Considerations	Diabetes insipidus possible

References

1. Guyton AC, Hall JE. The pituitary hormones and their control by the hypothalamus. In: Guyton AC, Hall JE, eds. *Textbook of Medical Physiology*. 9th ed. Philadelphia, PA: W.B. Saunders; 1996:933–944.
2. Schwartz JJ, Akhtar S, Rosenbaum SH. Endocrine function. In: Barash PG, Cullen BF, Stoelting RK, et al., eds. *Clinical Anesthesia*. 6th ed. Philadelphia, PA: Lippincott Williams & Wilkins, 2009:1279–1304.
3. Stoelting RK, Dierdorf SF. Endocrine diseases. In: Stoelting RK, Dierdorf SF, eds. *Anesthesia and Co-Existing Disease*. 4th ed. Philadelphia, PA: Churchill Livingstone, 2002:395–440.
4. Lim M, Williams D, Maartens N. Anaesthesia for pituitary surgery. *J Clin Neurosci* 2006;13:413–418.
5. Inder WJ, Hunt PJ. Glucocorticoid replacement in pituitary surgery: guidelines for perioperative assessment and management. *J Clin Endocrinol Metab* 2002;87:2745–2750.

85

Parathyroid Disorders

Andrea J. Fuller, MD

The parathyroid glands regulate intravascular calcium concentrations. One common disorder of these glands is hyperparathyroidism, usually caused by an adenoma. Removal of the parathyroid glands can lead to hypocalcemia. Patients with this condition must be properly assessed before administering anesthesia.

1) Anatomy/Normal Function of the Parathyroid Glands
   a) **Anatomy**
      i) Parathyroid glands are in the neck posterior to the thyroid gland.
      ii) Most people have four parathyroid glands.
   b) **Normal Function**
      i) Parathyroid glands secrete parathyroid hormone (PTH), which regulates intravascular calcium concentrations. (Fig. 85-1)
      ii) **Calcium**
         (1) Provides the foundation for bone.
         (2) It is a key neurotransmitter and plays a role in intracellular signaling and coagulation.
         (3) Exists as protein bound (to albumin) or ionized divalent cations.
            (a) The free, ionized calcium (Ca^{2+}) exerts physiologic effects (2).
         (4) **Extracellular (intravascular) calcium concentration depends on the albumin concentration.**
            (a) **Normal calcium levels = 8.6 to 10.4 mg/dL (3)**
2) Disorders of the Parathyroid Glands
   a) **Disorders causing** hyperparathyroidism
      i) **Primary hyperparathyroidism**
         (1) Most commonly caused by an **adenoma**.
            (a) Other causes include hyperplasia and parathyroid carcinoma (rare).
            (b) May also be associated with Multiple Endocrine Neoplasia syndrome (MEN).
      ii) **Secondary hyperparathyroidism**
         (1) **Causes**
            (a) Chronic renal failure
            (b) Sarcoidosis
            (c) Multiple myeloma
            (d) Vitamin D intoxication
         (2) **Diagnosis of hyperparathyroidism**
            (a) **High serum calcium or elevated serum ionized calcium in the presence of high serum PTH.**

The cardiovascular manifestations of hypercalcemia include hypertension and shortened PR and QT intervals.

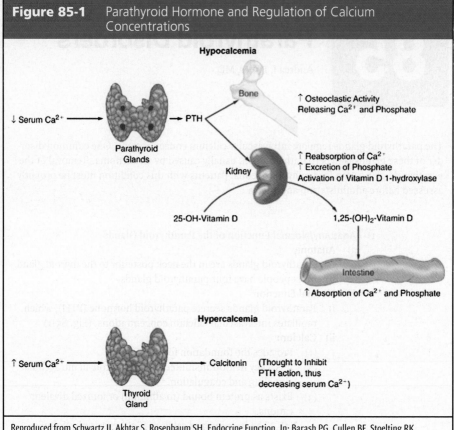

Figure 85-1 Parathyroid Hormone and Regulation of Calcium Concentrations

Reproduced from Schwartz JJ, Akhtar S, Rosenbaum SH. Endocrine Function. In: Barash PG, Cullen BF, Stoelting RK, et al, eds. *Clinical Anesthesia*. 6th ed. Philadelphia: Lippincott Williams & Wilkins, 2009: 1285, with permission.

      (b) Other laboratory abnormalities include
          (i) Hypophosphatemia
          (ii) Phosphaturia
          (iii) Hyperchloremia
          (iv) Hypercalciuria
          (v) Increased serum alkaline phosphatase
   iii) Increased circulating PTH causes **hypercalcemia (Table 85-1)**
 b) **Hypoparathyroidism**
   i) Most commonly caused by removal of parathyroid during thyroid or parathyroid surgery.
   ii) Results in hypocalcemia.
 c) **Other causes of hypocalcemia**
   i) Hypoalbuminemia
   ii) Chronic renal failure
   iii) Rapid blood transfusions
   iv) Clinical manifestations of **hypocalcemia**
      (1) **Acute**
         (a) Perioral paresthesias
         (b) Restlessness

Table 85-1
Signs and Symptoms of Hypercalcemia

Organ System	Manifestation
Musculoskeletal	Profound muscle weakness, bone pain
Gastrointestinal	Nausea, decreased appetite, vomiting, constipation, increased gastric ulcer formation, pancreatitis
Neurologic	Depression, lethargy, impaired memory, and confusion
Cardiovascular	Decreased intravascular volume, hypertension, shortened PR and QT intervals, myocardial calcification (long-term)
Renal	Polyuria, nephrolithiasis, proximal renal tubular acidosis

      (c)   Neuromuscular irritability
      (d)   Laryngospasm
      (e)   Apnea
   (2) **Trousseau Sign**
      (a)   Carpopedal spasm after 3 minutes of tourniquet-induced limb ischemia.
   (3) **Chvostek Sign**
      (a)   Facial muscle twitching elicited by tapping the facial nerve at the angle of the mandible.
   (4) **Chronic**
      (a)   Fatigue
      (b)   Skeletal muscle cramps
      (c)   Decreased mentation
      (d)   Prolonged ST segment
      (e)   QT interval
      (f)   Decreased inotropy
3) Medical treatment of hypercalcemia
   a) **Bisphosphonates** (pamidronate, etidronate, clodronate)
     i) Prevent calcium reabsorption
     ii) Rapid onset with long lasting effects
   b) **Calcitonin**
     i) Decreases skeletal release of calcium
     ii) Short duration limits use
   c) **Emergency correction of Ca^{2+}**
     i) Necessary with serum concentrations >15 mg/dL (2).
     ii) **Volume expansion** with intravenous fluid
        (1)   4 to 6 L may be required in 24 hours.
     iii) **Increased Ca^{2+} excretion** with loop diuretics

(1) Risks include
  (a) Cardiac decompensation
  (b) Hypophosphatemia
  (c) Hypokalemia
  (d) Hypomagnesemia
  iv) Dialysis (for patients with renal failure)
4) **Surgical treatment of primary hyperparathyroidism**
  a) Minimally invasive radio guided approach is gaining popularity.
    i) Involves localizing the parathyroid adenoma and removal through a small incision (4).
  b) Open neck exploration
    i) Involves removal of the adenoma but potentially removal of most parathyroid tissue.
5) **Anesthetic management of patients with primary hyperparathyroidism**
  a) Most patients presenting with primary hyperparathyroidism will be undergoing parathyroidectomy.
  b) **Preoperative**
    i) Attention should be paid to potential dysfunction of the cardiac, neurologic, and renal systems.
      (1) Evaluation should include
        (a) Electrolyte levels
        (b) ECG
        (c) Neurologic exam
      (2) Medical correction of extremely high serum Ca^{2+} levels may be necessary prior to elective surgery.
  c) **Intraoperative**
    i) No induction or maintenance agents are preferred over any others.
    ii) Careful titration of muscle relaxants with a nerve stimulator is necessary as patients may be more sensitive to their effects (5)
  d) **Postoperative**
    i) Serum Ca^{2+} levels return to normal 1 to 3 days postoperatively and are not usually checked in the immediate postoperative period.
      (1) Acute hypocalcemia (see above) may occur immediately postoperatively.
        (a) If suspected, serum Ca^{2+} should be checked.

    ii) **Recurrent laryngeal nerve injury**
      (1) The recurrent laryngeal nerve innervates the intrinsic muscles of the larynx.
        (a) Partial injury is more likely to affect abductor fibers.
      (2) **Unilateral recurrent laryngeal nerve palsy.**
        (a) Vocal cord is in paramedian position and cannot abduct or adduct.
        (b) Presents as hoarseness and stridor.
      (3) **Bilateral recurrent laryngeal nerve palsy (3)**
        (a) Results in inability to abduct or adduct the vocal cords, with both vocal cords in the paramedian position.
        (b) May be life threatening and require reintubation

Postoperative hypocalcemia may occur after parathyroidectomy and manifest as neuromuscular irritability and laryngeospasm.

Chapter Summary for Parathyroid Disorders

Causes of Hyperparathyroidism	Parathyroid adenoma, rarely associated with MEN syndrome
Manifestations	Hypercalcemia
Anesthetic Management	
Preoperative	May need to correct hypercalcemia with IV fluid and/or loop diuretics Assess cardiac, neurologic, and renal function
Intraoperative	May be sensitive to neuromuscular blockade
Postoperative	Recurrent laryngeal nerve injury possible and may result in airway compromise Acute hypocalcemia can present as laryngeospasm, apnea, restlessness, and neuromuscular irritability

MEN, multiple endocrine neoplasia; IV, intravenous.

References
1. Barash, Paul G. *Clinical Anesthesia*. 6th ed. Philadelphia, PA: Wolters Kluwer/Lippincott Williams & Wilkins; 2009.
2. Mihai R, Farndon JR. Parathyroid disease and calcium metabolism. *Br J Anaesth* 2000;85(1):29–43.
3. Miller RD. *Miller's Anesthesia*. 7th ed. Philadelphia, PA: Churchill Livingstone/Elsevier; 2009.
4. Lee WJ, Ruda J, Stack BC. Minimally invasive radioguided parathyroidectomy using intraoperative sestamibi localization. *Otolaryngol Clin North Am* 2004;37(4):789–798.
5. Roland EJL, Wierda JMKH, Turin BY, et al. Pharmacodynamic behavior of vecuronium in primary hyperparathroidism. *Can J Anaesth* 1994;41:694–698.

86 Obesity

Andrea J. Fuller, MD

Obesity is a growing clinical challenge for anesthesiologists. The incidence of obesity has risen in the past few decades and is estimated to be approximately 27% (1). Obesity increases the risk of many diseases, including diabetes mellitus (DM), coronary artery disease (CAD), obstructive sleep apnea (OSA), hypertension (HTN), and degenerative joint disease. As such, the anesthesiologist must understand the unique challenges, both practical and physiologic, that are faced in this population.

1) Introduction
   a) **Ideal body weight (IBW)**
      i) Defined as the weight associated with the lowest mortality for a given height
      ii) IBW can be calculated by the formula

   > IBW (kg) = height (cm) − x, where x =100 for men and 105 for women (2).

   b) **Body mass index (BMI)**
      i) The BMI is the weight in kg divided by the height in meters squared (**wt/ht²**).
      ii) Normal BMI is 18 to 24, overweight is 25 to 29, and obese is >30.
      iii) **Morbid obesity is defined as a BMI >40.**
   c) **Epidemiology**
      i) Approximately 27% of the US population is considered obese (1).
      ii) The rate of obesity varies with geographic region, with the Southern United States having the highest prevalence.

2) **Co-existing diseases**: Morbid obesity is associated with many physiologic derangements and can lead to multiple co-existing diseases, all of which should be optimized prior to elective surgery and managed appropriately intraoperatively.

    READ MORE

   Diabetes mellitus, Chapter 81, page 592

   Essential hypertension and anesthetic considerations, Chapter 58, page 424

   Obstructive sleep apnea, Chapter 74, page 524

   a) **Diabetes mellitus**
      i) The incidence of DM is 21% in patients weighing >300 lb (3).
      ii) Patients with DM have a higher incidence of CAD, kidney disease, and cerebrovascular disease.
      iii) DM increases the risk of surgical complications such as poor wound healing and infection.
   b) **Arterial HTN**
      i) The incidence of HTN in patients weighing >300 lb is 44% (3).
      ii) HTN further increases the cardiac workload and can contribute to left ventricular hypertrophy and failure.
   c) **Obstructive sleep apnea**
      i) Pharyngeal airway tissue enlargement is extremely common in the obese population and can cause OSA.

ii) It is estimated that 60% to 90% of patients with OSA are obese and most cases are undiagnosed (4).

iii) A history of snoring is highly suspicious for OSA (4).

iv) **Obesity hypoventilation syndrome (5)**

  (1) The end result of long term OSA

  (2) Due to desensitization of respiratory centers to hypercarbia, which results in central apnea

  (3) Characterized by Pickwickian syndrome: hypercarbia, hypoxemia, polycythemia, hypersomnolence, pulmonary HTN, biventricular failure

  (4) Patients with this syndrome are at extremely high risk for apnea, acidosis, respiratory failure, and potentially right heart failure ether postoperatively or with minimal sedation (e.g., monitored anesthesia care cases).

READ MORE

Gastrointestinal and hepatobiliary surgery, Chapter 132, page 921

Arthritis, Chapter 92, page 663

d) **Gastroesophageal reflux disease**

  i) The increased intra-abdominal pressure in morbidly obese individuals is often considered to increase the risk for gastroesophageal reflux although this is controversial.

  ii) Aspiration precautions should be strongly considered.

e) **Osteoarthritis**

  i) Increased weight places stress on joints and leads to the development of osteoarthritis. Many patients have chronic back and/or joint pain.

f) **Thromboembolic disease**

  i) Obesity increases the risk of thromboembolic events.

  ii) The increased incidence is likely due to polycythemia, increased abdominal pressure, and venous stasis from immobility (5).

  iii) Early ambulation and thromboprophylaxis are paramount in the obese surgical patient.

3) **Physiologic changes (Table 86-1)**

a) **Increased airway tissue and neck circumference**

b) **Increased blood flow to adipose tissues**

  i) In the obese patient blood flow increases significantly, with 20 to 30 mL blood flow/1 kg adipose tissue (2).

  ii) This leads to increased cardiac output and blood volume, which increases myocardial oxygen demand.

c) **Respiratory**

  i) Respiratory physiology changes dramatically in the obese population, making these patients at high risk for hypoxemia and possibly death.

  ii) **Functional residual capacity (FRC) is reduced (2).**

    (1) The reduction in lung volumes may be so severe that normal breathing approaches closing capacity and leads to ventilation-perfusion (V/Q) mismatch (2).

    (2) The supine position is often not well tolerated due to extreme V/Q mismatch.

Obese patients may not tolerate the supine position due to extreme decreases in FRC.

  iii) Obese patients have decreased respiratory compliance due to chest wall adipose tissue.

  iv) Chronic hypoxemia can lead to pulmonary HTN and right ventricular failure.

d) **Gastrointestinal** (see Table 86-1).

e) **Endocrine**

  i) Morbid obesity leads to impaired glucose tolerance and increases the risk of DM.

Table 86-1

Physiologic Derangements in Obese Patients and Their Anesthetic Implications

Organ System	Physiologic Derangements	Anesthetic Implications
Respiratory	↑ Oxygen consumption ↑ pharyngeal tissue possible ↓ ventilatory response to CO_2	Rapid arterial desaturation ↑ risk of OSA ↑ sensitivity to narcotics
	↓ FRC and ERV	Rapid arterial desaturation, ventilation-perfusion (VQ) abnormalities, possibly causing right to left shunt and pulmonary HTN Assumption of the supine position can worsen VQ mismatch
Cardiovascular	↑ blood volume and cardiac output ↑ risk for CAD ↑ risk for arterial HTN	LVH May need cardiac evaluation to determine presence of CAD
Endocrine	Impaired glucose tolerance leading to DM	Require intraoperative monitoring and control of glucose
Gastrointestinal	↑ intra-abdominal pressure ↑ gastric volume	↑ Risk for acid aspiration Consider premedication to reduce risk of pulmonary injury if aspiration occurs
Airway	↑ neck circumference ↑ Mallampatti score	Possible increased risk of difficult airway

OSA, obstructive sleep apnea; LVH, left ventricular hypertrophy; CAD, coronary artery disease; HTN, hypertension; DM, diabetes mellitus.

4) The perioperative approach to the obese patient
   a) **Preoperative considerations**
      i) **Surgical procedures**
         (1) Morbidly obese patients present to the operating room for a variety of surgical procedures.
         (2) Procedures performed to treat obesity include bariatric procedures such as gastric bypass or banding.
         (3) Others common procedures include uvulopalatopharyngoplasty or orthopedic surgeries due to joint degeneration, although the obese patient may require any type of surgical procedure.
      ii) **Preoperative assessment**
         (1) Should focus on comorbid conditions, with special attention to respiration, OSA, and airway assessment.
         (2) Preoperative laboratory evaluations will vary with the patient and procedure but may include

(a) Chemistry panel to evaluate electrolytes, blood glucose, and kidney function

(b) ECG to evaluate for ventricular (left or right) hypertrophy and evidence of ischemia

(c) CBC to evaluate for polycythemia

(d) Other studies such as cardiac stress tests and more extensive laboratory analysis may be indicated but are not routine.

iii) **Airway assessment**

(1) It is controversial whether airway management is more difficult in obese patients (6,7).

(2) Risk factors for difficult intubation in obese patients are large neck circumference and high Mallampati score (6,7).

iv) With a neck circumference of 60 cm or greater, the incidence of problematic intubation in one study was 35% (6)

v) Equipment to aid in management of a difficult airway should always be available and plans for difficult intubation should be made in high-risk patients

READ MORE

Combined spinal-epidural technique, Chapter 33, page 252

b) **Regional anesthesia**

i) Obese patients may benefit from regional anesthesia due to improved postoperative pain control and decreased use of narcotic analgesics.

ii) A recent study showed that the odds ratio of failed regional anesthesia in obese patients was 1.6, presumably due to technical difficulties (8).

iii) Decreased cerebral spinal fluid volume, high intra-abdominal pressure, and altered respiratory physiology may increase the risk of high spinal anesthesia.

(1) Careful monitoring is necessary in obese patients when spinal anesthesia is administered.

(2) A combined spinal epidural with a lower than average spinal dose may be considered when the optimal spinal anesthetic dose is unknown.

While most modern OR beds and equipment are designed with a high weight limit, it is important to verify the weight limits of the OR table prior to caring for a morbidly obese patient.

Intubation in obese individuals can be facilitated by placement of blankets under the head and shoulders until the sternal notch and external auditory meatus are aligned (9).

iv) **Preparing the OR for a morbidly obese patient**

(1) **OR table and gurneys**

(a) Check the weight limits of the operating room table and gurneys.

(b) Ensure that the table is wide enough to accommodate the patient. Table extensions may be necessary.

(c) If special positions (e.g., Trendelenburg position) will be required, one must ensure that the table is able to accommodate this position with the increased weight of the patient.

c) **Intraoperative management**

i) **Positioning**

(1) **Airway management**

(a) Intubation is often easier when the patient is placed on a "ramp" to align the sternal notch and external auditory meatus (7).

(b) If a "ramp" is used to facilitate airway management one must ensure that there are not pressure-inducing bumps in the bedding.

(c) Furthermore, the arms must be at the same level as the patient's shoulders to avoid a stretch injury to the brachial plexus.

(d) For long cases, it is prudent to remove the material used for the ramp.

READ MORE

Endotracheal intubation, Chapter 20, page 137

(2) **Padding**

    (a) Obesity places patients at risk of developing decubitus ulcers.

    (b) The heels, buttocks, and shoulders are at particular risk and should be checked and padded (2).

ii) **Preoxygenation**

    (1) Because the FRC approaches closing volume in obese individuals, they are at risk for hypoxemia on assumption of the supine position and induction of anesthesia.

    (2) Adequate preoxygenation to adequately denitrogenate the lungs is required and can be invaluable in cases of difficult airway.

iii) **Aspiration precautions**

    (1) The morbidly obese patient is at risk for gastric acid aspiration and appropriate precautions, including premedication with a nonparticulate antacid and H_2 receptor antagonist are usually necessary.

    (2) A rapid sequence induction should be strongly considered but may need to be modified if the patient experiences hypoxia on induction of anesthesia.

iv) **IV access**

    (1) IV access can be difficult in the presence of excess adipose tissue.

    (2) If adequate peripheral IV access is not possible the patient may require a central venous catheter.

When caring for an obese patient, ensure that the blood pressure cuff is adequately sized. Too small a cuff will overestimate blood pressure.

v) **Monitoring**

    (1) **BP management**

        (a) Many patients present with arterial HTN, which must be managed intraoperatively.

        (b) A large blood pressure cuff should be used. The measurement can be overestimated with a cuff that is too small for the patient.

        (c) If noninvasive blood pressure measurement is inaccurate or impossible and arterial line should be placed.

READ MORE

Ischemic heart disease, Chapter 51, page 359

    (2) **Cardiac considerations**

        (a) LVH and CAD may be present.

        (b) Invasive monitoring of central venous pressure or use of TEE is not routine but may be considered based on the patient's underlying cardiac disease and the surgical procedure.

Obese patients have both an increased risk of hypoventilation and decreased elimination of benzodiazepine drugs and extreme care should be taken with their administration.

vi) **Pharmacology (10)**

    (1) Can be complex due to changes in elimination and enzymes (e.g., pseudocholinesterase) which occur as body weight increases.

    (2) **Obese patients have an increased volume of distribution for lipid soluble drugs (e.g., benzodiazapines)**

        (a) Initial dosing should be based on actual body weight.

        (b) Clearance may be the same or increased with obesity but elimination may be prolonged due to the large volume of distribution (10).

            (i) Extreme caution should be taken with any lipid-soluble sedative/hypnotic drug is administered to an obese individual at risk for hypoventilation (i.e., those with OSA)

    (3) For **hydrophilic drugs** (e.g., muscle relaxants) the volume of distribution is unchanged and dosing should be based on IBW (10).

        (a) Pseudocholinesterase is increased and therefore **succinylcholine should be dosed closer to total body weight.**

    (4) **Volatile anesthetics**

        (a) The newer, more water-soluble volatile anesthetics (sevoflurane, desflurane) have very negligible differences in emergence times for obese versus lean individuals (10).

        (b)   More lipid-soluble anesthetics have much greater differences in emergence between obese and lean patients.

        (5)   Drugs with extensive extra-hepatic metabolism (e.g., remifentanil) appear to have similar pharmacokinetics in obese and lean individuals (10).

  d) **Anesthetic emergence**

     i)   Obese patients are at high risk of airway obstruction on emergence and should be extubated awake with intact airway reflexes

     ii) Due to altered respiratory mechanics, it may be helpful to place the patient semi-upright prior to extubation

     iii) Careful postoperative respiratory monitoring is required

5) Postoperative pain management

  a) **Risk of airway obstruction**

     i)   Any patient with a history suspicious for OSA is at risk for postoperative airway obstruction.

     ii) At the end of the procedure, patients should be awake with muscle relaxants fully reversed on extubation.

     iii) An oro or nasopharyngeal airway is helpful to prevent airway obstruction.

     iv) The patient should be transported with oxygen, preferably via a facemask.

     v) Retaining the endotracheal tube for postoperative ventilation may be preferable to extubation at the end of the procedure, depending on the risk of airway difficulty, length of surgery, and fluid shifts.

  b) **Sensitivity to opioid medications**

     i)   Any patient with a history suspicious for OSA is at risk for a decreased ventilatory response to increasing CO_2.

     ii) Respiratory monitoring should be considered when post-operative pain control includes use of opioids (4).

  c) **Neuraxial analgesia**

     i)   Obese patients may benefit from neuraxial opioid analgesia.

     ii) However, careful monitoring is imperative due to the risk of delayed respiratory depression.

The pharma-cokinetics of remifentanil are not significantly altered in obese patients.

Chapter Summary for Obesity

Definition	Obesity = BMI >30; Morbid Obesity = BMI >40
Coexisting Diseases	Diabetes, HTN, OSA, GERD, Osteoarthritis, Thromboembolic Disease, Cardiac Disease All should be optimized prior to elective surgery
OR Preparation	May require special beds and other equipment Noninvasive BP may be inaccurate Presssure points must be padded
Anesthetic Considerations	Airway management may be improved by aligning the sternal notch with the external auditory meatus Patients are at risk for hypoxemia in the supine position; IV access may be difficult Co-existing diseases may necessitate additional monitoring; Patients are at risk for airway obstruction on extubation and in PACU
Drug Dosing	Patients may be sensitive to lipid-soluble sedative hypnotic drugs (such as benzodiazapines)

BMI, body mass index; HTN, hypertension; OSA, obstructive sleep apnea; GERD, gastroesophageal reflux disease.

References

1. Center for Disease Control and Prevention. Vital signs: Obesity prevalence among adults—United States 2009. *MMWR Morb Mortal Wkly Rep* 2010;59:951–5.
2. Ogunnaike BO, Whitten CW. Anesthesia and obesity. In: Barash PG, Cullen BF, Stoelting RK, eds. *Clinical Anesthesia*. Philadelphia, PA: Lippincott Williams & Wilkins; 2006:1040–1052.
3. Mondolfi RN, Jones TM, Hyre AD, et al. Comparison of percent of United States adults weighing > or = 300 pounds (136 kilograms) in three time periods and comparison of five atherosclerotic risk factors for those weighing > or = 300 pounds to those < 300 pounds. *Am J Cardiol* 2007;100:1651–1653.
4. Benumof JL. Obesity, sleep apnea, the airway, and anesthesia. *Curr Opin Anes* 2004;17:21–30.
5. Wall RT. Endocrine disease. In: Hnes RL, Marschall KE, eds. *Stoelting's Anesthesia and Co-existing Disease*. 5th ed. Philadelphia, PA: Churchill Livingstone; 2008:365–406.
6. Brodsky JB, Lemmens HJM, Brock-Utne JG, et al. Morbid obesity and tracheal intubation. *Anesth Analg* 2002;94:732–736.
7. Juvin P, Lavaut E, Dupont H, et al. Difficult tracheal intubation is more common in obese than in lean patients. *Anesth Analg* 2003;97:595–600.
8. Nielsen KC, Guller U, Steele SM, et al. Influence of obesity on surgical regional anesthesia in the ambulatory setting: an analysis of 9,038 blocks. *Anesthesiology* 2005;102:181–187.
9. Brodsky JB, Lemmens HJM, Brock-Utne JG, et al. Anesthetic considerations for bariatric surgery: proper positioning is important for laryngoscopy. *Anesth Analg* 2003;96:1841–1842.
10. Casati A, Putzu M. Anesthesia in the obese patient: pharmacokinetic considerations. *J Clin Anesth* 2005;17:134–145.

87

Part E: Hematology and Oncology
Anemia

Wesley Liao, MD • Jamie Murphy, MD • Andrea J. Fuller, MD

Anemia is a deficiency in red blood cell (RBC) concentration caused by decreased production or peripheral loss. Perioperative anemia is associated with increased morbidity and mortality (1). Preoperative hemoglobin (Hgb) levels of <8 g/dL are associated with a 16-fold increase in mortality rate as compared with nonanemic patients (2,3). Blood transfusions due to perioperative anemia increase health care resource utilization and expose patients to increases in length of stay, need for ICU admission, infection risk, and immunosuppressive effects (2). Diagnosis and treatment of perioperative anemia has been demonstrated to improve overall patient outcomes and decrease the need for perioperative blood transfusions and its associated risks.

1) Definition
   a) The key characteristic of anemia is low oxygen transport capacity of the blood, either due to decreased RBC number or function.
   b) There is no absolute value to define anemia because the RBC number may vary with different physiologic states.
   c) However, anemia is generally defined in adults as a hemoglobin level <12.5 g/dL in males, <11.5 g/dL in females (4).

2) The oxyhemoglobin dissociation curve (5)
   a) The relationship between the arterial oxygen tension and the saturation of hemoglobin molecules with oxygen is described by the oxyhemoglobin dissociation curve (Fig. 87-1)
   b) The P50 value is the arterial oxygen concentration at which hemoglobin is 50% saturated with oxygen.
   c) A shift to the left occurs in the presence of alkalosis, hypothermia, decreased 2,3 diphosphoglygerate (DPG), and high concentrations of fetal hemoglobin. It indicates that oxygen is more tightly bound and there is less unloading of oxygen in the tissues.
   d) A right shift occurs in the presence of acidosis, hyperthermia, and increased 2,3 DPG. **Hemoglobin is less tightly bound to oxygen, which facilitates tissue oxygen delivery.**

3) Causes of Anemia
   a) **Blood Loss**
      i) May be chronic or acute
      ii) If blood loss is the suspected cause of anemia, the source of bleeding should be ascertained
   b) **Bone Marrow Failure**
      i) Drug toxicity from medications such as myelosuppressive drugs, chloramphenicol, and sulfonamides
      ii) Bone marrow suppression due to neoplasms, infections, irradiation, toxins, or idiopathic causes

↑ 2,3 DPG, acidosis, and hyperthermia shift the oxyhemoglobin dissociation curve to the right, which facilitates tissue oxygen delivery.

Figure 87-1   The Oxyhemoglobin Dissociation Curve

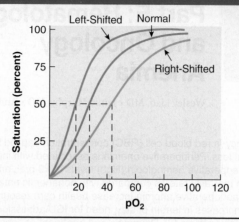

The relationship between arterial saturation of hemoglobin and oxygen tension is represented by the sigmoid-shaped oxyhemoglobin dissociation curve. When the curve is left shifted, the hemoglobin molecule binds oxygen more tightly. Reproduced from Greenberg SB, Murphy GS, Vender JS. Standard monitoring techniques. In: Barash PG, Cullen BF, Stoelting RK, et al., eds. *Clinical anesthesia*. 6th ed. Philadelphia, PA: Lippincott Williams & Wilkins, 2009:701, with permission.

---

c) **Hematopoetic Input Deficiencies**
  i) Deficiencies of the building blocks of RBC such as iron, folate, and B_{12}
  ii) Thalassemias
     (1) Genetic diseases that result in deficiency in the synthesis of normal hemoglobin
  iii) Anemia of Chronic Disease (6)
     (1) Occurs with chronic inflammation, tissue injury, infections, and cancer
     (2) Due to inadequate iron delivery to the bone marrow despite normal or increased iron stores
d) **Peripheral RBC destruction (6)**
  i) Autoimmune/antibody mediated
     (1) Causes include drugs and diseases such as Systemic Lupus Erytheratosus, Non-Hodgkin Lymphoma, Chronic Lyphocytic Leukemia
  ii) Nonimmune mediated
     (1) Causes include microangiopathic hemolytic anemia, hypersplenism, prosthetic heart valves, infections, burns, drugs, toxins
  iii) Hemolysis due to congenital defects
     (1) Thalassemias, sickle cell disease, hereditary spherocytosis, elliptocytosis, enzymopathies (G6PD/G6PDH deficiency)
e) **Defects in RBC Membrane Proteins or Components**
  i) Causes include Paroxysmal Nocturnal Hemoglobinemia, Wilson's Disease
f) **Hemodilution due to fluid resuscitation**

4) Physiologic changes associated with anemia
a) Severity and clinical manifestations of anemia are related to the speed of onset
b) **Acute Anemia (Table 87-1)**
  i) Sudden decrease in blood O_2 content and decreased O_2 delivery lead to a brisk sympathetic response.

Anemia decreases oxygen-carrying capacity and the physiologic response is to preserve oxygen delivery to the tissues.

Table 87-1	
Compensatory Response to Anemia (8)	
Anemia	**Compensatory Response**
Acute	↑HR, ↑SV, ↑O$_2$ extraction
Chronic	↑2.3 DPG, ↑CO, ↑PV, ↑P-50, ↓blood viscosity, rightward shift O$_2$-Hgb curve

HR, heart rate; SV, stroke volume; DPG, diphosphoglycerate; CO, cardiac output; PV, plasma volume; Hgb, hemoglobin.

    ii)   The response to acute blood loss is multifactorial. It depends on the volume and timing of blood loss, as well as patient's age, comorbidities, pre-existing volume status, and starting hemoglobin level.

    iii) There is an inverse relationship between hemoglobin levels and cardiac output (7).

    iv) Most patients begin to experience symptoms of tissue hypoxia, such as fatigue, headache, lightheadedness, dypsnea, or angina when hemoglobin levels reach 7 g/dL or lower.

  c) **Chronic anemia (Table 87-1)**

    i)   Compensation includes

      (1) Increased production of 2,3-diphosphoglycerate, which increases the P50 of hemoglobin binding, resulting in a right shift in the oxyhemoglobin dissociation curve to facilitate easier unloading of oxygen to tissues

      (2) Increased cardiac output and plasma volume

      (3) Decreased blood viscosity (8).

5) **Treatment**

  a) Treatment of anemia is based upon the underlying cause.

  b) Correction of perioperative anemia has the potential to decrease the need for blood transfusions perioperatively.

  c) Slow correction of hemoglobin levels, such as with oral supplementation or supplement injections, is generally favored.

READ MORE
Hematologic agents, Chapter 49, page 344

  d) Anemia from nutritional deficiencies (iron, folate, B$_{12}$) should be treated with appropriate replacement therapy.

  e) In cases of anemia of chronic disease (e.g., chronic renal insufficiency, malignancy, infections, inflammatory conditions, autoimmune disorders), treatment often involves erythropoietic agents (including recombinant human erythropoietin) and supplemental iron.

6) **Perioperative approach to the patient with anemia**

  a) **Preoperative Considerations**

    i)   **History should focus on potential causes for anemia**

      (1) Inquire about prior history of anemia or other hematologic, hepatic, renal, or endocrine disorders that may be associated with anemia

      (2) A thorough blood transfusion history is important

      (3) Poor diet can lead to B$_{12}$, folate, and iron deficiency

      (4) Medications such as aspirin and NSAIDs

      (5) History of alcohol and/or drug abuse may lead to nutritional deficiencies and/or chronic disease

      (6) Family history may reveal sickle cell anemia or thalassemia

      (7) History of splenectomy

      ii)   Symptoms may include fatigue, headaches, palpitations, shortness of breath, or angina.

      iii) Patients with B_{12} deficiency may have dementia and neuropathy

      iv) If symptoms of myocardial ischemia are present, further cardiac workup is indicated.

  b) **Physical Exam**

      i)   Patients may present with jaundice, mucous membrane pallor, hepatosplenomegaly, glossitis, petechia, purpura, koilonychia, neurologic abnormalities, tachycardia, or orthostatic hypotension.

  c) **Laboratory and other studies (4,6)**

      i)   A complete blood count (CBC) should be obtained and if anemia is present, further workup should be done

      ii)   Other tests may include

Iron-deficiency anemia and anemia of chronic disease are the two most common causes of anemia.

Increased mean cell volume (MCV) is seen in B12 deficiency anemia, while decreased MCV is seen with iron deficiency anemia.

          (1) Reticulocyte count measures the amount of RBC production by the bone marrow

             (a) Increases reflect increased production by the bone marrow in response to acute blood loss or hemolysis

             (b) Decreases reflect inability of the bone marrow to mount an appropriate response to decreased O_2 delivery

          (2) Peripheral blood smear will aid in the diagnosis of anemias with abnormal RBC morphology

          (3) Iron studies

             (a) Include ferritin, transferrin, and total iron binding capacity (TIBC)

             (b) Low ferritin, high transferrin, high TIBC, and low serum iron are seen with iron deficiency anemia

          (4) B_{12} and folate levels

          (5) Liver and renal function tests

          (6) Stool guiaic to evaluate for chronic gastrointestinal bleeding

      iii) For patients with known preoperative anemia who are scheduled for elective surgery, workup and treatment of anemia is ideally started at least 1 to 2 months prior to the date of surgery for maximal optimization.

      iv) Anemic patients undergoing emergency surgery may require blood transfusion prior to surgery, depending on the symptoms and underlying cause

Preoperative assessment of the anemic patient should focus on the underlying cause and intravascular volume status.

      v)   Careful consideration should be given to the patient's intravascular volume status and hypovolemia should be corrected if possible prior to proceeding with surgery

      vi) Patients with anemia may have thrombocytopenia or coagulopathy, which may contraindicate neuraxial anesthesia

  d) **Intraoperative Considerations**

      i)   The decision to transfuse RBC should be made based on the patient's symptoms, coexisting disease, and the surgical procedure.

READ MORE

Alternatives to blood product replacement, Chapter 28, page 215

      ii)   The current guidelines outlined by the American College of Physicians, the American Society of Anesthesiologists, and the Canadian Medical Association include a **transfusion threshold Hgb level of 6 to 8 g/dL (3,9–12)**.

          (1) Patients with a Hgb >10 are unlikely to benefit from blood transfusion.

          (2) Other potential indications for transfusion include otherwise stable patients with Hgb <7 g/dL, patients with Hgb <9 or 10 g/dL and preexisting cardiovascular disease, patients with acute bleeding (with anticipated blood loss resulting in hemoglobin

levels falling below recommended transfusion thresholds), and patients exhibiting symptomatic anemia (3,7,8).

  (3) In patients with preoperative chronic anemia, the decision to transfuse may be made earlier than in patients without anemia.

iii) **Monitoring**

  (1) In addition to Standard ASA monitors, invasive monitors such as arterial BP monitoring and central venous pressure may be helpful

iv) **Induction**

  (1) The goal at induction should be to maintain tissue O_2 delivery.

  (2) In euvolemic anemic patients, there is no preferred induction agent provided hemodynamic stability is maintained.

  (3) Etomidate may be preferable to other induction agents in the presence of hypovolemia.

v) **Efforts should be made to maintain O_2 delivery** during the anesthetic

vi) Conditions that would shift the oxyhemoglobin dissociation curve to the left should be avoided (e.g., alkalosis from hyperventilation, hypothermia) (4)

vii) **Prevention strategies to decrease perioperative blood loss should be considered**

  (1) This includes minimizing blood sampling frequency, using lower volume sampling tubes, employing surgical techniques that reduce intraoperative blood loss, intraoperative cell salvage, and autotransfusion.

e) **Postoperative Considerations**

  i) Careful postoperative monitoring of hemodynamics, volume status, and laboratory values is necessary

  ii) Transfusion may be required

Chapter Summary for Anemia

Definition	Deficiency in O_2-carrying capacity of the blood due to decreased RBC Generally defined as Hgb <12 g/dL in women and <13 g/dL in men
Causes	May be acute or chronic and include blood loss, nutritional deficiencies, chronic disease, bone marrow failure, hemolysis, and congenital abnormalities
Acute Anemia	Sudden decrease in blood O_2 content and decreased O_2 delivery leads to a brisk sympathetic response
Chronic Anemia	↑ 2,3-diphosphoglycerate produces a right shift in the oxyhemoglobin dissociation curve to facilitate tissue O_2 delivery ↑ cardiac output and plasma volume ↓ blood viscosity
Preoperative Considerations	Patients with preoperative anemia scheduled for elective surgery should ideally have workup and treatment 1–2 mo prior surgery for maximal optimization Attempt to ascertain cause of anemia if unknown Treatment is based on underlying cause Consider preoperative blood transfusion IF patient is symptomatic and/or indicated based on surgical procedure
Intraoperative Considerations	Maintain hemodynamic stability, O_2 delivery, and euvolemia Invasive monitoring may be required Transfusion may be indicated bearing in mind that there is no universal or absolute transfusion threshold Avoid conditions that will shift O_2-Hgb dissociation curve to the left such as alkalosis and hypothermia
Postoperative Considerations	Carefully monitor for blood loss, myocardial ischemia, and hemodynamic instability

References

1. Hare GMT, Baker JE, Mazer CD. Perioperative management of acute and chronic anemia: has the pendulum swung too far? *Can J Anesth* 2009;56:183–189.
2. Dunne JR, Malone D, Tracy JK, et al. Perioperative anemia: an independent risk factor for infection, mortality, and resource utilization in surgery. *J Surg Res* 2002;102:237–244.
3. Napolitano LM. Perioperative anemia. *Surg Clin North Am* 2005;85:1215–1227.
4. Hines RL, Marschall KE. *Anesthesia and Co-existing Disease*. Philadelphia, PA: Churchill Livingstone; 2008.
5. Barash PG, Cullen BF, Stoelting RK, et al., eds. *Clinical Anesthesia*. Philadelphia, PA: Lippincott Williams & Wilkins; 2009.
6. Kasper DL, Afuci AS, Longo DL, et al., eds. *Harrison's Principles of Internal Medicine*. New York, NY: McGraw Hill; 2005.
7. Madjdpour C, Spahn DR, Weiskopf RB. Anemia and perioperative red blood cell transfusion: a matter of tolerance. *Crit Care Med* 2006;34:S102–S108.
8. Armas-Loughran B, Kalra R, Carson JL. Evaluation and management of anemia and bleeding disorders in surgical patients. *Med Clin N Am* 2003;87:229–242.
9. Shander A, Knight K, Thurer R, et al. Prevalence and outcomes of anemia in surgery: a systematic review of the literature. *Am J Med* 2004;116:S58–S69.
10. Perioperative red blood cell transfusion. *JAMA* 1988;260:2700–2703.
11. Practice strategies for elective red blood cell transfusion. American College of Physicians. *Ann Intern Med* 1992;116:403–406.
12. Practice guidelines for perioperative blood transfusion and adjuvant therapies: an updated report by the American Society of Anesthesiologists Task Force on Perioperative Blood Transfusion and Adjuvant Therapies. *Anesthesiology* 2006;105:198–208.

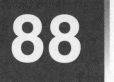

Sickle Cell Disease, Hemogloblinopathies, and Polycythemia Vera

Caleb Ing, MD

Sickle cell disease (SCD) is caused by an inherited structural disorder of the hemoglobin β-globin chain with a wide range of severity and variable speed of progression. Clinical consequences range from a benign sickle cell trait to homozygous (SS) patients with **chronic hemolytic anemia** and recurrent **vaso-occlusive crises** (VOC) causing **pain**, **tissue injury**, and **organ failure**. Other hemoglobinopathies include thalassemias, methemoglobinemia, and sulfhemoglobinemia. Polycythemia vera is a chronic myeloproliferative disorder producing an abundance of red cells, white cells, and platelets resulting in increased blood viscosity and risk of thrombosis.

1) **Sickle cell disease**
   a) **Etiology**

   READ MORE

   Anemia, Chapter 87, page 631

   i) Sickle cell disease (SCD) is caused by an inherited structural disorder of the hemoglobin β-globin chain with a wide range of severity and variable speed of progression.

   b) **Pathophysiology**
      i) Normally adult red blood cells contain three types of hemoglobin:
         (1) **HbA:** α and β chains, 96% to 98% of total hemoglobin.
         (2) **HbA₂:** α and δ chains, 1.5% to 3.2% of total hemoglobin.
         (3) **HbF:** α and γ chains, 0.5% to 0.8%; 90% of total hemoglobin during the first 10 weeks of life(1).
            (a) As **HbF** levels decrease in the first months of life, patients with homozygous (SS) disease almost exclusively produce **HbS**.
            (b) **Deoxygenation** causes insoluble HbS strands to polymerize and distort the shape of RBCs.
            (c) A PaO_2 of <40 mm Hg is likely to result in formation of sickle cells in a homozygous HbSS patient, but sickle polymer can also be found in well-oxygenated SS cells.
            (d) **Acidosis, dehydration, and hypothermia with vasoconstriction** also favor the formation of sickle cells.

   c) **Prevalence**
      i) The sickle cell trait occurs in 10% to 30% of people in Equatorial Africa and is also found in populations in the Mediterranean, Middle East, and India.
      ii) Approximately 8% of African Americans carry the sickle cell trait and 0.3% to 1.3% have sickle cell disease (2).

   d) **Diagnosis**
      i) Early diagnosis is by neonatal screening with Hb electrophoresis.

637

ii) Later in life, patients present with anemia, (Hb: 6 to 9 g/dL) elevated mean corpuscular volume, and leukocytosis (10,000–20,000/mm^3). Sickle-shaped erythrocytes are seen on peripheral blood smear.

e) **Signs and symptoms**

Vaso-occlusive crises (VOC) are treated with rest, warming, analgesia, and fluid replacement therapy.

i) Sickling results in decreased survival of RBCs and a chronic hemolysis with baseline anemia.

ii) Acute exacerbations can manifest as hemolytic, aplastic, or splenic sequestration crises, all resulting in a rapid fall in hemoglobin and are treated with blood transfusions.

iii) VOC are treated with **rest**, **warming**, **analgesia**, and **fluid replacement**.

iv) **Hydroxyurea** has been found to increase levels of HbF and decrease the incidence of VOC.

v) **Acute chest syndrome** (ACS) is responsible for up to 25% of sickle cell–related deaths and has an incidence as high as 10% postoperatively, on average developing 3 days after surgery. Patients with ACS present with **fever**, **cough**, **tachypnea**, **pleuritic chest pain**, **hypoxemia**, **pulmonary hypertension**, and radiological evidence of **lung infiltrates**.

f) **Physiologic changes**

i) Biventricular hypertrophy and a hyperdynamic circulation are frequently found in sickle cell patients.

ii) Patients may show signs of pulmonary fibrosis and restrictive lung disease from past episodes of ACS with 30% of adults developing pulmonary hypertension (3).

iii) CVAs and renal insults are common with renal damage causing a decrease in urine concentrating ability, and if severe, progressing to renal failure.

iv) Decreased or absent splenic function predisposes patients to infections.

v) Patients are at risk for priapism.

g) **Perioperative considerations**

i) **Preoperative considerations**

(1) Knowledge of a patient's history of VOC, severity of illness, and chronic organ damage allows for assessment of an individual's perioperative risk.

(2) Pregnant women tend to have greater perioperative morbidity, with increased age and infection also generating additional risk (4).

(3) Preoperative medications that can depress spontaneous ventilation should be used with caution and supplemental oxygen should be considered.

(4) **Transfusions:**

Consultation with hematology is recommended for complicated patients.

(a) Routine use of preoperative blood transfusions is controversial.

(b) Transfusion regimens range from aggressive (lowering the HbS to <30%), to conservative (only correcting the anemia), to not transfusing at all.

(c) A large-scale RCT involving low-to-moderate risk procedures showed no worse outcome with a conservative technique of maintaining a Hb of 10 g/dL regardless of HbS level, and showed a decrease in transfusion-related complications (5).

(d) **Consultation with hematology is recommended for complicated patients.**

Hypoxia, acidosis, dehydration, and hypothermia favor formation of sickle cells.

ii) **Intraoperative concerns**

(1) To avoid an acute occlusive crisis, maintain **hydration, oxygenation, normothermia,** and **avoid acidosis and hypovolemia**.

(2) End-organ function assessment should focus on cardiac, pulmonary, renal function, and neurological deficits.

(3) Controversy exists over the use of general versus regional anesthesia with some studies showing worsened outcomes with regional anesthesia (6) while others show no difference (7).

(4) The use of **tourniquets** for orthopedic surgery is controversial and the risk of precipitating an acute event with the benefit of decreased bleeding must be assessed.

(5) In cases requiring contrast dye, the use of hypertonic dye is associated with increased sickle cell formation, and isotonic contrast is a safer alternative (8).

(6) Induced hypothermia for CPB can potentially precipitate VOC, but has been performed safely.

iii) **Postoperative concerns**

(1) Patients should be observed for **postoperative pain, pulmonary compromise, and hypovolemia.**

(2) Early mobilization with aggressive chest physiotherapy is recommended.

(3) Supplemental oxygen should be weaned as abrupt withdrawal has been anecdotally associated with VOC (9).

2) **Variant sickle cell syndromes**

a) **Hemoglobin SC**

i) Etiology

(1) HbSC disease involves the presence of HbC, which is a variant hemoglobin that does not polymerize with HbS, but can cause red cell dehydration and increased sickling.

ii) Signs and symptoms

(1) HbSC patients exhibit symptoms that are more severe than sickle cell trait and less severe than sickle cell disease.

(2) Patients usually have a mild anemia (Hb >9).

(3) Patients who have homozygous HbC usually have a mild hemolytic anemia.

3) **Other hemoglobinopathies**

a) **Thalassemia**

i) Etiology

(1) The thalassemias are inherited diseases characterized by the inability to produce structurally normal hemoglobin.

   (a) **β-thalassemia** - no β chains, excess α chains

   (b) **α-thalassemia** - no α chains, excess β chains

ii) Signs and symptoms

(1) β-thalassemia major patients develop severe anemia, splenomegaly, and bone changes from marrow hypertrophy.

(2) Facial bones can be involved, resulting in difficult intubation.

(3) These patients are dependent on blood transfusion and have complications from iron overload.

(4) A high cardiac output state is often seen due to the anemia as well as a dilutional coagulopathy due to frequent transfusions.

(5) Cardiac failure and ventricular arrhythmias are frequent causes of death.

(6) β-thalassemia minor patients are generally asymptomatic with a microcytic anemia (Hb > 10 g/dL).

(7) Thalassemia intermedia patients have intermediate clinical severity (Hb: 7 to 10 g/dL) and are typically not transfusion dependent.

(8) Homozygous forms of α-thalassemia are incompatible with life and the surviving heterozygous patients seldom require transfusions or splenectomy.

ANESTHESIA AND COMORBID DISEASES

b) **Methemoglobinemia**

  i) Mechanism

Methemoglobinemia patients will have an SPO$_2$ of 85% regardless of PaO$_2$.

(1) Methemoglobin (Met-Hb) occurs when the iron in HbA is oxidized from a ferrous (Fe^{2+}) to ferric (Fe^{3+}) state, resulting in an inability to bind oxygen.

(2) The remaining nonoxidized heme groups develop an increased affinity to oxygen (a leftward shift in the O$_2$-Hb dissociation curve) resulting in more difficulty with release of bound oxygen. This severely limits oxygen delivery and can cause tissue hypoxia.

(3) Acquired methemoglobinemia can be induced by oxidizing agents such as **nitrites, nitroprusside, nitroglycerin, nitric oxide, dapsone, chloroquine, sulfonamides, chlorates, aniline dyes, metoclopramide**, and local anesthetics such as **benzocaine (Hurricane spray), lidocaine, and prilocaine.**

  ii) **Diagnosis**

(1) Patients are cyanotic in the presence of **normal PaO$_2$ levels**, but a **low measured SaO$_2$ concentration.**

(2) **SpO$_2$ measured by pulse oximetry shows a value of 85% regardless of PaO$_2$.**

(3) Cyanosis and blood with a chocolate-colored appearance occur when methemoglobin levels reach 15%, but healthy patients without anemia may be asymptomatic.

(4) Mental status changes, dizziness, and headache occur at 20% to 30%, while levels of 50% can cause dysrhythmias, seizures, coma, and death.

  iii) **Treatment**

(1) Cyanosis is treated with **methylene blue** (1 mg/kg IV over 5 minutes), which acts as an electron donor reducing oxidized hemoglobin.

(2) This dose can be repeated every 60 minutes, but doses above 7 mg/kg and rapid administration can paradoxically cause oxidization of Hb to Met-Hb.

(3) Methylene blue should not be given to patients with G6PD deficiency as it can cause hemolysis.

c) **Sulfhemoglobinemia**

  i) **Etiology**

(1) Caused by the oxidation of iron in hemoglobin and by similar drugs that cause methemoglobinemia. It is unknown why some patients develop sulfhemoglobinemia over methemoglobinemia.

(2) Patients have a normal PaO$_2$ value with decreased measured SpO$_2$.

(3) Sulfhemoglobin cannot bind oxygen, but contrary to Met-Hb, it causes a **rightward shift in the oxyhemoglobin dissociation curve aiding in release of bound oxygen**, so even high concentrations are well tolerated.

(4) No pharmacologic treatment is known.

4) **Polycythemia vera**

a) **Pathophysiology**

  i) Polycythemia vera (PV) is a chronic myeloproliferative disorder characterized by the **proliferation of red cells, white cells, and platelets.**

  ii) PV is distinguished from other myeloproliferative disorders by an increased red cell mass, and diagnosis generally involves a **hematocrit above 60% in men and 55% to 60% in women.**

b) **Signs and symptoms**
   i) Associated with **increased blood viscosity resulting in decreased cerebral blood flow** (headache, cognitive dysfunction) and **thrombotic complications** (ischemic stroke, myocardial infarction, peripheral arterial and deep vein thrombosis).
c) **Treatment**
   i) Chronic treatment involves phlebotomy with a target hematocrit of <45%, myelosuppressive drugs, low-dose aspirin, and possible splenectomy (10).
d) **Perioperative considerations**
   i) Preoperative considerations
      (1) Assess any coexisting bleeding disorder or coagulopathy and patients should be optimized with phlebotomy and myelosuppressive agents.
      (2) Aspirin and perioperative anticoagulation discontinuation should be discussed with the surgery and hematology services.
   ii) **Intraoperative and postoperative considerations**
      (1) Patients have an increased risk of **thrombosis, hemorrhage, and infection.**
      (2) Bleeding complications arise in 10% to 14% of patients.
      (3) DVT after major surgery occurs at a fivefold greater rate in PV patients (11,12).

Chapter Summary for Sickle Cell Disease, Hemogloblinopathies, and Polycythemia Vera

Sickle Cell Disease	Is caused by a disorder of the hemoglobin β-globin chain with a wide range of severity and variable speed of progression. Patients can have chronic hemolytic anemia and recurrent VOC causing pain, tissue injury, and organ failure. To avoid a VOC, maintain hydration, oxygenation, normothermia, and avoid acidosis. VOC are treated with rest, warming, analgesia, and fluid replacement. Complicated patients can benefit from a hematology consult.
Methemoglobinemia	Methemoglobin has an increased affinity for oxygen resulting in more difficulty with release of bound O_2. Patients are cyanotic in the presence of normal PaO_2 levels, but a low measured SaO_2 concentration. Methemoglobinemia is treated with methylene blue.
Polycythemia Vera	A myeloproliferative disorder of red cells, white cells, and platelets. Patients have increased blood viscosity leading to decreased cerebral blood flow. Patients are at increased risk for thrombosis, hemorrhage, and infection.

References

1. Marchant WA, Walker I. Anaesthetic management of the child with sickle cell disease. *Paediatr Anaesth* 2003;13(6):473–489.
2. Serjeant GR. Sickle-cell disease [see comment]. *Lancet* 1997;350(9079):725–730.
3. Gladwin MT, Sachdev V, Jison ML, et al. Pulmonary hypertension as a risk factor for death in patients with sickle cell disease [see comment]. *N Engl J Med* 2004;350(9):886–895.
4. Firth PG, Head CA. Sickle cell disease and anesthesia [see comment]. *Anesthesiology* 2004;101(3):766–785.
5. Vichinsky EP, Haberkern CM, Neumayr L, et al. A comparison of conservative and aggressive transfusion regimens in the perioperative management of sickle cell disease. The Preoperative Transfusion in Sickle Cell Disease Study Group [see comment]. *N Engl J Med* 1995;333(4):206–213.
6. Koshy M, Weiner SJ, Miller ST, et al. Surgery and anesthesia in sickle cell disease. Cooperative Study of Sickle Cell Diseases. *Blood* 1995;86(10):3676–3684.

7. Gross ML, Schwedler M, Bischoff RJ, et al. Impact of anesthetic agents on patients with sickle cell disease. *Am Surg* 1993;59(4):261–264.
8. Losco P, Nash G, Stone P, et al. Comparison of the effects of radiographic contrast media on dehydration and filterability of red blood cells from donors homozygous for hemoglobin A or hemoglobin S. *Am J Hematol* 2001;68(3):149–158.
9. Charache S. Preoperative transfusion in sickle cell anemia. *Am J Hematol* 1991;38(2):156–157.
10. Tefferi A. Polycythemia vera: a comprehensive review and clinical recommendations [see comment]. *Mayo Clin Proc* 2003;78(2):174–194.
11. Mesa RA, Nagorney DS, Schwager S, et al. Palliative goals, patient selection, and perioperative platelet management: outcomes and lessons from 3 decades of splenectomy for myelofibrosis with myeloid metaplasia at the Mayo Clinic. *Cancer* 2006;107(2):361–370.
12. Ruggeri M. Rodeghiero F, Tosetto A, et al. Postsurgery outcomes in patients with polycythemia vera and essential thrombocythemia: a retrospective survey. *Blood* 2008;111(2):666–671.

89

Coagulopathies

Ruth Fanning, MB, MRCPI, FFARCSI • Larry F. Chu, MD, MS

A coagulopathy is any condition that impairs the blood's ability to clot. Impaired hemostasis requires careful evaluation and timely treatment. It can be congenital or acquired and may lead to significant perioperative morbidity and mortality.

1) **Pathophysiology**

   a) Bleeding disorders typically involve the coagulation cascade, platelet function, or both (Fig. 89-1).

   b) **Congenital coagulation factor defects**

      i) Any coagulation factor may be deficient or have reduced activity, in isolation or in combination.

      ii) Hemophilia A (Factor VIII deficiency) is the most common congenital coagulation factor defect.

      iii) Hemophilia B (Factor IX deficiency) is less common and is clinically indistinguishable from Hemophilia A (Table 89-1) (2).

   c) **Acquired coagulation factor defects**

      i) **Immune-mediated factor defects**

         (1) Autoantibodies may cause an acquired hemophilia.

         (2) Acquired hemophilia A, the most common type, is typically seen in older patients and may cause severe bleeding. About one third of patients will have underlying disorders (autoimmune diseases such as SLE or rheumatoid arthritis) or lymphoproliferative disorders.

         (3) Alloantibody factor inhibitors in hereditary hemophilia patients occur in 4% to 30% of hemophilia A and 5% of hemophilia B patients receiving factor replacement (2).

         (4) Alloantibody factor inhibitors neutralize the infused factor and may crossreact with endogenous factor, sometimes increasing the severity of the clinical disease.

      ii) **Nonimmune-mediated factor defects**

         (1) **Decreased factor production** such as in liver disease and newborn infants.

         (2) **Abnormal production**

            (a) Warfarin treatment interferes with the ability of vitamin K–dependent coagulation factors to bind the surfaces where coagulation reactions occur.

         (3) **Vit K deficiency**

         (4) **Factor loss and sequestration (e.g., Nephrotic syndrome)**

         (5) **Increased factor destruction**

            (a) Destruction of fibrinogen in disseminated intravascular coagulation (DIC)

The functional activity of the factor determines the clinical presentation of a factor deficiency.

Acquired coagulation factor deficiencies are common, and may be immune or nonimmune mediated (3,4).

READ MORE

Hematologic agents, Chapter 49, page 344

Warfarin treatment is the most common cause of nonimmune-mediated acquired coagulation factor defects.

Figure 89-1 Coagulation—Role of Platelets and Coagulation Cascade in Clot Formation Activation (1)

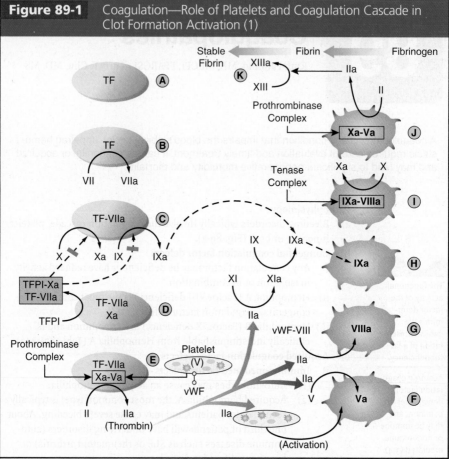

(A) Tissue factor (TF) is a protein expressed in extravascular tissue that is exposed after vascular injury. TF activates factor VII (B), which then activates factor X (C) Creating a TF-VIIa-Xa complex. TF-VIIa also produces a small amount of activated factor IXa. Factor Xa forms a prothrominase complex by binding to factor Va (E), which then catalyzes the conversion of prothrombin to thrombin (E). The activation process is inhibited by tissue factor pathway inhibitor, which binds to and inhibits factor Xa (D). **Amplification**: Platelets amplify the coagulation process that was activated by TF in four ways: Activating protease-activated surface receptors on platelets (F), activating plasma factor V (F), activating factor Viii by releasing it from the VWF carrier (G), and finally thrombin activates factors XI and IX (H). **Propagation**: Large amounts of thrombin are produced by two coagulation factor complexes on the phospholipids surface of platelets: Tenase complex (I) and prothrombinase complex (J). Thrombin catalyzes the formation of fibrin from fibrinogen that crosslinks platelets and stabilizes the clot. Thrombin also activates factor XIII (Fibrin-stabilizing factor) that mediates covalent bonding between fibrin monomers and thrombin activatable fibrinolysis inhibitor (TAFI) to prevent destruction of the clot (K). Reproduced from Drummond JC, Petrovitch CT, Lane TA. Hemostasis and transfusion medicine. In: Barash PG, Cullen BF, Stoelting RK, et al., eds. *Clinical Anesthesia*. 6th ed. Philadelphia, PA: Lippincott Williams & Wilkins; 2009:387, with permission.

Table 89-1
Coagulation Factor Defects (2)

Factor Deficiency	Incidence	Inheritance	Bleeding Severity
F8	1:10,000	X-linked recessive Xq28	Mild<5%, mod1—5%, severe <1%
F9	1, 30,000	X-linked recessive Xq27	Mild-severe
F11	Rare, Ashkenazi Jews	Autosomal recessive, 4q32q3	Mild-severe
F 2, 5, 7, 10	Rare	Variable inheritance	Mild-severe

Afibrinogenemia, dysfibrinogenemia, hypofibrinogenemia are rare abnormalities with variable clinical presentations. In addition, there are multiple congenital combinations of coagulation factor deficiencies and decreased activity.

VWD should be suspected in patients with a personal or a family history of menorrhagia, postpartum hemorrhage, or excessive bleeding after minor surgical procedures.

VWD is highly variable with many different subtypes. Patients with Type I VWD respond to desmopressin treatment, others may not. Consultation with a hematologist to determine the type of patients VWD is suggested.

(6) **Inactivation** by drugs used for thrombolytic therapy (e.g., tissue plasminogen activator) and direct thrombin inhibitor use (e.g., hirudin, argatroban) (2)

d) **Abnormalities of platelet function**

i) Von Willebrand disease (an abnormality of Von-Willebrand (VW) factor) is the most common congenital bleeding disorder, having a prevalence of approximately 1%. There are three main types.

ii) Difficult to diagnose because of variable inheritance and clinical presentation

iii) Should be suspected in patients with a history of menorrhagia or postpartum hemorrhage.

(1) **Type 1**, which has reduced VW factor levels, is a mild disease, inherited in an autosomal dominant manner. These patients usually respond with a two- to fivefold increase in factor VIII-VWF within 30 minutes of desmopressin (DDAVP) treatment (0.3 μg/kg in 50 mL infused over 30 minutes, consult hematologist for dosing) (5).

(2) **Type 2,** is caused by abnormal VWF, and has several subtypes including 2A, 2B, and 2N. DDAVP has variable effects on factor VIII and VWF release in these patients; consult a hematologist.

(3) **Type 3** (severe vWD), these patients have very little or no plasma or platelet vWF and **are not responsive to DDAVP**. Consider factor VIII-VWF concentrate (50 IU/daily major surgery, 40 IU/daily or every other day minor surgery, consult hematologist for dosing) (5).

e) **Abnormal or deceased platelet production**

i) Hypocellular bone marrow, e.g. aplastic anemia, drug, alcohol, or viral-induced aplasia

ii) Hypercellular Bone marrow—B$_{12}$ or folate deficiency

iii) Myelodysplastic diseases

iv) Myelofibrosis

v) Metastatic disease

f) **Increased peripheral platelet destruction (Table 89-2)**

g) **Platelet dysfunction (Table 89-3)**

h) **Dilutional** coagulopathy due to massive blood transfusion

i) **Sequestration** due to liver disease, splenic disease

Table 89-2
Causes of Increased Platelet Destruction

Sepsis	Platelet antibodies
Disseminated Intravascular Coagulation	Drug induced (e.g., Penicillin)
	Posttransfusion HLA directed
Thrombotic Thrombocytopenia Purpura (TTP/HUS)	Collagen vascular disease
	Idiopathic thrombocytopenic purpura (ITP)
Cardiopulmonary Bypass (CPB)	Mechanical heart valves

A bleeding abnormality typically manifests as moderate bleeding over a prolonged period, not as bleeding at an excessive rate.

2) **Evaluation and Treatment**
   a) **Family history**
      i) A family history of bleeding disorder may be seen in hemophilia patients and patients with inherited platelet disorders.
      ii) Up to 30% of cases of hemophilia A are spontaneous mutations with no family history. Von Willebrand disease, the commonest bleeding abnormality, is difficult to diagnose because of the variability in inheritance and clinical presentation.
   b) **Personal history**
      i) Personal history of surgical, dental bleeding, or easy bruising.
      ii) If abnormal bleeding occurs, note the frequency and the duration.
      iii) Location of abnormal bleeding
         (1) Bleeding from skin and mucous membranes tends to occur with platelet disorders.
         (2) Bleeding in joints and muscles tends to occur with the hemophilias.

Table 89-3
Causes of Platelet Dysfunction

Cause	Clinical Example
Disorders of platelet adhesion	Von Willebrand disease
Abnormalities of platelet receptors	Glanzmann thrombasthenia α-Adrenergic defects
Abnormalities of platelet granules	Quebec platelet disorder
Defects in platelet surface receptor agonists	Collagen defects
Platelet cytoskeletal defects	Wiskott-Aldrich
Drug induced	Aspirin, clopidogrel, fish oil

Table 89-4

Medical Diseases Associated with Abnormal Bleeding

Liver disease
Hematological Malignancy (e.g., leukemia or myeloproliferative disease)
Solid organ Malignancies (e.g., prostate, lung, colon)
Vitamin K or C Deficiency
Kidney Disease

c) **Medical diseases associated with bleeding abnormalities (Table 89-4)**
d) **Medication history**
   i) Aspirin, warfarin, heparin, clopidogrel
   ii) Herbal/dietary supplements that may interfere with clotting include fish oil, flax seed oil, garlic, ginger, gingko, saw palmetto
   iii) In the case of **known bleeding disorders**, a full history of the severity of the disease and required medications/blood products and previous surgical experience should be elicited.
e) **Physical examination**
   i) Assess the patient for bruising or petechiae. In particular, note if petechiae appear after application of BP cuff or tourniquet. Be aware of increased bleeding at IV cannula placement or blood testing.
f) **Laboratory testing**
   i) Various laboratory tests may be available at your institution. Consultation with a hematologist will best aid you in test selection and interpretation (Table 89-5).
   ii) **Blood tests of coagulation**
      (1) Full blood count and examination, including cell count and morphology.
      (2) Whole blood clotting time (rarely performed)

Table 89-5

Test Abnormalities Seen in Common Coagulopathies

Disorder	Platelet No.	Bleeding	PT	APTT
Hemophilia A	⇔	⇔	⇔	⇑
Hemophilia B	⇔	⇔	⇔	⇑
Vit K def	⇔	⇔	⇑	⇑
DIC	⇓	⇑	⇑	⇑
Von Willebrand	⇔	⇑	⇔	⇑/⇔
Bernard-Soulier	⇓	⇑	⇔	⇔
Glanzmann thrombasthenia	⇔	⇑	⇔	⇔

Deficiencies in factors VII or XIII will not be detected with aPTT test.

(a) A clot should occur in 5 to 15 minutes. A weak friable clot suggests hypofibrinogenemia. Early dissolution of the clot suggests enhanced fibrinolysis

(3) **APTT** (activated Partial Thromboplastin Time)

    (a) Measures the "intrinsic" and common coagulation pathways.

    (b) Normal PTT times require the presence of the following coagulation factors: I, II, III, IV, V, VI, VIII, IX, X, XI, and XII.

    (c) Normal: 25 to 39 seconds

(4) **PT, INR** (Prothrombin Time, International Normalized Ratio)

    (a) Prothrombin time and its derived measure, international normalized ratio (INR), are measures of the extrinsic pathway.

    (b) Normal PT: 12 to 15 seconds, INR: 0.8 to 1.2.

    (c) PT measures factors I, II, V, VII, and X.

(5) **TT** (Thrombin time)

    (a) Thrombin time compares a patient's rate of clot formation to that of a sample of normal pooled plasma.

    (b) Reflects fibrinogen activity

    (c) Normal: 10 to 15 seconds

(6) **ACT (Activated Clotting Time)**

    (a) Activated clotting time is a point of care test, used to monitor the effect of heparin.

    (b) A sample of whole blood is added to a tube containing negatively charged particles and time for the formation of a clot

    (c) Normal values are Kaolin: 90 to 150 seconds, Celite: 100 to 170 seconds, Glass: 110 to 190 seconds.

    (d) Platelet dysfunction and factor deficiencies may prolong the ACT

iii) **Coagulation factor assays**

    (1) **Coagulation factors** are defined by their **functional activity** rather than absolute value (i.e., the functional activity of the factor in the patient's plasma compared with that of a calibrator or standard plasma, the latter with a defined assayed activity of 100%) (2).

iv) **Factor inhibitor assay**

    (1) Measures antibodies to factors, which may reduce the activity of both intrinsic and administered factors.

v) **Platelet function tests**

    (1) **CBC** gives platelet number and size

    (2) **Blood film** shows platelet morphology

vi) **Assessment of platelet function**

    (1) **Bleeding time**

        (a) Involves making a standardized incision, or lance on the ventral forearm. A BP cuff is inflated above the wound. The time it takes for bleeding to stop is measured.

        (b) Normal bleeding time is 2 to 9 minutes.

        (c) Rarely performed

    (2) Aggregometry

        (a) Addition of an agonist (thrombin, ADP, epinephrine, collagen, ristocetin) to platelet-rich plasma to assess platelet aggregation

    (3) **Flow cytometry**

        (a) Assesses platelet membrane receptor functional status.

vii) **Thromboelastography**

    (1) Thromboelastography is a method of testing the coagulation system by measuring clot formation (Fig. 89-2) (1).

Figure 89-2   Diagram of a Normal Thromboelastogram and Commonly Derived Values

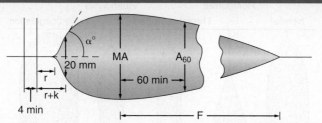

Reproduced from Drummond JC, Petrovitch CT, Lane TA. Hemostasis and transfusion medicine. In: Barash PG, Cullen BF, Stoelting RK, et al., eds. *Clinical Anesthesia.* 6th ed. Philadelphia, PA: Lippincott Williams & Wilkins, 2009:394, with permission.

  (2) It involves either rotating or oscillating a blood sample to initiate clot formation. It is available as a point-of-care test, and is particularly suited for managing transfusion therapy in the operative setting (6,7).

  (3) **The thromboelastogram (TEG)** measures a number of parameters

    (a) **R value or Reaction time**—the time in minutes from the start of a sample run until the first detectable levels of fibrin clot formation.

      (i) Reaction time generally reflects coagulation factor levels.

    (b) **K value**—the measure of time from the beginning of clot formation until the amplitude of the TEG reaches 20 mm.

      (i) k factor in conjunction with the alpha angle reflects coagulation factor amplification.

    (c) **Alpha angle**—the size in degrees of the angle formed by the tangent line to TEG tracing measure at the reaction time.

      (i) The angle reflects the acceleration of fibrin build up and crosslinking.

    (d) **Maximum amplitude (MA)**—the greatest amplitude of the TEG tracing. It reflects the maximum strength of the final hemostatic plug. MA assesses the combination of platelet count and function plus fibrinogen activity. Amplitude at 60 minutes is the amplitude of the TEG tracing 60 minutes after the MA is recorded and reflects the stability of the clot.

    (e) **Clot lysis index**—the amplitude at 60 minutes expressed as a percentage of the maximal amplitude (Fig. 89-3) (1).

3) **Anesthetic concerns**

 a) **Preoperative**

  i) The involvement of the patient's hematologist is imperative in the creation of a perioperative management plan. In the case of patients receiving anticoagulants or antiplatelet drugs, particularly in the setting of a recent revascularization, consultation should be made with their cardiologist.

  ii) Thorough history and physical exam should be elicited

  iii) Appropriate laboratory tests for the patient depending on their history should be performed.

  iv) Many patients with bleeding abnormalities may have had multiple blood product transfusions in the past and may have developed antibodies. Be sure you know the status of your patient and the length of time it may take to cross match blood.

  v) A comprehensive care plan should be constructed between the clinicians involved, surgeons, anesthesiologist, hematologist, intensivist as appropriate.

Figure 89-3   Examples of Normal and Abnormal Thromboelastograms

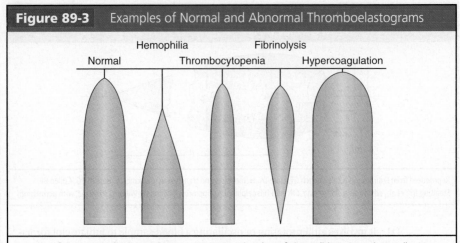

Reproduced from Drummond JC, Petrovitch CT, Lane TA. Hemostasis and transfusion medicine. In: Barash PG, Cullen BF, Stoelting Rk, et al., eds. *Clinical Anesthesia*. 6th ed. Philadelphia, PA: Lippincott Williams & Wilkins; 2009:394, with permission.

vi)   The type of procedure, location it is performed (e.g., suitability of surgery center, ICU facilities, blood bank capabilities) should be considered.

vii)   The patient and the family must be counseled regarding potential complications.

viii)   Consider the appropriate anesthetic technique for the procedure in the setting of the patient's coagulopathy: regional, general anesthesia, monitored anesthesia care, or neuraxial blockade.

ix)   Consider the need for pre-emptive therapy with coagulation factors, platelets, or FFP.

x)   Evaluate the patient's medications to determine if any need to be stopped prior to surgery (e.g., aspirin).

xi)   Consider the need for additional monitoring, for example, arterial line, CVP, PA catheter.

xii)   Ensure adequate IV access and plan for the possibility of large volume resuscitation in the event uncontrolled bleeding.

xiii)   Communicate with the Blood Bank to ensure appropriate resources

b)   **Intraoperative management**

i)   **Monitor blood loss**

(1)   **Visual** cues, swabs, suction, surgical field.

(2)   **Communicate** with the surgical team to get an accurate idea of ongoing blood loss; venous/arterial, speed of bleeding, the likelihood of controlling bleeding.

(3)   **Laboratory monitoring** for coagulopathy should include determination of ACT, platelet count, prothrombin time (PT) or INR, and aPTT. Other tests may include fibrinogen level, assessment of platelet function, thromboelastogram, d-dimers, and thrombin time as indicated (8).

ii)   **Monitor for adequate perfusion and oxygenation of vital organs.**

iii)   **Monitor for transfusion indications** relative to patient status, and intraoperative course.

iv)   **Therapies**

Be vigilant—bleeding disorders may become apparent or develop at any point during the case.

(1) Know the transfusion policies in your institution, in particular whether a "Massive Transfusion" policy exists. Know the location of the Blood transfusion services.

(2) Maintain adequate intravascular volume and BP with crystalloids or colloids. When appropriate, intraoperative or postoperative blood recovery and other means to decrease blood loss (e.g., deliberate hypotension) may be beneficial.

(3) Transfusion of allogeneic red blood cells or autologous blood

(4) **Transfusion of platelets**

    (a) If possible, a platelet count should be obtained before transfusion of platelets in a bleeding patient, and a test of platelet function should be done in patients with suspected or drug-induced platelet dysfunction (e.g., clopidogrel).

    (b) Bleeding and the surgical procedure (e.g., intracranial surgery) rather than absolute platelet count will determine the need for platelet transfusion.

    (c) Prophylactic platelet transfusion is rarely indicated.

(5) **Transfusion of fresh frozen plasma.**

    (a) If possible, coagulation tests (i.e., PT or INR and aPTT) should be obtained before the administration of FFP (8)

(6) **Single coagulation factor administration**

    (a) Factor replacement is dosed relative to the activity of the factor and its half-life (e.g., fibrinogen $T_{1/2}$ approximately 96 hours, 50% activity required. Factor VIII $T_{1/2}$ is approximately 12 hours, 50% activity required, Factor IX, $T_{1/2}$ is approximately 24 hours, 30% activity required.)

(7) **Transfusion of cryoprecipitate.**

    (a) If possible, a fibrinogen concentration should be obtained before the administration of cryoprecipitate in a bleeding patient.

    (b) Transfusion of cryoprecipitate is rarely indicated if fibrinogen concentration is greater than 150 mg/dL (8).

(8) **Multiple coagulation factor deficiency therapy**

    (a) FFP and platelets are indicated when there are demonstrable multifactor deficiencies associated with severe bleeding and/or DIC.

(9) **Drugs to treat excessive bleeding**

    (a) **DDAVP**

        (i) Increases Factor VIII and Von Willebrand Factor. Useful for uremia-induced platelet dysfunction, aspirin, Von Willebrand disease.

    (b) **Aprotinin**

        (i) Protease inhibitor w improves platelet function, blocks fibrinolysis.

    (c) **Antifibrinolytic agents-** E-Aminocaproic acid, Transexamic acid

(10) **Supportive Measures** are extremely important in maintaining organ function and preventing further exacerbation of the coagulopathy and may include:

    (a) Maintenance of normothermia

    (b) Use of blood warmers

    (c) Ensure adequate acid-base balance

    (d) Replacement of calcium and other electrolytes

    (e) Maintenance of hemodynamic stability and oxygenation.

READ MORE

Alternatives to blood product replacement, Chapter 28, page 215

Massive transfusion and resuscitation, Chapter 29, page 220

READ MORE

Hematologic agents, Chapter 49, page 344

c) **Postoperative management**

i) Postoperative considerations are related to the underlying disease processes and surgical procedure

ii) Consider the appropriate facilities for postoperative care, including regular ward, step down unit, ICU, or Coronary Care Unit.

iii) Consider postoperative intubation if large volumes of fluid and blood products have been given and airway edema is suspected.

iv) A thorough handover to PACU staff is essential in order to inform them of possible issues such as rebleeding, transfusion of remaining blood products, and monitoring of the patient's vital signs.

v) A pain management plan should be formulated and discussed with the surgical or acute pain management services, especially with regard to neuraxial catheters left in situ.

vi) **Follow up with your patient.** Postoperative rounds on coagulopathic patients are important to insure optimal postoperative patient management.

Chapter Summary for Coagulopathies

Definition	A coagulopathy is any condition that impairs the blood's ability to clot.
Pathophysiology	Bleeding abnormalities are typically coagulation-factor or platelet related. Acquired coagulation abnormalities are more common than congenital. A significant number of congenital abnormalities occur as spontaneous mutations and thus have no family history.
Management Strategies	1) Bleeding abnormalities can develop/become apparent at any time in patient care. 2) Be aware of available tests at your institution and their interpretation. 3) Be aware of the processes and protocols regarding blood product availability. 4) Ensure consultation with a hematologist. 5) Have a multidisciplinary plan for the patient's care. 6) "ASK FOR HELP" early.

References

1. Drummond JC, Petrovitch CT, Lane TA. Hemostasis and transfusion medicine. In: Barash PG, Cullen BF, Stoelting RK, et al., eds. *Clinical Anesthesia*. 6th ed. Philadelphia, PA: Lippincott Williams & Wilkins; 2009:369–412.
2. Wagenman BL, Townsend KT, Mathew P, et al. The laboratory approach to inherited and acquired coagulation factor deficiencies. *Clin Lab Med* 2009;29:229–252.
3. Watson HG, Chee YL, Greaves M. Rare acquired bleeding disorders. *Rev Clin Exp Hematol* 2001;5:405–429.
4. Franchini M, Veneri D. Acquired coagulation inhibitor-associated bleeding disorders: an update. *Hematology* 2005;10:443–449.
5. Hoffman. *Hematology: Basic Principles and Practice*. 5th ed. Philadelphia, PA: Churchill Livingstone; 2009. ISBN: 978-0-443-06715-0.
6. Depotis GJ, Joist JH, Goodnough LT. Monitoring of hemostasis in cardiac surgical patients: impact of point-of-care testing on blood loss and transfusion outcomes. *Clin Chem* 1997;43(9):1684–1696.
7. Shore-Lesserson L, Manspeizer HE, DePerio M, et al. Thromboelastography-guided transfusion algorithm reduces transfusion in complex cardiac surgery. *Anesth Analg* 1999;88(2):312–319.
8. Practice Guidelines for Perioperative Blood Transfusion and Adjuvant Therapies An Updated Report by the American Society of Anesthesiologists Task Force on Perioperative Blood Transfusion and Adjuvant Therapies. *Anesthesiology* 2006;105(1):198–208.

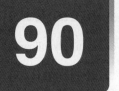

90

Part F: Skin and Musculoskeletal Diseases Malignant Hyperthermia

T. Kyle Harrison, MD

Malignant hyperthermia is a rare and potentially lethal condition associated with the administration of volatile anesthetics and/or depolarizing paralytic agents (succinylcholine). With appropriate treatment, the mortality from MH has decreased from >70% to <5%.

1) Pathophysiology
   a) **Molecular mechanism**
      i) Etiology is thought to be secondary to a genetic mutation in the ryanodine receptor, which affects calcium release in skeletal muscle sarcoplasmic reticulum.
      ii) The abnormal ryanodine receptor is stimulated from exposure to volatile anesthetics or a depolarizing paralytic.
         (1) Uncontrolled calcium release occurs, producing a hypermetabolic state within the skeletal muscle.
         (2) This hypermetabolic state produces the signs and symptoms associated with MH.
   b) **Prevalence**
      i) The prevalence of MH has been reported to be 1:12,000 for pediatric anesthetics and 1:40,000 adult anesthetics (1).
      ii) MH is most commonly a condition of children and young adults.
         (1) However, cases of MH have been reported for all ages from infants to the elderly.
         (2) Although two-thirds of MH-susceptible individuals will have an MH event during their first anesthetic, it can occur after several uneventful prior anesthetics (2).

2) **Signs and symptoms**
   a) Early signs and symptoms
      i) The signs and symptoms associated with MH are related to the hypermetabolic state that occurs in MH.

The earliest sign of MH is increased CO_2 production.

      ii) The **earliest sign is increased CO_2 production** with the resultant increase in respiratory rate in the spontaneously breathing patient or a rising $ETCO_2$ in a mechanically ventilated patient.
      iii) As cellular metabolism outstrips supply, **a metabolic acidosis develops,** and in fulminant cases hypoxia can develop from the massive consumption of oxygen in the skeletal muscle.
   b) **Late signs and symptoms**
      i) As the condition progresses, **muscle damage occurs releasing potassium** and eventually the **core body temperature begins to rise** from the sustained muscle activity.

653

ii)   Cardiac arrhythmias can develop secondary to the **hyperkalemia** and **acidosis.**

iii) Myoglobin released from the damaged muscle can result in acute renal failure and DIC.

iv)   The signs and symptoms of MH can occur quickly following a trigger or take hours to fully develop (2).

Cardiac arrhythmias can develop due to acidosis and hyperkalemia.

c) **Associated findings**

i)   An associated finding with MH is **masseter muscle spasm (MMS).**

ii)   Although mild jaw stiffness can be detected in all patients receiving succinylcholine, an exacerbated response with sustained spasm may develop in some patients especially children.

iii) It has been reported that up to **50% of children that experience MMS go on to develop MH.**

iv)   Isolated MMS is not enough to warrant treatment of MH without further signs of hypermetabolism but it would be prudent to change to a nontriggering anesthetic and monitor closely for sign of MH if MMS is noted (3).

3) **Treatment**

a) **Initial treatment and resuscitation**

READ MORE

Crisis management: malignant hyperthermia, Chapter 211, page 1328

i)   **Mobilize help**

(1)   Call for help

(2)   Once a presumptive diagnosis of MH has been made, one should quickly mobilize additional help and have an **MH cart brought to the room.**

(3)   Consult MH cognitive aid

ii)   **Stop triggering agent(s)**

(1)   After calling for help and turning off the volatile, one should increase the flow rates on the anesthesia machine to 10 L/min of 100% O_2.

The most important management step after turning off triggering agent is rapidly administering Dantrolene.

(2)   The **anesthesia machine and the circuit need not be changed.** The surgeon should be notified to complete the surgery as quickly as possible.

iii) **Administer dantrolene**

(1)   The most important treatment step in treating MH, **after turning off the triggering agent**, is the rapid administration of Dantrolene.

(2)   A 20-mg vial of Dantrolene should be mixed in 60 mL of sterile water. Because of its poor water solubility, it takes some time to get each vial into solution.

(3)   Assign one team member the sole task of mixing the Dantrolene as quickly as possible.

(4)   The loading dose is 2.5 mg/kg and should be repeated up to 10 mg/kg until clinical signs of improvement are noted.

iv)   **Monitor and treat signs and symptoms**

(1)   **An ABG should be sent** to monitor the acid/base and electrolyte status.

    (2) **Cardiac arrhythmias** should be treated as hyperkalemia with CaCl, insulin-glucose, and sodium bicarbonate.

    (3) **Institute hyperventilation**

        (a) Increase minute ventilation to eliminate excess CO_2 caused by hypermetabolism.

           (i) Monitor patient's peak inspiratory pressures for signs of air trapping due to insufficient expiratory time because of increased respiratory rate.

    (4) **Cooling should be instituted.**

        (a) The patient's core body temperature may rise significantly and can result in central nervous system injury.

        (b) In conjunction with arresting the MH event with dantrolene, the **patient should be actively cooled to prevent severe hyperthermia.**

        (c) Consider the use of

           (i) Chilled saline for the intravenous infusions.

           (ii) Gastric, peritoneal, and bladder lavage with cold saline may also help decrease the patient's body temperature.

           (iii) Packing the patient in ice can be an effective way to cool the patient.

    v) Maintenance of anesthesia

        (1) The patient's anesthetic should be maintained with either propofol or benzodiazepine/opioids.

        (2) Urinary output should be maintained with fluids, mannitol, and lasix to prevent acute renal failure from the myoglobin release.

  b) **Postoperative care**

    i) The patient should continue to receive treatment for MH for 36 hours with a dose of 1 mg/kg of Dantrolene every 6 hours in an ICU setting.

    ii) In addition, urinary output should be maintained with aggressive IV fluids and diuretics.

    iii) The patient should have frequent arterial blood gases including electrolytes, creatine kinase levels every 6 hours, and they should be monitored for possible DIC.

  c) **Follow-up**

    i) **Further diagnostic testing**

        (1) Patients who have had a suspected MH event should be referred for a **caffeine-halothane muscle biopsy test** at one of the regional MH testing centers.

        (2) Contact Malignant Hyperthermia Association of American for more information on test sites.

  4) **Future anesthetic care**

    a) All MH-susceptible patients should receive a **nontriggering anesthetic**.

    b) All anesthetic agents **with the exception of all volatile anesthetics and succinylcholine** are safe for the use in MH-susceptible individuals.

    c) An anesthesia machine without vaporizers attached and a clean circuit with fresh CO_2 absorbent flushed for 10 minutes at 10 L/min should be used for all MH-susceptible patients (4).

Patients suspected of MH should have follow-up testing performed to confirm the diagnosis.

Chapter Summary for Malignant Hyperthermia

Definition	A rare and potentially lethal condition where certain anesthetic agents cause a hypermetabolic state in skeletal muscle due to a genetic defect in the ryanodine receptor.
Triggering Anesthetic Agents	Depolarizing neuromuscular blocking agent (succinylcholine) Volatile anesthetic gases
Signs	Early: $\uparrow CO_2$ production, metabolic acidosis Late: Hyperthermia, cardiac arrhythmia, renal failure
Treatment	Call for help! Stop triggering anesthetic agent. Administer Dantrolene immediately Monitor and treat associated signs and symptoms
Postoperative Care	Continue Dantrolene in a monitored clinical setting (ICU) Aggressive IV fluids and diuretics Refer for further testing (caffeine-halothane muscle biopsy)

References

1. Ording H. Incidence of malignant hyperthermia in Denmark. *Anesth Analg* 1985;64:700–704.
2. Stoelting RK, Dierdorf SF. Diseases presenting in pediatric patients. In: *Anesthesia and Co-existing Disease*. 4th ed. New York, NY: Churchill Livingstone; 2002:716–721.
3. Saddler JM. Jaw stiffness: and ill understood condition. *Br J Anaesth* 1991;67:515–516.
4. Beebe JJ, Sessler DI. Preparation of anesthesia machines for patients susceptible to malignant hyperthermia. *Anesthesiology* 1988;69:395–400.

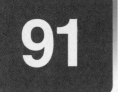

91 Burn Injuries

Alma N. Juels, MD

There are about 1.2 million people with burn injuries per year resulting in about 5,000 deaths. The majority of burns are thermal injuries, which hospitalize approximately 45,000 people in the United States each year. 70% of burn patients are men. Scalds are the most common type of burn in children below 5 years of age (1).

1) Classification of thermal burns
   a) **Superficial**
      i) Upper layers of the dermis
      ii) Skin appears red and slightly edematous.
   b) **Superficial partial thickness**
      i) Damage extends into the superficial layer of the dermis.
      ii) Blisters develop and the skin is red or whitish.
   c) **Deep partial thickness**
      i) Extends into the deep layer of the dermis
      ii) Marked edema and altered skin sensation
   d) **Full thickness**
      i) Extends through the epidermis, dermis, and subcutaneous tissue layer
      ii) Every body system may be affected.
   e) Subdermal
      i) Damages muscle, bone, and interstitial tissue
2) Pathophysiology
   a) Burns can affect all physiologic functions and organs.
      i) **Skin**: all skin functions are disrupted by burns.
         (1) Loss of sensory function of the skin
         (2) Hypothermia can occur due to extensive evaporative heat and water losses, and loss of thermoregulation.
         (3) Increased risk of infection and sepsis
      ii) **Cardiovascular** (2)
         (1) Acute phase
            (a) Cardiac output decreases as much as 50%, causing decreased organ and tissue perfusion.
            (b) An increase in capillary permeability occurs with loss of fluid and protein and is greatest in the first 12 hours.
         (2) Second phase (metabolic phase)
            (a) Begins 48 hours after the burn and involves increased blood flow
            (b) Older patients may have a delayed or nonexistent second phase.
            (c) Profound hypertension is common.

657

b) **Respiratory (4)**
   i) Early complications (up to 24 hours):
      (1) Carbon monoxide poisoning
      (2) Airway obstruction
      (3) Pulmonary edema
   ii) 2 to 5 days postinjury:
      (1) Patients may develop adult respiratory distress syndrome.
   iii) Late complications (days to weeks later):
      (1) May include pneumonia, atelectasis, and pulmonary emboli

c) **Gastrointestinal (3)**
   i) Acute complications
      (1) Ileus
      (2) Curling ulcer (Acute peptic ulcer of the duodenum)
      (3) Acute necrotizing enterocolitis.
   ii) 2 to 3 weeks postinjury
      (1) Acalculous cholecystitis

d) **Renal (3)**
   i) Diminished blood flow activates the renin-angiotensin-aldosterone system
      (1) Antidiuretic hormone is released, which results in retention of sodium and water with loss of potassium, calcium, and magnesium.
   ii) Acute renal failure can develop and has a very high mortality.
   iii) Acute tubular necrosis can develop secondary to hemoglobinuria and myoglobinuria.

e) **Hepatic (4)**
   i) Decreased hepatic function occurs due to hypoperfusion.

f) **Endocrine (4)**
   i) Massive release of catecholamines, glucagon, adrenocorticotropic hormone, antidiuretic hormone, renin, angiotensin, and aldosterone.
   ii) Patients can develop nonketotic hyperosmolar coma and adrenal insufficiency.

g) **Hematologic (4)**
   i) Anemia
   ii) Consumption of coagulation factors
   iii) Thrombocytopenia
   iv) Decreased platelet function
   v) Antithrombin deficiency

h) **Immunologic (1)**
   i) Increased susceptibility to infection, causing most morbidity and mortality

3) **Electrical burn patients may have more extensive injuries (6)**
   a) Areas of damaged skin may be present under "normal looking" skin, causing fluid requirements to be underestimated.
   b) Complications include:
      i) Myoglobinuria
      ii) Peripheral neuropathies
      iii) Spinal cord damage
      iv) Apnea

     v)   Late cataract formation

     vi) Cardiac dysrhythmias may occur up to 48 hours postinjury.

4) **Treatment**

  a) The primary goal is to resuscitate the patient, using the "ABCs" (4).

  b) **Airway/breathing**

Small amounts of airway edema may occlude a pediatric airway. Early endotracheal intubation should be considered in patients with inhalational injury even in the absence of respiratory distress.

     i)   Management is generally supportive.

     ii) Includes administration of supplemental O_2, inhaled β-agonist, and pulmonary toilet.

     iii) Intubation or tracheotomy may be necessary and should be considered **early;** it might be very difficult later due to edema and excessive secretions.

  c) **Circulation (5)**

     i)   Aggressive **fluid resuscitation** corrects **hypovolemia and organ hypoperfusion.**

     ii) **Therapy can be guided by** urine output

        (1) Should be maintained at 0.5 mL/kg/h.

        (2) In the presence of myoglobinuria, urine output should be at approximately 2 mL/kg/h.

     iii) **The Parkland formula** is the most common formula used to guide (6) fluid requirements.

        (1) **The Parkland formula** involves giving **4 mL of lactated Ringer/ kg/total body surface area (TBSA) burned (Tables 91-1 and 91-2).**

        (2) Half is given during the first 8 hours and the remainder over the next 16 hours.

           (a) This fluid requirement is in addition to daily maintenance.

     iv) Another formula is the **Modified Brooke formula,** which uses 2 mL/ kg/% burn (2).

     v)   Bicarbonate may be used to alkalinize the urine in the setting of pigment-related acute tubular necrosis (2).

     vi) **Colloid administration**

        (1) **No colloid should be used in the first 24 hours due to increased risk of edema formation**

Table 91-1

Total Body Surface Area Burned as Calculated by the "Rule of Nines" (2)

	Percentage of Body Surface Area
Head and neck	9%
Upper extremities	9% each
Chest (anterior and posterior)	9% each
Abdomen	9% each
Lower back	9% each
Lower extremities	18% each
Perineum	1%

Table 91-2
Rule of Nines for Children (2)

	Percentage of Body Surface Area According to Age		
	Newborn (%)	3 Y (%)	6 Y (%)
Head	18	15	12
Trunk	40	40	40
Arms	16	16	16
Legs	26	29	32

    (2) 24 hours after colloid is added (4)
        (a) 0% to 30% TBSA—no colloid
        (b) 30% to 50% TBSA—0.3 mL/kg/%/24 h
        (c) 50% to 70% TBSA—0.4 mL/kg/%/24 h
        (d) 70% to 100% TBSA burned—0.5 mL/kg/%/24 h

5) **Wound care**
  a) Early surgical intervention is crucial to improving outcome.
  b) Procedures usually involve decompression, such as
    i) Escharotomies
    ii) Fasciotomies
    iii) Excision
    iv) Reconstruction
  c) Supportive surgical procedures include (1)
    i) Tracheostomy
    ii) Gastrostomy
    iii) Cholecystectomy
    iv) Bronchoscopy
    v) Vascular access

6) **Anesthetic considerations (4)**
  a) **Preoperative considerations**
    i) History
      (1) Inquire about the time of burn and extent of burn for fluid replacement, type of burn, airway involvement, and associated injuries.
      (2) A standard preoperative history is obtained including current medical conditions, medications, and allergies.
    ii) Standard preoperative exam
      (1) Assess airway damage, wheezing, and decreased breaths sounds.
      (2) Include cardiac exam, vital signs, urine output, and neurologic exam.

Electrical burns may result in more extensive tissue damage than is appreciated from physical exam.

Pulse oximetry may overestimate the oxygen saturation in a patient with carbon monoxide poisoning (6).

        iii) Lab tests
- (1) ABG, electrolytes, and carboxyhemoglobin levels to determine the presence of carbon monoxide poisoning (6).

b) **Monitors (4)**
- i) Adequate monitoring can be difficult depending on the skin damage.
- ii) Needle electrodes or ECG pads sewn on may be needed.
- iii) BP cuff may be effective on a burned area but usually an arterial line is preferred.
- iv) Temperature monitoring is essential.
- v) Large bore IVs or central lines are needed for fluid and blood administration.

c) **Intraoperative considerations (2)**
- i) **Induction**
  - (1) Propofol is used if the patient is hemodynamically stable and euvolemic.
  - (2) Ketamine may be considered if hemodynamics are not normal. It is also the drug of choice for sedation for dressing changes due to its analgesic properties.
  - (3) Etomidate is a good choice for induction in an unstable patient and offers the advantage of not having the dysphoric reaction associated with ketamine.
  - (4) **All induction agents could cause hypotension due to hypovolemia or depleted catecholamines.**

Succinylcholine should be avoided after the first 24 hours in patients with thermal injuries due to the risk of hyperkalemia.

d) **Muscle relaxants (4)**
- i) **Succinylcholine is not to be used after the first 24 hours.**
  - (1) Hyperkalemia may result after administration of succinylcholine due to proliferation of extrajunctional acetylcholine receptors.
  - (2) Succinylcholine should not be used until the burn is healed, or within 6 months to 2 years after a burn.
- ii) **Nondepolarizing muscle relaxants**
  - (1) Burn patients tend to be resistant to nondepolarizing muscle relaxants, needing up to five times the normal dose.

e) **Drug metabolism**
- i) All drugs not administered IV have delayed absorption in the acute phase.
- ii) After 48 hours, albumin-bound drugs and drugs metabolized by oxidative metabolism have a prolonged effect.
- iii) Drugs metabolized by conjugation are not affected.
- iv) Opioid requirements are increased.
- v) Inhalation agents may be poorly tolerated due to hypovolemia.

f) **Regional anesthesia may be contraindicated in patients with electric burns** due to delayed neurological sequelae of the burn injury (2).

7) **Postoperative concerns**
- a) Postoperative care may best be done in a dedicated burn intensive care unit.
- b) Pain control may be difficult and large doses of opioids may be required.

Chapter Summary for Burns

Burns	Burns are thermal injury to the skin and tissues Multiple organ systems are affected
Initial Assessment	Perform history and physical exam Assess risk of airway compromise and extent of injuries Hypovolemia is likely
Fluid Management	Based on urine output May use Parkland or other formulae
Anesthetic Management	Choice of induction agent depends on risk of hypovolemia Monitoring may be difficult due to injury Patients are resistant to nondepolarizing neuromuscular blocking agents and may require higher doses Avoid succinylcholine after the first 24 h
Postoperative Management	Pain control may be difficult; increased doses of opioids may be required

References

1. American Burn Association: www.ameriburn.org
2. Levin P, Juels A. Anesthetic concerns in the burned patient. In: Duke J, ed. *Anesthesia Secrets*. 4th ed. Philadelphia; Mosby 2011.
3. Pham TN, Cancio LC, Gibran NS. American Burn Association Practice Guidelines burn shock resuscitation. *J Burn Care Res* 2008;29(1):257–266.
4. Capan LM, Miller SM. Trauma and burns. In Barash PG, Cullen BF, Stoelting RK, eds. *Clinical Anesthesia*. 5th ed. Philadelphia; Lippincott Williams & Wilkins, 2005.
5. Monafo WW. Initial Management of burns. *N Engl J Med* 1996;335(21);1581–1586.
6. Tintinalli JE, Kelen GD, Stapczynski JS. Thermal burns. In: *Emergency Medicine-A Comprehensive Study Guide*. 6th ed. McGraw Hill, 2004.

92 Arthritis

Andrea J. Fuller, MD • T. Kyle Harrison, MD

Arthritis is a general term referring to inflammation of joints. Rheumatoid arthritis (RA) and ankylosing spondylitis are systemic autoimmune diseases that affect primarily the joints and also multiple organ systems. Osteoarthritis (OA) is a degenerative process due to stress and trauma on joints over time and is not autoimmune. The perioperative approach to the patient with arthritis will be discussed in this chapter.

1) **Rheumatoid arthritis**
   a) **Pathophysiology and Characteristics (1)**
      i) RA is a systemic autoimmune disease that is characterized by both inflammation and destruction of synovial membranes with the resultant articular destruction.
      ii) Any joint can be affected, but RA tends to affect the small to medium-sized joints, especially in the hands and feet.
      iii) The thoracic and lumbar spine is usually spared.
      iv) Arthritis is usually symmetric
      v) Occurs more often in women
      vi) In addition to joint involvement, multiple organ systems may be affected, including the cardiovascular, pulmonary, and hematological systems.
   b) **Associated organ system involvement.** RA is a systemic disease affecting many organ systems.
      i) **Musculoskeletal (joint involvement)**
         (1) RA can involve the cervical spine, temporomandibular joints (TMJ), and the cricoarytenoid joints.
            (a) Cervical spine involvement has been reported to be as high as 86% in RA patients, and the severity of peripheral joint involvement correlates to the degree of cervical involvement (2).
            (b) Patients may have severely diminished joint range of motion secondary to progressive fibrosis and ankylosis.
            (c) Instability of the atlantoaxial and subaxial joints may lead to subluxation (3).
               (i) This subluxation can cause spinal cord compression with flexion or extension of the cervical spine.
      ii) **Cardiovascular (3,4)**
         (1) Cardiovascular involvement is common in RA patients and is the leading cause of death.
         (2) Cardiac granulomas can occur, which can cause conduction defects. In addition nodules can form on valves which may lead to valvular destruction.
         (3) Patients can also have pericardial disease with effusions.

RA patients are at risk for cervical spine subluxation and spinal cord injury with neck manipulation.

663

    iii) **Respiratory**

        (1) The chronic inflammatory state can cause restrictive and obstructive respiratory lung disease.

           (a) Fibrosis, small airway disease, and pulmonary hypertension are all possible.

    iv) **Hematologic**

        (1) RA patients are often anemic.

        (2) Immunosuppression is common due to immunosuppressive drugs and steroids used for treatment of the disease.

    v) **Renal**

        (1) RA patients often have decreased renal function, usually due to medications.

    vi) **Hepatic**

        (1) Elevated liver enzymes are often observed.

  c) **Treatment**

    i) Immunosuppressive drug therapy often includes steroids and other medications such as methotrexate.

    ii) Nonsteroidal anti-inflammatory drugs (NSAIDs) are often used to treat pain and inflammation.

  d) **Anesthetic considerations (1)**

    i) Atlantoaxial instability is a serious concern in patients with RA and places them at risk for spinal cord injury, possibly resulting in quadriplegia, with neck manipulation.

    ii) In any patient with RA, especially those with symptoms of pain or radiculopathy on neck movement, consider cervical spine x-rays to evaluate for atlantoaxial subluxation.

    iii) Cervical spine instability may also interfere with vertebral artery blood flow, so the patient should be queried about syncope or dizziness on neck movement.

        (1) If there is any question about the cervical spine stability, awake fiberoptic intubation should be performed.

    iv) The fact that RA is a multisystem disease should be considered when formulating the anesthetic plan.

2) **Ankylosing spondylitis**

  a) **Pathophysiology and characteristics**

    i) Ankylosing spondylitis is an autoimmune condition similar to RA that affects the spine.

    ii) Chronic inflammation of the vertebral articular surfaces leads to fusion of the spine.

        (1) The characteristic finding is a "bamboo spine" on x-ray.

  b) **Anesthetic considerations**

    i) These patients are at risk for difficult airway due to severely limited cervical spine range of motion.

        (1) Even trivial amounts of spine movement may cause fractures (5).

        (2) A thorough preoperative history and physical should be done, paying particular attention to neck range of motion.

        (3) Consider awake fiberoptic intubation.

    ii) In addition, patients with ankylosing spondylitis appear to be at increased risk of developing an epidural hematoma following neuraxial anesthesia (7).

    iii) Cardiac involvement is possible and may include aortic regurgitation, conduction abnormalities, and cardiomegaly (1).

3) **Osteoarthritis**

  a) **Pathophysiology and characteristics (1,6)**

    i) Degenerative changes in the joints caused by previous injury, repetitive use, and age

    ii) Characterized by pain, stiffness, and limited movement

    iii) Knees and hands are most commonly affected

iv) Degenerative arthritis of the spine may be present and lead to intervertebral disc herniation and nerve root compression.

v) OA is not an autoimmune disease.

vi) Most patients are not treated with systemic corticosteroids.

b) **Anesthetic considerations**

i) Obesity is a common comorbidity. Increased weight causes strain on joints, which causes difficulty with exercise and leads to weight gain.

ii) Cervical spine involvement is rare.

4) **Anesthetic management considerations for patients with arthritis**

a) **Preoperative considerations (1,3,4,6)**

i) A thorough history and physical should be performed, bearing in mind RA and ankylosing spondylitis affect multiple organ systems.

ii) Patients should be asked in the preoperative evaluation if they have pain radiating into the occiput, paresthesias, or sensory loss with head and neck movement.

(1) Flexion and extension cervical spine x-rays can help to determine the presence and severity of the subluxation in the cervical spine

iii) Patients with RA and ankylosing spondylitis may have pulmonary fibrosis

iv) Medications should be reviewed

(1) Patients with autoimmune arthritis may be treated with chronic steroid therapy.

(2) Consider the possibility of medication-induced kidney dysfunction

(3) Many patients have chronic pain requiring multiple medications, including opioids.

v) **Laboratory and other testing**

(1) Functional status is often difficult to determine due to limited mobility. Therefore, consider preoperative stress testing in appropriate patients.

(2) ECG should be obtained to evaluate for concomitant coronary artery disease, pericarditis, and conduction abnormalities.

(3) Chemistries may be helpful to determine the extent of any kidney dysfunction and electrolyte abnormalities.

(4) Blood counts should be obtained as anemia is common.

b) **Intraoperative considerations**

i) **Airway management**

(1) RA and ankylosing spondylitis patients should be considered high risk for difficult airway.

(a) As a general rule, these patients should be assumed to have an unstable neck unless proven otherwise.

(b) RA patients undergoing cervical spine surgery may experience less postoperative airway obstruction with fiberoptic intubation when compared with standard airway management (5).

(2) The temporomandibular joint is often affected in RA and can cause severe mouth opening limitations.

(3) The cricoarytenoid joint is also very commonly involved in RA.

(a) Hoarseness, weak voice, stridor, and laryngeal obstruction can result (3).

OA is the most common joint disease.

RA patients with a history of hoarseness, pain on swallowing, and stridor may have involvement of the cricoarytenoid joint, which places them at risk for difficult airway and postextubation laryngeal obstruction.

READ MORE

Challenges in anesthesia: the patient with chronic low back pain presenting for total knee replacement surgery, Chapter 146, page 1065

Fiberoptic intubation should be considered in RA and ankylosing spondylitis patients.

(4) Patients with ankylosing spondylitis may have extremely limited cervical range of motion.

ii) **IV access and invasive monitors**

(1) May be difficult to place if the patient has significant bone deformities or obesity

(2) Invasive monitors should be placed based on the procedure and the patient's coexisting organ dysfunction.

iii) **Positioning**

(1) Careful positioning and padding of all extremities are important to prevent nerve and soft tissue injuries.

(2) Some extremities may have limited movement. Do not force any position but instead carefully position the extremity with padding.

iv) **Blood loss**

(1) May be significant, especially in patients with RA or on chronic NSAIDs who have not had adequate time to discontinue medications

(2) Blood availability should be strongly considered for major surgeries, including orthopaedic cases.

v) **Perioperative stress dose steroids**

(1) May be indicated if the patient has been treated with long-term steroids

c) **Postoperative considerations**

i) Many patients have chronic pain, which may make postoperative pain management difficult.

ii) Peripheral nerve blocks and neuraxial analgesia should be considered. However, a preblock neurologic exam should be performed and documented.

READ MORE

Steroids, Chapter 46, page 326

Neuraxial block placement may be extremely difficult in patients with ankylosing spondylitis.

Chapter Summary for Arthritis

Consideration	Rheumatoid Arthritis	Ankylosing Spondylitis	Osteoarthritis
Pathophysiology	Autoimmune	Autoimmune	Degenerative
Commonly Affected Joints	Neck; TMJ; cricoarytenoid; hands and feet	Neck, spine, and sacroiliac joint; TMJ	Knees and hands
Other Manifestations	LV dysfunction, pericarditis; pulmonary fibrosis; anemia	Chest wall rigidity; bowel dysfunction	Obesity; advanced age
Preoperative Considerations	Evaluate for coexisting disease and systemic manifestations; attempt to determine functional status; consider blood product availability; reconcile medications and evaluate for medication-induced disease		
Intraoperative Considerations	High risk for difficult airway and neurologic damage due to unstable cervical spine	High risk for difficult airway; neck fractures possible with manipulation; neuraxial anesthesia may be difficult	Neck and airway typically normal
	Positioning and IV access may be difficult		
Postoperative Considerations	Pain management may be difficult due to opioid tolerance, respiratory problems, and chronic pain		

References

1. Hines RL, Marschall KE. *Anesthesia and Co-existing Disease*. Philadelphia, PA: Churchill Livingstone; 2008.
2. Macarthur A, Kleiman S. Rheumatoid cervical joint disease—a challenge to the anaesthetist. *Can J Anaesth* 1993;40:154–159.
3. Matti MV, Sharrock NE. Anesthesia on the rheumatoid patient. *Rheum Dis Clin North America* 1998;24:19–34.
4. Koota K, Isomäki IH, Mutru O. Death rate and causes of death in RA patients during a period of five years. *Scand J Rheumatol* 1977;6:241–244.
5. Wattenmaker I, Concepcion M, Hibberd P, et al. Upper-airway obstruction and perioperative management of the airway in patients managed with posterior operations on the cervical spine for rheumatoid arthritis. *J Bone Joint Surg Am* 1994;76:360–365.
6. Roizen MF, Fleisher LA. *Essence of Anesthesia Practice*. Philadelphia, PA: WB Saunders; 2002.
7. Robins K, Saravanan S, Watkins EJ. Ankylosing spondylitis and epidural haematoma. *Anaesthesia* 2005;60:624–625.

93

Systemic Lupus Erythematosus

T. Kyle Harrison, MD

Systemic lupus erythematosus (SLE) is a multisystem chronic inflammatory disease characterized by the presence of autoantibodies against nuclear structures, particularly DNA. Virtually any organ system can be involved, and the disease can be mild to severe.

1) Overview
    a) Epidemiology
        i) The overall incidence in the United States is 1 in 2000.
        ii) African-Americans and Hispanics have four times the incidence of whites.
        iii) Women are affected seven times as often as men, and SLE is the most frequently encountered autoimmune disease in pregnancy (1,2).
        iv) The stress of surgery may exacerbate SLE.
    b) Pathophysiology
        i) The deposition of autoantibodies results in inflammation and end-organ damage.
    c) Drug-induced SLE
        i) Drugs associated with the development of SLE include hydralazine, isoniazid, procainamide, and α-methyldopa.
            (1) Drug-induced SLE is usually more mild and characterized by rash, fever, arthralgias, anemia, and leukopenia.

2) Organ involvement
    a) **Cardiac:** Over half of all patients with SLE have some cardiac involvement. SLE can involve the pericardium, endocardium, myocardium, coronary arteries, and conduction system (3).
        i) Pericardial disease is one of the most common cardiac manifestations but hemodynamic compromise is rare.
        ii) Valvular abnormalities
            (1) Mitral and aortic valves are the most frequently affected.
            (2) Libman-Sacks endocarditis is a nonbacterial vegetation on the mitral valve.
            (3) Embolic complications are more common than hemodynamically significant lesions (4).
        iii) Myocardial dysfunction can occur secondary to acute myocarditis or related pathologies such as hypertension, renal disease, valvular lesions, and coronary artery disease (CAD).
        iv) CAD: Patients with SLE are at increased risk of CAD with a four to eight times higher incidence than the general population.
            (1) Young women have a 50-fold increased risk of developing CAD compared to age-matched controls (5).

Drug-induced SLE is associated with hydralazine, isoniazid, procainamide, and α-methyldopa.

Patients with SLE are at increased risk of CAD with a four to eight times higher incidence than the general population.

    v) Dysrhythmias: Sinus tachycardia is common. Rarely, atrioventricular and buddle branch blocks can occur (3).

b) **Neurologic:** SLE can affect both the central and the peripheral nervous system.

    i) Cognitive dysfunction, mood disorders, headaches, seizures, transverse myelitis, and cerebrovascular accidents have all been reported.

    ii) Sensory and autonomic neuropathy can also develop (6,7).

c) **Renal:** Virtually, all patients with SLE have some renal involvement, and 50% will develop renal disease.

    i) The most common cause is immune complex deposition resulting in complement activation and inflammation.

    ii) Patients may have proteinuria, hematuria, and pyuria.

    iii) Patients with SLE can progress to end-stage renal disease (1, 6).

d) **Pulmonary**

    i) Pleuritis and autoimmune pneumonitis result in cough, dyspnea, and arterial hypoxemia.

    ii) Restrictive lung disease can develop due to the chronic inflammatory process.

    iii) Pulmonary hypertension and right heart strain may be present.

e) **Hematologic**

    i) Thrombocytopenia, leukopenia, and anemia are commonly seen.

    ii) There is a strong association with SLE and **antiphospholipid antibody syndrome**, which is associated with arterial and venous thrombus formation.

    iii) Patients may also be on **chronic immunosuppressive medications**.

3) **Treatment**

a) The treatment involves decreasing inflammation and suppressing the immune system to prevent further end-organ damage.

b) Patients are frequently on nonsteroidal anti-inflammatory drugs as well as more potent anti-inflammatory agents such as corticosteroids, hydroxychloroquine, methotrexate, azathioprine, and cyclophosphamide.

c) Patients with a history of antiphospholipid antibody syndrome may be on anticoagulant medications

4) **Anesthetic concerns**: A thorough understanding of the diverse and complex nature of the disease is important for the anesthesiologist caring for a patient with SLE.

a) **Preoperative:** A complete preoperative evaluation with particular focus on the cardiopulmonary as well as neurological and renal systems is warranted. Disease severity and organ systems involved should be assessed.

    i) Assess the patient's exercise tolerance, with particular emphasis on any episodes of dyspnea or angina.

    ii) Check an ECG for conduction abnormalities and signs of ischemia.

        (1) A stress cardiac study may be indicated.

        (2) Echocardiography should be considered if there are findings on the cardiac exam suggestive of valvular disease or myocardial dysfunction.

    iii) Pulmonary function test and a chest x-ray are indicated in patients with dyspnea (rest or with mild exercise) to rule out pulmonary disease.

    iv) A careful neurological exam should be performed to determine the extent of central or peripheral nervous system involvement.

    v) Laboratory studies

        (1) Complete blood count

        (2) Coagulation studies

        (3) Basic metabolic panel to determine the extent of renal disease and electrolyte status

vi) Patients who have been receiving steroids for the past six months may require **perioperative stress dose steroids.**

b) **Intraoperative**

i) **Monitoring**

Most SLE patients are immunosuppressed, and strict sterile technique should always be used for procedures.

(1) Standard monitors should be used.

(2) Other monitors, such as invasive BP monitoring, should be used as warranted by the patient's systemic disease and the surgical procedure.

(3) Five-lead ECG monitoring should be considered based on the patient's risk for cardiac ischemia.

ii) **Induction agents.** The choice of induction agent should be determined by the extent of the patient's systemic disease and the hemodynamic goals of the procedure.

(1) Nephrotoxic medications should be avoided.

(2) If the patient has renal impairment, drug clearance may be decreased.

iii) Strict sterile technique should be used for any procedure, as SLE patients are immunosuppressed.

iv) Patients with thrombocytopenia are at risk for hemorrhage.

c) **Postoperative**

i) Monitor for signs of infection as patients may be immunosuppressed.

ii) Continue to monitor for signs of cardiac ischemia.

iii) Patients may be at increased risk of developing deep vein thrombus and pulmonary embolism.

Chapter Summary for SLE

Definition	SLE is a multisystem inflammatory disease affecting predominantly the cardiac, neurologic, hematologic, renal, and pulmonary systems.	
Potential SLE Manifestations	Cardiac	Conduction abnormalities, pericarditis, valvular disease, premature CAD
	Neurologic	Cognitive dysfunction, CVAs, vasculitis
	Pulmonary	Restrictive lung disease, possible pulmonary HTN
	Renal	Glomerulonephritis can result in renal failure
	Hematologic	Thrombocytopenia, Anemia, Immunosuppression
	Endocrine	Adrenal suppression possible, consider stress dose steroids
Preoperative Concerns	Preoperative evaluation, with particular focus on the cardiopulmonary, neurological, and renal systems. Careful neurological exam to determine the extent of central or peripheral nervous systems effects. Blood chemistry to evaluate degree of renal disease, and check electrolyte balance prior to surgery.	
Intraoperative Concerns	Consider invasive monitoring based on presence of systemic disease and surgical procedure. Nephrotoxic medications should be avoided. Sterile technique for invasive procedures due to immunosuppression.	
Postoperative Concerns	Monitor for signs of cardiac ischemia or infection. May be at increased risk of developing DVTs and PEs.	

CAD, coronary artery disease; CVA, cerebrovascular accident; HTN, hypertension.

References

1. Warren JB, Silver RM. Autoimmune disease in pregnancy: systemic lupus erythematosus and antiphospholipid syndrome. *Obstet Gynecol Clin North Am* 2004;31:345–72, vi–vii.
2. Kotzin BL. Systemic lupus erythematosus. *Cell* 1996;85:303–306.
3. Doria A, Iaccarino L, Sarzi-Puttini P, et al. Cardiac involvement in systemic lupus erythematosus. *Lupus* 2005;14:683–686.
4. Omdal R, Lunde P, Rasmussen K, et al. Transesophageal and transthoracic echocardiography and Doppler-examinations in systemic lupus erythematosus. *Scand J Rheumatol* 2001;30:275–281.
5. Manzi S, Meilahn EN, Rairie JE, et al. Age-specific incidence rates of myocardial infarction and angina in women with systemic lupus erythematosus. *Am J Epidemiol* 1997;145:408–415.
6. Dall'Era, Davis JC. Systemic lupus erythematosus. *Postgrad Med* 2003;114:31–40.
7. Boumpas DT AHI, Fessler BJ, et al. Systemic lupus erythematosus: emerging concepts. *Ann Intern Med* 1995;122:940–950.

ANESTHESIA AND COMORBID DISEASES

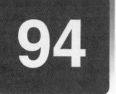

94 Myasthenia Gravis

Sabin Oana, MD

Due to recent advances in pharmacology and anesthetic care, myasthenia gravis (MG) has become better understood and safer to manage in the perioperative setting.

1) **Overview** (1)
   a) Affects approximately 20 people per 100,000 in the United States, mostly young women and older men
   b) Myasthenia Gravis Foundation of America (MGFA) Clinical Classification has replaced older schemes (Table 94-1).

2) **Pathophysiology**
   a) **MG is an autoimmune disease** (2) (Fig. 94-1).
      i) A breakdown in tolerance toward self-antigens through a T-cell–dependent process (that is mediated at least in part by the thymus) generates Acetylcholine receptor (AChR) antibodies (80% to 90% of the patients).
      ii) The resulting complement activation destroys the postsynaptic surface.
      iii) Decreased functional AChR limits muscle cell depolarization by decreasing the probability that a nerve impulse will be followed by an action potential (i.e., decreased safety factor).
      iv) Repetitive stimulation of the neuromuscular junction (NMJ) decreases the quantity of ACh released (normal phenomenon), decreasing even further the action potentials initiated in the muscle. This is the pathophysiological basis of fatigue in MG.

Table 94-1
MGFA Clinical Classification

MGFA Class I	Ocular MG
MGFA Class II[a]	Mild generalized MG
MGFA Class III[a]	Moderate generalized MG
MGFA Class IV[a]	Severe generalized MG
MGFA Class V	MG cases requiring intubation

[a]Classes II, III and IV have subgroups "a" for limb/axial or "b" for oropharyngeal/respiratory involvement.

Figure 94-1   Normal **(A)** and Myasthenic **(B)** NMJs

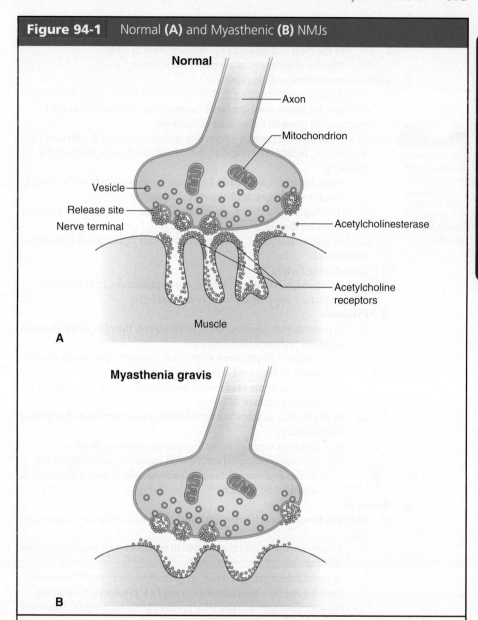

Normal

— Axon

— Mitochondrion

Vesicle —
Release site —
Nerve terminal —
— Acetylcholinesterase
— Acetylcholine receptors

Muscle

A

Myasthenia gravis

B

Nerve action potential arrives at the NMJ → Release of acetylcholine (ACh) quanta mediated by calcium → ACh binds to AChR on the postsynaptic (muscle) membrane → Sodium/potassium-mediated depolarization and contraction of the muscle → ACh is degraded by AChE. In MG, the muscle membrane has less folds, less ACh receptors, and the synaptic space is wider than normal. Adapted from Drachman DB. Myasthenia Gravis. *N Engl J Med*. 1994;330(25):1797–1810.

<ul>
<li>v) 7% of the patients don't have antibodies against AChR, but against muscle specific kinase (MuSK), a receptor for agrin (protein secreted by the axon and essential for the formation of NMJ).</li>
<li>vi) The rest of the patients are truly seronegative.</li>
</ul>

3) **Clinical presentation and diagnosis (3)**

MG is frequently associated with other autoimmune diseases such as hyperthyroidism and rheumatoid arthritis.

a) Main symptom is fluctuating skeletal muscle weakness, localized to specific muscles, often associated with fatigue (increased weakness after exercise) but not with a sensation of tiredness.

b) 50% of the patients present with ocular symptoms and 15% with oropharyngeal (i.e., bulbar, innervated by the cranial nerves) symptoms of the following:
   i) Dysarthria, which indicates laryngeal muscle weakness with possible ensuing extrathoracic **obstructive** flow pattern
   ii) Dysphagia is a common exacerbating factor for MG, and its presence increases the risk of **aspiration.**

c) Cardiac disease is typically not present, although thymomas may result in myocarditis.

d) **Exacerbating factors**
   i) Infections, medications, trauma, hot temperature, hypokalemia, pregnancy, hyperthyroidism, emotional upset

e) **Diagnosis**
   i) In patients with obvious ocular involvement, the **edrophonium test** is a bedside test useful for diagnosis.
      (1) 2 mg of edrophonium given every 1 minute up to 10 mg should result in decreased muscle weakness.
      (2) Side effects are bradycardia and bronchospasm due to the muscarinic effects of ACh.
   ii) In all patients, diagnostic confirmation should be obtained including the following:
      (1) Serologic testing checks for specific serum antibodies.
      (2) Electrophysiological testing with repetitive nerve stimulation studies and single-fiber electromyography is especially useful in seronegative patients.

4) **Treatment**
   a) **Acetylcholinesterase inhibitors (AChEIs)** are used to treat the symptoms of MG
      i) Allows for ACh accumulation, which improves neuromuscular transmission
      ii) Approximate equivalent doses are: neostigmine 15 mg PO = neostigmine 1.5 mg IM = neostigmine 0.5 mg IV = pyridostigmine 60 mg PO = pyridostigmine 2 mg IM = pyridostigmine 0.7 mg IV. Most common side effects are muscarinic.

   b) **Immunomodulators**
      i) Most MG patients require immunomodulators in addition to AChEI to control the disease.
      ii) Chronic treatment includes steroids and other immunosuppressants
         (1) Most commonly used are azathioprine, cyclosporine, and mycophenolate.
      iii) Plasmapheresis
         (1) Directly removes AChR antibodies from circulation
         (2) Reserved for myasthenic crisis (MC), preoperative or as an adjuvant.

      (3) Removes plasma AChE, so it can affect the metabolism of various drugs

      (4) Side effects include electrolyte imbalances, coagulopathies, and thrombotic events.

    iv) **Intravenous immune globulin** suppresses harmful inflammation and is proven effective in MG.

  c) **Surgical treatment**

    i) Thymectomy is generally effective and can be performed via a transsternal, transcervical, thoracoscopic, or robotic approach.

5) Differential diagnosis

  a) Differential diagnosis of the chronic weakness includes the myasthenic syndrome, motor neuron disease, and various myopathies and neuropathies.

  b) Cholinergic crisis

    i) Caused by excessive AChEI medication

    ii) Manifested as weakness, which may or may not be accompanied by cholinergic symptoms (bradycardia, miosis, hypersalivation)

    iii) The edrophonium test is not reliable at differentiating between the two conditions and is not recommended.

    iv) Treatment is symptomatic with antimuscarinic agents (glycopyrrolate and atropine).

6) **Preoperative evaluation (4,5)**

  a) History and physical should be performed with careful attention paid to

    i) Bulbar and respiratory muscle dysfunction, which increase the risk of aspiration and respiratory failure

    ii) Vascular or airway obstruction caused by an enlarged thymus

    iii) Chronic pulmonary disease, which increases the risk of postoperative ventilation (6)

      (1) Consider pulmonary function studies and plan for intensive care admission in these patients.

    iv) Associated autoimmune disorders

  b) Consider **preoperative neurologic optimization**, possibly including preoperative plasmapheresis, if patient not at baseline and in severe cases.

  c) **Medication reconciliation**

    i) Doses, adherence to regimen, and side effects should be ascertained.

    ii) **AChEI drugs should not be interrupted, especially in symptomatic patients.**

    iii) Steroid use is common.

      (1) Assess need for perioperative supplementation.

      (2) In patients treated with high-dose steroids and nondepolarizing neuromuscular blockers (NMBs), quadriplegic myopathy may occur (7).

    iv) Azathioprine-induced hepatotoxicity or bone marrow suppression

    v) Cyclosporine-associated nephrotoxicity

  d) MG patients should receive minimal sedation as hypoventilation could precipitate respiratory failure or aspiration. However, care should be taken to avoid stress and hyperventilation which could also worsen the clinical picture.

Central anticholinergic syndrome is produced by the inhibition of the central nervous system muscarinic receptors (e.g., atropine), manifested by confusion and treated with central acting AChEI (physostigmine).

READ MORE

Anterior mediastinal mass, Chapter 59, page 430

Remifentanil, propofol, desflurane, sevoflurane, and cisatracurium are modern anesthetic agents that can be used with confidence in patients with MG.

Table 94-2

Interaction of Anesthetic Agents with MG. T1 and T4 Represent Amplitudes of the First and the Fourth Twitches in a Train of Four Stimulation

Agent	Action	Comments Regarding Patients with MG
Volatile anesthetics	Suppression of T1 and a 40%–70% decrease in T4/T1 ratio at 2 MAC(8)	
Succinylcholine	Increase in ED95 from 0.31 mg/kg to 0.82 mg/kg, i.e., 2.6 times(9)	Resistant Prolonged duration of action
Atracurium and cisatracurium	ED95 of atracurium is decreased from 0.24 mg/kg to 0.07 mg/kg(13)	Sensitive Advantageous due to their unique mechanisms of elimination

  e) Strongly consider aspiration prophylaxis and precautions with rapid sequence induction and intubation.
7) Intraoperative management
  a) **Anesthetic agents in MG**
    i) **Volatile anesthetics** can profoundly decrease neuromuscular transmission in MG (8). In fact, the combination of weakness from disease and muscle relaxation from volatile anesthesia may obviate the need for muscle relaxation during surgery.
    ii) **Succinylcholine** (Table 94-2) (9).
      (1) The dose given should be increased to approximately 2 mg/kg.
      (2) Onset of action may be delayed.
      (3) Patients are more likely to exhibit signs of phase II block.
      (4) There is no contraindication to succinylcholine in MG in terms of risks of hyperkalemia or hypercatabolic syndromes.
    iii) **Nondepolarizing NMBs** (10)
      (1) Faster onset and prolonged duration of action in MG patients (11)
      (2) Sensitivity can be maintained in patients thought to be in remission and in those with isolated ocular myasthenia.
      (3) All the agents have been used with safe results if appropriate precautions in dosing and monitoring are taken (12,13).
      (4) If necessary, reversal of fade in neuromuscular block can be successfully accomplished using the usual medications in the usual doses.
      (5) Although not available in the United States, sugammadex has been used successfully in reversal of intense NMB in MG without any interference with ACh pathways (14).
    iv) **Narcotics are associated with higher risk of respiratory depression** even after epidural administration. Should be carefully titrated.
      (1) Remifentanil has been used successfully in association with both propofol and volatile anesthetics (15).

All MG patients should be monitored intraoperatively with a nerve stimulator.

      v) Local anesthetics depress neuromuscular transmission through both presynaptic and postsynaptic effects.

        (1) Amides local anesthetics are preferred (see below).

      vi) Interactions with AChE inhibitor therapy

        (1) Succinylcholine, mivacurium, and ester local anesthetics have impaired metabolism (i.e., prolonged duration of action).

        (2) Remifentanil and cisatracurium are unaffected.

b) Monitoring with peripheral nerve stimulator

    i) When eye muscles are affected, the usual pattern of the facial nerve being more resistant than ulnar nerve to the actions of NMBs could be reversed.

      (1) Consider double neuromuscular monitoring at both sites in those patients (16).

c) Anesthetic plan

Severe bradycardia is possible with spinal or epidural anesthesia and also after administration of remifentanil in a patient with MG treated with AChEI (17–19).

    i) Whenever feasible, local or regional anesthesia should be the first choice.

      (1) Spinal anesthesia may be preferable to epidural due to the lesser quantities of local anesthetics required.

      (2) Regional anesthesia does not eliminate the risk of MG exacerbation.

      (3) High levels of sensory blockade are more likely to precipitate respiratory distress in MG patients with a baseline compromised respiratory status.

      (4) In the presence of significant respiratory muscle involvement, general anesthesia may be necessary for aspiration prevention and respiratory support.

    ii) If general anesthesia is indicated, avoidance of NMBs is recommended.

      (1) Total intravenous anesthesia and the use of less soluble volatile anesthetics are the preferred techniques.

The possibility of postoperative mechanical ventilation should be discussed with MG patients.

A comprehensive and updated list of medications that exacerbate MG can be found at the MGFA website at http://www. myasthenia.org/.

      (2) In cases where the use of NMBs is mandatory, doses should be adjusted accordingly and their effects checked more frequently with a peripheral nerve stimulator.

d) Induction and intubation methods in order to avoid NMBs (only to be used if feasible with regard to cardiovascular stability):

    i) Increase the dose of IV induction agent.

    ii) Use volatiles to deepen anesthesia prior to attempting intubation.

    iii) Use remifentanil in induction doses.

e) For maintenance, a balanced anesthetic is the most common choice. Immobility can be obtained either with remifentanil or maintaining a deeper plane of anesthesia.

f) Anesthetic emergence

    i) Processed EEG monitoring might be useful to titrate agents toward the completion of surgery.

    ii) Immediate postoperative extubation can be accomplished in most cases.

    iii) Standard extubation criteria should be fulfilled.

      (1) Sustained head lift for 5 seconds is the gold standard to assess for neuromuscular strength (10).

      (2) Optimize patient's general condition (normothermia, normovolemia, electrolyte imbalance).

      iv) In the most severe cases, admission to intensive care and delayed extubation until the patient is awake and as close to his baseline as possible is the preferred approach (5).
- g) **Avoid medications that can exacerbate MG (20).**
  - i) Antibiotics that impair neuromuscular transmission include aminoglycosides, fluoroquinolones (ciprofloxacin), clindamycin, erythromycin.
  - ii) Cardiovascular drugs such as quinidine, β-adrenergic antagonists, calcium-channel blockers, procainamide, statins
  - iii) Neuropsychiatric drugs such as phenytoin, lithium
  - iv) Magnesium sulfate
8) **Postoperative considerations**
   - a) Patients require a monitored setting able to provide continuous pulse oximetry, supplemental O$_2$, more frequent nursing interventions, and physician checks.
   - b) The hand offs should be elaborate, with emphasis on resumption/titration of AChEI (IV or orally as tolerated) and avoidance of detrimental medication.
   - c) Due to increased work of breathing and increased postoperative stress, MG patients may deteriorate for several days after surgery.
9) **Special types of MG**
   - a) Neonatal MG
     - i) Caused by transfer of AChR antibodies from mother to infant
     - ii) Characterized by generalized weakness, which resolves spontaneously within 6 weeks of birth
   - b) Iatrogenic MG
     - i) Caused classically by D-penicillamine and also by alpha-interferon and bone marrow transplantation
   - c) Congenital MG
     - i) Genetically determined and includes congenital AChR deficiency and congenital choline acetyl transferase deficiency (1)
10) **Myasthenic crisis (MC) corresponds to MGFA class V (21)**
    - a) Defined by respiratory muscle weakness and impending respiratory failure
    - b) Most commonly precipitated by infections
    - c) Outcomes have improved due to advances in artificial ventilation but the overall duration of the crisis is still around 2 weeks.
    - d) Management includes the following:
      - i) Optimization and treatment of the precipitating factors
      - ii) Supportive care usually includes artificial ventilation and ICU care.
      - iii) Treatment of neuromuscular dysfunction, usually with plasmapheresis
    - e) When intubated, AChEI may be discontinued due to excess respiratory secretions, mucous plugging, and increased risk of arrhythmias.
11) **MG during pregnancy (22,23)**
    - a) Fluctuating course due to altered hormonal levels ante- and postpartum. Close monitoring and aggressive treatment are essential.
    - b) AChEI considerations in pregnancy
      - i) Associated with increased uterine contractility secondary to uterine cholinergic receptor stimulation
      - ii) During labor, parenteral doses should be considered.
      - iii) There is minimal placental and breast milk transfer.
    - c) Tocolytic and preeclamptic medications (magnesium sulfate, terbutaline, and ritodrine) could be associated with an excessive amount of muscle weakness.
    - d) Stage two of labor could be impaired due to muscle fatigue. Forceps delivery might be necessary.
    - e) For vaginal delivery and cesarean section, epidural or combined spinal-epidural are preferred if tolerated from a respiratory standpoint.

Lambert-Eaton Myasthenic Syndrome (LEMS)

1) **Overview (24)**

    a) **Presynaptic** acquired autoimmune disease characterized by antibody to the voltage-gated calcium channels at the motor nerve terminal.

        i) Results in decreased ACh release from the vesicles

    b) **Signs/symptoms**

        i) **Nonfluctuating weakness**, more frequently proximal in the lower limbs

        ii) **Rare bulbar or ocular symptoms**

        iii) **Tendon reflexes are maintained.**

        iv) Associated with **autonomic failure** and sensory neuropathy

        v) Weakness **improves with exercise.**

    c) Associated with **small-cell lung cancer**, other tumors, and autoimmune diseases

Weakness worsens with exercise in MG, but in Lambert-Eaton syndrome, weakness improves with exercise.

    d) **Treatment**

        i) 3,4-diaminopyridine (3,4 DAP), a potassium channel blocker at the motor nerve terminal, prolongs the action potential and enhances ACh release.

        ii) 3,4 DAP is an orphan drug in the United States. Overdose has been associated with seizures and one report of cardiac arrest.

        iii) Acute or chronic immunomodulation is achieved using the same approach as in MG.

        iv) Anticholinesterase drugs used in MG are not effective in LEMS.

2) **Anesthetic management**

    a) Most of the considerations from MG discussion apply to patients with LEMS with the notable differences that LEMS patients are **sensitive** to succinylcholine and **extremely** sensitive to nondepolarizing agents.

    b) Avoidance of NMB is preferred due to patient's extreme sensitivity.

    c) If NMB are used, doses should be reduced and the patient carefully monitored.

    d) Reversal of NMB may be insufficient with AChEI and extreme care should be taken to ensure muscular strength compatible with successful extubation.

Chapter Summary for Myasthenia Gravis and Myasthenic Syndrome

	Myasthenia Gravis	Lambert-Eaton Myasthenic Syndrome
Pathophysiology	Autoimmune disease where antibodies are formed to ACh receptor	Autoimmune disease affecting voltage-gated calcium channels at motor nerve terminal; results in decreased ACh release
Preoperative Evaluation	Optimization of weakness; plasmapheresis; continue AChEI; assessment of risks of aspiration and postoperative respiratory failure	AChEI not effective for treatment; associated with small-cell carcinoma of the lung
Intraoperative Management	Perform regional or avoidance of NMBs; minimal sedation; resistance to succinylcholine; sensitivity to nondepolarizing NMBs; "stress dose" of steroids; bradycardia risk; interference with the metabolism of drugs at esteratic sites	Sensitive to succinylcholine *and* sensitive to nondepolarizing NMB; other considerations similar to MG
Postoperative Considerations	Careful titration of narcotics, close monitoring of respiratory status	Careful titration of narcotics, close monitoring of respiratory status

AChEI, acetylcholinesterase inhibitor; ACh, acetylcholine; NMB, neuromuscular blocker; MG, myasthenia gravis.

References

1. Jaretzki A 3rd, Barohn RJ, Ernstoff RM, et al. Myasthenia gravis: recommendations for clinical research standards. Task Force of the Medical Scientific Advisory Board of the Myasthenia Gravis Foundation of America. *Ann Thorac Surg.* 2000 Jul;70(1):327–34.
2. Hughes BW, Moro De Casillas ML, Kaminski HJ. Pathophysiology of myasthenia gravis. *Semin Neurol* 2004;24(1):21–30.
3. Bird SJ. Clinical manifestations of myasthenia gravis. In: Rose BD, ed. *UpToDate.* Waltham: UpToDate; 2010.
4. Barrick B, Kyle R. Anesthesia issues. In: Howard JF, ed. *Myasthenia Gravis: A Manual for the Health Care Provider.* St. Paul: Myasthenia Gravis Foundation of America; 2008:54–59.
5. Dillon FX. Anesthesia issues in the perioperative management of myasthenia gravis. *Semin Neurol* 2004;24(1):83–94.
6. Naguib M, el Dawlatly AA, Ashour M, et al. Multivariate determinants of the need for postoperative ventilation in myasthenia gravis. *Can J Anaesth* 1996;43(10):1006–1013.
7. Murray MJ, Brull SJ, Bolton CF. Brief review: nondepolarizing neuromuscular blocking drugs and critical illness myopathy. *Can J Anaesth* 2006;53(11):1148–1156.
8. Nitahara K, Sugi Y, Higa K, et al. Neuromuscular effects of sevoflurane in myasthenia gravis patients. *Br J Anaesth* 2007;98(3):337–341.
9. Eisenkraft JB, Book WJ, Mann SM, et al. Resistance to succinylcholine in myasthenia gravis: a dose-response study. *Anesthesiology* 1988;69(5):760–763.
10. Baraka A. Anaesthesia and myasthenia gravis. *Can J Anaesth* 1992;39(5 Pt 1):476–486.
11. Baraka A. Onset of neuromuscular block in myasthenic patients. *Br J Anaesth* 1992;69(2):227–228.
12. De Haes A, Proost JH, Kuks JB, et al. Pharmacokinetic/pharmacodynamic modeling of rocuronium in myasthenic patients is improved by taking into account the number of unbound acetylcholine receptors. *Anesth Analg* 2002;95(3):588–596.
13. Mann R, Blobner M, Jelen-Esselborn S, et al. Preanesthetic train-of-four fade predicts the atracurium requirement of myasthenia gravis patients. *Anesthesiology* 2000;93(2):346–350.
14. Unterbuchner C, Fink H, Blobner M. The use of sugammadex in a patient with myasthenia gravis. *Anaesthesia* 2010;65(3):302–305.
15. Gritti P, Carrara B, Khotcholava M, et al. The use of desflurane or propofol in combination with remifentanil in myasthenic patients undergoing a video-assisted thoracoscopic-extended thymectomy. *Acta Anaesthesiol Scand* 2009;53(3):380–389.
16. Devys JM, Debaene B, Plaud B. Anesthesia for urgent abdominal surgery and myasthenia gravis. *Can J Anaesth* 2002;49(2):215–216.
17. Nauphal M, Baraka A. Bradycardia, hypotension and bronchospasm following remifentanil-propofol in a myasthenic patient treated by pyridostigmine—a case report. *Middle East J Anesthesiol* 2008;19(6):1387–1390.
18. Inoue S, Shiomi T, Furuya H. Severe bradycardia in a patient with myasthenia gravis during transurethral ureterolithotripsic procedure under spinal anaesthesia. *Anaesth Intensive Care* 2002;30(3):387.
19. Lin TC, Hsu CH, Kong SS, et al. Ventricular asystole and complete heart block after thoracic epidural analgesia for thymectomy. *Eur J Anaesthesiol* 2002;19(6):460–462.
20. Bershad EM, Feen ES, Suarez JI. Myasthenia gravis crisis. *South Med J* 2008;101(1):63–69.
21. Fernandes Filho JA, Suarez JI. Neurocritical care of myasthenic crisis. In: Kaminski HJ, ed. *Myasthenia Gravis and Related Disorders.* 2nd ed. New York: Humana Press; 2008:175–183.
22. Bader AM. Neurologic and neuromuscular disease. In: Chestnut DH, Polley LS, Tsu LC, Wong CA, eds. *Chestnut's Obstetric Anesthesia: Principles and Practice.* 4th ed. Philadelphia: Mosby; 2009:1053–1078.
23. Rolbin WH, Levinson G, Shnider SM, et al. Anesthetic considerations for myasthenia gravis and pregnancy. *Anesth Analg* 1978;57(4):441–447.
24. Petty R. Lambert Eaton myasthenic syndrome. *Pract Neurol* 2007;7(4):265–267.

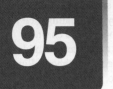

Part G: Psychiatric Disease and Substance Abuse Psychiatric Diseases

Dominique Schiffer, MD

The prevalence of depression in the United States is 5% to 9% and that of bipolar disorder is 2% to 4%. Depression is associated with poorer outcomes in patients with comorbidities such as coronary artery disease, diabetes, and stroke. "There is a bidirectional relationship between depression and medical illness, each having a negative impact on prognosis and treatment of the other condition" (1).

1) **Depression**

   a) A complex and heterogeneous disorder that comprises disorders of mood, cognitive function, and neurovegetative functions (i.e., energy, sleep, appetite, and sexual function)

   b) **Treatment** may use a multimodal approach that includes behavioral therapy, pharmacotherapy, and education. In those with treatment-resistant depression, electroconvulsive therapy (ECT) may be helpful (2).

     i) **Behavioral therapy**

       (1) Psychotherapy is a nonpharmacologic method for treating depression.

       (2) It includes supportive counseling, cognitive therapy, and problem-solving therapy.

     ii) **Pharmacological**

       (1) Nearly half of moderate to severe episodes of depression will respond to medication.

       (2) When a depressed patient presents for surgery, he or she may be taking one or more antidepressants with different mechanisms of action depending on their drug class.

       (3) **Antidepressants** act by altering noradrenergic and/or serotonergic neurotransmission. They increase the amount of norepinephrine and serotonin in synapses (3).

       (4) It is imperative that the anesthesiologist be familiar with the various classes of antidepressant medication.

         (a) **Selective serotonin reuptake inhibitors (SSRIs)**

           (i) SSRIs are the most broadly prescribed class of antidepressants for mild to moderate depression

           (ii) SSRIs and some of their metabolites inhibit certain cytochrome P-450 enzymes, with fluoxetine (Prozac) being the most potent inhibitor.

(iii) Some β-adrenergic antagonists and several cardiac antidysrhythmic drugs (Type 1C, e.g., propafenone) are metabolized by the same enzyme system that SSRIs inhibit, thereby potentiating their effects.

(iv) Other drugs metabolized by the Cytochrome P-450 enzymes that could potentially interact with SSRIs are diazepam, midazolam, tricyclics, omeprazole, warfarin, phenytoin, theophylline, haloperidol, carbemazapine, tolbutamide, and clozapine (4).

(v) A rare complication of SSRI treatment is SIADH with hyponatremia (4).

(b) **Tricyclic antidepressants (TCAs)**

   (i) **Mechanism of action**

     1. Block reuptake of epinephrine and serotonin in nerve cells (3).

     2. Alter both noradrenergic and serotonergic systems.

     3. Anticholinergic properties may cause orthostatic hypotension.

     4. Cardiac conduction delay can result in dysrhythmias and heart block.

     5. Response to sympathomimetics is unpredictable in patients taking TCAs.

      a. In patients recently started on TCAs, an exaggerated pressor response can be expected with both direct- and indirect-acting sympathomimetics, though the response may be more exaggerated with an indirect-acting sympathomimetic, such as ephedrine (5).

      b. For those who are chronically treated, either sympathomimetic is acceptable, although one should start with a smaller dose.

(c) **Monoamine oxidase inhibitors (MAOIs)**

   (i) **Mechanism of action**

     1. Inhibit the activity of monoamine oxidase, thereby preventing the breakdown of monoamine neurotransmitters.

     2. Use of this class of drugs has significantly declined recently because of a wide spectrum of side effects, drug-drug interactions, and toxicities.

     3. In patients taking MAOIs, the administration of propofol, barbiturates, and benzodiazepines **can result in hypotension and potentiate their CNS and respiratory depressant effects (3)**.

     4. A **hypertensive crisis** can be induced by giving indirect sympathomimetics (ephedrine), methyldopa, and levodopa, in patients taking MAOIs (3).

A hypertensive crisis can be induced by giving indirect sympathomimetics (ephedrine), methyldopa, and levodopa, in patients taking MAOIs.

2) **Bipolar disorder (manic-depressive illness)**

  a) Characterized by cyclical disturbances in mood, cognition, and behavior, with episodes of mania and hypomania

  b) **Treatment**

    i) **Lithium** is one of the most common drugs used for the treatment of bipolar disorder.

     (1) **Mechanism of action**

      (a) May be related to its effects on dopaminergic and noradrenergic transmission or on complex transduction pathways (5).

      (b) Lithium acts presynaptically to inhibit neuromuscular transmission (5).

      (c) Prolongation of neuromuscular blockade is possible with both depolarizing and nondepolarizing neuromuscular blockers. These drugs should be given in reduced doses. Monitoring the depth of neuromuscular blockade is essential (3).

(2) Plasma concentration levels must be measured to ensure safe and effective use. The therapeutic range is 1.0 to 1.2 mEq/L (5).

(3) Lithium can affect renal function; thus, renal function tests should be done every 6 months (5).

(4) ECG changes may be observed with lithium treatment.

    (a) Flattening of the T wave without any clinical consequences is common (5).

    (b) Toxicity may result in QRS complex widening (5).

    (c) Sinoatrial node dysfunction has been described (5).

(5) Hypothyroidism develops in 5% of patients (5).

3) Schizophrenia

  a) A group of disorders that are characterized by delusions, hallucinations, behavioral disturbances.

  b) **Antipsychotic medications** are chemically diverse compounds.

    i) Typical antipsychotics (chlorpromazine, haloperidol) block the dopamine D2 receptor.

    ii) Atypical antipsychotics (clozapine, olanzapine) act as 5-HT 2A antagonists.

    iii) Antipsychotic medication may enhance the effects of CNS depressants. The combination of antipsychotics and ECT is well tolerated (3).

4) Electroconvulsive therapy

  a) ECT provokes a generalized epileptic seizure.

  b) It is safe and effective and at times can be life saving.

  c) The average ECT course is about eight to nine treatments, usually administered three times a week. ECT also may be performed anywhere from once a week to once a month in order to prevent relapses.

  d) ECT can be safely done in both in-patient and out-patient settings (2).

  e) **Indications**

    i) Treatment-resistant depression

    ii) Schizophrenia with affective disorder

    iii) Psychotic depression

    iv) Catatonia

    v) Bipolar depression

    vi) Acute mania

    vii) The need for a rapid response due to psychosis or risk of suicide (2)

  f) **Mechanism**

    i) The mechanism is unknown, but effects may be secondary to alterations in neurophysiologic, neuroendocrinological, and neurochemical systems (3).

  g) **Description of ECT procedure**

    i) The psychiatrist places an EEG monitor and either unilateral or bilateral electrodes to deliver the ECT stimulus.

    ii) An additional BP cuff is placed on an available extremity, used to monitor seizure duration.

    iii) After preoxygenation with 100% oxygen, anesthesia is induced and the patient is ventilated via a facemask.

    iv) After inflating the second BP cuff above the systolic BP, a muscle relaxant is administered.

    v) A bite block is gently placed between the patient's teeth, and the electrical stimulus is applied to induce a seizure.

    vi) The seizure is monitored by both EEG and the tonic clonic activity in the extremity with the second blood pressure cuff.

    vii) Generally, anesthesia is required for only about 3 to 5 minutes.

viii) When the seizure is over, and spontaneous respirations return, the patient is taken to a recovery area and monitored for at minimum, 30 minutes. Standard discharge criteria are used for release from the PACU.

h) **Physiologic responses to ECT**

ECT induces a large parasympathetic surge followed by increased sympathetic nervous system activity.

i) Within seconds after the electrical current is applied, a **parasympathetic surge** occurs (15 to 20 seconds of bradycardia).

ii) Thereafter, a sympathetic surge ensues, with an increase in heart rate and BP.

(1) The rate pressure product may increase two- to fourfold, **increasing myocardial oxygen demand**. The anesthesiologist must understand this unique situation and be ready to treat the cardiovascular responses when necessary.

(2) Cerebral blood flow also increases after electrical stimulation. The maximal blood flow velocity in the middle cerebral artery more than doubles.

5) Anesthetic considerations with ECT

a) **Preoperative evaluation**

Reviewing old anesthetic records is especially helpful when caring for ECT patients.

i) The quality of the preoperative evaluation should be the same as for any surgical procedure (6).

(1) A thorough review of systems and targeted physical exam, with an emphasis on cardiac, respiratory, and neurological systems, should be done in order to identify possible risk factors.

(2) Additional tests, laboratory exams, and imaging studies may be requested based on the patient's history and physical examination.

(3) Since most patients require multiple ECT treatments, it is very helpful to review previous anesthetic records. Once this is done, asking the patient and/or caregivers about complications or problems with the previous anesthetic can help guide anesthetic management.

ii) **Contraindications**

(1) There are not any absolute contraindications to ECT.

(2) Conditions that increase a patient's risk of complications include:

(a) Unstable cardiac disease

(b) Cerebral vascular disease

(c) Recent cerebral hemorrhage or stroke

(d) Increased intracranial pressure

(3) ECT is safe for those who:

(a) Have cardiac pacemakers

(b) Have implantable cardiac defibrillators

(c) Are pregnant

(4) The anesthetic must be tailored appropriately for these conditions as would be for any surgical procedure (6).

iii) Written informed consent should be obtained for ECT (6).

(1) Patients who cannot give consent because of severe psychosis or catatonia may have consent be given by a family member (6).

(2) A government agency may become involved if there is no health care proxy (6).

b) **Intraoperative considerations**

i) ECT requires a complete general anesthetic, providing loss of consciousness, analgesia, amnesia, and muscle relaxation.

ii) The challenge is to provide the anesthetic without suppressing the seizure.

iii) At the same time, one must also manage the airway and the physiologic consequences of the electrically induced seizure.

iv) **Monitoring and equipment**
   (1) ECG, BP monitor, pulse oximeter, capnography.
   (2) Invasive BP monitoring is only necessary in unique cases such as in a patient with a cerebral aneurysm.
   (3) Facemask appropriate for assisted ventilation
   (4) Standard circle system or bag-valve-mask system
   (5) Resuscitative equipment
   (6) Laryngoscope
   (7) Endotracheal tube
   (8) Laryngeal mask airway for management of an airway emergency
   (9) Extra BP cuff to isolate circulation to an extremity
   (10) Bite block
   (11) BIS monitoring has been used in ECT with mixed results (6).

v) **Induction**
   (1) The efficacy of ECT is based on seizure duration, with the goal of 25 to 50 seconds to produce an antidepressant effect.
   (2) Many induction agents have anticonvulsant properties.
      (a) **Methohexital** is considered the "gold standard" induction agent for ECT.
         (i) The American Psychiatric Association recommends a dose of 0.75 mg to 1.0 mg/kg.
      (b) **Thiopental** shortens the seizure duration when compared to methohexital; there is an increase in bradycardia and PVCs. **It is not a preferred agent.**
      (c) **Propofol** at minimally hypnotic doses (0.75 mg/kg) is associated with similar seizure duration as methohexital. Larger doses (up to 1.5 mg/kg) can still lead to clinically acceptable seizure durations.
      (d) **Etomidate** in doses of 0.15 to 0.3 mg/kg has little impact on seizure threshold.
         (i) Associated with longer seizure duration than methohexital, thiopental, and propofol
         (ii) Associated with fewer hemodynamic changes than other induction agents
         (iii) Drawbacks include myoclonus, emetic symptoms, and increased confusional states post-ECT.
      (e) **Ketamine's** potential use as an induction agent for ECT remains controversial and some recommend further study.
         (i) A recent publication suggests that it may have excellent antidepressant properties (7).

vi) **Muscle relaxants**
   (1) Succinylcholine is the muscle relaxant of choice for ECT, due to quick the onset and fast recovery that result.
      (a) The recommended dose is 0.5 to 1.0 mg/kg.
      (b) Contraindications to the use of succinylcholine include:
         (i) Pseudocholinesterase deficiency
         (ii) Malignant hyperthermia
         (iii) Neuroleptic malignant syndrome
         (iv) Organophosphate poisoning
         (v) Conditions that render patient sensitive to the potassium-releasing effects of succinylcholine

(2) **Nondepolarizing muscle relaxants** can be used when succinylcholine is contraindicated.

    (a) In a recent crossover comparison study of rocuronium versus succinylcholine:

        (i) A 0.3 mg/kg dose of rocuronium was compared to succinylcholine 1 mg/kg for muscle relaxation at induction of anesthesia.

        (ii) Reversal agent (10 µg/kg of atropine and 20 µg/kg neostigmine) was given immediately after completion of the ECT procedure when rocuronium was used.

        (iii) Time to first spontaneous breath was 9.46 minutes with rocuronium and 8.07 minutes with succinylcholine **(8)**.

vii) **Respiratory management**

  (1) Control of the airway during ECT is paramount.

  (2) **Hypocarbia induced by hyperventilation can be used to enhance seizure duration.**

  (3) After induction, if mask ventilation is difficult, airway devices including LMAs can be used to achieve adequate ventilation.

  (4) Intubation may be indicated in certain circumstances such as late pregnancy or a full stomach.

  (5) Oxygen consumption and CO_2 production are increased by seizure activity. Ventilation must be increased appropriately.

    (a) Hypoxia and hypercarbia can aggravate tachycardia and hypertension.

viii) **Managing the hemodynamic effects of ECT**

  (1) **Anticholinergic agents**

    (a) Recommended for patients with bradycardia or heart block, or in those where a prolonged bradycardia may occur (i.e., patients on β-adrenergic antagonists)

    (b) Routine use of an anticholinergic agent results in increased tachycardia after ECT.

  (2) **β-adrenergic antagonists**

    (a) Both esmolol and labetolol have been extensively studied in the management of ECT-induced hemodynamic responses, including attenuating the rise in blood pressure and heart rate.

    (b) Esmolol is the drug of choice in ECT due to its rapid onset.

  (3) **Calcium channel antagonists**

    (a) Intravenous nifedipine (0.1 mg/kg) and nicardipine (40 µg/kg) have been reported to reduce mean arterial pressure and heart rate after ECT.

  (4) Other agents

    (a) Clonidine, nitroprusside, nitroglycerin, and trimethaphan have all been used successfully to control the hemodynamic response in ECT.

c) **Postoperative concerns**

  i) The most common side effects of ECT are confusion, agitation, amnesia, myalgias, nausea, and headache.

    (1) The confusional state can last up to an hour post-ECT.

    (2) Headaches and myalgias can be successfully treated with both NSAIDs and narcotic analgesics. Intranasal sumatriptan is also effective (2).

  ii) ECT can cause transient memory deficits.

  iii) The death rate from ECT is approximately 4 in 100,000 treatments, similar to that of general anesthesia.

Chapter Summary for Psychiatric Diseases

Indications	Treatment-resistant depression, schizophrenia, or psychotic depression.
Preoperative Evaluation	Thorough history and physical. Evaluation of prior ECT records. Informed consent.
Anesthetic Plan	Efficacy is determined by production of adequate seizure. Consider patient's comorbidities.
Intraoperative Management	
Equipment	Standard monitors and equipment for general anesthesia.
Induction Agents	Methohexital (gold standard), propofol, etomidate.
Muscle Relaxants	Succinylcholine is preferred.
Hemodynamic Management	Anticholinergic, antihypertensive agents are frequently required.
Postoperative Management	Treat possible headache, nausea, myalgias, or confusion.

References

1. Iosifescu D. Treating depression in the medically Ill. *Psych Clin North America* 2007;30(1):77–90.
2. Tess A, Smetana G. Medical evaluation of patients undergoing electroconvulsive therapy. *N Engl J Med* 2009;360:1437–1444.
3. Naguib M, Koorn R. Interactions between psychotropics, anaesthetics and electroconvulsive therapy. *CNS Drugs* 2002;16(4):229–247.
4. Kam P, Chang G. Review article: selective serotonin reuptake inhibitors. *Anaesthesia* 1997;52:982–988.
5. Stoelting RK. *Pharmacology and Physiology of Anesthetic Practice*. 3rd ed. Philadelphia, PA: Lippincott Williams & Wilkins;1999.
6. Deiner S, Frost EA. Electroconvulsive therapy and anesthesia. *Int Anesthesiol Clin* 2009;47(2):81–92.
7. MacPherson R, Loo C. Cognitive impairment following electroconvulsive therapy, does the choice of anesthetic agent make a difference? *J ECT* 2008;24:52–56.
8. Turkkal DC, Gokmen N, et al. A cross-over, post-electroconvulsive therapy comparison of clinical recovery from Rocuronium versus succinylcholine. *J Clin Anesth* 2009;20:589–593.
9. Ding Z, White PF. Anesthesia for electroconvulsive therapy. *Anesth Analg* 2002;94(5):1351–1364.

96 Alcohol and Substance Abuse

James Duke, MD, MBA

Substance abuse is commonly encountered in anesthetic practice. Intoxication may be acute, chronic, or one superimposed on the other, and withdrawal from intoxicants can also prove problematic. Many organ systems may be affected.

1) **Ethyl alcohol (EtOH)**—With the possible exception of nicotine, EtOH is the most common substance of abuse. The acute effects of EtOH lead to impairment in judgment, balance, and motor control, predisposing the user to traumatic injury. Chronic effects are listed in Table 96-1.
   a) **Effects on organ systems (see Table 96-1)**
      i) **Central nervous system (CNS)**
         (1) Depresses the CNS by augmenting inhibitory GABAergic synaptic transmission and by inhibiting excitatory NMDA transmission
         (2) Results in generalized blunting and loss of higher motor, sensory, and cognitive function and a depressive effect on inhibitory pathways (disinhibition)

Table 96-1

Chronic Effect of Alcohol Abuse

Organ System	Physiologic and Clinical Effects
Neurologic	Neuropsychiatric disorders, peripheral nerve palsies, Korsakoff psychosis, seizures, Wernicke's encephalopathy, delirium tremens
CV	Autonomic dysfunction, hypertension, dysrhythmias, congestive cardiomyopathy
Pulmonary	Pulmonary hypertension, right-heart failure, decrease in lung capacities, pneumonia
Gastrointestinal	Delayed gastric emptying, susceptibility to aspiration, esophagitis, gastritis, pancreatitis,
Hepatic	Impaired hepatic synthetic function, coagulation disturbances, unpredictable drug metabolism, hypoglycemia
Renal	Numerous electrolyte abnormalities
Immunologic	Decreased bone marrow function, susceptibility to infection

(3) Chronic EtOH use is associated with peripheral nerve and neuropsychiatric disorders, which may be due to neurotoxic effects or to nutritional deficiencies (e.g. Wernicke encephalopathy and Korsakoff psychosis).

    (a) Neuropathies have many features, including weakness of intrinsic muscles of the foot as well as proximal limb weakness, pain and numbness in the lower extremities (often in a stocking foot distribution), and decreased or absent deep tendon reflexes.

    (b) Autonomic dysfunction, manifesting as postural hypotension and delayed gastric emptying are also risks.

    (c) The EtOH-withdrawing patient may experience delirium and seizures, which can be fatal.

ii) **Cardiovascular (CV) system**

  (1) **Acute**

    (a) Moderate acute ingestion of EtOH produces no significant changes in blood pressure (BP) or myocardial contractility.

    (b) Heart rate increases and flushing results from cutaneous vasodilatation.

    (c) At toxic levels of acute EtOH ingestion, a decrease in central vasomotor activity causes respiratory and cardiac depression.

    (d) Acute intoxication may have negative inotropic effects.

  (2) **Chronic**

    (a) Hypertension

    (b) Cardiac dysfunction is the leading cause of death.

    (c) Tachycardia and dysrhythmias (e.g. acute atrial fibrillation, atrial flutter, ventricular ectopy and tachycardia) may indicate alcohol-related cardiac dysfunction, and a 12-lead electrocardiogram (ECG) should be evaluated.

    (d) May cause conduction delays

    (e) Severe use over an extended period may result in congestive cardiomyopathy with associated pulmonary hypertension and right-heart failure.

iii) **Respiratory system**

  (1) **Acute**

    (a) May cause depression of the ventilatory response to CO_2 and increases in dead-space ventilation

    (b) There is a generalized decrease in vital, functional residual, and inspiratory capacity.

    (c) Aspiration of gastric contents is a risk as laryngeal reflexes may be blunted.

    (d) EtOH users are susceptible to pulmonary infections.

iv) **Gastrointestinal and hepatobiliary systems**

  (1) Alterations in glucose homeostasis are common.

    (a) **Hypoglycemia** should be considered if the patient has an altered mental status not explained by intoxication.

    (b) The patient subsisting mostly on EtOH calories may experience an adverse reaction to glucose infusions, including Wernicke encephalopathy and acute phosphate depletion with rhabdomyolysis and neurologic dysfunction.

  (2) EtOH use may cause esophagitis, gastritis, and pancreatitis.

  (3) Delayed gastric emptying and the risk of aspiration have been mentioned.

  (4) Chronic severe consumption of EtOH leads to irreversible cirrhosis and alcohol-induced hepatitis.

    (a) Hepatic synthetic function is impaired, as manifested by hypoalbuminemia and decreased production of coagulation factors II, V, VII, X, and XIII.

(b) Distribution, metabolism, and excretion of drugs can be altered, so effects can be unpredictable.

(c) Esophageal varices develop as portal pressure increases, and the value of placement of a nasogastric tube in such patients should be carefully considered due to the risk of severe variceal bleeding.

  v) **Fluid and electrolyte abnormalities**

    (1) Hyponatremia, hypokalemia, hypophosphatemia, hypocalcemia, and hypomagnesemia are common.

    (2) EtOH inhibits ADH acutely and can result in dehydration.

    (3) Chronic use results in an edematous state due to secondary hyperaldosteronism. Ketoacidosis has been noted.

  vi) **Hematopoiesis**

    (1) Bone marrow is depressed and may be reflected in anemia, leukopenia, and thrombocytopenia.

    (2) Patients are prone to infections, especially pneumonia.

  vii) **Nutritional deficiencies**

    (1) Thiamine deficiency

      (a) Wernicke's encephalopathy (nystagmus, ocular palsy, ataxia)

      (b) Polyneuropathy

      (c) Cardiac failure characterized by high cardiac output, low systemic vascular resistance, and loss of vasomotor tone

    (2) Folic acid deficiency

      (a) Causes bone-marrow depression

b) **Effects on anesthetic agents**

  i) **Volatile anesthetics**

    (1) **Acute intoxication**

      (a) Minimal alveolar concentration (MAC) of inhalational agents is reduced by 40% or more, depending on the blood alcohol level.

    (2) **Chronic use**

      (a) MAC for inhalational agents is increased.

  ii) **Intravenous anesthetics**

    (1) **Acute intoxication**

      (a) Increased sensitivity to the effects of barbiturates, benzodiazepines, and opioids

READ MORE

Diseases of the liver and biliary tract, Chapter 77, page 551

    (2) **Chronic use**

      (a) May require larger-than-normal anesthetic doses

      (b) Intravascular volume status and autonomic dysfunction may complicate management.

        (i) Decisions as to drug dosing and fluid management must be individualized and based on response.

  iii) **Muscle relaxants**

    (1) Cirrhotic patients are edematous and have a greater V_D for water-soluble drugs such as muscle relaxants.

Patients who abuse alcohol may be at risk for hypothermia due to peripheral vasodilation and altered thermoregulation.

    (2) A larger initial dose of nondepolarizing relaxants may be needed, though drugs that rely on hepatic clearance may have a prolonged duration of action.

    (3) Repeated dosing should be based on nerve stimulation.

    (4) Impaired hepatic synthetic function may result in decreased levels of plasma cholinesterase, prolonging the effects of succinylcholine.

    (5) Muscle relaxants that are metabolized independent of organ function (e.g. cisatracurium) are good choices for patients with severe liver disease.

iv) **Sympathomimetic medications**
  (1) Patients may be less sensitive to endogenous or parenteral catecholamines, and direct-acting medications are suggested.

c) **Withdrawal states**
  i) Early withdrawal symptoms include tachycardia, anxiety, tremor, agitation, and hallucinations.
  ii) Delirium tremens and seizures are risks and are potentially fatal.
  iii) It should be noted that while medications such as clonidine decrease the symptoms of withdrawal, they are not protective for seizures.
    (1) Benzodiazepines should be administered to EtOH-dependent inpatients.

2) **Marijuana**
  a) When used as a solo agent used to alter consciousness it does not pose particular problems for the anesthesiologist, but it may be used in concert with other, more problematic, drugs of abuse. Marijuana cigarettes may be dipped in any number of substances, such as phencyclidine (PCP), creating toxicity issues from these substances.
  b) Like tobacco, marijuana has the potential to cause chronic lung disease, though most individuals do not smoke as much marijuana as tobacco cigarettes.

3) **Opioid abuse**
  a) This problem ranges from the patient who has abused prescription opioids to the patient who obtains injectable street drugs such as heroin.
  b) Patients with acute and legitimate requirements for opioids may become tolerant to the effects of these medications, requiring increasing doses, but do not tend to develop addictive behaviors.
  c) **Effects on organ systems** (Table 96-2)
    i) **Central nervous system**

Alcohol withdrawal can be fatal and should be treated aggressively.

The perioperative period is no time to control opioid use in the dependent patient and might be considered inhumane.

Nalaxone can precipitate withdrawal, severe hypertension, and pulmonary edema in habituated patients.

Table 96-2
Chronic Effects of Opioid Abuse

Organ System	Effect
CNS	Coma, respiratory arrest, hypoventilation
CV	Valvular disease, pulmonary edema
Pulmonary	Aspiration, atelectasis, hypoventilation, infections
Infectious	Sepsis, human immunodeficiency virus, tetanus, opportunistic infections
Dermatologic	Cellulitis, abscess formation
Gastrointestinal	Hepatitis
Endocrine	Adrenal suppression

(1) Excessive doses may result in oversedation, apnea, and death from respiratory depression.

(2) Pinpoint pupils in the setting of coma suggest opioid effect.

(3) The opioid antagonist, naloxone, delivered in divided doses, will reverse an opioid-induced coma.

ii) **Cardiovascular**

(1) Pulmonary embolism, pulmonary hypertension, cardiogenic pulmonary edema, endocarditis, and valvular disease have been described.

iii) **Pulmonary**

(1) Aspiration, pneumonia, atelectasis, respiratory depression, and noncardiogenic pulmonary edema are risks.

iv) **Hematologic**

(1) Predilection toward infectious diseases

(a) Mainly seen in users of **injectable** opioids

(i) Contaminated needles and nonsterile injection practices render these patients prone to diseases including hepatitis B and C, human immunodeficiency virus, bacterial endocarditis, pneumonia, cellulitis, abscess formation, sepsis, tetanus, fungal infections, etc.

Postoperative pain control is often challenging for patients with chronic opioid use, and regional anesthesia should be considered whenever possible.

d) **Effects on anesthesia**

i) Acute intoxication

(1) Opioids reduce volatile anesthetic requirements.

ii) Chronic use

(1) May have greater-than-expected volatile anesthetic or opioid requirements

(2) Providing adequate postoperative analgesia may be challenging.

(a) Consider the merits of peripheral nerve blocks for peripheral procedures.

(3) Obtaining intravenous access is often problematic.

4) **Opioid withdrawal**

a) **Symptoms**

i) Restlessness, sweating, nausea, rhinorrhea, abdominal cramping, and lacrimation. Overt withdrawal results in piloerection, emesis, diarrhea, muscle spasms, fever, chills, tachycardia, and hypertension.

b) **Onset and duration of withdrawal varies with the drug used.**

i) For example, meperidine withdrawal symptoms peak in 8 to 12 hours and last for 4 to 5 days. Heroin withdrawal symptoms usually peak within 36 to 72 hours and may last for 7 to 14 days.

c) **Treatment**

i) Includes slow-onset, long-duration medications (e.g., methadone, half-life 15 to 25 hours) that tend not to provide the euphoric feeling drug abusers crave (1)

(1) Methadone has been associated with torsade de pointes in patients with prolonged QT syndrome, so an ECG is necessary prior to its administration.

(2) Sympathetic symptoms may be treated with β-adrenergic antagonists or α_2-agonists such as clonidine.

(3) Withdrawal is not usually life threatening.

5) Cocaine can be administered through nasal inhalation or injection of its powdered form or smoking a highly addictive lipid soluble formulation known as crack.

   a) **Mechanism of action**

      i) Inhibition of the norepinephrine (NE), epinephrine, dopamine, and serotonin neuronal uptake

      ii) NMDA receptor agonist

   b) **Physiologic effects**

      i) Mainly due to increases in NE

      ii) Increases in serum NE levels increases systolic, diastolic and mean arterial pressure, heart rate, and body temperature

   c) **Metabolism**

      i) Hydrolyzed by plasma and liver esterases

      ii) Metabolites excreted by the kidney and can be detected in the urine for up to sixty hours

      iii) Patients with qualitative or quantitative cholinesterase deficiencies may be prone to cocaine toxicity at lower serum levels.

   d) **Effects on organ systems (Table 96-3)**

      i) **Central nervous system**

         (1) The patient may be euphoric or experience boundless energy but in excessive doses may become agitated, combative, or hallucinate.

Hyperthermia is a serious complication of cocaine intoxication and can cause death (2).

Table 96-3
Effects of Cocaine Abuse

Organ System	Effect
CNS	Euphoria, increased energy agitation Seizures CVA
CV	↑HR, ↑BP Chest pain Myocardial ischemia/infarction Dilated cardiomyopathy Aortic dissection Ventricular arrhythmias Sudden death
Pulmonary	Pneumothorax Pulmonary edema Pulmonary hemorrhage and infarction
Hematologic	Disseminated intravascular coagulation
Kidney	Acute renal injury Rhabdomyolysis
Other	Perforated nasal septum Severe hyperthermia

Selective β$_2$-adrenergic blockade should be avoided in the cocaine-intoxicated patient as it can lead to unopposed α$_1$-mediated coronary and peripheral vasoconstriction.

(2) Cocaine is hypermetabolic and blocks the thermoregulatory process of vasodilation and sweating.

  ii) **CV system**

    (1) Hypertension and tachycardia are common.

    (2) Patients may develop chest pain, myocardial ischemia or infarction, and dilated cardiomyopathies.

      (a) Treatment of cocaine-induced chest pain includes the use of selective β$_1$-adrenergic blockade, nitrates, calcium channel blockers, and α-adrenergic blockers.

      (b) Avoid selective β$_2$ agents because it may lead to unopposed α$_1$-mediated coronary and peripheral vasoconstriction (3).

      (c) Cocaine blocks sodium channels in cardiac conducting tissue and is proarrhythmic.

  e) **Anesthetizing the cocaine-intoxicated patient**

    i) **Preoperative considerations**

      (1) Prolongation of the QT interval predisposes the patient to torsades de pointes.

        (a) An ECG must be obtained preoperatively.

      (2) Elective surgery is safe in a cocaine-ingesting patient who is not acutely intoxicated and does not have significant alterations in vital signs or myocardial ischemia (4).

Fatal ventricular arrhythmias and sudden death have been associated with cocaine use.

    ii) **Intraoperative considerations**

      (1) The patient should be well anesthetized prior to airway instrumentation to avoid severe tachycardia and hypertension.

      (2) Ketamine and pancuronium potentiate the CV toxicity of cocaine and should be avoided.

      (3) The MAC of inhalational anesthetic agents is increased when acutely intoxicated.

      (4) Should hypotension require pressor therapy, direct-acting agents such as phenylephrine may be better as these patients may be catecholamine depleted.

      (5) Lidocaine may potentiate its proarrhythmic effects.

      (6) Hyperpyrexia may require active cooling measures.

      (7) Benzodiazepine administration is important to prevent seizures.

Cocaine abuse can cause catecholamine depletion and render patients unresponsive to indirect-acting sympathomimetics such as ephedrine.

    iii) **Postoperative considerations**

      (1) Cocaine withdrawal may be problematic.

        (a) Symptoms include agitation, anxiety, depression, fatigue, disturbed sleep, tremors, and myalgias.

  6) **Amphetamine and its derivatives (Methamphetamine, Crystal Meth, Ecstasy, MDMA)**

    a) Historically used to suppress appetite in obese patients and is now used for patients with attention deficits, etc.

    b) As a drug of abuse, amphetamines and the derivatives such as methamphetamine and ecstasy (3,4-methylenedioxymethamphetamine—MDMA) are used to induce euphoria, alertness, and enhance energy.

    c) Because of its relative ease of preparation and cost, Crystal "Meth" has become a significant drug of abuse in rural communities.

      i) Effects are similar to cocaine.

      ii) Result in release and block reuptake of NE, dopamine, and serotonin

    d) **Effects on organ systems**

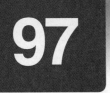
97

Part H: Diseases Associated with Pregnancy
Amniotic Fluid Embolus

Edward T. Riley, MD

Amniotic fluid embolism (AFE) is a rare obstetrical event that presents with cardiopulmonary dysfunction or collapse and altered mental status, followed by disseminated intravascular coagulation. This is a poorly understood phenomenon and hence is a diagnosis of exclusion. Treatment is supportive and requires access to major hospital resources such intensive care, operating rooms, massive transfusion of red cells and other blood products, and possibly extracorporeal life support (1).

READ MORE

Crisis management: amniotic fluid embolism, Chapter 209, page 1325

AFE is a serious pregnancy-related condition and is a diagnosis of exclusion.

1) **Incidence**
   a) The incidence and case fatality of AFE are inconsistently reported since it is a **diagnosis of exclusion.** The incidence varies depending on diagnostic criteria and what is reported through case series, governmental agencies, and registries.
   b) A pooled estimate of various population studies from North America and Europe revealed an incidence of 1 in 53,800 in Europe and 1 in 15,200 in North America (2).
   c) Case fatality rate
      i) Early estimates of case fatality were extremely high (86% and 61%), but later estimates are much lower (13% to 44%).
      ii) Diagnostic criteria, reporting bias, or improvements in care may explain these changes.
   d) Morbidity is high with many patients developing permanent neurologic sequelae.

2) **Signs and symptoms**
   a) **Initial phase**
      i) AFE usually presents with **sudden dyspnea and decreased oxygen saturation** occurring during labor or a cesarean delivery.
      ii) Hypotension is common and may lead to cardiac arrest.
         (1) The initial symptoms will be related to right heart failure, with hypoxemia and hypotension being the first symptoms.
         (2) In less severe cases, the hypotension is mild and the hypoxemia is transient.
         (3) In severe cases, complete cardiac arrest may occur due to acute right heart failure.
         (4) If the right heart failure is survived by the patient, there is danger of left heart failure in the second phase of the disease process.
      iii) AFE has been associated with tumultuous deliveries during the second stage, but this is not a clearly established finding.

697

READ MORE

Coagulopathies,
Chapter 89,
page 643

AFE typically
presents intra-
partum with
hypoxemia and
hypotension fol-
lowed by severe
coagulopathy.

     iv) Patients may appear to be having a seizure.

     v) AFE is often accompanied by evidence of acute fetal asphyxia (changes in fetal heart rate pattern).

     vi) May be accompanied by hypertonic contractions

b) **Secondary phase**

     i) Includes a severe consumptive coagulopathy characterized by

        (1) Low fibrinogen

        (2) Low Platelets

        (3) High D-dimer

        (4) Prolonged PT and PTT

        (5) The clinical picture is usually very clear. There is diffuse bleeding, and clotting studies are highly abnormal.

c) **The differential diagnosis of AFE includes (3):**

     i) Other obstetrical emergencies such as placental abruption, uterine rupture, uterine atony, or eclampsia

     ii) Anesthetic causes such as high spinal anesthesia or local anesthetic toxicity

     iii) Nonobstetric causes such as air or pulmonary embolism, anaphylaxis, or sepsis

3) Pathophysiology

READ MORE

Obstetrical
emergencies,
Chapter 100,
page 727

a) There is no clear understanding of the mechanism that leads to the AFE syndrome. This is a diagnosis of exclusion.

b) However, common features that aid in the diagnosis include

     i) An episode of respiratory distress or oxygen desaturation

     ii) Cardiovascular compromise ranging from hypotension to cardiac arrest

     iii) Coagulopathy

     iv) The presence of fetal squamous cells in the lungs of the patient in a postmortem exam or on the maternal side of the placental circulation suggests, but does not confirm, an amniotic fluid embolus.

c) Although the pathophysiology is not known, it is commonly agreed upon that there is some type of systemic response to mediators released in response to an unknown trigger.

d) Whether this is related directly to amniotic fluid is unknown.

e) Clinical responses to the syndrome include

Patients with
suspected AFE
may require
immedi-
ate airway
management.

     i) An initial period of pulmonary hypertension secondary to intense vasoconstriction in the pulmonary vasculature in response to the mediators

     ii) Relatively short-lived right heart failure and hypoxemia due to ventilation/perfusion mismatching

        (1) The pulmonary hypertension component of the syndrome is not a physical plugging of the vessels by amniotic fluid. Suggested, but not proven, mechanisms include:

            (a) Anaphylaxis to fetal material in the maternal circulation

            (b) Complement activation initiated by the amniotic fluid

     iii) The right heart failure and hypoxemia lead to left heart failure.

4) Treatment

READ MORE

Crisis manage-
ment: amniotic
fluid embolism,
Chapter 209,
page 1325

a) Treatment is supportive and includes

     i) Delivery of the fetus

     ii) Oxygen supplementation and ventilation if needed

        (1) May require immediate intubation with cricoid pressure if the patient is not maintaining her airway

iii) Invasive monitoring
   (1) An arterial line is absolutely indicated for blood pressure monitoring and frequent blood sampling.
   (2) Central monitoring (CVP or Pulmonary artery catheter) may be useful but not as important as the arterial line.
iv) Appropriate fluid resuscitation to maintain preload
v) Vasopressor medications as needed to maintain blood pressure
vi) Packed red blood cell replacement
vii) Blood product replacement for coagulopathy
viii) Newer modalities that may be useful, but are unproven
   (1) Cardiopulmonary bypass or extracorporeal membrane oxygenation should be considered if there is cardiovascular collapse, and pharmacologic treatment alone is inadequate to provide adequate blood pressure (4,5).
   (2) The right heart failure is transient, but anything that can be done to off-load the heart during the evolution of the disease may help survival. Treatment modalities to consider may include
      (a) Inhaled aerosolized prostacyclin
      (b) Inhaled nitric oxide
      (c) A right ventricular assist device (6)

b) Other treatments that theoretically make sense but are of no proven benefit and may be harmful include the following:
   i) **Steroids**
      (1) Some experts view AFE as an allergic reaction.
      (2) Steroids may help resolve the reaction, but at this time, this is of unproven value.
   ii) **Recombinant factor VIIa (RFVIIa)**
      (1) RFVIIa is a useful treatment adjunct during a major obstetric hemorrhage, and its use has been reported in patients with presumed AFE (3,6).
      (2) The bleeding in AFE is a consumptive coagulopathy that may include massive fibrinolysis with high levels of circulating tissue factor.
      (3) RFVIIa may have the effect of triggering thromboses and fibrosis (3).

Chapter Summary for Amniotic Fluid Embolus

Diagnosis	AFE is a diagnosis of exclusion. Nothing is pathomnemonic, but sudden dyspnea, decreased oxygen saturation, hypotension, followed by heart failure and a coagulopathy are highly suggestive.
Clinical Pathophysiology	Right heart failure secondary to pulmonary hypertension that is short lived Left heart failure Profound coagulopathy
Treatment	Delivery of the fetus Supplemental oxygen with intubation and mechanical ventilation if needed. Supportive care with fluid resuscitation, transfusion of packed cells and other blood products, vasopressors, as needed. Cardiopulmonary bypass if need there is cardiovascular collapse.

References

1. Clark SL. Amniotic fluid embolism. *Clin Obstet Gynecol* 2010;53(2):322–328.
2. Conde-Agudelo A, Romero R. Amniotic fluid embolism: an evidence-based review. *Am J Obstet Gynecol* 2009;201(5):445 e1–445 e13.
3. Gist RS, Stafford IP, Leibowitz AB, et al. Amniotic fluid embolism. *Anesth Analg* 2009;108(5):1599–1602.
4. Esposito RA, Grossi EA, Coppa G, et al. Successful treatment of postpartum shock caused by amniotic fluid embolism with cardiopulmonary bypass and pulmonary artery thromboembolectomy. *Am J Obstet Gynecol* 1990;163(2):572–574.
5. Shen HP, Chang WC, Yeh LS, et al. Amniotic fluid embolism treated with emergency extracorporeal membrane oxygenation: a case report. *J Reprod Med* 2009;54(11–12):706–708.
6. Nagarsheth NP, Pinney S, Bassily-Marcus A, et al. Successful placement of a right ventricular assist device for treatment of a presumed amniotic fluid embolism. *Anesth Analg* 2008;107(3):962–964.

Pregnancy and Hypertension

Amy Evers, MD

Hypertension (HTN) during pregnancy is one of the leading causes of maternal mortality in the United States, second only to embolism (1). It accounts for 18% of maternal deaths (2) and occurs in 12% to 22% of pregnancies (3). Risk factors include nulliparity, maternal age >40, family history, and associated chronic HTN or kidney disease. The complications associated with HTN in pregnancy are outlined in this chapter (4–6).

1) **Classifications of HTN during pregnancy (1)**
   a) **Chronic HTN (7)**
      i) Diagnosed at **<20 weeks gestational age** and/or continues >12 weeks postpartum
      ii) Patients typically are on antihypertensive medications prior to pregnancy
      iii) **Mild** systolic BP (SBP) ≥ 140 but <180, Diastolic BP (DBP) ≥ 90 but <110
      iv) **Severe** SBP ≥ 180 or DBP ≥ 110
   b) **Preeclampsia (Table 98-1)**
      i) HTN with **proteinuria**
      ii) Usually diagnosed after 20 weeks gestation
      iii) Can be diagnosed without proteinuria if the patient exhibits other symptoms such as headache, blurry vision, abdominal pain, abnormal liver function tests (LFTs), or thrombocytopenia
      iv) **Mild**
         (1) **SBP ≥ 140 but <160 or DBP ≥ 90 but <110**
         (2) Proteinuria ≥ 0.3 g over 24 hours, which usually correlates to ≥ 1+ on dipstick

While peripheral edema is a frequent finding in preeclampsia, it is not a criterion for diagnosis.

Table 98-1
Risks Associated with Preeclampsia (4)

	Increased Risk of...	Management Suggestions
Mild preeclampsia	Labor induction Caesarean delivery	Consider early epidural in case of urgent delivery. May also aid in BP management.
Severe preeclampsia	Abruptio placentae Preterm delivery Small for gestational age infants Maternal mortality Maternal morbidities	Prepare for the possibility of urgent delivery and postpartum hemorrhage. Consult neonatal team to counsel mother regarding neonatal resuscitation and critical care.

Table 98-2

Complications Associated with Severe Preeclampsia

Complication	Clinical Considerations
Cerebral vascular accident	Most common cause of death in patients with preeclampsia. BP management critical.
Pulmonary edema	Carefully monitor volume replacement and urine output.
Renal dysfunction	May require invasive monitoring for assessment of intravascular volume. Check electrolytes.
Liver dysfunction or rupture	Monitor coagulation, LFTs, and hemoglobin.
Hemorrhage	Type and crossmatch; carefully monitor blood loss.
Disseminated intravascular coagulopathy	Consider early preparation of clotting factors (e.g., FFP); monitor surgical field and other sites for microvascular bleeding.
HELLP (Hemolysis, Elevated Liver enzymes, Low Platelets) syndrome	Assess platelet count in severe preeclampsia prior to placing or removing epidural catheter. Prepare for general anesthesia for cesarean delivery.
Seizures (eclampsia)	Supportive care (see treatment plan below).

    v) **Severe (8) (Table 98-2)**
       (1) **SBP ≥ 160 or DBP ≥ 110**
       (2) Proteinuria ≥ 5 g/24 hours or 3+ on dipstick
       (3) Oliguria <500 mL/24 hours, creatinine >1.2 mg/dL
       (4) Blurry vision, headache, pulmonary edema, cyanosis, epigastric or right upper quadrant abdominal pain, abnormal LFTs, thrombocytopenia <100,000 cell/mm (4), or fetal growth restriction
  c) **Eclampsia**
    i) Preeclampsia with new-onset **seizures**
  d) **Preeclampsia superimposed on chronic HTN:** Diagnosis of chronic HTN and new-onset proteinuria, worsening proteinuria or BP, thrombocytopenia, or abnormal LFTs
  e) **Gestational HTN**
    i) **HTN without proteinuria**
    ii) Diagnosed after 20 weeks gestation in a previously normotensive patient
    iii) Resolves before 12 weeks postpartum
2) Treatment
  a) **Delivery of fetus** is the only cure for preeclampsia or eclampsia.
  b) **Treatment goals** are prevention of maternal complications and delivery of a mature neonate (4).
    i) **BP control**
       (1) Decrease DBP to just under 100 mm Hg (9).
       (2) Cerebral autoregulation may be altered, and normal BP may decrease blood flow to the brain, uterus, or other vital organs (10).
3) **Antihypertensives**
  a) **Vasodilators** (11)
    i) **Hydralazine**

          (1)   One of the most commonly used agents by obstetricians

          (2)   5 to 10 mg IV is given and has an effect in 20 minutes; lasts 2 to 3 hours.

          (3)   May cause a reflex tachycardia

   ii) **Sodium nitroprusside**

          (1)   May be useful for severe intractable HTN

          (2)   Administered by IV infusion

          (3)   **Very rapid onset**

          (4)   Be aware of possible cyanide toxicity in the mother or the neonate.

   iii) **Nitroglycerin**

          (1)   May be useful for severe intractable HTN

          (2)   Administered by IV infusion

          (3)   Very rapid onset

   iv) **α-Adrenergic agonists**

          (1)   **Methyldopa**

             (a)   Often used for outpatient BP control

   v) **β-Adrenergic antagonists (11)**

          (1)   **Esmolol**

             (a)   Generally avoided due to the potential for fetal bradycardia

          (2)   **Labetalol**

             (a)   Widely used by obstetricians

⌐ READ MORE

Adrenergic agents,
Chapter 45,
page 320

             (b)   10 to 20 mg boluses are given with onset in approximately 2 minutes, lasting 2 to 3 hours and has a maximum dose of 300 mg and a faster onset than hydralazine.

             (c)   Use caution in asthmatics since it is not cardioselective.

   vi) **Calcium channel blockers**

          (1)   Decrease SVR

          (2)   Can cause uterine relaxation

          (3)   May potentiate magnesium toxicity (11)

          (4)   **Nicardipine**

             (a)   May be useful in severe intractable HTN

             (b)   IV administration

          (5)   **Nifedipine**

             (a)   Also used for tocolysis

             (b)   Administration is oral or sublingual, 10 mg, q15–30min, up to 30 mg (9)

3) **Maintain adequate intravascular volume**

   a)   Despite being hypertensive, preeclamptic patients often have low intravascular volume and require fluid resuscitation.

   b)   Patients are at risk for pulmonary edema, so fluids must be given judiciously.

4) **Decrease Central Nervous System hyperactivity with magnesium sulfate (12)**

   a)   Magnesium functions as an **anticonvulsant, tocolytic, and mild vasodilator.**

      i) It is the choice anticonvulsant for prophylaxis in preeclampsia and treatment in eclampsia (13).

   b)   **All patients with severe preeclampsia and eclampsia should be treated with magnesium,** but controversy continues in those with mild preeclampsia (1).

   c)   Dosing

      i) 4 g bolus over 20 minutes, followed by a continuous infusion of 2 to 3 g/h

      ii) Continue the infusion for 24 hours postpartum (4).

          (1)   Use caution in patients with renal dysfunction as magnesium is excreted by the kidneys.

   d)   **Anesthetic concerns in patients on magnesium therapy**

Table 98-3

Clinical Effects of Magnesium Therapy

Magnesium Level (mg/dL)	Clinical Effect
4–8	Therapeutic range
5–10	EKG changes (widened QRS, prolonged QT)
>10	↓ Deep tendon reflexes
15–18	SA and AV nodal block
25–30	Cardiac arrest

      i) The intubating dose of succinylcholine is the same when a patient is receiving magnesium.

      ii) Nondepolarizing neuromuscular blockade will be potentiated by magnesium.

        (1) Doses should be dramatically reduced, and neuromuscular blockade should be monitored.

    e) **Toxicity (Table 98-3)**

      i) Deep tendon reflexes are followed clinically, and toxicity is suspected when they are decreased.

      ii) Treat overdoses with 10 mL of 10% calcium gluconate or calcium chloride.

5) **Anesthetic management**

    a) **Preoperative**

      i) **History and physical exam**

        (1) A thorough history and physical should be performed.

        (2) **Patients with preeclampsia are at high risk for difficult airway due generalized edema.**

      ii) Patients are at high risk for cesarean delivery due to decreased uteroplacental perfusion. The provision of anesthesia for cesarean delivery should be discussed with the patient.

        (1) Early epidural catheter placement will help with pain control and BP management, and should be in place should urgent or emergent cesarean delivery be necessary (14).

      iii) **Laboratories**

        (1) **Hematocrit**

        (2) **Platelet count (14)**

          (a) **There is no recommended threshold for platelet values prior to placement of neuraxial blockade.**

          (b) Evidence suggests that patients with **HELLP syndrome are at high risk for epidural hematoma (15).**

          (c) Those with a low but stable platelet count may be at less risk for complications from a neuraxial block than patients with rapidly decreasing platelet counts.

          (d) In the presence of preeclampsia, it is advisable to **monitor serial platelet counts** and have a recent (within 6 hours) value prior to placement of a neuraxial block and/or removal of an epidural catheter (16).

(e) Most practitioners would not place a neuraxial block in a preeclamptic patient with a platelet count <80,000 cells/mm³, although it may be appropriate in very selected cases (16).

(f) Most practitioners would perform neuraxial blockade with a platelet count >100,000 cells/mm³.

(g) The decision to perform neuraxial blockade in patients who fall into the "gray area" should be individualized based on the patient's airway exam, coexisting disease, and rate of platelet drop.

(h) If neuraxial blockade is performed, consider the following:
(i) Small needles such as those used for spinal anesthesia are probably less traumatic than larger epidural needles (15).
(ii) Strongly consider having the most experienced practitioner place the block. The risk of hematoma increases with the number of passes of the needle.

(3) **Liver function tests (LFTs)**
(a) Patients with elevated LFTs are at high risk for coagulation abnormalities.

(4) **Blood type and screen**
(a) Type and crossmatch should be done in the presence of liver dysfunction, thrombocytopenia, or if estimated blood loss is expected to be high.

(5) **Urine protein**

iv) **Treatment of eclampsia (Table 98-4)**
(1) **Seizures are usually self-limited**, lasting a few minutes.
(2) Fetal bradycardia is common but usually resolves.
(3) Can occur antepartum (38% to 53%), intrapartum (18% to 36%), or postpartum (11% to 44%) (5).
(4) **Deliver the baby** after the seizure and BP is controlled.
(a) If the mother is stable, allow the placental unit to resuscitate the baby prior to delivery (5).

b) **Intraoperative considerations**
i) **Monitoring**
(1) **Blood pressure**
(a) Noninvasive monitoring is usually adequate.
(b) Consider an **arterial line** if the patient has pulmonary edema, requires an infusion of antihypertensives or frequent blood draws.

Table 98-4
Treatment of Eclampsia

Stop the seizure with:
  Magnesium (bolus additional 2–4 g or 6 g loading dose if infusion not running)
  Benzodiazepines, barbiturates, or propofol as appropriate
Maintain adequate oxygenation/ventilation
  Monitor SpO₂
  Administer 100% O₂
  Monitor ventilation and assist if necessary
  Intubate only to protect against hypercarbia or aspiration
Ensure adequate left uterine displacement
Control BP
Consult with Obstetrician regarding delivery plan
Always rule out other causes (e.g., hypoglycemia, seizure disorder)

(2) **Central venous pressure (CVP) monitor/pulmonary artery catheter**

   (a) There is no data to support routine use of invasive monitors (1,8,17).

   (b) Patients with severe preeclampsia may require a pulmonary artery catheter, especially those with (17) pulmonary edema, severe renal or cardiac disease, oliguria unresponsive to fluids, and severe refractory HTN (1,8).

(3) **Fluid management**

   (a) Pulmonary capillary wedge pressure should be kept at 5 to 8 mm Hg (11).

   (b) If a CVP catheter is used to guide volume expansion, the CVP should be kept ≤ 4 mm Hg (11).

   (c) If no invasive monitoring is used, administer volume based on the patient's clinical condition, estimated blood loss, and vital signs.

c) **Postoperative considerations**

   i) Patients are at risk for seizures for 24 to 48 hours postpartum.

   ii) Continue magnesium.

   iii) Check platelet counts prior to removal of epidural catheter.

   iv) The catheter should not be removed if the patient is thrombocytopenic.

6) Management of labor analgesia in patients with preeclampsia

a) **Neuraxial analgesia**

   i) Preferred for patients with preeclampsia to blunt the sympathetic response to labor pain

   ii) Contraindicated in the presence of thrombocytopenia or abnormal coagulation (1)

b) **IV analgesia**

   i) Appropriate in patients who are unable or unwilling to receive neuraxial analgesia

7) Management of anesthesia for cesarean delivery

a) **Neuraxial anesthesia**

   i) **Epidural**

      (1) **If a well-functioning epidural catheter is in place (e.g., from labor),** it can be used if time permits.

      (2) **Preferred by some to prevent rapid drop in BP that may occur with spinal anesthesia**

   ii) **Spinal**

      (1) More recent studies indicate spinal anesthesia is safe (18) and causes less hypotension than in healthy parturients (19).

   iii) Combined spinal-epidural technique has also been shown to have minimal hemodynamic effects (20).

b) **General anesthesia**

   i) Appropriate when regional anesthesia is not performed due to time constraints or contraindications.

   ii) Patients are at risk for severe HTN on airway instrumentation.

      (1) Lidocaine, remifentanil, or nitroglycerin may be used during induction to blunt the BP response to intubation.

READ MORE

Obstetrical anesthesia, Chapter 144, page 1047

Spinal anesthesia may be safer than epidural anesthesia for cesarean delivery in patients with severe preeclampsia due to the use of smaller needles and lack of indwelling catheter should the platelet count drop.

Cerebrovascular accident due to uncontrolled HTN is the leading cause of death in patients with preeclampsia.

iii) If the airway is nonreassuring secondary to airway edema or other causes, awake fiber optic intubation may be necessary.

c) **Avoid methylergonovine** as a uterotonic agent as profound HTN can occur, possibly leading to a hypertensive crisis.

Chapter Summary for HTN in Pregnancy

Classification	Diagnosis	Clinical Considerations
Chronic HTN	HTN present prior to pregnancy or earlier than 20 weeks	Be aware of possible comorbidities
Gestational HTN	HTN during pregnancy without proteinuria	Monitor for the development of preeclampsia
Preeclampsia	Mild = SBP > 140, DBP > 90 plus proteinuria >0.3 g/24 h Severe = SBP >160, DBP > 110 Proteinuria > 5 g/24 h Associated symptoms such as headache, visual changes, abdominal pain, HELLP syndrome	Severe disease typically treated with magnesium sulfate Regional analgesia and anesthesia preferred in absence of contraindications Monitor platelet count regularly Delivery based on maternal and fetal status Prepare for possible emergent delivery
Eclampsia	Preeclampsia with seizures	Supportive care Difficult airway possible Consult OB team about delivery plan

All patients with HTN in pregnancy need to have adequate BP control. Treatment and clinical concerns vary depending on the type of HTN.

References

1. Report of the National High Blood Pressure Education Program Working Group on high blood pressure in pregnancy. *Am J Obstet Gynecol* 2000;183(1):S1–S22.
2. Koonin LM, MacKay AP, Berg CJ, et al. Pregnancy-related mortality surveillance—United States, 1987–1990. *Mor Mortal Wkly Rep CDC Surveill Summ* 1997;4694:17–36.
3. Walker JJ. Pre-eclampsia. *Lancet* 2000;356:1260–1265.
4. Sibai BM. Diagnosis and management of gestational hypertension and preeclampsia. *Obstet Gynecol* 2003;102(1):181–192.
5. Sibai BM. Diagnosis, prevention, and management of eclampsia. *Obstet Gynecol* 2005;105(2):402–410.
6. Hauth JC, Ewell MG, Levine RJ, et al. Pregnancy outcomes in healthy nulliparas who developed hypertension. Calcium for Preeclampsia Prevention Study Group. *Obstet Gynecol* 2000;95(1):24–28.
7. ACOG Practice Bulletin. Chronic hypertension in pregnancy. ACOG Committee on Practice Bulletins. *Obstet Gynecol* 2001;98(1 Suppl): 177–185.
8. ACOG practice bulletin. Diagnosis and management of preeclampsia and eclampsia. Number 33, January 2002. *Obstet Gynecol* 2002;99(1):159–167.
9. Vidaeff A, Carroll M, Ramin S. Acute hypertensive emergencies in pregnancy. *Crit Care Med* 2005;13(10 Suppl):S307–S312.
10. Coppage KH, Sibai BM, Treatment of hypertensive complications in pregnancy. *Curr Pharmaceut Des* 2005;11:749–757.
11. Ramanathan J, Bennett K. Pre-eclampsia: fluids, drugs, and anesthetic management. *Anesthesiol Clin North America*. 2003;21(1):145–163.
12. Hughes SC, Levinson G, Rosen MA, eds. *Shnider and Levinson's Anesthesia for Obstetrics*, 4th ed. Philadelphia: Lippincott Williams & Wilkins, 2002.
13. The Eclampsia Trial Collaborative Group. Which anticonvulsant for women with eclampsia? Evidence from the Collaborative Eclampsia Trial. *Lancet* 1995; 345:1455–1463.
14. American Society of Anesthesiologists Task Force on Obstetric Anesthesia. Practice guidelines for obstetric anesthesia: an updated report by the American Society of Anesthesiologists Task Force on Obstetric Anesthesia. *Anesthesiology* 2007;106(4):843–863.
15. Moen V, Dahlgren N, Irestedt L. Severe neurological complications after central neuraxial blockades in Sweden 1990–1999. *Anesthesiology* 2004;101(4):950–959.

16. Abramovitz S, Beilin Y. Thrombocytopenia, low molecular weight heparin, and obstetric anesthesia. *Anesthesiol Clin North America*. 2003;21(1):99–109.
17. American Society of Anesthesiologists Task Force on Obstetric Anesthesia. Practice guidelines for pulmonary artery catheterization: an updated report by the American Society of Anesthesiologists Task Force on Pulmonary Artery Catheterization. *Anesthesiology*. 2003;99(4): 988–1014.
18. Cisalyaputra S, Rodanant O, Somboonviboon W, et al. Spinal versus epidural anesthesia for cesarean section in severe preeclampsia: a prospective randomized, multicenter study. *Anesth Analg* 2005;101:862–868.
19. Aya AGM, Mangin R, Vialles N, et al. Patients with severe preeclampsia experience less hypotension during spinal anesthesia for elective cesarean delivery than healthy parturients: a prospective cohort comparison. *Anesth Analg*. 2003;97:867–872.
20. Ramanathan J, Vaddadi AK, Arheart KL. Combined spinal and epidural anesthesia with low doses of intrathecal bupivacaine in women with severe preeclampsia: a preliminary report. *Reg Anesth Pain Med* 2001;26:46–51.

99 Pregnancy and Coexisting Disease

Amy Gagnon, MD • Camille Hoffman, MD • Bronwen Kahn, MD • Andrea J. Fuller, MD

Increasing numbers of women are becoming pregnant in the presence of preexisting illnesses. Coexisting disease states have significant implications for pregnancy outcome and the care these patients require. In addition to the normal physiologic changes of pregnancy, the pathophysiology of individual conditions must be considered during assessment and treatment of pregnant women. Fetal well-being is dependent upon maternal hemodynamic stability and perfusion, and the acutely ill mother must be treated aggressively in order to maintain maternal health and fetal viability.

Pregnancy can be considered a stress test that may reveal a woman's underlying predisposition to develop a variety of chronic diseases.

1) **Introduction**
   a) **Definition**
      i) Coexisting disease in pregnancy is any medical condition that occurs in the pregnant patient. The disease may be unique to pregnancy or present prior to pregnancy. Often, pregnancy exacerbates preexisting disease.
   b) **Epidemiology**
      i) The most common diseases associated with pregnancy are hypertension (HTN) and diabetes mellitus.
      ii) The incidence and complexity of coexisting disease in pregnancy is increasing.
         (1) Women are delaying childbearing to an older age.
         (2) Improved treatment of pediatric diseases, especially congenital heart disease, allows these patients to reach childbearing age and achieve pregnancy.
   c) **The approach to the pregnant patient with coexisting illness should include**
      (i) **A thorough understanding of the underlying disease process and the physiologic consequences of pregnancy because more specialized care may be necessary in the peripartum period**
      (ii) Discussion with obstetrician about mode of delivery
      (iii) Multidisciplinary conference with the physicians involved in the care of the patient to discuss potential peripartum complications and to develop a clear plan that includes management of potential emergencies
2) **Endocrine disease**
   a) **Gestational diabetes mellitus (GDM) (1,2)**
      i) **Epidemiology**
         (1) Affects 2% to 12% of pregnancies
         (2) Prevalence has doubled in the last 10 years, driven by the rising incidence of obesity, the rise in mean maternal age, and changing diagnostic criteria.

709

Insulin has typically been prescribed for GDM, but recently oral hypoglycemic agents have become accepted for use during pregnancy (3).

READ MORE

Obstetrical emergencies, Chapter 100, page 727

Mothers with GDM have a 25% to 40% risk of cesarean delivery.

READ MORE

Diabetes mellitus, Chapter 81, page 592

ii) **Definition (Table 99-2)**
   (1) **Glucose intolerance of variable severity with onset or first recognition during pregnancy**

iii) **Pathophysiology**
   (1) **GDM is caused by a combination of metabolic abnormalities including increased insulin resistance, impaired insulin secretion, and increased hepatic glucose production.**
   (2) **Physiologic insulin resistance of pregnancy**
     (a) Under normal circumstances, human placental lactogen and human placental growth hormone increase maternal glucose levels, creating a glucose gradient from mother to fetus.
   (3) When glucose intolerance related to obesity or predisposition already exists, and pancreatic β-cell reserve is insufficient, maternal hyperglycemia results.
   (4) Fetal hyperglycemia occurs due to maternal hyperglycemia, which results in fetal hyperinsulinemia, which places the infant at risk for **life-threatening hypoglycemia** in the neonatal period.

iv) **Adverse pregnancy outcomes associated with GDM (Table 99-1)**
   (1) GDM confers a 50% risk of developing Type 2 DM within 5 to 10 years and a long-term risk of 70% (2).

v) **Intrapartum management**
   (1) Maintenance of maternal glucose between 70 and 120 mg/dL with the use of IV insulin and dextrose infusions as necessary

b) **Diabetes mellitus (DM) (Table 99-2)**
i) Preexisting DM complicates as many as 2% of all pregnancies, and the proportion of Type 2 DM is increasing with the prevalence of obesity.
ii) DM in pregnancy is described by the White classification system, which is based upon duration of diabetes and the presence of end-organ damage.
iii) Hyperglycemia and hyperinsulinemia carry the same risks to mother and fetus as GDM.

Table 99-1
Adverse Pregnancy Outcomes Associated with GDM

Preeclampsia	Shoulder dystocia
Intrauterine fetal demise	Birth trauma
Polyhydramnios	Operative delivery
Fetal macrosomia	Perinatal mortality
Neonatal metabolic complications (hypoglycemia, hyperbilirubinemia, erythrocytosis, hypocalcemia)	Preterm labor
Polyhydramnios	

Table 99-2
White Classification of DM in Pregnancy

Gestational Diabetes	
A1	GDM; diet controlled
A2	GDM; medication (usually insulin) controlled
Diabetes Present Prior to Pregnancy	
B	Onset at age 20 y or older and duration <10 y
C	Onset at age 10–19 y or duration of 10–19 y
D	Onset before 10 y of age, duration over 20 y, benign retinopathy or HTN (not preeclampsia)

Other subtypes of D and classification types are based on associated end-organ disease

Source: Rosene-Montella K, Keely E, Barbour L, et al. *Medical Care of the Pregnant Patient*. Philadelphia, PA: American College of Physicians Press; 2008.

During pregnancy, DKA can occur with less provocation or at lower levels of hyperglycemia than one might expect.

    iv) **Type I DM**
- (1) Associated with increased incidence of other autoimmune conditions
- (2) Increased risk for hypoglycemia in the first trimester due to an early increase in insulin sensitivity, especially in the fasting state
- (3) Diabetic ketoacidosis (DKA) is more commonly associated with Type 1 DM but can occur in Type 2 and rarely with GDM.

    v) **Type II DM**
- (1) Incidence has increased dramatically among women of younger age groups due to the epidemic of obesity
- (2) Associated with HTN, hyperlipidemia, obesity, and polycystic ovarian disease

c) **Thyroid disease (4,5)**
    i) Physiologic changes in thyroid function tests occur during normal pregnancy.
- (1) Decrease in thyroid-stimulating hormone (TSH) mediated by β-hCG
- (2) Increase in thyroid-binding globulin causes increased total T3 and T4.
- (3) Free T3 and T4 remain the same as nonpregnant values.

    ii) **Hypothyroidism**
- (1) **Causes**
  - (a) Iodine deficiency is the leading cause of hypothyroidism globally.
  - (b) Hashimoto thyroiditis is the most common in United States.
- (2) Associated with infertility and pregnancy loss
- (3) Children exposed to hypothyroxinemia during gestation are at risk for a range of neurodevelopmental delays.
- (4) Pregnant women with even mild subclinical hypothyroidism have higher rates of stillbirth, preterm birth, preeclampsia, breech presentation, intrauterine growth restriction (IUGR), and placental abruption.
- (5) **Treatment**
  - (a) Thyroxine replacement doses are increased beginning early in pregnancy.
  - (b) After delivery, prepregnancy dose is resumed and followed frequently for the first year, due to risk of postpartum thyroiditis.

iii) **Hyperthyroidism**
  (1) **Causes**
    (a) Graves disease
      (i) Most common cause of pregnancy-related hyperthyroidism
      (ii) Due to thyroid autoantibodies, which can cross the placenta and place the fetus at risk of fetal or neonatal Graves disease
      (iii) Manifests as fetal tachycardia, high-output failure and hydrops, IUGR, and fetal goiter
  (2) **Treatment**

READ MORE

Thyroid disease, Chapter 82, page 598

    (a) **Subclinical hyperthyroidism**
      (i) Defined by low TSH with normal free T4
      (ii) Not associated with adverse pregnancy outcomes
      (iii) Should not be treated because of the risk of suppression of the developing fetal thyroid gland.
    (b) **Overt hyperthyroidism**
      (i) Diagnosed by low TSH and elevated free T4 and/or T3
      (ii) Treated with a thionamide, preferably propylthiouracil
      (iii) The goal of treatment is a free T4 in the high-normal range.

Thyroid storm in hyperthyroid patients can be precipitated by labor, infection, preeclampsia, trauma, and cesarean delivery.

      (iv) β-adrenergic antagonists may be used to control symptoms (i.e., tachycardia, tremor).
  (3) Pregnancy complicated by poorly controlled hyperthyroidism is associated with increased rates of spontaneous abortion, preterm labor, low birth weight, stillbirth, preeclampsia, and heart failure.
  (4) **Thyroid storm** may occur in hyperthyroid pregnant patients in response to labor, infection, preeclampsia, trauma, and cesarean delivery.

d) **Pituitary disease**
  i) **Pituitary adenomas**
    (1) Treated with dopamine agonists, which may be required for conception but are discontinued once pregnancy achieved due to fetal risks
    (2) Maternal complications are due to tumor enlargement stimulated by estrogen.

READ MORE

Pituitary disorders, Chapter 84, page 615

      (a) Macroadenomas have a higher chance of enlarging enough to cause neurologic symptoms than microadenomas.
      (b) Patients should be followed for the development of headache or visual symptoms.
  ii) **Hypopituitarism**
    (1) Caused by various conditions whose mechanisms fall into the categories of tumor, infiltrative disease, congenital insufficiency, or surgical destruction.
  iii) **Sheehan syndrome**
    (1) Pituitary necrosis in the setting of shock or massive peripartum hemorrhage resulting in panhypopituitarism
    (2) Patients often present with infertility.
    (3) During pregnancy, the diagnosis should be suspected in the presence of headache, visual field changes, diabetes insipidus, or prolonged hypotension

Sheehan Syndrome is a cause of panhypopituitarism unique to pregnancy. The risk increases in patients with shock due to peripartum hemorrhage.

    (4) **Treatment**
      (a) Appropriate hormone replacement (cortisol, thyroid hormone, DDAVP), including stress dose glucocorticoids when indicated
      (b) Periodic measurements of BP and electrolytes and monitoring fetal growth by ultrasound.
    (5) **If acute hypopituitarism is suspected**

READ
MORE

Adrenal
disorders,
Chapter 83,
page 608

        (a)   Management includes fluid resuscitation, IV dextrose, stress dose steroids (hydrocortisone: 100 mg IV q8h)

        (b)   Diagnostic workup includes measuring prolactin, ACTH, cortisol, TSH, free T4, electrolytes, glucose, and MRI when stable

  e) **Adrenal conditions**

      i)   **Pheochromocytoma (5)**

          (1)   High maternal and fetal mortality rates

          (2)   It should always be considered in the differential diagnosis of labile, severe HTN.

          (3)   Proteinuria occurs in 20% of cases, making it difficult to distinguish from preeclampsia.

          (4)   Most sensitive diagnostic test is urinary or plasma metanephrines.

          (5)   Once diagnosed, α-adrenergic blockade should be instituted immediately, followed by β-adrenergic blockade titrated with a goal of maternal heart rate between 80 and 100 (5).

          (6)   If diagnosed in the first two trimesters, the tumor should be surgically removed.

          (7)   If the patient is in the third trimester and medical therapy is adequate, surgery may be delayed until postpartum.

          (8)   Cesarean delivery is associated with lower maternal mortality (5).

3) Hematologic diseases

  a) **Thrombocytopenia in pregnancy**

      i)   Thrombocytopenia in pregnancy is a frequent concern for anesthesiologists.

      ii)   The first step in evaluating any thrombocytopenic parturient is to determine the cause of thrombocytopenia.

      iii) Other important factors to consider are the rate of platelet drop and whether the patient is on any medications that may affect platelet function (e.g., aspirin).

The approach to the parturient with thrombocytopenia includes consideration of the cause of thrombocytopenia, rate of platelet drop, and medication use.

      iv)   Thrombocytopenia occurs in approximately 5% of pregnancies and is usually without consequence when the diagnosis is **gestational thrombocytopenia**

      v)   **Gestational thrombocytopenia has five diagnostic criteria (Table 99-3) (6,7).**

          (1)   **Anesthesia considerations for gestational thrombocytopenia**

              (a)   Usually no change in routine obstetric or anesthetic care is necessary.

              (b)   The decision to perform neuraxial analgesia/anesthesia is individualized but is generally considered safe in patients with uncomplicated gestational thrombocytopenia **(8)**

Table 99-3

Diagnostic Criteria for Gestational Thrombocytopenia

Thrombocytopenia is mild (platelets are usually >70,000/μL and average 130–150,000/μL) and the patient is asymptomatic

No past history of thrombocytopenia outside of pregnancy

Occurs late in gestation—in the midthird trimester or beyond

Resolves postpartum

No associated fetal thrombocytopenia

b) **HELLP syndrome and/or severe preeclampsia (9)**

READ MORE

Pregnancy and hypertension, Chapter 98, page 701

   i) Thrombocytopenia complicates approximately 15% of preeclampsia cases
   ii) May be seen when disseminated intravascular coagulation is associated with severe preeclampsia/HELLP syndrome
   iii) **Anesthesia considerations**
      (1) Assess platelet count, coagulation studies before placement of regional anesthetic.
      (2) The decision to perform neuraxial procedures will be based on the patient's airway exam, rate of platelet drop, and coexisting illnesses
      (3) Assess patient's airway, renal function, and IV access to formulate anesthetic plan for delivery.

c) **Idiopathic thrombocytopenia (ITP) (10,11)**

<5% of patients with preeclampsia will have a platelet count <50,000 cells/ mm³.

   i) ITP is difficult to differentiate from gestational thrombocytopenia.
      (1) Usually presents earlier in pregnancy
      (2) Platelet counts are more commonly < 50,000 cells/mm³.
   ii) Neonatal hemorrhage is a risk with ITP and is more common when ITP patients have undergone splenectomy, and platelets are <50,000 cells/mm³ at some point during pregnancy.
   iii) **Anesthesia considerations**
      (1) Maintenance of platelet counts >50,000 cells/mm³ is considered safe for vaginal or cesarean delivery.
      (2) Hemorrhage does not appear related to the degree of thrombocytopenia.
         (a) Blood and products should be available for cesarean delivery.
      (3) NSAIDs should be avoided in the postpartum period.
      (4) In a study of 118 deliveries in women with ITP, 42 received neuraxial anesthesia with no complications reported in those with platelet counts: <100,000 cells/mm³ (62%), <75,000 cells/mm³ (17%), or <50,000 cells/mm³ (2%) (10).
         (a) Based on these data and the rarity of neuraxial bleeding complications, **no absolute platelet number may be determined safe or unsafe**. The decision to place a neuraxial block must be individualized.

d) **Thrombotic thrombocytopenia purpura-hemolytic uremic syndrome (TTP-HUS) (12)**
   i) Rare condition in pregnancy (1/25,000)
   ii) Acute renal failure is common, and treatment includes plasma exchange, hemodialysis, and transfusion.
   iii) If disease is severe, fetus viable, and preeclampsia cannot be excluded, delivery is appropriate.
   iv) Unlike preeclampsia/HELLP, hematologic abnormalities may progress beyond 3 days postpartum.

e) **Disseminated intravascular coagulation**

READ MORE

Hemorrhage in the parturient, Chapter 101, page 740

   i) May occur in the setting of severe preeclampsia/HELLP syndrome or as a sequelae of hemorrhage
   ii) Anesthesia considerations
      (1) Blood product replacement, supportive care, general endotracheal anesthesia if necessary
      (2) Avoid removal of epidural catheters until coagulopathy is corrected.

f) **Acute thromboembolism (2,8)**
   i) Teleologically, the hypercoagulable state of pregnancy can be seen as preparation for blood loss of delivery, but it presents a challenge to the carefully balanced system of clotting.

ii) Most pregnancy-related venous thromboembolism (VTE) occurs in the antenatal period with the highest risk 6 to 8 weeks following delivery.

Pregnancy is a hypercoagulable state mediated by an increase in many procoagulant factors, a decrease in fibrinolytic activity, and the presence of venous stasis and increased endothelial damage (Virchow triad).

iii) **Diagnosis (2)**

   (1) Symptoms and physical findings of deep venous thrombosis (DVT) and pulmonary embolus (PE) are relatively nonspecific and common during normal pregnancy, making the diagnosis challenging.

   (2) No findings on physical exam, ECG, or arterial blood gas have sufficient sensitivity to rule in or out the diagnosis of VTE.

   (3) Radiologic studies required for the diagnosis and treatment of thromboembolic disease should be used during pregnancy.

   (4) Venous ultrasound is the procedure of choice to evaluate suspected DVT.

   (5) V/Q scan, starting with perfusion studies, is useful if clinical suspicion is either low or high.

   (6) CT scans may be used to evaluate for PE but carry higher radiation exposure than other methods and should be combined with lower extremity Doppler ultrasound.

   (7) D-dimer, although normally elevated in late pregnancy and postpartum, may also be useful in assigning pretest probability.

VTE is one of the most common causes of maternal death (2).

iv) **Treatment of thromboembolic disease in pregnancy (2)**

   (1) Immediate therapeutic anticoagulation should be initiated with either unfractionated heparin or low molecular weight heparin (LMWH).

   (2) **Full therapeutic anticoagulation should be provided for a total of 3 to 6 months, including prophylaxis for the duration of pregnancy and postpartum.**

   (3) There are no randomized controlled trials to guide dosing or monitoring of anticoagulation in pregnant patients.

Pregnancy increases the volume of distribution and renal clearance of heparin and LMWH, necessitating increased dose and frequency when used for therapeutic anticoagulation.

     (a) Compared to heparin, LMWH has a longer half-life and therefore longer dosing interval.

     (b) During pregnancy, the pharmacokinetics are altered such that twice daily dosing and frequent PTTs or anti-Xa levels are required.

     (c) Warfarin is contraindicated in pregnancy because of its association with congenital malformations and fetal and neonatal hemorrhage, but it may be used while breast-feeding.

     (d) Prophylaxis using either unfractionated heparin or LMWH should be recommended for women at high risk of VTE.

Table 99-4

Causes of Thrombophilia in Pregnancy

Factor V Leiden
Prothrombin gene mutation
Deficiency of protein S, C, and/or antithrombin
Systemic lupus erythematosus
Antiphospholipid antibody syndrome
Methyltetrahydrofolate reductase mutations

READ MORE

Sickle cell disease, hemoglobinopathies, and polycythemia vera, Chapter 88, page 637

g) **Inherited and acquired thrombophilias** (Table 99-4)
   i) May predispose women to adverse pregnancy outcome and thromboembolic disease
   ii) Complications are related to altered uteroplacental blood flow and include IUGR, preeclampsia, stillbirth, placental abruption.
   iii) Women with histories of VTE, recurrent miscarriages, and/or placental-mediated adverse pregnancy outcomes should be evaluated for the presence of identifiable thrombophilia.

h) **Sickle cell anemia**
   i) Complications

READ MORE

Coagulopathies, Chapter 89, page 643

   ii) Higher risk of vasoocclusive complications because of the pregnancy-related increase in RBC-adhesive proteins
   iii) This manifests in the placental circulation causing areas of infarction, fibrosis, and villous necrosis and may cause IUGR or stillbirth.
   iv) Maternal complications include more frequent urinary tract infections (UTI), painful crises, acute chest syndrome, splenic infarction.
   v) May also have higher rates of preeclampsia, preterm labor, low birthweight, and placental abruption
   vi) Management during pregnancy
       (1) Careful prevention of dehydration and frequent screening for UTI
       (2) Prompt treatment of painful crises with hydration, O_2, and analgesia

Patients with vWD may have a postpartum hemorrhage days to weeks after delivery, when Factor VIII levels begin to fall to prepregnancy levels.

       (3) Transfusion should be reserved for severe anemia or acute indications such as preeclampsia, sepsis, renal failure, acute chest syndrome, or anticipated surgery.

i) **von Willebrand disease (13)**
   i) Genetic disease affecting von Willebrand Factor (vWF) and Factor VIII quality and quantity
   ii) Several different types exist, with Type I the most common.
   iii) Many patients have normal vWF and Factor VIII levels during pregnancy, but levels fall postpartum and **bleeding may occur days to weeks later.**
   iv) Treat with DDAVP, which increases vWF and Factor VIII levels
       (1) May be given to patients prior to surgery or delivery to decrease bleeding risk
       (2) Most effective for patients with Type I vWD
   v) **Anesthetic concerns**
       (1) Every effort must be made to determine the type of vWD.

Patients with thrombophilias are often anticoagulated during pregnancy, labor, and delivery and require communication between care providers regarding the best plan for anesthesia and analgesia.

       (2) Laboratory studies should include bleeding time, Factor VIII level, vWF level, platelet count, PT, aPTT, and vWF function studies.
       (3) **Neuraxial analgesia is not necessarily contraindicated**, especially in Type I patients, but therapy should be individualized in consultation with a hematologist.

4) **Neurologic diseases**

a) **Multiple sclerosis (MS)**
   i) MS is a chronic demyelinating disease affecting the central nervous system.
   ii) Two thirds of MS patients are women of childbearing age, and 10% have the disease during pregnancy.
   iii) Pregnancy may have a beneficial effect.

READ MORE

Anesthesia and diseases of the nervous system, Chapter 76, page 534

Patients with MS do not have higher rates of pregnancy complications (16).

(1) Recent studies suggest pregnancy reduces the likelihood of acquiring MS (14).

(2) Nulliparous women have more disability due to MS than women who become pregnant, regardless of when MS presents (15).

iv) Relapse rate is higher in the first 3 months postpartum and is not associated with breast-feeding or epidural analgesia.

v) Treatment of MS during pregnancy includes the use of corticosteroids, azathioprine, and interferon in select cases.

vi) **Anesthetic considerations**

   (1) Increased temperature is associated with relapse in MS (17). Every effort should be made to monitor temperature, especially in patients with epidural analgesia.

   (2) There is a theoretical risk of damage to demyelinated nerves with spinal anesthesia, and most practitioners prefer epidural over spinal analgesia and anesthesia.

vii) It is important to document any preexisting neurologic defects and use clinical judgment when determining if regional anesthesia is appropriate.

b) **Paraplegia (8)**

   i) Women with spinal cord injury remain fertile and have specialized issues during pregnancy.

   ii) Risk of problems depends on the level of injury.

      (1) Pulmonary function may be affected and should be serially assessed with pulmonary function tests.

      (2) Thermoregulation may be impaired, resulting in either hypothermia or hyperthermia.

READ MORE

Spine surgery, Chapter 137, page 959

      (3) May require operative assistance to achieve vaginal delivery in the absence of maternal expulsive effort

      (4) Ability to perceive labor pain is impaired in women with cord injuries below T5-10 (18).

      (5) **Autonomic dysreflexia**

         (a) The principal concern in labor in paraplegic or quadriplegic women

         (b) Occurs in 85% of women with spinal cord injuries in labor

         (c) Patients with lesions above T8 are at highest risk.

         (d) Results in sympathetic hyperactivity in response to noxious stimuli below the level of the lesion.

Hemodynamic instability associated with autonomic dysreflexia may threaten uteroplacental perfusion and necessitate emergent delivery if not treated (19).

         (e) Signs and symptoms

            (i) Labile, severe HTN, arrhythmia, headache, loss of consciousness, facial erythema, diaphoresis

            (ii) May wax and wane with contractions

         (f) Anesthetic considerations (8)

            (i) Epidural analgesia to the T10 level is recommended to prevent this syndrome.

            (ii) Antihypertensive medications may be required.

               1. In refractory cases, nitroprusside or IV magnesium may be considered.

c) **Seizure disorders (20)**

   i) Most patients with epilepsy have uncomplicated pregnancies.

      (1) The rate of obstetric complications including spontaneous abortion, hyperemesis gravidarum, anemia, eclampsia, placental abruption, IUGR, stillbirth, and preterm delivery is twofold higher.

   ii) Medication therapy

(1) Preconception counseling is necessary to determine the best medication regimen due to the significant increase in fetal malformations seen with antiepileptic drugs (AEDs).

(2) Fetal effects

(a) Infants of mothers with epilepsy are at higher risk for seizure disorder and birth defects.

(b) All AEDs can cause similar fetal dysmorphic features.

(c) Major malformations are doubled compared to the general population.

Seizure after 20 weeks of pregnancy in the absence of a known seizure disorder is considered eclampsia until proven otherwise. Treat with supportive measures and IV magnesium (21).

(3) The physiologic changes of pregnancy lead to subtherapeutic levels of AEDs during pregnancy.

(a) Levels and therapeutic effect must be monitored and doses increased to prevent breakthrough seizures.

(b) Folate metabolism may be altered by AEDs, necessitating increased supplementation.

(c) Many AEDs inhibit vitamin K transport across the placenta, placing exposed neonates at risk for vitamin K deficiency and neonatal hemorrhage.

iii) **Management of acute seizure during pregnancy**

(1) If patient has a known seizure disorder, provide supportive care, use a first-line AED, and investigate precipitating cause.

(2) The use of IV benzodiazepines is first-line therapy in status epilepticus.

(3) Always consider the possibility of hypoglycemia causing the seizure and check blood glucose when appropriate

iv) **Intrapartum concerns (20)**

(1) During labor and delivery, women with primary generalized epilepsy may have a seizure.

(2) Sleep deprivation and meperidine should be avoided as they lower the seizure threshold.

READ MORE

Asthma and reactive airway disease, Chapter 72, page 512

(3) Treat seizures with IV benzodiazepines during active labor.

(4) Administer O_2 and place patient in left lateral position.

(5) Generalized seizures during labor may cause prolonged fetal bradycardia.

(6) Cesarean delivery should be performed if frequent, uncontrolled seizures occur or if the mother is unable to cooperate with labor.

c) Postpartum considerations include insuring safety in caring for a new infant.

5) **Pulmonary disease in pregnancy**

a) **Asthma (8,22)**

i) Most common pulmonary disease in pregnancy with 20% to 36% of pregnant asthmatics experiencing at least one exacerbation during pregnancy

(1) Managed with β-adrenergic agonists, inhaled corticosteroids, and mast cell inhibitors

(a) Systemic steroids are used in severe exacerbations.

Respiratory compromise in the mother results in fetal heart tracing changes consistent with hypoxia and acidosis in the fetus.

ii) Exacerbations leading to acid-base changes with pCO_2 > 35 mm Hg or pO_2 < 70 mm Hg represent more severe compromise due to the normal physiologic changes of pregnancy that enable O_2 shunting to the fetus.

iii) Respiratory support, including intubation, must be considered to maintain maternal and fetal oxygenation.

b) **Obstructive sleep apnea (OSA) (23,24)**
  i) OSA may be precipitated or exacerbated during pregnancy and impaired fetal growth may result from chronic hypoxia.
  ii) OSA is associated with hypertensive disorders during pregnancy.
  iii) Pregnant patients with known OSA should undergo a cardiac evaluation to rule out pulmonary HTN, which may include an echocardiogram.
  iv) CPAP should be prescribed.

⟲ READ MORE

Obstructive sleep apnea, Chapter 74, page 524

6) **Obesity and pregnancy after bariatric surgery (25,26)**
  a) Bariatric surgery in women of childbearing age is becoming more common.
  b) Rates of GDM and preeclampsia are lower following bariatric surgery.
  c) Cesarean delivery rates are lower, and neonatal outcomes are similar or better in women who undergo bariatric surgery versus obese women.
  d) Surgical complications such as bowel obstruction and intestinal hernias are a concern in pregnancies following bariatric surgery.
  e) **Anesthetic considerations**
    i) Compared to lean women, obese women have a higher rate of anesthetic complications such as epidural failure (42% vs. 6% of nonobese patients), inadvertent dural puncture, and more placement attempts (27).
    ii) As obese women are also at risk for difficult intubation, early placement of an epidural or an intrathecal catheter may obviate the need for emergent intubation.

OSA patients who receive opiates after cesarean delivery are at risk for respiratory depression postoperatively and must be monitored closely.

7) **Pregnancy after transplant (28,29)**
  a) Posttransplant patients are at risk for hypertensive disease and preeclampsia.
  b) Patients may require steroid therapy.
    i) Patients receiving steroids may develop GDM, increasing the risk of wound infection or breakdown following cesarean delivery
    ii) Stress dose steroids are recommended at the time of cesarean delivery but may also be considered with vaginal delivery.
  c) Organ rejection does not appear to be exacerbated by pregnancy.
  d) Surgeons must be mindful of an abdominal kidney at the time of cesarean delivery.
  e) Fetal concerns include early pregnancy loss, congenital malformation due to teratogenic antirejection drugs, stillbirth, immunosuppression, prematurity, and low birth weight.
  f) Epidural labor analgesia is recommended to control pain and minimize a pain-induced sympathetic responses.

In obese patients, it is helpful to place the patient in the lateral supine position prior to securing an epidural catheter in order to prevent catheter migration (27).

8) Dermatologic disorders (dermatoses of pregnancy) (8)
  a) **Pruritic urticarial papules and plaques of pregnancy**
    i) Occurs first in abdominal striae but may spread to extremities and cause hives
    ii) The face, palms, and soles are usually spared.
    iii) Typically does not alter anesthetic management. Consideration should be given to avoidance of affected areas to decrease the potential for bacterial contamination.
  b) **Intrahepatic cholestasis of pregnancy (8,30)**
    i) A disorder of intense pruritus, most commonly of the palms and soles, occurring in second and third trimesters of pregnancy

ii) Results in an elevation in serum bile acid concentrations and may cause elevated transaminases

iii) Coagulation abnormalities are not typically observed and, if present, may represent vitamin K deficiency due to cholestasis or bile acid sequestrants.

iv) Ursodiol (ursodeoxycholic acid) is the most commonly prescribed medication to reduce symptoms and bile salts.

v) Spontaneous in utero death is a fetal complication of this disease.

    (1) Risk correlates with the level of bile acid elevation.

    (2) Amniocentesis to confirm fetal lung maturity and then induction of labor between 36 and 37 weeks is recommended to reduce the risk of term fetal demise (30).

9) **Cardiac disease in pregnancy (2,8)**

  a) **General principles**

READ MORE

Aortic valvular disease, Chapter 54, page 383

    i) In caring for gravid patients with heart disease, one must determine the New York Heart Association (NYHA) functional class.

      (1) In patients with NYHA class I or II lesions, maternal and fetal mortality is approximately 0.4% and 2%, respectively.

      (2) The risk rises up to 7% in women and 30% in fetuses with class III or IV lesions.

      (3) Generally, regional anesthesia is appropriate for most patients with cardiac disease. Adequate pain control can decrease cardiac work, help avoid maternal tachycardia, and allow operative vaginal delivery.

      (4) Each cardiac lesion has unique requirements, and a multidisciplinary team, including obstetricians, anesthesiologists, and cardiologists, should formulate a detailed delivery plan for each patient with heart disease.

Passive second stage of labor (i.e., no "pushing") with operative vaginal delivery can assist in decreasing the cardiovascular stress associated with the delivery process.

    ii) Labor increases cardiac output by approximately 45% above prelabor values, which can be extremely problematic in patients with poorly compensated cardiac disease (8).

    iii) After delivery, increases in preload due to the autotransfusion from the contracting uterus can add further stress on the heart, making **the immediate postpartum period an extremely high-risk time for patients with cardiac disease** (8).

    iv) Guidelines for antimicrobial prophylaxis against endocarditis have recently changed, with the majority of patients no longer requiring antibiotic prophylaxis (31).

      (1) Patients with complex congenital heart disease require antimicrobial prophylaxis for endocarditis for vaginal or cesarean delivery.

      (2) Consultation with the patient's cardiologist and/or the ACC/AHA guidelines is recommended (31).

  b) **Valvular heart disease**

    i) Due to the physiologic 30% to 50% increase in plasma volume with gestation, regurgitant lesions are better tolerated than stenotic lesions.

    ii) **Patients with severe stenotic heart defects will not tolerate sudden drops in systemic vascular resistance.**

      (1) If used, epidural medications must be administered very slowly.

READ MORE

Mitral valve disease, Chapter 55, page 394

      (2) Intrathecal local anesthetics are typically avoided due to the possibility of rapid sympathectomy and tendency to result in rapid loss of preload. Careful consideration should be given to the use of a neuraxial opioid only technique.

      (3) For cesarean delivery, most patients receive carefully controlled epidural anesthesia or general anesthesia.

iii) **Mitral stenosis** (8, 32)

   (1) Pregnancy considerations

      (a) Risks associated with pregnancy are greatest in the third trimester or the puerperal period, correlating with the increased plasma volume. They include atrial arrhythmias, thromboembolic events, and pulmonary edema.

   (2) Maternal risks directly correlate to the severity of stenosis, based upon the area of the mitral valve.

   (3) One third of patients with NYHA class I or II heart failure experience adverse cardiac complications (pulmonary edema, arrhythmias), while two thirds experience such complications if their functional class is III or IV.

   (4) Rate of maternal and fetal mortality in patients with NYHA class III-IV is up to 20% and 30%, respectively.

The immediate postpartum period is an extremely high risk time for patients with cardiac disease. Patients should have close monitoring with consideration for admission to the Intensive Care Unit.

   (5) **Treatment of mitral stenosis**

      (a) β-Adrenergic blockade, gentle diuresis, and restriction of physical activity can help control heart rate and symptoms in moderate to severe mitral stenosis.

      (b) Atrial fibrillation should be aggressively treated with digoxin or β-adrenergic antagonists to control heart rate, as well as anticoagulation to prevent embolization.

      (c) In patients refractory to medical treatment, percutaneous balloon valvuloplasty with pelvic shielding can be considered.

   (6) **Intrapartum management goals**

      (a) Avoid tachycardia and maintain preload by avoiding hypotension.

   (7) **Anesthetic considerations**

      (a) Adequate pain control can help prevent tachycardia.

      (b) Intrathecal and epidural anesthesia carry a risk of rapid decrease in SVR, leading to hypotension. These risks can be minimized by careful titration and use of very dilute local anesthetics or opioid-only solutions.

READ MORE

Aortic valvular disease, Chapter 54, page 383

      (c) If hypotension develops, phenylephrine is preferred to avoid tachycardia.

iv) **Aortic stenosis (AS)**

   (1) Often due to congenital bicuspid aortic valve

   (2) Bicuspid aortic valves can be associated with coarctation of the aorta, which can predispose patients to aortic aneurysms and dissection.

   (3) **Pregnancy considerations**

      (a) Patients have a fixed stroke volume, so variation in cardiac output is determined by heart rate only.

         (i) Bradycardia leads to hypotension, and tachycardia decreases ventricular filling time and coronary perfusion, leading to hypotension, syncope, and risk of myocardial ischemia.

   (4) Severity of AS defined by valve area and/or the peak gradient across the valve

   (5) **Treatment of aortic stenosis**

      (a) Severe AS is associated with increased maternal and fetal morbidity and mortality.

      (b) Ideally, the aortic valve should be replaced or repaired prior to conception, but intervention can be considered midgestation if the patient is symptomatic and resistant to medical therapy.

(6) **Intrapartum management**

    (a) Passive second stage with operative vaginal delivery is preferred.

    (b) Hemorrhage prevention and treatment should be aggressive in order to avoid the detrimental effects of tachycardia and hypotension.

(7) **Anesthetic considerations**

    (a) Regional anesthesia is generally avoided in severe cases. The decision to use neuraxial techniques should be individualized to the patient. If regional anesthesia is used, hypotension should be strictly avoided.

    (b) Avoid vasodilatory agents.

v) **Mitral regurgitation**

READ MORE

Mitral valve disease, Chapter 55, page 394

READ MORE

Aortic valve disease, Chapter 54, page 383

(1) Mitral valve prolapse, affecting approximately 5% to 15% of women of childbearing age, is the most common etiology.

(2) **Pregnancy considerations**

    (a) Increased blood volume during pregnancy promotes forward flow across the regurgitant valve.

    (b) Pregnancy is generally well tolerated, and most patients require no medications.

    (c) Severe cases can be associated with markedly dilated left atrium, atrial fibrillation, and pulmonary edema, which can be treated with diuretics.

vi) **Aortic regurgitation**

(1) **Pregnancy considerations**

    (a) A sudden increase in afterload, such as that seen in preeclampsia with severe HTN, can lead to acute cardiac decompensation.

READ MORE

Valvular heart disease, Chapter 53, page 375

(2) **Treatment**

    (a) Hydralazine is the antihypertensive medication of choice.

    (b) Treatment of heart failure involves digoxin, diuretics, and hydralazine. Angiotensin-converting enzyme (ACE)-inhibitors are contraindicated in pregnancy but can be used postpartum.

vii) **Mechanical heart valves**

(1) When a valve is replaced, mechanical valves are often used in younger patients (as opposed to bioprosthetic valves) because of their prolonged durability.

(2) **Pregnancy considerations**

    (a) Mechanical heart valves carry a very high risk of thrombotic disease, especially in association with the hypercoaguable state of pregnancy.

(3) **Treatment (33)**

    (a) Warfarin is a known teratogen and controversy surrounds its use in pregnancy, even in these very high-risk patients.

    (b) Patients with first-generation mechanical heart valves are at particularly increased risk of clots and may be offered warfarin (to maintain an INR of 2.5 to 3.5) for 35 weeks of gestation, followed by IV unfractionated heparin. Another option may include subcutaneous heparin (unfractionated or low molecular weight) for the first 12 weeks of pregnancy, followed by warfarin until 35 weeks, when they are transitioned to intravenous heparin

        (i) Cesarean delivery should be performed if delivery is indicated while on warfarin.

    (c) A second-generation prosthesis presents a slightly lower risk of thrombosis, and patients may be offered the option of subcutaneous heparin (unfractionated or LMWH) throughout gestation.

READ MORE

Regional anesthesia in the anticoagulated patient, Chapter 172, page 1171

(4) **Intrapartum management**
   (a) Most authorities recommend discontinuing anticoagulation during labor, with reinitiation of IV heparin 4 to 6 hours following an uncomplicated delivery.
   (b) In rare cases, reversal of anticoagulation may be required in patients who require emergent cesarean delivery. Consultation with a hematologist and potentially a cardiac surgeon is suggested in this situation.

(5) **Anesthetic considerations**

READ MORE

Congenital heart disease, Chapter 112, page 798

   (a) The decision to perform neuraxial procedures on patients who require anticoagulation should be individualized based on laboratory data, and the risks and benefits to a particular patient.
   (b) Many patients on chronic anticoagulation will not be candidates for regional anesthesia/analgesia. For labor, these patients should be offered IV opioids, and preparations should be made for general anesthesia should cesarean delivery be necessary.

c) **Congenital heart disease**
   i) **Coarctation of the aorta**
      (1) **Pregnancy considerations**
         (a) Severity of aortic coarctation is based upon the difference in BP between the upper and the lower extremities, with a gradient >20 mm Hg, indicating a severe lesion.
         (b) Risks of pregnancy include worsening HTN, heart failure, aortic dissection and rupture, as well as rupture of any associated cerebral aneurysms.
         (c) Patients with unrepaired aortic coarctation have a mortality rate up to 9%.
      (2) **Intrapartum management**
         (a) Severe fluctuations in BP should be prevented by providing adequate pain control.
         (b) Consideration for passive second stage and operative vaginal delivery if cesarean delivery is not performed
   ii) **Left-to-right shunting lesions**
      (1) **Pregnancy considerations**
         (a) Due to volume expansion associated with pregnancy, left-to-right heart shunts (ventricular septal defects [VSDs], atrial septal defects, and patent ductus arteriosus) are generally well tolerated during pregnancy.
         (b) Risks of pregnancy are related to shunt size and degree of pulmonary HTN.
         (c) Paradoxical embolization across the shunt can cause stroke, so these patients are typically prescribed low-dose aspirin.
         (d) Postpartum hemorrhage can lead to acute hypotension with transient shunt reversal and cyanosis.

READ MORE

Pulmonary hypertension Chapter 62, page 447

      (2) **Eisenmenger syndrome**
         (a) Longstanding left-to-right shunt can lead to pulmonary HTN and shunt reversal (Eisenmenger syndrome).
         (b) Maternal mortality in the setting of Eisenmenger syndrome is up to 50%, with the greatest risk of death within the immediate postpartum period.
         (c) Antepartum management of these patients involves bedrest, supplemental O_2, anticoagulation and prolonged hospitalization.

(d) **Intrapartum management**

    (i) These patients are at extremely high risk for maternal death, and a multidisciplinary approach is required for their care.

    (ii) There is no benefit to cesarean delivery, and vaginal delivery is preferred.

    (iii) Patients should receive slow epidural anesthesia or intrathecal narcotics and aggressive avoidance of postpartum hemorrhage.

    (iv) If cesarean delivery is required, patients typically receive general anesthesia, possibly with inhaled nitric oxide. An individualized plan should be made for each patient.

iii) Right-to-left shunting lesions

    (1) **Tetralogy of fallot (TOF) (33)**

      (a) **Pregnancy considerations**

        (i) Patients with corrected TOF and good residual functional status usually tolerate pregnancy well.

READ MORE

Cardiac arrhythmias and pacemakers, Chapter 57, page 412

        (ii) Cardiac complications in corrected lesions during pregnancy can include symptomatic right-sided heart failure and arrhythmias.

      (b) **Uncorrected TOF (33)**

        (i) May have clinical deterioration during pregnancy with associated maternal and fetal morbidity and mortality

        (ii) Cardiac complications can include increased right-to-left shunting via a residual VSD with worsening cyanosis, biventricular heart failure, arrhythmias, and cerebral vascular accidents from paradoxical emboli.

      (c) Prophylaxis for bacterial endocarditis is recommended (31).

d) **Complete heart block (2)**

    i) Patients with complete heart block, with or without a pacemaker, may become symptomatic, particularly during labor and delivery.

    ii) Due to the physiologic increase in heart rate during pregnancy, the pacing heart rate is typically increased by 10% to 20% in pregnant women.

e) **Ischemic heart disease (2)**

READ MORE

Ischemic heart disease, Chapter 51, page 359

Delivery within 2 weeks of an acute MI has been associated with a 50% maternal mortality due to heart failure or arrhythmias.

    i) Becoming more common in pregnancy as women choose to delay childbearing

    ii) Maternal mortality rate for acute myocardial infarction (MI) is 7% to 35%.

    iii) Medical therapy is the same in the pregnant patient and includes O_2, aspirin, β-adrenergic antagonists, heparin, and nitrates.

    iv) Thrombolytic agents have been used successfully in pregnancy but are associated with placental abruption and hemorrhage, especially when used in the peripartum period.

    v) Management of the pregnant patient with previous MI can include limiting physical activity and continuation of most cardiovascular medications.

    vi) Up to 50% of these patients will experience some cardiac complications during pregnancy, ranging from angina to heart failure.

    vii) Vaginal delivery, with adequate pain control and passive/assisted second stage, is the delivery method of choice.

f) **Peripartum cardiomyopathy**

i) The diagnosis of peripartum cardiomyopathy is made when a patient develops **new-onset heart failure (defined as an ejection fraction of <45%) during pregnancy or within 5 months of delivery, in the absence of a determinable cause of heart failure.**

ii) The etiology remains elusive, but known risk factors include advanced maternal age, multiple gestation, and African descent.

iii) Treatment includes medications to reduce preload (diuretics), reduce afterload (vasodilators such as hydralazine or nitroglycerin), and inotropes (digoxin or dobutamine).

  (1) ACE-inhibitors are contraindicated in pregnancy but can be initiated postpartum.

  (2) Anticoagulation should also be considered.

iv) Approximately 50% of patients have marked improvement in clinical symptoms and left ventricular function within 6 months of diagnosis.

Chapter Summary for Pregnancy and Coexisting Disease

General Principles	Understand underlying disease process and how it is affected by physiologic changes of pregnancy. Consultation with obstetrician and possibly multiple specialists may be required for optimal care. Mode of delivery should be discussed as most patients benefit from vaginal delivery but may require a passive second stage.
Diabetes Mellitus	One of the most common coexisting diseases Patients are at high risk for pregnancy complications and cesarean delivery.
Other Endocrine Disease	Thyroid disorders carry significant fetal risks if untreated. Pituitary disorders may cause hormonal imbalances and require stress dose steroids. Adrenal disorders may include pheochromocytoma.
Neurologic Disease	Paraplegia increases the risk of autonomic dysreflexia MS patients are sensitive to hyperpyrexia but generally tolerate pregnancy well. Epilepsy medications increase the risk of fetal anomalies.
Hematologic Disease	Thrombophilias are common in pregnancy. VTE is one of the leading causes of maternal death worldwide. Patients may present with long-term anticoagulation. In patients with thrombocytopenia, determine cause and individualize management plans.
Pulmonary Disease	"Normal" $PaCO_2$ levels in a pregnant asthmatic patient may represent severe respiratory compromise due to the physiologic changes of pregnancy. OSA is common and should be treated with CPAP. Patients with OSA should be carefully monitored after neuraxial opioid administration.
Cardiac Disease	Increasing in frequency in the pregnant population. Patients may present with valvular disease, congenital heart disease, and/or ischemic disease. Management plans should consider the increased cardiac work with labor and the immediate postpartum period. Individualized management often includes a multidisciplinary approach.

References

1. Getahun D, Nath C, Ananth CV, et al. Gestational diabetes in the United States: temporal trends 1989 through 2004. *Am J Obstet Gynecol* 2008;198:e1–e5
2. Rosene-Montella K, Keely E, Barbour L, et al. *Medical Care of the Pregnant Patient*. Philadelphia, PA: American College of Physicians Press; 2008.
3. Rowan JA, Hague WM, Gao W, et al. Metformin versus insulin for the treatment of gestational diabetes. *N Engl J Med* 2008;358:2003–2015.
4. Abalovich M, Amino N, Barbour LA, et al. Management of thyroid dysfunction during pregnancy and postpartum: an Endocrine Society Clinical Practice Guideline. *J Clin Endocrinol Metab* 2007;92:S1–S47.
5. Botchan A, Hauser R, Kupfermine M, et al. Pheochromocytoma in pregnancy: case report and review of the literature. *Obstet Gynecol Surv* 1995;50:321–327.
6. Anteby E, Shalev O. Clinical relevance of gestational thrombocytopenia of <100,000/microliter. *Am J Hematol* 1994;47:118–122.
7. Letsky EA, Greaves M. Guidelines on the investigation and management of thrombocytopenia in pregnancy and neonatal alloimmune thrombocytopenia. *Br J Haematol* 1996;95:21–26.
8. Gambling DR, Douglas MJ, McKay RSF, eds. *Obstetric Anesthesia and Uncommon Disorders*. Cambridge: Cambridge University Press; 2008.
9. Burrows RF, Kelton JG. Fetal thrombocytopenia and its relation to maternal thrombocytopenia. *N Engl J Med* 1993;329:1463–1466.
10. Webert KE, Mittal R, Sigouin C, et al. A retrospective 11 year analysis of obstetric patients with idiopathic thrombocytopenic purpura. *Blood* 2003;102:4306–4311.
11. George JN, Woolf SH, Raskob GE, et al. Idiopathic thrombocytopenic purpura: a practice guideline developed by explicit methods for the American Society of Hematology. *Blood* 1996;88:3–40.
12. Dashe JS, Ramin SM, Cunningham FG. The long-term consequences of thrombotic microangiopathy (thrombotic thrombocytopenic purpura and hemolytic uremic syndrome) in pregnancy. *Obstet Gynecol* 1998;91:662–668.
13. Butwick AJ, Carvalho B. Neuraxial anesthesia for cesarean delivery in a parturient with type 1 von Willebrand Disease and scoliosis. *J Clin Anesth* 3007;19:230–233.
14. Stenager E, Stenager EN, Jensen K. Effect of pregnancy on the prognosis for multiple sclerosis. A 5-year follow up investigation. *Acta Neurol Scand* 1994;90:305–308.
15. Runmarker B, Andersen O. Pregnancy is associated with a lower risk of onset and a better prognosis in multiple sclerosis. *Brain* 1995;118:253–261.
16. Dahl J, Myhr KM, Daltveit AK, et al. Pregnancy, delivery, and birth outcome in women with multiple sclerosis. *Neurology* 2005;65:1961–1963.
17. Argyriou AA, Makris N. Multiple sclerosis and reproductive risks in women. *Reprod Sci* 2008;15:755–764.
18. Pereira L. Obstetric management of the patient with spinal cord injury. *Obstet Gynecol Surv* 2003;58:678.
19. ACOG Committee Opinion: Number 275, September 2002. Obstetric management of patients with spinal cord injuries. *Obstet Gynecol* 2002;100:625.
20. So EL. Update on epilepsy. *Med Clin North Am* 1993;77:203–214.
21. Sibai BM, Spinnato JA, Watson DL, et al. Eclampsia. IV. Neurological findings and future outcome. *Am J Obstet Gynecol* 1985;184–192.
22. Namazy JA, Schatz M. Pregnancy and asthma: recent developments. *Curr Opin Pulm Med* 2005;11:56–60.
23. Maasilta P, Bachour A, Teramo K, et al. Sleep-related disordered breathing during pregnancy in obese women. *Chest* 2001;120:1448–1454.
24. Boushra NN. Anaesthetic management of patients with sleep apnoea syndrome. *Can J Anaesth* 1996;43:599–616.
25. Maggard MA, Yermilov I, Li Z, et al. Pregnancy and fertility following bariatric surgery: a systematic review. *JAMA* 2008;300:2286–2296.
26. Soens MA, Birnbach DJ, Ranasinghe JS, et al. Obstetric anesthesia for the obese and morbidly obese patient: an ounce of prevention is worth more than a pound of treatment. *Acta Anaesthesiol Scand* 2008;52:6–19.
27. Hamilton CL, Riley ET, Cohen SE. Changes in the position of epidural catheters associated with patient movement. *Anesthesiology* 1997;86:776–784.
28. Fuchs KM, Wu D, Ebcioglu Z. Pregnancy in renal transplant recipients. *Sem Perinatol* 2007;31:339–347.
29. Bonanno C, Dove L. Pregnancy after liver transplantation. *Sem Perinatol* 2007;31:348–353.
30. Rioseco AJ, Ivankovic MB, Manzur A, et al. Intrahepatic cholestasis of pregnancy: a retrospective case-control study of perinatal outcome. *Am J Obstet Gynecol* 1994;170:890–895.
31. Nishimura RA, Carabello BA, Faxon DP, et al. ACC/AHA 2008 Guideline Update on Valvular Heart Disease: Focused Update on Infective endocarditis: A Report of the American College of Cardiology/American Heart Association Task Force on Practice Guidelines. *J Am Coll Cardiol* 2008;53:676–685.
32. Klein L, Galan H. Cardiac Disease in Pregnancy. *Obstet Gynecol Clin North Am* 2004;31:429–459.
33. Creasy R, Resnik R, Iams J, et al. *Maternal-Fetal Medicine*. Philadelphia, PA: WB Saunders; 2009.

100 Obstetrical Emergencies

Andrea J. Fuller, MD • Elisabeth A. Aron, MD

Emergencies can arise at any point during labor and delivery and may be life threatening. While certain high-risk conditions may raise the incidence of delivery complications, many obstetrical emergencies can occur in any delivery at any time. It is the anesthesia provider's responsibility to understand obstetric complications and respond to them in a timely and appropriate manner.

1) Umbilical cord prolapse
   a) **General principles**
      i) Umbilical cord prolapse (UCP) is a rare obstetric emergency that requires immediate delivery, generally by cesarean section. The incidence is 0.14% to 0.62 % (1).
   b) **Pathophysiology**
      i) UCP occurs when the umbilical cord presents prior to the presenting part of the fetus or alongside the fetus.
      ii) Results in compression of the umbilical cord and can lead to fetal hypoxia
      iii) UCP can be classified as *overt* (where the cord is palpated) or *occult* (where the cord is not palpated but fetal bradycardia is observed).
      iv) The first indication of a UCP is palpation of the cord following a procedure, fetal bradycardia, or moderate to severe variable decelerations following a normal fetal tracing.
   c) **Risk factors**
      i) Include prematurity, fetal malpresentation, multiple gestation, polyhydramnios, multiparity, and rupture of membranes
   d) **Treatment and management**
      i) The standard treatment of UCP is immediate cesarean delivery (CD).
         (1) Maneuvers such as elevating the head with a hand, change in maternal position, and distention of the bladder using a Foley catheter may be useful to elevate the presenting part off the cord while a cesarean section can be begun.
   e) **Anesthetic management**
      i) CD must be immediate.
      ii) Usually, general anesthesia is required due to the urgency of the situation.
      iii) If the patient's airway is not favorable, regional anesthesia or awake intubation may be necessary.
      iv) It must be emphasized that time is of the essence for a favorable neonatal outcome, and one must carefully weigh the benefit to the mother of taking more time to achieve optimal regional anesthesia.

Sudden fetal bradycardia after rupture of membranes is concerning for umbilical cord prolapse.

727

2) **Uterine inversion**
   a) **Pathophysiology**
      i) Uterine inversion is a partial or full inversion of the body of the uterus.
         (1) Puerperal uterine inversion is rare with an incidence of 1/500 to 1/20,000 (2).
      ii) **Diagnosis**
         (1) Patients present with postpartum hemorrhage, shock, shock out of proportion to blood loss, or palpation of pelvic mass during bimanual exam.
         (2) When the uterus does not protrude out of the vagina, the diagnosis can be missed, leading to a subacute or chronic inversion.
   b) **Risk factors**
      i) Fundal placenta (10% of pregnancies have fundal placentas), adherent placenta, a short umbilical cord, excess traction on the cord, fundal pressure, and use of oxytocin
      ii) The greatest risk appears to be in primaparous women with fundal placenta (3).
      iii) Active management of the third stage of labor (placental delivery) may decrease the incidence of uterine inversion (4).
   c) **Treatment and management**
      i) Treatment depends on prompt recognition.
      ii) Postpartum hemorrhage and shock should be managed with IV fluids and blood product replacement.

READ MORE
Hemorrhage in the parturient, Chapter 101, page 740

      iii) The uterus must be replaced into the pelvic cavity.
         (1) Oxytocin should not be given.
         (2) The placenta should be left in situ until the uterus is replaced.
         (3) The obstetrician will attempt to grasp the uterus and push it back into the vagina and pelvis (Johnson maneuver).
         (4) If this is not successful, uterine relaxation is necessary.
            (a) Options for uterine relaxation include
               (i) Terbutaline 0.125 to 0.25 mg IV, Magnesium sulfate 2 g IV, nitroglycerin 25 to 100 μg IV, or nitroglycerin 0.4 mg SL (5)
            (b) General anesthesia with high-dose volatile agent can be used but requires intubation and airway protection (6).

Nitroglycerin, administered IV or sublingual, is helpful for uterine relaxation for many obstetrical emergencies.

         (5) Once the uterus is repositioned
            (a) The physician's hand should be kept inside until oxytocin is started and the uterus contracts
            (b) The placenta can be removed following uterine replacement
            (c) The uterine cavity should be manually inspected for retained placenta and uterine rupture
         (6) Rarely, the uterus cannot be manually returned to the pelvis, and an operative approach is indicated.
   d) **Anesthetic management considerations**
      i) Uterine inversion can be associated with hemorrhage and shock.
      ii) Attention should be paid to IV access, blood product replacement if necessary, uterine relaxation to facilitate replacement into the pelvis, and patient comfort during the procedure.
      iii) If the uterus is not easily replaced, transport to the operating room should be considered to facilitate monitoring and visualization.
3) **Shoulder dystocia**
   a) General principles

    i) The incidence of shoulder dystocia is 0.6% to 1.4% of all deliveries and increases with increased birth weight (7). The incidence of shoulder dystocia is 3% to 10% when neonatal weight is between 4,000 to 4,500 g, and 8% to 24% when >4,500 g (8).

b) **Pathophysiology**

    i) Following the delivery of the neonatal head, the shoulders become impacted against the symphysis pubis and umbilical cord compression occurs. Increased shoulder-to-head and chest-to-head proportions are associated with shoulder dystocia (9).

    ii) **Fetal complications**

        (1) Asphyxia, meconium aspiration, plexus injuries (Erb, Duchene, Klumpke), and injuries to clavicle or humerus

    iii) **Maternal complications**

        (1) Postpartum hemorrhage, vaginal lacerations, and ruptured uterus

c) **Risk factors**

    i) Many patients have no identifiable risk factors.

    ii) Risk factors

        (1) Include large gestational weight and gestational diabetes mellitus, increased maternal age, maternal obesity, post-term pregnancy, history of prior dystocia, multiparity, post-term gestation, history of macrosomic infant, labor induction, and prolonged second stage of labor

        (2) Forceps and vacuum assistance may also increase the risk of shoulder dystocia.

d) **Treatment and management**

    i) Prompt recognition followed by initiation of the following steps by the obstetrician to relieve the impacted fetal shoulder

        (1) Get help, perform episiotomy (controversial), drain maternal bladder.

        (2) Suprapubic pressure and McRobert maneuver. McRobert maneuver is hyperflexion and abduction of hips causing cephalodad rotation of symphysis pubis and flattening of the lumbar lordosis that frees the impacted shoulder.

        (3) Maneuvers attempted at disimpacting the anterior shoulder. These include the corkscrew maneuver that involves rotating the anterior shoulder posteriorly to release the impacted shoulder.

        (4) Zavanelli maneuver. The Zavanelli maneuver is an attempt to replace the fetal head into the uterus followed by cesarean section.

e) **Anesthetic considerations**

    i) Attention should be paid to minimizing second-stage motor block and optimal pain management.

    ii) In patients with high estimated fetal weight (EFW), the anesthesia provider should be prepared for the possibility of CD.

f) **Prevention**

    i) Prevention may not always be possible.

    ii) A multidisciplinary management plan is helpful to efficiently treat dystocia.

    iii) Elective CD is considered for EFW 4,500 g in diabetic women (10,11), EFW >5,000 g, and women with a prior history of shoulder dystocia.

4) **Vaginal birth after cesarean section (VBAC)/uterine rupture**

a) General principles

    i) Incidence of VBAC

        (1) Has varied over time with an increase from 3% in 1980 to 31% in 1998 and back down to 9.2% in 2004 (12–14)

        (2) These changes in incidence reflect political, medical, legal, and patient/practitioner preferences.

Patients with a prior midline or T-shaped uterine incision have a significantly higher rate of uterine rupture with labor and those with a prior low transverse incision.

Since a uterine rupture is a life-threatening emergency for mother and baby, constant communication with obstetricians and nurses regarding progress of labor and adequacy of the epidural catheter is essential for any patient attempting a VBAC.

In any VBAC patient with an epidural having severe breakthrough pain, a uterine rupture should be suspected.

      ii)   The incidence of uterine rupture due to a prior CD. Depends upon uterine scar type
         (1)   Rate of rupture with a prior classical or T-shaped uterine incision is 4% to 9%
         (2)   A prior low vertical incision is 1% to 7%, and a low transverse incision is 0.2% to 1.5% (15–17).

 b)   **Pathophysiology**
      i)   **Uterine rupture may occur at any time during the pregnancy but most commonly during labor.**
      ii)   With rupture of the scar and the uterus, the placenta may separate causing fetal hypoxia.
         (1)   Generally, the first recognizable sign of uterine rupture is fetal variable decelerations, but may also include maternal pain, maternal hypotension, loss of fetal station, and bleeding.
      iii)   Candidates for a trial of labor (TOL) include history of one prior CD, clinically adequate pelvis, no other uterine scars or previous rupture, physicians immediately available to perform CD, and immediate availability of anesthesia (15).

 c)   **Risk factors for uterine rupture during a TOL**
      i)   Age >30, more than one prior CD, history of postpartum fever and/or chorioamnionitis with prior CD, interdelivery interval <18 to 24 months from prior CD, dysfunctional labor, and prior one layer uterine closure

 d)   **Treatment and management**
      i)   Treatment involves prompt recognition followed by immediate CD.
      ii)   If the rupture is large and associated with hemorrhage, cesarean hysterectomy may be required.

 e)   **Prevention**
      i)   Prevention may not always be possible.
      ii)   Patients should be appropriately counseled prior to undergoing a TOL.
      iii)   Prostaglandins should not be used in induction of labor during VBAC as this has shown to increase the rate of uterine rupture.
      iv)   VBAC should only be performed in hospitals where cesarean section is immediately available.

 f)   **Anesthetic considerations**
      i)   Early anesthetic evaluation is recommended with special attention paid to the airway exam and counseling regarding early epidural placement.
      ii)   Although a well-functioning epidural catheter is optimal, there may not be time to dose the catheter for cesarean section and emergent general anesthesia may be necessary.
      iii)   If a cesarean hysterectomy is required, bleeding could be profuse and require invasive monitoring, large bore IV access, and blood transfusion.

5)   Nonreassuring fetal heart rate (FHR) tracing (fetal distress)
 a)   Fetal well-being is often determined by FHR monitoring.
 b)   **Criteria to determine fetal status**
      i)   Historically, providers have not used the same criteria or definitions to describe fetal distress and FHR.
      ii)   There has been dispute over the use of the term *fetal distress*, resulting in ACOG recommending using the term *nonreassuring FHR tracing*.

iii) The National Institute of Child Health and Human Development (NICHD) Research Planning Workshop on electronic fetal monitoring has developed guidelines for the interpretation of fetal monitoring (18,19).

c) **Pathophysiology**

   i) The purpose of fetal monitoring is to distinguish FHR patterns associated with abnormal fetal acid-base status and which are associated with a physiologically compensated fetus.

   ii) The fetus responds to acute hypoxia by redistributing its blood flow to maintain cardiac output while protecting vital organs, decreasing its consumption of O2, and undergoing anaerobic glycolysis.

   iii) This condition is readily reversible and may sustain a fetus for 30 minutes.

   iv) After 30 minutes or during more severe hypoxia, cardiac output will decrease, resulting in decreased blood flow to the brain and the heart and hypoxic tissue damage may occur.

d) **Categories of FHR tracings (Figs. 100-1 to 100-3)**

   i) The NICHD has broken down FHR patterns into three categories: I, II, and III (20,21)

   ii) **Category I FHR tracings**

   (1) Normal

   (2) Predict normal fetal acid-base status

   (3) Characteristics include:
       (a) Baseline rate of 110 to 160 bpm
       (b) Moderate baseline FHR variability
           (i) Variability is defined as fluctuations in baseline of two cycles per minute or greater and can be determined visually as the amplitude of the peak to trough in beats per minute.
       (c) Absence of late or variable decelerations
       (d) Early decelerations may or may not be present.
       (e) Accelerations may or may not be present.

   iii) **Category II FHR tracings (Fig. 100-4)**

   (1) Indeterminant

   (2) Not always predictive of fetal acid-base status

   (3) Encompasses all FHR tracings not category I or III, including:
       (a) Bradycardia not accompanied by absent baseline variability
       (b) Tachycardia
       (c) Minimal or marked baseline variability; absent baseline variability without recurrent decelerations
       (d) Absence of accelerations following fetal scalp stimulation
       (e) Recurrent variable decelerations with minimal or moderate baseline variability
       (f) Prolonged decelerations (>2 minutes but <10 minutes), recurrent late decelerations with moderate baseline variability, variable decelerations with a slow return to baseline, overshoots, or "shoulders"

   iv) **Category III FHR tracings (Fig. 100-5)**

   (1) Abnormal

   (2) Predictive of abnormal fetal acid-base status.

   (3) Characteristics include:
       (a) Absent baseline FHR variability and any of the following:
           (i) Recurrent late decelerations
           (ii) Recurrent variable decelerations
           (iii) Bradycardia
       (b) Sinusoidal pattern

Figure 100-1 Characteristics of a Category I (Reassuring) FHR Tracing

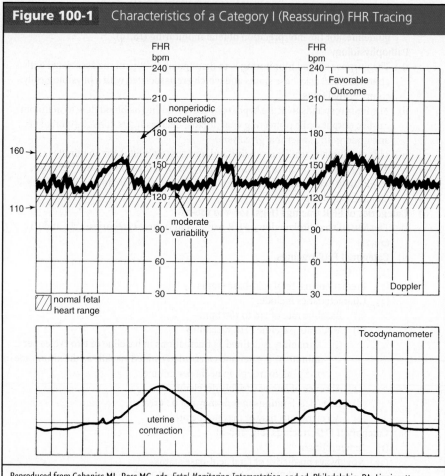

Reproduced from Cabaniss ML, Ross MG, eds. *Fetal Monitoring Interpretation*. 2nd ed. Philadelphia, PA: Lippincott Williams & Wilkins; 2010, with permission.

Figure 100-2 Category I (Reassuring) FHR Tracing

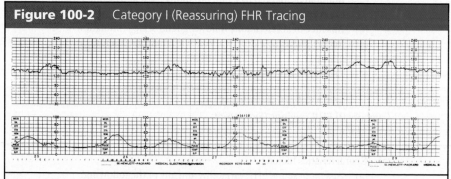

FHR is at the top and uterine contractions are recorded at the bottom.
Reproduced from Cabaniss ML, Ross MG, eds. *Fetal Monitoring Interpretation*. 2nd ed. Philadelphia, PA: Lippincott Williams & Wilkins; 2010, with permission.

Figure 100-3   Category I: Early Decelerations

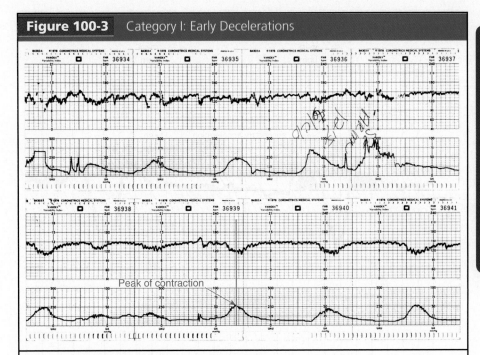

The nadir of the deceleration is at the peak of the uterine contraction (*line drawn*).
Adapted from Cabaniss ML, Ross MG, eds. *Fetal Monitoring Interpretation*. 2nd ed. Philadelphia, PA: Lippincott Williams & Wilkins; 2010.

e) **Risk factors for fetal distress**

  i) Preterm infants, multiple pregnancies, induction of labor, oligohydramnios, and pregnancies complicated by intrauterine growth restriction (IUGR), HTN, or type I DM

f) **Treatment and management**

  i) Most practitioners advise using either continuous or intermittent fetal monitoring throughout labor.

  ii) Resuscitative measures aimed at increasing O2 delivery can be performed.

   (1) Repositioning the patient, increasing IV fluids, treating hypotension (especially after epidural or spinal analgesia), administering tocolytic agents to stop contractions, and administering O_2.

  iii) If delivery is remote, cesarean section is performed when a nonreassuring FHR is diagnosed.

  iv) If possible, delivery may be expedited with forceps or vacuum the setting of non-reassuring FHR.

g) **Prevention**

  i) **Optimizing the maternal condition is the best way to prevent fetal distress.** This includes avoiding aortocaval compression, hypotension, and acidosis.

  ii) Consider early epidural placement in high-risk pregnancies.

  iii) Continuous fetal monitoring is generally recommended when labor induction medications are administered (oxytocin and/or prostaglandins) in order to avoid iatrogenic causes.

It is in the anesthesia provider's best interest to become familiar with normal and nonreassuring FHR tracings. This allows for better communication on the labor ward and decision making in urgent situations.

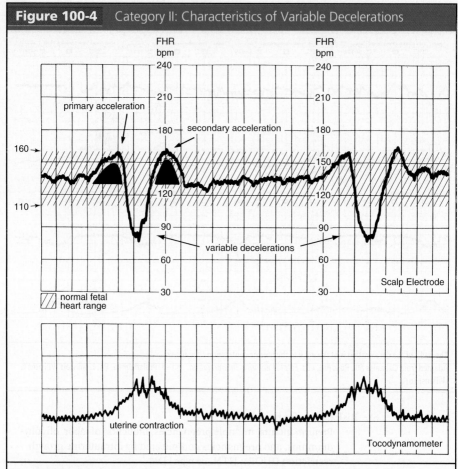

Figure 100-4 Category II: Characteristics of Variable Decelerations

Reproduced from Cabaniss ML, Ross MG, eds. *Fetal Monitoring Interpretation*. 2nd ed. Philadelphia, PA: Lippincott Williams & Wilkins; 2010, with permission.

6) Retained placenta
   a) **Pathophysiology**
      i) The third stage of labor is defined as the time from delivery of the infant to the delivery of the placenta.
         (1) A normal third stage of labor is <30 minutes.
         (2) After 30 minutes, manual removal of the placenta may be attempted.
         (3) Removal should be attempted prior to 30 minutes in the presence of postpartum hemorrhage.
      ii) If the majority of the placenta has delivered, but uterine bleeding continues, the patient must be evaluated for retained placental fragments.
   b) **Risk factors for retained placenta**
      i) Advanced maternal age, previous uterine curettage, premature rupture of membranes, preterm delivery (especially in the second trimester), history of retained placenta (22,23)
   c) **Treatment/management**
      i) Initial treatment is gentle umbilical cord traction and uterine massage.

Figure 100-5 — Category III: Late Decelerations

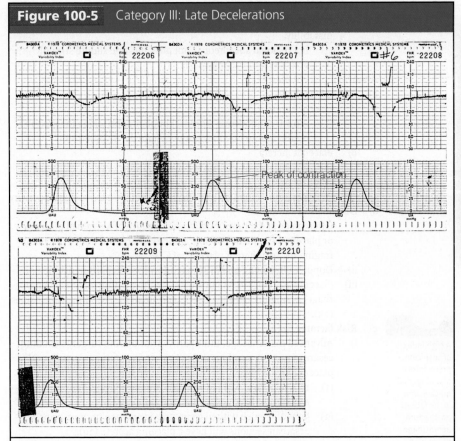

The nadir of the deceleration is *after* the peak of the uterine contraction (*line drawn*).
Adapted from Cabaniss ML, Ross MG, eds. *Fetal Monitoring Interpretation*. 2nd ed. Philadelphia, PA: Lippincott Williams & Wilkins; 2010.

ii) Ocytocin and/or prostaglandins may also be administered IM, IV, or vaginally.

iii) If initial treatment is unsuccessful, the placenta may be removed manually.

    (1) A tocolytic or nitrogylcerin may be required for uterine relaxation

iv) Ultrasound may be performed to look for placental fragments.

    (1) If suspicious for placental fragments, a uterine curettage may be performed using a large curette or a manual sweep may be attempted.

In cases of retained placenta, special consideration must be given to the patient's hemodynamic status.

d) **Anesthetic considerations**

i) The patient may require additional pain control for removal of retained placenta.

ii) It is advisable to transport the patient to the operating room for monitoring and optimal visualization by the obstetrician.

iii) If an epidural catheter is in place, a bolus of local anesthetic with or without narcotic should be given.

        iv)   It is difficult to adequately titrate sedative medications in these patients due to the risk of aspiration and possible hemodynamic instability.

           (1)   If a regional anesthetic is not possible, one should strongly consider general anesthesia.

  7) **Abnormal placentation (24)**

    a) Pathophysiology

       i)   Placenta accreta

          (1)   A form of abnormal placental implantation where the placenta is adherent to but does not penetrate the myometrium

       ii)   Placenta increta

          (1)   Placental invasion into the myometrium

       iii)   Placenta percreta

          (1)   Invasion beyond the uterine serosa and into the abdominal cavity

    b) **Diagnosis**

       i)   Often made at the time of delivery in the face of a retained placenta or placental fragments, sonographic evidence of retained placental fragments, or adherent placenta at CD

       ii)   Doppler ultrasound and MRI may allow for antepartum diagnosis.

       iii)   Placenta accreta is associated with life-threatening maternal hemorrhage, premature delivery, IUGR, and small for gestational age babies (25).

    c) **Risk factors**

       i)   Advanced maternal age, multiparity, prior uterine surgery including cesarean section, previous uterine curettage, uterine scarring, and placenta previa.

          (1)   10% to 20% of women with placenta previa and one prior cesarean section have a placenta accreta.

          (2)   50% of women with placenta previa and two or more prior cesarean sections will have a placenta accreta (26).

    d) **Treatment/management**

       i)   Placenta accreta should be suspected based on risk factors.

       ii)   A focal placenta accreta may be managed conservatively by oversewing or excising the implantation site at the time of delivery.

       iii)   Hysterectomy is usually required to remove the placenta in situ and control bleeding.

       iv)   In rare cases, the placenta is left in situ with the administration of methotrexate postpartum.

       v)   Blood products and/or consultations with other services including Interventional Radiology, Surgery, Urology, and Oncology may be indicated.

    e) **Anesthetic considerations**

       i)   **Patients are at high risk for massive blood loss.**

       ii)   One should have a high index of suspicion in patients with placenta previa and multiple previous cesarean sections.

       iii)   The anesthetic plan should include large bore IV access, blood product availability, and provisions for long surgical time. Invasive arterial monitoring is often helpful for blood pressure monitoring and frequent blood draws.

A high index of suspicion, preoperative planning, and quick action in the face of postpartum hemorrhage can lead to fewer complications in patients with placenta accreta.

READ MORE

Hemorrhage in the parturient, Chapter 101, page 740

Massive transfusion and resuscitation, Chapters 29 and 215, pages 220 and 1336

      iv) An epidural catheter is useful for repeated dosing (27).

      v) General anesthesia is not mandatory but should be considered if multiple transfusions are required (27).

      vi) Interventional radiology procedures can preserve fertility and may decrease blood loss, but the patient must be hemodynamically stable for safe transport.

8) **Operative vaginal delivery**

  a) Operative vaginal delivery is the delivery of the fetus with the aid of forceps or a vacuum

  b) Pathophysiology

    i) Operative delivery may be performed when fetal station is outlet, low, or mid.

      (1) High forceps should not be attempted due to the increased risk of neonatal morbidity and mortality.

    ii) In vacuum-assisted deliveries, pressure to the fetal scalp is used to assist in delivery.

    iii) In forceps-assisted deliveries, pressure is applied to the fetal skull to assist in delivery.

    iv) Selection of vacuum versus forceps is generally provider driven (28).

  c) **Indications for assisted vaginal delivery**

    i) Include prolonged second stage, fetal compromise or nonreassuring FHR, and shortening the second stage for maternal benefit

  d) **Complications**

    i) Both vacuum and forceps have been associated with maternal complications including hematomas, lacerations, and pelvic floor injury.

    ii) Fetal complications include scalp laceration, cephalohematomas, subgaleal hematomas, intracranial hemorrhage, hyperbilirubinemia, and retinal hemorrhages.

    iii) The incidence of shoulder dystocia is increased with operative vaginal delivery.

  e) **Contraindications to operative vaginal delivery**

    i) Vacuum prior to 34 weeks secondary to the increased risk of cerebral hemorrhage, known fetal bone demineralization or bleeding disorder, unengaged fetal head, unknown position of fetal head.

  f) **Treatment/management**

    i) Patients should meet ACOG criteria for operative vaginal delivery (29).

    ii) Immediate CD should be available.

    iii) Operator experience should determine which instrument is used in each situation.

    iv) Neonatal care providers should be made aware of operative deliveries to assess for neonatal complications.

  g) **Anesthetic considerations**

    i) Pain control is necessary for operative vaginal delivery.

    ii) A well-functioning epidural catheter is optimal.

    iii) A bolus (~5 mL) of higher concentration local anesthetic (0.25% bupivacaine or 1% to 1.5% lidocaine) with or without opioid is recommended.

    iv) One must be prepared for emergent CD, ideally with epidural anesthesia, but general anesthesia may be required if an epidural is not in place or the situation is too emergent.

READ MORE

Obstetrical anesthesia, Chapter 144, page 1047

Chapter Summary for Obstetrical Emergencies

Clinical Problem	Considerations	Recommended Action
Umbilical Cord Prolapse	Life-threatening fetal emergency	Emergent CD required, usually with GA.
Uterine Inversion	Potential for hemorrhage and shock	Treat with uterine relaxant and hemodynamic support.
Uterine Rupture	Life-threatening maternal and fetal emergency. Potential for hemorrhage.	Urgent CD usually required. T&C blood and prepare for potential hemorrhage
Placenta Accreta/ Increta/Percreta	Massive blood loss and hysterectomy possible.	T&C blood and products, consider invasive monitoring. Plan for postoperative care.
Shoulder Dystocia	More common with maternal diabetes and large babies. May require CD.	Minimize motor block with epidural analgesia. Prepare for CD.
Nonreassuring FHR Tracing	Category III tracings may be associated with fetal hypoxemia and acidosis.	Prepare for urgent delivery. Consult with obstetrician. May use regional or general anesthesia depending on the situation.
Operative Vaginal Delivery	Forceps or vacuum assistance required. If unsuccessful, may require emergent CD.	Ensure patient comfort, preferably by dosing epidural catheter. Prepare for CD.

GA, general anesthesia; CD, cesarean delivery; T&C, type and cross.

References

1. Koonings PP, Paul RH, Campbell K. Umbilical cord prolapse. A contemporary look. *J Reprod Med* 1990;35:690.
2. Watson P, Besch N, Bowes WA. Management of acute and subacute puerperal inversion of the uterus. *Obstet Gynecol* 1980;55(1):12.
3. Kochenour NK. Intrapartum obstetric emergencies. *Crit Care Clin* 1991;7(4):851–864.
4. Baskett TF. Acute uterine inversion: a review of 40 cases. *J Obstet Gynecol Can* 2002;24(12):953–956.
5. Abouleish E., Ali V, Joumaa B, et al. Anaesthetic management of acute puerperal uterine inversion. *Br J Anaesth* 1995;75(4):486–487.
6. Riley ET, Flanagan B, Cohen SE, et al. Intravenous nitroglycerin: a potent uterine relaxant for emergency obstetric procedures. Review of the literature and report of three cases. *Int J Obstet Anesth* 1996;5(4):264–268.
7. ACOG Practice Bulletin: Shoulder dystocia. Nov 2002; number 40. *Obstet Gynecol* 2002; 100: 1045–50.
8. Al-Najashi S, Al-Suleiman A, El-Yahia A, et al. Shoulder dystocia—a clinical study of 56 cases. *Aust N Z J Ostet Gynaecol* 1988;28:107.
9. Modanlou HD, Komatsu G, Dorchester W, et al. Large-for-gestation-age neonates: Anthropometric reasons for shoulder dystocia. *Obstet Gynecol* 1982;60:417.
10. Kjos SL, Henry OA, Montoro M, et al. Insulin-requiring diabetes in pregnancy: a randomized trial of active induction of labor and expectant management. *Am J Obstet Gynecol* 1993;169:611–615.
11. Rouse DJ, Owen J, Goldenberg RL, et al. The effectiveness and costs of elective cesarean delivery for fetal macrosomia diagnosed by ultrasound. *JAMA* 1996;276:1480–486.
12. Centers for Disease Control and Prevention. www.cdc.gov.
13. International Cesarean Awareness Network, Inc. www.ican-online.org/resources/statistics.php (Accessed 3/10/05).
14. Landon, MB, Spong, CY, Thom. E, et al. Risk of uterine rupture with a trial of labor in women with multiple and single prior cesarean delivery. *Obstet Gynecol* 2004;104:203.
15. ACOG Practice Bulletin: Vaginal birth after previous cesarean delivery. July 2004; number 54. *Obstet Gynecol* 2004; 104:203.
16. DeCosta C. Vaginal birth after classical cesarean section. *Aust N Z J Obstet Gynecol* 2005;45:182.
17. Macones, GA, Peipert, J, Nelson, DB, et al. Maternal complications with vaginal birth after cesarean delivery: a multicenter study. *Am J Obstet Gynecol* 2005;193:1656.
18. The National Institute of Child Health and Human Development Research Planning Workshop. Electronic Fetal heart rate monitoring: research and guidelines for interpretation. *Am J Obstet Gynecol* 1997;177:1385–1390.
19. Macones GA, Hankins GDV, Spong CY. Current xommentaries. The 2008 National Institutes of Health and Human Development Workshop Report on Electronic Fetal Monitoring. *Obstet Gynecol* 2008;112:661–666.
20. Cabaniss ML, Ross MG, eds. *Fetal Monitoring Interpretation*. 2nd ed. Philadelphia, PA: Lippincott Williams & Wilkins; 2010.

21. ACOG Practice Bulletin. July 2009; number 106.
22. Titiz H, Wallace A, Voaklander DC, et al. Manual removal of the placenta: a case control study. *Aust N Z Obstet Gynaecol* 2001;41(1):41–44.
23. Panpaprai P, Boriboonhirunsarn D, et al. Risk factors of retained placenta in Siriraj hospital. *J Med Assoc Thai* 2007;90(7):1293–1297.
24. Hughes SC, Levinson G, Rosen MA, eds. *Anesthesia for Obstetrics*. 4th ed. Philadelphia, PA: Lippincott Williams & Wilkins; 2002.
25. Gielchinsky Y, Mankuta D, Rojansky N, et al. Perinatal outcome of pregnancies complicated by placenta accreta. *Obstet Gynecol* 2004;104: 527–530.
26. Creasy RK, Resnik R. *Maternal-Fetal Medicine*. 4th ed. Philadelphia, PA: WB Saunders Company; 1999:620.
27. Fuller AJ, Carvalho B, Brummel C, et al. Epidural anesthesia for elective cesarean delivery with intraoperative arterial occlusion balloon catheter placement. *Anesth Analg* 2006;102(2):585–587.
28. Bofill JA, Rust OA, Perry KG, et al. Operative vaginal delivery: a survey of fellows of ACOG. *Obstet Gynecol* 1996;88:1007–1010.
29. ACOG Practice Bulletin: Operative vaginal delivery. June 2000; number 17. *Obstet Gynecol* 2000; 95:6.

101 Hemorrhage in the Parturient

Andrea J. Fuller, MD

Postpartum hemorrhage (PPH) is the leading cause of ICU admission in the United States and one of the leading causes of maternal death worldwide. Morbidity from hemorrhage includes loss of fertility, shock, coagulopathy, adult respiratory distress syndrome, and pituitary necrosis (Sheehan syndrome).

1) Definition of PPH
   a) Blood loss in excess of 500 mL for a vaginal delivery and 1,000 mL for cesarean delivery is suspicious for PPH.
   b) Exact amount of blood loss is difficult to determine and often underestimated due to the presence of amniotic fluid and lack of containment of the blood.
   c) Signs of poor perfusion, including tachycardia, decreased pulse pressure, decreased BP, tachypnea, decreased urine output, and altered mental status, should alert the practitioner to the possibility of PPH.
   d) **Primary PPH**
      i) Hemorrhage occurring within 24 hours postdelivery
   e) **Secondary PPH**
      i) Hemorrhage occurring between 24 hours and 6 to 12 weeks postdelivery (1)
2) Risk factors for PPH (1)
   a) Prolonged, augmented, and/or rapid labor
   b) Overdistention of the uterus
   c) Episiotomy
   d) Previous history of PPH
   e) Preeclampsia
   f) Chorioamnionitis
   g) Operative delivery (forceps or vacuum)
   h) Asian or Hispanic descent
3) Causes of hemorrhage
   a) **Uterine atony**
      i) Uterine atony is the most common cause of PPH (1).
      ii) Characterized by a soft, poorly contracted uterus
      iii) **Risk factors** for uterine atony
         (1) Prolonged, augmented, or rapid labor
         (2) Infection (such as chorioamnionitis)
         (3) Overdistention of the uterus from macrosomia, multiple gestations, or polyhydramnios
         (4) General anesthesia can contribute to atony because volatile agents decrease uterine contractility.
   b) **Placental abnormalities (previa, accreta, increta)**

READ MORE

Obstetrical emergencies, Chapter 100, page 727

i) Placental abnormalities include placenta previa, placenta accreta, placenta increta, and placenta percreta.

ii) Placenta previa occurs when the placenta covers the cervical os.

    (1) The other placental abnormalities depend on the depth of invasion into the uterine myometrium, with placenta percreta extending through the myometrium and into the peritoneal cavity.

iii) **Risk factors**

    (1) **Previous uterine surgery** (especially cesarean section)

        (a) For example, the risk of placenta accreta is 40% in the presence of a placenta previa and three previous cesarean sections (2).

    (2) Advanced maternal age

    (3) Assisted reproductive technology (3)

c) **Coagulation defects**

i) **Inherited**

    (1) **Von Willebrand Disease (VWD)**

        (a) Most common inherited coagulation defect

        (b) Patients with VWD are at risk for PPH and commonly have delayed hemorrhage as their coagulation factors reach prepregnancy levels in the weeks following delivery (4).

        (c) May require treatment with desmopressin acetate, cryoprecipitate, or fresh frozen plasma during and after delivery (4)

        (d) Because there are several different forms of VWD, it is best to consult a hematologist when caring for these patients.

ii) **Acquired Coagulation Defects**

    (1) Causes

        (a) Syndrome of hemolysis, elevated liver enzymes, and low platelets (HELLP)

        (b) Disseminated intravascular coagulation (DIC)

            (i) DIC can occur as a result of placental abruption, prolonged intrauterine fetal demise, and amniotic fluid embolism.

        (c) Sepsis

            (i) Due to chorioamnionitis, retained products of conception, surgical infection, or systemic infection from nonobstetric causes

d) **Uterine inversion**

i) Characterized by rapid onset of hemorrhage and shock during the third stage of delivery

ii) Uterus must be restored to its normal position, which may require nitroglycerin, β-agonist agents, magnesium sulfate, or general anesthesia to relax the uterus.

iii) Once in its normal position, uterotonic agents should be administered to facilitate uterine contraction (5).

e) **Retained products of conception**

i) Can cause primary or secondary PPH

ii) Treatment

    (1) Manual removal of the placenta, which can be performed under regional or general anesthesia depending on the hemodynamic stability of the patient (5)

    (2) Nitroglycerin has been reported effective in providing uterine relaxation for removal of retained placenta (6).

Patients with abnormal placentation are at risk for massive blood loss at delivery.

READ MORE

Coagulopathies, Chapter 89, page 643

READ MORE

Obstetrical emergencies, Chapter 100, page 727

Nitroglycerin may be useful during a uterine inversion to facilitate replacement of the uterus into the pelvis.

Methylergo-
navine can
cause severe
hypertension
and should
not be given to
patients with
hypertension.

Prostaglandin
$F_{2\alpha}$ can increase
pulmonary vas-
cular resistance
and should
be avoided
in patients
with asthma
or pulmonary
hypertension.

f) **Genital tract or uterine lacerations/hematomas**
  i) Lacerations and/or hematomas are the most common cause of injury during childbirth and should be suspected as a cause of hemorrhage in a patient with persistent vaginal bleeding despite adequate uterine tone (5).
  ii) Patients who have VWD or who have had a vacuum or forceps delivery are at highest risk (4,5).
4) **Treatment of hemorrhage**
  a) **Pharmacologic treatment of uterine atony**
    i) The anesthesia provider is commonly asked to administer utero-tonic agents.
    ii) The route of administration, dosage, and side effects of the various agents are outlined in Table 101-1.
    iii) It is important to be aware of the side effects and contraindications of uterotonic medications (see Table 101-1)
    iv) Methylergonavine and prostaglandin $F_{2\alpha}$ should always be administered intramuscularly (1).
    v) **Surgical techniques to control uterine atony include uterine massage, balloon tamponade (Bakri balloon), B-Lynch sutures, and bilateral uterine or hypogastric artery ligation (1).**
    vi) In cases of placental abnormality and/or extreme uterine atony, hysterectomy may be required.

Table 101-1
Medical Management of Postpartum Hemorrhage

Drug[a]	Dose/Route	Frequency	Comment
Oxytocin (Pitocin)	IV: 10–40 units in 1 L normal saline or lactated Ringer solution IM: 10 units	Continuous	Avoid undiluted rapid IV Infusion, which causes hypotension.
Methylergonovine (Methergine)	IM: 0.2 mg	Every 2–4 h	Avoid if patient is hypertensive.
15-Methyl PGF$_{2\alpha}$ (Carboprost) (Hemabate)	IM: 0.25 mg	Every 15–90 min, 8 doses maximum	Avoid in asthmatic patients; relative contraindication if hepatic, renal, and cardiac disease. Diarrhea, fever, tachycardia can occur.
Dinoprostone (Prostin E$_2$)	Suppository: vaginal or rectal 20 mg	Every 2 h	Avoid if patient is hypotensive. Fever is common. Stored frozen, it must be thawed to room temperature.
Misoprostol (Cytotec, PGE$_1$)	800–1,000 µg rectally		

[a]All agents can cause nausea and vomiting.
IM, intramuscularly: IV, Intravenously; PG, prostaglandin.
Reused from ACOG Practice Bulletin: Clinical Management Guidelines for Obstetrician-Gynecologists Number 76, October 2006: postpartum hemorrhage. *Obstet Gynecol* 2006;108:1042, with permission.

READ MORE

Blood component therapy, Chapter 27, page 209

Alternatives to blood product replacement, Chapter 28, page 215

In the bleeding obstetric patient, constant communication with the surgeon about ongoing blood loss is imperative.

In an OB patient with PPH, regional anesthesia is an option, but one must carefully consider general anesthesia with endotracheal intubation in patients who are hemodynamically unstable or requiring large amounts of fluids and blood products.

b) In cases of hemorrhage where the patient is relatively hemodynamically stable, the **uterine arteries can be embolized (7)**.
  i) **Advantages of this technique**
     (1) Potential avoidance of surgery, decreased blood transfusion, and preservation of fertility
     (2) In patients at risk for hemorrhage, uterine artery catheters and balloons can be placed preoperatively (8).
  ii) **Disadvantages**
     (1) Include possibility of infection, vascular injury, or thrombosis

c) **Blood component therapy**
  i) Many patients with obstetric hemorrhage will require treatment with blood components.
  ii) Evaluation of clotting is important, and the patient may require treatment with platelets and clotting factors in addition to red blood cells.

d) **Pharmacologic treatment of OB hemorrhage**
  i) Activated recombinant factor VII (rFVIIa) can be used to treat intractable obstetric hemorrhage.
     (1) **Mechanism of action** is augmentation of the intrinsic clotting pathway by binding with tissue factor and directly activating factors IX and X (9)
     (2) The most effective dose is 90 to 100 μg/kg IV (9).
     (3) Side effects in the obstetrical population are rare but include thrombosis of vessels or indwelling devices.

Chapter Summary for Hemorrhage in the Parturient

Implications	OB hemorrhage is common. It is the leading cause of ICU admission and one of the leading causes of maternal death worldwide.
Definition	>500 mL EBL for vaginal delivery and >1,000 mL for cesarean delivery.
Causes	Uterine atony most common. Other causes include coagulation defects, lacerations, retained products of conception, placental abnormalities.
Treatment	Treat uterine atony with uterotonics or surgical techniques. Avoid large boluses of oxytocin IV. Avoid methylergonavine in patients with hypertension. Avoid prostaglandin $F_{2\alpha}$ in asthmatics or pulmonary hypertension. General treatment includes volume resuscitation, airway management, and blood product replacement.
Postoperative Care	Consider the possibility for ongoing blood loss and/or coagulopathy. Patients may require postoperative intubation and care in an ICU.

References

1. ACOG Practice Bulletin: Clinical Management Guidelines for Obstetrician-Gynecologists Number 76, October 2006: postpartum hemorrhage. *Obstet Gynecol* 2006;108:1039–1047.

2. Clark SL, Koonings PP, Phelan JP. Placenta previa/accreta and prior cesarean section. *Obstet Gynecol* 1985;66:89–92.

3. Wu S, Kocherginsky M, Hibbard JU. Abnormal placentation: Twenty-year analysis. *Am J Obstet Gynecol* 2005;192:1458–1461.

4. James AH. Von Willebrand disease. *Obstet Gynecol Surv* 2006;61:136–144.

5. Mayer DC, Spielman FJ, Bell EA. Antepartum and postpartum hemorrhage. In: Chestnut DH, ed. *Obstetric Anesthesia: Principles and Practice*. Philadelphia, PA: Elsevier Mosby; 2004:662–682.

6. Riley ET, Flanagan B, Cohen SE, et al. Intravenous nitroglycerin: a potent uterine relaxant for emergency obstetric procedures. Review of literature and report of three cases. *Int J Obstet Anesth* 1996;5:264–268.

7. Hansch E, Chitkara U, McAlpine J, et al. Pelvic arterial embolization for control of obstetric hemorrhage: a five-year experience. *Am J Obstet Gynecol* 1999;180:1454–1460.

8. Fuller AJ, Carvalho B, Brummel C, et al. Epidural anesthesia for elective cesarean delivery with intraoperative arterial occlusion balloon catheter placement. *Anesth Analg* 2006;102:585–587.

9. Karalapillai D, Popham P. Recombinant factor VIIa in massive postpartum haemorrhage. *Int J Obstet Anesth* 2007;16:29–34.

102 Neonatal Resuscitation

Echo Rowe, MD

As anesthesiologists, most often our clinical focus resides in the mother during labor or Cesarean delivery, while other medical providers provide neonatal care. According to the American Academy of Pediatrics, approximately 10% of newborns require some assistance to begin breathing after birth, but 1% will require extensive resuscitation to survive (1). It is the responsibility of the anesthesiologist to understand the basic principles of neonatal resuscitation and be prepared to provide this life-saving care when necessary.

Anesthesiologists are most likely to provide neonatal resuscitation when other providers are unavailable or unexpected events occur, such as emergent delivery or difficult neonatal airway.

It is helpful to familiarize yourself with the equipment for neonatal resuscitation before an emergency occurs.

1) Introduction
   a) **Neonatal resuscitation** primarily consists of basic life support with a focus on airway, breathing, and circulation (ABCs) (2).
   b) The ABCs are the heart of our everyday practice and such skills may be called upon when other medical personnel are not available or during certain neonatal emergencies, whether anticipated or not.

2) **Risk factors:** A number of antepartum and intrapartum factors may increase the likelihood of positive-pressure ventilation or endotracheal intubation at the time of delivery, including gestational age, multiple gestation pregnancy, and meconium stained amniotic fluid (3).
   a) Important information to obtain when responding to a resuscitation
      i) Estimated gestational age
      ii) Presence of meconium
      iii) Maternal diseases and/or pregnancy complications
      iv) Any fetal anomalies such as congenital heart disease, congenital diaphragmatic hernia, gastroschisis, or syndromes associated with difficult intubation such as Pierre Robin

3) Treatment
   a) Equipment: Having appropriate supplies and equipment ready and available can save invaluable time.
   b) The anesthesiologist caring for the mother's primary responsibility is to the mother. If called upon to assist with resuscitation of the infant, the benefit to the child must be compared to the risk to the mother (4).
   c) Restoring oxygenation and ventilation is the utmost priority as the infant transitions from intrauterine to extrauterine life. Equipment used for this purpose is listed in Table 102-1.

4) Assessment
   a) The initial assessment should take <30 seconds and includes checking for meconium, respiratory effort, color, heart rate (HR), and muscle tone.
      i) These are the clinical factors that guide further resuscitation and reassessment.

745

Table 102-1

Neonatal Resuscitation Equipment

	Equipment/Supplies	Sizes
General	Sterile gown and gloves (if CD) Warm blankets Infant warmer with timer	
Suction	Bulb syringe Suction catheter with meconium aspirator	6, 8, 10, 12 Fr
Bag-mask ventilation	Neonatal resuscitation bag O_2 source Pressure manometer Cushioned face mask	Newborn and premature
Intubation	Laryngoscope blades and handle ETT—uncuffed Thin stylets CO_2 detector	Miller 0 (premature) Miller 1 (term) 2.5 mm < 1,000 g/28 wk 3.0 mm 1,000–2,000 g/28–34 wk 3.5 mm 2,000–3,000 g/34–38 wk 4.0 mm > 3,000 g/>38 wk
Medications	Epinephrine Nalaxone Normal saline	

CD, cesarean delivery; ETT, endotracheal tube; Fr, French; mm, millimeter; wk, weeks.

b) **Apgar scores** (Table 102-2)
    i) Assigned at 1, 5, and 10 minutes of life
   ii) APGAR scores are a retrospective measure of an infant's need for and response to resuscitative measure
  iii) Not particularly useful as an assessment tool to guide resuscitative efforts

Table 102-2

Apgar Scoring

	0	1	2
Color	Blue or pale	Body pink, Extremities blue	Completely pink
Respiratory effort	Absent	Slow, irregular	Good, crying
Heart rate	Absent	<100 bpm	>100 bpm
Reflex irritability	No response	Grimace	Cough, sneeze, cry
Muscle tone	Limp	Some flexion	Good, active motion

5) **Resuscitation: The Neonatal Resuscitation Program (NRP) algorithm is widely available with key points as follows (Fig. 102-1):**
   a) After initial assessment, provide warmth, drying, and stimulation.
   b) Position and clear the airway if necessary.
   c) Provide supplemental O_2 as needed.
   d) If apnea, poor respiratory effort, or HR < 100 bpm → begin effective ventilation either by bag-mask or placing endotracheal tube.
   e) Higher pressures may be required when initiating ventilation to open alveoli. Watch level of chest rise to assess adequate ventilation.
   f) If HR still <100 bpm after 30 to 60 seconds of effective ventilation, start chest compressions.
   g) Chest compressions should occur at a rate of 100 bpm with a breath given after every third compression.
      i) "One and Two and Three and Breathe...."
   h) If HR remains <100 bpm, administer epinephrine.

6) **Resuscitation tips**
   a) Place infant in sniffing position (shoulder roll may be helpful) and apply gentle chin lift into mask to obtain a proper seal. Avoid downward force onto the mask.
   b) Watch for chest rise as primary endpoint to adequate ventilation.
      i) Keep in mind that higher peak inspiratory pressures up to 40 mm Hg may be initially required to open closed alveoli. A pressure manometer is helpful along with clinical indicators such as chest rise.
   c) Avoid insufflation of the stomach as it may further impair ventilation. Decompress if needed.
   d) Chest compressions can be done by encircling the infant with both hands and placing both thumbs on lower sternum or by placing two fingers perpendicular to the chest.
   e) Chest compressions should depress the sternum one third the depth of the chest while the fingers remain in place at all times.
   f) Compressions to ventilation ratio should be 3:1 at a rate of 90 compressions and 30 breaths per minute.
   g) It can be helpful to keep cadence out loud with "One-and-Two-and-Three-and-Breathe."
   h) When the HR is >100 bpm and ventilation is adequate, resuscitation may be stopped.

7) **Special considerations**
   a) Meconium
      i) Occurs in approximately 7% to 20% of live births with up to 10% of these infants developing meconium aspiration syndrome (MAS) (5)
         (1) MAS can lead to hypoxic respiratory failure, persistent pulmonary hypertension, pneumonia, and sepsis all with significant potential for long-term morbidity and mortality.
      ii) Current NRP guidelines call for **intubation and suctioning** of the trachea only if the infant is **not vigorous**, defined as **depressed respirations, decreased muscle tone, or HR <100 bpm** (1).
         (1) In this case, the infant should be intubated and the trachea suctioned while ETT is withdrawn.
         (2) Repeat until lower airways cleared or additional resuscitation should be undertaken (1).

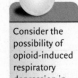

Consider the possibility of opioid-induced respiratory depression in any neonate whose mother has received IV narcotics close to delivery.

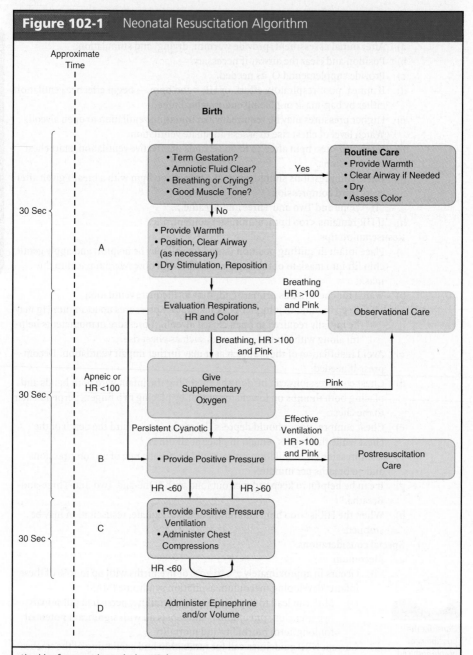

Figure 102-1 Neonatal Resuscitation Algorithm

Algorithm for neonatal resuscitation. HR, heart rate.
Reprinted from 2005 american heart association [AHA] guidelines for cardiopulmonary resuscitation [CPR] and emergency cardiovascular care [ECC] of pediatric and neonatal patients: Neonatal resuscitation. *Pediatrics* 2006; 117:E1029, with permission.

Do not give naloxone to infants of mothers on methadone maintenance or with chronic addiction.

b) **Maternal opioid administration** within 4 hours of delivery may contribute to respiratory depression in the neonate.

   i) If respiratory depression persists after PPV and normal HR, consider administering naloxone; however, PPV and supportive care should continue.

   ii) Keep in mind that the half-life of naloxone may be shorter than that of the circulating opioid and therefore may need to be redosed.

8) Medications

a) **Epinephrine** should be given when the HR remains <100 bpm after 30 seconds of assisted ventilation and an additional 30 seconds of chest compressions.

   i) Can be administered via the endotracheal tube, umbilical vein, or IV

     (1) Regardless of route of administration, dose is **10 to 30 µg/kg.**

   ii) A quick way to make an epinephrine solution for administration is to dilute one ampule (1 mg) into a 100-mL bag of normal saline for a final concentration of 10 µg/mL. The resuscitation dose is then 1 to 3 mL/kg. However, commercial preparations of epinephrine are available in a 1:10,000 solution (100 µg/mL), and the dose would then be 0.1 to 0.3 mL/kg. It is always best to check what will be available at your institution before an emergency arises.

b) **Naloxone**

   i) Administration can also be via endotracheal or IV routes.

   ii) Recommended dose is **0.1 mg/kg.**

Chapter Summary for Neonatal Resuscitation	
General Considerations	A large number of infants will require assistance with breathing and/or resuscitation at birth. Neonatal resuscitation should ideally be provided by a provider whose primary responsibility is the infant.
Preparation	Equipment should be prepared prior to an emergency. Doses of medications should be posted and easily accessible.
Primary Goals	Restoring oxygenation and ventilation is the first priority. Infant should be stimulated and the airway cleared, with PPV if necessary. Neonatal resuscitation algorithm may be required in cases of depressed infants.
Special Considerations	Meconium aspiration can cause significant morbidity. In cases of depressed infants, in the presence of meconium, the trachea should be intubated and suctioned. Consider naloxone administration in infants who had acute in utero exposure to opioid medications during maternal labor.

PPV, positive pressure ventilation.

References

1. Kattwinkel J, ed. *Textbook of Neonatal Resuscitation*. 5th ed. Elk Grove Village, IL: American Academy of Pediatrics and American Heart Association; 2006.
2. Rajani AK, Chitkara R, Halamek LP. Delivery room management of the newborn. *Pediatr Clin North Am* 2009;56;515–535.
3. Aziz K, Chadwick M, Baker M, et al. Ante- and intra-artum factors that predict increased need for neonatal resuscitation. *Resuscitation* 2008;79:444–452.
4. American Society of Anesthesiologists Guidelines for Regional Anesthesia in Obstetrics at http://www.asahq.org/publicationsAndServices/ standards/45.pdf. Accessed 6/23/2010.
5. Dargaville PA, Copnell BC. The epidemiology of meconium aspiration syndrome; incidence, risk factors, therapies, and outcome. *Pediatrics* 2006;117:1712–1721.

103 Overview of Pediatric Anesthesiology

Christopher L. Ciarallo, MD

Children are not just little adults. Anesthesiologists must not only be comfortable with wide variation in anatomy and physiology, from the tiny premature infant to the adult with congenital diseases, but also have an understanding of psychological state and developmental issues throughout childhood. Finally, the care of children requires appropriately sized equipment and personnel experienced in the preoperative assessment and postoperative recovery of children.

1) **Ethical and legal considerations**

   a) Minors, with the notable exceptions of emancipated and court-determined mature minors, are not competent to provide **informed consent** for their medical care.

   b) Typically, a surrogate decision maker for the minor (e.g., parent, guardian, or the court) is solicited to provide **informed permission** on behalf of the minor.

   c) Childhood cognitive and moral development suggest a **"rule of sevens" guideline** in pediatric decision-making capacity.

      i) In general, decisions made on behalf of children <7 years old should employ their **best-interests standard**.

      ii) Children 7 to 14 years old can likely differentiate right and wrong and should be involved in **informed assent** to their medical care.

      iii) **Informed assent** is vital in the medical care of the adolescent, but it may be superseded in the event of a life- or limb-threatening emergency.

   d) Confidentiality between the anesthesiologist and the pediatric patient

      i) Must be maintained unless nondisclosure may result in serious harm to the patient or others.

      ii) Minor patients and their guardian should be notified that a preoperative pregnancy test is being performed, but a **positive result should be reported only to the patient**. The patient should be strongly encouraged to discuss this result with her guardian.

   e) **Children of Jehovah's Witnesses**

      i) Require early and open preoperative discussion of blood transfusion.

      ii) Children without cardiovascular disease **will tolerate a serum hemoglobin of 7 g/dL** without significant acidosis or organ dysfunction (1).

      iii) In the situation of potentially critical anemia and guardian refusal of blood products, a **court order must be obtained preoperatively** to make the "neglected child" a ward of the court for the perioperative period. A hospital ethics service consultation should be considered.

A straight laryngoscope blade (Miller, Wisconsin, Wis-Hipple) is recommended for endotracheal intubation in children <2 years old.

2) **Anatomy and physiology**

a) **Airway**

READ MORE

Management of the pediatric difficult airway, Chapter 126, page 873; Practical pediatrics, Chapter 129, page 873

i) Pediatric patients have a proportionately larger occiput and shorter neck than adults. As a result, a **shoulder roll rather than a head pillow may improve airway patency** during mask ventilation and endotracheal intubation.

ii) **Infants <6 months old are obligate nasal breathers.**

iii) The pediatric epiglottis is long and floppy, and the pediatric larynx is more anterior and cephalad (at the level of the C3-4 vertebral body rather than C5-6 as in adults).

iv) Modern bronchoscopic data suggest that the pediatric cricoid cartilage is ellipsoid rather than round and that the pediatric subglottic area is cylindrical with the narrowest portion at the glottis rather than at the cricoid cartilage (2).

v) Uncuffed endotracheal tubes (ETTs) may not provide effective occlusion for positive-pressure ventilation and may lead to repeated laryngoscopy and intubation for tube exchanges.

Insertion of LMA backward with partially inflated cuff and then rotating 180 degrees to the anatomic position provides the highest success rate.

(1) Poorly fitted tubes result in unreliable ventilation and capnography, anesthetic gas pollution, and increased fresh gas waste.

vi) **Pediatric cuffed ETTs**

(1) **Can be safely used for children as young as full-term neonates.**

(2) Have smaller internal diameters and increase the work of breathing during spontaneous ventilation.

(3) The cuff should be positioned entirely below the glottis, and the pressure checked frequently when using nitrous oxide.

vii) **Appropriate ETT depth**

(1) May be approximated by the various formulae (e.g. 4+[age(in years)/4] for uncuffed; 3.5+[age(in years)/4] for cuffed) or by aligning the ETT double black line markers at the vocal cords.

The most critical factor in selecting the appropriate ETT size is the ability to maintain an air leak at <20 to 25 cm H_2O pressure to minimize the risk of mucosal ischemia and subsequent subglottic stenosis.

(2) **The most reliable method of determining correct tube depth is to deliberately mainstem the ETT and withdraw it until bilateral breath sounds are heard.** The ETT should be secured at a position 1 to 2 cm (depending on age) proximal to this point above the carina (3).

viii) **Single-lung ventilation**

(1) Children under the age of 6 years old require a single-lumen mainstem intubation or a 5-Fr bronchial blocker.

(2) The smallest double-lumen ETT (26 Fr) has an outer diameter of 9.3 mm and is likely not appropriate for children under 8 years old.

READ MORE

Practical pediatric anesthesia, Chapter 129, page 899

ix) **Laryngeal mask airways (LMAs)**

(1) Sized primarily based on patient weight and can be utilized in infants as small as 3 to 5 kg.

(2) In children 6 months to 6 years old, **inserting the LMA backward** with a partially inflated cuff and then rotating 180 degrees to an anatomic position provides the highest success rate and the lowest incidence of airway complications (4).

The most reliable method of determining correct ETT depth is to deliberately mainstem the ETT and withdraw until bilateral breath sounds are heard.

READ MORE
Practical pediatric anesthesia, Chapter 129, page 899

All intravenous tubing and injectates must be meticulously deaired, as the incidence of intracardiac shunt and relative intravascular air volumes are higher in the pediatric population.

Bradycardia is poorly tolerated in pediatric patients. Have a low threshold to treat with atropine, glycopyrrolate, or epinephrine early.

b) **Respiratory**

   i) Children have pliable ribs and increased chest wall compliance along with smaller airways, a reduced number of alveoli, and reduced parenchymal lung compliance.

     (1) **The resulting higher closing volumes and a relative increase in intra-abdominal contents lead to significantly reduced functional residual capacity.**

   ii) **Children have twice the oxygen consumption** of adults (6 to 8 cc/kg/min compared to 3 to 4 cc/kg/min), providing limited reserve during periods of apnea.

     (1) Accordingly, **true rapid sequence induction is rarely utilized** in pediatric anesthesia (e.g., pyloric stenosis, small-bowel obstruction).

   iii) Neonates, particularly premature neonates, have an underdeveloped central respiratory drive and may **react to hypercarbia and hypoxemia with apnea.**

     (1) Opioids should be used judiciously in this population, and questionable neonates should be admitted to the intensive care unit for apnea monitoring.

c) **Cardiovascular**

   i) The **pediatric autonomic nervous system is parasympathetic dominant**, and children frequently respond to noxious stimuli with bradycardia.

   ii) Infants and neonates have a relatively noncompliant left ventricle that cannot increase contractility to increase cardiac output.

   iii) Hypocalcemia should be considered and corrected in hypotensive pediatric patients.

   iv) Hypovolemic pediatric patients may not manifest tachycardia before systemic hypotension.

d) **Vascular access**

   i) Intravenous access can be challenging in pediatric patients, and "blind" techniques may be necessary.

   ii) Reliable locations for "blind" access are the **saphenous vein** just anterosuperior to the medial malleolus, the **median cubital vein** in the antecubital fossa, and the **dorsal hand vein** between the fourth and the fifth carpal bones.

   iii) Intraosseous access is more precarious but may be obtained with an intraosseous or Touhy needle in the **proximal tibia, distal tibia, or distal femur**.

   iv) Central venous access can also be difficult in pediatric patients, but the use of ultrasound has been shown to markedly increase success rates while reducing complications (5).

   v) The Valsalva maneuver is the most effective technique to increase the cross-sectional area of the internal jugular or the femoral veins in children (6), while inguinal compression will also effectively augment the femoral vein (7).

   vi) Guidewire-assisted radial artery cannulation may be more efficient and successful than a direct cannulation technique in pediatric patients (8).

e) **Hepatorenal**

   i) Neonates have relatively increased total body water and reduced plasma protein concentration.

READ
MORE

Practical pediatric anesthesia, Chapter 129, page 899

Maintenance fluids are slightly hypotonic at a rate per hour as calculated by the "4-2-1 rule" (4 mL/kg for the first 10 kg, 2 mL/kg for the subsequent 10 kg, and 1 mL/kg for each kg thereafter).

READ
MORE

Practical pediatric anesthesia, Chapter 129, page 899

    ii) Total protein and albumin binding do not reach adult values until 10-12 months old.

    iii) Hepatic P-450 enzymes mature over months to years, and glucuronidation does not mature until 6 months of life.

    iv) Importantly, amide local anesthetics, morphine, barbiturates, and diazepam are cleared more slowly in infants than older children (9).

    v) **Morphine should be used with caution in unmonitored infants <6 months old**.

    vi) Glomerular filtration and renal concentrating ability do not mature until 5 to 6 months of life, and excessive intravascular sodium cannot be effectively excreted. **Intraoperative fluid resuscitation should be made with an isotonic balanced salt solution.**

    vii) As hepatic glycogen stores are minimal during the first few months of life, prolonged fasting in neonates mandates blood glucose testing and/or **supplemental IV dextrose at a rate of 6 to 8 mg/kg/min.**

    viii) In general, **all children <3 months old and those with significant liver disease, sepsis, or prolonged parenteral nutrition should have intraoperative glucose supplementation.**

f) **Hematologic**

    i) **Physiologic anemia occurs between the second and the third months of life, with a hemoglobin nadir around 11 to 11.5 g/dL.**

    ii) Estimated blood volumes are around 100 mL/kg for premature neonates, 90 mL/kg for term neonates, 80 mL/kg for infants, and 70 to 75 mL/kg for small children.

    iii) Red blood cell transfusions in neonates and immunocompromised children should be crossmatched, leukoreduced, and irradiated. Other children require only cross-matched and leukoreduced red blood cells.

    iv) Stored blood may have elevated plasma potassium levels, but small-volume transfusions very rarely cause hyperkalemia.

        (1) In the event of anticipated massive transfusion, **fresh (<7 days from collection)** or **washed red blood cells** may be requested from the blood bank.

g) **Gastrointestinal**

    i) Compared with adults, pediatric fasting gastric contents are of larger volume (on a mL/kg basis) and of lower pH (10).

    ii) The overall incidence of pediatric perioperative pulmonary aspiration is approximately 1:2,000 to 1:3,000 anesthetics, with 80% occurring during induction of anesthesia (11). Surprisingly, morbidity associated with pediatric pulmonary aspiration is very low, and **patients not requiring supplemental O_2 within 2 hours of an aspiration event may be safely discharged home without sequelae (11)** (Table 103-1).

h) **Dermatologic**

    i) Pediatric patients dissipate heat readily during anesthesia as a result of their relative large body surface area, thin skin, and insufficient fat stores.

    ii) Forced air warmers, heating lamps, and warmed IV fluids are important in pediatric temperature maintenance. Operating room temperatures may be raised to 75°F to 80°F.

Table 103-1

Pediatric NPO Guidelines

	American Society of Anesthesiologists Fasting Guidelines	Children's Hospital of Philadelphia Fasting Guidelines (12)
Clear liquids	2 h	2 h
Breast milk	4 h	3 h
Infant formula	6 h	4 h if < 6 mo old 6 h if ≥ 6 mo old
Nonhuman milk	6 h	6 h
Light snack	6 h	6 h
Large meal, fats, meats	8 h	8 h

Hypothermia may lead to delayed awakening, apnea, coagulopathy, insufficient reversal of neuromuscular blockade, and delayed drug metabolism.

3) Preoperative evaluation

  a) **Separation anxiety**

    i) During normal development, children become distressed when removed from their caregivers at around 8 to 9 months of life.

    ii) **Oral midazolam at a dose of 0.3 to 0.5 mg/kg (maximum 20 mg)** is an effective sedative and anxiolytic when given 10 to 30 minutes before induction.

    iii) Parental presence at induction

      (1) Surprisingly, as compared with midazolam, **parental presence during induction of anesthesia does not appear to alleviate the objective or the subjective anxiety in either the parent or the child** (13).

      (2) Appears to increase parental satisfaction with the anesthetic, provided they are forewarned of the peculiar ocular and body movements observed during Stage II anesthesia. (Table 103-2)

  b) **Preoperative labs (9)**

    i) Routine preoperative laboratory testing of pediatric patients is not indicated. However, certain disease states warrant further evaluation.

    ii) **Former premature infants** <56 weeks postconceptual age (PCA) should have a preoperative hematocrit, as a value <30 may be associated with apnea after anesthesia.

    iii) Pediatric patients with **sickle cell disease** should have a preoperative hemoglobin electrophoresis and hematocrit, as percentage of hemoglobin S HbS > 40% or Hct < 30 are risk factors for sickle crisis.

    iv) **Hemophiliac patients** should have preoperative factor VIII or IX level drawn to assist in factor replacement therapy.

    v) Patients with **diabetes mellitus** should have preoperative glucose checked.

    vi) Patients with **diabetes insipidus** should have preoperative electrolytes documented.

PEDIATRIC ANESTHESIA

Table 103-2
Pediatric Premedication

Premedication	Suggested Dose (mg/kg)
Midazolam (oral)	0.25–0.5
Midazolam (intranasal)	0.2–0.3
Midazolam (intravenous)	0.05–0.1
Ketamine (oral)	3–6
Ketamine (intramuscular)	2–3
Ketamine (intravenous)	0.5
Clonidine (oral)	0.002–0.004
Methohexital (rectal)	25

READ
MORE

Congenital
heart disease,
Chapter 112,
page 798

c) **Congenital heart disease**
  i) Preoperative consultation with a pediatric cardiologist or a pediatric cardiac anesthesiologist is strongly recommended to address the cardiac anatomy, function, and altered physiology in congenital heart disease.
  ii) Recent (i.e., within the last 3 to 6 months) cardiac catheterization and echocardiography reports should be obtained.
d) **Asthma**
  i) The patient's home medication schedule, known triggers, and overall control should be assessed.
  ii) Prior emergency room visits, endotracheal intubation or intensive care admissions, and corticosteroid use are markers of more severe disease.
  iii) Parents should be questioned about familiarity with nebulizer masks or metered-dose inhalers.
  iv) **Home medications should be taken preoperatively, even in asymptomatic patients.**
  v) Airway management may consist of an LMA or ETT.
    (1) Laryngeal masks may be less likely to induce bronchospasm, but will be ineffective in delivering high positive airway pressures, if required.
    (2) Adequate anesthesia is critical during intubation, and consideration should be given to deep extubation.
  vi) In children with reactive airways, **sevoflurane is a more effective bronchodilator than desflurane** at 1 minimal alveolar concentration (MAC) (14).
  vii) Inhaled β-agonists and IV corticosteroids should be readily available.

Laryngeal
masks may
reduce the
incidence of
respiratory
complications
as compared to
endotracheal
intubation and
may be safely
utilized 2 or
more weeks
following a URI
(16).

e) **Upper respiratory infection (URI)**
  i) **Recent (within 4 weeks) or concurrent URI** in children increases the perianesthetic risk of oxygen desaturation, breath holding, laryngospasm, bronchospasm, and coughing.
  ii) Independent risk factors for respiratory complications include **endotracheal intubation in a child <5 years old, history of prematurity, history of reactive airway disease, paternal smoking, airway surgery, presence of copious secretions, and presence of nasal congestion** (15) (Fig. 103-1).

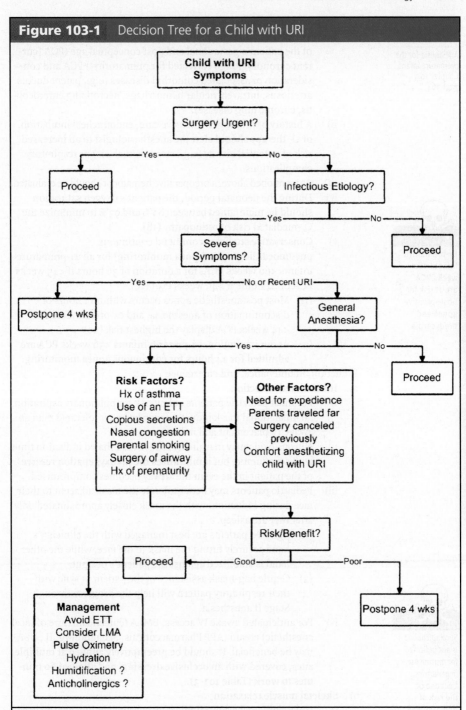

Figure 103-1   Decision Tree for a Child with URI

Suggested algorithm for the assessment and the anesthetic management of the child with an URI.
ETT, endotracheal tube; Hx, history; LMA, laryngeal mask airway; URI, upper respiratory infection.

READ MORE

Anesthesia for the premature infant, Chapter 104, page 764

f) **Ex-premature infant**

   i) The care of an ex-premature infant must include documentation of the patient's gestational and post conceptual age (PCA [current chronologic age corrected for prematurity]) PCA and consideration of associated comorbid diseases (e.g., patent ductus arteriosus, intraventricular hemorrhage, necrotizing enterocolitis, chronic lung disease).

   ii) A history of prolonged intensive care, endotracheal intubation, or O_2 therapy should alert the anesthesiologist to an increased risk of potential airway (e.g., stenosis/malacia) or respiratory complications.

   iii) As mentioned above, a preoperative hematocrit should be evaluated.

   iv) During the neonatal period, the patient's **oxygen saturation should be maintained between 88% and 93%** to minimize the O_2-mediated risk of retinopathy (18).

Ex-premature infants <60 weeks PCA are at risk for postoperative apnea and bradycardia.

   v) **Conservative studies recommend continuous pneumocardiography (apnea monitoring) for all ex-premature infants <60 weeks PCA, for a duration of 36 hours if <45 weeks PCA or 24 hours if >45 weeks PCA** (19).

   (1) Most postanesthetic apnea occurs within 12 hours of discontinuation of anesthesia, and ex-preterm infants <44 weeks PCA display the highest risk (20).

   (2) At our institution, **ex-preterm infants <56 weeks PCA are admitted for 24 hours for continuous apnea monitoring.**

4) **Induction, maintenance, and emergence**

   a) **Inhalational induction**

   i) For most pediatric patients at low risk for pulmonary aspiration, an inhalational mask induction may be better tolerated than an awake IV placement and induction.

   ii) Nitrous oxide may marginally reduce the inhaled induction time with sevoflurane, but it **minimizes the preoxygenation reserve** of the patient in the event the airway becomes compromised.

   iii) Pediatric patients may better tolerate the mask adjacent to their face during induction, with the mask closely approximated only after they are asleep.

   (1) Agitated patients are best managed with the clinician's hand securely fitting the mask to the face, while the other hand is stabilized against the patient's occiput.

   (2) Gentle bag-mask assistance of the patient in sync with their respiratory pattern will help the progress through Stage II anesthesia.

Succinylcholine is not indicated for routine use in pediatrics, because of the risk of undiagnosed myopathy and hyperkalemic cardiac arrest.

   iv) For anticipated awake IV access, EMLA (eutectic mixture of local anesthetic) cream (APP Pharmaceuticals, Schaumburg, IL, USA) may be beneficial. It should be **preemptively applied at multiple sites, covered with an occlusive dressing, and allowed 60 minutes to work** (Table 103-3).

   b) **Skeletal muscle relaxation**

   i) Unless otherwise contraindicated, succinylcholine may be used for rapid sequence intubations and for the treatment of refractory laryngospasm.

   ii) The **pediatric intubating dose of succinylcholine** is 2 mg/kg IV or 4 mg/kg IM.

Table 103-3

% Vapor to Achieve One Minimum Alveolar Concentration (MAC) as a Function of Age (21)

Age	Approximate Sevoflurane (%)	Approximate Isoflurane (%)	Approximate Desflurane (%)
Preterm	<2.5	1.3	<9.3
Neonate	3.2	1.6	9.3
6 mo old	2.5	1.8	9.9
12 mo old	2.6	1.7	8.7
2 y.o.	2.5	1.6	8.5
6 y.o.	2.5	1.5	8.2

iii) The **laryngospasm dose for succinylcholine is 0.1 mg/kg** IV (22).

iv) As children are particularly prone to bradycardia, succinylcholine should be coadministered with **atropine 0.01 to 0.02 mg/kg IV or IM.**

v) Pediatric patients are routinely intubated without skeletal muscle relaxation.

   (1) Deepening an inhaled anesthetic with intravenous **propofol (1 to 3 mg/kg) OR remifentanil (3 to 5 µg/kg for neonates/infants, 1 to 2 µg/kg for older children) AND atropine (0.01 to 0.02 mg/kg) or glycopyrrolate (0.004 to 0.01 mg/kg)** are appropriate choices to assist with laryngoscopy.

vi) **Topical lidocaine (2 to 4 mg/kg)** to the vocal cords and subglottis may blunt the coughing and laryngospasm reflexes during intubation.

vii) As in adults, nondepolarizing muscle relaxants are dosed according to weight, and should be monitored and reversed according to train-of-four monitoring.

viii) Neuromuscular reversal of all nondepolarizing relaxants is strongly encouraged, as children are at an increased risk of postoperative complications.

Laryngospasm should be aggressively treated with *sustained positive airway pressure,* followed by deepening of anesthesia with IV agents, muscle relaxation, and possible tracheal intubation (24).

   (1) Of note, **vecuronium is a long-acting muscle relaxant in neonates and infants,** with only 10% recovery of neuromuscular function at 60 minutes (9).

c) **Deep extubation**

i) Unless contraindicated by aspiration risk, altered mental status, or difficult intubation, deep tracheal extubation may be appropriate for pediatric patients.

ii) The clinician should be comfortable with managing a pediatric airway, and **appropriate personnel and equipment should be immediately available to monitor and assist with complications during emergence.**

iii) No difference in supplemental O_2 requirements or airway-related complications was apparent between awake and deep tracheal extubation in elective cases (23).

iv) Laryngospasm has an incidence of 0.1% to 1.7%. Failure to effectively recognize and treat laryngospasm may result in hypoxemia, bradycardia, or negative pressure pulmonary edema.

PEDIATRIC ANESTHESIA

d) **Stridor**

i) Postextubation stridor may be a result of edema (i.e., sustained coughing or an inappropriately sized ETT), inflammation (i.e., URI), or glottic secretions/foreign body.

ii) Initial management should include supplemental O_2 (consider positive pressure) and **dexamethasone (0.5 mg/kg IV)**.

iii) Nebulized racemic epinephrine (0.5 mL of 2.25% solution in 2.5 mL normal saline) may help reduce tissue edema but mandates a **4-hour post-treatment observation period** because of the risk of rebound edema and stridor.

iv) **Refractory stridor may necessitate tracheal reintubation with a smaller ETT** and possible otolaryngology evaluation.

e) **Emergence agitation**

i) Across multiple studies, emergence agitation in pediatric patients receiving volatile anesthesia is approximately 30%.

ii) Desflurane, sevoflurane, and isoflurane appear to be of higher risk than halothane or propofol (25,26).

iii) **Propofol (1 mg/kg IV) at the end of surgery may reduce the incidence of emergence agitation** (27).

iv) Hypoxemia, hypercarbia, and urinary retention should be excluded as contributing factors to emergence agitation.

v) Addressing this issue preoperatively with the family may help preempt escalation of parental anxiety in this situation.

f) **Postoperative nausea and vomiting**

i) Postoperative vomiting is rare in neonates and infants.

ii) School-aged children have a higher incidence of nausea and vomiting than adults (34% to 50%), and prophylaxis should be considered (9).

iii) The **combination of dexamethasone (0.15 to 0.5 mg/kg IV) and 5-hydroxytryptamine receptor antagonist (e.g., ondansetron 0.1 mg/kg IV)** provides a 50% to 60% relative risk reduction (28). Metoclopramide (0.1 to 0.15 mg/kg IV) may be an effective rescue antiemetic.

5) **Pain management**

a) **Non-narcotic analgesics**

i) **Acetaminophen may be given orally (15 mg/kg every 6 hours) or rectally (35 to 40 mg/kg one-time loading dose THEN 15 mg/kg/dose)** and is a mild to moderately effective analgesic. An intravenous formulation of acetaminophen is now available for use in children in the US. Refer to the commonly used drug table in Chapter 129 practical pediatrics for dosing.

ii) Maximum dosages of acetaminophen are 60 mg/kg/24 hours in infants under 3 months old and 90 mg/kg/24 hours for older children.

iii) Acetaminophen suppositories are uniformly distributed medications and may be manually divided, but clinicians are notoriously inaccurate in their estimation.

iv) Other effective adjunct analgesics include
(1) **Ibuprofen (10 mg/kg PO)**
(2) **Ketorolac (0.5 mg/kg IV, maximum 30 mg)**

Propofol 1 mg/kg IV given at the end of surgery may reduce the incidence of emergence agitation.

Acetaminophen may be given rectally 35 to 40 mg/kg as a one-time loading dose.

To avoid overdosing, families must be alerted to combination medications that contain acetaminophen (e.g., Tylenol No. 3, Tylenol No. 4, Lortab, Vicodin, Percocet, and other over-the-counter products).

Clinician should decide appropriate interval for redosing medication based on clinical situation and patient condition.

READ MORE

Caudal epidural anesthesia, Chapter 125, page 867, Section XIII, Atlas of peripheral nerve block procedures, Chapters 172–184

The maximum subcutaneous dose of bupivacaine in infants <3 months old is 1.5 to 2 mg/kg. After 3 months, the maximum is 2.5 mg/kg.

For epidural placement, the distance from skin to epidural space in the lumbar spine for children 6 months to 10 years old is approximately 1 mm/kg of body weight.

v) Aspirin and aspirin-containing products should not be routinely given to children under the age of 19 years old because of the risk of developing Reye's syndrome.

b) **Narcotics**

i) Most synthetic and semisynthetic opioids have been successfully used in pediatric patients.

ii) **Methadone and morphine should be used cautiously in unmonitored neonates and infants due to their impaired clearance.**

iii) Continuous opioid infusions in intubated neonates should be **preservative-free** formulations.

iv) Commonly administered parenteral opioids include

(1) **Morphine (0.05 to 0.1 mg/kg IV)**

(2) **Fentanyl (0.0005 to 0.001 mg/kg IV = 0.5 to 1 microgram/kg IV)**

(3) **Hydromorphone (0.01 to 0.015 mg/kg IV)**

v) Commonly administered oral opioids include

(1) **Codeine (with acetaminophen) (0.5 to 1 mg/kg)**

(2) **Oxycodone elixir (0.05 to 0.15 mg/kg)**

(3) **Hydrocodone (with acetaminophen) elixir (0.15 mg/kg)**

c) **Regional anesthesia**

i) Regional anesthesia has been employed with increasing frequency in pediatric patients, particularly since the introduction of ultrasound-guided techniques.

ii) The documented regional anesthesia complication rate in pediatric patients is 0.09% evaluated over 24,000 anesthetics (29).

iii) Local anesthetic toxicity must be considered in all pediatric patients. **The weight-based acceptable doses of local anesthetic must be calculated.**

iv) Neonates and infants have lower serum levels of alpha-1-acid glycoprotein than adults and thus have higher unbound amide local anesthetic levels for equivalent doses. In addition, the time to peak serum levels after injection is prolonged in infants and small children.

v) As in adults, continuous epidural infusions may be performed at the caudal, lumbar, and thoracic levels.

(1) Radiographic or ultrasound confirmation of the final catheter location is recommended.

(2) **The distance from skin to epidural space in the lumbar spine of children 6 months to 10 years old is approximately 1 mm/kg body weight (30).**

(3) Epidural test dose should be performed with 0.5 mcg/kg epinephrine.

(4) Bolus dose should be approximated at 0.04-0.05 mL/kg/dermatome level.

vi) Peripheral nerve blocks are safe and efficacious in pediatric patients.

(1) The dose for individual blocks varies greatly by location and technique (e.g., loss of resistance, ultrasound guided, stimulator guided)

(2) Most peripheral nerves can be successfully anesthetized with **0.2 to 0.3 cc/kg or less of local anesthetic.**

(3) In general, pediatric nerve blocks are shorter in duration than adult blocks.

PEDIATRIC ANESTHESIA

Chapter Summary for Pediatric Anesthesia Overview

Overview	Pediatric anesthesia is a specialized practice of anesthesiology that requires specific skills and knowledge of anatomy, pathophysiology, and procedures unique to children and infants.
Ethical and Legal Issues	Minors are usually not competent to provide informed consent for their medical care. Unique issues of informed permission from surrogate decision makers and informed assent for older children apply.
Airway Anatomy	Pediatric patients can have long and floppy epiglottis and the larynx is more anterior and cephalad. Using a straight blade and having patient in a sniffing position can help with intubation.
Preoperative Issues	Separation anxiety begins after 8 to 9 months of life. Consider oral midazolam 0.3–0.5 mg/kg (max 20 mg) for sedation and anxiolysis. Presence of a parent at induction does not appear to reduce anxiety compared to midazolam but may increase parental satisfaction provided they are given appropriate preparation.
Intraoperative Issues	Most pediatric patients have a low risk of pulmonary aspiration. Inhalational mask induction is generally better tolerated than awake IV placement and IV induction. Succinylcholine is contraindicated for routine use in pediatrics.
Postoperative Issues	Postextubation stridor may be due to edema, inflammation, or glottic secretions/foreign body and may be treated with steroids, nebulized racemic epinephrine, and supplemental oxygen. Laryngospasm should be aggressively treated with sustained positive airway pressure, deepening anesthesia with IV agents, and muscle relaxation. Endotracheal intubation may be necessary.

References

1. Lacroix J, Hebert PC, Hutchison JS, et al. Transfusion strategies for patients in pediatric intensive care units. *N Engl J Med* 2007;356(16): 1609–1619.
2. Dalal PG, Murray D, Messner AH, et al. Pediatric laryngeal dimensions: an age-based analysis. *Ped Anesth* 2009;108:1475–1479.
3. Mariano ER, Ramamoorthy C, Chu LF, et al. A comparison of three methods for estimating appropriate tracheal tube depth in children. *Ped Anesth* 2005;15:846–851.
4. Ghai B, Makkar JK, Bhardwaj N, et al. Laryngeal mask airway insertion in children: comparison between rotational, lateral, and standard technique. *Ped Anesth* 2008;18:308–312.
5. Chuan WX, Wei W, Yu L. A randomized-controlled study of ultrasound prelocation vs. anatomical landmark-guided cannulation of the internal jugular vein in infants and children. *Ped Anesth* 2005;15:733–738.
6. Verghese ST, Nath A, Zenger D, et al. The effects of the simulated Valsalva maneuver, liver compression, and/or Trendelenberg position on the cross-sectional area of the internal jugular vein in infants and young children. *Anesth Analg* 2002;94:250–254.
7. Kim JT, Park CS, Kim HJ, et al. The effect of inguinal compression, Valsalva maneuver, and reverse Trendelenberg position on the cross-sectional area of the femoral vein in children. *Anesth Analg* 2009;108:1493–1496.
8. Yildirim V, Ozal E, Cosar A, et al. Direct versus guidewire-assisted pediatric radial artery cannulation technique. *J Cardiothorac Vasc Anesth* 2006;20:48–50.
9. Holzman RS, Mancuso TJ, Polaner DM, eds. *A Practical Approach to Pediatric Anesthesia*. 1st ed. Philadelphia, PA: Wolters Kluwer; 2008.
10. Manchikanti L, Colliver JA, Marrero TC, et al. Assessment of age-related acid aspiration risk factors in pediatric, adult, and geriatric patients. *Anesth Analg* 1985;64:11–17.
11. Warner MA, Warner ME, Warner DO, et al. Perioperative pulmonary aspiration in infants and children. *Anesthesiology* 1999;90:66–71.
12. Cook-Sather SD, Litman RS. Modern fasting guidelines in children. *Best Pract Res Clin Anaesthesiol* 2006;20:471–81.
13. Chundamala J, Wright JG, Kemp SM. An evidence-based review of parental presence during anesthesia induction and parent/child anxiety. *Can J Anesth* 2009;56:57–70.
14. von Ungern-Sternberg BS, Saudan S, Petak F, et al. Desflurane, but not sevoflurane impairs airway and respiratory tissue mechanics in children with susceptible airways. *Anesthesiology* 2008;108:216–224.
15. Tait AR, Malviya S, Voepel-Lewis T, et al. Risk factors for perioperative adverse respiratory events in children with upper respiratory tract infections. *Anesthesiology* 2001;95:299–306.

16. von Ungern-Sternberg BS, Boda K, Schwab C, et al. Laryngeal mask airway is associated with an increased incidence of adverse respiratory events in children with recent upper respiratory tract infections. Anaesthesiology 2007;107:714-9.
17. Tait AR, Malviya S. Anesthesia for the child with an upper respiratory tract infection: still a dilemma? *Anesth Analg* 2005;100:59–65.
18. Saugstad OD. Optimal oxygenation at birth and in the neonatal period. *Neonatology* 2007;91:319–322.
19. Kurth CD, Spitzer AR, Broennie AM, et al. Postoperative apnea in preterm infants. *Anesthesiology* 1987;66:483–488.
20. Malviya A, Swartz J, Lerman J. Are all preterm infants younger than 60 weeks postconceptual age at risk for postanesthetic apnea? *Anesthesiology* 1993;78:1076–1081.
21. Eger EI. Age, minimum alveolar anesthetic concentration, and minimum alveolar anesthetic concentration-awake. *Anesth Analg* 2001;93:947–953.
22. Chung DC, Rowbottom SJ. A very small dose of suxamethonium relieves laryngospasm. *Anaesthesia* 1993;48:229–230.
23. Patel RI, Hannallah RS, Norden J, et al. Emergence airway complications in children: a comparison of tracheal extubation in awake and deeply anesthetized patients. *Anesth Analg* 1991;73:266–270.
24. Burgoyne LL, Anghelescu DL. Intervention steps for treating laryngospasm in pediatric patients. *Paediatr Anaesth* 2008;18:297–302.
25. Meyer RR, Munster P, Werner C, et al. Isoflurane is associated with a similar incidence of emergence agitation/delirium as sevoflurane in young children—a randomized controlled study. *Paediatr Anaesth* 2007;17:56–60.
26. Welborn LG, Hannallah RS, Norden JM, et al. Comparison of emergence and recovery characteristics of sevoflurane, desflurane, and halothane in pediatric ambulatory patients. *Anesth Analg* 1996;83:917–920.
27. Abu-Shahwan I. Effect of propofol on emergence behavior in children after sevoflurane general anesthesia. *Paediatr Anaesth* 2008;18:55–59.
28. Engelman E, Salengros J, Barvais L. How much does pharmacologic prophylaxis reduce postoperative vomiting in children: calculation of prophylaxis effectiveness and expected incidence of vomiting under treatment using Bayesian meta-analysis. *Anesthesiology* 2008;109:1023–1035.
29. Giaufre E, Dalens B, Gombert A. Epidemiology and morbidity of regional anesthesia in children: a one-year prospective survey of the French-Language Society of Pediatric Anesthesiologists. *Anesth Analg* 1996;83:904–912.
30. Bosenberg AT, Gouws E. Skin-epidural distance in children. *Anaesthesia* 1995;50:895–897.

PEDIATRIC ANESTHESIA

104

Part A: Diseases in Pediatric Patients
Anesthesia for the Premature Infant

Julie L. Williamson, DO

Premature birth is defined as birth prior to 37 weeks' gestational age and is an important cause of morbidity and mortality in children. In the United States, the rate of premature birth is 12.7% and has increased 36% over the last 25 years, largely due to late pre-term (34 to 36 weeks' postgestational age) births (1). Premature babies are more likely to have underlying congenital disorders (3% to 7% in very low birth weight infants). Eighty-five percent of neonates with a birth weight >500 g will survive and represent a substantial proportion of children presenting for anesthesia (2). Even in the absence of underlying anomalies or with later preterm infants, careful anesthetic management is needed to optimize their vulnerable physiologic state.

Awake intubations are commonly performed by neonatologists and may be the most prudent method of securing the airway of a premature infant with a potentially difficult airway.

1) **Physiology and implications of prematurity**
   a) **Airway**
      i) Endotracheal tubes (ETTs)
         (1) Tiny ETTs (2.0 to 3.0) are at increased risk for obstruction due to kinking and secretions.
         (2) Inspired gasses should be warmed and humidified.
         (3) Frequent suctioning may be required.
      ii) **Subglottic stenosis** is common in previously intubated infants. Smaller-than-anticipated ETTs should be prepared.
      iii) Tracheomalacia or bronchomalacia may cause airway collapse on exhalation. This can be overcome with continuous positive airway pressure (CPAP) or positive end expiratory pressure (PEEP).
      iv) While **awake intubation** by direct laryngoscopy is not common in anesthesiology, it is common in the NICU and may be the most prudent method in this patient population if a difficult airway is suspected.
   b) **Central nervous system (3)**
      i) Periventricular leukomalacia and hemorrhagic infarction are common in premature infants of 27 weeks' gestational age and younger.
         (1) Grade I **intraventricular hemorrhage (IVH)** is bleeding into the fragile germinal matrix of the ventricles and is the most common site of bleeding in prematures. Does not correlate to neurologic outcome.
         (2) Grade II IVH indicates bleeding into the ventricle.
         (3) Grade III IVH causes enlargement of the ventricle.
         (4) Grade IV IVH involves intraparenchymal bleeding and may require placement of a ventricular peritoneal shunt, and is associated with adverse neurologic outcomes.

Avoid extreme swings in blood pressure to minimize risk of intraventricular bleeding.

Coagulopathy should be aggressively treated to minimize risk of intracranial bleeding.

Supplemental O_2 should be avoided when possible in infants until 44 weeks' postgestational age.

Parasympathetic tone predominates in the neonate, so atropine may be used to prevent bradycardia on induction.

Apnea is both centrally mediated and obstructive in premature infants and neonates.

ii) Cerebral autoregulation and complications
  (1) The limits of cerebral autoregulation in the premature infant are unknown; therefore a key anesthetic goal is avoidance of extreme swings in blood pressure.
    (a) Hypotension is a risk factor for cerebral ischemia.
    (b) Hypertension may increase risk of IVH.
  (2) Coagulopathy should be aggressively treated prior to undergoing surgery.
iii) **Retinopathy of prematurity (ROP)** is pathology of retinal vasculature in which aberrant vascular development can cause retinal tears and detachment and may ultimately lead to blindness.
  (1) Risk factors for ROP include **prematurity, low birth weight, and exposure to supplemental O_2**. Up to 70% of neonates weighing <1,000 g will be affected.
  (2) Supplemental O_2 should be avoided when possible in infants until 44 weeks' postgestational age (4).
  (3) Supplemental O_2 should be given with a goal SpO_2 for the neonate above 90%.
iv) **Parasympathetic tone predominates in the neonate.** Removal of sympathetic tone with anesthetic agents can cause profound bradycardia and hypotension.
  (1) It is common to premedicate infants with vagolytic drugs prior to induction or to manipulation of the peritoneum or the eyes.
  (2) **Atropine 10 μg/kg with a minimum dose of 100 μg can be used to prevent bradycardia on induction.**

c) **Respiratory system**
  i) Central response to hypoxia and hypercapnia is dysregulated in the premature infant. Although ventilation may initially increase, the infant quickly may become apneic.
  ii) Anesthetic agents will suppress the response to hypoxia or hypercapnia, placing the emerging or the postoperative infant at increased risk for apnea.
    (1) **Apnea is both centrally mediated and obstructive in premature infants and neonates.**
      (a) Central apnea may result from hypoxia, hypercarbia, intracranial hemorrhage, hypothermia, airway stimulation, or without any apparent inciting event.
      (b) Obstructive apnea is associated with oropharyngeal incoordination and hypotonia and is commonly due to obstruction from the tongue.
    (2) **Oral airways are often needed to mask ventilate premature infants.**
    (3) Postoperative apnea >15 seconds or associated with bradycardia or desaturation is common in the premature infant, and its occurrence is proportional to early gestational age and is associated with anemia (HCT < 30%) and invasive surgical procedures (5).
  iii) Functional residual capacity is 30 cc/kg, similar to that of an adult. However, alveolar ventilation is two to three times that of an adult (100 to 150 cc/kg/min), reflecting the greater O_2 consumption of the infant.

Oral airways are often needed to mask ventilate premature infants.

Preoxygenate the patient to mitigate the rapid desaturation during induction.

iv) Preoxygenate whenever feasible to mitigate the rapid desaturation of the infant during induction.

v) **Surfactant is not endogenously produced until 34 weeks of gestation.**

    (1) Respiratory distress syndrome is a consequence of inadequate (premature infants) or delayed (infants of diabetic mothers) surfactant production. Lung volumes and compliance are decreased and intrapulmonary shunt, V/Q mismatching, and risk of pneumothorax are increased in this disease state (5).

    (2) **Continuous PEEP may aid oxygenation.** Decreased lung compliance may require high peak inflating pressures that risk pneumothorax and interstitial emphysema.

    (3) Pressure control ventilation and monitoring of peak pressures and tidal volumes are needed to avoid lung damage.

    (4) Decompensation of a ventilated infant should raise concern for pneumothorax, which can be evacuated with a 22-gauge IV catheter placed at the second intercostal space in the anterior axillary line.

    (5) Continued supplemental O_2 requirement at 36 weeks' gestational age is referred to as **chronic lung disease**. These children are at increased risk of perioperative laryngospasm and bronchospasm into the early school age years.

d) **Cardiovascular system**

i) A poorly organized myocardium, poor diastolic function, and increased amount of connective tissue lead to decreased compliance in the neonatal heart.

Goal SpO2 for the neonate should be >90%.

ii) Premature infants have limited ability to augment stroke volume; therefore, **cardiac output is strongly dependent on heart rate.**

iii) Circulating blood volume is also quite limited in the small premature infant.

iv) **The combination of high resting heart rate, decreased stroke volume reserve, and low blood volume predisposes the premature infant to cardiovascular collapse during induction of anesthesia or major surgical events (3).**

v) Vasodilation, myocardial dysfunction, and bradycardia from volatile agents are poorly tolerated in premature infants.

Vasodilation, myocardial dysfunction, and bradycardia from volatile agents are poorly tolerated in premature infants.

vi) The transition to extrauterine physiology is often delayed in these infants. Failure of the ductus arteriosus and the foramen ovale to close is common.

    (1) **Strict attention should be paid to avoid air bubbles in IV tubing and injections to prevent "paradoxical" shunting of air emboli from the right to the left atrium.**

    (2) **Patent ductus arterious (PDA)** can cause pulmonary hypertension and even congestive heart failure.

        (a) Infants in the neonatal intensive care unit (NICU) with PDA are often treated with fluid restriction and diuretics, which may lead to a hypovolemic infant with electrolyte derangements presenting for surgery.

        (b) Fluid resuscitation and sodium and potassium imbalance may need to be corrected prior to induction.

READ MORE
congenital heart disease, Chapter 112, page 798

e) **Gastroenteric system**

i) Hyperbilirubinemia requiring phototherapy is ubiquitous in prematures and treatment with "bili lights" will **increase insensible fluid losses.**

ii) NPO times are generally the same as older children: 2 hours for clears, 4 hours for breast milk, and 6 hours for formula.

f) **Fluid, electrolytes, and nutrition**

Use dextrose-containing fluid as a maintenance solution and then replace losses with non–dextrose-containing isotonic fluids.

For hypoglycemia (<40 mg/dL), bolus 2 to 4 cc/kg of 10% dextrose over 1 minute IV.

i) Glucose requirement is relatively high. Infusion of 5 mL/kg/h of 10% dextrose-containing solution will provide the 6 to 8 mg/kg/min glucose infusion rate that the premature infant needs.

ii) If a concentrated dextrose solution (e.g., total parental nutrition with 15% dextrose) is changed to a lower concentration or rate, hypoglycemia can occur rapidly. Regular monitoring of serum glucose levels intraoperatively is recommended.

iii) **Use dextrose-containing fluid as a maintenance solution and then replace losses with non–dextrose-containing isotonic crystalloid, colloid, or blood product as needed.**

iv) For hypoglycemia below 40 mg/dL of glucose, bolus 2 to 4 cc/kg 10% dextrose over 1 minute to provide 200 mg/kg of glucose (5).

v) The neonatal myocardium is relatively dependent on extracellular calcium release, so an ionized calcium level greater than 1.0 mmol/L will aid cardiac output.

(1) **Calcium chloride should be infused via a central line. Calcium gluconate may be slowly infused peripherally (6).**

vi) Sodium and potassium are not repleted in the first day of life. Daily requirements thereafter are similar to adults.

vii) Newborn premature infants may have up to 90% of total body water as extracellular fluid volume.

(1) Spontaneous diuresis over the first few days of life is often augmented by diuretic therapy to treat the respiratory distress syndrome.

(2) These infants often present to the OR with intravascular volume depletion requiring fluid resuscitation prior to induction.

viii) Immature hepatic and renal function, altered volume of distribution, and decreased protein binding **all lead to altered pharmacokinetics in prematures**. It is important to carefully titrate doses of medications to effect (e.g., use a train-of-four stimulator to redose neuromuscular blockade).

g) **Hematologic system**

Blood products for premature infants should be irradiated to prevent graft versus host reaction.

i) Estimated blood volume of the premature infant is 90-100 cc/kg.

ii) **The normal hematocrit of a term newborn is 60%, but an early preterm neonate may have an Hct of 40%.**

iii) Hct below 30% is poorly tolerated and is associated with apnea.

iv) Blood should be filtered, warmed and administered slowly to avoid hyperkalemia.

v) **Blood products for infants should be irradiated to prevent graft versus host reaction, a lethal complication of transfusion in neonates (7).**

vi) **Newborn premature infants commonly have vitamin K deficiency and thrombocytopenia.**

h) **Temperature regulation** is important in small infants.

i) The room should be warmed to 27°C/80°F to avoid metabolic stress.

ii) Radiant warmers can be used.

iii) Inhaled gases should be heated and humidified; transfused fluids and irrigation fluids should be warmed.

2) **Preanesthetic evaluation**

a) History and physical should include assessment of cardiac anatomy if hypoxia or other congenital malformations exist.

b) Volume status should be carefully assessed as preoperative fluid resuscitation may be needed; a sunken fontanelle, decreased skin turgor, or decreasing weight are signs of hypovolemia in the infant.

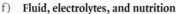

PEDIATRIC ANESTHESIA

3) **Anesthetic management**

a) Anesthesia has been safely delivered to these small, fragile children for decades using both regional and general techniques.

b) **Induction**

MAC of isoflurane is reduced in the premature infant, and even low levels of volatile agent may lead to hemodynamic decompensation.

i) Preoxygenate infant with 100% FiO$_2$.

ii) Consider aspirating gastric contents by orogastric or nasogastric tube prior to induction.

iii) Assure that peripheral IV is patent if IV induction planned.

iv) Consider atropine or glycopyrrolate to decrease secretions and prevent bradycardia.

v) Opioids, midazolam, ketamine, and propofol are commonly used induction agents, though propofol can cause disproportionate hemodynamic decompensation in hypovolemic or sick infants.

vi) Paralysis is obtained with 0.6 mg/kg of rocuronium (up to 1.2 mg/kg for rapid sequence intubation).

c) **Maintenance**

Premature infants currently younger than 60 weeks' postgestational age should be admitted for monitoring postoperatively.

i) MAC (minimum alveolar concentration) of isoflurane is reduced in the premature infant; even low levels of volatile agent may lead to hemodynamic decompensation.

ii) **Ketamine** in doses of 2 to 4 mg/kg every 20 to 30 minutes provides analgesia and anesthesia and maintains circulatory tone in most circumstances.

iii) Opioids are well tolerated with regard to hemodynamics, and titration of high dose opioids (e.g., 10 to 20 micrograms per kilogram of fentanyl) may be used for maintenance if postoperative ventilation is planned.

iv) **Remifentanil infusion** is also well tolerated and allows for early postoperative extubation. Doses of 0.06 to 1 µg/kg/min in combination with volatile agent or up to 2 µg/kg/min have been used to maintain anesthesia (8).

d) **Postoperative management/disposition**

i) **Postanesthetic observation is recommended even in the absence of comorbidities and even if no surgical procedure is performed, (e.g. imaging studies).**

ii) **Apnea is possible even without opioid use and has been reported even when solely regional anesthesia was performed.**

iii) **Current recommendations are to defer surgery and anesthesia until after 60 weeks' postgestational age when possible.**

iv) Anemia (Hct < 30%) increases risk of postoperative apnea.

v) Conservative recommendations are to admit infants less than 60 weeks gestational age after regional or general anesthesia for postoperative monitoring.

vi) At our institution, infants born at less than 37 weeks gestational age who are less then 48 weeks gestational age at the time of the anesthetic will be admitted overnight.

vii) Infants who were born earlier than 37 weeks and who are between 48-60 weeks PCA at the time of anesthetic will be admitted for monitoring if they have any significant comorbidities.

Chapter Summary for Anesthesia for Premature Infants

Definitions	Prematurity: gestational age < 37 weeks. Small for gestational age (aka intrauterine growth restricted) are those <10%tile for gestational age.
Airway	Humidify and warm gases to prevent occlusions. Watch for kinking and obstruction in small ETTs.
Neurologic	Monitor postoperatively for central apnea. Avoid swings in BP causing IVH. Avoid supplemental O_2 causing ROP. High parasympathetic tone—consider pretreatment with atropine.
Respiratory	Increased alveolar ventilation leads to rapid desaturation. Surfactant deficiency leads to high peak inspiratory pressures and risk of pneumothorax.
Cardiovascular	Cardiac output is heart rate dependent. Avoid air bubbles due to presence of shunts.
Fluids, Electrolytes, Nutrition	Deliver adequate glucose infusion rate. Supplement calcium if hemodynamically unstable. Assess for hypovolemia and resuscitate prior to induction.
Hematologic	PRBCs should be warmed, filtered, and irradiated. Hct < 30% is associated with apnea.
Induction	Preoxygenate with 100% oxygen. Pretreat with vagolytic agent.
Maintenance	Volatile agents and propofol may cause hemodynamic instability. Monitor neuromuscular blockade due to variable pharmacokinetics. Maintain thermal environment >80°F.
Postoperative	High risk for apnea. Monitor infants <60 wk postgestational age overnight.

ETT, endotracheal tube; IVH, intraventricular hemorrhage; ROP, retinopathy of prematurity; PRBCs, packed red blood cells.

PEDIATRIC ANESTHESIA

References

1. March of Dimes White Paper on Preterm Birth: The Global and Regional Toll. White Plains, NY2009 [January 24, 2009]; Available from: www.marchofdimes.com/files/66423_MOD-Complete.pdf?src=mod.com
2. Fanaroff AA, Stoll BJ, Wright LL, et al. Trends in neonatal morbidity and mortality for very low birthweight infants. *Am J Obstet Gynecol* 2007;196(2):147.e1–147.e8.
3. Mancuso T. Anesthesia for the preterm newborn. In: Holzman RS MTaPD, ed. *A Practical Approach to Pediatric Anesthesia*. Philadelphia, PA: Lippincott Williams and Wilkins; 2008:601–609.
4. Hauser MW, Valley, Robert D, et al. Anesthesia for pediatric ophthalmic surgery. In: Motoyama EK, Peter J, eds. *Smith's Anesthesia for Infants and Children*. 7th ed. Philadelphia, PA: Mosby Inc.; 2006:781–782.
5. Brett CM, Davis PJ, Bikhazi G. Anesthesia for neonates and premature infants. In: Motoyama EK, PJ, eds. *Smith's Anesthesia for Infants and Children*. 7th ed. Philadelphia, PA: Mosby Elsevier; 2006:521–579.
6. Banasiak KJaC, Thomas O. Disorders of calcium, magnesium and phosphate. In: Nichols DG, ed. *Rogers' Textbook of Pediatric Intensive Care*. 4th ed. Philadelphia, PA: Lippincott Williams & Wilkins; 2008:1641.
7. Litty CA. Neonatal red cell transfusions. *Immunohematology* 2008;24(1):10–14.
8. Galinkin JL, Davis PJ, McGowan FX, et al. A randomized multicenter study of remifentanil compared with halothane in neonates and infants undergoing pyloromyotomy. II. Perioperative breathing patterns in neonates and infants with pyloric stenosis. *Anesth Analg* 2001;93(6):1387–1392.
9. Walther-Larsen S, Rasmussen LS. The former preterm infant and risk of postoperative apnoea: recommendations for management. *Acta Anaesthesiol Scand* 2006;50(7):888–893.

105 Congenital Diaphragmatic Hernia

Julianne M. Mendoza, MD

Congenital diaphragmatic hernia (CDH) occurs in 1:2,000 to 5,000 live births. **Population-based mortality rates among live-born infants with CDH is approximately 50% (1),** though some tertiary pediatric surgical centers have reported much lower mortality rates of 20%.

1) Pathophysiology
   a) A failure of diaphragmatic development during the 7th to 10th weeks of gestation allows for herniation of abdominal viscera into the thorax that compresses developing lung tissue resulting in pulmonary hypoplasia.
   b) **Over 80% of CDH occur at the left posterolateral diaphragm, known as the** *foramen of Bochdalek,* resulting in a left-sided herniation.
   c) The hypoplastic lungs have decreased compliance and surface area for gas exchange resulting hypoxemia and impaired ventilation with acidosis and persistent pulmonary hypertension.
   d) Morbidity and mortality are related to the severity of lung hypoplasia and pulmonary hypertension.

2) Signs/symptoms/clinical findings
   a) **Neonates present at birth in respiratory distress with acute hypoxemia.**
   b) **Physical exam** findings include a scaphoid abdomen, barrel-shaped chest, and absent breath sounds on the ipsilateral side.
   c) Associated findings
      i) **Cardiac anomalies are found in 25% of CDH patients,** including persistent ductus arteriosus, and atrial septal defects and ventricular septal defects.
      ii) Intestinal malrotation and gastroesophageal reflux disease are common.
   d) CXR confirms diagnosis by demonstrating herniated viscera in the thorax often with the cardiac silhouette deviated to the contralateral side.

3) Surgical treatment
   a) Delayed surgical repair until after respiratory and hemodynamic stabilization increases survival (2).
   b) Surgical repair may be performed with the patient on high-frequency oscillatory ventilation (HFOV) when mean airway pressures have been weaned to <12 cm H_2O, or with patient on extracorporeal membrane oxygenation (ECMO) (3).
   c) Surgical approach is usually via a subcostal incision on the ipsilateral side, followed by reduction of the herniated viscera into the abdomen and closure of the diaphragmatic defect primarily or with a synthetic patch.

Congenital cardiac disease occurs in 25% of patients with CDH—echocardiogram is recommended preoperatively.

PEDIATRIC ANESTHESIA

d) Surgical repair usually occurs in the operating room, but some centers have the capability to do the procedure in the neonatal intensive care unit (NICU) for neonates who are unable to be safely transported such as those on ECMO or HFOV.

4) Anesthetic management

  a) **Preoperative considerations**

    i) Assessment of patient

      (1) Care should be taken to note which side of the thorax is involved.

        (a) Right-sided hernias with herniation of liver into the thoracic cavity have been associated with increased morbidity (4).

      (2) Signs of persistent pulmonary hypertension such as hypoxemia and increasing ventilatory requirements may necessitate delay in surgical repair.

      (3) **Hypotension may be secondary to intrathoracic compression from distended herniated viscera.**

    ii) Labs

      (1) Type and cross should be completed, and blood should be immediately available during surgical procedure. Significant blood loss is unusual, unless patient is anticoagulated on ECMO.

      (2) Hemoglobin/hematocrit and platelet count may be obtained for baseline measurement and for comparison during procedure if there is significant bleeding or coagulopathy.

      (3) Other labs depending on clinical condition of patient

        (a) Electrolytes

        (b) Blood gases

    iii) Studies

      (1) **Echocardiogram should be completed prior to surgery to evaluate for structural congenital heart disease and examine function.** Pulmonary artery pressures may be estimated as an indication of possible pulmonary hypertension.

      (2) Cranial ultrasound may be indicated to rule out intracranial hemorrhages in premature infants, or patients anticoagulated on ECMO.

      (3) Renal ultrasound may be indicated to evaluate for structural kidney disease.

  b) **Monitors/lines**

    i) Standard ASA monitors

    ii) Additional pulse oximeters are recommended.

      (1) In case of failure of single oximeter due to poor perfusion.

      (2) May consider placing preductal and postductal monitors for patients with congenital heart disease.

    iii) Arterial line is usually indicated as lung disease will warrant frequent monitoring of arterial blood gases, in addition to beat-to-beat blood pressure monitoring.

    iv) Central venous line is usually indicated to provide high concentration dextrose solutions, calcium replacement, or other inotropic infusions.

    v) Additional peripheral IVs may be necessary, especially if central venous access is not available.

    vi) If patient is on ECMO, then additional line placement may be contraindicated because of increased risk to an anticoagulated patient.

  c) **Intraoperative management**

    i) **Induction**

Avoid positive-pressure MASK ventilation—to prevent gastric insufflation and expanding herniated bowel in lung. Use low PIP if mask ventilation is necessary.

(1) Symptomatic patients are usually already in the NICU intubated, with umbilical arterial lines and umbilical venous access on sedatives, analgesics, or muscle relaxants.

(2) Historically, neonatologists may perform an awake intubation in the delivery room or on hemodynamically unstable patients; however, this is not recommended for patients with severe respiratory distress as it may exacerbate pulmonary hypertension.

(3) **An orogastric or a nasogastric tube inserted preoperatively may help decompress the herniated contents and improve ventilation.**

(4) For patients who are more stable and may not be intubated

    (a) Patient should be preoxygenated with 100% FiO_2 barring any congenital cardiac physiologic contraindications.

    (b) Secure airway immediately with endotracheal tube (ETT) while minimizing positive-pressure mask ventilation, which may cause gastric distension and increase pulmonary compression.

    (c) N_2O should not be used as it limits the FiO_2 and may exacerbate lung compression.

(5) The use of muscle relaxants facilitates intubation and may decrease need for high peak pressures when mask ventilating.

(6) If patient is on HFOV or ECMO, paralytic for muscle relaxation and narcotics may be added to the sedation regimen already in place.

ii) **Maintenance**

(1) **Unless there are cardiac contraindications, 100% O_2 should be maintained throughout the procedure to minimize pulmonary vascular resistance.**

(2) N_2O should not be used as it limits the FiO_2 and may distend bowel contents making repair more difficult.

(3) The use of muscle relaxants facilitates mechanical ventilation, surgical reduction of the herniated viscera, and closure of the diaphragmatic defect.

(4) Adequate analgesia with opioids should be used to alleviate pain and prevent increase in sympathetic tone causing increased pulmonary vascular resistance.

(5) In patients on ECMO, the increased volume of distribution within the circuit necessitates an increased dose of opioids.

(6) Inhaled anesthetics may be used depending on hemodynamic status.

iii) **Special anesthetic considerations**

(1) Place an orogastric or a nasogastric tube after intubation to decompress intestinal contents.

(2) Cardiovascular

    (a) In patients with small abdominal cavities, reduction of the hernia contents into the abdomen may cause hypotension and increased peak inspiratory pressures as the diaphragm is displaced cephalad and the inferior vena cava is compressed by hernia contents.

    (b) Inotropic drugs may be necessary for hemodynamically unstable patients.

(3) Pulmonary/ventilation

    (a) **Use of ICU ventilator instead of anesthesia machine should be considered for patients with severe lung disease or prematurity.**

Place gastric tube to decompress intestinal contents after intubation.

Consider ICU ventilator for patients with severe lung disease or prematurity.

Consider contralateral pneumothorax if patient has acute decompensation.

Table 105-1

Goals of "Gentle Ventilation" and Permissive Hypercapnea

Accept postductal arterial pCO_2 levels of 55–60 mm Hg
Goal pH > 7.35
Accept preductal oxygen saturation >85%
Limit peak inspiratory pressure to <25 cm H_2O

PEDIATRIC ANESTHESIA

(b) Avoid hypoxia and acidosis, which may increase pulmonary vascular resistance or worsen myocardial function.

(c) Avoid barotrauma

  (i) Barotrauma may contribute to 25% of CDH deaths (5).

  (ii) **Consider the presence of a contralateral pneumothorax if the patient demonstrates a sudden decrease in cardiac output, lung compliance, or oxygenation.**

  (iii) **"Gentle ventilation" with permissive hypercapnea** strategies aim to limit peak inspiratory pressure and minimize barotrauma (Table 105-1).

(d) **High-frequency oscillatory ventilation (HFOV)** is used when conventional ventilation modes fail to adequately oxygenate or ventilate patient.

  (i) HFOV allows ventilation at higher mean airway pressures with lower peak inspiratory pressures.

  (ii) HFOV delivers small volumes of air that approximate the anatomic dead space at a rapid rate to maintain alveolar recruitment and improve oxygenation with less barotrauma.

  (iii) Positioning and transport of patient on HFOV are complicated by the limited length of circuit to ETT and the need to keep the circuit in a straight line.

(e) **Extra corporeal membrane oxygenation (ECMO)** may be used in patients with pulmonary hypertension as a temporizing measure until the reactive component of increased pulmonary resistance resolves.

  (i) Requires anticoagulation, which limits the ability to place new lines and increases risk of both surgical and intracranial bleeding.

  (ii) Requires experienced personnel to operate and troubleshoot the circuit.

  (iii) Transport to the OR is complicated, so procedures may be done at the bedside in the NICU.

(f) **Inhaled nitric oxide** can improve oxygenation and decrease intrapulmonary shunt in patients with pulmonary hypertension.

d) **Postoperative management/disposition**

  i) Patients are usually left intubated in the NICU.

  ii) Though the herniation has been repaired, the lungs are still hypoplastic and the risk of pulmonary hypertension is still present.

  iii) Patients should be maintained on sedatives/analgesics to prevent catecholamine release from pain exacerbating pulmonary vascular resistance.

Chapter Summary for Congenital Diaphragmatic Hernia

General Considerations	CDH is a failure of diaphragmatic development that results in herniation of abdominal viscera into the thorax and pulmonary hypoplasia. Over 80% of CDH occur at the left posterolateral diaphragm, known as the *foramen of Bochdalek*, resulting in a left-sided herniation.
Preoperative Considerations	Neonates present at birth in respiratory distress with acute hypoxemia, scaphoid abdomen, barrel-shaped chest, and absent breath sounds on the ipsilateral side. Hypoplastic lungs have decreased compliance and surface area for gas exchange resulting hypoxemia and impaired ventilation with acidosis and persistent pulmonary hypertension. Cardiac anomalies are found in 25% of CDH patients, so echocardiogram recommended preoperatively. Intestinal malrotation and gastroesophageal reflux disease are common. Delayed surgical repair until after respiratory and hemodynamic stabilization increases survival.
Intraoperative Considerations	The airway should be secured immediately with an endotracheal intubation while avoiding positive-pressure ventilation. Hypotension may be secondary to intrathoracic compression from distended herniated viscera. An orogastric or a nasogastric tube inserted preoperatively may help decompress the herniated contents and improve ventilation. Unless there are cardiac contraindications, 100% O_2 should be maintained throughout the procedure to minimize pulmonary vascular resistance. Use of ICU ventilator instead of anesthesia machine should be considered for patients with severe lung disease or prematurity. Consider the presence of a contralateral pneumothorax if the patient demonstrates a sudden decrease in cardiac output, lung compliance, or oxygenation. "Gentle ventilation" with permissive hypercapnea strategies aims to limit peak inspiratory pressure and minimize barotrauma.

References

1. Colvin J, Bowers C, Dickinson JE, et al. Outcomes of congenital diaphragmatic hernia: a population-based study in Western Australia. *Pediatrics* 2005;116(3):e356–e363.
2. Reickart CA, Hirschl RB, Schumacher R, et al. Effect of very delayed repair of congenital diaphragmatic hernia on survival and extracorporeal life support use. *Surgery* 1996;120(4):766–772.
3. Chiu P, Hedrick HL. Postnatal management and long-term outcome for survivors with congenital diaphragmatic hernia. *Prenat Diagn* 2008;28:592–603.
4. Fisher JC, Jefferson RA, Arkovitz MS, et al. Redefining outcomes in right congenital diaphragmatic hernia. *J Pediatr Surg* 2008;43:373.
5. Wilson JM, Lund DP, Lillehei CW, et al. Congenital diaphragmatic hernia—a tale of two cities: the Boston experience. *J Pediatr Surg* 1997;32(3):401–405.

106 Tracheoesophageal Fistula

Julianne M. Mendoza, MD • Calvin Kuan, MD

Tracheoesophageal fistula (TEF) occurs in 1:3,000 births. A survival rate of 90% is often achieved in TEF patients who do not have other congenital anomalies. However, up to 50% of TEF patients have other associated congenital anomalies, and 35% have associated cardiac anomalies.

The most common combination of congenital anomalies seen with TEF is termed the vertebral, anal, cardiac, tracheo-oesophageal fistula, radial aplasia or renal defects, and limb association (VACTERL).

1) Pathophysiology/anatomy
   a) The median pharyngeal groove develops into the respiratory and digestive tubes during gestation. Failure of the mesenchyme between the tubes to separate results in TEF.
   b) There are five types of congenital TEF as described by Gross (3,4) (Fig. 106-1).
      i) **Gross Type C: distal TEF with proximal atretic esophageal pouch is the most common type and accounts for 85% of cases.**
      ii) Gross Type A: isolated esophageal atresia, accounts for 6% of cases.
      iii) Gross Type E: also known as H-type consists of TEF without esophageal atresia and accounts for 6% of cases.
      iv) Gross Type B: proximal TEF with distal esophageal atresia, occurs with a frequency of 2%.
      v) Gross Type D: proximal and distal fistulas, is the least common type with a frequency of 1%.
   c) The usual location of the fistula is one to two tracheal rings above the carina; however, it is not always visible.

2) Signs/symptoms/clinical findings
   a) Neonates often present with regurgitation of the first feeding and coughing, choking and cyanosis.
   b) Abdominal radiograph may show absent bowel gas.
   c) Aspiration and subsequent pneumonia are not uncommon.

Diagnosis of TEF (except H-type) can be confirmed by placing a catheter in the esophagus and visualizing it in a blind upper esophageal pouch on chest radiograph.

3) Surgical treatment
   a) Most infants have surgical repair in the neonatal period that consists of division of the fistula and primary esophageal anastomosis ("short gap atresia").
   b) Patients with a wide separation between the proximal and the distal esophagus, known as **long-gap TEF**, may require cervical esophagostomy with delayed esophageal repair after time is allowed for sufficient esophageal growth or interposition with jejunum or colon.
   c) Surgical approach may be through a right thoracotomy or thoracoscopically in the left lateral position.
   d) Rigid bronchoscopy may be required at the beginning of the case to identify the position of the fistula.

Figure 106-1   Types of Esophageal Atresia and Tracheoesophageal Fistula

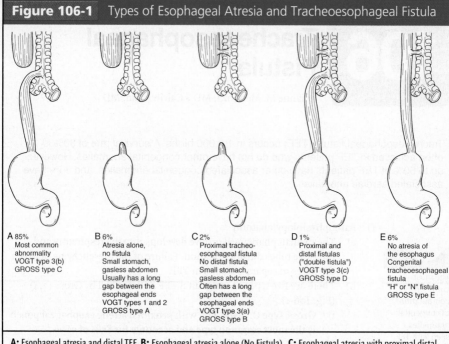

A 85%
Most common
abnormality
VOGT type 3(b)
GROSS type C

B 6%
Atresia alone,
no fistula
Small stomach,
gasless abdomen
Usually has a long
gap between the
esophageal ends
VOGT types 1 and 2
GROSS type A

C 2%
Proximal tracheo-
esophageal fistula
No distal fistula
Small stomach,
gasless abdomen
Often has a long
gap between the
esophageal ends
VOGT type 3(a)
GROSS type B

D 1%
Proximal and
distal fistulas
("double fistula")
VOGT type 3(c)
GROSS type D

E 6%
No atresia of
the esophagus
Congenital
tracheoesophageal
fistula
"H" or "N" fistula
GROSS type E

A: Esophageal atresia and distal TEF. **B:** Esophageal atresia alone (No Fistula). **C:** Esophageal atresia with proximal distal fistula. **D:** Esophageal atresia with double fistula. **E:** "H" Fistula—Percentage reflects approximate incidence. Reproduced from Beasley SW. Esophageal Atresia and Tracheoesophageal Fistula. In: Oldham KT, Colombani PM, Foglia RP, Skinner MA, eds. *Principles and Practice of Pediatric Surgery.* Vol 2. Philadelphia, PA: Lippincott Williams & Wilkins, 2005:1042, with permission.

Up to 50% of patients with TEF have other congenital anomalies, and 35% have congenital heart disease. Preoperative echocardiogram is recommended.

e) Some children may have staged repairs with initial placement of gastrostomy tube to vent the stomach and so that patient may grow before the definitive esophageal repair is performed.

4) **Anesthetic management**

a) **Preoperative considerations**

i) The presence of other congenital anomalies should be sought before surgical repair is undertaken—especially VACTERL association.

(1) Cardiac

(a) **Echocardiographic evaluation should be completed prior to surgery to evaluate for cardiac anomalies.**

(b) Cardiac anomalies that require maintained patency of the ductus arteriosus by prostaglandin infusion, such as hypoplastic aortic arch, have been associated with increased mortality of 57% versus 10% in patients with non–ductal-dependent cardiac lesions (2).

(2) Renal ultrasound should be obtained preoperatively to rule out structural kidney disease.

ii) **Understanding the specific subtype of TEF as well as the location of the fistula is necessary for appropriate airway management.**
- (1) Gross Types A and B are not at risk for gastric inflation.
- (2) Gross Type D has more than one fistula.

iii) An orogastric or a nasogastric tube should be inserted into the stomach or the blind esophageal pouch to remove secretions and prevent aspiration.

iv) Low birth weight <1,500 g has been associated with increased morbidity and mortality though surgical repair is generally not delayed.

v) Labs
- (1) Type and cross should be completed, and blood should be immediately available during the procedure.
- (2) Electrolytes should be checked and dehydration corrected with volume resuscitation.

b) **Monitors/lines**
- i) Standard ASA monitors
- ii) Additional pulse oximeters
  - (1) In case of failure of single oximeter due to poor perfusion.
  - (2) May consider placing preductal and postductal monitors for patients with congenital heart disease.
- iii) Arterial line is usually indicated for blood gas monitoring and for patients with cardiac anomalies, especially if the lesions are ductal-dependent.
- iv) Central venous line is usually indicated to provide high-concentration dextrose solutions, calcium replacement, or other inotropic infusions.

c) **Intraoperative management**
- i) Induction
  - (1) **Copious secretions** tend to be present in TEF patients, and frequent suctioning is required. A preinduction dose of glycopyrrolate 10 µg/kg IV may assist in decreasing the secretions for intubation.
  - (2) Historically, neonatologists might perform an awake intubation with the patient spontaneously breathing to secure airway without mask ventilation.
  - (3) Inhalational induction is not contraindicated.
  - (4) **Mask ventilation**
    - (a) **Positive-pressure ventilation prior to intubation should be avoided** because air will go down the path of least resistance, which may be the fistula instead of the trachea.
    - (b) If positive-pressure mask ventilation is required, keep peak inflation pressures as low as possible. No greater than 10 to 15 cm H_2O is recommended.
  - (5) **Intubation**
    - (a) **Ideally, the tip of the endotracheal tube (ETT) should be positioned below the fistula above the carina,** so breaths will be directed into lungs rather than through the fistula. This will not be possible if fistula is at carina or in a mainstem bronchus (5).
    - (b) After intubation, the ETT should be advanced initially into the right mainstem bronchus.
    - (c) While listening with a stethoscope over the left chest, the ETT is pulled back until air is heard in the stomach and then advanced slightly until bilateral breath sounds are heard with no air heard in the stomach.
    - (d) Alternatively, the ETT can be pulled back until breath sounds are audible in the left chest. If bilateral breath sounds are equal, and no air is heard in the stomach, the ETT can be assumed to be positioned between the carina and fistula.

PEDIATRIC ANESTHESIA

ii) Maintenance

    (1) Total IV anesthetic may be indicated because leaking of anesthetic vapor is common during surgical repair of fistula.

        (a) An analgesic and anesthestic/hypnotic should be used such as fentanyl or ketamine with midazolam or propofol.

        (b) Paralysis should be employed to assist in ventilation and exposure during surgical repair.

iii) **Special anesthetic considerations**

With positive-pressure ventilation (mask or ETT), keep PIP as low as possible (<10 to 15 cm H_2O) to avoid gastric inflation.

Ideal position of ETT is below fistula and above carina.

    (1) **Ventilation**

        (a) The infant should be ventilated on 100% inspired oxygen during the surgical repair.

            (i) Single left lung ventilation may be desired for optimal exposure during during surgical repair but may not be possible secondary to the neonate's small size and inability to adequately oxygenate with single lung ventilation.

            (ii) The right lung is often compressed with retractors to obtain exposure, and a decrease in SpO_2 indicates that the retracted lung needs to be reexpanded.

            (iii) If the fistula is located at the carina or the mainstem bronchus, adequate ventilation may be problematic or impossible.

                1. Adjust settings to achieve desired minute ventilation with low peak inspiratory pressures, low tidal volumes, and increased respiratory rates.

                2. Occlusion of the fistula or venting of stomach may be necessary to ventilate.

    (2) **Gastrostomy**

Gastrostomy or occlusion of fistula with balloon-tipped catheter may be necessary if gastric inflation interferes with adequate ventilation.

        (a) The surgeon may place gastrostomy before surgery to allow intermittent venting to ameliorate gastric distension.

        (b) Emergent gastrostomy may be rarely necessary.

    (3) **Occlusion of fistula**

        (a) Under bronchoscopic guidance, a balloon-tipped catheter can be passed down the trachea to occlude the fistula.

        (b) If gastrostomy is in place, a balloon-tipped catheter can be passed retrograde from the stomach into the esophagus to occlude the fistula.

iv) **Emergence/analgesia**

    (1) Decision about extubation should weigh pulmonary status, hemodynamic stability, anesthetic, and surgical/airway concerns.

    (2) Children who have had aspiration events or pneumonia may require mechanical ventilatory support after a thoracotomy.

    (3) Thoracic epidural catheter threaded up from caudal space will provide excellent analgesia postoperatively.

5) **Postoperative management**

    a) Care should be taken to avoid disrupting the esophageal anastomosis by extending the neck or suctioning the esophagus.

    b) **Postoperative complications**

i) Anastomotic leaks and esophageal strictures may develop.
ii) A right chest tube is often left in place to detect leaks and treat pneumothorax in the immediate postoperative period.
iii) Gastroesophageal reflux may develop with increased risk of aspiration.

Chapter Summary for TEF

General Considerations	The most common type of TEF is Type C defined as distal TEF with proximal atretic esophageal pouch. The most common combination of congenital anomalies seen with TEF is termed the VACTERL.
Preoperative Considerations	Up to 50% of patients with TEF have other associated congenital anomalies, and 35% have congenital cardiac defects. Preoperative echocardiogram is recommended. Understanding the specific subtype of TEF as well as the location of the fistula is necessary for appropriate airway management.
Intraoperative Considerations	Positive pressure (via mask or ETT) should employ as low peak pressures as possible to avoid gastric insufflation. Position tip of ETT below the fistula and above carina for optimal ventilation. Gastrostomy or occlusion of fistula with balloon may be necessary if gastric inflation interferes with adequate ventilation.
Postoperative Considerations	A right chest tube is often left in place to detect leaks and treat pneumothorax in the immediate postoperative period.

References

1. Cote CJ, Lerman J, Todres ID, eds. *A Practice of Anesthesia for Infants and Children*. Philadelphia, PA: Saunders Elsevier; 2009.
2. Diaz LK, Akpek EA, Dinavahi R, et al. Tracheoesophageal fistula and associated congenital heart disease: implications for anesthetic management and survival. *Pediatr Anesth* 2005;15:862–869.
3. Gross, RE. The surgery of infancy and childhood. Philadelphia, PA: WB Saunders; 1953.
4. Kovesi T, Rubin S. Long-term complications of congenital esophageal atresia and/or tracheoesophageal fistula. *Chest* 2004;126(3):915–925.
5. Andropoulos DB, Rowe RW, Betts JM. Anaesthetic and surgical airway management during tracheo-oesophageal fistula repair. *Pediatr Anesth* 8(4):313–319.

PEDIATRIC ANESTHESIA

107 Meningomyelocele

Julianne M. Mendoza, MD

Meningomyelocele is the most common form of **spina bifida**, or **neural tube defect**, occurring in 1 in 1,000 live births. There is a 25% mortality, usually in infancy, with the majority of patients surviving to adulthood albeit with significant comorbidities.

In myelomeningocele, exposure of neural tissue to the intrauterine environment causes direct trauma to the spinal cord.

1) Pathophysiology
   a) A failure of spinal neural tube to close by 28 days' postconception results in a defect in the vertebral column with protrusion of meninges and spinal cord.
   b) **Spinal dysraphism** results from an abnormal or incomplete formation of the midline structures over the back.
   c) **Spina bifida occulta** occurs in the absence of herniation of neural tissue or its coverings so that the overlying skin is intact but may have a hairy patch or dermal sinus that communicates with the meninges or spinal cord.
   d) **Spina bifida cystica** has an obvious lesion on the back and is further delineated into **meningocele** if the spinal cord is covered by meninges or **myelomeningocele** if it is not.

2) Signs/symptoms/clinical findings
   a) Diagnosis is often made prenatally by ultrasound or at birth on physical exam.
   b) 80% of lesions involve the lumbar or the sacral region.
   c) Neurologic deficits are present at birth and are dictated by the level of the lesion. Paralysis and sensory deficits are common below the level of the lesion. Urinary and fecal incontinence affect up to 97% of patients.
   d) Other anomalies are often associated with meningomyelocele.
      i) **Chiari II malformation** is an abnormality of the posterior fossa and the cervical spine that causes caudal displacement of the cerebellar tonsils and medulla and associated hydrocephalus.
      ii) **Hydrocephalus** develops from overproduction or impaired drainage of cerebrospinal fluid.
      iii) **Cranial nerve dysfunction** can cause vocal cord paralysis and diminished gag reflex with increased risk of aspiration.
      iv) **Brainstem dysfunction** can cause an abnormal response to hypoxia and hypercarbia resulting in patients being prone to apnea.

3) Surgical treatment
   a) Repair is performed in the first 24 to 48 hours of life to minimize the risk of infection.
   b) **Approximately 60% of patients will require a ventriculoperitoneal shunt** that may be placed at the time of repair or upon development of symptoms of hydrocephalus.

4) **Anesthetic management**

   a) **Preoperative considerations**

      i) Premedication is usually not necessary in neonates.

      ii) Labs

         (1) Type and cross should be completed, and blood should be immediately available during surgical procedure. Large blood loss may accompany the repair if extensive dissection is required to close the defect.

         (2) Hemoglobin/hematocrit/platelet count may be obtained for baseline measurement and for comparison during procedure if there is significant bleeding or coagulopathy.

         (3) With large exposed lesions, there may be increased insensible fluid loss, dehydration, and electrolyte abnormalities.

   b) **Monitors/lines**

      i) Standard ASA monitors, including core temperature monitoring for large, exposed lesions.

      ii) Good peripheral IV access to administer medications and blood as needed.

      iii) Arterial line access may be indicated for extensive repairs or hemodynamically unstable patients.

      iv) Central venous access may be indicated to administer high-concentration dextrose solutions, calcium chloride replacement, or other inotropic infusions.

   c) **Intraoperative management**

      i) **Induction**

         (1) Mask induction with volatile agent is not contraindicated though most patients will have an IV catheter in place.

         (2) Patients may be given a sedative/hypnotic and muscle relaxant for IV induction.

         (3) **Succinylcholine is not contraindicated** in the newborn period in these patients as there is no association with hyperkalemia (1).

         (4) LMA and other airway aids should be immediately available in case of an unexpected difficult airway.

      ii) **Special anesthetic considerations**

         (1) **Positioning patient during induction and endotracheal intubation should be performed with great care to avoid trauma to the herniated sac.**

            (a) Avoid direct pressure on the meningomyelocele by padding the back.

            (b) Consider induction and intubation in the left lateral position for patients with large lesions.

            (c) Patients will usually be prone for the surgical repair.

         (2) **Latex exposure and sensitivity**

            (a) Latex allergy is common and care should be taken to avoid latex exposure from birth (2).

            (b) Latex allergy under general anesthesia may manifest as hypotension and wheezing. Treatment should include volume resuscitation and epinephrine.

         (3) Intraoperative neuromuscular monitoring may be utilized during dissection.

            (a) Muscle relaxants should be avoided during such monitoring.

Careful positioning of the patient is important for intubation and during the case to avoid injury to exposed tissue.

 READ MORE

Read more on latex sensitivities in chapter 67: Allergy and anaphylaxis, page 484.

These patients are at high risk of developing life-threatening latex sensitivity throughout life. Care must be taken to avoid exposure from birth.

Latex allergy under general anesthesia may manifest as hypotension and wheezing. Treatment should include epinephrine and volume resuscitation.

PEDIATRIC ANESTHESIA

(b) Discussion with the neuromonitoring team should take place to determine what level of volatile anesthetic is possible without interference with the neuromonitoring. IV infusions of remifentanil may be used to supplement the volatile anesthetic.

iii) **Emergence/analgesia**

(1) Extubation may be performed in the operating room if the patient is deemed appropriately awake and with good pulmonary function.

(2) Patients with other comorbidities (e.g., hydrocephalus) or who have required large volume resuscitation may require prolonged intubation postoperatively.

(3) Surgeon may infiltrate surgical site with local anesthetic; however, the extent of actual analgesia will vary.

(4) The patient will likely require systemic opioids or other analgesics such as fentanyl, morphine, acetaminophen.

d) **Postoperative management/disposition**

i) Neonatal patients are often returned to the neonatal intensive care unit for postoperative care.

ii) A neurological examination to document lower extremity movement should be completed as soon as possible after surgical repair.

Chapter Summary for Meningomyelocele

General Considerations	Meningomyelocele is a protrusion of meninges and spinal cord through a defect, most often in the lumbar or the sacral vertebral column. Neurologic deficits present at birth may include paralysis and sensory deficit below the lesion, Chiari II malformation, and hydrocephalus. Surgical repair occurs within 24–48 h after birth in the prone position with care taken during intubation and positioning to protect the herniated sac.
Preoperative Considerations	Electrolyte disturbances and dehydration may be present if a large defect is present. Type and cross should be completed and blood should be available in the operating room at time of repair.
Intraoperative Considerations	Consider intubating in the lateral decubitus position to avoid applying direct pressure to the herniated sac. Development of latex allergy is common in this patient population and care should be taken to avoid latex exposure from birth. Intraoperative neuromuscular monitoring may be utilized during dissection.
Postoperative Considerations	A neurological examination to document lower extremity movement should be completed as soon as possible after surgical repair.

References

1. Cote CJ, Lerman J, Todres ID, eds. *A Practice of Anesthesia for Infants and Children*. Philadelphia, PA: Saunders Elsevier; 2009.
2. Bowman RM, McLone DG, Grant JA., et al. Spina bifida outcome: a 25-year prospective. *Pediatr Neurosurg* 2001;34(3):114–120.

108

Patent Ductus Arteriosus

Calvin Kuan, MD

The patent ductus arteriosus (PDA) is a remnant from fetal circulation extending from the main pulmonary artery to the descending aorta usually immediately distal to the origin of the left subclavian artery. **Functional closure** usually occurs within the first day of life. **Anatomic closure**, where the DA loses the ability to reopen, may not occur for several weeks. Up to 60% of preterm infants weighing <1,500 g may have a PDA; the incidence is even higher in infants weighing <1,000 g (Figure 108-1).

Functional closure of DA usually occurs within the first day of life. Anatomic closure may occur several weeks later.

A PDA shunting left to right will cause pulmonary overcirculation. A PDA shunting right to left will cause cyanosis.

Cardiovascular problems may include low diastolic blood pressure and systemic hypo-perfusion requiring inotropic support.

Pulmonary problems may include pulmonary overcirculation and inability to wean off the ventilator.

1) Pathophysiology
   a) A patent DA results in left-to-right shunting from descending aorta to pulmonary artery once pulmonary vascular resistance (PVR) has decreased.
   b) Left-to-right shunt results in pulmonary overcirculation and volume overload of left heart.
   c) If PVR remains high, blood may shunt right to left, resulting in **cyanosis**.
2) Signs/symptoms/clinical findings
   a) Cardiovascular
      i) Harsh systolic ejection murmur that may be continuous at left upper sternal border (LUSB).
      ii) Bounding pulses, hyperdynamic precordium, and palmar pulses may also be present.
      iii) In young children, particularly premature infants, the shunt effectively steals blood flow from aorta resulting in relative hypotension (especially low diastolic pressures) and hypoperfusion of coronary arteries and abdominal viscera that may require inotropic support.
      iv) Older children may develop pulmonary vascular changes and CHF.
   b) Respiratory
      i) Isolated PDA usually with left to right shunt and therefore SpO_2 should be normal.
      ii) With complex congenital heart disease, shunt may be right to left or bidirectional, so patient may be cyanotic.
      iii) Pulmonary overcirculation may result in increased ventilation and O_2 requirements, and inability to wean off ventilator.
   c) Others
      i) Intraventricular hemorrhage
      ii) Necrotizing enterocolitis
      iii) Renal failure
      iv) Chronic lung disease
   d) **Older children/adults may be asymptomatic.**
   e) EKG may be normal or show left ventricular hypertrophy in small to moderate PDA. Bilateral ventricular hypertrophy in large PDA.

Figure 108-1 Patent Ductus Arteriosus

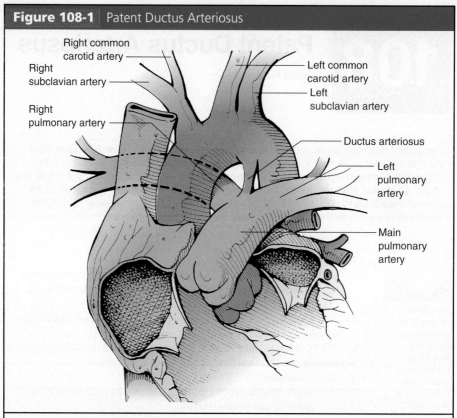

The ductus arteriosus connects the junction of the main and left pulmonary arteries to the descending aorta adjacent to the origin of the left subclavian artery. Reproduced from Rouine-Rapp K, Miller-Hance WC. Transesophageal echocardiography for congenital heart disease in the adult. In: Perrino AC, Reeves ST, eds. *A Practical Approach to Transesophageal Echocardiography*. 2nd ed. Philadelphia, PA: Lippincott Williams & Wilkins; 2008:381, with permission.

   f) Chest radiograph (CXR) may show cardiomegaly and increased pulmonary vascular markings with large shunts.

3) **Treatment**
   a) **Medical**
      i) Management may include diuretics and fluid restriction.
      ii) Indomethacin/cyclooxygenase inhibitors may be administered to stimulate closure (2).
         (1) Risk of renal and platelet dysfunction and intestinal perforation.
         (2) Relatively contraindicated in infants with a history of single kidney, renal dysfunction, intracranial hemorrhage, or necrotizing enterocolitis.
   b) **Surgical**
      i) Ligation of PDA usually through left thoracotomy either at bedside in neonatal intensive care unit (NICU) or in OR.
   c) Interventional cardiac catheter insertion of occlusion device may be attempted in older children.

4) Anesthetic management
   a) **Preoperative evaluation**
      i) Assess overall cardiovascular status and degree of pulmonary overcirculation and shunting.
      ii) Assess pulmonary status and arterial blood gas results if available.
      iii) Cross-matched blood should be available at bedside.

Use 2 pulse oximeters: one on preductal right hand and second on lower extremity to catch inadvertent clamping of aorta.

   b) **Monitors/lines**
      i) Standard monitors with 2 pulse oximeters—one on right hand (preductal) and second one in lower extremity (postductal).
         (1) Loss of waveform in lower extremity monitor will help identify inadvertent clamping of aorta.
         (2) If the pulmonary artery is ligated accidentally, SpO_2 in both extremities and end-tidal CO_2 will decrease.
      ii) Invasive BP monitoring is desirable but may not be necessary depending on hemodynamic status of the individual patient.

If arterial line not available, NIBP should be measured in right arm to best estimate cerebral perfusion.

      iii) If arterial line not present, noninvasive BP should be measured in the **right arm to best estimate cerebral perfusion.**
   c) **Intraoperative management**
      i) **Induction**
         (1) Patients are usually intubated in the NICU and do not require premedication.
         (2) If patient is hemodynamically unstable and/or on inotropic support, consider waiting until surgeon is ready to make incision before administering anesthetic agents.
      ii) **Maintenance**
         (1) Analgesia
            (a) Fentanyl 1 to 2 mg/kg IV q5–10min as needed
            (b) Ketamine 1 to 2 mg/kg IV q5–15min as needed
         (2) Muscle relaxation
            (a) pancuronium 0.1 to 0.2 mg/kg IV
            (b) vecuronium 0.1 to 0.2 mg/kg IV
            (c) rocuronium 0.5 to 1 mg/kg IV

Surgical retraction of lungs during procedure may cause endobronchial intubation and desaturation or bradycardia.

      iii) **Special anesthetic considerations**
         (1) Continue dextrose containing IV fluids or parenteral nutrition at basal rate.
         (2) Airway/ventilation
            (a) Know the location of the ETT as **surgical retraction during surgery may cause endobronchial intubation with desaturation or bradycardia.**
            (b) Ventilation strategy of mild hypoventilation and minimizing FiO_2 may avoid lowering PVR and reduce pulmonary overcirculation.
         (3) With successful PDA ligation, arterial diastolic and mean pressure increase and PDA murmur disappears.

Ventilation strategy of mild hypoventilation and minimizing FiO2 may avoid lowering PVR and reduce pulmonary overcirculation.

   d) **Postoperative management**
      i) Patients are usually left intubated to recover in the NICU.
      ii) Extubation readiness should be left to the discretion of the neonatologist as other medical issues may need to be resolved.
      iii) For postoperative analgesia, an intercostal nerve block may be performed by surgeon.

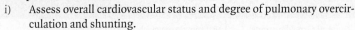

PEDIATRIC ANESTHESIA

Chapter Summary for PDA Ligation

General Considerations	Patients are commonly premature infants in the NICU
Preoperative Considerations	Cardiovascular status—blood pressure and peripheral perfusion and pulmonary overcirculation. Pulmonary status—degree of cyanosis and ventilatory settings. Also assess renal function and acid-base status.
Intraoperative Considerations	Have 2 pulse oximeters—one on right hand and second on lower extremity. Lung retraction may cause endobronchial intubation and desaturation or bradycardia. Ventilation strategy and FiO_2 may affect degree of left to right shunting.
Postoperative Considerations	Patients usually left intubated and sedated in NICU.

References

1. Perrino AC, Reeves ST. *A Practical Approach to Transesophageal Echocardiography*. 2nd ed. Philadelphia, PA: Lippincott Williams & Wilkins; 2008:381.
2. Malviya MN, Ohlsson A, Shah SS. Surgical versus medical treatment with cyclooxygenase inhibitors for symptomatic patent ductus arteriosus in preterm infants. The Cochrane Library, Issue 4, 2009.

Suggested Readings

1. Coté CJ, Lerman J, Todres ID. *A Practice of Anesthesia for Infants and Children*. 4th ed. Philadelphia, PA: WB Saunders; 2009.
2. Holzman RS, Mancuso TJ, Polaner DM. *A Practical Approach to Pediatric Anesthesia*. Philadelphia, PA: Lippincot Williams & Wilkins; 2008.

Omphalocele and Gastroschisis

Calvin Kuan, MD

Omphalocele and gastroschisis are congenital abnormalities of the anterior abdominal wall. These abdominal wall defects (AWD) are a significant source of morbidity and mortality in the neonatal population despite advances in neonatology and surgical care. They are considered surgical emergencies due to the risk for major fluid deficits, bowel obstruction, ischemia, and sepsis.

Omphalocele is covered by a membranous sac. Gastroschisis is not covered.

1) Pathophysiology/embryology
   a) **Omphalocele**
      i) The herniation of abdominal contents through a defect at the base of the umbilicus; **extruded contents are covered by a membranous sac.**
      ii) Speculated to result from the incomplete return of bowel into the abdominal cavity after physiologic umbilical herniation during embryonic development.
   b) **Gastroschisis**
      i) An isolated full-thickness defect lateral (usually to the right) of the normally inserted umbilicus; **extruded contents are uncovered.**
      ii) Likely results from a vascular accident involving the omphalomesenteric artery during gestation or failed development of one of the lateral folds of the embryo.
2) Signs/symptoms/clinical findings (Table 109-1)
   a) **Omphalocele**
      i) Depending upon the size of defect, extruded viscera may include small or large bowel, stomach, spleen, or liver.
      ii) The herniated viscera are covered with a membranous sac composed of fused layers of the amnion and peritoneum, and the bowel is usually morphologically and functionally normal.

PEDIATRIC ANESTHESIA

Table 109-1
Abdominal Wall Defects

	Incidence (Live Births)	Gender	Associated Anomalies	Prematurity Incidence
Omphalocele	1:3,000–10,000	M > F	High association with other anomalies (50%–76%); Cardiovascular 15%–25%	33%
Gastroschisis	1:30,000	M = F	Rare	58%

Reproduced from Holzman RS, Mancuso TJ, Polaner DM. *A Practical Approach to Pediatric Anesthesia*. Philadelphia, PA: Lippincott Williams & Wilkins; 2008:295–298, with permission.

iii) **Omphaloceles have a high association with other anomalies.**
  (1) Chromosomal anomalies
  (2) Congenital heart disease
  (3) Pulmonary hypoplasia
  (4) Genitourinary anomalies
  (5) Neural tube defects
  (6) Beckwith-Wiedemann syndrome
  (7) Pentalogy of Cantrell

  b) **Gastroschisis**
    i) The herniated viscera and intestines are not covered and are exposed to amniotic fluid and then air at time of delivery leading to inflammation, edema, and functionally abnormal bowel.
    ii) Animal models suggest that amniotic fluid is directly toxic to exposed bowel and may lead to thickened peel and dysmotility (1).
    iii) Although there are less associated anomalies with gastroschisis, **nearly 25% of cases have associated gastrointestinal problems** including atresia, volvulus, stenosis, and compromised bowel function (2).
    iv) Intrauterine growth retardation is noted in a significant number of gastroschisis cases (3).

3) **Surgical treatment**
  a) Primary or complete surgical reduction is carried out if the abdomen is large enough to accommodate return of viscera without excessive intra-abdominal pressure that may compromise organ perfusion and decrease ventilatory reserve.
  b) Staged reduction involves covering viscera with prosthetic Silon pouch and gradually reducing the size of the pouch in stages allowing for the abdominal cavity to accommodate to the increased mass over 1 to 2 weeks (4).

4) **Anesthetic management**
  a) **Preoperative considerations**
    i) Management of these lesions from birth until surgical repair is directed at **minimizing heat and fluid loss from exposed surfaces, normalizing intravascular fluid status, and preventing development of sepsis and hypothermia.**
    ii) Cover mucosal surfaces with sterile, saline-soaked dressing; plastic wrap further decreases evaporative losses.
    iii) Nasogastric tube placement helps to prevent intestinal distention.
    iv) Assessment of intravascular fluid status.
    v) Empiric antibiotics are administered given high risk of infection from peritonitis, ischemia and parenchymal disease.
    vi) Identification of associated anomalies (e.g., cardiac, chromosomal, Beckwith-Wiedemann) (4).
  b) **Monitors/lines**
    i) Standard ASA monitors
    ii) Additional pulse oximeters recommended for upper and lower extremities as lower extremity perfusion may be compromised after closure.
    iii) Arterial line recommended for hemodynamic monitoring and blood gases to gauge effects of abdominal pressure on ventilation.
    iv) Central venous line recommended for additional access and/or postoperative parenteral nutrition.

c) **Intraoperative management**
   i) **Induction**
      (1) **Orogastric tube should be placed prior to induction to empty stomach contents.**
      (2) Decision of method of induction should be determined based on clinical condition of patient including factors such as airway, degree of obstruction, and hemodynamic stability.
      (3) Choose an endotracheal tube (ETT) size that will allow for ventilation with higher peak inspiratory pressures that may be required after closure.
      (4) Consider using a cuffed ETT.

Choose an ETT that will allow for ventilation with higher peak inspiratory pressures that may be required after abdominal closure. Consider using a cuffed ETT.

   ii) **Maintenance**
      (1) Avoid nitrous oxide.
      (2) Anesthetic with vapor versus TIVA versus balanced techniques depend on clinical situation and availability of access.
      (3) Muscle relaxation is highly advised and may be requested by surgeon to facilitate closure.
   iii) **Special anesthetic considerations**
      (1) **Higher peak inspiratory pressures may be required to maintain minute ventilation after closure.**
      (2) Use of PEEP may help minimize atelectasis after closure.
      (3) **Communicate with surgeons regarding neuromuscular blockade in order to evaluate intra-abdominal pressures** (5).
      (4) Assessment of intra-abdominal pressure; if <20 mm Hg, primary closure is likely possible.
      (5) Consider using peak inspiratory pressure or transduction of intra-gastric or bladder pressures as diagnostic adjuncts (4).
   iv) **Emergence**
      (1) Except for the most benign small-volume herniations, most patients will require postoperative ventilatory support and NICU care.
      (2) Many may require continued paralysis to minimize intra-abdominal pressure.

d) **Postoperative management**
   i) Perioperative risks include respiratory failure, ARDS, abdominal compartment syndrome, renal failure, infection, coagulopathy, and hypothermia (5).
   ii) Necrotizing enterocolitis has been reported to complicate the postoperative course of up to 20% of neonates with gastroschisis (6).
   iii) Patients with prolonged ileus may require parenteral nutrition.
   iv) Pain control may be achieved with epidural analgesia via caudal, lumbar, or thoracic approaches with radiographic confirmation (5).
   v) Outcomes in gastroschisis have improved over past few decades with contemporary overall survival rate as high as 90% to 95% (3).

Chapter Summary for Omphalocele and Gastroschisis

General Considerations	Omphalocele is the herniation of abdominal contents through a defect at the base of the umbilicus; extruded contents are covered by a membranous sac. Gastroschisis is a defect off midline (usually to the right); extruded contents are uncovered. AWDs are considered a neonatal surgical emergency due to the concern for major fluid deficits, bowel obstruction, ischemia, and sepsis.
Preoperative Considerations	Omphaloceles have a high association with other anomalies. Although there are less associated anomalies with gastroschisis, nearly 25% of cases have associated gastrointestinal problems including atresia, volvulus, stenosis, and compromised bowel function. Management of these lesions from birth until surgical repair is directed at minimizing heat and fluid loss from exposed surfaces, normalizing intravascular fluid status and preventing development of sepsis and hypothermia. Naso/oro-gastric tube placement to prevent intestinal distention.
Intraoperative Considerations	Choose an ETT size that will allow for ventilation with higher peak inspiratory pressures that may be required after closure. Consider using a cuffed ETT. Muscle relaxation highly advised and may be requested by surgeon to facilitate closure. Higher peak inspiratory pressures may be required to maintain minute ventilation after closure. Use of PEEP may help minimize atelectasis after closure.
Postoperative Considerations	Most patients will require postoperative ventilatory support and NICU care.

References

1. Vargun R, Aktug T, Heper A, et al. Effects of intrauterine treatment on interstitial cells of Cajal in gastroschisis. *J Pediatr Surg* 2007; 42:783–787.
2. Sadler T. *Langman's Medical Embryology*. 9th ed. Philadelphia, PA: Lippincott Williams & Wilkins; 2003.
3. Islam S. Clinical care outcomes in abdominal wall defects. *Curr Opin Pediatr* 2008;20:305–310.
4. Coté CJ, Lerman J, Todres ID. *A Practice of Anesthesia for Infants and Children*. 4th ed. Philadelphia, PA: Saunders; 2009:763–764.
5. Holzman RS, Mancuso TJ, Polaner DM. *A Practical Approach to Pediatric Anesthesia*. Philadelphia, PA: Lippincott Williams & Wilkins; 2008:295–298.
6. Dierdorf SF, Krishna G. Anesthetic management of neonatal surgical emergencies. *Anesth Analg* 1981;60:204–213.

110 Intussusception

Nicholette Kasman, MD

Intussusception is the most common cause of intestinal obstruction in children between 3 months and 6 years. Only 10% to 25% of cases occur after age 2, with the majority of cases (61%) occurring during the first year of life (1). There is a higher incidence in males over females (3 to 2). Many of the management principles discussed here also apply to any child with a bowel obstruction.

1) **Pathophysiology**
   a) Intussusception occurs when a more proximal portion of bowel invaginates into more distal bowel (1,2).
   b) **90% of pediatric intussusceptions are ileocolic and idiopathic** (1).
   c) The most commonly associated diseases are cystic fibrosis, Henoch-Schönlein purpura, and Meckel's diverticulum (1).
   d) Lymphoid hyperplasia, possibly induced by a viral infection, also can act as a "**lead point**" in the pathogenesis of intussusception. During this process, the intestine propagates itself distally and with it draws the blood vessels (1).
   e) Initially, compression of the vessels causes venous congestion and bowel edema; however as the obstruction progresses, the arterial supply may become compromised leading to ischemia, bowel necrosis, and gangrene.

2) **Signs/symptoms/clinical findings**
   a) The classic presentation of intussusception includes (1,3)
      i) **Colicky abdominal pain**
      ii) **"Red currant jelly" stools**
      iii) **Vomiting**
   b) **Neonates with acquired lesions rarely present with all symptoms**.
   c) Other symptoms include abdominal distension, a palpable abdominal mass, late passage of meconium, lethargy, hypotonia, and fluctuating consciousness (1–3).
   d) Associated findings may include aspiration pneumonia, dehydration, hypovolemia, and metabolic abnormalities.

Classic presentation of intussusception is (a) colicky abdominal pain, (b) red currant jelly stools, and (c) vomiting.

3) **Treatment**
   a) The preferred method for reduction of intussusception is radiologic reduction by either barium or air enema.
   b) These procedures have 70% and 84% success rates, respectively (1).
   c) Absolute contraindications to radiologic reduction include peritonitis, perforation, and profound shock.
   d) Recurrence after a radiologic reduction ranges between 10% and 15% (1).
   e) If the intussusception requires surgery, the preferred method is via a laparoscopic repair followed by an open repair.
   f) Recurrence after surgical reduction is unusual occurring in 1% to 3% of cases (1).

4) Anesthetic management
   a) **Preoperative considerations**
      i) Evaluation of fluid status
         (1) Hypovolemia secondary to vomiting may cause an initial contraction alkalosis followed by a metabolic acidosis (4).
         (2) Distributive or relative hypovolemia may occur from sepsis due to infection or ischemic bowel.
         (3) Baseline electrolytes should be obtained; however, there may not be time to wait to correct abnormalities prior to surgery.
      ii) Anemia may be present secondary to intra-abdominal bleeding. Type and cross should be sent.
      iii) **Full stomach precautions should be taken.** The patient may benefit from placement of a preoperative nasogastric or orogastric tube.
   b) **Monitors/lines**
      i) Standard ASA monitors may be adequate in patients who have been medically optimized.
      ii) A preoperatively placed IV may be adequate for access unless patient is hemodynamically unstable or septic.
      iii) In hemodynamically unstable patients, an additional IV, an arterial line, and possibly a central venous line for evaluation of fluid status may be necessary.
   c) **Intraoperative management**
      i) **Induction**

Suction out the stomach prior to induction to minimize risk of aspiration. Then proceed with rapid sequence induction.

         (1) Surgical correction of intussusception requires a general anesthetic.
         (2) Children may be actively vomiting and are at high risk of aspiration. It is recommended to empty the child's stomach with a nasogastric or orogastric tube prior to induction with the patient awake to decrease the risk of aspiration on induction.
         (3) Induction should then proceed with a **rapid sequence induction**. All of the concurrent risks of rapid sequence induction in children need to be considered.
         (4) Agents
            (a) Induction
               (i) Ketamine, etomidate, propofol, or other agent at the anesthesiologist's discretion depending on patient stability.
            (b) Muscle relaxants
               (i) The use of succinylcholine or high-dose rocuronium for rapid sequence induction in children is appropriate and indicated in acute bowel obstruction.
            (c) Narcotics
               (i) Midazolam may be considered for preoperative sedation.
               (ii) Fentanyl, morphine, or hydromorphone for analgesia.
            (d) Inhaled agents
               (i) Mask induction is contraindicated as a first choice, but if IV access is lost or not available, it may be considered with concurrent cricoid pressure and suctioning immediately available.
      ii) **Maintenance**
         (1) Choice of drugs for maintenance of anesthesia depends on the clinical situation.

    (2)   If the patient is too hemodynamically unstable to tolerate enough inhalational agent, a ketamine infusion (0.5 to 2 mg/kg/h IV) may provide adequate anesthesia without depressing blood pressure (5,6).

    (3)   There is conflicting evidence about the occurrence and significance of bowel distension after application of N_2O. Many surgeons prefer that it be avoided due to concerns about clinically significant bowel distension that would impair the working space (4).

  iii) **Special anesthetic considerations**

    (1)   In severe cases, there may be significant fluid losses from evaporation during open procedures and through third spacing (1,4).

    (2)   Gangrenous bowel may result in severe metabolic acidosis and require correction of electrolyte abnormalities.

    (3)   Vigilance must be maintained for developing sepsis.

    (4)   Blood product transfusion may be indicated with bleeding and/or fluid shifts.

  iv) **Emergence**

    (1)   The decision whether to proceed with extubation should be based on the stability of the patient as determined by the anesthesiologist.

d) **Postoperative management/analgesia**

  i) There is a risk of persistent postoperative ileus, venous thrombosis, infection, and abdominal compartment syndrome.

  ii) If the repair was done laparoscopically, systemic analgesics combined with injections of local anesthetic at the trochar sites may be sufficient for postoperative pain control (7).

  iii) If the repair was done as an open procedure, placement of a postoperative epidural or single-shot caudal may assist patient recovery.

  iv) If there is significant edema or third spacing, the surgeon may not be able to close the abdomen. Postoperative mechanical ventilation in a pediatric intensive care unit may be necessary.

Chapter Summary for Intussusception

General Considerations	Intussusception occurs when a more proximal portion of bowel invaginates into more distal bowel. Initially, compression of the vessels causes venous congestion and bowel edema; however, as the obstruction progresses, the arterial supply may become compromised, leading to ischemia, bowel necrosis, and gangrene.
Preoperative Considerations	The classic presentation of intussusception includes colicky abdominal pain, "red currant jelly" stools, and vomiting. Neonates with acquired lesions rarely present with classic symptoms.
Intraoperative Considerations	Full stomach precautions should be taken. Stomach should be suctioned out with a preinduction orogastric tube prior to rapid sequence induction. In severe cases, there may be significant fluid losses from evaporation during open procedures and through third spacing.
Postoperative Considerations	If the repair was done laparoscopically, systemic analgesics combined with local anesthetic at trochar sites may be sufficient for postoperative pain control. A repair done as an open procedure may benefit from placement of a postoperative epidural or single-shot caudal to assist patient recovery. Patients are at risk for persistent postoperative ileus, venous thrombosis, infection, and abdominal compartment syndrome.

References

1. Waseem M, Rosenberg HK. Intussusception. *Pediatr Emerg Care* 2008;24(11):793–800.
2. Kleizen KJ, Hunck A, Wijnen MH, et al. Neurological symptoms in children with intussusception. *Acta Paediatr* 2009;98(11):1822–1824.
3. Bhowmick K, Kang G, Bose A, et al. Retrospective surveillance for intussusception in children aged less than five years in a South Indian tertiary-care hospital. *J Health Popul Nutr* 2009;2(5):660–665.
4. Roberts J, Romanelli T, Todres I. Neonatal emergencies. In: Cote, Lerman, Todres, eds. *A Practice of Anesthesia for Infants and Children*. 4th ed. Chap 36: 760–766.
5. Stowe DF, Bosnjak ZJ, Kampine JP. Comparison of etomidate, ketamine, midazolam, propofol, and thiopental on function and metabolism of isolated hearts. *Anesth Analg* 1992;74(4):547–558.
6. Zausig YA, Busse H, Lunz D, et al. Cardiac effects of induction agents in the septic rat heart. *Crit Care* 2009;13(5):R144.
7. Lonnqvist P, Lerman J. General abdominal and urologic surgery. In: Cote, Lerman, Todres, eds. *A practice of Anesthesia for Infants and Children*. 4th ed. Chap 27: 583–594.

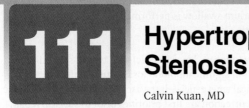

111 Hypertrophic Pyloric Stenosis

Calvin Kuan, MD

The classic presentation of pyloric stenosis is a 3-week-old male infant with acute non-bilious emesis after feeding who is still hungry afterwards. Most patients present between 2 and 12 weeks of age. The incidence is approximately 1 in 500 live births with a male to female ratio of 4:1. Of interest, 30% of patients with pyloric stenosis are firstborn males.

The classic electrolyte abnormality in patients with pyloric stenosis is a hypochloremic, hypokalemic metabolic alkalosis.

1) **Pathophysiology**
   a) Gradual hypertrophy of muscularis layer of pylorus resulting in progressive gastric outlet obstruction.
   b) Persistent vomiting leads to loss of fluids and electrolytes (e.g., hydrochloric acid from stomach), resulting in classic **hypovolemia with hypochloremic, hypokalemic metabolic alkalosis.**
   c) Increased aldosterone induces a renal response to hold on to sodium and hydrogen by secreting potassium instead, normalizing serum pH initially.
   d) Upon depletion of electrolytes (e.g., total body potassium), kidneys secrete hydrogen (paradoxic aciduria), further increasing metabolic alkalemia.
   e) Continued emesis can result in prerenal azotemia, hypovolemic shock, and metabolic acidosis.
2) **Signs/symptoms/clinical findings**
   a) Early
      i) Nonbilious emesis after feeding, with infant still hungry afterwards.
      ii) Persistent episodic projectile vomiting develops in 70% of patients.
   b) Later: evidence of hypovolemia
      i) Tachycardia
      ii) Decreased urine output
      iii) Poor skin turgor
      iv) Decreased activity
   c) Much later: severe dehydration
      i) Weight loss
      ii) Altered mental status
      iii) Shock
3) **Diagnosis**
   a) Clinical
      i) History of emesis as described above.
      ii) Palpation of "olive-shaped mass" in right upper quadrant near the midline in the abdomen.
      iii) Infants are usually diagnosed earlier now than in the past, so many will not present with signs of severe dehydration or electrolyte abnormalities.
   b) Radiographic

PEDIATRIC ANESTHESIA

795

i) The modality of choice is abdominal ultrasound.

ii) Upper GI barium swallow is performed when the ultrasound is nondiagnostic.

4) **Surgical treatment**

a) Surgical myotomy (open vs. laparoscopic) with typical surgical time 0.5 to 1 hour without significant blood loss or fluid shifts.

b) **This is not a surgical emergency**—intravascular volume and metabolic stabilization and correction are first priorities prior to surgical repair.

5) **Anesthetic management**

a) **Preoperative considerations**

i) Clinical evaluation of hydration status

(1) Adequate urine output of at least 0.5 cc/kg/h.

(2) Normal skin turgor, skin color, and capillary refill time.

(3) Normal tear production and moist mucus membranes.

(4) Normal mental status and activity level.

ii) Laboratory evaluation

(1) Goal of plasma chloride > 100 mEq/L.

(2) Goal of plasma bicarbonate < 29 mEq/L.

(3) Goal of urine chloride > 20 mEq/L.

(4) Treatment of hypokalemia should be initiated only after alkalemia resolved and urine output verified.

b) **Monitors/lines**

(1) Standard ASA monitors

(2) Single functioning peripheral IV should be in situ preoperatively.

(3) Invasive monitoring (arterial or central venous) is not usually necessary.

c) **Intraoperative management**

i) **Induction**

(1) **Prior to induction, perform awake orogastric suctioning in supine and left and right lateral positions** with large-bore orogastric tube (OG) to minimize the risk of aspiration.

(2) Preoxygenate with 100% O_2.

(3) **Awake intubation** may be performed if there is a concern for a difficult airway.

(4) **Rapid sequence induction with cricoid pressure**

(a) Succinylcholine $\pm$ atropine OR

(b) Rocuronium

(5) Replace OG tube following intubation.

ii) **Maintenance**

(1) Inhalational agent or TIVA with propofol or balanced technique.

(2) Minimize opiates given risk of post-op apnea in minimally painful laparoscopic cases.

iii) **Special anesthetic considerations**

(1) Aspiration risk is high due to nature of disease despite appropriate fasting time, so gastric suctioning in many positions is advised before induction.

(2) Surgical time may be very short with either open or laparoscopic procedures, so timing of muscle relaxants and analgesics with emergence must be considered.

Surgical repair of pyloric stenosis is not an emergency. Correction of volume and metabolic disturbances should be first priority.

Prior to induction, perform awake orogastric suctioning of stomach contents in supine and lateral positions.

iv) **Emergence**

    (1) Awake extubation is recommended.

    (2) Full reversal of nondepolarizing blockade is recommended.

d) **Postoperative management**

i) Analgesia

    (1) Local anesthetics may be infiltrated by the surgeon into wound.

    (2) Acetaminophen may be given rectally preoperatively or postoperatively.

    (3) Opioids may be necessary with open procedures; however, the patient (especially ex-premature infants) should be monitored for post-op apnea.

ii) Disposition

    (1) Patients should not be discharged home immediately postoperatively.

    (2) **Patients should be monitored for apnea for at least 12 hours following surgery due to abnormal CO_2 response caused by the preoperative metabolic alkalosis (1).**

Patients should be monitored for apnea for at least 12 hours following surgery due to abnormal CO_2 response caused by the preoperative metabolic alkalosis (1).

Chapter Summary for Hypertrophic Pyloric Stenosis

General Considerations	Hypertrophy of muscularis layer of pylorus resulting in high-grade gastric outlet obstruction. Classic findings are of hypovolemia with hypochloremic, hypokalemic metabolic alkalosis.
Preoperative Considerations	Surgical repair is not an emergency. Patients should wait until volume resuscitated and electrolyte abnormalities corrected prior to surgery.
Intraoperative Considerations	Suction out stomach with orogastric tube in supine and lateral positions prior to induction. Preoxygenate with 100% FiO_2. Rapid sequence induction with succinylcholine or rocuronium recommended.
Postoperative Considerations	Patients should be monitored for apnea for at least 12 hours following surgery.

PEDIATRIC ANESTHESIA

Reference

1. Coté CJ, Lerman J, Todres ID. *A Practice of Anesthesia for Infants and Children.* 4th ed. Philadelphia, PA: WB Saunders; 2009.

Suggested Reading

Holzman RS, Mancuso TJ, Polaner DM. *A Practical Approach to Pediatric Anesthesia.* Philadelphia, PA: Lippincott Williams & Wilkins; 2008.

112

Congenital Heart Disease

Calvin Kuan, MD

Pediatric congenital heart diseases (CHD) encompass a wide spectrum of anatomic lesions some of which are relatively benign and are definitively repaired with minimal sequelae, while others can only be palliated and result in a lifetime of medical care.

1) **Introduction**
   a) To safely manage patients with congenital heart lesions, the anesthesiologist must thoroughly understand:
      i) The individual patient's anatomy (visualizing the path of blood flow throughout the body including any abnormal pathways and shunts).
      ii) How the lesion(s) affects the patient's physiology.
      iii) Be able to predict the interactions of surgery and anesthesia—including pain, blood loss, fluid management, positive pressure ventilation, as well as the effects of oxygen and anesthetic agents.

Patients with CHD are at significantly increased risk of morbidity and mortality for all types of anesthetics.

   b) **It is strongly recommended that children with CHD be treated at institutions with experienced multidisciplinary teams, and that there is adequate communication between all the services involved**—primary care physician, pediatric cardiologist, neonatologist, pediatric intensivist, surgeon, anesthesiologist, and any relevant subspecialist.

2) **Risks of anesthesia**
   a) **Children, particularly neonates and infants, with major cardiac anomalies have significantly increased risk of both cardiac arrest and mortality for noncardiac surgeries** (1–4).
      i) Children with CHD are more likely to have cardiac arrest compared to children without CHD.
      ii) In one study, 54% of cardiac arrests in children with CHD occurred in the general operating rooms for noncardiac surgeries (4).
      iii) Outcomes appear significantly better for the patient with CHD when cared for by teams with experience managing such patients (3).
   b) With rare exceptions, patients with the following lesions are at low risk and do not require special care.
      i) repaired patent ductus arteriosus (PDA)
      ii) repaired or unrepaired secundum atrial septal defect (ASD)
      iii) repaired or unrepaired asymptomatic, small ventricular septal defects (VSD)
      iv) asymptomatic pulmonary stenosis (PS)

Knowledge of the specific lesion and history, and communication with the patient's cardiologist are essential to implementing a safe anesthetic plan.

   c) Patients with the following lesions are at highest risk and should be treated at a comprehensive pediatric cardiac center:
      i) Any patient with single ventricle physiology
         (1) Hypoplastic left heart syndrome (HLHS)
         (2) Tricuspid atresia
         (3) Double outlet right ventricle (DORV)

        (4)   Unbalanced atrioventricular canal (AVC)

        (5)   Double inlet left ventricle (DILV)

        (6)   Severe Ebstein anomaly

    ii) pulmonary hypertension (PH)

    iii) ventricular dysfunction or heart failure, particularly cardiomyopathies

    iv) moderate-to-severe valvular obstruction or regurgitation (particularly aortic stenosis)

    v) systemic to pulmonary artery surgically placed shunt (BT shunt, central shunt, aortopulmonary window)

    vi) status post recent heart transplantation

  d) Patients with other lesions/conditions fall in between the two categories and should be assessed individually as there is wide range of symptoms with varying pathophysiology.

3) Preoperative evaluation

  a) **Know the diagnosis**

    i) **It is absolutely essential to know the correct cardiac anatomy** as each lesion has different implications for anesthetic care.

  b) **Get accurate information**

    i) It is not uncommon for patients and parents to have an incomplete understanding of a patient's physiology and complex medical history.

    ii) Accurate information should be obtained directly from the patient's cardiologist, and from thorough review of medical records and studies.

  c) **Past medical/surgical history**

    i) **Anatomy/physiology:** Understanding the natural history of the individual lesions is essential. For example:

        (1)   A child with a lesion that depends on a PDA to deliver blood may deteriorate when the duct closes a few days after birth.

        (2)   A child with a large VSD may be minimally symptomatic at 1 year old but develop Eisenmenger physiology at 20 years of age.

    ii) **Surgical history.** The anatomy and physiology may change significantly with each surgical procedure. For example:

        (1)   A child with a history of a Blalock Taussig shunt may have inaccurate blood pressure readings on the ipsilateral arm.

        (2)   A child who has had a heart transplant may not respond to atropine given for bradycardia and may require epinephrine instead.

    iii) **Past medical history/review of systems:** Review the patient's past medical history and how illnesses of other organ systems may affect the anesthetic management. For example:

        (1)   A child with severe aortic stenosis may not tolerate the tachycardia caused by albuterol given to treat bronchospasm.

        (2)   A child with heterotaxy/asplenia should be treated as being relatively immuno-compromised.

  d) **Physical exam**

    i) **Vital signs:** Know the normal values at rest for the individual patient with the particular lesion. For example:

        (1)   A patient on β-adrenergic blockade should be expected to have a slower-than-normal heart rate.

        (2)   A teenager with an unrepaired coarctation of aorta may be expected to have baseline hypertension.

    ii) **Oxygen saturation:** It is essential to know what the oxygen saturation measurement should be for each patient whether cyanotic or acyanotic, and to know whether the patient has an O_2 requirement at rest to maintain the saturation. For example:

        (1)   A neonate with an unrepaired hypoplastic left heart syndrome (HLHS) may have baseline saturations of 75% to 85%, which is optimal. Saturations of 95% may actually be too high and indicate pathologic pulmonary overcirculation.

(2) A child with pulmonary hypertension who requires an FiO_2 of 40% at baseline should be induced with an FiO_2 of at least 40% to avoid the risk of an increase in pulmonary vascular resistance due to hypoxia.

iii) **Cardiovascular/fluid/volume status:** It is important to evaluate the fluid status of children with heart disease as they may not tolerate relative hypovolemia especially under anesthesia. For example:

(1) The patient's blood pressure may be in the normal range when awake, but administration of anesthetic agents may lower systemic vascular resistance (e.g., inhaled agents, propofol) and result in hypotension.

(2) Children with systemic to pulmonary artery shunts are at an increased risk of clotting the shunt off when hypovolemic.

iv) **Exercise tolerance:** When one does not have documented recent echocardiography exams or cardiac catheterizations, **the subjective reporting of exercise ability is a useful assessment tool of cardiac function.** Recent changes should raise the concern for deterioration in cardiac function. Examples of questions for parents or patients are:

(1) "Does the child do physical exercise at school? If so, what sort of activities or sports can she do?"

(2) "Can the child run, jump, and play? And can he keep up with other children his age?"

(3) "How long can she play before she gets tired, short of breath, or turn blue?"

(4) "Has the child's ability to do any of the above changed noticeably recently?"

v) Recent changes should raise the concern for deterioration in cardiac function and should prompt additional investigation prior to anesthesia and surgery.

e) **Studies**

i) **Electrocardiogram**

(1) All children with a history of cardiac disease should have a baseline EKG done as close to anesthetic date as possible.

(2) Having a baseline to compare with intraoperative changes may avoid unnecessary interventions.

ii) **Echocardiography exam**

(1) Except for children who have had a complete repair of their lesions, are asymptomatic, and have regular follow-up with their cardiologist, **a recent echocardiogram (within 3 to 6 months) by the child's pediatric cardiologist is recommended**.

A recent echocardiogram (within 3 to 6 months) by the child's pediatric cardiologist is recommended.

(2) Decision whether to proceed with anesthesia without a recent exam should be made on an individual basis depending on the changes in cardiac physiology expected since the last exam and the information that would be gained.

iii) **Cardiac catheterization findings**

(1) Cardiac catheterization is not required for all patients.

(2) Severity of pulmonary hypertension (PH) affects perioperative outcomes and a more recent cardiac catheterization may be required if the patient is known to have significant PH.

(3) If the patient has had a catheterization, useful information may be available:

(a) Measuring gradients across valves or shunts

(b) Measuring systolic and diastolic pressures that may indicate degree of ventricular function or failure

    (c)   Identifying stenoses not seen on echocardiogram

    (d)   Identifying occluded vessels that might be chosen for venous or arterial access.

    (e)   Evaluating anatomy and patency of coronary arteries

    (f)   Measuring the **Qp:Qs** (ratio of pulmonary to systemic blood flow), which may give information on the hemodynamic effects of O_2.

        (i)   Qp/Qs < 1: indicates right left shunt and cyanosis.

        (ii)   Qp/Qs = 1: indicates no shunt, or balanced shunt. Usually asymptomatic.

        (iii)   Qp/Qs > 1: indicates left-to-right shunt, with pulmonary overcirculation and potential congestive heart failure CHF.

f) **Labs**

  i) **CBC (complete blood count)**

    (1)   Know the **goal hemoglobin/hematocrit (Hgb/Hct)** for the patient.

      (a)   Some children may require much higher than normal baseline Hct. For example, cyanotic children in general have a high Hct to increase O_2 content of blood.

      (b)   Our institutional practice is to keep the Hgb ≥ 15 g/dL (Hct > 45% to 50%) for cyanotic children in the perioperative period to optimize O_2-carrying capacity.

    (2) **Baseline platelet count**

      (a)   Patients on long-term aspirin therapy may have decreased platelet *function* despite normal platelet counts.

      (b)   Patients on left ventricular assist devices are often placed on antiplatelet medications, so thrombocytopenia and abnormal platelet function should be anticipated.

  ii) **Type and cross**

    (1)   Patients who have had multiple surgeries and transfusions may develop antibodies to blood products. Additional time may be required for the blood bank to crossmatch blood.

  iii) **Chemistries**

    (1)   Potassium

      (a)   **Hyperkalemia is a much greater concern and risk of morbidity than hypokalemia** in the pediatric population.

      (b)   An exception to the above recommendation is that patients on digoxin should have K + ≥ 3.5. Digoxin competes with K + in the myocardium; hypokalemia increases risk of digoxin toxicity.

      (c)   **Consider using washed RBC or freshest RBC if large-volume transfusion is anticipated.**

    (2)   Calcium

      (a)   **Children, particularly neonates, are dependent on calcium for myocardial function and do not tolerate hypocalcemia.**

      (b)   Patients with DiGeorge syndrome may have relative hypocalcemia and require additional supplementation.

      (c)   Administration of blood products or albumin may cause hypocalcemia.

  iv) **Coagulation studies**

    (1)   Patients may be anticoagulated for prosthetic valves or a history of thromboses. Negotiation may be necessary between a surgeon who wants to do a craniotomy and a cardiologist who wants to prevent clots on the aortic or the mitral valve.

PEDIATRIC ANESTHESIA

A bubble in the IV tubing is a bullet to the brain or the heart.

Oxygen is a drug. Know how it may affect your patient's physiology.

Consultation with a pediatric cardiologist or pediatric cardiac anesthesiologist is strongly recommended before initiating anesthesia.

4) Special anesthetic considerations

   a) **"A bubble is a bullet to the brain/heart:"** It is absolutely critical to ensure that all fluids entering the patient are cleared of air bubbles that may embolize to the brain or the coronary arteries.

   b) **"Oxygen is a drug:"** O_2 causes pulmonary vascular vasodilation.

      i) For a patient with pulmonary hypertension, it may be beneficial in lowering pulmonary vascular resistance.

      ii) For a child with single ventricle physiology whose cardiac output depends on a balance between systemic vascular resistance (SVR) and pulmonary vascular resistance (PVR), even a slight increase in FiO_2 may cause a decrease in PVR and result in systemic hypoperfusion and myocardial ischemia.

   c) **Postoperative care/disposition**

      i) Patients should be closely monitored postoperatively by PACU personnel experienced with taking care of patients with CHD.

      ii) Patients who are young, unrepaired, cyanotic, or have single ventricle physiology might require monitoring overnight depending on the surgical procedure.

      iii) Special care should be taken when administering narcotics due to effects on respiratory drive, oxygenation and ventilation, and their effects on cardiac physiology.

   d) **Vascular access**

      i) Vascular access (venous and arterial) may be extremely difficult in patients who have undergone several major surgeries, or have been hospitalized for a long time.

      ii) It is not uncommon for vessels to be stenotic or occluded and therefore unusable.

      iii) Some patients may require very specific placement of lines. For example, the patient with a coarctation will require an arterial line in the right arm.

5) **Selected lesions and anesthetic concerns:** The purpose of this section is to provide some basic understanding of select congenital cardiac lesions. Please refer to recommended references for additional information.

Anesthetic Considerations for Selected Congenital Lesions

Lesion: describes the anatomy of the defect(s)

Clinical findings: describes signs, symptoms, and pathophysiology.

Repair: describes the usual surgical repair

PRE repair concerns: describes some of the major anesthetic concerns for patients with an UNrepaired lesion.
  What is the expected oxygen saturation on room air?
  Can 100% oxygen be used during induction?
  Is there a need for SBE prophylaxis?
  Other special considerations

POST repair concerns: describes some of the major anesthetic concerns for patients outside of the immediate period of surgical repair.
  Does the patient have normal anatomy and circulation?
  What is the expected oxygen saturation on room air?
  Can 100% oxygen be used during induction?
  Is there a need for subacute bacterial endocarditis (SBE) prophylaxis?
  Other special considerations

Atrial Septal Defect (Fig. 112-1)

Lesion: Defect in the atrial septum. There are four types that may occur individually or in combination:
Primum: (5%–7%) Associated with AV canal (AVC) defect.
Secundum: most common (85%). Asymptomatic.
Sinus venosus: (2%–5%) associated with partial anomalous pulmonary venous return (PAPVR).
Coronary sinus: associated with persistent left SVC.

Clinical findings
Usually asymptomatic in children
Usually left-to-right shunt; may have bidirectional shunt but does not result in cyanosis
Over time (i.e., decades), right heart volume overload may lead to CHF and pulmonary hypertension (PH)

Repair
Device closure in cath lab
Primary closure via sternotomy with cardiopulmonary bypass

Prerepair concerns
SpO_2 should be normal.
No restrictions on O_2 use
SBE prophylaxis not required (7)
Special anesthetic considerations
　Care must be taken to avoid air bubbles in all lines and injections
　Otherwise, there are no significant hemodynamic concerns

Postrepair concerns
Anatomy is considered normal after repair.
Expect normal SpO_2 on room air.
No restrictions on O_2 use
SBE prophylaxis required only for first 6 mo after repair (7)
No other special anesthetic considerations

PEDIATRIC ANESTHESIA

Figure 112-1 Location of Atrial Septal Defects

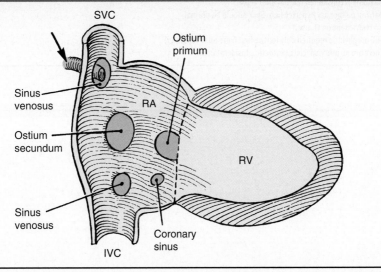

View of the atrial septum showing locations of the different types of atrial septal defects. Superior Vena Cava (SVC) Inferior Vena Cava (IVC), Anomalous pulmonary venous return associated with sinus venosus location (*Arrow*). RA, Right Atrium; RV, Right Ventricle. Reused from Rouine-Rapp K, Miller-Hance WC. Transesophageal echocardiography for congenital heart disease in the adult. In: Perrino AC Jr, Reeves ST, eds. *A Practical Approach to Transesophageal Echocardiography*. 2nd ed. Philadelphia, PA: Lippincott Williams & Wilkins; 2008:372, with permission.

Ventricular Septal Defect (Fig. 112-2)

Lesion: Defect in the ventricular septum. There are multiple types that may occur individually or in combination:
Perimembranous, or membranous, are the most common (70%) (6)
Muscular (5%–20%) may be single or multiple (e.g., "Swiss cheese" type).
Inlet (5%–8%) are also known as AV canal type and are associated with primum ASDs.
Supracristal are also known as infundibular, conoventricular, conal, subpulmonary, subarterial, or doubly committed
VSD. These account for 5%–7% of all VSDs in the Western world, and up to 30% of VSDs in the East.

Clinical findings
Depends on location of defect, size and age of patient.
Primary problem is pulmonary overcirculation due to a left-to-right shunt.
If left untreated, this may eventually lead to pulmonary vascular changes and Eisenmenger physiology, which is
pulmonary hypertension causing a reversal of shunt and severe cyanosis.
A large, unrestrictive VSD may result in congestive heart failure earlier in life due to volume overload of the left
ventricle.

Repair
Device closure in cath lab.
Primary closure via sternotomy with cardiopulmonary bypass.

Prerepair concerns
Expected SpO_2 depends on amount and direction of shunt.
SpO_2 should be normal with left-to-right shunts.
SpO_2 may be as low as 75%–80% with right-to-left shunts.
O_2 may be used for induction with the caveat that it may decrease pulmonary vascular resistance, increasing the left to
right shunt, and exacerbating pulmonary overcirculation.
SBE prophylaxis is not required unless patient is cyanotic.
Special anesthetic considerations
Care must be taken to avoid air bubbles in all lines and injections.
Anesthetic plan should take into consideration the degree of cyanosis and heart failure. If the patient is a teenager or
an adult, there should be suspicion for pulmonary hypertensive changes.

Postrepair concerns
Anatomy is considered normal after repair.
Barring pulmonary hypertension, SpO_2 should be normal.
No restrictions on O_2 use.
SBE prophylaxis required only for the first 6 mo after repair. (7)
There are no other special anesthetic considerations.

Figure 112-2   Location of Ventricular Septal Defects

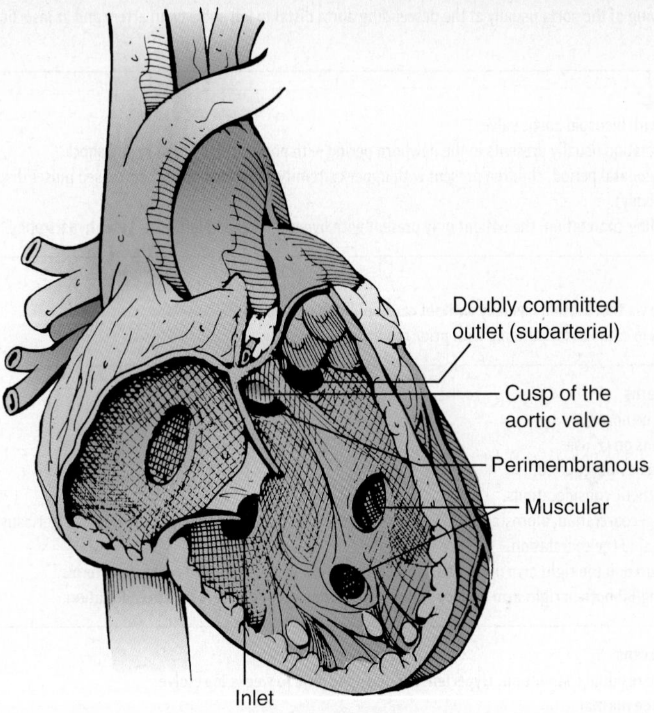

View of the interventricular septum from the right ventricle showing common locations of the different types of VSDs. Reused from Rouine-Rapp K, Miller-Hance WC. Transesophageal echocardiography for congenital heart disease in the adult. In: Perrino AC Jr, Reeves ST, eds. *A Practical Approach to Transesophageal Echocardiography*. 2nd ed. Philadelphia, PA: Lippincott Williams & Wilkins; 2008:377, with permission.

Coarctation of Aorta (Fig. 112-3)

Lesion: Narrowing of the aorta usually at the descending aorta distal to left subclavian artery and at insertion site of ductus arteriosus.

Clinical findings
Associated with bicuspid aortic valve.

Critical coarctation usually presents in the newborn period with poor cardiac function and shock.

Outside of neonatal period, children present with upper extremity hypertension and decreased pulses distal to narrowing (e.g., lower body).

In longstanding coarctation, the patient may present with hypertension and left ventricular hypertrophy.

Repair
Primary closure via thoracotomy usually without cardiopulmonary bypass.

Balloon dilation in cath lab for patients with prior repair.

Prerepair concerns
SpO_2 should be normal.

No restrictions on O_2 use.

SBE prophylaxis not required.

Special anesthetic considerations:

For critical coarctation, alprostadil (PGE_1) may be needed to maintain patency of the ductus arteriosus to perfuse the body distal to the coarctation.

BP measured in the right arm more accurately reflects flow to the brain and coronary arteries.

Measuring BP both in right arm and legs allows measurement of gradient across coarctation.

Postrepair concerns
There may be residual coarctation. Hypertension may take days to weeks to resolve.

SpO_2 should be normal.

No restrictions on O_2 use.

SBE prophylaxis is not required. (7)

There are no other special anesthetic considerations.

Figure 112-3 Coarctation of the Aorta

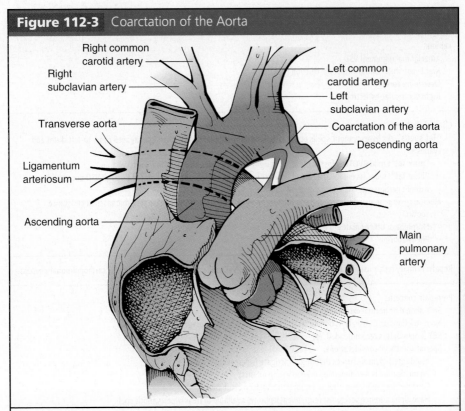

Most common location of aortic coarctation- juxtaductal distal to the left subclavian artery. Reused from Rouine-Rapp K, Miller-Hance WC. Transesophageal echocardiography for congenital heart disease in the adult. In: Perrino AC Jr, Reeves ST, eds. *A Practical Approach to Transesophageal Echocardiography*. 2nd ed. Philadelphia, PA: Lippincott Williams & Wilkins; 2008:382, with permission.

PEDIATRIC ANESTHESIA

Tetralogy of Fallot (Fig. 112-4)

Lesions
Anterior malalignment VSD
Right ventricular outflow tract obstruction (RVOTO)
Overriding aorta
Right ventricular hypertrophy

Clinical findings
"Tet spells" aka hypercyanotic spells occur with RVOT infundibular spasm causing increased right-to-left shunt and cyanosis.
"pink Tet": mild RVOTO. Most of blood from right ventricle goes into pulmonary artery.
"blue Tet": more severe RVOTO. Blood flow to lungs is obstructed, and gets shunted through VSD out to body without getting oxygenated.
Medical treatment includes maneuvers to relax infundibular spasm and/or increase systemic vascular resistance.
100% O_2
Morphine or other opiates
Phenylephrine

Repair: Primary repair usually as neonate includes closure of VSD and enlargement of RVOT under cardiopulmonary bypass.

Prerepair concerns
SpO_2 should be normal except during a hypercyanotic spell.
No restrictions on O_2 use. O_2 is beneficial and patients should be preoxygenated with 100% O_2.
SBE prophylaxis is recommended. (7)
Special anesthetic considerations:
Avoid catecholamine surges that might instigate hypercyanotic spell.
Premedication is recommended even in young infants.
Consider deep induction prior to intubation and deep extubation.
Have alpha adrenergic agonist (e.g., phenylephrine) available to treat hypercyanotic spell.

Postrepair concerns
Anatomy and physiology:
Surgeon may leave a patent foramen ovale (PFO) as a "pop-off valve" if there is RV dysfunction.
There may be residual pulmonary insufficiency that may lead to RV volume overload, especially if the repair was with a transannular patch.
Pulmonary stenosis may develop over time.
SpO_2 should be normal unless there is shunting through a PFO.
No restrictions on O_2 use.
SBE prophylaxis recommended for 6 mo after repair and may be required afterward if prosthetic material was used.
There are no other special anesthetic considerations.

Figure 112-4 | Tetralogy of Fallot

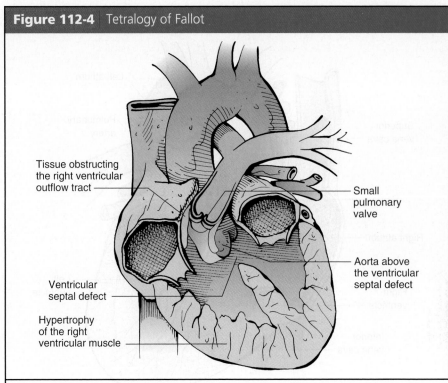

Tissue obstructing the right ventricular outflow tract

Small pulmonary valve

Aorta above the ventricular septal defect

Ventricular septal defect

Hypertrophy of the right ventricular muscle

Components of Tetralogy of Fallot: right ventricular outflow tract obstruction; ventricular septal defect; right venticular hypertrophy; and overriding aorta. Reused from Rouine-Rapp K, Miller-Hance WC. Transesophageal echocardiography for congenital heart disease in the adult. In: Perrino AC Jr, Reeves ST, eds. *A Practical Approach to Transesophageal Echocardiography*. 2nd ed. Philadelphia, PA: Lippincott Williams & Wilkins; 2008:387, with permission.

PEDIATRIC ANESTHESIA

Glossary of Congenital Heart Disease Terms

Aorto-pulmonary window (aka APW or aortopulmonary septal defect): May be a pathological congenital lesion or a surgical procedure performed to increase pulmonary blood flow resulting in side-to-side connection of ascending aorta to main pulmonary artery. Physiologically similar to central shunt.

Arterial switch procedure (aka Jatene procedure): Surgical procedure to repair D-TGA (see entry below and Fig. 112-5) by switching malpositioned aorta and pulmonary artery. Requires moving the coronary arteries to new location (Fig. 112-6).

Blalock-Taussig shunt (BTS): Surgical procedure that creates a shunt between the subclavian artery and the pulmonary artery to supply additional pulmonary blood flow in some congenital lesions.

  Classic BTS: End to side anastomosis of native subclavian artery to ipsilateral pulmonary artery.

  Modified BTS: Artificial shunt placed side to side between the subclavian artery and the ipsilateral pulmonary artery.

Central shunt: Artificial shunt placed side to side between ascending aorta and the main pulmonary artery to increase pulmonary blood flow. Physiologically similar to aortopulmonary window.

Complete transposition of the great arteries (aka D-TGA): Congenital lesion where aorta arises from right ventricle and pulmonary artery arises from left ventricle resulting in two parallel

Figure 112-5   D-Transposition of the Great Arteries

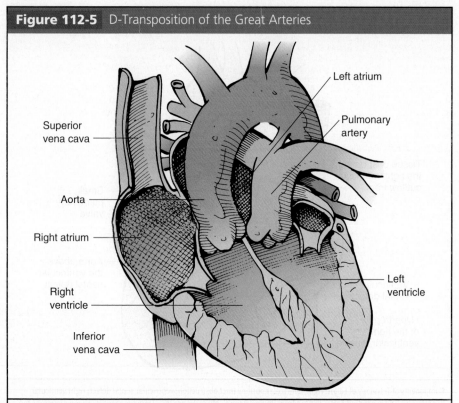

Left atrium

Superior
vena cava

Pulmonary
artery

Aorta

Right atrium

Left
ventricle

Right
ventricle

Inferior
vena cava

D-TGA: aorta arises from right ventricle carrying deoxygenated blood. Pulmonary artery arises from left ventricle carrying oxygenated blood. Parallel circulation requires mixing of blood for patient to survive. Reused from Rouine-Rapp K, Miller-Hance WC. Transesophageal echocardiography for congenital heart disease in the adult. In: Perrino AC Jr, Reeves ST, eds. *A Practical Approach to Transesophageal Echocardiography*. 2nd ed. Philadelphia, PA: Lippincott Williams & Wilkins; 2008:390, with permission.

circulations. Survival depends on adequate mixing of oxygenated and deoxygenated blood. (Fig. 112.5).

Damus-Kaye-Stansel (DKS): Surgical procedure used for various congenital lesions with systemic outflow tract hypoplasia or obstruction. Main pulmonary artery is transected and connected end to side to ascending aorta to allow blood to go systemically. An alternative source of pulmonary blood flow is created (see entries for BT shunt, Sano, or RV to PA conduit).

Double outlet right ventricle (DORV): Congenital lesion where both the aorta and the pulmonary artery arise from the right ventricle. A VSD is present for exit of blood from left ventricle. Pathophysiology depends on position of VSD and other factors. May result in single or dual ventricle physiology.

Double switch procedure: Surgical procedure to repair L-TGA (see entry below, and Fig. 112-7) with an atrial level switch (see entries for Mustard or Senning) and arterial switch procedure. Usually requires preconditioning with pulmonary artery banding (PAB).

Ebstein anomaly: "Atrialization" of the right ventricle. Abnormal and downward displacement of tricuspid valve with spectrum of clinical manifestations from asymptomatic to single ventricle pathway. Often associated with dysrhythmias.

Figure 112-6   Arterial Switch Procedure

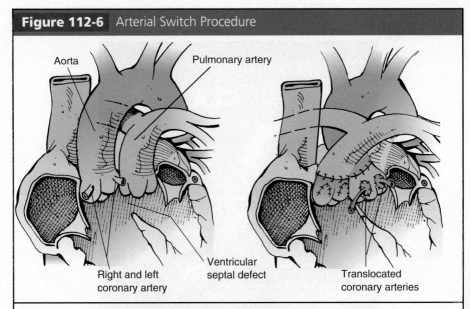

Arterial switch procedure: aorta and pulmonary arteries are transected and switched to normal positions. Coronary artery buttons must be moved to new aortic position. ASD/VSD must be closed. Reused from Rouine-Rapp K, Miller-Hance WC. Transesophageal echocardiography for congenital heart disease in the adult. In: Perrino AC Jr, Reeves ST, eds. *A Practical Approach to Transesophageal Echocardiography*. 2nd ed. Philadelphia, PA: Lippincott Williams & Wilkins; 2008:391, with permission.

Endocardial cushion defect (ECD aka AV canal, aka atrioventricular septal defect (AVSD)): Congenital lesion with a spectrum of manifestations including primum ASD, inlet VSD, and mitral and tricuspid valve abnormalities. Often associated with Trisomy 21.

Fontan procedure: Surgical procedure that is the final stage of palliation for single ventricle lesions usually done at 12 to 24 months of age. The goal of this procedure is to direct all venous return (now the IVC, in addition to the SVC return that was already redirected during the Glenn procedure) to the pulmonary circulation, bypassing the heart completely, depending on passive drainage into pulmonary arteries. After this surgery, the patient will ideally have 100% SpO_2.

   Original Fontan: End-to-end connection of SVC to right pulmonary artery, separation of right and left pulmonary arteries at confluence, anastamosis of right atrial appendage to the proximal separated end of right pulmonary artery RPA, closure of ASD, and ligation of main pulmonary artery. Not performed any longer.

   Extracardiac Fontan: Use of Dacron tube conduit to connect the IVC to the RPA. Has fewer complications from dysrhythmias.

   Lateral tunnel Fontan (aka intracardiac): Use of the patient's native right atrial tissue to create a tunnel connecting the IVC to the PA, without any blood flow to right ventricle. Associated with higher risk of dysrhythmias.

Glenn procedure (aka cavopulmonary shunt): In patients with single ventricle physiology, a surgical procedure that connects the SVC to the pulmonary artery allowing venous drainage from upper body to bypass the heart. Usually done to volume unload the heart and to increase pulmonary blood flow.

   Classic Glenn: In the original surgery, the right pulmonary artery was transected and anastamosed end to end to the SVC. The left pulmonary artery (now discontinuous from the right) continued to get flow from heart via main pulmonary artery.

Figure 112-7   L-TGA or Congenitally Correct Transposition (CC-TGA)

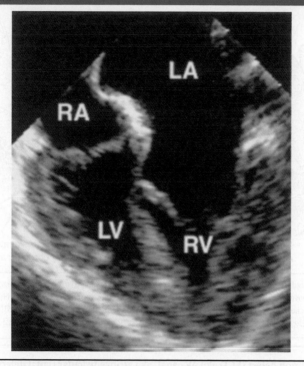

Transesophageal echo showing heart with L-TGA. Note ventricular inversion with left ventricle on right; and right ventricle on left. Reused from Rouine-Rapp K, Miller-Hance WC. Transesophageal echocardiography for congenital heart disease in the adult. In: Perrino AC Jr, Reeves ST, eds. *A Practical Approach to Transesophageal Echocardiography.* 2nd ed. Philadelphia, PA: Lippincott Williams & Wilkins; 2008:392, with permission.

Bidirectional Glenn. The current modification connects the SVC to the right PA, but allows venous blood to drain both to right and left pulmonary arteries, hence "bidirectional."
Bilateral bidirectional Glenn. For patients with right and left SVCs, both SVCs must be connected to ipsilateral pulmonary arteries, hence "bilateral" shunts.
Jatene procedure—see Arterial switch procedure.
Levotransposition of the great arteries (aka L-TGA or congenitally corrected TGA [cc-TGA]): Congenital lesion of ventricular inversion where the right-sided ventricle (that pumps to the pulmonary artery) is morphologically a left ventricle, and the left-sided ventricle (that pumps to the aorta) is morphologically a right ventricle. Functionally normal anatomy, but often associated with dysrhythmias, other cardiac lesions, and potential failure of the systemic ventricle (Fig. 112-7).
Mustard procedure: Surgical procedure using pericardial or artificial material to create a baffle (i.e., rerouting of blood flow) in the atria to palliate D-TGA. Similar to Senning procedure (Fig. 112-8).
Norwood procedure: First-stage surgical procedure in the pathway to palliate hypoplastic left heart syndrome. Repair includes creation of neoaorta using native main pulmonary artery that is transected. Alternative source of pulmonary blood flow is created—for example, Sano RV to PA shunt. Subsequent stages include Glenn and Fontan procedure (Fig. 112-9).

Figure 112-8 Dextro-Transposition of the Great Arteries Following an Atrial Redirection Procedure

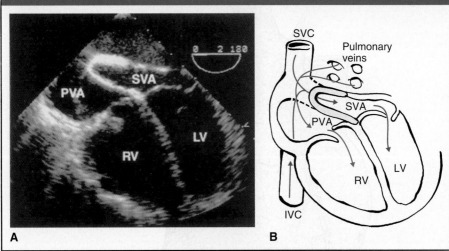

A: two-dimensional transesophageal echocardiographic midesophageal four-chamber view that demonstrates the features of an atrial redirection procedure. In this procedure, venous return from the systemic and pulmonary circulations is rerouted through a baffle. Following placement of a baffle, desaturated blood from the superior and inferior vena cavae drains into the systemic atrium (SVA) then through the mitral valve into the left ventricle (LV) then into the pulmonary artery. Blood from the pulmonary veins drains into the pulmonary atrium (PVA) then through the tricuspid valve into the right ventricle (RV) then into the aorta. The RV remains the systemic ventricle. B: illustration is included to clarify the route of blood flow following an atrial redirection procedure. (SVC, superior vena cava; IVC, inferior vena cava). Reproduced from Rouine-Rapp K, Miller-Hance WC. Transesophageal echocardiography for congenital heart disease in the adult. In: Perrino AC, Reeves ST, eds. *A Practical Approach to Transesophageal Echocardiography*. 2nd ed. Philadelphia, PA: Lippincott Williams & Wilkins; 2008:391, with permission.

Partial anomalous pulmonary venous return (PAPVR): Congenital lesion where some of the pulmonary veins do not drain into the left atrium, but drain into the right atrium or some other part of the venous system. When none of the pulmonary veins drain normally into the left atrium, the lesion is termed total anomalous pulmonary venous return (TAPVR).

Potts shunt: Surgical procedure creating a shunt between the descending aorta and the left pulmonary artery. No longer performed.

Pulmonary atresia with intact ventricular septum (PA/IVS): Congenital lesion with an atretic pulmonary valve and no VSD for exit of blood from the right ventricle. An atrial shunt (PFO or ASD) is necessary for survival. Coronary sinusoids may develop from the elevated RV pressures, resulting in increased risk of right ventricular ischemia.

Pulmonary artery banding (PAB): Surgical procedure to tighten the pulmonary artery to decrease amount of pulmonary blood flow and/or to strengthen the ventricle.

Rashkind procedure: Procedure performed at bedside or in the cardiac cath lab to enlarge a patent foramen ovale or ASD in lesions that require increased mixing of systemic and pulmonary circulation, e.g., D-TGA with an intact atrial septum.

Rastelli procedure: Surgical procedure used to correct certain lesions with pulmonary artery abnormalities. The pulmonary artery is transected. The VSD is closed with a patch that simultaneously directs blood from the LV to the aorta. Finally, an RV to PA conduit is created to supply pulmonary blood flow.

Sano modification (Fig. 112-9): Surgical procedure creating a valved RV to PA conduit as a modification of the Norwood procedure.

Figure 112-9 Norwood Procedure with Sano Modification

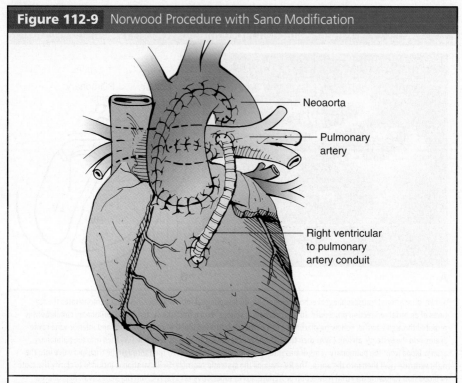

Neoaorta

Pulmonary
artery

Right ventricular
to pulmonary
artery conduit

Norwood procedure consists of using native pulmonary artery to create neo-aorta. Sano modification is valved conduit from RV to PA to provide pulmonary blood flow. Reused from Rouine-Rapp K, Miller-Hance WC. Transesophageal echocardiography for congenital heart disease in the adult. In: Perrino AC Jr, Reeves ST, eds. *A Practical Approach to Transesophageal Echocardiography*. 2nd ed. Philadelphia, PA: Lippincott Williams & Wilkins; 2008:395, with permission.

Senning procedure. Surgical procedure using native atrial tissue to create a baffle in the atria to palliate D-TGA. Similar to Mustard procedure.

Tetralogy of Fallot: See TOF entry in chapter above.

Tetralogy of Fallot with absent pulmonary valve (TOF/APV): Congenital lesion that is a small subset of TOF where the pulmonary valve is completely absent resulting in severe pulmonary regurgitation. A pulmonary artery aneurysm may develop that may be so large as to compress the trachea and bronchi, causing severe airway problems.

Tetralogy of Fallot with pulmonary atresia and MAPCAs (major aortopulmonary collateral arteries) (TOF/PA/MAPCA's): Congenital lesion previously described as truncus arteriosus type IV. An extreme form of TOF with complete pulmonary atresia. Pulmonary blood flow is from PDA or multiple aortopulmonary collateral arteries (MAPCAs). Surgical repair with unifocalization procedure.

Total anomalous pulmonary venous return (TAPVR): None of the pulmonary veins drain into the left atrium. The specific anatomy determines the physiology and the urgency of repair. Obstructed TAPVR is a surgical emergency.

Tricuspid atresia: Congenital lesion with absent or atretic tricuspid valve and hypoplastic right ventricle. Repair of this single ventricle lesion eventually leads to Fontan procedure.

Truncus arteriosus: Congenital lesion where only one great vessel leaves the heart and supplies blood flow to pulmonary arteries, aorta, and coronary arteries. A VSD is necessary for survival. Associated with interrupted aortic arch and DiGeorge syndrome.

Unifocalization procedure: Complex surgical procedure for treatment of patients with TOF/PA/ MAPCA's where aortopulmonary collaterals are separated from the aorta and connected to the pulmonary artery to supply deoxygenated blood to lungs. May be done as single surgery or staged procedure depending on degree of pulmonary hypoplasia.

Waterston shunt: Surgical procedure creating a shunt between the ascending aorta and the right pulmonary artery. No longer performed.

Chapter Summary for Congenital Heart Disease (CHD)

Overview	CHD comprises a wide spectrum of lesions with varying manifestations.
	Children with CHD are at significantly higher risk of morbidity and mortality with anesthesia.
	Communication with patient's caregivers, cardiologist, and surgeon is critical.
Preoperative	Understanding the anatomy and physiology is essential to providing safe anesthesia.
	Know what the baseline oxygen saturation should be at rest.
	Assess the patient's exercise tolerance as an indication of cardiac function.
	Evaluate recent studies and consider getting new ones if studies are outdated.
	Consultation with a pediatric cardiologist or a pediatric cardiac anesthesiologist is strongly recommended before initiating anesthesia.
Intraoperative	A bubble is a bullet to the brain or the heart. Take great care not to inject any air into intravenous lines.
	Oxygen is a drug. Know whether increased FiO_2 may adversely affect the patient.
Postoperative Issues	Patients should be closely monitored postoperatively by PACU personnel experienced with taking care of patients with CHD.
	Special care should be taken when administering narcotics due to effects of respiratory drive, oxygenation and ventilation, and their effects on cardiac physiology.

References

1. Baum VC, Barton DM, Gutgesell HP. Influence of congenital heart disease on mortality after noncardiac surgery in hospitalized children. *Pediatrics* 2000;105:332–335.
2. Flick RP, Sprung J, Harrison TE, et al. Perioperative cardiac arrests in children between 1988 and 2005 at a tertiary referral center. *Anesthesiology* 2007;106: 226–237.
3. Odegard KC, DiNardo JA, Kussman BD, et al. The frequency of anesthesia-related cardiac arrests in patients with congenital heart disease undergoing cardiac surgery. *Pediatric Anesth* 2007;105(2):335–343.
4. Ramamoorthy C, Haberkern CM, Bhananker SM, et al. Anesthesia-related cardiac arrest in children with heart disease: data from the Pediatric Perioperative Cardiac Arrest (POCA) Registry. *Anesth Anal* 2010;10(5):1376–1382.
5. Coté CJ, Lerman J, Todres ID. *A Practice of Anesthesia for Infants and Children*. 4th ed. Philadelphia, PA: WB Saunders; 2009.
6. Park MK, *Pediatric Cardiology for Practitioners*. 5th ed. Philadelphia, PA: Mosby Elsevier; 2008.
7. Wilson W, Taubert KA, Gewitz M, Prevention of infective endocarditis: guidelines from the American Heart Association. *Circulation* 2007;116:1736–1754.
8. Perrino AC, Reeves ST. *A Practical Approach to Transesophageal Echocardiography*. Philadelphia, PA: Lippincott Williams & Wilkins; 2008.

Additional reading/references

1. Park MK, *Pediatric Cardiology for Practitioners*. 5th ed. Philadelphia, PA: Mosby Elsevier; 2008.
2. Andropoulos DB, Stayer SA, Russell IA, et al. *Anesthesia for Congenital Heart Disease*. 2nd ed. West Sussex, UK: Wiley-Blackwell; 2010.
3. The Congenital Heart Information Network website: http://tchin.org

PEDIATRIC ANESTHESIA

113 Cerebral Palsy

Jeannie Seybold, MD

Cerebral palsy (CP) is a heterogeneous group of motor and posture impairment disorders resulting from injury to the central nervous system during early brain development (antenatally to 2 years of age). CP is the leading cause of motor disability in childhood. Prevalence in the developed world is 1 to 2.5 per 1,000 live births of normal birth weight (1). Prevalence is increased in premature or low birth weight infants, who account for more than 25% of the children with CP (2).

1) Pathophysiology
    a) Brain injury is caused by leukomalacia from periventricular hemorrhage and manifests as spastic diplegia (1,3).
    b) The identified etiologies are multifactorial and include intrapartum hypoxia, cerebral maldevelopment, perinatal stroke or infection, congenital abnormalities, trauma, and genetic predisposition.
2) Signs/symptoms/clinical findings
    a) **Motor defect: A motor defect is always present.** Impairment depends on the site of the defect (1–3).
        i) **Spasticity**—a motor cortex (cerebral) abnormality found in 70% of patients.
            (1) Major subtypes include **spastic diplegia** (21%), **hemiplegia** (21%), and **quadriplegia** (27%).
            (2) Spastic quadriplegia is associated with feeding problems, aspiration, epilepsy, and intellectual disability.
            (3) Patients with spastic diplegia and hemiplegia are most likely to have normal intelligence and functional improvement.
            (4) Contractures develop over time.
        ii) **Ataxia**—cerebellar defect (10%); associated with epilepsy, cognitive disability, and poor prognosis for functional improvement.
        iii) **Dyskinesia**—basal ganglia injury (10%); associated with drooling, epilepsy and dysarthria, with low–to–normal intelligence.
        iv) **Mixed disorder** (10%); combination of 2 or more of the above CP types.
    b) **Associated findings**
        i) The degree of functional and cognitive impairment varies widely depending on the type and severity of CP. Most patients with CP will also have at least one of the following (3):
        ii) Speech, sensory, or cognitive impairment
        iii) Behavioral problems
        iv) Seizures (30% of patients)
        v) Reactive airway disease
        vi) Gastroesophageal reflux disease (GERD)
        vii) Pulmonary morbidity from chronic aspiration, impaired cough, and feeding difficulties

3) Treatment

    a) Is multimodal and integrates medical, surgical, and physical therapy to maintain function and to reduce pain.

    b) Common surgeries include tendon transfer and release to improve mobilization, spine surgery to limit progression of scoliosis, dental rehabilitation, imaging, feeding gastrostomies/endoscopy, antireflux surgery, tracheostomy, and neurosurgical procedures.

4) Anesthetic management

    a) **Preoperative considerations**

        i) Difficulty in communication may be due to dysarthria, impaired vision, hearing, speech or cognition, or lack of cooperation. **Some patients with speech impairment have normal intelligence.** Caregivers can describe how the child communicates and previous responses to premedication.

        ii) Restrictive lung disease or cardiac disease may be present in patients with scoliosis.

        iii) Patients with CP often have **complex outpatient pharmacologic regimens:**

            (1) Antispasmodics may increase sensitivity to anesthetic medications. These include baclofen (centrally acting GABA-beta receptor agonist), benzodiazepines, vigabatrin (GABA transaminase inhibitor), tizanidine (clonidine derivative), and dantrolene, which acts peripherally on skeletal muscle.

            (2) Anticonvulsants, such as valproic acid, can cause platelet dysfunction or thrombocytopenia.

        iv) **Latex allergy risk** may be increased if the patient has had multiple medical and surgical interventions from an early age.

    b) Premedication may be necessary to reduce anxiety and spasm.

        i) Heavy premedication should be used with caution in patients who are predominantly hypotonic and at risk for aspiration due to decreased airway tone.

        ii) Common agents include midazolam or ketamine.

    c) **Monitors/lines/positioning**

        i) **PIV placement may be difficult** due to contractures and chronic low fluid intake exacerbated by preoperative fasting. The use of EMLA/warming devices may be helpful.

        ii) Special care should be taken when positioning patients with contractures. They have **an increased risk of nerve damage and pressure sores** due to decreased fat pads and exposed bony structures. Injuries will be slow to heal if the nutritional status is poor.

        iii) **Temperature regulation:** At baseline, most patients with CP have borderline hypothermia and warming/temperature conservation measures may be necessary (1–3).

    d) **Intraoperative management**

        i) **Induction**

            (1) Inhalational induction may be challenging due to hyperactive salivary glands and difficulty handling secretions secondary to pseudobulbar palsy or poor head control. An antisialogogue and frequent suctioning will reduce oral secretions.

            (2) A rapid sequence induction may be indicated for patients with severe GERD symptoms.

The degree of functional and cognitive impairment varies widely in patients with CP. Patients with CP may have normal cognition but have difficulty communicating.

Special care should be taken when positioning patients with contractures who have an increased risk of nerve damage and pressure sores.

Inhalational induction may be challenging due to hyperactive salivary glands and difficulty handling secretions secondary to pseudobulbar palsy or poor head control.

PEDIATRIC ANESTHESIA

(3) Patients with CP have been reported to have a clinically insignificant sensitivity to succinylcholine and mildly increased resistance to nondepolarizing neuromuscular blockers. There was no difference in serum potassium levels after succinylcholine administration in children with CP compared with normal controls (2).

    (4) Successful use of laryngeal mask airways and tracheal tubes has been described.

ii) **Maintenance**

    (1) Children with CP may be more sensitive to anesthetic agents and opioids.

    (2) Minimum alveolar concentration (MAC) is decreased in patients with CP.

        (a) MAC of halothane is 0.9 in healthy children, 0.71 in children with CP, and 0.63 in children with CP on chronic anticonvulsant medication (2).

        (b) MAC of other anesthetic gases has not been studied. It may be prudent to use short-acting inhalational or IV agents to facili- tate extubation at the end of the case.

iii) **Special anesthetic considerations**

    (1) Antiseizure medications such as phenobarbital, phenytoin, and val- proic acid may be dosed intravenously. If there is major blood loss, recheck levels and redose as necessary.

    (2) Blood loss

        (a) Risks from bleeding are increased if the patient is anemic at baseline due to poor nutritional status.

        (b) Patients with CP can have subnormal levels of clotting factors, platelet dysfunction, or borderline thrombocytopenia from chronic anticonvulsant therapy.

        (c) Patients with CP experience greater blood loss per spinal seg- ment in scoliosis surgery than patients with idiopathic scolio- sis. Early use of aminocaproic acid has been reported to reduce blood loss during spine surgery in patients with CP (4).

iv) **Emergence**

    (1) Consider postoperative ventilation if large-volume resuscitation is required to keep up with blood loss.

    (2) Patients with severe chronic lung disease, oxygen dependence at baseline, or an inability to maintain a patent airway may also require postoperative ventilation, CPAP or BIPAP, especially if analgesic requirements are high.

e) **Postoperative management/disposition**

i) Pain control

    (1) Effective analgesia is necessary to reduce postop spasms.

    (2) Regional and neuraxial anesthesia used in combination with GA is effective for surgery on children with CP and can reduce painful postop muscle spasms.

    (3) **Epidural clonidine has been reported to be a useful antispasmodic agent (1).**

    (4) Patients with CP may be more sensitive to narcotic medication (2) and doses should be titrated to effect.

    (5) Patients should be monitored continuously in the PACU for airway obstruction and hypoventilation.

ii) Disposition: Availability of monitored bed or critical care unit bed is recommended for patients with severe underlying pulmonary, cardiac, or neurologic disease.

Chapter Summary for CP

General Considerations	CP encompasses a group of diverse motor system disorders with an accompanying wide spectrum of functional and cognitive impairment.
Preoperative Considerations	Patients with problems communicating may have normal intelligence, and the practitioner should be sensitive to the patient's limitations. The preoperative workup should address current medications and comorbidities, which may include GERD, epilepsy, chronic pulmonary disease, aspiration, and behavioral problems.
Intraoperative Considerations	Special attention should be paid to patient positioning and temperature conservation. Surgical blood loss may be greater than expected.
Postoperative Considerations	Adequate analgesia is required to prevent painful postoperative spasms.

References

1. Wongprasartsuk P, Stevens J. Cerebral palsy and anaesthesia. *Paediatr Anaesth* 2002:12:296–303.
2. Theroux MC, Akins RE. Surgery and anesthesia for children who have cerebral palsy. *Anes Clin N Am* 2005;23:733–743.
3. Nolan J, Chalkiadis GA, Low J, et al. Anaesthesia and pain management in cerebral palsy. *Anaesthesia* 2000;55:32–41.
4. Thompson GH, Florentino-Pineda I, Poe-Kochert, et al. Role of Amicar in surgery for neuromuscular scoliosis. *Spine* 2008;33(24):2623–2629.

PEDIATRIC ANESTHESIA

Muscular Dystrophy

Evan Serfass, MD, PhD

The muscular dystrophies are a group of inherited disorders of muscle that have in common progressive weakness of involved muscle groups. Although thought of primarily as affecting skeletal muscle, cardiac and smooth muscle also can be severely affected. Common surgeries for patients with muscular dystrophy include release of contracture and correction of scoliosis. Patients with severe manifestations of a muscular dystrophy are at significantly greater risk of morbidity during and after anesthesia and sedation.

1) Pathophysiology: This group of diseases is caused by defective or absent proteins in the cytoskeleton of muscle cells. Connections between the cytoskeleton and the extracellular matrix are weak, resulting in damage to muscle cell membranes and degeneration of muscle fibers. **There is progressive development of skeletal weakness, contractures, and involvement of cardiac, respiratory, and smooth muscle.**

2) Types of muscular dystrophy
   a) **Duchenne muscular dystrophy (DMD)** is the most severe type. It is sex linked, affecting 1 in 3,500 male births. DMD usually presents by 5 years of age; 75% of patients are nonambulatory by age 10, and 75% die before age 20 (1).
   b) **Becker muscular dystrophy (BMD)** presents similarly to DMD but with slower progression. It affects 1 in 30,000 male births, and patients usually present in early adolescence (1).
   c) **Myotonic dystrophy (MyoD)** is the most prevalent muscular dystrophy in Caucasians, affecting 1 in 8,000, and is usually transmitted in an autosomal dominant fashion. The age of onset and disease severity is highly variable, with many patients remaining undiagnosed into adulthood (2,3).
   d) **Emery-Dreifuss muscular dystrophy** has mild skeletal muscle manifestations, but cardiac conduction defects are prominent and may cause sudden death (2,4).
   e) Other muscular dystrophies include limb-girdle, fascioscapulo-humeral, and oculopharyngeal muscular dystrophy, with the names indicating the primary muscle groups affected (1).

3) Signs/symptoms/clinical findings
   a) Early
      i) DMD and BMD: The earliest sign is often **difficulty running, jumping, or ascending steps.** Waddling gait, lumbar lordosis, and calf enlargement are also signatures. **Gowers' sign** (the use of arms to help rise from a sitting position) is characteristic (1,2).
      ii) MyoD: Hands, forearms, facial muscles, and ankle dorsiflexors (→ foot drop) are the commonly affected muscle groups. **Muscle pain** is common. **Myotonia**—best appreciated in the hand—is prominent in the early stages (2,3).

b) Late

   i) Respiratory function (5)

      (1) Decreased vital capacity, maximal inspiratory pressure (MIP), and maximal expiratory pressure (MEP) are common.

      (2) **Pharyngoesophageal weakness** develops, resulting in aspiration.

      (3) In DMD and BMD, progressive **scoliosis** results in restrictive lung disease.

   ii) Cardiac dysfunction (5)

Succinylcholine is *absolutely* contraindicated in patients with DMD or BMD. Succinylcholine is *relatively* contraindicated in pediatric patients due to risk of undiagnosed myopathies.

      (1) MyoD: **Atrial fibrillation and flutter** are the most common arrhythmias, but ventricular arrhythmias can also occur. Cardiomyopathies are unusual, but left ventricular hypertrophy or dilatation is not uncommon.

      (2) DMD: Primary **dilated cardiomyopathy** and conduction abnormalities develop in the teenage years. Significant mitral regurgitation may be present. Patients may not have cardiac symptoms, as their skeletal muscle weakness makes exercise impossible. Cardiac consultation prior to anesthesia is strongly advised.

      (3) BMD: Similar to DMD but may have earlier onset as their ability to exercise puts strain on the heart.

      (4) Emery-Dreifuss muscular dystrophy: Conduction abnormalities are common and are associated with a significant risk of **sudden death**; a permanent pacemaker or implantable defibrillator may be necessary. Weakness progresses slowly compared to other forms.

Inhalational anesthetics may cause rhabdomyolysis and cardiac arrest in muscular dystrophy patients. TIVA is recommended.

   iii) Smooth muscle involvement is most common in MyoD, with irritable bowel syndrome–like symptoms, dysphagia, and possibly aspiration pneumonia (3,5).

c) Associated findings

   i) **Elevated creatine kinase** (often 10 to 100 times normal in DMD patients) (2)

   ii) Mental retardation (30% of DMD patients)

   iii) Side effects of steroid use, as chronic steroid therapy is becoming common (1)

4) Anesthetic management

a) **Succinylcholine can lead to rhabdomyolysis and hyperkalemia, precipitating cardiac arrest.** The black box warning on succinylcholine is due to deaths in undiagnosed DMD children who received this medication. **DMD and BMD are absolute contraindications to the use of succinylcholine (5).**

b) **Inhalational anesthetics** may also precipitate rhabdomyolysis and cardiac arrest, even in the absence of succinylcholine. A total intravenous anesthetic (TIVA) is suggested (2,5,6).

c) **Cardiac arrest may even occur postprocedurally in the post-anesthesia care unit (PACU) due to ongoing rhabdomyolysis and potassium release (7).**

Both onset of and recovery from nondepolarizing neuromuscular blockers are prolonged.

d) **Rhabdomyolysis is most common in patients <8 years old**, as these patients have large numbers of fragile regenerating muscle fibers (2).

e) There is **no increased risk of malignant hyperthermia** (7), although rhabdomyolysis and other complications can present a similar clinical picture.

f) Careful use of nondepolarizing neuromuscular blockers is required, as **both the onset and the recovery are prolonged** (5).

Respiratory weakness is common: expect difficulties with spontaneous ventilation intraoperatively and postoperatively.

Myocardium is often affected: life-threatening cardiomyopathies and dysrhythmias are common.

g) Possible **difficult mask ventilation** may occur due to macroglossia and limited mandibular and C-spine mobility in DMD, BMD. No increased risk of unanticipated difficult intubation has been reported (5).

h) Patients are at risk for respiratory complications due to muscle weakness, such as obstruction, hypoventilation, atelectasis, respiratory failure, and difficulty weaning from mechanical ventilation (2,5).

i) Patients are at risk for cardiac complications, including arrhythmias and heart failure due to myocardial depression or fluid overload (5).

j) **Chronic steroid use** in DMD may lead to obesity, glucose intolerance, and osteoporosis and may necessitate stress-dose steroids (8).

5) **Summary of DMD management guidelines** from the American College of Chest Physicians consensus statement (5). Use clinical judgment in applying these to BMD, MyoD, or other muscular dystrophy patients.

a) Preprocedure

   i) Anesthesia pre-op evaluation with a detailed review of systems, focusing on strength and motor capabilities. Family medical and anesthetic history may point to undiagnosed muscular dystrophy (especially myotonic dystrophy, which is often undiagnosed due to its varying severity); however, spontaneous mutations are responsible for at least 30% of cases of muscular dystrophy (2).

   ii) Pulmonary consultation should be obtained in any muscular dystrophy patient with suspected respiratory compromise. **Spirometry** should include forced vital capacity (FVC), MIP, MEP, peak cough flow (PCF), and SpO_2 on room air.
      (1) If FVC < 50% predicted → increased risk of respiratory complications
      (2) If FVC < 30% predicted → high risk of respiratory complications
      (3) If SpO_2 < 95%, $PaCO_2$ or $EtCO_2$ should be measured prior to surgery.
      (4) Training in noninvasive positive pressure ventilation (NPPV) is suggested if FVC < 50% predicted.
      (5) Training in assisted cough if PCF < 270 L/min or MEP < 60 cm H_2O

   iii) Cardiology consultation should be obtained for evaluation and medication optimization.

   iv) Nutritional assessment and optimization

   v) Discussion of increased risk of anesthesia or sedation, resuscitation parameters, and advance directives (if appropriate) should occur prior to the procedure.

b) Intraoperative management

   i) Setting and personnel may need to be of higher acuity or training than for the same procedure in a patient without muscular dystrophy.
      (1) Procedures normally performed outside the OR may need to be performed in the OR or PACU.
      (2) A respiratory therapist and an anesthesiologist with experience with muscular dystrophy patients may be required for intraprocedure and postprocedure care.

    ii) If FVC < 50% of predicted, use assisted or controlled ventilation for procedures normally done with spontaneous ventilation alone.

    iii) Closely monitor cardiac and fluid status due to risk of congestive heart failure; consider using arterial lines, central lines, and trans-esophageal echocardiography.

  c) Postoperative management

    i) Strongly consider an ICU bed for postprocedure care, especially in DMD or older BMD patients.

    ii) Consider extubation to NPPV if FVC < 50% predicted or the patient is on NPPV preoperatively. If possible, use the patient's home NPPV device.

    iii) Extubation in the ICU avoids the risk of transporting a spontaneously ventilating patient with respiratory compromise.

    iv) Supplemental O_2 may mask problems with ventilation. Common causes of hypoxemia include hypoventilation, atelectasis, secretions, and obstruction.

    v) Consider manually or mechanically assisted coughing.

    vi) Optimize postop pain control.

      (1) Continuous NPPV or delayed extubation may be necessary.

      (2) **Strongly consider local, regional, or neuraxial techniques.**

6) Follow-up

  a) Previously diagnosed patients: Appropriate postprocedure care is dictated by disease progression. Severely affected patients may require ICU recovery even for minor procedures using solely sedation (5).

  b) In undiagnosed patients who experience rhabdomyolysis or cardiac arrest due to hyperkalemia, ICU care will be necessary. Geneticists can establish the diagnosis and test family members; neurology, pulmonology, and cardiology follow-up are all appropriate (7) .

Chapter Summary for Muscular Dystrophy

General Considerations	The muscular dystrophies (MD) are inherited disorders that result in weakness of skeletal, cardiac, and smooth muscles. Succinylcholine and volatile anesthetics (alone or together) can precipitate rhabdomyolysis and cardiac arrest due to hyperkalemia in those with MD. Diagnosis of MD is often not made until 3–5 y of age or later. Succinylcholine is therefore relatively contraindicated in all pediatric patients.
Preoperative Considerations	Preoperative consultation with pulmonologists and cardiologists should be sought due to weakness of respiratory muscles, cardiomyopathies, and arrhythmias.
Intraoperative Considerations	Onset and recovery from nondepolarizing neuromuscular blockers may be significantly prolonged.
Postoperative Considerations	Recovery in the ICU may be necessary for patients with compromised respiratory or cardiac function.

PEDIATRIC ANESTHESIA

References

1. Darras BT. Patient information: overview of muscular dystrophies (Beyond the Basics). In: *UpToDate*, Basow DS (Ed), UpToDate, Waltham, MA, 2011.
2. Coté CJ, Lerman J, Todres ID. *A practice of Anesthesia for Infants and Children*. 4th ed. Philadelphia, PA: WB Saunders; 2009:503–505.
3. Darras BT, Chad D. Myotonic dystrophy: etiology, clinical features, and diagnosis. In: *UpToDate*, Basow DS (Ed), UpToDate, Waltham, MA 2011.
4. Dierdorf SF, Walton JS. Anesthesia for patients with rare and coexisting diseases. In: *Clinical Anesthesia*. 5th ed. Barash PG, Cullen BF, Stoelting RF (Eds). Philadelphia, PA: Lippincott Williams & Wilkins; 2006:502–505.
5. Birnkrant DJ, Panitch HB, Benditt JO, et al. American College of Chest Physicians consensus statement on the respiratory and related management of patients with Duchenne muscular dystrophy undergoing anesthesia or sedation. *Chest* 2007; 132:1977–1986.
6. Doyle E. *Paediatric Anaesthesia*. Oxford: Oxford University Press; 2007:564–566.
7. Gurnaney H, Brown A, Litman RS. Malignant hyperthermia and muscular dystrophies. *Anesth Analg* 2009; 109:1043–1048.
8. Darras BT. Treatment of Duchenne and Becker muscular dystrophy. In: *UpToDate*, Basow DS (Ed), UpToDate, Waltham, MA, 2011.

115 Epidermolysis Bullosa

Jeannie Seybold, MD

Epidermolysis Bullosa (EB) encompasses a group of rare inherited skin disorders. Patients with EB present many unique challenges to the anesthesiologist. Preparation is essential for delivering anesthetic care to these fragile patients, who often require multiple surgical procedures. Although EB is a rare disease, many of the principles discussed in this chapter apply to patients with delicate skin and/or other skin diseases.

1) **Pathophysiology**—All types of EB involve mutations in proteins that anchor the dermal and the epidermal layers of the skin. There are three major types and over 20 subtypes described (1,2).

   a) **EB simplex** (1 to 2:100,000 prevalence)—It is characterized by intraepidermal blistering. This is usually the most benign form with rare oral involvement.

   b) **Junctional EB** (<1:1,000,000 prevalence)—Blistering occurs in the lamina lucida. Almost all are autosomal recessive and have severe blistering with perioral lesions. Patients may have tracheal lesions with involvement of columnar epithelium. Death often occurs before 2 years of age.

   c) **Dystrophic EB** (2:100,000 prevalence)—Blistering occurs in the dermis and is more severe in the recessively inherited form than in the less common autosomal dominant form. Patients are prone to scarring, stricture formation, gastroesophageal reflux disease (GERD), dental caries, and the development of squamous cell carcinomas in adulthood. These patients present most frequently for surgical procedures.

2) Signs/symptoms/clinical findings

   a) **Painful bullae form with minor friction or shearing forces to the skin or squamous epithelium of oral, pharyngeal or esophageal mucosa. All adhesives (e.g., EKG pads, eye tape, endotracheal tube (ETT) tape, IV tape, Tegaderm or Opsite) are strictly contraindicated.**

   b) Common sequelae include scarring and stricture formation, feeding difficulties, dehydration, failure to thrive, anemia, difficult airway, joint contractures, and pseudosyndactyly.

   c) Chronic wound healing results in a **hypermetabolic state with increased caloric demands and in chronic infections.**

   d) **Patients with EB have normal pain sensation**. Many live with severe chronic daily pain and anxiety.

3) **Surgical treatment**

   a) Patients with EB present for frequent surgical procedures to improve function that is limited by strictures, scarring or aberrant wound healing, for dental care, or to treat malnutrition.

   b) Common surgeries: Esophageal dilation, syndactyly release and subsequent dressing changes, gastrostomy tube placement, dental rehabilitation, and excision of skin cancers.

4) **Anesthetic management**
   a) **Preop considerations**
      i) Review anesthetic records for previous care and complications, airway assessment, patient's anxiety level and response to premedication.
         (1) Adequate premedication with oral midazolam or ketamine should be given to children to prevent struggling, which may lead to injury during induction.
      ii) Interview patient and family about previous anesthesia experiences and comorbidities. Patients with severe EB may have **cardiomyopathy** from selenium deficiency or chronic renal disease (1).
      iii) Patients often arrive wrapped in protective dressings from home, and caregivers should be interviewed about current areas of skin erosion and the best places for venous cannulation.
         (1) EMLA cream may be useful if covered with nonadhesive cling film, and care is taken not to apply any shear forces when removing the cream.
      iv) Patients may be **anemic and hypoalbuminemic** from chronic malnutrition or blood loss from skin erosions.
   b) **Monitors/lines/positioning**
      i) It is helpful to preassemble an **EB kit** for such cases. Contents may include

Avoid all adhesives on skin. Remove adhesives from electrodes and probes or cover adhesives with a clear dressing such as Tegaderm so that it is no longer sticky.

         (1) **Steroid or petroleum-based lubricant cream** (e.g., Albolene unscented moisturizing cleanser, DSE Healthcare Solutions, LLC) for generously lubricating any equipment that will contact the patient's skin, including masks, nasal cannulae, ETT ties, and the care provider's hands or gloves.
         (2) **Water-based lubricant** (e.g., Surgilube, UniMed-Midwest, or KY Jelly, Johnson & Johnson) for lubricating instruments to be placed in the mouth or airway.
         (3) **Nonadherent silicone dressings** (e.g., Mepitel, Molnlycke Health Care) or Petrolatum gauze (e.g., Xeroform, Covidien) for covering IV catheters.
         (4) **Soft cotton dressings** (e.g., Webril, Covidien) to further secure IV catheters and for padding under NIBP cuffs.
         (5) **Self-adherent wrap** (e.g., Coban, 3M) and elastic netting (e.g., Surg-o-flex, Surg-o-flex of America) to secure covered catheters or monitoring probes.
         (6) **Sterile ophthalmic ointment** (e.g., Lacrilube, Allergan) to prevent drying of the eyes.
         (7) **ETT ties (described below)**
         (8) **Prepared monitoring probes** (described below)

Avoid all shearing forces on skin. Use downward pressure rather than lateral pressure when touching skin. Pad NIBP cuff.

      ii) Clip-on type pulse oximetry probes or the disposable type with the adhesive removed or covered with a transparent film (Tegaderm, 3M) may be used on a digit or ear. This may be wrapped in Vaseline gauze or a silicone dressing and further secured with Coban or Surg-o-flex netting.
      iii) **Adhesives will tear off skin.** All adhesives on ECG electrodes must be removed or covered prior to placement on skin. The patient may lie on top of the electrodes or alternatively, the electrodes and the grounding pads can be placed on the back of a water-based gel defibrillator pad (3M Defib pad) (3), and the nonadherent gel pad can then be placed on the patient's skin.
      iv) NIBP cuffs may be used as long as the extremity underneath is padded with Webril dressing to avoid direct contact and shearing. Consider placing an arterial catheter if frequent blood pressure monitoring is necessary or for long cases.

v) It is safe to use a lubricated axillary probe for temperature monitoring.

vi) **Peripheral IV placement**

(1) May be extremely difficult if there is extensive scarring or contractures of extremities.

(2) Prep the skin by spraying or gently dabbing on alcohol or sterile saline solution. To distend the vein, manually apply gentle downward pressure with a lubricated gauze or fingers.

(3) All lines should be padded with silicone or Vaseline gauze dressing at places of contact with the skin. Lines can be secured with sutures, cotton underdressings, and wrapped with Coban/Surg-o-flex.

vii) **Positioning**

(1) The patient should be kept on a **sheepskin pad**. When transferring patients, allow the patients to move themselves (if cooperative and not heavily sedated) or gently lift the sheepskin pad with the patient on it.

(2) **All pressure points should be well padded, and all contact areas should be checked for folds and wrinkles in sheets or drapes that can cause blistering.**

(3) After induction of anesthesia, the eyes may be protected with an ocular ointment or lubricated eye pads. **EB patients are at high risk for corneal abrasions.**

c) **Intraop management**

i) **Induction/airway management**

(1) **Progressive perioral scarring resulting in limited mouth opening and neck immobility may result in difficulty visualizing the airway.** A fiberoptic intubation may be the preferred method for securing the airway in certain EB patients and should always be available as a backup. A tracheostomy may be considered and discussed preoperatively in severe cases.

(2) **A gently applied mask that has been well lubricated may be used for an inhalational induction.** (When a mask induction is contraindicated, IM ketamine may be given if it is not possible to place an IV catheter.) Lubricate your hands well. Tilt the head by placing a lubricated hand under the occiput.

(3) Succinylcholine has been used uneventfully in many reports. Nondepolarizing muscle relaxants may have a prolonged effect due to hypoalbuminenia. An antisialogogue may be helpful for reducing secretions.

(4) Gentle direct laryngoscopy may be possible with a well-lubricated laryngoscope blade. **Oral intubation is preferable to nasal intubation.**

(5) **ETTs are generally safe** as the larynx, which is pseudostratified columnar epithelium, is rarely involved unless the patient has junctional EB. It is important to have ETTs in a range of smaller-than-expected sizes available.

(6) **Secure the prelubricated ETT with lubricated ties.** Umbilical ties or the ties from a surgical mask encircling the back of the head have been used.

(7) Successful use of well-lubricated and padded laryngeal mask airways has been reported but may lead to lingual bullae formation.

(8) When appropriate, regional or neuraxial anesthesia in a sedated patient may be used to avoid airway manipulation. Sterile prep can be sprayed or dripped on the skin without rubbing. Subcutaneous infiltration of local anesthesia has been performed without complications (4).

ii) **Maintenance**

(1) Total intravenous anesthesia (TIVA) with nasal cannula oxygen delivery should be considered when appropriate to avoid manipulating the airway.

EB patients have increased insensible losses and increased risk of infection from skin breakdown.

PEDIATRIC ANESTHESIA

    (2) Constant vigilance is required to make sure there is no skin or mucosal damage.

    (3) There may be increased insensible losses of fluid and body heat if the patient has large areas of skin erosion.

  iii) **Emergence**

    (1) A controlled extubation is preferred to avoid application of positive pressure ventilation in response to laryngospasm or bronchospasm.

    (2) Secretions should be suctioned only under direct vision. Do not touch the mucosa with the catheter tip.

d) **Postoperative management**

  i) PONV should be anticipated and managed with appropriate perioperative antiemetic medications. Vomiting can cause esophageal erosions.

  ii) Appropriate analgesia and patient comfort are necessary to prevent writhing, which can cause injury. Early parental presence may be helpful.

Chapter Summary of EB

General Considerations	Avoid all shearing forces and adhesives of any kind on the skin or mucosa. Preparation of equipment and positioning is critical to providing a safe anesthetic. Assemble an EB kit with all of the necessary supplies and prepared monitoring devices prior to starting the case.
Preoperative Considerations	Pediatric patients may require ample premedication/parental presence to prevent struggling. Extra care should be taken in padding, transporting, and positioning the patient.
Intraoperative Considerations	Lubricate anything that will contact the skin or mucosa. A fiberoptic intubation setup and a range of smaller ETTs must be available as backup.
Postoperative Considerations	Adequate analgesia and prophylaxis for PONV will minimize postoperative complications.

EB, epidermolysis bullosa; ETT, endotracheal tube; PONV, postoperative nausea and vomiting.

References

1. Herod J, Denyer J, Goldman A, et al. Epidermolysis bullosa in children: pathophysiology, anaesthesia and pain management. *Paediatr Anaesth* 2002;12(5):388–397.
2. Culpepper TL. Anesthetic implications in epidermolysis bullosa dystrophica. *AANA J* 2001;69(2):114–118.
3. Edler AA, Ramamurthi RJ, Valenzuela GA. Improving electrical safety for patients with Epidermolysis bullosa. *Paediatr Anaesth* 2008; 18(11) 1107–1109, 2008.
4. Lin YC, Golianu B. *J Clinical Anes* 2006;18:267–271.
5. Ames WA, Mayou BJ, Williams K. Anaesthetic management of epidermolysis bullosa. *Br J Anaesth* 1999;82(5):746–751.

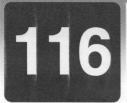

116 Down Syndrome

Jeannie Seybold, MD

Down syndrome (DS) is the most common chromosomal abnormality. Also known as *Down's syndrome* in the United Kingdom, this disorder affecting chromosome 21 manifests as **a spectrum of cardiac, airway, craniofacial, and musculoskeletal abnormalities that can increase the risks of complications during anesthesia.**

1) Introduction
   a) Epidemiology
      i) DS occurs in 1 out of approximately 732 live births in the United States (1).
      ii) The risk of having a child with DS increases with advancing maternal age and chromosome 21 nondisjunction.
      iii) Maternal ages and incidences of DS (in parentheses) are 25 (1:1,200), 35 (1:350), and 45 (1:30) (2).
   b) Pathophysiology
      i) 95% are due to trisomy 21, and approximately 4% are due to an unbalanced translocation or mosaicism involving chromosome 21 (3).
2) Signs/symptoms/clinical findings
   a) Craniofacial/neurologic
      i) Characteristic facial features include microbrachycephaly, flat occiput, small low-set ears, Brushfield spots, palpebral fissures, and microdontia.
      ii) **Atlantoaxial instability** is common. 1% to 2% of patients are symptomatic, and up to 15% have radiologic evidence but no symptoms (4).
      iii) Stenotic ear canals can lead to hearing loss.
      iv) Developmental and growth delay are characteristic.
   b) Pulmonary
      i) **Chronic airway obstruction and obstructive sleep apnea (OSA) are more common in patients with DS** due to hypertrophy of the lingual tonsils and adenoids, macroglossia, and midfacial hypoplasia with smaller oral and nasal cavities.
      ii) There may be lower airway problems due to pulmonary hypoplasia with a decreased number of alveoli.

Congenital cardiac disease and chronic pulmonary disease must be ruled out and evaluated preoperatively.

   c) Cardiac
      i) **40% to 50% have congenital heart disease (3,5) (Table 116-1).**
      ii) Pulmonary hypoplasia in patients with DS and cardiac disease may contribute to the development of pulmonary hypertension and Eisenmenger syndrome.
      iii) Adults with DS have a higher incidence of mitral valve prolapse and aortic regurgitation.
   d) Gastrointestinal/other
      i) Duodenal atresia occurs 300 times more frequently in individuals with DS than in normal individuals (5).

Table 116-1

Congenital Cardiac Defects in DS

Endocardial cushion (aka atrioventricular canal) defects (40%)
Ventricular septal defects (32%)
Atrial septal defects (10%)
Patent ductus arteriosus (4%–12%)
Tetralogy of Fallot (6%–8%)

      ii)   Obesity is common and can make IV access challenging.

      iii) DS may be associated with immune dysfunction, increasing the risk of infection.

      iv) 1% of patients with DS will develop leukemia (5).

      v)   Patients with DS can have overreactive vagal tone, muscle hypotonia, and extreme joint laxity. Other structural characteristics include a single palmar crease, and middle finger dysplasia.

  3) **Surgical treatment**

    a) Patients will present for surgical correction of choanal atresia, cleft lip and palate, cataracts, strabismus, OSA, airway and cardiac anomalies.

  4) **Anesthetic management**

    a) **Preoperative considerations**

      i)   It is important to interview caregivers about the patient's communication skills, anxiety level, comorbidities including cardiac history, cervical spine and neurological problems, and previous experiences with anesthesia, premedication, and postoperative nausea and pain control.

      ii) Head extension during laryngoscopy may result in spinal cord injury in patients with atlantoaxial instability.

DS patients may have atlanto-axial instability. Avoid extreme neck flexion, extension or rotation, which may lead to neurological injury.

        (1) Routine radiographic screening of all patients with DS has not been shown to be predictive of neurologic injury and is not recommended unless the patient shows signs of spinal cord compression such as torticollis, neck pain, easy fatigability, hyperreflexia, clonus, abnormal gait, Babinski sign, or other upper motor neuron or posterior column signs.

        (2) In these cases, lateral neck radiographs in the flexed, extended, and neutral positions may be warranted to determine if the patient will require cervical spine stabilization prior to elective surgery.

      iii) A recent echocardiogram or cardiac evaluation may be necessary if the patient has a history of heart disease, if cardiac disease is suspected, or after surgical correction of cardiac lesions. Anesthetic management should be tailored to the pathophysiology of the lesion present.

      iv) Prophylactic antibiotics may be required.

    b) **Premedication**

      i)   Developmental delay can lead to an unpredictable response to sedative medications. Patients with OSA may be more sensitive to premedication and experience airway obstruction.

      ii) A 0.5 to 0.75 mg/kg PO dose of midazolam is recommended to facilitate inhalational induction or peripheral IV catheter placement.

      iii) Intramuscular ketamine or midazolam may be necessary if patients are uncooperative with taking oral medications.

      iv) Anticholinergics may be useful to decrease oral secretions.

c) **Intraoperative management**

i) Avoid a rapid inhalational induction. Incremental increases in vapor delivery will minimize the risk of bradycardia, which can occur in patients with high vagal tone.

ii) Great care must be taken to **avoid extreme flexion, extension, or rotation of the neck in all patients with DS.** Stabilization with a soft collar should be considered if there is evidence of atlantoaxial instability.

iii) Airway management may be more difficult as upper airway obstruction is likely after induction of anesthesia due to large tongue, and hyperextension of the neck must be avoided during laryngoscopy.

iv) **A smaller-than-expected endotracheal tube (ETT) may be required** if there is subglottic narrowing.

v) Patients with DS do not have a higher incidence of bronchospasm when compared with the general pediatric population.

vi) A smaller cricoid ring and larynx predispose to postextubation stridor and subglottic stenosis. The risk of postextubation stridor may be diminished by a tracheal tube leak test and the administration of dexamethasone, especially in ENT cases with a high risk of postsurgical edema.

d) **Emergence**

i) Awake extubation is recommended as there is an increased likelihood of airway obstruction.

ii) Adequate postoperative analgesia is necessary as the patients may have difficulty communicating. Patients with OSA may be more sensitive to narcotic medications.

e) **Postoperative management**

i) Continuous monitoring should be performed postoperatively in the PACU as airway obstruction or stridor may be present. The appropriate emergency airway equipment must be readily available.

ii) Post-extubation stridor should be treated with humidified O_2 and aerosolized racemic epinephrine. A monitored bed may be required on the ward if there is risk of tongue edema (i.e., post-airway surgery).

A smaller-than-expected ETT size may be required due to subglottic stenosis. Be sure to check for a leak around the ETT.

PEDIATRIC ANESTHESIA

Chapter Summary for Down Syndrome

General Considerations	Trisomy 21 manifests as a spectrum of cardiac, airway, craniofacial, and musculoskeletal abnormalities that can increase the risks of complications during anesthesia.
Preoperative Considerations	It is important to ask about symptomatic atlantoaxial instability, congenital cardiac defects, pulmonary hypertension, airway problems including upper airway obstruction and subglottic tracheal stenosis, cognitive and communication skills. Routine radiographic screening for neck instability is not recommended if the patient is asymptomatic. Recent cardiology evaluation is recommended for patients with congenital heart disease.
Intraoperative Considerations	A smaller-than-expected ETT may be necessary due to subglottic stenosis. Higher vagal tone may increase the risk of bradycardia.
Postoperative Considerations	Obesity and craniofacial anatomy may increase the likelihood of postop airway obstruction and stridor.

References

1. Sherman SL, Allen EG, Bean LH, et al. Epidemiology of Down Syndrome. *Ment Retard Dev Disabil Res Rev* 2007;13:221–227.
2. National Down Syndrome Society Incidences and Maternal Age data, ndss.org
3. Borland LM, Colligan J, Brandom BW. *Paediatr Anesth* 2004;14:733–738.
4. Braganza SF, Adam HM. Atlantoaxial Dislocation. *Pediatr Rev* 2003;24:106.
5. Stoelting RK, Dierdorf SF. *Anesthesia and Co-existing Disease.* 4th ed. Churchill Livingstone Philadephia, PA; 2002:706–707.
6. Meitzner MC, Skurnowicz JA. Anesthetic considerations for patients with Down syndrome. *AANA J* 2005;73(2):103–107.

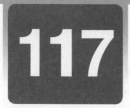

117

Cystic Fibrosis

Samuel Mireles, MD

Cystic fibrosis (CF) is an autosomal recessive disease caused by a dysfunctional trans-membrane chloride channel in epithelial cells of the airway, intestine, sweat, pancreatic and biliary ducts, and vas deferens. It is the most common lethal inherited disorder among Caucasians, with an incidence of 1:2,000 white births, but it can affect all racial groups (1). Due to advances in medical management, median predicted survival is now >35 years (2).

1) Signs/symptoms/clinical findings
   a) **Pulmonary**

Chronic lung disease may lead to pulmonary hypertension and cor pulmonale.

   i) Although disease manifestations vary widely, CF is progressive with pulmonary disease being the main cause of morbidity and mortality.
   ii) Patients have **viscous mucous and impaired ciliary clearance,** which leads to mucus plugging, chronic infection, inflammation, and epithelial injury.
   iii) **Chronic infections** lead to bronchiectasis, increased airway resistance and bullae, but there is also evidence of impaired airway function in infants prior to clinically recognized infections (3).
   iv) Pulmonary function tests are consistent with **obstructive disease with increased functional residual capacity but decreased forced expiratory volume, peak expiratory flow, and vital capacity.**
   v) Tachypnea often leads to hypocapnea, but in severe disease, hypercapnea may prevail.
   b) **Cardiac**
   i) Chronic hypoxemia **can lead to pulmonary hypertension** and right ventricular enlargement in CF patients, although the incidence is unclear (4).
   ii) **End-stage pulmonary disease** may be associated with cor pulmonale, right ventricular failure, and fluid retention, which are associated with poor prognosis (5).
   c) **Gastrointestinal**

Malnutrition, malabsorption, and liver dysfunction may lead to coagulopathies.

   i) **Malnutrition secondary to malabsorption** is a common manifestation of the disease.
   ii) Low weight and body mass index are closely associated with poor lung function (6).
   iii) Gastroesophageal reflux is common.
   d) **Hematologic**
   i) CF patients have malabsorption of vitamin K and decreased synthesis of factors II, VII, IX, and X.

e) **Hepatic**
   i) CF patients have **decreased plasma cholinesterase**.
   ii) Patients with end-stage disease and cor pulmonale may also have hepatomegaly and gastroesophageal varices.

f) **Pancreatic**
   i) **>12% of patients over 13 years have insulin-dependent diabetes mellitus**. CF-related diabetes may contribute to lung disease and worse outcome (7).

2) **Surgeries/procedures commonly performed in CF patients**
   a) Nasal polypectomy, endoscopic sinus surgeries
   b) Bronchoscopy, pulmonary lavage, management of pneumothoraces
   c) Investigation or correction of gastrointestinal disease such as meconium ileus in the neonate, gastroesophageal endoscopy, cholecystectomy, and sclerosis of varices due to portal hypertension in end-stage disease.
   d) Insertion of venous access devices
   e) Organ transplantation, especially lung

3) **Anesthetic management**
   a) **Preoperative evaluation**
      i) Focus on the severity and optimization of pulmonary disease since this is the primary cause of morbidity and mortality in CF patients and the most common cause of perioperative complications.
      ii) **History** should assess
         (1) Extent of multisystem involvement
         (2) Recent hospitalizations
         (3) Recent infections and antimicrobial sensitivities
         (4) Quality and quantity of secretions
         (5) Response to bronchodilators
         (6) Exercise tolerance
      iii) **Physical exam** should include
         (1) Weight and body mass index
         (2) Baseline SpO_2
         (3) Cardiopulmonary assessment
      iv) **Studies**
         (1) Routine studies are not indicated.
         (2) Depending on the severity of disease and the extent of multisystem involvement the following may be appropriate:
            (a) Arterial blood gas
            (b) Chest radiograph
            (c) Pulmonary function tests
            (d) Electrocardiogram
            (e) Echocardiogram
            (f) Glucose
            (g) Liver function tests
            (h) Coagulation studies
         (3) As with all preoperative assessment, invasive studies need only be obtained when the results are expected to alter management decisions.
      v) **Pulmonary optimization**
         (1) Pulmonary function should be optimized with chest physiotherapy, bronchodilators, and humidified nebulizer treatments.
         (2) Nebulized saline treatments may be administered up until induction.
         (3) Nebulized hypertonic saline (7% sodium chloride) has been shown to improve mucous clearance and lung function (8).
         (4) **Dornase alfa (DNase)** has been shown to reduce air trapping, improve FEV_1, and decrease pulmonary exacerbation rate (9).

Optimize pulmonary function preoperatively with bronchodilators, hypertonic saline treatment, and DNase.

b) **Monitoring/lines**
    i)   Standard ASA monitors are usually all that is required
    ii) Invasive lines are rarely necessary but may be indicated depending on the severity of disease and the surgical procedure.
    iii) In patients with severe lung disease, cor pulmonale, or intermediate-to high-risk procedures, invasive monitoring may be indicated.

c) **Intraoperative management**
    i)   General anesthesia may be necessary due to patient age, coagulopathy, or surgical procedure.
    ii) Regional anesthesia offers the advantage of improved respiratory mechanics and is preferred over general anesthesia when not contraindicated.
    iii) **Induction**
        (1) Anxiolysis with benzodiazepines is appropriate with anxious pediatric patients.
        (2) Inhalation induction may be prolonged due to increased functional residual capacity, small tidal volumes, and V/Q mismatch (10).
        (3) IV induction and aspiration prophylaxis should be considered in patients with significant gastroesophageal reflux.
        (4) A cuffed endotracheal tube is preferred because of the higher airway pressures needed to ventilate poorly compliant lungs.

Humidify all gases during the anesthetic, and consider suctioning ETT to prevent plugging of airways.

    iv) **Maintenance**
        (1) A deep anesthetic should be employed to prevent airway hyperreactivity.
        (2) Short-acting agents, local anesthetics, and nonopioid analgesics should all be considered to prevent postoperative respiratory depression.
        (3) **Humidification of anesthetic gases is extremely important to reduce inspissated secretions and mucus plugging.**
    v) **Emergence**
        (1) Ideally, the patient will be spontaneously breathing and extubated at the end of the procedure.
        (2) Complete reversal of neuromuscular blockers must be assured.
        (3) Deep extubation, when not contraindicated by difficult airway or gastroesophageal reflux, may decrease airway hyperreactivity in patients who are able to demonstrate adequate spontaneous respirations prior to emergence.
        (4) A head-up position will improve respiratory mechanics.
    vi) **Complications**
        (1) Most common are bronchospasm, laryngospasm, obstruction from inspissated secretions, hypoxemia, and atelectasis.
        (2) Less common complications include pneumothorax, pneumonia, postoperative respiratory failure, and opioid induced ileus.

d) **Postoperative management/disposition**
    i)   The goals are to provide adequate analgesia without respiratory depression, improve clearance of secretions, and minimize atelectasis.
    ii) Early ambulation, chest physiotherapy, nebulized saline treatments, and bronchodilators as needed should be utilized in postoperative care.
    iii) Monitored wards or ICU should be considered for severely affected patients.

PEDIATRIC ANESTHESIA

Chapter Summary for Cystic Fibrosis

General Considerations	Cystic fibrosis is a multisystem disease with pulmonary, cardiac, gastrointestinal, endocrine and hematologic manifestations.
Preoperative Considerations	**Optimize pulmonary function preoperatively** by the use of chest physiotherapy, bronchodilators, and humidified nebulizer treatments.
Intraoperative Considerations	**Maintain deep anesthetic** to prevent airway hyperreactivity and **humidify anesthetic gases** to improve mucous clearance.
Postoperative Considerations	**Avoid postoperative respiratory depression** by the use of regional techniques when feasible, short-acting anesthetics/opioids and nonopioid analgesics.

References

1. Della Rocca G. Anaesthesia in patients with cystic fibrosis. *Curr Opin Anaesthesiol* 2002;15:95–101.
2. Marshall BC, Hazle L. Cystic Fibrosis Foundation Patient Registry: Annual Data Report 2007;3–4.
3. Ranganathan SC, Dezateux C, Bush A, et al. Airway function in infants newly diagnosed with cystic fibrosis. *Lancet* 2001;358(9279):1964–1965.
4. Bright-Thomas RJ, Webb AK. The heart in cystic fibrosis. *J R Soc Med* 2002;95(Suppl 41):2–10.
5. Moss AJ. The cardiovascular system in cystic fibrosis. *Pediatrics* 1982;70(5):728–741.
6. Pedreira CC, Robert RG, Dalton V, et al. Association of body composition and lung function in children with cystic fibrosis. *Pediatr Pulmonol* 2005;39(3):276–280.
7. Accurso FJ. Update in cystic fibrosis. *Am J Respir Crit Care Med* 2006;173:944–947.
8. Donaldson SH, Bennett WD, Zeman KL, et al. Mucus clearance and lung function in cystic fibrosis with hypertonic saline. *N Engl J Med* 2006;354:241–250.
9. Huffmyer JL, Littlewood KE, Nemergut EC. Perioperative management of the adult with cystic fibrosis. *Anesth Analg* 2009;109(6):1952.
10. Cote CJ, Lerman J, Todres DI, eds. *A practice of Anesthesia for Infants and Children*. 4th ed. Philadelphia, PA: Saunders; 2009:234.

118 Part B: Anesthetic Concerns and Procedures in Pediatric Anesthesia
Adenotonsillectomy

Dondee Almazan, MD • Calvin Kuan, MD

Adenotonsillectomy, or tonsillectomy and adenoidectomy (T&A), was a nearly universal procedure for children in the early 1900s for a wide range of medical conditions. It is still one of the most commonly performed pediatric surgical procedures in the world. The indication for surgery is now limited to recurrent tonsillitis or obstructive sleep apnea (OSA).

1) **Pathophysiology**
   a) Nasal and pharyngeal upper airway obstruction can cause chronic hypoxemia and hypercarbia, which may lead to pulmonary vascular changes resulting in pulmonary hypertension, right ventricular hypertrophy, and even cor pulmonale—all of which significantly increase risks of anesthesia.
   b) Chronic or recurrent infections are not associated with cardiopulmonary changes.
2) **Signs/symptoms/clinical findings**
   a) History
      i) Sleep problems
      ii) Loud snoring
      iii) Daytime somnolence
      iv) Observed pauses during sleep
      v) Irritability
      vi) Speech problems
   b) Physical exam
      i) BMI > 95%tile for age/gender
      ii) Craniofacial abnormalities affecting the airway (e.g., Treacher Collins)
      iii) Upper airway obstruction
      iv) Coughing
      v) Halitosis
      vi) Acute or recurrent otitis media and/or adenoiditis or tonsillitis
   c) Less common or more serious findings include:
      i) Failure to thrive
      ii) Hypoxemia, hypercarbia
      iii) Cardiac abnormalities
         (1) left ventricular dysfunction
         (2) right ventricular hypertrophy

(3) pulmonary hypertension
(4) cor-pulmonale

iv) Peritonsillar abscess
v) Repeated lower respiratory tract infections

3) **Surgical treatment**
a) **Tonsillectomy** is the surgical excision of the palatine tonsils.
b) **Adenoidectomy** is usually performed in conjunction with tonsillectomy, especially if there are associated chronic adenoiditis, recurrent otitis media, and nasal obstruction.
c) Many different surgical techniques are employed, including dissection, ultrasound ablation and electrocautery, each with its own advantages and disadvantages.

4) **Anesthetic management**

Refer to the American Society of Anesthesiologists (ASA) and the American Academy of Pediatrics (AAP) guidelines for more information about the perioperative management of children with OSA (2–5).

a) **Preoperative considerations**
i) Determine the indication for surgery and include review of medical records and previous anesthetics, medical history, physical exam, and sleep studies.
ii) Focus on airway, cardiac, pulmonary, and hematologic systems.
(1) It is most important to identify children with sleep-disordered breathing or OSA because they are at greater risk of developing perioperative complications (1–3).
(a) There is no official definition for diagnosis of OSA in children.
(b) Many children may be referred for surgery without formal or extensive workup, but they are still at risk for OSA-associated complications.
(c) The practitioner must have a high index of clinical suspicion and need for workup to determine severity of disease.

Assess patients for risk of OSA because of increased perioperative complications—airway obstruction, respiratory depression.

(2) Patients with obstructive symptoms may have underlying craniofacial abnormalities that are associated with difficult airways.
(3) **Recent upper respiratory infections may necessitate postponing surgery due to increased respiratory complications (6) and increased risk for postoperative bleeding (7).**
(4) **Any history of easy bleeding or bruising must be investigated to rule out underlying coagulopathy.**
iii) **Additional labs/studies** prior to surgery for the otherwise healthy child are not necessary and should be ordered on a case-by-case basis depending on the individual medical history and physical exam (e.g., easy bleeding).
iv) **Premedication** should be individualized, rather than routine.

Premedication should not automatically be given to patients with OSA without adequate monitoring preoperatively.

(1) **Children with sleep-disordered breathing or OSA have increased sensitivity to sedatives and opiates**—a dose of midazolam 0.5 mg/kg PO may result in hypoxia or even apnea.
(2) **If premedication is given, children should be closely monitored for obstruction and hypoxemia.**

b) **Intraoperative considerations**
i) **Monitors/lines/position**
(1) Standard ASA monitors with a single IV line are sufficient for routine T&A cases.

(2) Patients with cardiac or pulmonary involvement may require invasive monitors.

(3) The patient is typically turned 90 degrees away from the anesthesiologist.

ii) **Induction**

  (1) Inhalational induction is typically initiated with sevoflurane and $O_2 \pm N_2O$.

    (a) Use of 100% O_2 will allow greater oxygen reserve in case of airway problems.

  (2) Patients with OSA have a greater incidence of respiratory problems (e.g., laryngospasm, breath holding and desaturation) on induction compared to children with tonsillitis (8).

  (3) IV induction may be safer for children with significant cardiac or pulmonary comorbidities.

iii) **Airway** may be secured either with ETT or LMA

  (1) Reinforced or armored LMA

    (a) Classic or nonreinforced LMAs are likely to kink or dislodge.

    (b) Spiral reinforced LMA Flexible™ can be positioned safely under the Dingman retractor without kinking or dislodging.

    (c) The smallest size Flexible™ currently available is size 2 for children of 10 to 20 kg.

    (d) Use may depend on surgeon preference and familiarity.

    (e) LMA use is associated with decreased incidence of postoperative stridor and laryngospasm (9), but does not protect airway in case of laryngospasm.

    (f) There is no evidence that LMA decreases morbidity over an ETT.

  (2) **Cuffed oral RAE ETT**

    (a) Cuffed ETT are preferred to minimize number of intubations and to minimize leak of O_2 or anesthetic gases.

    (b) Oral RAE tubes are preferred due to the preformed angle for better surgical exposure and decreased risk of kinking.

    (c) Armored cuffed ETT may also be used as they are also less likely to kink.

    (d) Advantages of the ETT over the LMA include:

      (i) Provision of a secured airway

      (ii) Ability to safely paralyze and ventilate a patient if necessary

      (iii) Isolation of trachea with cuffed ETT from blood/fluids

      (iv) Ability to minimize leak of O_2 into surgical field, decreasing risk of airway fire

iv) **Maintenance**

  (1) **Volatile versus IV anesthesia**

    (a) Volatile anesthetics

      (i) Sevoflurane is associated with a smoother induction and a slightly longer emergence compared to desflurane.

      (ii) Desflurane has a faster offset compared to sevoflurane when used for maintenance but can cause tachycardia and severe laryngospasm during emergence.

      (iii) Both have similar incidence of emergence delirium and time to patient discharge.

    (b) IV anesthetics may be used to supplement volatile anesthetic or as a TIVA.

Children with OSA have greater incidence of respiratory problems on induction compared to children with tonsillitis.

(i) Propofol as bolus or infusion can decrease amount of volatile agent needed, help decrease postoperative nausea and vomiting (PONV), and may help for a smoother emergence.

(ii) Opioids should be titrated in during case as needed.

(2) Controlled versus spontaneous ventilation

(a) Controlled ventilation

(i) May be necessary for patients who require muscle relaxation for induction/intubation or treatment of airway obstruction.

(ii) Advantages

1. The ability to use paralytic agent to guarantee immobility during surgery.

(iii) Disadvantages

1. Need to administer reversal agents with associated risks of nausea/vomiting and residual neuromuscular blockade.

2. Unable to gauge titration of postoperative analgesia.

(b) Spontaneous ventilation

(i) Advantages

1. Respiratory rate and ETCO2 level can be used as a guide for titration of opioid or other analgesics during the case to achieve a smoother emergence.

2. Theoretically faster emergence as there is no need to wait for return of spontaneous respirations.

(ii) Disadvantages

1. May require deeper level of anesthesia to prevent movement interfering with surgery.

2. May not be an option if paralysis was necessary on induction.

c) **Special anesthetic considerations**

i) Anesthesia for T&A has a high incidence of upper airway obstruction and airway reactivity.

ii) **A mouth gag is usually placed by the surgeon and must be removed at the end of the case.**

iii) Be vigilant for tube kinking and lips/tongue being pinched especially during Dingman insertion.

iv) **Airway fire**

READ MORE
ENT and laser surgery, Chapter 138, page 969

(1) Risk depends on surgical technique.

(2) Use the lowest tolerated FiO$_2$.

(3) Use of cuffed ETT with minimal leak around cuff.

(4) N$_2$O is noncombustible but will accelerate burning of combustible material in a fire.

(5) Discuss with surgeon and nursing staff regarding a treatment plan if airway fire should occur.

v) **Acute postobstructive pulmonary edema (2)**

(1) Acute upper airway obstruction in spontaneously breathing patient may result in **negative pressure pulmonary edema.**

(2) Relief of chronic upper airway obstruction may cause noncardiogenic pulmonary edema.

(3) Treatment of both includes endotracheal intubation with higher than normal PEEP, and supportive care.

(4) Since the problem is not primarily fluid overload, diuresis is contraindicated and may be detrimental.

vi) **Emergence/analgesia**

Spontaneous ventilation during case allows for titration of narcotics/analgesics to respiratory rate to achieve adequate analgesia prior to emergence.

A mouth gag is typically placed by the surgeon and must be removed at the end of the case.

Due to risk of airway fire, keep FiO$_2$ as low as tolerated by patient.

a) **Extubation**
   i)   Historically recommended to extubate patients awake, but many practitioners do choose to extubate patients deep.
   ii)   Full reversal of neuromuscular blockade is recommended.
   iii) **Deep extubation**
       (1) Advantages
            (a) Theoretically less risk of postoperative bleeding from coughing or bucking on emergence.
            (b) In children whose indication is infection rather than OSA, the risk of airway problems is less.
       (2) Disadvantages
            (a) Increased risk of airway obstruction and laryngospasm.
       (3) Strategies to decrease risk of airway obstruction
            (a) Use propofol for maintenance over vapor anesthetic.
            (b) Select older/larger patients with less severe obstructive histories for deep extubation.
   iv) **Awake extubation**
       (1) Advantages
            (a) Ability to protect airway from blood/secretions prior to extubation.
       (2) Disadvantages
            (a) Coughing and straining on emergence may cause bleeding from surgical sites.

Turn patient on side prior to extubation to allow secretions/blood to pool out of mouth and decrease risk of laryngospasm.

b) **Positioning patient for emergence**
   i)   Tonsil or recovery position: **patient in lateral position to allow fluid to pool away from and out of mouth.**
   ii)   Patient may be kept in this position for transport to recovery.

c) **Analgesic management**
   i)   Adenotonsillectomy is very stimulating during the surgery and can be very painful postoperatively.
   ii)   Goal of complete analgesia must be weighed against risk and side effects of drugs used (airway obstruction and hypoventilation).
   iii) **Dexamethasone**
       (1) A single dose 0.5 to 1 mg/kg IV (maximum dose: 20 mg) given intraoperatively is effective for procedures using electrocautery.
       (2) May also help decrease risk of PONV.
   iv) **Acetaminophen**
       (1) Effective adjunct analgesic may be given during surgery.
       (2) Loading dose of 30 to 40 mg/kg rectally and then 15 to 20 mg/kg every 4 to 6 hours orally or rectally.
   v)   **Opioids**
       (1) Associated with increased incidence of PONV and respiratory depression.
       (2) Weigh risk/benefits of giving long-acting versus short-acting agents in children.
       (3) **Codeine should not be given to children with OSA who are not monitored due to risk of active metabolites causing respiratory depression (10).**
       (4) Children with OSA
            (a) **Smaller-than-expected opioid dose may produce exaggerated respiratory depression (11).**
            (b) Titrate doses to effect while watching analgesic response and respiratory rate and avoiding overdosing.

Children with OSA are extra sensitive to narcotics—give incremental doses titrating to respiratory rate and analgesic effect.

PEDIATRIC ANESTHESIA

        vi)   **Nonsteroidal anti-inflammatory drugs (NSAIDs)**
- (1) Effective postoperative opioid sparing adjunct.
- (2) Reported increase in postoperative bleeding, but systematic reviews have not supported this finding.
- (3) Aspirin increases bleeding risk, but other NSAIDs do not.
- (4) Should only be used after consulting with the surgeon.

        vii) **Ketamine**
- (1) May decrease need for opiates and have preemptive analgesic properties.

    d) **Recommendations to decrease PONV**
- i) Suction out stomach and oropharynx prior to extubation.
- ii) Consider use of propofol for maintenance.
- iii) Ondansetron is more effective than metoclopramide.
- iv) Dexamethasone is effective in preventing PONV as well as treating pain.
- v) Minimize use of opioids and avoid neuromuscular reversal agents if possible.

6) **Postoperative considerations**
    a) **Disposition**
- i) The need for postoperative admission and monitoring depends on the severity of preoperative illness.
- ii) Even though the offending anatomy has been removed, the risk of obstruction may remain, and in some instances be exacerbated immediately postoperatively.
- iii) Children with the following clinical features of OSA may require overnight admission to ward or PICU for postoperative management (2,8).

Children with severe OSA and other criteria must be admitted for observation postoperatively.

        1) Age < 3 years
        2) History or concern of obstructive breathing with apnea
        3) Morbid obesity
        4) Severe desaturation or obstruction on induction or postoperatively
        5) Coexisting neuromuscular, cardiac, pulmonary, or other systemic illness
        6) Pulmonary hypertension
        7) Low weight/failure to thrive

    b) Other interventions that may help to avoid reintubation postoperatively include CPAP, BIPAP, and high-flow nasal cannula.

7) **Post-tonsillectomy bleeding is a surgical emergency (Fig. 118-1)**
- a) Approximately 75% of bleeding occurs within 6 hours of surgery with the remainder occurring 5 to 10 days after surgery when the scar over the surgical site retracts (3).
- b) Assess severity of hypovolemia and anemia and initiate aggressive volume resuscitation with isotonic crystalloid and/or colloid solution before the operation.
- c) Type and Crossmatch (T&C) for RBC should be obtained, and blood sent to the operating room.
- d) Patients will have likely swallowed a significant amount of blood and must be considered to have full stomachs and aspiration risk.
- e) **Ensure adequate large bore suction is available.**
- f) **Induction**
  - i) **Preoxygenate in the lateral position** so blood can drain out of the oral cavity.
  - ii) Perform **rapid sequence induction with cricoid pressure** (in lateral or supine position) using reduced induction dosages of rapid-onset agents.
    - (1) **Etomidate** 0.3 mg/kg IV
    - (2) **Ketamine** 1 to 2 mg/kg IV or 2 to 4 mg/kg IM
    - (3) Titrated doses of **propofol** 1 mg/kg IV
  - iii) Rapid-onset muscle relaxation is indicated.

| Figure 118-1 | Post-Tonsillectomy Bleeding |

Preop:
1. Assess hemodynamic/volume status
2. Obtain IV access
3. Volume resuscitation with isotonic crystalloid/colloid
4. Send type and cross
5. Suction out stomach
6. If patient stable and IV access difficult, may consider inhalational induction with cricoid pressure

↓

Intraop—Preparation:
1. Preoxygenation with 100% FiO_2 in lateral position
2. Have working large bore suction available

↓

Intraop—Induction/intubation:
1. Induction in supine or lateral position
2. Rapid sequence induction (RSI) with cricoid pressure
3. Anticipate difficult visualization due to bleeding
4. Use cuffed ETT with stylet

↓

Intraop—Induction/medication:
1. Induction agent
   a. Etomidate 0.3 mg/kg IV **OR**
   b. Ketamine 1–2 mg/kg IV, 2–4 mg/kg IM
2. Rapid onset paralytic
   a. Succinylcholine 2 mg/kg IV, 2–4 mg/kg IM **OR**
   b. Rocuronium 1–1.2 mg/kg IV, 2 mg/kg IM

↓

Emergence/Postop management:
1. Suction stomach and oropharynx prior to extubation
2. Extubate in lateral position when fully awake
3. If aspiration suspected, and/or lung compliance is poor, consider leaving intubated and transfer to ICU

PEDIATRIC ANESTHESIA

(1) **Succinylcholine** 2 mg/kg IV or 4 mg/kg IM
(2) **Rocuronium** 1.2 mg/kg IV or 2 mg/kg IM
iv) Anticholinergic agents may be given simultaneously to preempt bradycardia and act as antisialogogue.
   (1) **Atropine** 0.02 mg/kg IV
   (2) Glycopyrrolate 0.01 mg/kg IV
v) **Anticipate a difficult intubation due to bleeding and full stomach.**
   (1) **Cuffed ETT** should be used to minimize aspiration risk and to avoid the need to reintubate for inappropriate size.
   (2) Stylet recommended because of potentially difficult visualization

For post-tonsillectomy bleeding, assume that patient is hypovolemic and anemic, and will have a full stomach and difficult intubation.

g) **Maintenance**
   i)   Surgery not as painful as initial T&A repair, so analgesic needs will likely be less.
   ii)   Anesthetic with volatile or TIVA supplemented with opiates as tolerated by patient hemodynamics.

h) **Emergence**
   i)   Have surgeon suction out stomach and oropharynx completely.
   ii)   Fully reverse muscle relaxation.
   iii) Turn patient to side for emergence.
   iv)   Extubate only when the child is awake with full return of airway reflexes.

i) **Postoperative management/disposition**
   i)   Follow up Hgb/Hct.
   ii)   If aspiration suspected and/or lung compliance is poor, consider leaving patient intubated and transfer to ICU.

Chapter Summary for Tonsillectomy and Adenoidectomy

General Considerations	Indications are now limited to recurrent infection or OSA.
Preoperative Considerations	Evaluation should focus on OSA symptoms including CO_2 retention, hypoxemia, and pulmonary hypertension. Pts with severe OSA are at risk for postop complications. Consider risk of respiratory depression with preoperative anxiolytic medications .
Intraoperative Considerations	Spontaneous breathing allows titration of narcotics to respiratory rate and $ETCO_2$. Aggressive PONV prophylaxis recommended. Consider extubation and recovery in the lateral position.
Postoperative Considerations	Severe OSA symptoms may require postoperative admission for respiratory observation.
Postoperative Bleeding	Life-threatening emergency. Patients may be severely hypovolemic and are at high risk for aspiration. Anticipate difficult airway and have adequate help available.

OSA, obstructive sleep apnea; PONV, postoperative nausea and vomiting; $ETCO_2$, end tidal carbon dioxide.

References

1.   Rosen GM, Muckle RP, Mahowald MW, et al. Postoperative respiratory compromise in children with obstructive sleep apnea syndrome: can it be anticipated? *Pediatrics* 1994;93:784–788.
2.   Schwengel DA, Sterni LM, Tunkel DE, et al. Perioperative management of children with obstructive sleep apnea. *Anesth Analg* 2009:109:60–75.
3.   Cote CJ, Lerman J, Todres DI, eds. *A Practice of Anesthesia for Infants and Children*. 4th ed. Philadelphia, PA: Saunders; 2009.
4.   ASA Practice guidelines for the perioperative management of patients with obstructive sleep apnea. *Anesthesiology* 2006:104:1081–1093.
5.   Clinical practice guideline: diagnosis and management of childhood obstructive sleep apnea syndrome. *Pediatrics* 2002;109:704–712.
6.   Cohen MM, Cameron CB. Should you cancel the operation when a child has an upper respiratory tract infection? *Anesth Analg* 1991;72:282–288.
7.   Schloss MD, Tan AKW, Schloss B, et al. Outpatient tonsillectomy and adenoidectomy: complications and recommendations. *Int J Pediatr Otorhinolaryngol* 1994;30:115–122.
8.   Sanders JC, King MA, Mitchell RB, Kelly JP. Perioperative complications of adenotonsillectomy in children with obstructive sleep apnea syndrome. *Anesth Analg* 2006;103:1115–1121.
9.   Webster AC, Morley-Forster PK, Dain S, et al. Anaesthesia for adenotonsillectomy: a comparison between tracheal intubation and the armoured laryngeal mask airway. *Can J Anaesth* 1993;40:1171–1177.
10. Ciszkowski C, Madadi P, Phillips MS, et al. Codeine, ultrarapid-metabolism genotype, and postoperative death. *N Engl J Med* 361;8;827–828.
11. Waters KA, McBrien F, Stewart P, et al. Effects of OSA, inhalational anesthesia, and fentanyl on the airway and ventilation of children. *J Appl Physiol* 2002;92:1987–1994.

119 Myringotomy and Ventilation Tubes

Dondee Almazan, MD · Calvin Kuan, MD

Myringotomy and placement of ventilation tubes are one of the most common surgical procedures for children requiring general anesthesia. It is typically an ambulatory surgery for infants and toddlers.

1) **Indication**
   a) Failed medical management of **chronic serous otitis media** to prevent consequent hearing loss and cholesteatoma formation.
2) **Signs and symptoms** are typically a constellation of upper respiratory symptoms.
   a) Persistent rhinorrhea
   b) Congestion
   c) Coughing
   d) Low-grade fever
   e) Recurrent respiratory infections that often resolve with fluid drainage.
3) **Surgical treatment**
   a) **Myringotomy** refers to the creation of an opening in the tympanic membrane to allow fluid drainage.
   b) **Tympanostomy tubes** or **bilateral tympanostomy tubes (BTTs)** (aka *ventilation tubes* or *pressure equalization* **[PE]** *tubes* in the United States and *grommets* in the United Kingdom) are small plastic tubes inserted in the tympanic membrane as a stent to allow fluid drainage from the middle ear.
   c) Surgery typically lasts only a **few minutes for each ear**, with the patient supine and head turned to the contralateral side.
4) **Anesthetic management**
   a) **Preoperative evaluation**
      i) Labs or other studies are not routinely indicated for patients without significant comorbidities.
      ii) History and physical
         (1) Children presenting for this procedure often have a history of recent upper respiratory tract infection (URI).
         (2) Though controversial, **canceling surgery for symptoms of only rhinorrhea or mild URI is usually not warranted.**
            (a) There is not an increased risk of perioperative complications, provided airway manipulation is avoided and/or an LMA is used and the patient is not endotracheally intubated (1,2).
         (3) Patients with lower respiratory infections and possible pneumonia (high-grade fever, productive cough, hypoxia, and CXR findings) should have surgery postponed for 4 to 6 weeks.

Children with upper respiratory infection may safely proceed with surgery. Consider postponing surgery for children with lower respiratory infections or severe symptoms.

PEDIATRIC ANESTHESIA

845

b) **Intraoperative management**
   i)   Premedication is typically omitted, especially if parental presence is permitted for induction.
   ii) Standard ASA monitors
   iii) Lines
      (1) Many practitioners will perform this anesthetic without an IV.
      (2) An IV may be indicated for children with significant comorbidities who may require postoperative analgesia or fluids or who may be at increased risk of airway complications.
      (3) An IV may also be placed at any time during the case for postoperative use if significant laryngospasm has occurred.
c) **Induction**
   i)   Inhalation induction with sevoflurane, O_2 ± nitrous oxide (N_2O)
d) **Maintenance**
   i)   Maintenance of anesthesia is typically achieved with the patient spontaneously breathing with a combination of sevoflurane/O_2/N_2O.
   ii) If an IV is in place, anesthetic may be supplemented with IV agents as indicated.
   iii) A propofol maintenance IV infusion may be beneficial for children at high risk for emergence delirium.
e) **Special anesthetic goals/issues**
   i)   Due to the very short duration, most anesthesiologists will maintain the anesthetic through mask ventilation with one hand, while the other hand is charting or administering medications.
   ii) An oral airway may assist in maintaining a patent airway and minimizes head movement during spontaneous respirations.
   iii) An LMA may be utilized for expected prolonged surgeries (e.g., Down syndrome patients with narrowed ear canals).
f) **Emergence**
   i)   **Postoperative pain** is usually minimal but not completely absent, so some combination of supplemental analgesia is recommended.
      (1) **Acetaminophen** (10 to 20 mg/kg PO) preoperatively or (30 to 40 mg/kg PR as a one-time loading dose) immediately after induction is usually sufficient.
      (2) **Fentanyl** (1 to 2 μg/kg intranasal, IM, or IV) can also be given intraoperatively to provide postoperative analgesia.
         (a) Intranasal fentanyl can potentially drip into the pharynx and cause airway irritation.
      (3) **Ketamine** (0.5 to 2 mg/kg IV or 1 to 4 mg/kg IM) may be used for patients with tolerance to opioids or with other contraindications.
      (4) **Ketorolac** (0.5 to 1 mg/kg IV) has been shown to reduce rescue analgesic requirement (4).
   ii) **Emergence delirium**
      (1) Be aware of emergence delirium, especially when using pure volatile anesthetic technique.
      (2) Supplementation with propofol, short-acting opioids (e.g., fentanyl) or ketorolac can be helpful with postoperative agitation.
5) **Disposition**
   a) Most patients are discharged home when standard criteria are met.

Chapter Summary for Myringotomy and Ventilation Tubes

General Considerations	Myringotomy and ventilation tubes are one of the most common ambulatory surgical procedures in children.
Preoperative Considerations	Children typically present with URI symptoms that often resolve after surgery. Canceling surgery is usually not warranted unless the patient has a lower respiratory tract infection or severe symptoms.
Intraoperative Considerations	General anesthesia using mask induction and maintenance with volatile anesthetics without endotracheal tube or IV is most common technique. Pain management with rectal acetaminophen, fentanyl, or other analgesics per provider's discretion.
Postoperative Considerations	Minimal postoperative pain.

References

1. Tait AR, Knight PR. The effects of general anesthesia on upper respiratory tract infections in children. *Anesthesiology* 1987;67:930–935.
2. Tait AR, Pandit UA, Voepel-Lewis T, et al. Use of the laryngeal mask airway in children with upper respiratory tract infections: a comparison with endotracheal intubation. *Anesth Analg* 1998; 86:706–711.
3. Cote CJ, Lerman J, Todres DI, eds. *A Practice of Anesthesia for Infants and Children*. 4th ed. Philadelphia, PA: Saunders; 2009.
4. Davis PJ, Greenberg JA, Gendelman M, et al. Recovery characteristics of sevoflurane and halothane in preschool-aged children undergoing bilateral myringotomy and pressure equalization tube insertion. *Anesth Analg* 1999;88:34–38.

PEDIATRIC ANESTHESIA

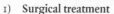

Cleft Lip/Cleft Palate

120

Nicholette Kasman, MD

Cleft lip and cleft palate are the most common craniofacial disorders, occurring in 1:750 births and are the fourth most common birth defect (2). It is more common in boys and only 30% occur in conjunction with other anomalies (3).

There are over 300 syndromes associated with cleft lip and palate, but the most common are Pierre Robin sequence, Down syndrome, Klippel-Feil, and Treacher Collins syndrome (1).

1) **Surgical treatment**
   a) Usually staged, the first procedure done for repair of cleft palate closes the anterior part of the hard palate- the alveolar defect; corrects the alar base; and provides symmetrical closure of the lip.
      i) Usually occurs around 3 months of age.
      ii) This allows the baby to feed and demonstrate normal facial expressions (1,2).
   b) The second procedure involves closure of the posterior hard palate and the soft palate before the development of speech.
      i) Usually occurs around 6 to 12 months of age.
      ii) This allows the infant to develop speech (1,2).
   c) Surgery for lip, nose, and palatal revisions as well as alveolar bone grafts occur in early childhood (1).
   d) Rhinoplasties and maxillary osteotomies done to complete the repair occur at 17 to 20 years of age (1).

2) **Anesthetic management**
   a) **Preoperative considerations**
      i) The most important part of the preoperative workup is evaluation of the airway. In one study (4):
         (1) The incidence of failed intubation was only 1%.
         (2) **There were no occurrences of "cannot intubate and cannot ventilate" by mask.**
         (3) Of the patients who were classified as difficult laryngoscopic views (initially grade III or IV), 45% had bilateral cleft lip, 35% had isolated cleft palate with retrognathia, and only 3% had unilateral cleft lip.
         (4) The characteristics most associated with difficult laryngoscopy were:
            (a) Extensive clefts
            (b) Retrognathia
            (c) Age <6 months
      ii) Patients with associated syndromes may present greater challenges:
         (1) **Pierre Robin sequence:** Mandibular hypoplasia as well as downward displacement and retraction of the tongue (3,4).
         (2) **Klippel-Feil syndrome:** Severe limitation of flexion and extension of the neck as a result of the fusion of cervical vertebrae, spinal canal stenosis, and scoliosis (3).

The presence of a cleft lip or a palate does not necessarily indicate that the patient will have a difficult airway.

  (3) **Down syndrome:** Narrowed nasopharynx and a relatively large, protuberant tongue in addition to the cleft lip and the palate (3).

  (4) **Treacher Collins syndrome** or mandibulofacial dysostosis: Maxillary, zygomatic, and mandibular hypoplasia (3).

Patients with associated craniofacial syndromes may present greater challenges in part from the presence of retrognathia.

b) **Monitors/lines/positioning**

 i) Standard ASA monitors and a single IV are generally adequate.

 ii) The patient is generally positioned at 180 degrees from the anesthesiologist.

 iii) Care should be taken in securing the endotracheal tube (1,2).

c) **Intraoperative management**

 i) **Induction**

  (1) Premedication with oral midazolam decreases both patient and parental anxiety (5).

  (2) Induction of anesthesia via face mask is generally uncomplicated.

  (3) The tongue may fall back into the cleft, obstructing the nasal passage. This can be corrected by placement of an oral airway (3,4).

  (4) During laryngoscopy, care should be taken to prevent the blade from entering the cleft.

  (5) Use of an oral RAE tube facilitates surgical access. Use of cuffed ETT minimizes risk of blood or secretions going into lungs (1).

  (6) Throat packs usually impinge on the surgical field and are not generally required for cleft palate repair; however, **communication between surgeon and anesthesiologist regarding placement of throat packs must be clear.**

Communicate with the surgeon about placement and removal of throat packs.

 ii) **Maintenance**

  (1) Maintenance with inhaled agents or TIVA is appropriate.

  (2) Muscle relaxation may be required to expedite induction or facilitate intubation but is usually not necessary during the procedure.

 iii) **Special anesthetic considerations**

  (1) Vigilance should be maintained for obstruction or kinking of the ETT by surgical retractors.

  (2) Allowing the patient to breathe spontaneously after induction and during the surgery allows titration of narcotics to achieve adequate analgesia prior to emergence.

   (a) Giving narcotics prior to spontaneous respirations risks apnea and delayed emergence.

   (b) Waiting until emergence to give narcotics risks inadequate analgesia.

   (c) Titrate opioids are to keep the respiratory rate in the low normal range and the $ETCO_2$ in the high normal range.

 iv) **Emergence**

  (1) Prior to emergence, it is important to ensure all throat packs are removed.

  (2) **Ask the surgeon to place an orogastric tube to suction under direct visualization to avoid disturbing suture lines by blind suctioning.**

  (3) A nasopharyngeal airway can be inserted by the surgeon prior to extubation to permit suctioning of the airway without damaging the palatal repair and to provide a patent airway (1).

  (4) An emergence without coughing or bucking is ideal to avoid bleeding and laryngospasm. Techniques that can be helpful include:

PEDIATRIC ANESTHESIA

(a) Deep extubation

(b) Making sure adequate analgesia/narcotics have been given

(c) Lidocaine 1 mg/kg IV prior to extubation

(d) Clonidine 1 to 2 µg/kg IV for postoperative anxiolysis and to decrease emergence delirium

Turning the patient on the side for extubation allows blood to pool out of the airway.

(5) Some practitioners prefer to extubate the patient awake to minimize risk of laryngospasm and airway obstruction.

(6) **Turning patient on the side prior to extubation** allows blood to pool out of the airway and may decrease the risk of laryngospasm.

d) **Postoperative management**

i) **Analgesia**

(1) Postoperative pain is usually managed with opioids and acetaminophen; however, the residual depressant effect of opioids is a major concern as blood, edema, and unfamiliar suture lines can make postoperative laryngoscopy and emergency reintubation difficult.

(2) Placement of **bilateral infraorbital nerve blocks** with 0.25% Bupivicaine has been shown to improve postoperative pain control as well as parental satisfaction (6).

(3) Postoperative mouth breathing may be stressful for young children apart from the pain of surgery, and some practitioners use clonidine 1 to 2 µg/kg IV for postoperative anxiolysis.

ii) **Disposition**

(1) Patients are at risk for acute upper airway obstruction due to upper airway narrowing, edema, and residual anesthetic and must be monitored in an appropriate setting (1).

(2) Ongoing evaluation for signs of postoperative airway obstruction must continue even at home for the first 48 hours (1).

Chapter Summary for Cleft Lip/Cleft Palate

General Considerations	The presence of a cleft lip or a palate is not an indication that the child will have a difficult airway.
Preoperative Considerations	The characteristics most associated with difficult laryngoscopy include extensive clefts, retrognathia, and age <6 mo.
Intraoperative Considerations	Use of a cuffed oral RAE tube facilitates surgical access and minimizes aspiration risk of blood or secretions. The placement and the removal of throat packs need to be clearly communicated between surgeon and anesthesiologist. Ask the surgeon to suction the stomach and the oropharynx under direct visualization to avoid disturbing suture lines by blind suctioning. A nasopharyngeal airway can be inserted by the surgeon prior to extubation to permit suctioning of the airway without damaging the palatal repair and to provide a patent airway.
Postoperative Considerations	Postoperatively patients are at risk for acute upper airway obstruction due to upper airway narrowing, edema and residual anesthetic and must be monitored in an appropriate setting. Ongoing evaluation for signs of postoperative airway obstruction must continue even at home for the first 48 h.

References

1. Engelhardt T, Crawford MW, Lerman J. Plastic and reconstructive surgery. In: Cote CJ, Lerman J, Todres ID, eds. *A Practice of Anesthesia for Infants and Children*. 4th ed. Philadelphia, PA: Saunders/Elsevier; 2009:chap 33.
2. Hardcastle T. Anaesthesia for repair of cleft lip and palate. *J Perioper Pract* 2009;19(1):20–23.
3. Nargozian C. The airway in patients with craniofacial abnormalities. *Pediatr Anesth* 2004;14:53–59.
4. Gunawardana RH. Difficult laryngoscopy in cleft lip and palate surgery. *Br J Anaesth* 1996;76:757–759.
5. Fazi L, Jantzen EC, Rose JB, et al. A comparison of oral clonidine and oral midazolam as preanesthetic medications in the pediatric tonsillectomy patient. *Anesth Anal* 2001;92(1):56–61.
6. Takmaz SA, Uysal HY, Usal A, et al. Bilateral extraoral, infraorbital nerve block for postoperative pain relief after cleft lip repair in pediatric patients: a randomized, double-blind controlled study. *Ann Plast Surg* 2009;63(1):59–62.

PEDIATRIC ANESTHESIA

121 Foreign Body Aspiration

Naiyi Sun, MD

Foreign body aspiration occurs most commonly in toddlers from 1 to 3 years of age (1). The most commonly retrieved objects are peanuts, which are problematic as they release oil, causing a chemical inflammation (1). Nonorganic objects that are particularly challenging and require urgent removal include needles, batteries, and magnets. Removal of all aspirated items is essential due to risk of atelectasis, bronchiectasis, chronic pneumonia, and inflammatory granulation tissue formation (2).

1) **Pathophysiology**
   a) Objects are found in the right bronchus more frequently than in the left.
   b) Less than 5% of objects are found in the trachea and hypopharynx. Two third of the objects lodge in the mainstem bronchi and remainder are found in the distal bronchi (3).

2) **Signs/symptoms/clinical findings**

   In patients who present with refractory wheezing, there should be a high index of suspicion for aspirated foreign body.

   a) Most airway foreign bodies do not cause acute respiratory distress and often they have been in situ for days prior to medical attention being sought. Occasionally, acute life-threatening airway obstruction may occur following an aspiration event.
   b) Presenting signs and symptoms may vary depending on the location and the size of the object. **Choking and wheezing following a witnessed aspiration event is the most common presentation.** In patients who present with refractory wheezing, there should be a high index of suspicion for aspirated foreign body.
   c) Objects lodged in the larynx and trachea are associated with high mortality rates and are considered an **airway emergency.** When objects are lodged in the mainstem bronchus or more distal airway, signs and symptoms include **cough, stridor, dyspnea, wheezing, unilateral decreased breath sounds, and occasionally cyanosis.**

3) **Diagnosis**
   a) CXR is commonly normal because most aspirated foreign bodies are organic and radiolucent (2).
   b) However, **CXRs may demonstrate localized area of hyperinflation, atelectasis, or pulmonary infiltrate.** The foreign body causing obstruction to the bronchus may create a unidirectional ball-valve phenomenon leading to distal hyperinflation from air trapping. With complete bronchial obstruction by a large foreign body, distal atelectasis or collapse may occur.
   c) Any object causing airway obstruction with acute respiratory distress requires emergent removal. Imaging studies are usually unnecessary and should not delay surgical treatment.

Button or cell batteries lodged in the esophagus can cause severe, life-threatening burns within 2 hours of ingestion, so they must be removed immediately.

4) Treatment
   a) Suspected foreign body aspiration requires prompt diagnostic and therapeutic rigid bronchoscopy. Removal of foreign objects with a rigid bronchoscopy is successful 95% to 98% of the time (3).
   b) **Button batteries (or button cell) in the esophagus can cause severe, life-threatening burns within 2 hours of ingestion**, so they must be removed immediately (4).

5) Anesthetic management
   a) **Preoperative management**
      i) Consider administering atropine or glycopyrrolate prior to induction to dry airway secretions.
      ii) Anxiolytics such as midazolam should be given with caution as it may exacerbate existing upper airway obstruction.

Anxiolytics such as midazolam should be given with caution as it may exacerbate upper airway obstruction.

   b) **Monitoring**
      i) A preoperative IV is useful for hydration and medication administration prior to induction. However, in an emergency or with a distressed child, IV access after inhalation induction is acceptable.
      ii) A precordial stethoscope in addition to standard ASA monitors can be useful in detecting any changes in ventilation intraoperatively. Invasive monitoring is not necessary for most cases.
   c) **Intraoperative management**
      i) **Induction**
         (1) **Gentle inhalation induction with 100% O_2 and sevoflurane is recommended** as it allows preservation of spontaneous ventilation and avoids the possibility of moving the foreign object more distally.
         (2) Nitrous oxide should be avoided as it reduces the FiO_2 and may increase significant gas volume and pressure if significant air trapping exists.
         (3) Following induction of general anesthesia, the surgeon may request that the OR table be turned 90 degrees.
      ii) **Maintenance**
         (1) There are two approaches to the anesthetic management for removal of aspirated foreign bodies: spontaneous ventilation and controlled ventilation.
            (a) A controlled ventilation technique relies on intermittent positive-pressure breaths between apneic periods when the surgeon instruments the airway. Advantages include rapid control of the airway and no patient movement. A significant disadvantage is that positive-pressure ventilation can unintentionally push the object further into the airway.
            (b) Spontaneous ventilation allows for uninterrupted ventilation; however, there is higher risk of patient movement, coughing, and laryngospasm.
         (2) In most cases, **the safest technique is to preserve spontaneous ventilation** at least until the nature and the location of the foreign body have been identified by bronchoscopy.
         (3) **A total IV anesthetic technique using propofol plus remifentanil or ketamine for maintenance is preferable** because it allows a steady level of anesthesia that is independent of ventilation.

PEDIATRIC ANESTHESIA

iii) **Special anesthetic considerations**

   (1) The anesthesiologist needs to achieve sufficient depth of anesthesia during the procedure to obliterate airway reflexes and prevent patient movement and coughing during instrumentation, while maintaining spontaneous ventilation and hemodynamic stability.

   (2) During bronchoscopy, the anesthesiologist needs to constantly monitor for chest excursion, breath sounds, and SpO_2. **Constant communication between surgical and anesthesia personnel regarding the child's airway status is crucial.**

iv) **Special surgical considerations**

   (1) Once adequate anesthesia depth is achieved, topical lidocaine 1% to 2% can be sprayed to laryngeal structures and tracheal mucosa prior to bronchoscopy. This is essential for suppression of airway reflexes and prevention of coughing and bronchospasm.

   (2) Once the ventilating bronchoscope is in the subglottis, the anesthesia circuit can be connected to the scope to allow O_2 delivery and positive-pressure ventilation if necessary.

   (3) When a large foreign body is removed, the forceps and the bronchoscope must be removed together through immobile vocal cords. Administration of a small dose of short-acting nondepolarizing muscle relaxant may be necessary to permit safe removal of the apparatus.

   (4) **Complete tracheal obstruction may occur during removal of the foreign body.** If the object cannot be immediately removed, it may be necessary to push the object down into a mainstem bronchus to allow ventilation of the lungs.

   (5) After the foreign body is safely retrieved, a follow-up bronchoscopy is immediately performed to look for any residual foreign bodies and to rule out airway injury.

   (6) Rarely, the foreign body is so disseminated that it cannot be easily removed; a thoracotomy, bronchotomy, or cardiopulmonary bypass may be necessary.

d) **Intraoperative complications**

  i) Hypoxia and hypercarbia may occur due to inadequate ventilation. Short periods of hypercarbia may be well tolerated. Hypoxia should be treated with removal of the bronchoscope and effective mask ventilation.

  ii) Bronchospasm during the procedure should be treated with increasing depth of anesthesia, inhaled albuterol, or IV bronchodilators.

  iii) Prophylactic steroid therapy with **dexamethasone** 0.5 mg/kg IV to a maximum dose of 20 mg is useful in preventing upper airway edema and secondary stridor from airway manipulation (5).

e) **Postoperative management**

  i) The patient should be placed in the head-up position. Respiratory status should be closely monitored because of the possibility of airway obstruction secondary to edema.

  ii) If stridor develops, administer humidified O_2 and racemic epinephrine inhalation (0.5 mL of 2.25% solution nebulized). **Heliox** (helium and oxygen mixture) may be considered if the degree of stridor is severe and the patient does not require more than 40% FiO_2 (3).

  iii) Postobstructive pulmonary edema can develop in children in the recovery room. Treatment is supportive with controlled ventilation and positive end-expiratory pressure.

Chapter Summary for Foreign Body Aspiration

Diagnosis	Signs and symptoms include cough, stridor, dyspnea, wheezing, unilateral decreased breath sounds, and cyanosis. Chest radiographs are commonly normal.
Treatment	Prompt diagnostic and therapeutic rigid bronchoscopy. Button or cell batteries must be removed from esophagus within 2 h of ingestion.
Preoperative Considerations	Consider anticholinergics to decrease secretions. Anxiolytics should be given with caution. Preinduction IV useful but not required.
Intraoperative Considerations	Gentle inhalation induction with 100% O$_2$ and sevoflurane. N$_2$O should be avoided. A total IV anesthetic technique for maintenance with propofol plus remifentanil or ketamine. Preserve spontaneous ventilation until the nature and the location of the foreign body have been identified.
Postoperative Considerations	Recover in head-up position. Watch for stridor and postobstructive pulmonary edema.

PEDIATRIC ANESTHESIA

References

1. Farrell PT. Rigid bronchoscopy for foreign body removal: anaesthesia and ventilation. *Paediatr Anesth* 2004;14:84–89.
2. Zur KB, Litman RS. Pediatric airway foreign body retrieval: surgical and anesthetic perspectives. *Paediatr Anesth* 2009;19:109–117.
3. Salcedo L. Foreign body aspiration. *Anesthesiol Clin N Am* 1998;16:885–892.
4. Litovitz T, Whitaker N, Clark L. Emerging battery-ingestion hazard: clinical implications. *Pediatrics* 2010;125:1168–1177.
5. Verghese ST, Hannallah RS. Pediatric otolaryngologic emergencies. *Anesthesiol Clin N Am* 2001;19:237–256.

122 Epiglottitis

Naiyi Sun, MD

Due to the small size of the airway in infants and small children, inflammation from epiglottitis can result in significant airway compromise that would otherwise not be seen in older children and adults. The management of these patients presents a unique challenge to any anesthesiologist.

1) Pathophysiology

a) Epiglottitis is a **life-threatening infection that causes severe edema of the supraglottic structures.** The swelling can progress rapidly and lead to complete airway obstruction.

b) It can affect children in all age groups, but most commonly occurs in children between 2 and 6 years of age.

c) Historically, the most frequent causative agent was *Haemophilus influenza* type B (Hib).

i) With the introduction of the Hib conjugate vaccine, epiglottitis secondary to *Neisseria meningitides*, Group A *streptococcus*, and *Candida albicans* is becoming more prevalent (1).

The typical presentation of epiglottitis is an acute onset with toxic appearance, high fever, respiratory distress, drooling, and sitting in tripod position with slow respiratory rate to minimize turbulence

2) Signs/symptoms/clinical findings

a) Epiglottitis is characterized by an **acute and rapid onset of respiratory distress.**

b) Symptoms can include severe sore throat, dysphagia, dysphonia, and dyspnea.

c) Signs

i) The patient may have a **toxic appearance**, fever, tachycardia, tachypnea, inspiratory stridor and, in extreme cases, hypoxia and cyanosis.

ii) **Drooling** is commonly seen due to difficulty and pain with swallowing.

iii) The child often assumes the **tripod position** of sitting forward with open mouth and tongue out to try to decrease work of breathing.

d) Respiratory pattern is often slow and quiet to minimize turbulence.

Acute epiglottitis is a clinical diagnosis. Do not delay securing the airway to obtain radiologic studies.

3) Diagnosis

a) **Acute epiglottitis is a clinical diagnosis.** Examination of the mouth and the oropharynx should be avoided until trained experts are ready to secure the airway with an endotracheal tube.

b) Imaging studies are usually unnecessary and should not delay definitive airway management. The "**thumbprint sign**", representing a swollen epiglottis on lateral cervical spine radiograph, is classically associated with epiglottitis.

4) **Anesthetic management**
   a) **Preoperative considerations**
      i) **Manipulation of the mouth and the oropharynx should be avoided** to minimize agitation of the child as it may precipitate an acute airway obstruction. For the same reason, venipuncture and painful injections should be avoided prior to securing the airway.
      ii) **Once the diagnosis of epiglottitis is made or strongly suspected, arrangements should be made immediately to secure the airway in the controlled setting of the operating room.**
      iii) **The child should be transported to the operating room by personnel skilled in pediatric airway management with appropriate airway equipment.**
      iv) The child should be kept calm sitting on a caretaker's lap breathing spontaneously with continuous SpO_2. Supplemental O_2 should be given if tolerated by the patient.
   b) **Monitors/lines**
      i) Standard ASA monitors
      ii) Single peripheral IV
      iii) Additional monitors and invasive lines as needed after patient is anesthetized and airway secured.
   c) **Intraoperative management**
      i) **Induction/airway**
         (1) A surgeon skilled in surgical airway management and rigid bronchoscopy should be present prior to induction with tracheostomy tray and bronchoscopy equipment in the operating room.
         (2) Anesthesia induction should be performed by mask with sevoflurane and **100% O_2** with the **child sitting up in his position of greatest comfort.**
         (3) When adequate depth of anesthesia is accomplished, the patient may be transitioned to the supine position and peripheral IV access secured. Continuous positive pressure by mask may be needed to overcome upper airway obstruction.
         (4) If an IV is in situ, IV induction may be considered with ketamine 1 to 3 mg/kg IV and may be titrated gradually along with glycopyrrolate 0.005 to 0.01 mg/kg IV to decrease secretions.

         (5) Lidocaine 1 mg/kg IV may be given on induction to minimize the risk of coughing and laryngospasm prior to laryngoscopy (2).
      ii) **Special anesthetic considerations**
         (1) It is crucial to **maintain spontaneous ventilation** due to the possibility of difficult intubation. The laryngeal structures may be difficult to visualize due to swelling and the glottic opening may be small or even occluded.
         (2) If the laryngeal structures are difficult to visualize, expiratory gas bubbles during spontaneous ventilation or bubbles induced by gentle pressure on the child's chest may reveal the glottic opening.

(3) Due to airway swelling, the endotracheal tube used should be 0.5 to 1 mm smaller in diameter than would be appropriate for the age and size of the patient. The endotracheal tube (ETT) should also be styletted to improve ability to direct the ETT and advance through the swollen glottic opening.

5) **Postoperative management**
   a) Once the airway is secured, IV antibiotics should be started immediately. **Ceftriaxone** 50 mg/kg IVq12–24h is the first-line antibiotic (1). IV antibiotics should be continued for at least 3 to 5 days followed by oral therapy.
   b) Supportive treatment includes IV hydration, sedation, and acetaminophen.
   c) Pulmonary edema can develop in 7% of children with severe epiglottitis (3). Treatment is supportively with controlled ventilation, positive end-expiratory pressure (PEEP), and diuretics.
   d) Flexible laryngoscopy under propofol sedation can be performed to visualize the epiglottis before extubation. The child is usually ready for extubation in 24 to 48 hours (4).

Chapter Summary for Epiglottitis

General Considerations	Life-threatening infection causing severe edema of the supraglottic structures. Acute onset of severe sore throat, high fever, dysphagia, dysphonia, and dyspnea.
Preoperative Considerations	It is crucial to minimize agitation of the child as it may precipitate acute airway obstruction by avoiding repeated exams and IV placement. The child should be transported to the operating room by personnel skilled in pediatric airway management with appropriate airway equipment.
Intraoperative Considerations	Mask induction with 100% O_2 and sevoflurane. Keep patient spontaneous breathing during induction. Secure critical airway with styletted ETT ½–1 size smaller. If the laryngeal structures are difficult to visualize, expiratory gas bubbles during spontaneous ventilation or bubbles induced by gentle pressure on the child's chest may reveal the glottic opening.
Postoperative Considerations	IV antibiotics, hydration, and sedation.

References

1. DeSoto, H. Epiglottitis and croup in airway obstruction in children. *Anesthesiol Clin N Am* 1998;16(4):853–868.
2. Steward DJ, Lerman J. Manual of pediatric anesthesia. 5th ed. Churchill Livingstone 2001. *Otorhinolaryngology* 254–256.
3. Davis HW, Gartener JC, Galvis AG, et al. Acute upper airway obstruction: croup and epiglottitis. *Pediatr Clin North Am* 1981;28(4):859–880.
4. Verghese ST, Hannallah RS. Pediatric otolaryngologic emergencies. *Anesthesiol Clin N Am* 2001;19(2):237–256.

MRI and CT

Rebecca Claure, MD

Children undergoing nonpainful diagnostic studies may require deep sedation or general anesthesia due to their inability to remain motionless for long periods of time and/or their inability to cooperate with requirements of the study (e.g., need for breath holding). Children with normal developmental maturity and age >7 years old for MRI or age >3 years old for CT can usually undergo the study without sedation (8). Unique challenges to delivering anesthesia in the MRI/CT suite include limited space, an unfamiliar environment, and the safety hazards associated with MRI.

1) **Anesthetic technique**—May be dictated by available equipment.
   a) **Special considerations**
      i) **Airway**

Special attention should be paid to ensure a stable, patent airway in every patient because of limited access to the patient in the MRI scanner.

   (1) Due to the child's position in the MRI scanner and the anesthesiologist's distance from the child (i.e., often in a separate control room), it may be impossible to access the airway quickly once the scan has started.
   (2) **Special attention should be made to establish a patent airway before the scan has started, and ensure adequate ventilation throughout the study.**

      ii) **Oral contrast**
   (1) Children may be required to ingest oral contrast prior to CT of the abdomen or pelvis in order to opacify the stomach and bowel.
   (2) The oral contrast material is given anywhere from 30 minutes to 3 hours prior to the scan depending on institutional protocol, **potentially violating traditional NPO requirements.**
   (3) Currently, there is no standard of care for airway management in these children. Many practitioners choose to mask induce the child and allow spontaneous ventilation with a natural airway; others choose to secure the airway with a rapid sequence induction and an endotracheal tube.

Consider NPO time requirements when timing administration for oral contrast.

   (4) The risk of aspiration of dilute oral contrast material with an unprotected airway seems to be minimal (1,10). One must weigh the risks of aspiration with a natural airway versus the risks of a rapid sequence intubation on a case-by-case basis.
      iii) Alternative techniques for short scans:
   (1) Timing of scan during a nap and after a feed.
   (2) Wrapping of young infants in warm blankets and giving them a pacifier dipped in dextrose water.

PEDIATRIC ANESTHESIA

b) **Preoperative evaluation**

   i) Overall assessment of medical condition

   ii) Consider "risk" factors that may be of special concern when anesthetizing patients in remote locations (8). These include history of difficult intubation, potentially difficult airway or IV access, or a history of serious complications such as cardiorespiratory failure or malignant hyperthermia (8).

   iii) If IV contrast is required, **adequate renal function should be verified by history and/or laboratory evaluation** (3).

   iv) Choice of an anesthetic with a natural airway versus LMA/ETT depends on the patient's medical condition, risk of aspiration, scan requirements (e.g., need for breath holding), and length of scan. Limitations of the MRI/CT environment must also be considered.

c) **Premedication**

   i) For younger children, midazolam PO may be given for anxiolysis.

   ii) For older children, placement of an IV after topical anesthesia (e.g., EMLA, Ela-max [or L-M-X], Synera patch) may be attempted, followed by midazolam IV for anxiolysis.

d) **Induction**

   i) For younger children, mask induction with sevoflurane+/-nitrous oxide if there are no contraindications.

   ii) For older children, IV induction with propofol.

   iii) If rapid sequence induction indicated, induction with propofol plus succinylcholine or rocuronium with cricoid pressure.

e) **Maintenance**

   i) When deciding on a maintenance plan, one should consider the length of the study. CT scans are usually <15 minutes, while MRI scans are at least 30 minutes and can last up to a few hours.

   ii) If the patient is not intubated, spontaneous ventilation with oxygen supplementation via nasal cannula or face mask maintained by inhalational anesthesia (2) or TIVA with propofol (9), dexmedetomidine (5) or dexmedetomidine plus midazolam (4).

   iii) If the patient is intubated, maintenance can be inhalational anesthesia or TIVA with propofol.

   iv) Advantages of using a propofol-based regimen may include a more rapid recovery from anesthesia, a decreased incidence of postoperative nausea and vomiting, and a decreased incidence of emergence delirium.

   v) When doing a TIVA with only one IV, consider how to maintain depth of anesthesia when the radiologist needs to stop TIVA to administer contrast agent.

   vi) **Breath holding or apnea** may be necessary for studies of the chest, heart, abdomen, or pelvis.

     (1) The number and the duration of breath holds will vary according to the study.

     (2) If patient oxygenation and safety are an issue, the anesthesiologist should discuss the situation with the radiologist because scan protocols can be altered to minimize frequency and/or duration of breath holds. The radiologist may also be satisfied with low tidal volume breathing and not require strict apnea.

     (3) Breath holds may be achieved with hyperventilation, deepening anesthesia, or a small dose of paralytic.

Heat loss can be a problem for young children for long scans in the magnet.

(a) Hyperventilation of ETCO$_2$ into the low 20 range often causes a long enough apnea for scans. Some patients may not tolerate the change in PaCO2/pH in which case other methods may be required.

(b) Deepening anesthesia (e.g., bolus of propofol) may be effective as long as the patient will hemodynamically tolerate the dose.

(c) Otherwise, small dose of short-acting muscle relaxant may be required.

f) **Complications**

i) Airway obstruction or respiratory depression

ii) Hypothermia

    (1) Temperature in the MRI suite is normally cold.

    (2) Accurate monitoring of body temperature may be difficult in the scanner.

    (3) There is a potential for significant heat loss particularly in infants and small children (3). Care should be taken to keep patients covered to minimize heat loss.

Strict adherence to MRI safety must be followed in order to avoid injury. All ferromagnetic objects must be kept out of the MRI scanner room.

iii) Reaction to IV contrast media

    (1) Fortunately, this is relatively rare in children (7).

    (2) Adverse reactions can range from nausea, vomiting, bronchospasm, pulmonary edema, to anaphylaxis with hypotension and cardiovascular collapse. Most life-threatening reactions occur immediately or within 20 minutes of contrast agent administration (1).

    (3) Risk factors for IV contrast media reactions include a previous reaction to contrast media, or a history of atopy or allergy (1,7).

2) **MRI safety—There are numerous safety considerations associated with the MRI environment (3).**

a) The strength of the magnetic field is described in Tesla (T) units.

i) Most scanners are either 1.5 or 3 T.

ii) A 1.5-T scanner is equal to 30,000 times the magnetic field of the earth's surface (1).

b) There are no known reports of harmful physiologic effects from magnetic fields (3).

c) Monitors and equipment must be adaptable to the MRI suite. In general, **all equipment must be nonferromagnetic.**

d) Significant morbidity and potential mortality can result from ferromagnetic objects brought into the MRI suite. Meticulous attention must be given to ensuring all ferromagnetic objects are removed from patient and patient care team. Common "forgotten" items include keys, watches, beepers, stethoscopes, and scissors.

e) Implanted devices such as aneurysm clips should be confirmed to be MRI safe in order to avoid injury from a dislodged implant (6).

f) Burns are possible from objects that heat during the MRI process, such as wires (e.g., EKG leads), or from the child's body touching the bore of the scanner (6). Leads should be wrapped and prevented from coiling.

g) **Acoustic injury** due to the noise of the MRI scanner is possible (6). Earplugs should be placed on all patients to prevent hearing damage.

Chapter Summary for MRI/CT Anesthesia

General Considerations	Children may require anesthesia for these nonpainful procedures.
Preoperative Considerations	Consider timing of oral contrast ingestion with appropriate NPO status. Assess renal function if IV contrast is required.
Intraoperative Considerations	Ensure a patent and stable airway in the MRI scanner due to limited access. Breath holding or apnea may be required. Monitor temperature.
Special Considerations	MRI safety rules must be followed at all times—only nonferromagnetic equipment can be used.

References

1. Cote CJ, Lerman J, Todres ID, eds. *A Practice of Anesthesia for Infants and Children*. 4th ed. Philadelphia, PA: Saunders Elsevier; 2009: 996–1003, 1007.
2. De Sanctis Briggs V. Magnetic resonance imaging under sedation in newborns and infants:a study of 640 cases using sevoflurane. *Paediatr Anaesth* 2005;15(1):9–15.
3. Gooden CK. The child in MRI and CT: considerations and technique. *Int Anesthesiol Clin* 2009;47(3):15–23.
4. Heard C, Burrows F, Johnson K, et al. A comparison of dexmedetomidine—midazolam with propofol for maintenance of anesthesia in children undergoing magnetic resonance imaging. *Anesth Analg* 2008;107(6):1832–1839.
5. Heard CM, Joshi P, Johnson K. Dexmedetomidine for pediatric MRI sedation: a review of a series of cases. *Paediatr Anaesth* 2007;17(9): 888–892.
6. The Joint Commission Website. Sentinel event alert: preventing accidents and injuries in the MRI suite. www.jointcommission.org/ SentinelEvents/SentinelAlert Issue 38. Published February 14, 2008.
7. Motoyama EK, Davis PJ, eds. *Smith's Anesthesia for Infants and Children*. 7th ed. Philadelphia, PA: Mosby Elsevier; 2006:846–848, 851–852.
8. Taghon TA, Bryan YF, Kurth CD. Pediatric radiology sedation and anesthesia. *Int Anesthesiol Clin* 2006;44(1):65–79.
9. Usher AG, Kearney RA, Tsui BCH. Propofol total intravenous anesthesia for MRI in children. *Paediatric Anesth* 2005;15(1):23–28.
10. Ziegler MA, Fricke BL, Donnelly LF. Is administration of enteric contrast material safe before abdominal CT in children who require sedation? Experience with chloral hydrate and pentobarbital. *Am J Roentgenol* 2003;180:13–15.

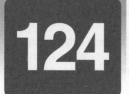

124 Nissen Fundoplication, Gastrostomy Tube Placement, and Laparoscopic Procedures

Nicholette Kasman, MD

Gastroesophageal reflux (GERD) is common in childhood. In otherwise healthy infants, symptoms of GERD occur in as many as 67% of infants around 4 to 5 months, decreasing to <5% by 12 months. The tone in the lower esophageal sphincter is low at birth and may take up to 4 to 6 weeks to achieve adult levels. Populations that are particularly vulnerable to the disease include preterm infants in whom episodes of reflux may be associated with apneas and bradycardias and neurologically impaired children with muscular discoordination such as those with cerebral palsy (3,4).

1) Pathophysiology
   a) GERD can be physiologic secondary to immature development of the lower esophageal sphincter.
   b) May occur secondary to cerebral palsy or developmental delay leading to dysmotility issues (3).
   c) May occur in patients who have a history of diaphragmatic hernia, trascheoesophageal fistula, or esophageal atresia repairs.
2) Signs/symptoms/clinical findings
   a) Early signs and symptoms
      i) In infants, the most common manifestation of GERD is spitting up with feeds.
      ii) Other signs include aspiration and cough.
   b) Late signs and symptoms
      i) Asthma
      ii) Chronic bronchitis and/or bronchiectasis
      iii) Pulmonary fibrosis
      iv) COPD
      v) Recurrent pneumonias
      vi) Laryngitis
      vii) Sinusitis
      viii) Vocal cord granulomas
      ix) Dental erosions
      x) Noncardiac chest pain
      xi) Sleep apnea (4)
3) Surgical treatment
   a) **Surgical technique**
      i) The most common technique is the **Nissen fundoplication**, a 360 degree wrap of the stomach around the esophagus (2).

READ MORE

Anesthesia for laparoscopic surgery, Chapter 133, page 927

      ii) The majority of cases are done laparoscopically. Specific considerations for these surgeries include the effects of pneumoperitoneum on respiratory and cardiac function.

      iii) The anesthesiologist must place a bougie into the esophagus to help the surgeon determine how tightly to wrap the muscles around the esophagus. For this reason, it is necessary to intubate the trachea, even if the procedure is not done laparoscopically.

  b) Overall surgical risk is low. However, risks may include esophageal or gastric perforation, hemorrhage from short gastric vessel or splenic vessel tear, pneumothorax, and CO_2 embolus (2).

  c) An open procedure may be indicated if the patient has had prior gastric surgeries or if there is a complication with an ongoing laparoscopic repair (2).

  d) The patient populations at high risk for GERD are also at risk for failure to thrive, from both the sequelae of chronic reflux disease and the often concomitant muscular dysmotility. In such patients, a percutaneous gastrostomy tube is often placed after completion of the fundoplication and can be used for gastric decompression as well as feeding.

4) **Anesthetic management**

  a) **Preoperative considerations**

      i) The patient may have a history of recurrent aspiration with subsequently impaired pulmonary function. Optimization with bronchodilators may be appropriate (2).

      ii) Patients with neurologic impairment may have impaired airway reflexes, seizure disorder, poor nutrition, contractures, and difficult venous access (3).

      iii) Proton pump inhibitors, antisecretory agents, and motility agents should be continued through the morning of surgery (2,3).

      iv) Blood should be available for the case. Although the need for transfusion is rare, there is the potential for catastrophic large-vessel disruption (1).

      v) Premedicaton with oral midazolam will lessen patient and parent anxiety in children old enough to experience separation anxiety. Premedication with antisialogogues, antacids, or promotility agents may also be considered (1).

  b) **Monitors/lines/positioning**

      i) Standard ASA monitors, ± urinary catheter are generally adequate (1,2).

      ii) A single peripheral IV is necessary both for intraoperative use and for postoperative fluids until the gastrostomy is usable.

      iii) The patient is usually supine. Access to the mouth is necessary for insertion of bougie during the procedure (1).

  c) **Intraoperative management**

      i) **Induction**

         (1) These children should be **considered "full stomachs,"** and a rapid sequence induction is ideal. However, difficulties obtaining preoperative IV access, challenges with preoxygenation, and lack of patient cooperation may make this impractical. The decision whether to proceed with mask induction or preinduction IV should be made on a case-by-case basis (1,3).

         (2) Place an orogastric tube after intubation to minimize risk of aspiration as well as to deflate the stomach and aid the surgeon's view of their field (1,2).

         (3) Muscle relaxation is appropriate and usually necessary for the laparoscopic or the open procedure (1,2).

      ii) **Maintenance**

         (1) Standard maintenance of anesthesia can be accomplished with a combination of air/O_2/inhaled agent and muscle relaxant (1,2).

Insufflation during laparoscopy may cause the ETT to enter the right mainstem bronchus. Care should be taken on intubation to position the ETT well above the carina.

(2) Patients with severe developmental delay or who are to be extubated in the OR may benefit from shorter acting agents, for example, TIVA with propofol ± remifentanil.

(3) N_2O is generally avoided in order to minimize intestinal distension (2).

iii) **Special anesthetic considerations**

(1) Increased abdominal pressure may lead to

(a) ↓ diaphragmatic excursion

(b) ↑ atelectasis

(c) ↓ FRC

(d) ↑ V/Q mismatch (2)

(2) Hypercarbia during laparoscopy may necessitate increased minute ventilation to compensate. However, most children tolerate the elevated CO2 unless they have increased intracranial pressure or pulmonary hypertension (1).

(3) Cephalad displacement of the carina during insufflation or Trendelenburg positioning may cause endobronchial intubation (1).

(4) With higher insufflation pressures, venous return may be impaired leading to decreased cardiac output (1).

(5) Trendelenburg positioning may exacerbate the effects of pneumoperitoneum (1).

A bougie must be inserted into esophagus during procedure. Care must be taken to avoid accidental extubation.

(6) The surgeon will ask the anesthesiologist to insert a bougie into the esophagus to maintain a patent esophagus for the wrap. Care must be taken to avoid accidental extubation. Direct access and visualization of the airway are necessary at all times.

(7) The surgeon may ask the anesthesiologist to insufflate air into the stomach during the procedure to determine if there are any leaks in the stomach (2).

iv) **Emergence**

(1) Emergence and extubation are generally uncomplicated and include reversal of neuromuscular blockers and administration of an antiemetic (1–3).

(2) The stomach and oropharynx should be suctioned out completely prior to extubation.

(3) The decision to extubate deep or awake depends on the individual patient's condition and risks.

d) **Postoperative management**

i) Analgesia

(1) For laparoscopic procedures, pain is generally adequately controlled with a combination of opioids and local anesthetic applied at trochar sites.

(2) For open procedures, a midthoracic epidural or caudal epidural threaded up
to the midthoracic level can be placed postoperatively (3).

ii) Disposition

(1) In the postoperative period, respiratory function may still be impaired, so patients should be watched closely (2).

(2) For laparoscopic procedures, patients can often resume feeds the following day and have minimal pain, so they may only be hospitalized 1 to 2 days.

(3) For open procedures, patients often have comorbidities and, combined with more pain, may require longer hospitalizations.

PEDIATRIC ANESTHESIA

Chapter Summary for Nissen Fundoplication, Gastrostomy Tube Placement, and Laparoscopic Procedures

General Considerations	Most children have significant comorbidities including developmental delay, cerebral palsy, GERD, failure to thrive, chronic lung disease. Nissen fundoplication and gastrostomy may be done as open procedure or laparoscopically.
Preoperative Considerations	Continue antacid medications in preoperative period. Although the risk of blood loss is low, the potential for large vessel disruption is possible. Blood should be available.
Intraoperative Considerations	As most will have GERD, a rapid sequence induction or modified rapid sequence is indicated. A bougie will need to inserted into esophagus during procedure, so care must be taken around the airway. Anesthetic concerns of laparoscopic procedures include hypercarbia, effects of pneumoperitoneum, necessity of endotracheal intubation, and inadvertent right mainstem intubation.
Postoperative Considerations	Procedures done laparoscopically generally have minimal to moderate pain. Opioids and local anesthetic at trochar sites are generally adequate. For open procedures, a thoracic epidural or a caudal epidural threaded to the thoracic level is helpful.

References

1. Hammer GB. Anesthesia for minimally invasive surgery in pediatric patients. In: Jaffe RA, Samuels SI, eds. *Anesthesiologist's Manual of Surgical Procedures*. 3rd ed. Philadelphia, PA: Lippincott Williams & Wilkins; 2004.
2. Curet MJ, Sastry SG. Laparoscopic esophageal fundoplication. In: Jaffe RA, Samuels SI, eds. *Anesthesiologist's Manual of Surgical Procedures*. 3rd ed. Philadelphia, PA: Lippincott Williams & Wilkins; 2004: 456–461.
3. Navaratnam M. Fundoplication. In: Doyle E, ed. *Paediatric Anaesthesia*. Oxford: Oxford University Press; 2007: 242–244.
4. Hassall E. Decisions in diagnosing and managing chronic gastroesophageal disease in children. *J Pediatr* 2005;146(3 Suppl):S3–S12.

125 Caudal Epidural Anesthesia

Dondee Almazan, MD • Calvin Kuan, MD

Caudal epidural anesthesia is the most commonly used regional technique in children. Single-shot techniques may be used for intraoperative and postoperative analgesia for surgeries up to the level of the umbilicus.

Mongolian spots are NOT a contraindication to caudal block.

Caudal epidural injection is a STERILE procedure. Proper aseptic techniques must be employed.

1) Indications
   a) Analgesia alone (e.g., skin grafting)
   b) Adjunct to general anesthesia (e.g., abdominal surgery)
   c) Surgical anesthesia (e.g., hypospadia, hernia repair)
   d) Postoperative analgesia (e.g., lower extremity orthopaedic cases)
   e) Treatment of chronic pain (e.g., CRPS)
2) Contraindications (Table 125-1)
3) Risks and complications
   a) Risks: No procedures are without risk. However, years of experience and published data have shown that placement of caudals in anesthetized children is safe when performed by experienced anesthesiologists (1).
   b) Complications
      i) Misplaced injection—IV, intraosseous, subcutaneous, or intrathecal
      ii) Rectal perforation
      iii) Urinary retention
      iv) Hematoma
      v) Absent or patchy block
      vi) Infection
      vii) Hypotension
      viii) Lower extremity weakness/paralysis

PEDIATRIC ANESTHESIA

Table 125-1
Contraindications to Pediatric Caudal Block

Absolute Contraindications	Relative Contraindications
Patient or parent refusal	Previous caudal surgery
Lack of consent	CNS abnormalities (e.g., multiple sclerosis and syringomyelia)
Coagulopathy and/or thrombocytopenia	Spina bifida/neural tube defects
Sepsis	Tethered spinal cord
Infection at site of injection	Scoliosis
Uncorrected hypovolemia	Local skin changes (e.g., dimples, hairy patches, abnormal pigmentation) that may be associated with undiagnosed vertebral abnormalities

The maximum safe dose for caudal bupivacaine is 3 mg/kg (equal to 1.2 mL/kg of 0.25% bupivacaine).

4) Equipment
   a) Sterilizing solution
   b) Sterile gloves and drapes
   c) Caudal needle or Angiocaths: short bevel, 22 gauge, needle with stylet
   d) Connector (e.g., T-piece or IV extension tubing) may be used to extend from the catheter to the syringe for easier injection.
5) Drug selection
   a) **Level of block desired and drug dose is primarily dependent on the volume of local anesthetic given, rather than the concentration of the local anesthetic.**
      i) Commonly used drugs and concentrations are
         (1) Bupivacaine or levobupivacaine 0.125%; 0.25%; or 0.5%
         (2) Ropivacaine 0.2%
   b) The maximum safe dose for caudal bupivacaine is 3 mg/kg (equal to 1.2 mL/kg of 0.25% bupivacaine) [2].
   c) There are various published formulae for calculating the appropriate dose of local anesthetic (Table 125-2):
      i) Armitage suggests the following dosing (3):
         (1) 0.5 mL/kg will block the sacral nerve roots.
         (2) 1 mL/kg will block lower thoracic and upper lumbar nerve roots.
         (3) 1.25 mL/kg will block the midthoracic (T6) nerve roots.
      ii) Takasaki developed the following formula (4):

Volume of drug infused = 0.05 mL/kg/dermatome to be blocked

      iii) A simplified formula commonly used is (5):

Volume of drug infused = 1 mL/kg of bupivacaine will block up to around T6-10 level.

Simple formula for determine amount of drug to give: 1 mL/kg will block up to umbilicus.

      iv) Maximum recommended volume for any patient is between 20 and 30 mL (5).
      v) Use of 0.25% or greater bupivacaine may result in prolonged motor blockade, which may delay discharge for day surgeries —so use of 0.125% or 0.25% bupivacaine is recommended.
6) Epidural adjuncts
   a) **All additives must be preservative free.**
   b) **Epinephrine** (2.5 to 5 μg/kg)

Table 125-2
Formulae for Drug Dosing for Caudals (3-5)

Author	Amount of Local Anesthetic (Desired Level of Block)
Armitage	0.5 ml/kg (Sacral) 1 ml/kg (Lumbar) 1.25 ml/kg (Thoracic)
Takasaki	0.05 ml/kg/dermatome
Simplified	1 ml/kg (T6-10)

i) May be included in the initial injection to rule out intravascular injection.

ii) Addition of epinephrine does not prolong the duration of caudal anesthesia.

c) **Opioids** should be used judiciously because of concerns for respiratory depression, urinary retention, and nausea.

i) Infants and children are at special risk, and **should be monitored for at least 12 hours up to 18 hours after administration.**

ii) Children who also receive systemic opioids are at additional risk due to a synergistic effect.

All additives must be preservative free.

Patients given epidural caudal opioids should be monitored for at least 12 to 18 hours.

d) **Clonidine** (1 to 2 µg/kg)

i) May prolong duration of anesthesia (6,7).

ii) Also has potentially undesirable systemic sedating effects.

e) **Ketamine** (0.5 mg/kg)

i) May prolong the duration of anesthesia.

ii) Preservative-free formulation is very difficult to find.

7) Technique

a) **Monitoring/lines**

i) Standard ASA monitors should already be in place as children will usually be receiving the caudal under general anesthesia.

ii) An IV line should be in place for fluid administration or resuscitation if necessary.

b) **Positioning and preparation (Fig. 125-1)**

i) The child is most commonly placed in the lateral decubitus position.

ii) The posterior superior iliac spines are identified, and the sacral cornu is palpated.

iii) Area is prepped using the sterilizing solution of choice.

c) **Placement of block (Fig. 125-2)**

i) An IV needle is advanced at a 45-degree angle through the sacral hiatus.

ii) A distinct "pop" is felt as the needle pierces the sacrococcygeal ligament.

iii) When using angiocath, a "pop" may not occur, but the catheter should advance without resistance.

iv) The angle of the needle is then lowered almost parallel to the skin and the catheter (but not the needle) advanced into the caudal space.

v) Verify negative aspiration of blood and CSF.

vi) Administer incremental doses of the medication every 20 to 30 seconds over a few minutes while monitoring vital signs for evidence of IV or intrathecal administration.

Any resistance to injection should raise concern of incorrect position of the catheter.

vii) Resistance with injection for a caudal block should be similar to that of injecting through peripheral IV. **Any resistance to injection should raise concern of incorrect position of the catheter.**

viii) During each medication administration, palpate for swelling/fullness at injection site to rule out subcutaneous infiltration.

8) Continuous epidural catheter

a) Continuous epidural infusions may be performed in the caudal or the lumbar space by insertion of a catheter up to the lumbar or the thoracic levels.

b) In children <9 to 12 months of age, a 20-gauge epidural catheter may be threaded through an 18-gauge angiocath as high as the thoracic level.

c) Confirmation of catheter position is recommended with chest radiograph, fluoroscopy, or ultrasound.

d) 1 mm/kg of body weight estimates the distance from skin to epidural space in the lumbar space for children 6 months to 10 years old (8).

PEDIATRIC ANESTHESIA

Figure 125-1 Positioning for Caudal Block

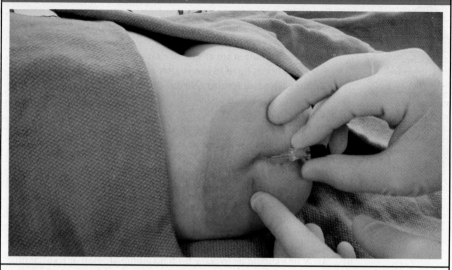

Lateral decubitus position for caudal block. Epidural catheter or venous angiocatheter may be used. Aseptic technique with skin prep, drapes, and gloves is necessary. Reused with permission from Hall SC, Suresh S. Neonatal Anesthesia. In: *Clinical Anesthesia*. Barash PG, Cullen BF, Stoelting RK, et al., eds. Philadelphia, PA: Lippincott Williams & Wilkins; 2009:1189.

Give incremental doses every 20 to 30 seconds to catch an inadvertent intravascular injection.

9) **Anesthetic considerations**
   a) Unlike adults, pediatric patients usually do not become hypotensive with the onset of block.
   b) Hypotension should be interpreted as sign of possible intravascular injection rather than sympathectomy from block.
   c) Intravascular injections may occur with a negative aspiration because local anesthetics may be quickly absorbed through intraosseous channels.
   d) The reliability of epinephrine causing tachycardia has also been questioned (10).
   e) Therefore, **the safest method to minimize risk of intravascular injection is to give incremental doses of drug.**

10) **Evaluation of the block**
    a) Since most caudals are done in children under general anesthesia, evaluation for sensory and motor blockade may not be possible.
    b) In addition, sympathectomy may also not be a reliable indicator of adequate anesthesia.
    c) Therefore, lack of response to surgical stimulation proves to be the best way to assess block efficacy.

11) **Postoperative management**
    a) Depending on duration of surgery, some motor blockade may be expected postoperatively.
    b) Motor and sensory blockade is commensurate with total dosage and type of local anesthetic and adjuvants used.
    c) Parents should be warned not to allow the child to ambulate without supervision.
    d) If opioids are used, patients should be monitored for at least 12 hours (and up to 18 hours) postoperatively for respiratory depression.

Figure 125-2   Technique for Caudal Block

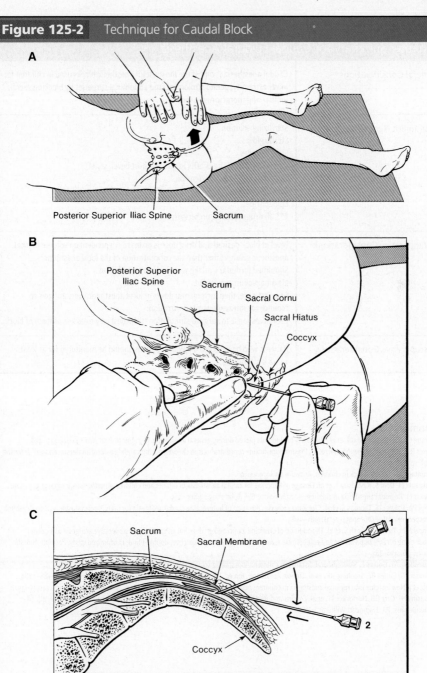

A Posterior Superior Iliac Spine   Sacrum

B Posterior Superior Iliac Spine   Sacrum   Sacral Cornu   Sacral Hiatus   Coccyx

C Sacrum   Sacral Membrane   Coccyx

PEDIATRIC ANESTHESIA

A: Lateral decubitus position for caudal block. **B:** Palpation of landmarks and insertion of catheter at sacral hiatus. **C:** Sagittal view of catheter insertion through sacral membrane then lowering of angle to thread catheter. Reproduced with permission from Veering BT, Cousins MJ. Epidural neural blockade. In: Cousins MJ, Carr DB, Horlocker TT, Bridenbaugh PO, eds. *Cousins & Bridenbaugh's Neural Blockade In Clinical Anesthesia and Pain Medicine.* 4th ed. Philadelphia, PA: Lippincott Williams & Wilkins; 2009:284.

Chapter Summary for Caudal Epidural Anesthesia

General Considerations	Caudal anesthesia is one of the most useful anesthetic blocks used in children for lower extremity, genito-urological, and abdominal surgeries by blocking sacral, lumbar and thoracic nerve roots.
Equipment Needed	Sterilizing solution Sterile gloves Sterile drapes Caudal needle or angiocath (22 gauge, short bevel, stylet) Optional connector as extension Local anesthetic Epinephrine *** all drugs must be preservative free
Intraoperative Considerations	Level of block desired and drug dose is primarily dependent on volume of local anesthetic given, rather than the concentration of the local anesthetic. Simplified formula: 1 mL/kg will block up to umbilicus. Maximal volume 20–30 mL. Give test dose, then incremental doses of local anesthetic every 20–30 s to monitor for intravenous administration. Lack of response to surgical stimulation is the best way to assess efficacy of block.
Postoperative Considerations	Patients who have received epidural opioids should be monitored for at least 12-18 h afterwards.

References

1. Krane EJ, Dalens BJ, Murat I, et al. The safety of epidurals placed during general anesthesia. *Reg Anesth Pain Med* 1998;23:433–438.
2. Eyres RL, Bishop W, Oppenheim R, et al. Plasma bupivacaine concentrations in children during caudal epidural analgesia. *Anaesth Intensive Care* 1983;11:20–22.
3. Armitage EN. Caudal block in children. *Anaesthesia* 1979;34:396.
4. Takasaki M, Dohi S, Kawabata Y, et al. Dosage of lidocaine for caudal anesthesia in infants and children. *Anesthesiology* 1977;47:527–529.
5. Zwass M. Regional anesthesia in children. *Anesthesiology Clin N Am* 2005;23:815–835.
6. Tripi PA, Palmer JS, Thomas S, et al. Clonidine increases duration of bupivacaine caudal analgesia for ureteroneocystostomy: a double-blind prospective trial. *J Urol* 2005;174(3):1081–1083.
7. Wheeler M, Patel A, Suresh S, et al. The addition of clonidine 2 microg.kg⁻¹ does not enhance the postoperative analgesia of a caudal block using 0.125% bupivacaine and epinephrine 1:200,000 in children: a prospective, double-blind, randomized study. *Paediatr Anaesth* 2005;15(6):476–483.
8. Bosenberg AT, Gouws E. Skin-epidural distance in children. *Anaesthesia* 1995;50:895–897.
9. Barash PG, Cullen BF, Stoelting RK, et al. *Clinical Anesthesia*. 6th ed. Philadelphia, PA: Lippincott Williams & Wilkins; 2006:1188–1189.
10. Tobias J. New insights into regional anesthesia in children: new techniques and new indications. *Curr Opin Anaesthesiol* 2001:14:345–352.
11. Cousins MJ, Carr DB, Horlocker TT, et al. *Cousins and Bridenbaugh's Neural Blockade in Clinical Anesthesia and Pain Medicine*. 4th ed. Philadelphia, PA: Lippincott Williams & Wilkins.

126 Management of the Pediatric Difficult Airway

Calvin Kuan, MD

To safely anesthetize the pediatric patient with a difficult airway, the practitioner must be familiar with pediatric anatomy, physiology, and pharmacology, and be facile with the equipment necessary to secure the pediatric airway.

The anesthesiologist caring for children should be knowledgeable about pediatric airway anatomy and the differences with adult anatomy.

Straight blades are usually better for young children (<2 to 3 years old).

1) **Introduction**
   a) Many congenital syndromes and acquired conditions are associated with having a difficult airway in children.
   b) The presence of a syndrome does not mean a patient will necessarily have a difficult airway, nor does absence of a syndrome guarantee a successful intubation.
   c) Patient's age and progression of the syndrome may influence airway difficulty. For example:
      i) Patients with Pierre-Robin sequence tend to become easier to manage with growth of their mandibles over time.
      ii) The airway management of patients with mucopolysaccharide storage diseases often becomes more difficult with age.

2) **Pediatric anatomy/physiology**
   a) There are six clinically significant anatomic and physiologic differences between normal pediatric and adult airways. These differences all contribute to the inherent difficulty of the pediatric airway (2).
   b) **Tongue**
      i) Compared to adults, the infant tongue is relatively large in proportion to the oral cavity.
      ii) Significance
         (1) Airway obstruction from the tongue occurs frequently in children, especially in the supine position and with loss of pharyngeal muscle tone under anesthesia.
         (2) The tongue is more likely to obscure the view under direct laryngoscopy.
      iii) Solutions:
         (1) Chin lift
         (2) Jaw thrust
         (3) Change in head position—tilt to side
         (4) Use of oral airway
         (5) Manually pulling the tongue out with clamp, gauze or a stitch to the tongue.
         (6) **A straight blade** may be better than a curved blade to achieve a direct line of sight to the larynx in younger children.
   c) **Position of larynx**
      i) The larynx may be as cephalad as C3 level for a premature infant, C3-4 for a newborn infant, and C4-5 for an adult (2).

PEDIATRIC ANESTHESIA

  ii) Significance
  (1) The **superior** location of the larynx means that there is a more acute angle from the oral axis to the tracheal axis and may result in more difficulty visualizing the larynx under direct laryngoscopy.
  iii) Solutions
  (1) External laryngeal manipulation or cricoid pressure may be employed to bring the larynx into view in order to insert the ETT.
  (2) If the above maneuver does not work, a stylet may be necessary to direct the ETT into the trachea.
 d) **Epiglottis**
  i) The adult epiglottis is broad, firm, and positioned parallel to the trachea.
  ii) The neonatal/pediatric epiglottis is relatively short, narrow, floppy, and angled posteriorly relative to the trachea (Fig. 126-1).
  iii) Significance
  (1) Because of this posterior angle, the epiglottis may block the entrance to the larynx.
  (2) Blind techniques (e.g., blind nasal intubation, or insertion of an ETT through an LMA without direct visualization of glottis) are likely to be less successful and more traumatic.
  iv) Solutions
  (1) Attempt to lift the epiglottis under direct laryngoscopic visualization to expose the glottis.
  (2) Use a styletted ETT to go around the epiglottis.
  (3) If there is resistance to insertion, try pulling out the stylet and sliding the ETT forward into the trachea. Without the stylet, the tip of the ETT is more malleable and less likely to hit the tracheal wall.
 e) **Vocal cords**
  i) Adult vocal cords are perpendicular to the axis of the trachea.
  ii) Pediatric vocal cords are slanted such that the anterior commissure is inferior, and the posterior commissure is superior (Fig. 126-1).
  iii) Significance
  (1) In children, the ETT may get caught at the junction of the anterior commissure and the epiglottis, and not pass into the trachea.

Figure 126-1   Orientation of Epiglottis and Vocal Cords

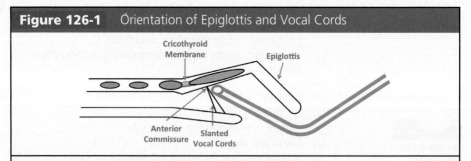

During direct laryngoscopy, the epiglottis may block visualization of the vocal cords. A stylet may be necessary to blindly direct the ETT underneath the epiglottis, but may still get caught at the anterior commisure. Photo by Shannon D. Schwartz.

- iv) Solutions
  - (1) Directing the ETT posteriorly and twisting it with a corkscrew motion may ease insertion and allow it to pass into the trachea.
- f) **Subglottic area**
  - i) The pediatric subglottic area is smaller than the adult subglottic area.
  - ii) Significance
    - (1) The practitioner must take care to ensure that the ETT chosen is the appropriate size and not so large that it will damage the tracheal tissue from sustained pressure.
  - iii) Solution
    - (1) The safest and most efficient way to accomplish this is to ensure that there is a leak around the ETT.
    - (2) Ideally, this leak will occur between pressures of 15 to 25 cm of H_2O, but a leak at a higher pressure may be desired if one expects a decrease in lung compliance.

To minimize risk of tracheal injury, ensure there is a leak around the ETT.

- g) **Oxygenation**
  - i) **A healthy child has at least a two to three times greater O2 consumption at baseline compared to a healthy adult (6 to 8 cc/kg/min vs. 3 cc/kg/min).**
  - ii) Significance
    - (1) A healthy 70-kg adult can maintain 100% SpO_2 for almost 10 minutes after adequate preoxygenation.
    - (2) A healthy 10-kg child can maintain 100% SpO_2 for only about 4 minutes—approximately the same amount of time as an obese 127-kg adult (3).
    - (3) This and other differences mean that **even in normal healthy children, there is less time to secure the airway before hypoxia occurs (1).**
  - iii) Solution
    - (1) Adequate preoxygenation with 100% FiO_2. Ensure a closed system to avoid entraining room air.
    - (2) If available, monitor expired O_2 level.
    - (3) Maintain oxygenation throughout induction until airway is secured.

Because children have higher O_2 consumption than adults, there is significantly less time to secure an airway prior to desaturation.

3) **Evaluation of pediatric airway**
  - a) Many techniques exist to assess the airway of adults. None of them have been shown to be sensitive or specific in predicting the degree of difficulty intubating children (1).
  - b) It is essential for the practitioner to evaluate the possibility of a difficult airway in every pediatric patient with a thorough past anesthetic history, medical history, and physical exam.

4) **Basic guidelines for management of the pediatric difficult airway**
  - a) Due to the heterogeneity of causes of difficult airways in pediatrics, it is impossible to discuss specific techniques that will be applicable to all pediatric patients. However, a few important guidelines should be mentioned:
  - b) **Preoxygenate and keep oxygenated.**
    - i) Except for the rare clinical situations where a higher FiO_2 may be contraindicated (e.g., single ventricle physiology), adequate preoxygenation of all patients will maximize time before desaturation in the case of a failed airway.

READ MORE

Congenital heart disease, Chapter 112, page 798

PEDIATRIC ANESTHESIA

c) Consider an antisialogogue to dry secretions prior to induction.

   i) Glycopyrrolate (5 to 10 μg/kg IV) is usually adequate and can be repeated as needed.

d) Maintain spontaneous ventilation.

   i) Allows for faster emergence if the decision is made to abort the anesthetic.

   ii) Minimizes the risk of airway obstruction due to loss of tone from deeper level of anesthesia.

   iii) Maintenance with an inhaled anesthetic or ketamine IV is a common technique because it is more likely to preserve respiratory drive.

e) **Always have an LMA immediately available as backup.**

   i) Even under optimal circumstances, children cannot maintain adequate SpO_2 for more than a few minutes after a failed attempt to secure the airway.

   ii) **There may not be enough time to attempt any technique other than an LMA. Appropriately sized LMAs should be immediately available in locations where children are anesthetized.**

   iii) It is worth noting that LMAs (especially those sized 2 or smaller) are more difficult to seat securely and easier to dislodge in children compared to adults.

      (1) Constant vigilance is necessary to ensure that the LMA is seated properly at all times.

f) Consider fiberoptic intubation early in the process while the airway is still patent rather than after multiple attempts to intubate the trachea have resulted in bleeding, swelling, and unrecognizable anatomy.

g) **Call for help early!**

   i) Many of the techniques that have been described for use in pediatrics require multiple steps and are most safely accomplished with experienced assistance.

h) **Alternative devices and techniques**

   i) Other airway devices (e.g., Glidescope, Trachlight, Fastrach intubating LMA, etc.) and techniques (e.g., blind nasal intubation, digitally assisted intubation) are available. The decision to use these alternatives should be made on a case-by-case basis by practitioners with experience with the specific techniques.

5) Difficult airway algorithm

  a) *Anticipated* difficult airway

   i) **Use your clinical judgment.** Keep in mind that children are not just little adults. They have different anatomy and physiology, and therefore require individual strategies for management. Most important to consider is that there is often significantly less time to accomplish what is usually a more difficult goal.

   ii) Devise a primary plan A and have a backup plan B, C, D, etc. as needed.

   iii) **Patients with clear evidence of a difficult airway and/or complex medical conditions for *elective* procedures should be referred to a tertiary pediatric center** with multidisciplinary services that have experience caring for pediatric patients intraoperatively and postoperatively.

   iv) There may be rare clinical situations where **elective use of extracorporeal membrane oxygenation (ECMO) or cardiopulmonary bypass** is the safest option.

      (1) These may include severe mediastinal mass (4), severe anatomical distortion due to burn injury (5), or significant distal tracheal obstruction or disruption where even an appropriately placed airway will not provide adequate oxygenation.

  b) *Unanticipated* difficult airway

   i) If the first attempt at direct laryngoscopy was unsuccessful, a second attempt may be made if at least one condition has been changed including repositioning the patient, using a different blade, and changing to a more experienced practitioner.

   ii) If the second attempt is also unsuccessful, the practitioner should call for help and then weigh the risks and benefits of continued attempts.

   iii) If oxygenation and airway patency are not assured, the speediest and safest option is to insert an LMA.

An LMA should be immediately available to be used to maintain a patent airway for oxygenation and as a conduit for fiberoptic intubation.

READ MORE

Wire Cricothyroidotomy cognitive aid, Chapter 157, page 1110

Verify that all equipment used for techniques described below will fit through each other as there may be variation in size between different manufacturers.

c) **Failed airway (cannot intubate/cannot ventilate)**
   i) In the situation of inability to mask ventilate or intubate, the most important goal of the anesthesiologist is to keep the patient oxygenated.
   ii) To this end, an LMA should be placed immediately.
   iii) If the LMA is unsuccessful, or if the obstruction is at the glottis, then a surgical airway should be considered.
      (1) For children over 10 to 12 years old, a surgical cricothyroidotomy or tracheostomy may be considered.
      (2) For children under 10 to 12 years old, a needle cricothyroidotomy is recommended.
         (a) Keep in mind that for younger children **the risk of complications with emergency surgical airway is extremely high** (2), so this should be attempted only in a true emergency.
         (b) If the obstruction is located in the subglottic region or lower (i.e., closer to the carina), a surgical airway at the cricothyroid membrane may not create a patent airway.

6) **Special techniques/situations**
   a) **Conversion of nonintubating LMA into endotracheal tube:**
      i) The smallest intubating LMA (Fastrach) is a size 3 for patients >30 kg (usually >9 to 10 years old).
      ii) The smallest accompanying extra-long ETT with a stabilizing rod is 6.0 mm (internal diameter).
      iii) Blind intubation of the trachea of a smaller child through an LMA is unlikely to be successful because the epiglottis frequently obstructs the glottic opening, and fiberoptic assistance may be necessary.
      iv) Additional problems should be anticipated:
         (1) **Problem no. 1: Aperture bars may block the advancement of the ETT.**
            (a) **Solution no. 1-A:** Cut out the aperture bars of the LMA prior to insertion (Fig. 126-2). The ETT may get caught on the bars if they are not cut short enough—especially the distal bars further away from the shaft of the LMA.

Figure 126-2   Special Considerations for Pediatric Airway Equipment

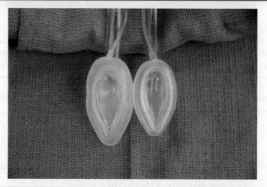

LMA on the left has aperture bars removed. Smaller LMA on right has bars intact for comparison. Note: If the bars are not cut short enough, the ETT may get caught on them during insertion. Photos by Shannon D. Schwartz.

PEDIATRIC ANESTHESIA

READ
MORE

Read more on
airway exchange
catheters in prac-
tical pediatrics
Chapter 112,
page 798

(b) **Solution no. 1-B:** An Air-Q (Mercury Medical, Clearwater, FL) intubating laryngeal airway, which does not have bars, or LMA Excel, which has mobile bars, may be used.

(2) **Problem no. 2: The ETT cuff will not fit through the connector of the LMA** (Fig. 126-3A)

  (a) **Solution A:** Use an UNcuffed ETT first then convert to a cuffed ETT with an airway exchange catheter (Fig. 126-3B)

  (b) **Solution B:** Use an LMA Excel or Air-Q intubating laryngeal airway, both of which have removable connectors.

Figure 126-3	Special Considerations for Pediatric Airway Equipment

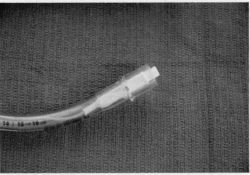

A

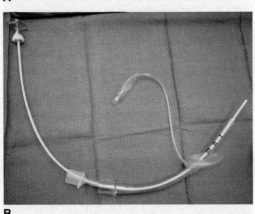

B

A: The cuff of the ETT will not fit through connector of LMAs smaller than Size 3. **B:** An airway exchange catheter may be inserted into an uncuffed ETT through the LMA to safely exchange it for a cuffed ETT. Photos by Shannon D. Schwartz.

(3) **Problem no. 3: The pediatric ETT is too short. The LMA cannot be removed safely without dislodging the ETT.**

  (a) **Solution A:** Elongate an ETT by connecting it end to end with another ETT that is one half size smaller (e.g., 4.0 with a 3.5 ETT) (Fig. 126-4A).

  (b) **Solution B:** Alternatively, the smaller end of an ETT 15-mm connector may be cut off and used as a male-male adaptor to connect two ETTs of the same size (Fig. 126-4B) (6).

  (c) **Solution C:** Leave the LMA with ETT in situ for the case.

Figure 126-4   Special Considerations for Pediatric Airway Equipment

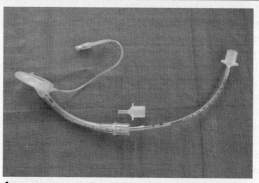

A

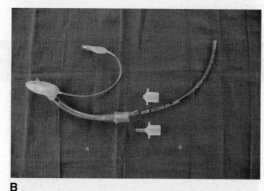

B

A: A 0.5 size smaller ETT may be used as a "Pusher" by fitting it into the end of an ETT with connector removed. This allows safe removal of the LMA. **B:** The smaller diameter end of an ETT connector may be cut and used to connect two equal-sized ETT to make them long enough to safely remove an LMA. Photos by Shannon D. Schwartz.

b) **Fiberoptic intubation of small child with adult bronchoscope**
   i) One can successfully intubate a small child or neonate even when the smallest fiberoptic scope available is an adult one.
   ii) **Necessary additional equipment**
      (1) **Guidewire** that will fit through the suction/working channel of the bronchoscope.
      (2) Guidewires smaller than 0.035 inches (0.89 mm) in diameter may be too flimsy to support an ETT without kinking.
      (3) It is important to verify that the wire is long enough to extend out of the bronchoscope prior to use. Cardiac catheterization or urological catheters (usually 100 to 150 cm long) are ideal.
      (4) **Airway exchange catheter** that is large enough to fit over the guidewire, and small enough to fit through the desired ETT.
   iii) **Procedure**
      (1) First locate the larygneal inlet with the adult fiberoptic scope directly through the mouth.
      (2) Then insert the guidewire through the working channel of the scope into the trachea under direct visualization.
      (3) Similar to a Seldinger technique: remove the fiberoptic scope (but leave the guidewire).

(4) Insert the airway exchange catheter (AEC) over the guidewire to stiffen it. Without the AEC, the guidewire may not remain in the trachea and may flip out when trying to pass the ETT.

(5) Then pass the ETT over the airway exchange catheter into the trachea.

(6) Confirm placement with ETCO$_2$ and auscultation.

c) **Emergency needle cricothyrotomy**

    i) In smaller children in whom surgical tracheostomy is not possible, insertion of an intravenous catheter may be lifesaving.

    ii) One must be able to attach the 15-mm adaptor of the standard breathing circuit to the Luer lock end of the catheter. Two options exist here:

        (1) The connectors of the standard 3.5 ETT (Sheridan CF, Hudson RCI, Durham, NC) fit directly onto the end of the intravenous catheter. (Fig. 126-5A)

        (2) A 3-mL Luer lock syringe (BD, Franklin Lakes, NJ) with the plunger removed can be connected to the catheter, and the connector from a 7.0 ETT (Mallinckrodt Intermediate Hi-Lo, Covidien, Hazelwood, MO) can fit directly into the syringe (Fig. 126-5B).

Figure 126-5   Adapting an Intravenous Catheter for Emergency Needle Cricothyrotomy

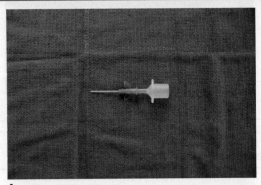

A

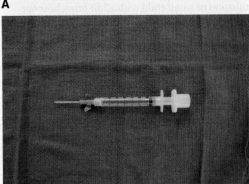

B

A: The connector from a 3.5 ETT fits into the end of a standard intravenous catheter to convert the Luer lock into a 15 mm adaptor. **B:** If a 3.5 ETT connector is not available, a 3 mL syringe with the plunger removed can be attached to the connector of a 7.0 ETT. Photos by Shannon Schwartz.

d) **Clinical pearls**
   i) **Distorted or indistinguishable anatomy:**

      (1) Patients may have laryngeal anatomy that is unrecognizable either by direct laryngoscopy or fiberoptic bronchoscopy.

      (2) Solution A: Identify the trachea by looking for bubbles and directing the ETT toward them.

      (3) Solution B: Bubbles may be created by having an assistant gently squeeze the chest.

If you cannot recognize any structures during direct laryngoscopy, look for air bubbles to locate trachea.

   ii) **Abdominal distention may impair ventilation**

      (1) Bag/mask ventilation may insufflate air into the stomach and intestines and limit the ability to ventilate or oxygenate—even to the point of causing a clinical picture like a tension pneumothorax.

      (2) Solution A: Minimize inflation by using only as high-peak inspiratory pressures as necessary to achieve adequate ventilate/oxygenate during bag/mask ventilation.

      (3) Solution B: Use cricoid pressure to minimize insufflation of air into esophagus and stomach.

      (4) Solution C: Place an orogastric or a nasogastric tube to release the air in the stomach. This may be repeated as necessary when high pressures are required.

Vigorous mask ventilation may insufflate air into the stomach and impair ventilation.

Chapter Summary for Management of the Pediatric Difficult Airway

Use your clinical judgment.
Preoxygenate and keep patient well oxygenated.
Use an antisialogogue to dry secretions.
Maintain spontaneous respirations.
Have LMA immediately available.
Call for experienced assistance early.
Consider fiberoptic bronchoscopy early.

PEDIATRIC ANESTHESIA

References

1. Gregory GA, Riazi J. Classification and assessment of the difficult pediatric airway. *Anaesth Clin N Am* 1998;16:729–741.
2. Wheeler M, Cote CJ, Todres ID. IN: Cote CJ, Lerman J, Todres ID. The pediatric airway. In: A *Practice of Anesthesia for Infants and Children*. 4th ed. Philadelphia, PA: Saunders; 2009:237–273.
3. Benumof JL, Dagg R, Benumof R. Critical hemoglobin desaturation will occur before return to an unparalyzed state following 1 mg/kg intravenous succinylcholine. *Anesthesiology* 1997;87:979–982.
4. Chung SL, Lerman J. Mediastinal masses and anesthesia in children. *Anaesth Clin N Am* 1998;16:893–910.
5. Sheridan RL, Goldstein MA, Stoddard FJ, et al. An 18-month-old girl with an advanced neck contracture after a burn. *N Engl J Med* 2008;358:729–735.
6. Muraika L, Heyman JS, Shevchenko Y. Fiberoptic tracheal intubation through a laryngeal mask airway in a child with Treacher Collins syndrome. *Anesth Analg* 2003;97:1298–1299.

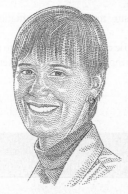

127

Challenges in Anesthesia: Emergent Management and Resuscitation in the Delivery Room of Newborn with a Difficult Airway

Anita Honkanen, MD

Clinical Vignette

You are working in a small community hospital with an active OB service, a class IIb NICU (1), and all general services. While you are on call, you are called STAT to assist with the airway management of a newborn in the OR delivery room. The mother is also in crisis and her anesthesiologist is unable to assist. When you arrive in the OR, you find a labor and delivery nurse and a respiratory therapist at the newborn incubator with a 3-kg infant. The patient is making occasional gasping respiratory efforts with marked retractions, has a heart rate of 80, and flaccid, blue extremities. It is now 5 minutes since birth, and APGAR score at 1 minute was 4. The respiratory therapist is holding a bag/mask over the infant's face while the nurse is vigorously massaging the patient. You are told that there was meconium staining of the amniotic fluid, and that the patient seems to have a "funny looking" face. You note meconium staining of the baby's face and the mask.

Any anesthesiologist approaching this situation must understand several basic elements of neonatal physiology in order to both understand the gravity of the circumstances and how to respond appropriately. The patient is in a near cardiorespiratory code status and will require rapid interventions to avoid long-term adverse outcomes.

The foundation of knowledge critical for understanding how to respond includes familiarity with the basic physiology of the newborn's circulatory and respiratory systems and how they transition from the fetus to the neonate. Knowledge of the pediatric airway and pediatric resuscitation is also essential. Finally, familiarity with the physical features associated with some of the common congenital abnormalities that can lead to airway compromise is helpful.

Normally, there is ONE umbilical vein (oxygenated blood) and TWO umbilical arteries (deoxygenated blood) in the umbilicus.

In the fetal circulation, blood travels through the umbilical vein to the heart via the ductus venosus through the liver to the inferior vena cava and right atrium (RA) (Fig 127-1, III). This oxygenated blood from the placenta comprises 70% of the flow into the heart. The other deoxygenated 30% comes from the superior vena cava. The oxygenated blood takes two routes, some passing through the foramen ovale to the left side of the heart while the rest flows through the right ventricle, to the pulmonary artery (PA). From the PA, <10% flows through the lungs, while the rest passes through the ductus arteriosus and

Figure 127-1 Diagram of Fetal Circulation

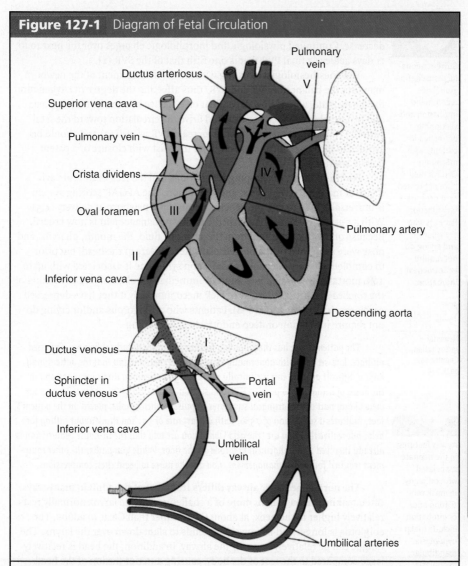

Pulmonary vein

Ductus arteriosus

V

Superior vena cava

Pulmonary vein

Crista dividens

IV

Oval foramen   III

Pulmonary artery

II

Inferior vena cava

Descending aorta

Ductus venosus   I

Sphincter in ductus venosus

Portal vein

Inferior vena cava

Umbilical vein

Umbilical arteries

From Sadler TW. *Langman's Medical Embryology*. 11th ed. Philadelphia, PA: Lippincott Williams & Wilkins; 2010:197, with permission.

into the descending aorta. With streaming of blood in the RA, the most highly oxygenated blood flows into the left atrium (Fig 127-1, IV) passing through the left ventricle into the aorta and up to the coronary arteries, head, and upper extremities (2). The paired umbilical arteries branch from the iliac arteries in the groin and join the single umbilical vein to take deoxygenated blood from the fetus to the placenta for gas exchange. (See Fig. 127-1)

The main factor responsible for maintenance of the fetal circulatory pattern is the balance between the pulmonary vascular resistance (PVR) and the systemic vascular resistance (SVR) (3). In the fetus, PVR is higher than SVR, creating a parallel circulatory pattern. Two events trigger the immediate transition to the neonatal circulation: (a) Systemic event: clamping of the cord with loss of the low resistance placental circuit, and (b) Pulmonary event: inflation of the

Current neonatal resuscitation guidelines recommend intubation and suctioning of trachea in patients with meconium ONLY if they have depressed cardiorespiratory function. Patients who are vigorous and crying do not require endotracheal intubation.

READ MORE

Neonatal resuscitation, Chapter 102, page 745

Airway features in the neonate associated with difficulty in mask ventilation and/or intubation include malar hypoplasia, mandibular hypoplasia, choanal atresia

READ MORE

Management of the pediatric difficult airway, Chapter 126, page 873

READ MORE

Practical pediatric anesthesia, Chapter 129, page 899

lungs with the first breath, dropping resistance. After the first few hours, with production of prostanoids, the PVR normally completes 80% of its ultimate decrease. Continued physiologic and morphologic changes over the next 10 to 11 days achieve a final PVR that is one fifth that of the SVR (2).

The anesthesiologist assisting with airway management of the newborn may alter the balance of PVR and SVR, thus affecting the degree of oxygenation for the neonate, who is now dependent on effective breathing. Both hypoxia and hypercarbia will increase PVR and drive the circulation toward the fetal pattern (3). Indomethacin will act to increase PVR as well (2) and should be avoided in these patients unless required to assist with closure of a patent ductus arteriosus.

For this patient, the gasping respirations and the lack of tone are evidence of marginal oxygenation and ventilation. The APGAR scoring system is universally used to rate the general status of the newborn at delivery (4,5). With a 5-minute APGAR of 3, expedient airway management is now crucial. Because of the thick meconium in the amniotic fluid, the mouth, pharynx, and nose were suctioned by the obstetrician after delivery of the head, but prior to complete delivery. Meconium aspiration syndrome is associated with up to 40% mortality (6). Guidelines support immediate intubation and suctioning of the trachea in patients born with thick meconium only if they have depressed cardiorespiratory function (6–8). Patients who are vigorous and/or crying do not require intubation or deep endotracheal suctioning.

The patient's face has the following features: slanting palpebral fissures, depressed midface, low-set ears with abnormally shaped pinna. Recognizing that the patient may have a difficult airway, but is clinically unstable, you attempt a direct laryngoscopy in the hopes of being able to pass an ETT and suction the trachea of this infant. There is no view of any part of the laryngeal structures. A pulse oximeter probe, placed on the patient's foot, indicates a saturation of 75%, with a heart rate of 55. You think about calling for help, but realize that you are "the help" when you are told that the in-house pediatrician is already involved in management of a code on the floor. While you gather the other equipment required for further management, you ask the nurse to begin chest compressions.

The normal pediatric airway differs from that of the adult in many ways, often making management more of a challenge (9). The larynx normally rests relatively higher in the neck, at about C3-4, rather than C6 as in adults. The epiglottis is longer and narrower and tends to slant down over the larynx. The tongue can be relatively large for the airway. In addition, the head is relatively large compared to the rest of the body, causing anterior flexion of the head on the neck if resting flat on a surface. Placement of a small roll behind the shoulders of the neonate can create improved positioning of the head relative to the neck. A straight blade when used to pick up the epiglottis is often easier to place in the mouth and achieves a better view of laryngeal structures than a curved blade (10). Choosing the appropriate-sized blade and airway adjuncts for the child is critical in maximizing the ability to effectively mask ventilate, obtain a view of the larynx, and place an ETT that seats without too much pressure while avoiding an air leak around the tube (5).

Apart from the increased challenge in intubation often encountered in the small child with normal anatomical features, there are several congenital syndromes and conditions associated with difficult airway management and compromise in the neonate. One of the common themes in many of these conditions is a relatively small oropharynx that may be unable to accommodate

READ MORE

Management of the pediatric difficult airway, Chapter 126, page 873

Intravenous high-dose epinephrine (100 μg/kg/dose) is no longer recommended.

READ MORE

Management of pediatric arrest and resuscitation, Chapter 128, page 890

IV glucose bolus is not recommended to be given automatically unless there is history of diabetes in mother, or documented hypoglycemia (<40–50 mg/dL in the newborn).

READ MORE

Practical pediatric anesthesia , Chapter 129, page 899

Neonates are obligate nasal breathers who may need assistance breathing if the nares are not patent.

the bulk of the tongue; there is either too small a bony cage or too large a tongue structure, with the end result being trouble developing a view of the laryngeal structures (10). The malformations described in the patient presented here are consistent with a diagnosis of **Treacher-Collins Syndrome** (11). These features include **malar hypoplasia**, down-slanting palpebral fissures, external ear abnormalities with low-set ears, **mandibular and pharyngeal hypoplasia,** and **choanal atresia** (The features in bold contribute to the difficulty in airway management). Other common syndromes are associated with difficult airway management in the newborn and pediatric patients include Down, Noonan, Pierre-Robin, Turner, Treacher-Collins, and DiGeorge syndromes.

The vast majority of cardiac arrests in children are related to airway and breathing issues, so a successful resuscitation of the neonate must start with effective airway management. However, **if the heart rate drops below 60 bpm, chest compressions should be initiated at a rate of 90 to 100 bpm** (5,8,12). High-dose (100 μg/kg) epinephrine is no longer recommended, as it is associated with poorer long-term outcomes (12–14). Epinephrine can be given at a dose of 10 μg/kg IM or via IV or via the ETT at a dose of 30 to 100 μg/kg (5,15). For ease of access, the umbilical vessels are often used in the neonate, with two arteries to one vein easily identifiable. Sterile procedure must be used, and proper depth of placement is critical in avoiding damage to the liver, heart, or other organs (16).

Immediate administration of glucose is not recommended (14,17) unless there is a history of diabetes in the mother or other condition that would predispose to fetal hyperinsulinemia or hypoglycemia (18). D10 in water, at 3 to 5 mL/kg, is an appropriate initial bolus dose followed by an infusion of D10 in ¼ NS at 4 mL/kg/h. This solution for ongoing maintenance ensures both adequate serum glucose levels despite the neonatal lack of glycogen stores in the liver with limited gluconeogenesis capacity, and avoids a heavy salt load to the immature kidneys.

It is important to keep the normal vital sign parameters in mind when involved in the resuscitation of neonates and infants. These parameters vary considerably by age group. Attempting to achieve vitals appropriate in an adult or older child could put the neonate at risk for circulatory failure or intracranial hemorrhage.

Adequate preparation is also critical, ensuring the necessary equipment, medications, supplies, and personnel are readily available to respond in a timely manner. Table 127-1 summarizes the various elements that should be immediately available at deliveries.

Another physiologic reality for neonates is that they are obligate nasal breathers. If the nares are not patent, as is suspected in this child due to his midface hypoplasia, an oral airway to separate the tongue and the roof of the mouth can be life saving. Patients with choanal atresia must have some means of creating an open channel through the mouth until definitive surgical correction can be achieved (19).

Bag mask ventilation is marginally successful in this patient, but after placement of a 50-mm oral airway, complete obstruction of the airway occurs. You remove the airway and place a size 1.0 LMA. With the first vigorous breath, you note a strong expiratory effort by the infant. Gentle sustained breaths with long inspiratory times to inflate the lungs and increase FRC are successful, and the oxygen saturation levels increase to 99% after 2 minutes using 100% oxygen. Heart rate gradually increases to 160 bpm.

It is not unusual to have difficulty fitting the appropriate sized oral airway in neonates with abnormal facial structure. In this child, placement of the oral

Table 127-1

Considerations and Equipment in Neonatal Resuscitation Emergencies

General Considerations	Equipment:
Temperature of room	Neonatal bed/warmer
Gestational age of infant/size	Suction: bulb and wall canister
Prenatal condition: fetal distress	Oral pharyngeal airway
Maternal condition: effects on fetus	Oxygen/air flow regulator
	Pressure manometer for airway
Personnel Resources	CO_2 monitor
Nurse	Pulse oximeter
Respiratory therapist	Stethoscope
Neonatologist/pediatrician	Laryngoscope
Anesthesiologist	ETTs
	Stylets
Meds and Fluids	LMA, LTS II
Epinephrine: 1:10,000 in dilution (=10 µg/mL)	Mask
Atropine: 0.4 mg/mL, TB syringe and 23 G needle	T-Piece bag device
Sodium bicarbonate: 0.1% = 1 mEq/mL	Self-Inflating Ambu Bag Device
D5 1/4 NS, D10 IV fluid, 5% albumin	IV catheters: 24 G, UA/UV catheter tray

The LMA is an effective airway rescue device but requires constant vigilance in young children/neonates as it does not seat as securely in children as in adults.

airway appeared to occlude the airway further. But when it was replaced with a size 1.0 laryngeal mask airway (LMA), a patent upper airway was achieved. Supraglottic airway devices, such as the LMA and the Laryngeal Tube Suction II (LTS II), have been shown to be very effective in management of the neonatal and infant airway (9,20). The LMA has also proven to be a very effective device to rescue a lost airway in neonates and infants (10). However, it is important to remember that the **LMA does not seat as definitively in children as compared to adults.** Thus, it may be necessary to adjust the depth of placement while ventilating the patient and observing the ease and degree of chest excursion. The LMA should be secured with tape at the appropriate depth and can be further supported by placement of small rolls of gauze to either side within the mouth.

Slow, sustained breaths at peak airway pressures of 30 to 40 serve to decrease atelectasis in the infant, increase FRC, improve lung compliance and tidal volumes. Caution must be taken to avoid overinflation of the lungs, which can cause long-term damage. Continuous observation of chest excursion during resuscitation is important to help avoid barotrauma and to ensure adequate ventilation (5). CPAP has been associated with avoidance of mechanical ventilation in neonates requiring some respiratory assistance and shown to improve response to surfactant in premature infants (21,22).

If oxygen saturation does not improve with 100% FiO_2, consider the possibility of congenital cyanotic heart disease.

The use of 100% O_2 is still controversial, as its use has been associated with the need for increased ventilation and higher levels of superoxide dismutase. Poorer long-term outcomes have been reported as well (23). In addition, maintaining an SpO_2 level in the low to mid 90s from birth is associated with a decreased incidence of retinopathy of prematurity (14). An acceptable approach during resuscitation is to start with 60% O_2 concentration, titrating up to 100% as needed to keep the SpO_2 above 85% to 90% (5). If the SpO_2 does not improve with increased FiO_2, consider the possibility of congenital cyanotic heart disease.

At this point, the pediatrician arrives and requests that you assist with securing of a definitive airway for this baby.

The airway of this child has temporarily been stabilized with the LMA, but there are two conditions that warrant a more definitive airway: (a) choanal atresia with abnormal jaw structure, which has compromised upper airway patency; and (b) meconium aspiration, which could compromise pulmonary function. As you have already demonstrated the inability to visualize the laryngeal structures with direct laryngoscopy, attempts to further manipulate the airway should be done in an OR with an ENT surgeon prepared to perform a bronchoscopy or a tracheostomy if needed (24).

Using inhalational anesthesia to maintain spontaneous respiration and topicalization of the laryngeal structures with 1% lidocaine prior to starting will improve conditions for a successful intubation. TIVA techniques (with propofol and/or ketamine) can be used as well, but whatever method is used should include maintenance of spontaneous respirations throughout the intubation attempt. Atropine or glycopyrrolate may be given to decrease secretions and help prevent possible vagal reflex reactions to airway manipulation (10).

A 2.2-mm fiberoptic scope, loaded with either a 2.5- or 3.0-mm ETT, with a second tube above as a "pusher," will pass through the LMA easily. The LMA acts as an effective guide directing the bronchoscope toward the laryngeal structures, greatly facilitating passage of the bronchoscope through the vocal cords. With the tip of the bronchoscope at the carina, the ETT can then be passed over the bronchoscope through the LMA into the trachea. The distal ETT is used as a pusher to allow removal of the LMA from the mouth after passage of the proximal ETT into the trachea (10). Note that it is important to have experienced assistance as it takes more than one set of hands to effectively guide the bronchoscope and facilitate passage of the ETT through the LMA into the trachea. Ideally, only experienced individuals should attempt this procedure. Thus, if the child is stable with the LMA in situ, transport should be arranged to a facility with experienced personnel and equipment. Ultimately, surgery to correct the choanal atresia and/or increase the size of the mandible will likely be necessary.

READ MORE

Practical pediatric anesthesia, Chapter 129, page 899 and Mangement of the pediatric difficult airway, Chapter 126, page 873

In summary, the management of the neonate at delivery requires familiarity with the normal physiology of the neonate transitioning from the fetal state, an understanding of the equipment and materials appropriate for use in the neonate, and an appreciation of the influences of both the maternal history and the neonatal conditions likely to be encountered that can affect the patient's acute pathophysiology and anatomical structures. Facility with the critical steps in both resuscitation of the neonate and effective airway management of the neonatal difficult airway can be life saving. Following is a table summarizing both the preparation and the steps to take, which can be used as a cognitive aid, for reference during this emergent circumstance (Table 127-2).

PEDIATRIC ANESTHESIA

Table 127-2

Cognitive Aid for Neonatal Resuscitation and Airway Management in the Delivery Room

Step	Action or Item	Goal or Gauge
General Preparation		
1	Infant warmer, drying towels	Maintain adequate warmth
2	Protective garb: gloves, masks, gowns, eye shields	Maintain personal protection
3	Medications, fluids, umbilical catheter tray, IV supplies	Resuscitation if required
4	Suction bulb	Allow gentle removal oropharyngeal secretions

(continued)

Table 127-2

Cognitive Aid for Neonatal Resuscitation and Airway Management in the Delivery Room (Continued)

Step	Action or Item	Goal or Gauge
Preparation: Airway Equipment, Materials, Supplies		
1	Oxygen/air source	Blender available for graded application
2	Bag/mask devices Neonatal mask Ambu or continuous flow circuits: neonatal size	Allow positive pressure ventilation
3	Intubating equipment: allow securing of airway Laryngoscopes: Miller 00, 0, 1 blades ETT's: 2.5, 3.0, 3.5 cuffed and uncuffed Stylet	Secure airway, allow positive pressure ventilation

4	Supraglottic devices
	   oropharyngeal airways (OPA): 40 mm, 50 mm
	   LMA: 1, 1.5
	   LTS II: 0
		If unable to mask ventilate and/or intubate

Assessment: Adequate Circulation and Respiration		**Positive signs**
1	Immediate review	HR > 100 Spontaneous respirations Absence of central cyanosis
2	Mechanics	Chest movement Absence of retractions
3	Vital signs	RR: 40–60 HR: 120–140 O_2 saturations > 90%
Steps in Assisting Respiration/Ventilation: Increase Level of Assistance Until Adequate Response Seen		
1	Assess patient's respiratory status	See respiratory assessment section above
2	Apply blow-by O_2, massage patient	Stimulate spontaneous respiratory effort
3	Apply CPAP	For HR < 100, cyanosis, O_2 saturations < 90%
4	Insert OPA, reapply CPAP, gentle bag-mask ventilation	Inadequate response to Step 3
5	Laryngoscopy and intubation: ventilate	Inadequate response to Step 4 or requires tracheal suction
6	Place LMA: ventilate	Unable to intubate

(continued)

Table 127-2

Cognitive Aid for Neonatal Resuscitation and Airway Management in the Delivery Room (*Continued*)

Step	Action or Item	Goal or Gauge
	Other Interventions: Access, Medications, Fluids	
1	Consider chest compressions	If patient's HR < 60
2	Obtain IV access: consider umbilical vein catheter	Requires administration of medication or fluids
3	Administer resuscitation medications Epinephrine: 10–30 µg/kg IV, 30–100 µg/kg via ETT Bicarbonate: 4 mL/kg of 0.5 mEq/L solution, slowly via UV	HR < 60, ensure adequate ventilation first if possible HR < 60 **despite adequate ventilation and epinephrine**
4	Administer fluids: NS, 5% albumin, blood: 10 mL/kg	Inadequate response to prior resuscitation steps

PEDIATRIC ANESTHESIA

References

1. Stark AR. Levels of neonatal care. *Pediatrics* 2004;114(5):1341–1347.
2. Clarke WR. The transitional circulation: physiology and anesthetic implications. *J Clin Anesth* 1990;2(3):192–211.
3. Stokes MA. Anesthetic and Preoperative Management. In: Lake CL, Booker PD, eds. *Pediatric Cardiac Anesthesia* 4th ed. Philadelphia, PA: Lippincott Williams & Wilkins; 2005:180–181; Chap 10.
4. Ahanya SN, Lakshmanan J, Morgan BL, et al. Meconium passage in utero: mechanisms, consequences, and management. *Obstet Gynecol Surv* 2005;60(1):45–56; quiz 73–74.
5. Ringer SA. Resuscitation in the delivery room. In: Cloherty J, Eichenwald E, Stark A, eds. *Manual of Neonatal Care*. Philadelphia, PA: Lippincott Williams & Wilkins; 2008:59–71; chap 4.
6. Bhutani VK. Developing a systems approach to prevent meconium aspiration syndrome: lessons learned from multinational studies. *J Perinatol* 2008;28 Suppl 3:S30–S35.
7. Whitfield JM, Charsha DS, Chiruvolu A. Prevention of meconium aspiration syndrome: an update and the Baylor experience. *Proc (Bayl Univ Med Cent)* 2009;22(2):128–131.
8. Kattwinkel J, Niermeyer S, Nadkarni V, Tibballs J, Phillips B, Zideman D, Van Reempts P, Osmond M. Resuscitation of the newly born infant: an advisory statement from the Pediatric Working Group of the International Liaison Committee on *Resuscitation*. Resuscitation 1999;40(2):71–88.
9. Infosino A. Pediatric upper airway and congenital anomalies. *Anesthesiol Clin N Am* 2002;20(4):747–766.
10. Walker RW, Ellwood J. The management of difficult intubation in children. *Paediatr Anaesth* 2009;19 Suppl 1:77–87.
11. Baum V, O'Flaherty J. *Anesthesia for Genetic, Metabolic, and Dysmorphic Syndromes of Childhood* 2nd ed. Philadelphia, PA: Lippincott Williams, & Wilkins; 2007.
12. ECC Committee, Subcommittees and Task Forces of the American Heart Association, 2005 American Heart Association (AHA) guidelines for cardiopulmonary resuscitation (CPR) and emergency cardiovascular care (ECC) of pediatric and neonatal patients: pediatric basic life support. *Pediatrics* 2006;117(5):e989–e1004.
13. Finer NN, Rich WD. Neonatal resuscitation: raising the bar. *Curr Opin Pediatr* 2004;16(2):157–162.
14. Wyllie J, Niermeyer S. The role of resuscitation drugs and placental transfusion in the delivery room management of newborn infants. *Semin Fetal Neonatal Med* 2008;13(6):416–423.
15. *PALS Provider Manual*, ed. A.H.A.a.A.A.o. Pediatrics. 2006: American Heart Association and American Academy of Pediatrics.
16. Yigiter M, Arda IS, Hicsonmez A. Hepatic laceration because of malpositioning of the umbilical vein catheter: case report and literature review. *J Pediatr Surg* 2008;43(5):E39–E41.
17. McGowan JE, Perlman JM. Glucose management during and after intensive delivery room resuscitation. *Clin Perinatol* 2006;33(1):183–196, x.
18. Stenninger E, Lindqvist A, Aman J, et al. Continuous Subcutaneous Glucose Monitoring System in diabetic mothers during labour and postnatal glucose adaptation of their infants. *Diabet Med* 2008;25(4):450–454.
19. Ibrahim AA, Magdy EA, Hassab MH. Endoscopic choanoplasty without stenting for congenital choanal atresia repair. *Int J Pediatr Otorhinolaryngol* 2010;74(2):144–150.
20. Scheller B, Schalk R, Byhahn C, et al. Laryngeal tube suction II for difficult airway management in neonates and small infants. *Resuscitation* 2009;80(7):805–810.
21. Verder H, Robertson B, Greisen G, et al. Nasal CPAP and surfactant for treatment of respiratory distress syndrome and prevention of bronchopulmonary dysplasia. *Acta Paediatr* 2009;98(9):1400–1408.
22. Rojas MA, Lozano JM, Rojas MX, et al. Very early surfactant without mandatory ventilation in premature infants treated with early continuous positive airway pressure: a randomized, controlled trial. *Pediatrics* 2009;123(1):137–142.
23. Gitto E, Reiter RJ, Karbownik M, et al. Oxidative stress in resuscitation and in ventilation of newborns. *Eur Respir J* 2009;34(6):1461–1469.
24. Wrightson F, Soma M, Smith JH. Anesthetic experience of 100 pediatric tracheostomies. *Paediatr Anaesth* 2009;19(7):659–666.

READ MORE

Neonatal resuscitation, Chapter 102, page 745

128 Management of Pediatric Arrest and Resuscitation

Samuel Mireles, MD

Cardiac arrest in adults and children usually presents differently due to dissimilar underlying etiology. As such, there are some important differences in the appropriate management of adult and pediatric cardiac arrest.

1) **Etiology of perioperative cardiac arrest**
   a) According to the Pediatric Perioperative Cardiac Arrest Registry (1), 49% of perioperative deaths during 1998 to 2004 were anesthesia related.
   b) Cardiovascular causes were the most common (41% of all perioperative arrests).
   c) Hypovolemia from blood loss and transfusion-related hyperkalemia were the most common identifiable cardiovascular causes (12% and 5%, respectively).
   d) Respiratory causes were the second most common cause (27% of arrests), with laryngospasm being the most common respiratory cause (6%).
   e) Medication-related arrests were the third most common cause at 18%.

2) **Airway**
   a) **Bag-valve-mask (BVM)**
      i) Appropriate initial maneuver before tracheal intubation is BVM ventilation with jaw thrust. The use of an oral airway may also be necessary.
      ii) **Gastric inflation due to excessive ventilation pressures can impede lung expansion** and impair oxygenation. It also carries significant risk of pulmonary aspiration.
      iii) Adequate ventilation should be judged by bilateral chest excursion, as well as auscultation.
   b) **Endotracheal intubation**
      i) The most reliable verification of successful endotracheal intubation is visualization of the endotracheal tube passing through the cords and bilateral auscultation of breath sounds.
      ii) End-tidal CO_2 (ETCO$_2$) confirmation of endotracheal intubation
         (1) **ETCO$_2$ will only be present in the setting of effective pulmonary circulation.**
         (2) ETCO$_2$ may not be detected, even with appropriate endotracheal intubation, if chest compressions are not effective.
      iii) Effective BVM ventilation without endotracheal intubation is preferable to multiple failed attempts at intubation by inexperienced personnel.

Initial management of pediatric arrest begins with the airway except in the case of known ventricular fibrillation (VF) or pulseless ventricular tachycardia (VT) when defibrillation is the priority.

ETCO$_2$ will only be present in the setting of effective pulmonary circulation. ETCO$_2$ may not be detected, even with appropriate endotracheal intubation, if chest compressions are not effective.

3) **Breathing** (Table 128-1)

   a) Excessive ventilation is common during resuscitation after cardiac arrest.

   b) Hyperventilation (even with normal peak inspiratory pressures) can lead to decreased venous return, decreased cardiac output, and decreased cerebral perfusion secondary to decreased $PaCO_2$.

   c) Once an artificial airway is placed, ventilation should be given at 8 to 10 breaths/min without any pause during chest compressions (Table 128-1).

4) **Circulation**

   a) **Chest compressions**

      i) In an intubated child, **sudden drop in $ETCO_2$ may indicate decreased cardiac output.** Once airway issues are ruled out, consider a cardiac cause of low or absent $ETCO_2$.

Excessive ventilation increases intrathoracic pressure and leads to decreased venous return, decreased cardiac output, decreased cerebral perfusion, and barotrauma.

Table 128-1

Summary of CPR Maneuvers Based on Age (2)

Maneuver	Adult (Adolescent or Older)	Child (1 y to Adolescence)[a]	Infant (<1 y)
Airway	Head tilt/chin lift (jaw thrust if trauma)		
Breathing: initial	Two breaths at 1 second/breath		
Breathing: subsequent (without advanced airway)	10–12 breaths/min	12–20 breaths/min	
Breathing: subsequent (with advanced airway)	8–10 breaths/min		
Foreign body	Abdominal thrusts		Back blows and chest thrusts
Circulation: pulse check	Carotid		Brachial or femoral
Compression landmarks	Lower half of sternum/between nipples		Lower half of sternum/just below nipples
Compression method	Heel of one hand, other hand on top	Heel of one hand, or as for adults	2 thumbs of encircled hands (2 providers) or 2–3 fingers
Compression depth[b]	11/2–2 inches	1/3–1/2 depth of chest	
Compression rate	~100/min		
Compression/ventilation ratio	30:2	30:2 (single rescuer) 15:2 (2 rescuers)	
Defibrillation AED	Adult pads	Use pediatric system for 1–8 y, if available	

[a]Note that pediatric hospitals and intensive care units may choose to continue the use of PALS for adolescents as well as younger children.
[b]If an arterial line is in place, use presence and shape of arterial waveform to judge effectiveness of compressions.

PEDIATRIC ANESTHESIA

To determine whether compressions are resulting in adequate cardiac output, assess for (a) presence of ETCO$_2$; (b) BP tracing on arterial line; and (c) palpable femoral, brachial, carotid pulses.

    ii)   Chest compressions are a critical part of resuscitation as they provide the only means of end-organ perfusion after an arrest.

    iii)   Attention should be paid to the rate (100/min) and depth of compressions, allowing time for adequate chest recoil. It is important to minimize interruptions to ensure optimal perfusion (Table 128-1).

    iv)   If an arterial line is in place, use presence and shape of arterial waveform to judge effectiveness of compressions.

  b) **Defibrillation**

    i)   Use **infant paddles for children <10 kg.**

    ii)   Use **adult paddles for children >10 kg.**

Table 128-2

Medications for Pediatric Resuscitation (5,6)

Medication	Dose	Comments
Adenosine	0.1 mg/kg (max. 6 mg), repeat dose 0.2 mg/kg (max. 12 mg)	Monitor ECG; Rapid IV/IO bolus.
Amiodarone	5 mg/kg IV/IO, repeat up to 15 mg/kg (max. 300 mg)	Monitor ECG and blood pressure; Caution when used with other QT-prolonging drugs.
Atropine	0.02 mg/kg IV/IO, 0.03 mg/kg ET	May need higher dose with organophosphate poisoning. A minimum dose of 0.1 mg is often reported, but is unsupported in literature and may be toxic for smaller patients. (7)
Calcium chloride	10–20 mg/kg IV/IO	Via large bore, preferably central line or IO.
Calcium Gluconate	60 mg/kg IV/IO	Central line preferred, peripheral IV OK.
Epinephrine	0.01 mg/kg IV/IO, 0.1 mg/kg ET; max. dose 1 mg IV/IO and 10 mg ET	May repeat q3–5min.
Glucose	0.5–1 g/kg IV/IO	D10 preferred over D50 in infants due to association between D50 and intraventricular hemorrhage.
Lidocaine	1 mg/kg IV/IO, followed by 20–50 µg/kg/min infusion IV/IO; 2–3 mg/kg ET	Consider decreased dose with hepatic disease, hypoproteinemia, or severely decreased cardiac output. Toxic metabolites may accumulate with renal insufficiency.
Magnesium sulfate	25–50 mg/kg IV/IO (max. dose 2 g)	
Naloxone	<5 y or ≤20 kg: 0.1 mg/kg IV/IO/ET	Lower doses recommended to reverse respiratory depression in nonarrest situation (1–15 µg/kg).
	≥5 y or >20 kg: 2 mg IV/IO/ET	
Sodium bicarbonate	1 mEq/kg IV/IO slowly	After adequate ventilation established.

IV, intravenous; IO, intraosseous; ET, endotracheal.

Medications that can be given via ETT: use the mnemonic "LANE" = Lidocaine, Atropine, Naloxone, Epinephrine.

    iii)   A dose of **2 J/kg is recommended for the first shock** (monophasic or biphasic) (2).

    iv)   A dose of **4 J/kg is recommended for subsequent shocks** (monophasic or biphasic) (2).

5)   **Medications for pediatric resuscitation and arrhythmias**

    a)   The following medications can be **administered via the ETT**: Lidocaine, Atropine, Naloxone, Epinephrine. Mnemonic = LANE.

    b)   The total volume administered through the ETT with each drug dose should not exceed 5 mL in the child and 10 mL in the adult. Drug concentrations should be adjusted with these volume limits in mind (3).

    c)   **High-dose epinephrine (100 µg/kg) has been shown to result in worse outcomes in pediatric arrest and should be avoided except via the endotracheal route** (4) (Table 128-2).

Chapter Summary for Management of Pediatric Arrest and Resuscitation

1) Respiratory insufficiency is the most common preexisting condition in children prior to cardiac arrest among pediatric inpatients.

2) Bradycardia, dysrhythmia, and shock can all occur secondary to respiratory failure.

3) The development of hypotension in a child with previously compensated shock is an ominous sign of impending arrest. The practitioner should be alert to signs of compensated shock and should not wait for hypotension to begin treatment (6).

References

1. Bhananker SM, Ramamoorthy C, Geiduschek JM, et al. Anesthesia-related cardiac arrest in children: update from the pediatric perioperative cardiac arrest registry. *Anesth Analg* 2007;105(2):344–350.

2. American Heart Association. Part 3: Overview of CPR. *Circulation* 2005;112;IV-12–IV-18; originally published online Nov 28, 2005.

3. Morris MC, Todres ID, Schleien CL. Cardiopulmonary resuscitation. In: Coté CJ, Lerman J, Todres ID, eds. *A Practice of Anesthesia for Infants and Children.* 4th ed. Philadelphia, PA: Saunders; 2009.

4. Perondi M, Reis A, Paiva E, et al. A comparison of high-dose and standard-dose epinephrine in children with cardiac arrest. *N Engl J Med* 2004;350:1722–1730.

5. American Heart Association. Part 12: Pediatric Advanced Life Support. *Circulation* 2005; 112;IV-167–IV-187; originally published online Nov 28, 2005.

6. American Heart Association. Pediatric Advanced Life Support: Provider Manual. 2006:65–68.

7. Barrington, KJ. The myth of a minimum dose for atropine. *Pediatrics* 2011:127 (4); 783–784.

PEDIATRIC ANESTHESIA

Following algorithms from Barash PG, Cullen BF, Stoelting RK, et al, eds. Handbook of Clinical Anesthesia. 6th Edition. Philadelphia, PA: Lippincott Williams & Wilkins, 2009. Adapted from American Heart Association: Guidelines 2000 for Cardiopulmonary Resuscitation and Emergency Cardiovascular Care: International Consensus on Science. Circulation 2000;102(8).

Basic Life Support Algorithm

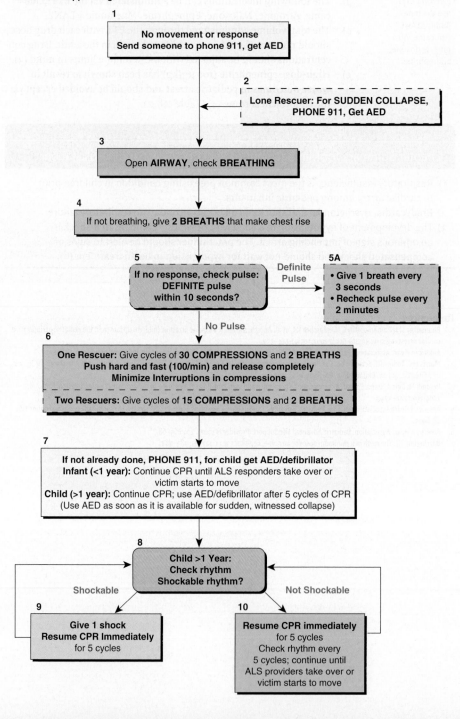

Pulseless Arrest Algorithm

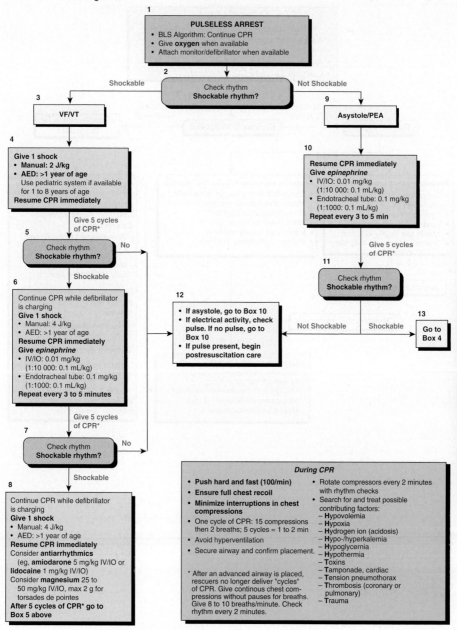

1
PULSELESS ARREST
- BLS Algorithm: Continue CPR
- Give **oxygen** when available
- Attach monitor/defibrillator when available

2
Check rhythm
Shockable rhythm?

Shockable → **3** VF/VT

Not Shockable → **9** Asystole/PEA

4
Give 1 shock
- **Manual: 2 J/kg**
- **AED: >1 year of age**
  Use pediatric system if available
  for 1 to 8 years of age
Resume CPR immediately

Give 5 cycles of CPR*

5
Check rhythm
Shockable rhythm?   No

Shockable

6
Continue CPR while defibrillator
is charging
Give 1 shock
- **Manual: 4 J/kg**
- **AED: >1 year of age**
Resume CPR immediately
Give *epinephrine*
- IV/IO: 0.01 mg/kg
  (1:10 000: 0.1 mL/kg)
- Endotracheal tube: 0.1 mg/kg
  (1:1000: 0.1 mL/kg)
Repeat every 3 to 5 minutes

Give 5 cycles of CPR*

7
Check rhythm
Shockable rhythm?   No

Shockable

8
Continue CPR while defibrillator
is charging
Give 1 shock
- **Manual: 4 J/kg**
- **AED: >1 year of age**
Resume CPR immediately
Consider **antiarrhythmics**
  (eg, **amiodarone** 5 mg/kg IV/IO or
  lidocaine 1 mg/kg IV/IO)
Consider **magnesium** 25 to
  50 mg/kg IV/IO, max 2 g for
  torsades de pointes
**After 5 cycles of CPR* go to
Box 5 above**

10
Resume CPR immediately
Give *epinephrine*
- IV/IO: 0.01 mg/kg
  (1:10 000: 0.1 mL/kg)
- Endotracheal tube: 0.1 mg/kg
  (1:1000: 0.1 mL/kg)
Repeat every 3 to 5 min

Give 5 cycles of CPR*

11
Check rhythm
Shockable rhythm?

Not Shockable

Shockable → **13** Go to Box 4

12
- If asystole, go to Box 10
- If electrical activity, check
  pulse. If no pulse, go to
  Box 10
- If pulse present, begin
  postresuscitation care

During CPR

- **Push hard and fast (100/min)**
- **Ensure full chest recoil**
- **Minimize interruptions in chest
  compressions**
- One cycle of CPR: 15 compressions
  then 2 breaths; 5 cycles ≈ 1 to 2 min
- Avoid hyperventilation
- Secure airway and confirm placement.

* After an advanced airway is placed,
rescuers no longer deliver "cycles"
of CPR. Give continous chest compressions without pauses for breaths.
Give 8 to 10 breaths/minute. Check
rhythm every 2 minutes.

- Rotate compressors every 2 minutes
  with rhythm checks
- Search for and treat possible
  contributing factors:
  – **H**ypovolemia
  – **H**ypoxia
  – **H**ydrogen ion (acidosis)
  – **H**ypo-/hyperkalemia
  – **H**ypoglycemia
  – **H**ypothermia
  – **T**oxins
  – **T**amponade, cardiac
  – **T**ension pneumothorax
  – **T**hrombosis (coronary or
    pulmonary)
  – **T**rauma

PEDIATRIC ANESTHESIA

Tachycardia with pulses and ADEQUATE perfusion algorithm

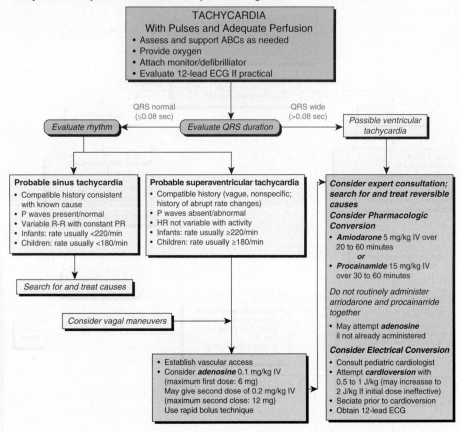

TACHYCARDIA
With Pulses and Adequate Perfusion
- Assess and support ABCs as needed
- Provide oxygen
- Attach monitor/defibrilliator
- Evaluate 12-lead ECG If practical

QRS normal (≤0.08 sec)   QRS wide (>0.08 sec)

Evaluate rhythm   *Evaluate QRS duration*   *Possible ventricular tachycardia*

Probable sinus tachycardia
- Compatible history consistent with known cause
- P waves present/normal
- Variable R-R with constant PR
- Infants: rate usually <220/min
- Children: rate usually <180/min

Probable superaventricular tachycardia
- Compatible history (vague, nonspecific; history of abrupt rate changes)
- P waves absent/abnormal
- HR not variable with activity
- Infants: rate usually ≥220/min
- Children: rate usually ≥180/min

Consider expert consultation; search for and treat reversible causes
Consider Pharmacologic Conversion
- *Amiodarone* 5 mg/kg IV over 20 to 60 minutes
      or
- *Procainamide* 15 mg/kg IV over 30 to 60 minutes

Do not routinely administer arriodarone and procainarride together
- May attempt *adenosine* il not already acmin;stered

Consider Electrical Conversion
- Consult pediatric cardiologist
- Attempt *cardioversion* with 0.5 to 1 J/kg (may increasse to 2 J/kg If initial dose ineffective)
- Seciate prior to cardioversion
- Obtain 12-lead ECG

Search for and treat causes

Consider vagal maneuvers

- Establish vascular access
- Consider *adenosine* 0.1 mg/kg IV (maximum first dose: 6 mg) May give second dose of 0.2 mg/kg IV (maximum second close: 12 mg) Use rapid bolus technique

Tachycardia with pulses and POOR perfusion algorithm

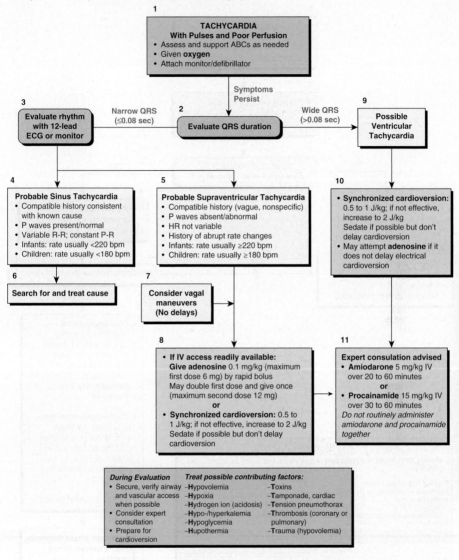

1

TACHYCARDIA
With Pulses and Poor Perfusion
- Assess and support ABCs as needed
- Given **oxygen**
- Attach monitor/defibrillator

Symptoms
Persist

3

Evaluate rhythm with 12-lead ECG or monitor

Narrow QRS
(≤0.08 sec)

2

Evaluate QRS duration

Wide QRS
(>0.08 sec)

9

Possible Ventricular Tachycardia

4

Probable Sinus Tachycardia
- Compatible history consistent with known cause
- P waves present/normal
- Variable R-R; constant P-R
- Infants: rate usually <220 bpm
- Children: rate usually <180 bpm

5

Probable Supraventricular Tachycardia
- Compatible history (vague, nonspecific)
- P waves absent/abnormal
- HR not variable
- History of abrupt rate changes
- Infants: rate usually ≥220 bpm
- Children: rate usually ≥180 bpm

10

- **Synchronized cardioversion:** 0.5 to 1 J/kg; if not effective, increase to 2 J/kg Sedate if possible but don't delay cardioversion
- May attempt **adenosine** if it does not delay electrical cardioversion

6

Search for and treat cause

7

Consider vagal maneuvers (No delays)

8

- If IV access readily available:
  Give adenosine 0.1 mg/kg (maximum first dose 6 mg) by rapid bolus May double first dose and give once (maximum second dose 12 mg)
  or
- **Synchronized cardioversion:** 0.5 to 1 J/kg; if not effective, increase to 2 J/kg Sedate if possible but don't delay cardioversion

11

Expert consulation advised
- **Amiodarone** 5 mg/kg IV over 20 to 60 minutes
  or
- **Procainamide** 15 mg/kg IV over 30 to 60 minutes
Do not routinely administer amiodarone and procainamide together

During Evaluation	*Treat possible contributing factors:*	
- Secure, verify airway and vascular access when possible	–**H**ypovolemia	–**T**oxins
	–**H**ypoxia	–**T**amponade, cardiac
	–**H**ydrogen ion (acidosis)	–**T**ension pneumothorax
- Consider expert consultation	–**H**ypo-/hyperkalemia	–**T**hrombosis (coronary or
	–**H**ypoglycemia	pulmonary)
- Prepare for cardioversion	–**H**uothermia	–**T**rauma (hypovolemia)

PEDIATRIC ANESTHESIA

Bradycardia with a pulse algorithm

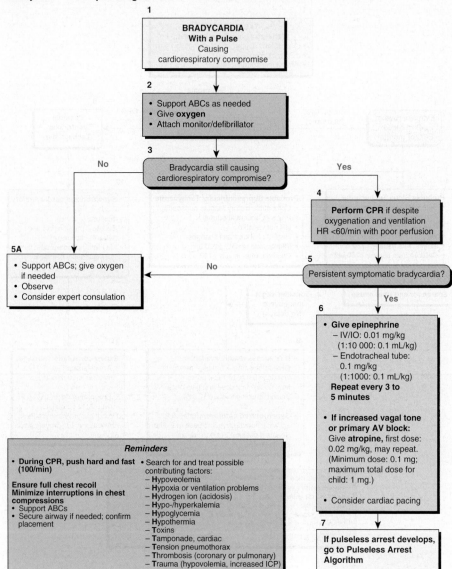

1

BRADYCARDIA
With a Pulse
Causing
cardiorespiratory compromise

2

- Support ABCs as needed
- Give **oxygen**
- Attach monitor/defibrillator

3

No ← Bradycardia still causing
cardiorespiratory compromise? → Yes

4

Perform CPR if despite
oxygenation and ventilation
HR <60/min with poor perfusion

5A

- Support ABCs; give oxygen
  if needed
- Observe
- Consider expert consulation

5

No ← Persistent symptomatic bradycardia?

Yes

6

- **Give epinephrine**
  – IV/IO: 0.01 mg/kg
    (1:10 000: 0.1 mL/kg)
  – Endotracheal tube:
    0.1 mg/kg
    (1:1000: 0.1 mL/kg)
  **Repeat every 3 to
  5 minutes**

- **If increased vagal tone
  or primary AV block:**
  Give **atropine**, first dose:
  0.02 mg/kg, may repeat.
  (Minimum dose: 0.1 mg;
  maximum total dose for
  child: 1 mg.)

- Consider cardiac pacing

7

If pulseless arrest develops,
go to Pulseless Arrest
Algorithm

Reminders

- **During CPR, push hard and fast
  (100/min)**

Ensure full chest recoil
**Minimize interruptions in chest
compressions**
- Support ABCs
- Secure airway if needed; confirm
  placement

- Search for and treat possible
  contributing factors:
  – Hypoveolemia
  – Hypoxia or ventilation problems
  – Hydrogen ion (acidosis)
  – Hypo-/hyperkalemia
  – Hypoglycemia
  – Hypothermia
  – Toxins
  – Tamponade, cardiac
  – Tension pneumothorax
  – Thrombosis (coronary or pulmonary)
  – Trauma (hypovolemia, increased ICP)

129 Practical Pediatric Anesthesia

Ellen Choi, MD • Calvin Kuan, MD

Vital Signs (Table 129-1)

Quick formula to estimate weight: weight (kg) = (age in years × 2) + 9

Rule of thumb for lowest acceptable mean arterial pressure (MAP) in the neonatal period = approximate gestational age, e.g., a 2-week-old full term (40 week) infant should have MAP around 42 mm Hg (= 40 + 2).

Table 129-1
Pediatric Vital Signs and Approximate Weight

Age	Weight (kg)	Heart Rate	Systolic Blood Pressure	Diastolic Blood Pressure	Respiratory Rate
Premature infant	<3.0	120–170	55–75	35–45	45–60
Term neonate	3.5	100–150	65–86	40–45	40–60
6 mo	7	90–120	70–90	50–65	30–50
1 y	10	80–120	80–100	55–65	30–50
2 y	12	70–110	90–100	55–70	25–40
3 y	14	70–110	90–110	55–70	25–35
4 y	16	65–110	90–110	60–75	25–35
5 y	18	65–100	90–110	60–75	20–30
6 y	20	65–100	90–110	60–75	20–30
8 y	25	60–90	100–120	60–75	20–30
10 y	30	60–90	100–120	60–75	20–25
12 y	40	60–90	100–120	60–75	<20
14 y	50	55–85	110–135	60–75	<20
Adult	70	55–85	110–135	60–75	<20

Airway

1) **Routine airway management**

   a) Endotracheal intubation (Table 129-3)

     i) Smallest cuffed ETT available is 3.0.

     ii) Smallest UNcuffed ETT available is 2.0.

     iii) **Formula for calculating approximate UNcuffed ETT size:**

> **(Age in years/4) + 4**

     iv) Formula for calculating approximate CUFFED ETT (= 0.5 size smaller than uncuffed for similar age) size:

> **(Age in years/4) + 3.5**

     v) Quick rule of thumb for appropriate size of ETT suction catheter and the depth at which to tape the ETT for premature infants and neonates: "Weight 1, 2, 3... Suction cather 4, 5, 6,... Distance 7, 8, 9." (Table 129-2)

     vi) **Formula for approximate ETT depth from lip/gums to midtrachea for oral intubation:**

> **Size of ETT × 3 = cm marking on ETT at lips/gums**

     vii) **The most reliable method for determining appropriate position for an oral or nasal ETT is the mainstem method (6).**

       (1) After intubation, advance the ETT into the right mainstem bronchus.

       (2) Listen over the left chest for return of breath sounds indicating the position of the ETT at the carina.

       (3) Then position the ETT above the carina 1 to 3 cm depending on patient age and surgical situation.

     viii) **Checking for a leak around ETT:**

       (1) For most healthy children, the leak around the ETT **should be no greater than 20 to 25 cm H_2O** to avoid tracheal mucosa ischemia.

       (2) A leak <10 to 15 cm H_2O with an UNcuffed ETT may necessitate a change to a larger size or a cuffed ETT to adequately ventilate.

       (3) To check for a leak:

         (a) With a stethoscope, auscultate the upper airway at the mouth or neck.

Formula for approximate UNcuffed ETT size: (age in years/4) + 4

Quick method for initial approximation of ETT depth: size of ETT × 3 = distance from lips/gums to midtrachea.

The most reliable method for determining correct ETT depth is the mainstem intubation method.

Table 129-2

Suction Catheter and Depth of ETT Placement for Premature Infants

Weight (kg)	Size of suction catheter for ETT (Fr)	Distance from gums to mid-trachea (cm)
1	4 (or 5)	7
2	5 (or 6)	8
3	6	9

For most children, the leak around ETT should be no greater than 20 to 25 cm H_2O. However, individual cases will depend on lung compliance and surgical needs.

    (b)   Turn the APL valve on the anesthesia machine to the maximal accepted peak pressure (30 to 40 cm H_2O).

    (c)   Allow the airway pressure rise.

    (d)   Watching the manometer, note the pressure at which air is first heard "leaking" around ETT in the airway.

  ix) **Special anesthetic considerations:**

    (1)   The ETT size and target leak for an individual case should take into consideration the patient's pulmonary compliance and the likelihood of change of compliance with surgery or disease process. For example, a child with worsening ARDS may require increased peak pressures to ventilate in the near future.

    (2)   Take care to ensure that gas flow is not too high relative to patient size to avoid overinflation of lungs.

    (3)   Take care not to close the APL valve completely.

    (4)   If patient is unstable, squeeze the anesthetic bag to accelerate lung inflation and allow for quicker leak check.

2)   **Alternative airway equipment (Table 129-4)**

  a) **Airway exchange catheters (AEC)** (Cook Medical, Inc. Bloomington, IN) (Table 129-5):

    i)   Used to facilitate exchange or replacement of ETT in an intubated patient.

READ MORE

Management of the pediatric difficult airway, Chapter 126, page 873

    ii)   Used to stiffen a guidewire that has been passed through a fiberoptic bronchoscope for intubation through an LMA.

    iii)   Sizes 8-19 French have an Luer lock adaptor for jet ventilation connection or 15-mm ETT connector (Rapi-Fit Adaptor) to connect to a breathing circuit or an ambu bag.

    iv)   Connector may also be used to attach to $ETCO_2$ monitor for verification of endotracheal vs esophageal position.

  b) Single-lung ventilation (Table 129-6):

    i)   Single-lung ventilation in the pediatric population can be challenging because of the difficulty in finding the appropriate tube or device for lung isolation in accordance with the patient's size without obstructing the upper airway.

PEDIATRIC ANESTHESIA

Table 129-3

Laryngoscope Blades and Sizes

Age	Miller	Wis-Hipple	MacIntosh
Preterm	0[a]		
Full term	0 or 1[a]	1	
1 y.o.	1	1 or 1.5[a]	1
2 y.o.	1 or 2	1.5[a]	1 or 2
3–5 y	2	1.5[a]	2[a]
6–10 y	2[a]		2 or 3
>10 y	2[a]		3[a]

[a]Recommended for first attempt.

Table 129-4

Difficult Airway Equipment: Laryngeal Mask Airway, Endotracheal Tube (ETT), and Fiberoptic Bronchoscopes

Patient weight (kg)	Classic or Unique LMA size[a]	Maximum Size ETT[b] that will fit through LMA (recommended by the manufacturer)	Maximum size ETT[b] that will fit through LMA (our recommendation)	Maximum fiberoptic bronchoscope size (mm)
<5.0	1.0	3.5 uncuffed	3.0 uncuffed	2.7
5.0–10.0	1.5	4.0 uncuffed	4.0 uncuffed[c]	3.0
10.0–20.0	2.0	4.5 uncuffed	4.5 uncuffed 4.5 cuffed[d]	3.5
20.0–30.0	2.5	5.0 uncuffed	5.0 uncuffed 5.0 cuffed[d]	4.0
30.0–50.0	3.0	6.0 cuffed	6.0 cuffed	5.0
50.0–70.0	4.0	6.0 cuffed	6.0 cuffed	5.0
70.0–100.0	5.0	7.0 cuffed	7.0 cuffed	5.0

[a]LMA Classic and LMA Unique (LMA North America, Inc., San Diego, CA).
[b]Mallinkrodt Intermediate Hi-Lo ETT (Covidien-Nellcor and Puritan Bennett, Boulder, CO).
[c]Generous amounts of lubrication required to pass easily.
[d]The cuffed 4.5 and 5.0 ETT will fit into the shaft of the LMA, but the balloon will not fit through the LMA connector. Refer to chapter 126: "Management of the Pediatric Difficult Airway" for more detailed discussion of alternative solutions.
Data from LMA Unique product brochure at www.lmana.com (LMA North America, Inc., San Diego, CA).

Table 129-5

Airway Exchange Catheters

Catheter Size (Fr)	Catheter Length (cm)	Catheter ID (mm)	Smallest ETT Size (ID mm)
5[a]	100[a]		2.0
8	45	1.6	3.0
11	83	2.3	4.0
14	83	3.0	5.0
19	83	3.4	7.0

[a]Not designed for airway exchange use. Adapted from interventional catheterization use.
Table adapted from Cook Medical website, Cook Airway Exchange Catheters- www.cookmedical.com

Table 129-6

Options for Single-Lung Ventilation

Age (y)	ETT (ID in mm)	Bronchial Blocker (Fr)	Univent (ID in mm)	Double-Lumen Tube (Fr)
0.5–1	3.5–4.0	2–3	Not available	Not available
1–2	4.0–4.5	3	Not available	Not available
2–4	4.5–5.0	5	Not available	Not available
4–6	5.0–5.5	5	Not available	Not available
6–8	5.5–6	5	3.5	Not available
8–10	6.0 cuffed	5	3.5	26
10–12	6.5 cuffed	5	4.5	26–28
12–14	6.5–7.0 cuffed	7	4.5	32
14–16	7.0 cuffed	7	6.0	35 to 41 **
16–18	8.0–8.5 cuffed	7–9	7.0	35 to 41 **

** For adult sized patients, double lumen tube sizing should be based on tracheal diameter. Adapted with permission from Golianu B, Hammer GB. Pediatric thoracic anesthesia. *Curr Opin Anaesthesiol* 2005;18:5–11.

ii) In many situations, endobronchial intubation may be easier and less time consuming than attempting to place and maintain a bronchial blocker when the patient is too small for a double-lumen tube.

iii) Fiberoptic bronchoscopy is useful to place and verify the position of bronchial blockers and double-lumen tubes, especially when access to auscultation is limited during surgery.

Vascular Access

1) Central venous cather insertion: Formulae to determine length of catheter to insert based on patient height for central venous catheters placement via RIJ or right subclavian vein (Table 129-7):

For patients <100 cm:

$$(\text{height [cm]}/10)-1 = \text{distance (cm) to SVC/RA junction}$$

For patients >100 cm:

$$(\text{height [cm]}/10)-2 = \text{distance (cm) to SVC/RA junction}$$

2) Size of central venous catheters for right internal jugular vein cannulation:
   a) patients <10 kg ⟶ 4 French (Fr)
   b) patients 10–30 kg ⟶ 5 Fr
   c) patients 30–50 kg ⟶ 7 Fr
   d) patients >50 kg ⟶ 9 Fr

PEDIATRIC ANESTHESIA

Table 129-7
Central Venous Catheter Insertion Depth

Weight (kg)	Length (cm) of catheter insertion from skin to SVC/RA junction
2.0–2.9	4
3.0–4.9	5
5.0–6.9	6
7.0–9.9	7
10–12.9	8
13.0–19.9	9
20.0–29.9	10
30.0–39.9	11
40.0–49.9	12
50.0–59.9	13
60.0–69.9	14
70.0–79.9	15
>80.0	16

Adapted with permission from Andropoulos D, Bent ST, Skjonsby B, et al. The optimal length of insertion of central venous catheters for pediatric patients. *Anesth Analg* 2001;93:883–886.

Use ultrasound to verify position, size, and patency of vessels prior to cannulation.

3) Special anesthetic considerations
   a) Visualization with an ultrasound prior to cannulation is recommended to assess size, verify patency of the vein, and check position of vein relative to artery.
   b) Position of catheter in vein should be confirmed with ultrasound visualization in vein or right heart, transducing a venous waveform, or confirmation with venous blood gas measurements.
   c) Confirmation of position of tip of catheter can be made by chest radiograph or transesophageal echocardiographic visualization of tip in SVC or RA.

Hematology (Table 129-8)

1) **Pediatric red cell transfusion** should be calculated according to the following formula (7):

$$\text{Volume of PRBC to transfuse (mL)} = 1.6 \times \text{weight (kg)} \times \text{desired rise in Hct (\%)}$$

Table 129-8
Transfusion Estimates

	Volume to transfuse	Expected change
PRBC	10–15 mL/kg	Increases Hgb by 2–3, or Hct by 6%–9%
Fresh frozen plasma	10–15 mL/kg	Increases factor level by 15%–20%
Platelets	10 mL/kg	Increases platelets by 50,000–100,000/μL
Cryoprecipitate	1–2 units/10 kg	Increases fibrinogen by 60–100 mg/dL

Table 129-9

Commonly used Drugs: Pediatric Dosing

Drug	Suggested Dose	Maximum Single Dose
Induction		
Propofol	2–3 mg/kg IV	
Ketamine	1–3 mg /kg IV 3–10 mg/kg IM	
Etomidate	0.2–0.3 mg/kg IV	
Muscle Relaxant		
Cisatracurium	0.1–0.2 mg/kg IV	
Rocuronium	0.6–1.2 mg/kg IV	
Vecuronium	0.1 mg/kg IV	
Succinylcholine	1–2 mg/kg IV 4–5 mg/kg IM	
Muscle relaxant reversal agents		
Neostigmine	0.05–0.07 mg/kg IV	
Glycopyrrolate	0.01–0.015 mg/kg IV	
Edrophonium	0.3–1 mg/kg	
Benzodiazepines		
Midazolam	0.1 mg/kg IV 0.5–1 mg/kg PO	20 mg PO
Opioids		
Fentanyl	1 µg/kg IV	
Morphine	0.1 mg/kg IV	
Hydromorphone	10–20 µg/kg IV	
Naloxone (opioid reversal)	0.25–0.5 µg/kg titrating to effect	2 mg; can give up to 100 µg/kg

(continued)

PEDIATRIC ANESTHESIA

Table 129-9

Commonly used Drugs: Pediatric Dosing (*Continued*)

Drug	Suggested Dose	Maximum Single Dose
Other Analgesics		
Ketorolac	0.5 mg/kg IV	60 mg
Acetaminophen	30–40 µg/kg PR single loading dose, then 15 mg/kg PO/PR New IV formulatIon (Ofirmev): Newborns and children < 2 yo: 15 mg/kg IV q8h or 12.5 mg/kg IV q6h Children > 2 yo: 15 mg/kg IV q6h or 12.5 mg/kg IV q4h	1000 mg; watch total daily dose
Ibuprofen	10 mg/kg PO q6h	800 mg
Antiemetics		
Dexamethasone	0.1–0.2 mg/kg IV	20 mg
Ondansatron	0.1 mg/kg IV	4 mg
Metoclopromide	0.15 mg/kg IV/PO	
Antibiotics		
Cefazolin	25 mg/kg IV	2,000 mg
Steroids		
Dexamethasone	*Airway edema*: 0.5–2 mg/kg/d IV, IM, or PO, divided into q6hr beginning 24 h before extubation and continuing for 4–6 dose afterward *Physiologic replacement*: 0.03–0.15 mg/kg/d divided into q6–12h dosing	
Hydrocortisone	*Acute adrenal insufficiency*: Older children: 1–2 mg/kg bolus and then 150–250 mg/d in q6–8h divided doses Younger children and infants: 1–2 mg bolus and then 25–150 mg/d divided into q6–8h doses	

2) Maximum allowable blood loss (MABL):

$$MABL = \frac{EBV \times (\text{starting Hct} - \text{minimal acceptable Hct})}{\text{starting Hct}}$$

EBV= estimated blood volume (approx 70-100 mL/kg depending on age).

Table 129-10

Vasoactive Drugs for Infusion[a]

Drug	Dose
Dopamine	1–20 µg/kg/min
Dobutamine	1–20 µg/kg/min
Epinephrine	0.05–1 µg/kg/min
Isoproterenol	0.05–1 µg/kg/min
Norepinephrine	0.05–1 µg/kg/min
Milrinone	25–50 µg/kg optional loading dose, 0.5–1 µg/kg/min infusion
Phenylephrine	0.1–1 µg/kg/min
Vasopressin	0.0001–0.0005 units/kg/min

[a]All drugs should be titrated to effect.

For propofol (or any drug) at 10 mg/mL concentration, taking patient's weight in kg as volume in mL will last 1 hour at a dose of 166 micrograms/kg/min.

How to determine the volume of propofol (or any other drug) to draw up for a case to minimize waste:

Method

1) Take the patient's weight in kg and convert to mL of propofol (e.g., for a 12-kg child, draw up 12 mL).
2) That amount will last 1 hour at a dose of 166 µg/kg/min.
3) Estimate the duration of the case, mulitply the hours times the volume per hour for the patient, and you can determine the amount needed.
4) Knowing the amount will help decide whether to open a large or small vial and may help to minimize wastage. This formula can also be used for other drugs as long as the concentration is prepared in multiples of 10. Using the same example: For remifentanil if prepared as 10 µg/mL, 12 mL will last 1 hour at a dose of 0.166 µg/kg/min. For a drug prepared as 1 mg/mL, 12 mL will last 1 hour at a dose of 16.6 µg/kg/min.

PEDIATRIC ANESTHESIA

Suggested Reading/References

1. Holzman RS, van der Velde ME, Kaus SJ, et al. *A Practical Approach to Pediatric Anesthesia*. Philadelphia, PA: Lippincott Williams & Wilkins; 2008.
2. Cote CJ, Lerman J, Todres ID. *A Practice of Anesthesia for Infants and Children*. Philadelphia, PA: Saunders Elsevier, 2009.
3. Andropoulos D, Bent ST, Skjonsby B, et al. The optimal length of insertion of central venous catheters for pediatric patients. *Anesth Analg* 2001;93:883–886.
4. LMA website. http://www.lmana.com.
5. Golianu B, Hammer GB. Pediatric thoracic anesthesia. *Curr Opin Anaesthesiol* 2005;18:5–11.
6. Mariano ER, Ramamoorthy C, Chu LF, et al. A comparison of three methods for estimating appropriate tracheal tube depth in children. *Ped Anesth* 2005;15:846–851.
7. Morris KP, Naqvi N, Davies P, et al. A new formula for blood transfusion volume in the critically ill. *Arch Dis Child* 2005;90:724–728.

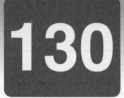

130 Outpatient Anesthesia

Steve Melton, MD • Stephen M. Klein, MD

The scope of ambulatory anesthesia and surgery is continually expanding. This chapter discusses issues important to providing successful ambulatory anesthesia, including surgery and patient risk factor evaluation, postanesthetic recovery and discharge, unanticipated inpatient admission, perioperative emergencies and transfer, and office-based anesthesia.

1) Overview

   a) Outpatient anesthesia, or ambulatory anesthesia, is an anesthesiology subspecialty encompassing the preoperative, intraoperative, and postoperative anesthetic care of patients undergoing elective, same-day surgical procedures.

   b) By definition, patients undergoing ambulatory surgery do not require admission to the hospital and are well enough to be discharged from the facility after the procedure.

   c) From 1996 to 2006, the number of outpatient surgery visits in the United States increased from 20.8 to 34.7 million, accounting for approximately half of all surgery visits in 1996 and two thirds of all surgery visits in 2006 (1).

   d) Advancements in surgical technique and technology resulting in less invasive surgery, and advancements in anesthesia care and postoperative pain management, are allowing patients and surgeries once requiring inpatient care and resources to be scheduled in the outpatient setting. These advancements have resulted in reduced expenses in a competitive, cost-conscious healthcare environment with improved patient satisfaction (2).

   e) The ASA Guidelines for Ambulatory surgery (3) encompass recommendations pertaining to physicians, staff, facility, equipment, and clinical care that apply to anesthesiology personnel administering ambulatory anesthesia in all settings.

READ MORE

Preanesthesia assessment Chapter 2, page 10

2) Risk evaluation for outpatient surgery

   a) **Risk identification** is the foundation for perioperative risk reduction.

   b) Conditions associated with increased risk in the outpatient population include (4–6):

     i) Congestive heart failure (CHF)

     ii) Coronary artery disease (CAD)

     iii) Hypertension

     iv) Asthma

     v) COPD

     vi) Pulmonary hypertension

     vii) Obesity

Risk identification is the foundation for perioperative risk reduction.

CONCERNS IN SUBSPECIALTY ANESTHESIA

909

Table 130-1

Pre-Existing Medical Conditions as Predictors of Adverse Events in Outpatient Surgery

Medical Condition (Predictor)	Event
Hypertension	Any intraoperative event Intraoperative cardiovascular event
Obesity	Intraoperative respiratory event Postoperative respiratory event
Smoking	Postoperative respiratory event
Asthma	Postoperative respiratory event
GERD	Intubation-related event

Reproduced from Chung F, Mezei G, Tong D. Pre-existing medical conditions as predictors of adverse events in day-case surgery. *Br J Anaesth* 1999;83:262–270.

      viii) Smoking
      ix) Sleep apnea
      x) Gastroesophageal reflux (GERD)

  c) Signs and/or symptoms of instability or insufficient management in any of these areas require further investigation, optimization and/or inpatient setting.

  d) It is important for the anesthesiologist to know which pre-existing medical condition predicts a specific intraoperative and/or postoperative adverse event (AE).

  e) Based on risk identification the anesthesiologist should be able to mitigate adverse events and provide optimal care for the case (7) (Table 130-1).

Table 130-2

Risk Factors in Ambulatory Surgery

Patient Related	Surgery Related	Anesthesia Related	Facility Related
Comorbidity and degree of stabilization	Site and duration	Need for general anesthesia	Freestanding surgery center
Age	Degree of invasiveness	Need for tracheal intubation	Hospital affiliated/integrated
Body mass index	Fluid balance		Office based
Social/cultural conditions	Expected postoperative pain		Distance from emergency service
Escort availability	Risk of complications		Social service availability

Modified from Bettelli G. High risk patients in day surgery. *Minerva Anestesiol* 2009;75:259–268.

When deciding whether a particular surgery and/or patient is suitable for the outpatient setting, it is necessary to identify whether the risk would be minimized in an inpatient environment and what hospital-based resources might be needed.

f) While an individual risk factor is important, it is the combination of different factors and their management that determines the final outcome, increasing or decreasing the risk of AEs (8) (Table 130-2).

g) When deciding whether a particular surgery and/or patient is suitable for the outpatient setting, it is necessary to identify whether the risk would be minimized in an inpatient environment and what hospital-based resources might be needed.

h) A multidisciplinary approach to handling concerning issues will optimize perioperative management and lead to system improvements (9).

i) While current evidence-based medicine can provide recommendations on some high-risk ambulatory issues, for others the evidence is still lacking and/or requires larger, well-designed studies (Table 130-3).

3) Postanesthetic recovery and discharge

a) Reasons for delays after ambulatory surgery are multifactorial (9) (Table 130-4).

b) Postoperative pain and postoperative nausea and vomiting (**PONV**)

    i) Commonly prolongs PACU stay after ambulatory surgery (14,15).

    ii) An aggressive plan for each of these issues must be addressed prior to surgery.

Table 130-3
High-Risk Ambulatory Issues

Cardiac	• After acute myocardial infraction, ambulatory surgery should be delayed at least 4–6 wk, provided angina symptoms have disappeared and patient functional status is adequate after that period (10). • Elective noncardiac surgery is not recommended within 4 wk of coronary revascularization with balloon angioplasty (10). • Following coronary stent placement, elective surgery should be postponed until patients have completed 4–6 wk of aspirin and thienopyridine therapy after bare-metal stents, and 12 mo after drug-eluting stents, if such therapy must be discontinued for surgery (10). • If possible, aspirin should be continued perioperatively (10).
Respiratory	• Patients without acute respiratory symptoms do not need preoperative spirometry (10). • Postoperative management of obstructive sleep apnea in the outpatient setting should include minimization of narcotics, regional anesthesia when appropriate, PACU protocols, and perioperative continuous positive airway pressure (11).
Pediatric	• Ex-premature infants at a postconceptual age of 52–60 wk are considered amenable for ambulatory surgery due to a low incidence of postoperative apnea and bradycardia; anemia should be excluded (12).
Geriatric	• While overall risk for elderly patients undergoing day surgery is low, in a study of patients >65 y of age, increased risk of inpatient hospital admission or death within 7 d was associated with age >85, prior inpatient hospitalization within 6 mo, surgical procedure performed in an office or outpatient setting, and invasiveness of surgery (13).

CONCERNS IN SUBSPECIALTY ANESTHESIA

Table 130-4

Factors Associated with Delayed Discharge after Ambulatory Surgery

Preoperative	Intraoperative	Postoperative
Female gender	Long-duration surgery	PONV
Increasing age	General anesthesia	Pain
History of congestive heart failure (CHF)	Spinal anesthesia	Drowsiness
		No escort

Reproduced from Awad IT, Chung F. Factors affecting recovery and discharge following ambulatory surgery. *Can J Anaesth* 2006;53:858–872.

READ MORE

Postoperative nausea and vomiting, Chapter 7, page 47

Postoperative pain control should be managed using a multimodal approach.

READ MORE

Peripheral nerve blocks, Chapter 34, page 256

PONV associated with ambulatory surgery increases health care costs due to delayed discharge and hospital admission.

c) **Pain**
   i)   Pain control should be managed using a multimodal coordinated approach.
        (1) Agents should be used in combination to provide analgesia with a focus on minimizing side effects
        (2) Frequently used medications may include some or all of the following to maximize analgesia and minimize side effects: nonsteroidal anti-inflammatory, acetaminophen, NMDA antagonists, and opioids.
   ii) **Peripheral nerve blocks (PNBs)** provide site-specific surgical anesthesia and postoperative analgesia, reducing opioid requirements and opioid-related side effects (16).
   iii) As part of a multimodal approach to postoperative pain management, PNBs with long-acting **local anesthetic (LA)** can provide prolonged analgesia.
        (1) The duration can be extended further with the placement of a perineural catheter and subsequent continuous LA infusion at home (16).
        (2) Discharging patients home prior to regression of motor and sensory block can be done safely (17).
        (3) Patients receiving lower-extremity PNBs should receive coaching on crutch walking.
        (4) Alternative care should be arranged for those identified as unsafe or without adequate home resources.
        (5) Patients receiving upper-extremity PNBs should have the affected extremity placed in a sling.
        (6) Instructions specific to protection and care of the blocked extremity should be provided.
        (7) If being discharged with a perineural catheter, additional instructions on catheter care and removal, and signs and symptoms of local anesthetic toxicity should be included.
        (8) Timing of PNB resolution and initiation of pain medications should be reviewed to minimize and anticipate pain when the PNB resolves.
        (9) Intravenous lipid emulsion 20% must be available as part of the treatment strategy for local anesthetic–induced cardiotoxicity if PNBs are utilized.

d) **PONV**

READ MORE

Post anesthesia care unit, Chapter 147, page 1069

   i) PONV associated with ambulatory surgery increases health care costs due to delayed discharge (pharmaceutical costs and nursing care) and hospital admission.

   ii) It accounts for 0.1% to 0.2% of unanticipated admissions, which is significant in the United States where more than 31 million patients undergo ambulatory anesthesia each year (18).

   iii) An aggressive PONV prophylaxis and treatment algorithm is prudent (18).

e) **Discharge criteria**

   i) The major accreditation bodies in the United States require that policies and procedures be implemented to ensure the safe recovery of patients after ambulatory anesthesia.

   ii) Various scoring systems have been devised to facilitate timely and safe patient postanesthesia care unit (PACU) discharge and home readiness after ambulatory surgery (9,19).

   iii) Discharge criteria of an outcome-based system.
      (1) Patient alert and oriented to time and place.
      (2) Stable vital signs.
      (3) Pain controlled by oral analgesics or peripheral nerve block.
      (4) Nausea or emesis controlled.
      (5) Able to walk without dizziness.
      (6) No unexpected bleeding from the operative site.
      (7) Oral fluid intake and voiding on case-by-case basis (9,20) (Table 130-5).
      (8) Discharge instructions and prescriptions received from surgeon and anesthesiologist.
      (9) Patient accepts readiness for discharge.

   iv) These systems maximize patient safety and avoid inappropriate or premature discharge.

   v) Responsible adult escorts are mandatory after ambulatory surgery (21).

4) **Unanticipated inpatient admission after ambulatory surgery**

   a) The reported incidence of unanticipated inpatient admission after ambulatory surgery is 1% to 2% (9).

   b) Reasons for unanticipated inpatient admissions are multifactorial including long duration of surgery, postoperative bleeding, pain, and PONV (9) (Table 130-6).

   c) The low incidence reflects that preoperative identification and management of identified factors is successful.

Table 130-5

Oral Fluid Intake and Voiding after Ambulatory Surgery

Oral fluid intake prior to d/c not mandatory, required only for select patients on case-by-case basis (9)

Low-risk patients can be d/c home without voiding; should be instructed to return to the hospital if unable to void within 6–8 h.ᵃ This includes patients undergoing short-acting spinal anesthetics for procedures at low risk for urinary retention (20)

Patients at high risk for urinary retention should be required to void prior to discharge with a residual volume <300 mL as measured by ultrasound. If bladder volume >500–600 mL, catheterization prior to discharge (20)

Table 130-6			
Most Common Factors Associated with Unanticipated Inpatient Admission			
Long duration of surgery			
Postoperative bleeding			
Pain			
PONV			

Modified from Awad IT, Chung F. Factors affecting recovery and discharge following ambulatory surgery. *Can J Anaesth* 2006;53:858–872.

Perioperative emergencies extending beyond the resources or available patient care of the ambulatory or office-based setting must be identified immediately.

  i)   Risk identification, including case selection
  ii)   Multidisciplinary approach to handling concerning problems
  iii)   Multimodal analgesia including regional anesthesia with PNBs
  iv)   Aggressive PONV prophylaxis and treatment algorithm

5) **Perioperative emergencies and transfer**

 a)   Anesthesiologist should be physically present until all patients have been discharged from anesthesia care.

 b)   Personnel with training in advanced resuscitative techniques (e.g., ACLS, PALS) should be immediately available.

 c)   Availability of these providers allows for acute stabilization of perioperative emergencies.

 d)   Perioperative emergencies extending beyond the resources or available patient care of the ambulatory or office-based setting must be identified immediately.

 e)   Emergency care and transfer protocols must be in place and activated without hesitation.

 f)   Options for transfer to the inpatient setting.
  i)   Activation of the 911 system.
  ii)   Hospital emergency medical services.
  iii)   Physically transporting the patient across a parking lot, hospital tunnel, etc. in a stretcher with oxygen, monitors, manual resuscitator, and any other resuscitative equipment.

 g)   Direct communication between the anesthesiologist, the admitting physician, and the emergency room or intensive care unit physician receiving the patient must occur, providing a thorough transfer of care.

 h)   Training for such emergencies should occur at frequent intervals to ensure that in the event of an emergency all personnel, both medical and administrative, can execute their roles, and that supplies are in order (22).

 i)   All outpatient centers should have the medications including Dantrolene, equipment, and written protocols available to treat malignant hyperthermia when triggering agents are used.

 j)   All outpatient centers should have intravenous lipid emulsion 20% available as part of the treatment strategy for local anesthetic–induced cardiotoxicity if PNBs are utilized.

 k)   Surgeons should have admitting privileges at nearby hospitals, a transfer agreement with another physician who has admitting privileges, or an emergency transfer agreement with a nearby hospital (22).

6) Office-based anesthesia
   a) Like surgery visits to freestanding outpatient surgery centers, office-based surgery visits are increasing in number.
   b) There are special problems that anesthesiologists must recognize when administering anesthesia in the office setting (23).
   c) In a comparative outcome analysis of procedures performed in physicians' offices and ambulatory surgery centers, the death rate per 100,000 procedures was 9.2 in offices and 0.78 in day surgery centers (8).
   d) **ASA guidelines for office-based anesthesia** encompass recommendations pertaining to physicians, staff, facility, equipment, and clinical care that apply to anesthesiology personnel administering ambulatory anesthesia in the office-based setting: (23)

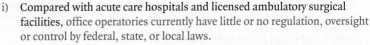

All office-based facilities should have oxygen, suction, resuscitation equipment, and emergency drugs including Dantrolene if triggering agents are used and intravenous lipid emulsion 20% if PNBs are used.

   i) Compared with acute care hospitals and licensed ambulatory surgical facilities, office operatories currently have little or no regulation, oversight or control by federal, state, or local laws.
   ii) Anesthesiologists must satisfactorily investigate. Anesthesiologists must satisfactorily investigate the office-based setting and structure
      (1) Governance
      (2) Organization
      (3) Construction
      (4) Equipment
      (5) Policies and procedures, including fire, safety, drugs, emergencies, staffing, training, and unanticipated patient transfers.
   iii) All office-based facilities should have a reliable source of oxygen, suction, resuscitation equipment, and emergency drugs including Dantrolene if triggering agents are used and intravenous lipid emulsion 20% if PNBs are utilized.
   iv) The anesthesiologist should adhere to the standards for pre- and post-anesthesia care, anesthetic monitoring, and guidelines for ambulatory anesthesia and surgery (3).

Chapter Summary for Outpatient Surgery

Risk Identification	Critical for risk reduction and for assessing appropriateness of ambulatory surgery.
Postoperative Pain and Postoperative Nausea and Vomiting (PONV)	Pain and nausea/vomiting commonly prolong stay after ambulatory surgery.
Ambulatory Anesthesia	Regional anesthesia with PNBs should be used when possible PONV prophylaxis is essential A multidisciplinary perioperative approach will optimize perioperative management and lead to system improvements The anesthesiologist should be physically present until the patient has been discharged from anesthesia care
Emergency Care, Medications, and Transfer Protocols	Must be in place in the ambulatory as well as office-based settings. Personnel with training in advanced resuscitative techniques (e.g., ACLS, PALS) should be immediately available until all patients are discharged home, allowing for acute stabilization of perioperative emergencies.

CONCERNS IN SUBSPECIALTY ANESTHESIA

References

1. Cullen KA, Hall MJ, Golosinskiy A. Ambulatory surgery in the United States, 2006. *Natl Health Stat Report* 2009;11:1–25.
2. White PF. Ambulatory anesthesia advances into the new millennium. *Anesth Analg* 2000;90:1234–1235.
3. www.asahq.org. Guidelines for Ambulatory Anesthesia and Surgery, October 22, 2008.
4. Bryson GL, Chung F, Finegan BA, et al. Patient selection in ambulatory anesthesia—an evidence-based review: part I. *Can J Anaesth* 2004;51:768–781.
5. Bryson GL, Chung F, Cox RG, et al. Patient selection in ambulatory anesthesia—an evidence-based review: part II. *Can J Anaesth* 2004;51:782–794.
6. Chung F, Mezei G. Adverse outcomes in ambulatory anesthesia. *Can J Anaesth* 1999;46:R18–R34.
7. Chung F, Mezei G, Tong D. Pre-existing medical conditions as predictors of adverse events in day-case surgery. *Br J Anaesth* 1999;83:262–270.
8. Bettelli G. High risk patients in day surgery. *Minerva Anestesiol* 2009;75:259–268.
9. Awad IT, Chung F. Factors affecting recovery and discharge following ambulatory surgery. *Can J Anaesth* 2006;53:858–872.
10. Fleisher LA, Beckman JA, Brown KA, et al. ACC/AHA 2007 guidelines on perioperative cardiovascular evaluation and care for noncardiac surgery: executive summary: a report of the American College of Cardiology/American Heart Association Task Force on Practice Guidelines (Writing Committee to Revise the 2002 Guidelines on Perioperative Cardiovascular Evaluation for Noncardiac Surgery) Developed in Collaboration With the American Society of Echocardiography, American Society of Nuclear Cardiology, Heart Rhythm Society, Society of Cardiovascular Anesthesiologists, Society for Cardiovascular Angiography and Interventions, Society for Vascular Medicine and Biology, and Society for Vascular Surgery. *J Am Coll Cardiol* 2007;50:1707–1732.
11. Chung SA, Yuan H, Chung F. A systemic review of obstructive sleep apnea and its implications for anesthesiologists. *Anesth Analg* 2008;107:1543–1563.
12. Cote CJ, Zaslavsky A, Downes JJ, et al. Postoperative apnea in former preterm infants after inguinal herniorrhaphy. A combined analysis. *Anesthesiology* 1995;82:809–822.
13. Fleisher LA, Pasternak LR, Herbert R, et al. Inpatient hospital admission and death after outpatient surgery in elderly patients: importance of patient and system characteristics and location of care. *Arch Surg* 2004;139:67–72.
14. Junger A, Klasen J, Benson M, et al. Factors determining length of stay of surgical day-case patients. *Eur J Anaesthesiol* 2001;18:314–321.
15. Chung F, Ritchie E, Su J. Postoperative pain in ambulatory surgery. *Anesth Analg* 1997;85:808–816.
16. Klein SM, Evans H, Nielsen KC, et al. Peripheral nerve block techniques for ambulatory surgery. *Anesth Analg* 2005;101:1663–1676.
17. Klein SM, Nielsen KC, Greengrass RA, et al. Ambulatory discharge after long-acting peripheral nerve blockade: 2382 blocks with ropivacaine. *Anesth Analg* 2002;94:65–70, table of contents.
18. Gan TJ, Meyer TA, Apfel CC, et al. Society for Ambulatory Anesthesia guidelines for the management of postoperative nausea and vomiting. *Anesth Analg* 2007;105:1615–1628.
19. Aldrete JA. The post-anesthesia recovery score revisited. *J Clin Anesth* 1995;7:89–91.
20. Mulroy MF, Salinas FV, Larkin KL, et al. Ambulatory surgery patients may be discharged before voiding after short-acting spinal and epidural anesthesia. *Anesthesiology* 2002;97:315–319.
21. Chung F, Imasogie N, Ho J, et al. Frequency and implications of ambulatory surgery without a patient escort. *Can J Anaesth* 2005;52:1022–1026.
22. Desai MS. Office-based anesthesia: techniques and procedures. In: Steele SM, ed. *Ambulatory Anesthesia and Perioperative Analgesia*. New York, NY: McGraw-Hill Companies, Inc.; 2005:345–355.
23. www.ashq.org. Guidelines for Office-Based Anesthesia. October 22, 2009.

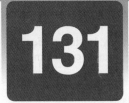

131

Robotic Surgery

Allison Long, MD

During recent years, there has been a surge in robotic surgery. With growing market pressures for minimally invasive procedures, the role of robotic-assisted surgery and its advantages of improved surgical precision over standard open and laparoscopic procedures will likely continue to grow (1). Anesthesiologists should have basic knowledge of these systems to formulate an anesthetic plan, recognize potential complications, and provide safe patient care.

1) **Robotic systems**
   a) The da Vinci surgical system is currently the only commercially available system in the United States.
   b) This system has three components: a console, an optical three-dimensional vision tower, and a surgical cart.
   c) **Advantages of computer-assisted robotic surgery over standard laparoscopy include**
      i) Improved operative field visibility with three-dimensional imaging systems
      ii) Computer-assisted scaling improves control of fine movements and reduces the "fulcrum effect" that amplifies unwanted motions such as hand tremor.
      iii) More ergonomic, anatomic control of instruments that closely mimics the movement of the human wrist
   d) **Pitfalls/limitations include**
      i) Several pieces of large, bulky equipment require large amounts of OR space.
      ii) The robot itself is quite large and care must be taken in positioning robotic arms.
      iii) Invasion of the anesthetic work space
      iv) Impaired access to patient once robotic arms are positioned and engaged

Some surgical procedures are easier to perform and result in less blood loss with a robot than standard techniques.

2) **Indications**: Although the da Vinci robotic systems were initially designed for cardiothoracic surgeries, there are an increasing number of other surgical procedures utilizing robots. These include
   a) **General surgery**: Virtually all gastrointestinal procedures have been performed safely by surgeons using this technology. Procedures most commonly performed include cholecystectomy, fundoplication, Heller myotomy, bariatric surgery, and colectomy (2).
   b) **Cardiac surgery**: Mitral valve surgery, atrial septal defect repair, internal mammary artery harvest, PDA ligation, coronary artery bypass grafting, atrial fibrillation surgery, and left ventricular pacemaker lead placement
   c) **Thoracic surgery**: Esophageal procedures, resection of mediastinal masses, and thymectomy

d) **Urologic surgery**: Radical prostatectomy, radical cystectomy, radical and simple nephrectomy, live donor nephrectomy, pyleoplasty, and adrenalectomy

e) **Gynecologic surgery**: Sacral colpopexy, myomectomy, treatment of endometriosis, hysterectomy, salpingo-oopherectomy, ovarian cystectomy, and repair of vesicovaginal fistula

f) **Pediatric surgery**

g) **Orthopedic surgery**: Total hip and knee arthroplasty

3) **Contraindications**

a) Poor pulmonary function test results may be a contraindication to robotically assisted cardiac surgery because single-lung ventilation may be poorly tolerated.

b) The prolonged Trendelenburg position required for robotically-assisted radical prostatectomy is relatively contraindicated in patients with a history of stroke or cerebral aneurysm (2).

4) **Anesthetic considerations: Patient safety during robot-assisted surgery requires advance planning and preparation.**

a) **Patient positioning**: robotic surgery with the da Vinci system does not allow for changes in patient position on the OR table once the robot has been docked.

↳ READ MORE

Positioning of the surgical patient, Chapter 5, page 34

  i) Pelvic procedures such as prostatectomy are usually done in lithotomy and steep Trendelenburg position, while upper abdominal surgeries are best done in the supine position with reverse Trendelenburg position.

  ii) Intrathoracic procedures often require the lateral position with variations of Trendelenburg and reverse Trendelenburg depending on the surgical site.

  iii) Mediastinal surgeries often require lateral positioning with lateral table tilt.

  iv) Before positioning the robotic cart, pressure points must be carefully padded.

  v) Close attention should be directed to the robot and the patient's head and chest during placement and removal of the robot to avoid injury.

  vi) **After robotic instruments are engaged, any patient movement can be disastrous.**

Any patient movement after the robot is docked can be disastrous.

The OR team should be trained for rapid removal of the robot in case of airway emergency or cardiac arrest.

b) **Limited intraoperative access to patient**

  i) Preparation and open communication between the anesthesiologist and the surgical team is essential.

  ii) Because of the proximity of the side cart to the patient's head, there is limited access to the patient's airway and neck, and the head must be protected against inadvertent collision with the robotic arms when moving.

c) **Patient preparation and monitoring**

  i) Bilateral peripheral IV access is valuable because the left upper extremity is not immediately available during surgery.

  ii) Neuromuscular blockade is very important in avoiding any patient movement while the robot is engaged.

  iii) Arterial and central venous catheterization, if necessary, should be placed prior to robotic docking.

  iv) Core temperature should be maintained with warm IV fluids and forced air warming.

Thoracic surgery and placement of double lumen tube, Chapters 140 and 156, pages 999 and 1107

Anesthesia for laparoscopic surgery, Chapter 133, page 927

Pay careful attention to patient positioning prior to robot docking in order to minimize the potential for nerve and other injuries.

d) Special considerations for **intrathoracic** robot-assisted surgery
   i) All robotic procedures that demand entrance into the thoracic cavity require single-lung ventilation.
   ii) Most commonly, the left-sided double lumen endotracheal tube is used for lung isolation.
   iii) CO_2 insufflation into the thoracic cavity to a pressure of 10 to 15 mm Hg maintains the lung away from the operative area.

e) Special considerations for **pediatric** robot-assisted surgery
   i) Confirming proper endotracheal tube depth with fluoroscopy after patient positioning may help prevent an airway emergency (3).
   ii) A left-sided precordial stethoscope monitors for inadvertent right main stem intubation.

5) **Potential complications**: The physiologic perturbations during robotic surgery are similar for both laparoscopic and thoracoscopic procedures.
   a) The presence of a pneumoperitoneum affects many organ systems (Table 131-1).
   b) Increased risk for nerve injury caused by
      i) Patient positioning required for optimal surgical conditions and
      ii) Possible prolonged operative times as surgeons gain experience with robotic assisted surgery.
   c) Anesthesia-related challenges in **thoracic** robotic surgery
      i) Prolonged one-lung ventilation
      ii) Hemodynamic instability due to obstruction of venous return and profound hypotension, associated with CO_2 insufflation of the hemithorax (1).
      iii) CO_2 insufflation in the chest cavity will lead to an increase in peak airway pressure, particularly during one-lung ventilation (4).

Table 131-1
Effects of Pneumoperitoneum on Organ Systems

Neurologic	↑ cerebral blood flow and ICP
Gastrointestinal	↓ portal and hepatic vein flow ↓ total hepatic blood flow and flow through hepatic microcirculation No change in hepatic artery flow ↓ gastric pH, mesenteric blood flow, and microcirculation blood flow
Renal	↓ renal artery and vein blood flow ↓ medullary and cortical flow
Cardiovascular	↓ venous return may result in lower extremity edema ↓ in cardiac index by up to 50% (especially when patient is in reverse Trendelenburg position)
Respiratory	↓ pulmonary compliance by 30%–50% ↓ FRC ↑ peak airway and plateau pressures **Maintenance of normocarbia and acid base status may be challenging in patients with poor preoperative pulmonary function**

ICP, intracranial pressure; FRC, functional residual capacity.

Chapter Summary for Robotic Surgery

Robotic Surgery	Several surgical advantages over standard laparoscopy. Large, bulky equipment presents anesthetic challenges.
Indications	Multiple surgical procedures are completed with the use of robots. Robot-assisted radical prostatectomy is currently the most common.
Contraindications	Poor pulmonary function may not allow for single-lung ventilation during thoracic surgery. History of stroke or aneurysm may prevent the use of prolonged Trendelenburg positioning.
Anesthetic Considerations	Patient safety requires advance planning, preparation, and open communication. All vascular access and positioning must be complete before robotic docking. Any patient movement after docking may be disastrous. The OR team must be trained for rapid removal of robot in case of airway emergency or cardiac arrest.
Potential Complications	Pneumoperitoneum affects multiple organ systems. Increased risk for nerve injury and edema exists.

References

1. Sullivan MJ, Frost EA, Lew MW. Anesthetic care of the patient for robotic surgery. *Middle East J Anesthesiol* 2008;19:967–982.
2. Goswami S, Nishanian E, Mets B. Anesthesia for robotic surgery. In: Miller RD, ed. *Miller's Anesthesia*. 7th ed. Orlando, FL: Churchill Livingstone; 2009.
3. Mariano ER, Furukawa L, Woo RK, et al. Anesthetic concerns for robot-assisted laparoscopy in an infant. *Anesth Analg* 2004;99:1665–1667.
4. Campos JH. An update on robotic thoracic surgery and anesthesia. *Curr Opin Anaesth* 2010;23:1–6.

132 Gastrointestinal and Hepatobiliary Surgery

Kellie Hancock, MD • Matthew J. Fiegel, MD

Gastrointestinal (GI) surgeries include procedures involving the esophagus, stomach, small and large intestines, pancreas, and gallbladder. Impairment of the GI tract can affect the balance of water, electrolytes, and nutrients in the body. Preoperative assessment of **volume status, serum electrolytes, acid base status, and nutrition** becomes critical in these cases (1).

I) Gastrointestinal (GI) surgery
   a) Procedures
      i) **Exploratory laparotomy** is performed to diagnose and treat various conditions including **inflammation, infection, perforation, and abnormal growths**. Patients presenting for exploratory laparotomy range from those with new-onset acute abdomen to those with abdominal sepsis and multiorgan failure, so careful preoperative evaluation with physical exam and review of laboratory data is important (2).
         (1) Cases are often performed emergently.
         (2) It is important to balance the need for optimization of the patient's pre-existing medical problems and correction of fluid deficits with the risk of a deteriorating surgical condition.
         (3) Additional intraoperative monitoring including arterial line and central line may be appropriate in patients with cardiovascular disease or hemodynamic instability.
      ii) **Cancer debulking** procedures can increase the efficacy of chemotherapy and radiation and help relieve symptoms caused by tumor bulk. Cytoreduction surgery is often long and complicated, requiring resection of multiple abdominal organs.
         (1) **Chemotherapy drugs** may have significant side effects, and it is important to review the toxicity and possible side effects of the patient's chemotherapeutics.
            (a) Bleomycin and Busulfan have pulmonary effects.
            (b) Doxorubicin causes dose-dependent cardiomyopathy.
            (c) Cisplatin, Paclitaxel, and Vincristine are associated with peripheral and/or autonomic neuropathies (1,3).
         (2) Management of anesthesia may be influenced by anemia, thrombocytopenia, electrolyte abnormalities, and the effects of metastatic lesions in liver, lung, bone, or brain (1,3).
      iii) **Whipple procedure** (pancreatoduodenectomy)
         (1) This is the most common operation performed for pancreatic cancer.

(2) Patients present a major challenge to the anesthesiologist due to the anatomical complexity of the surgery.

(3) Blood loss depends on metastatic involvement of hepatic and portal vessels, pre-existing coagulation abnormalities, and the presence of portal hypertension (4).

(4) All patients require large-bore IV access, type and cross (T&C), and fluid warmers.

(5) Invasive monitoring, including arterial line and central line, is recommended.

(6) Volume status and electrolytes must be followed closely.

(7) Thoracic epidural for postoperative pain should be considered.

(8) Complications

    (a) Hemorrhage from portal vein or vena caval injury, anastamotic leak, intra-abdominal abscess, and fistula (4).

iv) Hernia repair

    (1) Ventral hernias that occur due to defects in the abdominal wall include incisional, umbilical, epigastric, Spigelian, and hernias related to peritoneal dialysis.

    (2) There are many anesthetic options for hernia repairs including general anesthesia, local anesthesia with or without sedation, and regional anesthesia. Communication with the patient and the surgeon is important in developing the anesthetic plan.

2) Hepatobiliary surgery

    a) **Disorders of the liver and biliary tract can be categorized as parenchymal disease (hepatitis and cirrhosis) and cholestasis (involving the extrahepatic biliary pathway).**

    b) **Procedures**

      i) **Liver biopsy** is an important tool for diagnosis and staging of liver disease.

        (1) There are several methods for obtaining liver tissue including percutaneous, transjugular, laparoscopic, and ultrasound or CT-guided fine needle aspiration.

        (2) Coagulation defects

          (a) Coagulation status should be evaluated prior to procedure (5).

          (b) The American Association for the Study of Liver Diseases (AASLD) recommends platelet transfusion prior to biopsy for a **platelet count <50,000.** The AASLD also recommends a transjugular approach for patients with a **prothrombin time prolonged by more than 4 seconds** (5).

          (c) Consider DDAVP in patients with chronic renal failure as the interaction between platelets and factor VIII and vWF may be the primary hemostatic defect in uremia

        (3) Complications

          (a) Intraperitoneal hemorrhage, hematomas, hemobilia, bile peritonitis, and transient bacteremia

          (b) Adequate IV access and preparation of crossmatched blood is recommended due to the potential for blood loss.

      ii) Liver resection

        (1) Up to **80% to 85% of the liver can be safely resected** assuming good function of the remaining liver (6).

        (2) **Significant intraoperative blood loss is possible.**

READ MORE

Coagulopathies, Chapter 89, page 643

(a) Preoperative coagulation assessment is a mandatory part of the workup for major hepatic resection, as correction of coagulopathies can decrease perioperative bleeding.

(b) Sufficient vascular access to permit rapid transfusion, type and crossmatch (T&C), and fluid warmers are necessary; direct arterial and CVP monitoring are advisable.

(c) Use of the **thromboelastogram** helps guide coagulopathy correction and may reduce transfusion requirements during hepatobiliary operations (6).

(3) Preoperative jaundice is associated with perioperative renal impairment, so adequate renal protection is important in these patients (7).

(4) **Fluid management during major hepatic resection is controversial.**

(a) Reduction of CVP by restriction of fluid replacement may decrease intra-operative blood loss by reducing hepatic venous congestion.

(b) Other strategies include liberal fluid and blood administration early in the case as a buffer against sudden blood loss (8).

(5) Complications

(a) Significant third space fluid shifts, ongoing coagulopathy, bleeding, liver failure with encephalopathy, renal impairment, and biliary leak

iii) **Cholecystectomy**

(1) Gall stones are the most common cause of diseases of the gall bladder.

(2) The gall bladder can be removed via an open technique or laparoscopy, occasionally requiring cholangiogram to delineate the anatomy.

(3) Anesthetic considerations for laparoscopic cholecystectomy are similar to those for other laparoscopic procedures.

(4) Bile leakage, hemorrhage from the gall bladder bed, liver injury, and iatrogenic bile duct injury can occur.

READ MORE

Anesthesia for laparoscopic Surgery, Chapter 133, page 927

(5) **Opioid-induced sphincter of Oddi spasm**

(a) Incidence is very low and probably not a factor in the selection of pain management drugs.

(b) If spasm occurs, it can be treated with IV glucagon, naloxone, or nitroglycerin (9).

3) **General management principles**

a) **Thoracic epidural for postoperative pain**

i) Because a large incision may be necessary to adequately visualize the organs, blood vessels, and tissues in the abdominal cavity, an epidural for postoperative pain control should be considered.

ii) This is often used in elective gastrointestinal and hepatobiliary surgery and may even have a role in the emergency situation.

iii) Advantages of epidural analgesia

(1) A number of randomized controlled trials have shown a clear reduction in pain scores with epidural anesthesia when compared with intramuscular opioids or patient-controlled intravenous opioids (10–12).

(2) The sympathectomy created by thoracic epidural analgesia benefits bowel function by reducing systemic opioids requirements, reducing the duration of postoperative ileus, and improving gastric intramucosal pH (13,14).

(3) Other benefits may include decreased stress response, improved tissue oxygenation, improved spirometry parameters, and fewer thromboembolic events (15,16).

iv) Contraindications

(1) Hypovolemia and bacteremia are relative contraindications to neuraxial block.

(2) Coagulation deficits are a contraindication to neuraxial analgesia.

CONCERNS IN SUBSPECIALTY ANESTHESIA

  (a) Coagulation issues should be evaluated in the critically ill patient and in those with liver dysfunction.

  (b) Patients should also be questioned about any medications that affect coagulation.

  v) The insertion site should correspond to the middle or the top of the surgical incision for best pain coverage (Table 132-1).

  vi) Medications used for analgesia

  (1) A combination of local anesthetic and opioids provides the best analgesia and with fewer side effects

  (2) This combination causes less motor blockade than local anesthetic alone and decreases the duration of ileus compared with epidural opioid alone or patient-controlled analgesia.

b) **Monitoring**

  i) **Invasive arterial monitoring** is used for repeated blood sampling or where rapid changes in hemodynamic status are likely.

  ii) **Central line** placement is indicated in cases where large fluid shifts will occur that need to be followed on a timely basis.

  (1) A single CVP measurement offers little information in any circumstance, but this is especially true in the case of a tense abdomen.

  (2) Changes in CVP in response to fluid administration may provide helpful information (17).

  (3) May be needed for inotropic/vasopressive agents or postoperative TPN administration.

  iii) **Urine output**

  (1) An important indicator of fluid status

  (2) Measuring urine electrolytes can be helpful in cases of low urine output.

  iv) Newer monitors that may help guide blood/fluid therapy include cardiac index measurements taken from arterial lines and ScVO$_2$ measurements taken from central lines.

> CVP will be unreliable in cases with increased intra-abdominal pressure.

Table 132-1

Appropriate Epidural Levels for Surgical Procedures

Level	Procedures
T6-7	Gastrectomy, esophagectomy, cholecystectomy, Whipple, hepatic resection
T8-9	Ovarian cancer debulking
T9-10	Colectomy, bowel resection, laparoscopic cholecystectomy, A-P resection
T10-12	Pelvic exenteration

c) **Fluid replacement**
   i) Perioperative hypovolemia is associated with poorer clinical outcomes following elective abdominal surgery and can be even more detrimental in an emergency case (18). Depletion of fluid compartments is likely in patients with abdominal pathology, and large fluid and electrolyte shifts occur with major abdominal surgery.
   ii) Preoperative fluid deficits may be substantial in patients with diarrhea, vomiting, pyrexia, or increased nasogastric output. Dehydration is also seen in patients who underwent preoperative bowel preparation. Fluid deficits in excess of 4 L may occur.
   iii) **Third space fluid losses**
      (1) Elective intra-abdominal surgery = **6 to 8 mL/kg/h.**
      (2) For a lengthy laparotomy through a large abdominal incision, losses **can exceed 10 mL/kg/h.**
   iv) Recent work has suggested that a degree of fluid restriction may be beneficial in patients undergoing abdominal surgery with decreased complications and length of hospital stay (19). These studies looked at relatively well patients, and caution should be taken when extrapolating these results to a sicker population.

d) **Blood loss**
   i) Certain carcinomas, particularly right-sided colonic and gastric tumors, present with **iron-deficiency anemia from chronic blood loss.** Preoperative transfusion may be indicated to maintain O_2 carrying capacity and prevent intraoperative myocardial ischemia.
   ii) Intraoperative blood loss should be followed carefully, and transfusion may be indicated to insure adequate oxygen delivery. Hemodynamic stability, central venous O_2 saturation, lactate, and base deficit can be helpful guides (17).

e) **Postoperative care** plays an important role in the recovery of the patient.
   i) **Extubation**
      (1) Maintenance of temperature, use of rapidly metabolized anesthetic agents, and adequate reversal of muscle relaxation can improve extubation success.
      (2) If rapid sequence intubation was deemed necessary, care is required during emergence from anesthesia as the patient is at high risk of aspiration as they return to consciousness with impaired airway reflexes (20).
         (a) Waiting until the patient is fully awake and following commands, elevation of the head of the bed prior to extubation, and placement in left lateral position after extubation may reduce the risk of aspiration.
      (3) For patients with large fluid shifts, massive blood replacement, or requiring hemodynamic support during surgery, it may be prudent to postpone extubation and plan for postoperative ventilation.
   ii) **Respiratory complications** are common following abdominal surgery.
      (1) Thirteen to thirty-three percent of patients have postoperative respiratory problems.
      (2) Splinting, abdominal distension, diaphragmatic dysfunction, and acute lung injury all play a role in respiratory problems (21).
   iii) **ICU care** may be necessary for patients with large fluid shifts, cardiovascular instability, poor respiratory function, or inadequate urine output.

Chapter Summary for GI and Hepatobiliary Surgery

Overview	GI surgeries include procedures involving the esophagus, stomach, small and large intestines, pancreas, and gallbladder. Patients may have abnormalities with electrolyte and acid-base balance, and nutritional deficits.
Preoperative Considerations	Assess volume status, electrolytes, acid base status, and coagulation. Balance optimization of the patient's pre-existing medical problems and correction of fluid deficits and laboratory abnormalities with the risk of a deteriorating surgical condition.
Intraoperative Considerations	The degree of IV access and invasive monitoring is determined by the extent of surgery and the patient's underlying medical conditions. Vigilant monitoring of hemodynamic status, fluid and blood losses, coagulation, electrolytes, and acid base status is critical.
Postoperative Considerations	Thoracic epidurals for postoperative pain have many advantages in elective gastrointestinal and hepatobiliary surgery, but hypovolemia, bacteremia, and coagulopathy may preclude their use.

References

1. Hines RL, Marschall KE. *Stoelting's Anesthesia and Coexisting Disease*. 5th ed. Philadelphia, PA: Churchill Livingstone; 2008:280.
2. Cook TM, Day CJE. Hospital mortality after urgent and emergency laparotomy in patients aged 65 yr and over. Risk and prediction of risk using multiple logistic regression analysis. *Br J Anaesth* 1998;80:776–781.
3. Vadivelu N. Cancer. In: Hines RL, Marschall KE, eds. *Stoelting's Anesthesia and Coexisting Disease*. 5th ed. Philadelphia, PA: Churchill Livingstone; 2008:501–520.
4. Bottager TV, Junonger T. Factors influencing morbidity and mortality after pancreaticoduodenectomy. *Ann Surg* 2000;232(6):786–795.
5. Rockey DC, Caldwell SH, Goodman ZD, et al. Liver biopsy. *Hepatology* 2009;49:1017.
6. Kaufman BS, Roccaforte JD. Anesthesia and the liver. In: Barash PG, Cullen BF, Stoelting RK, eds. *Clinical Anesthesia*. 5th ed. Philadelphia, PA: Lippincott Williams & Wilkins; 2006.
7. Fogarty BJ, Parks RW, Rowlands BJ, et al. Renal dysfunction in obstructive jaundice. *Br J Surg* 1995;82:877–884.
8. Matsumata T, Itasaka H, Shirabe K, et al. Strategies for reducing blood transfusions in hepatic resection. *HPB Surg* 1994;8:1–6.
9. Barash P, Cullen B, Stoelting R. *Clinical Anesthesia*. 5th ed. Philadelphia, PA: Lippincott Williams and Wilkins; 2006:1066.
10. Rigg JRA, Jamrozik K, Myles PS, et al. MASTER Anaesthesia Trial Study Group. Epidural anaesthesia and analgesia and outcome of major surgery, a randomized trial. *Lancet* 2002;359:1276–1282.
11. Flisberg P, Tornebrandt K, Walther B, et al. Pain relief after esophagectomy. Thoracic epidural analgesia is better than parenteral opioids. *J Cardiothoracic Vasc Anesth* 2001;15:282–287.
12. Fotiadis RJ, Badvie S, Weston MD, et al. Epidural analgesia in gastrointestinal surgery. *Br J Surg* 2004;91:828–841.
13. Kabon B, Fleischmann E, Teschan T, et al. Thoracic epidural anesthesia increases tissue oxygenation during major abdominal surgery. *Anesth Analg* 2003;97:1812–1817.
14. Steinbrook RA. Epidural anesthesia and gastrointestinal motility. *Anesth Analg* 1997;86:837–844.
15. Kouraklis G, Glinavou A, Raftopoulos L, et al. Epidural analgesia attenuates the systemic response to upper abdominal surgery: a randomized trial. *Int Surg* 2000;85:353–357.
16. Rodgers A, Walker N, Schug S, et al. Reduction of post-operative mortality and morbidity with epidural or spinal anaesthesia: results from overview of randomised trials. *BMJ* 2000;321:1493–1497.
17. Grocott MPW, Mythen MG, Gan TJ. Perioperative fluid management and clinical outcome in adults. *Anesth Analg* 2005;100:1093–1201.
18. Nisanevish V, Felenstein I, Almogy G, et al. Effect of intraoperative fluid management on outcome after intraabdominal surgery. *Anesthesiology* 2005;103:25–32.
19. Gan TJ, Soppit A, Maroof M, et al. Goal-directed intraoperative fluid administration reduced length of hospital stay after major surgery. *Anesthesiology* 2001;97:820–826.
20. Miller R. *Miller's Anesthesia*. 6th ed. Philadelphia, PA: Elsevier; 2005:1649.
21. Lumb AB. *Nunn's Applied Respiratory Physiology*. 6th ed. London: Elsevier; 2005.

133 | Anesthesia for Laparoscopic Surgery

Pedro P. Tanaka, MD, PhD • John H. Nguyen, MD

Laparoscopic surgery is one of the principal techniques for minimally invasive surgery of the abdomen and is used for procedures that range across multiple surgical subspecialties. It describes a group of operations performed with the aid of a camera placed in the abdomen or the pelvis. Pneumoperitoneum and specific patient positions (e.g., Trendelenburg) are used to expose the abdominal organs for surgery.

1) Overview of laparoscopic surgery
   a) Indications include gynecologic, abdominal, and thoracic procedures
   b) **Advantages**
      i) When compared to open abdominal surgery, advantages include reduced surgical trauma, less pain, fewer postoperative pulmonary complications, and shorter recovery times.
   c) **Disadvantages**
      i) Longer surgical times and higher equipment costs (1)
   d) Prevalence of technique
      i) Because expertise and equipment have improved, laparoscopy has become one of the most common surgical procedures performed on an outpatient basis.
   e) Establishment of pneumoperitoneum
      i) Veress needle insertion
         (1) Inserted blindly, often into an intraumbilical incision through fascia into peritoneum.
         (2) CO_2 gas is insufflated through the needle to establish a pneumoperitoneum.
      ii) Trochar insertion
         (1) Trochars are ports through which laparoscopic instruments are inserted into the abdomen.
         (2) Trochars are inserted once a pneumoperitoneum has been established.
      iii) Minilaparotomy
         (1) Pneumoperitoneum can also be established by inserting an insufflation cannula surgically through an open minilaparotomy procedure.
2) Pathophysiologic effects and complications
   The pneumoperitoneum is achieved by insufflating the abdomen with CO_2. These maneuvers induce a number of clinically relevant pathophysiologic effects during surgery.
   a) **Cardiovascular system**
      i) **Hemodynamic effects**
         (1) Pneumoperitoneum *increases*
            (a) Systemic vascular resistance (SVR)

(b)   Mean arterial pressure (MAP)
(c)   Cardiac filling pressures
(2)   Pneumoperitoneum *decreases*
(a)   Venous return
(b)   Cardiac output (CO)
(3)   These effects are **proportional to the increase in intra-abdominal pressure** (IAP) and are significant with insufflation pressures >10 mm Hg.
(4)   Mechanism
(a)   Increased IAP causes compression of the abdominal organs and vessels.
(b)   Resistance to flow through arterial beds is increased due to both mechanical and neurohumeral factors.
(c)   Caval compression and increased venous resistance lead to decreased venous return.
(d)   Intrathoracic pressure transmitted to the heart causes increased cardiac filling pressures.
(e)   Decreased preload and increased afterload result in decreased CO.
(f)   MAP is increased overall because increases in SVR exceed decreases in CO_2.
(5)   Management
(a)   The lowest insufflation pressure required to achieve adequate surgical exposure (<15 mm Hg) should be used.
(b)   Increases in SVR may be treated with vasodilating agents, centrally acting α_2-agonists, or opioids.
(c)   Decreases in venous return and CO may be attenuated by appropriate preloading prior to the induction of pneumoperitoneum.

ii) **Complications**
(1)   **Cardiac arrhythmias**
(a)   Bradyarrhythmias, dysrhythmias, and asystole can occur during insertion of laparoscopic ports or during insufflation of the abdomen.
(b)   Mechanism
(i)   Sudden stretching of the peritoneum can precipitate a sudden and reflexive increase in vagal tone.
(c)   Management
(i)   Slow insufflation of CO_2 can decrease the risk of arrhythmias.
(ii)   Administration of anticholinergic medications may be appropriate for bradyarrhythmias.
(iii)   If the arrhythmia persists or results in hemodynamic compromise, prompt interruption of the surgery and release of pneumoperitoneum is indicated.

b) **Pulmonary and respiratory system**
i) **Ventilatory effects**
(1)   Mechanism
(a)   Pneumoperitoneum transmits pressure to the thorax and decreases pulmonary compliance by 30% to 50%.
(b)   Elevation of the diaphragm results in decreased functional residual capacity (FRC), leading to atelectasis, V/Q mismatching, and hypoxemia.
(c)   Hypercapnea results from systemic absorption of the CO_2 pneumoperitoneum (2).
(2)   Management
(a)   Institution of positive end-expiratory pressure (PEEP) can mitigate the decreases in FRC.
(b)   Hypercapnea can be managed with hyperventilation.

ii) **Complications**

(1) **CO_2 subcutaneous emphysema**

(a) This is the most common respiratory complication during laparoscopy.

(b) It is suggested by an increase in end-tidal CO_2 (ETCO$_2$) >25% or an increase that occurs >30 minutes after abdominal CO_2 insufflation.

CO_2 subcutaneous emphysema itself is not a contraindication to extubation at the end of surgery provided that other extubation criteria are satisfied (4).

(c) The cause is extraperitoneal insufflation of CO_2. Some cases are accidental. Others are intentional (e.g., in nephrectomies, where retroperitoneal exposure is required) (3).

(d) Management

(i) Hypercapnea can be treated with an increase in mechanical ventilation.

(ii) In cases where the degree of hypercapnea becomes unmanageable with hyperventilation alone, the pneumoperitoneum can be temporarily released to allow for CO_2 elimination.

(2) **Pneumothorax**

(a) Mechanism

(i) Movement of gas from the peritoneum into the thorax can occur under pressure through weak areas and defects in the diaphragm.

(ii) Pneumothorax may be asymptomatic.

(iii) Pneumothorax may manifest as increased peak airway pressures, decreased O_2 saturation, and hypotension.

(iv) In severe cases, profound hypotension and cardiac arrest can occur (3).

(b) Management

(i) Early diagnosis and treatment can be life saving.

(ii) Surgery should be stopped and the pneumoperitoneum released.

(iii) Supportive measures should be continued while confirming the diagnosis, either clinically or with chest radiograph.

(iv) Depending on the degree of cardiopulmonary compromise, the pneumothorax may be observed or treated with an intercostal cannula or a thoracostomy tube.

(v) After stabilization of the patient, conversion to an open procedure may be indicated (4).

(3) **Endobronchial intubation**

(a) Mechanism

(i) Elevation of the diaphragm during pneumoperitoneum can lead to endobronchial intubation.

(ii) Manifests as a decrease in O_2 saturation as a result of intrapulmonary shunt and increased airway pressure (3).

(b) Management

(i) The lungs should be auscultated and the endotracheal tube should be slightly withdrawn as needed.

(4) **Gas (CO_2) embolism**

(a) Mechanism

(i) Gas embolism, although rare, has a mortality rate of nearly 30%.

(ii) Profound hypotension, arrhythmias, or asystole can occur as a result of a "gas lock" in the vena cava or right ventricle (RV) that interrupts circulation.

(iii) **An increase in ETCO$_2$ is observed.** This may be followed by an **acute decrease in ETCO$_2$** if there is severe hypotension.

Gas embolism from misplacement of trocars or the Veress needle most frequently occurs on induction of pneumoperitoneum but can occur at any point during surgery (3).

      (iv) The major cause is intravascular insufflation of gas from misplacement of the Veress needle or trocar either directly into a vessel or into a parenchymal organ.

      (v) Risk factors include hysteroscopy, hypovolemia, and a history of prior abdominal surgeries.

  (b) Management

      (i) Initial steps include immediate deflation of the pneumoperitoneum, institution of 100% FiO_2.

      (ii) Place patient in the left lateral head-down position to remove air from the RV outflow track.

      (iii) Hyperventilate to eliminate the increased $PaCO_2$ caused by the sudden increase in pulmonary dead space.

      (iv) A central line may be required to aspirate gas from the RV.

      (v) CPR may be required.

      (vi) Hyperbaric O_2 treatment should be considered if there is suspicion of cerebral gas embolism (4).

  c) **Effects of positioning**

    i) Hemodynamic effects

      (1) The head-down position generally increases venous return and CO, whereas the head-up position has the opposite effect.

    ii) Ventilatory effects

      (1) The head-down position generally decreases FRC, overall lung volumes, and lung compliance.

3) Patient monitoring

  a) Routine ASA monitors are indicated.

  b) Neuromuscular monitors can be used to ensure adequate paralysis.

  c) In elderly ASA III and IV patients with cardiopulmonary comorbidities, consider invasive monitoring (5).

4) Anesthetic technique

  a) A wide variety of anesthetic drugs have been used for laparoscopic procedures, and most are satisfactory.

  b) **Induction of anesthesia**

    i) IV induction agents such as thiopental, propofol, and etomidate, and a variety of muscle relaxants including succinylcholine, mivacurium, rocuronium, and vecuronium have been reported.

    ii) Although the benefit of rapid sequence induction has been questioned, it is still standard of care in patients with risk of pulmonary aspiration.

    iii) Special attention should be given during pneumoperitoneum creation, due to occurrence of embolic episodes and dysrhythmias.

  c) **Maintenance of anesthesia**

    i) As more procedures are conducted on an outpatient basis, the choice of maintenance agent is likely to be reduced to short-acting drugs such as sevoflurane, desflurane, and infusions of propofol.

    ii) There is apparently no clinical advantage to omitting nitrous oxide.

    iii) Although ultrashort-acting opioid analgesics such as remifentanil have allowed bypassing Phase I recovery in ambulatory setting, this should be determined by your hospital policy.

    iv) Because laparoscopy surgery has generally been performed with tracheal intubation and controlled ventilation, short- or intermediate-acting neuromuscular blockers should be administered based on surgical length.

    v) General anesthesia has been performed without intubation safely and effectively with ProSeal laryngeal mask airway in nonobese patients (5).

(I) Careful attention for patients with high airway pressures (>30 cm H_2O) or where extreme head-down tilt will be applied.

vi) **Emergence from general anesthesia**

(I) Reversal of neuromuscular blockade

(a) Consider administering neuromuscular blocking reversal agents to patients who receive neuromuscular blocking drugs.

(b) The association between drugs such as neostigmine and glycopyrrolate and PONV is controversial.

(c) Even minor degrees of residual neuromuscular block can produce distressing symptoms and potentially increased risk of respiratory complications.

vii) Regional anesthesia (spinal, epidural) can be used in laparoscopic procedures (diagnostic, infertility, and tubal ligation) (6). Not widely done because the high thoracic sensory level required for patient comfort during pneumoperitoneum may result in respiratory impairment.

5) Postoperative recovery

a) **Nausea and vomiting**

i) Postoperative nausea and vomiting (PONV) is common after laparoscopic surgery, although its etiology is not clear.

ii) Ondansetron or other 5-HT3 antagonists given at the end of surgery result in a significantly greater antiemetic effect compared with preinduction dosing.

iii) Prophylactic dexamethasone decreases the incidence for nausea and vomiting after laparoscopic cholecystectomy relative to placebo and may decrease the severity of pain with no adverse effects noted from this single steroid dose (7).

b) **Pain**

i) Postoperative pain in laparoscopic surgery is less severe compared to an open procedure, but still considerable.

ii) Most effective pain relief can be obtained by combining opioids, local anesthetics, and NSAIDS into balanced analgesia.

iii) This approach at least allows reduced opioid dose by the use of other modalities, thereby limiting side effects, decreasing postoperative pain and analgesics, and facilitating an earlier return to normal activities.

iv) Rectus sheath block, local infiltration of the laparoscopy portals, and intraperitoneal local anesthesia can be used as regional techniques for pain relief (6).

Chapter Summary for Anesthesia for Laparoscopic Surgery

Laparoscopy	Minimally invasive surgery with important physiologic effects.
Insertion of Veress Needle	Watch for inadvertent intravascular placement and CO2 embolism
Insertion of Trocars	Watch for inadvertent intravascular placement, especially if minilaparotomy is not performed.
Pneumoperitoneum	Can cause hypertension ($\uparrow$ SVR due to $\uparrow$CO2), hypotension ($\downarrow$ venous return), arrhythmias, $\downarrow$ SpO2 (due to $\downarrow$ FRC, $\uparrow$ Peak pressure)
Trendelenburg Positioning	Ensure patient strapped to bed, mainstem intubation, $\downarrow$ FRC
Postoperative Concerns	PONV common and should be treated, decreased pain compared to similar procedures done with open approach

CONCERNS IN SUBSPECIALTY ANESTHESIA

References

1. Smith I. Anesthesia for laparoscopy with emphasis on outpatient laparoscopy. *Anesthesiol Clin N Am* 2001;19:21–41.
2. O'Malley C, Cunningham A. Physiology changes during laparoscopy. *Anesthesiol Clin N Am* 2001;19:1–19.
3. Joshi G. Complications of laparoscopy. *Anesthesiol Clin N Am* 2001;19:89–105.
4. Henny CP, Hofland J. Laparoscopic surgery. *Surg Endosc* 2005;19:1163–1171.
5. Hohlrieder M, Brimacombe J, Eschertzhuber S, et al. A study of airway management using the ProSeal LMA laryngeal mask airway compared with the tracheal tube on postoperative analgesia requirements following gynaecological laparoscopic surgery. *Anaesthesia* 2007;62(9):913–918.
6. Gerges FJ, Kanazi G, Jabbour-khoury S. Anesthesia for laparoscopy: a review. *J Clin Anesth* 2006;18:67–78.
7. Karanicolas P, Smith SE, Kanbur, et al. The impact of prophylactic dexamethasone on nausea and vomiting after laparoscopic cholecystectomy. A systematic review and meta-analysis. *Ann Surg* 2008;248:751–762.

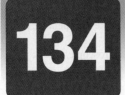

134 Anesthesia for Urologic Surgery

Cosmin Guta, MD • Bryan Maxwell, MD

Urologic surgery encompasses a variety of procedures to treat prostatic masses or tumors, urinary tract conditions, kidney stones, or testicular tumors. Many chronic or malignant diseases can benefit from urologic resection or surgery. Providing anesthesia for these surgical procedures can pose unique challenges for the anesthesiologist.

1) Overview
  a) Urologic surgery integrates operations of the pelvis that include the colon and urogenital and gynecologic organs.
    i) Common reasons for urologic surgery include malignancy, organ dysfunction or obstruction, pain, and inflammatory diseases.
    ii) Common operations include nephrectomy, bladder surgery, prostate surgery, testicular surgery, and surgery involving the urethra and ureters.
  b) **Anesthesia for urologic surgery presents many challenges, including**
    i) Potential for large amounts of surgical blood loss during surgery in the highly vascular pelvic region
    ii) Potential for fluid absorption during cystoscopic surgeries
    iii) Patient positioning in lateral or flexed positions
2) **Anesthetic considerations for urologic procedures**
  a) **Radical prostatectomy**
    i) **Indications**
      (1) Prostate cancer is the most common type of cancer in men, affecting 10% of all men at some point in their life.
      (2) Involves resection of large prostatic masses or, more commonly, tumors.
      (3) The procedure is performed by open laparotomy, but laparoscopic and robotic surgery are being used more frequently in many centers. The short-term results of these less invasive procedures appear to be comparable to standard open operations, at least for early malignancies (1).
      (4) Radical retropubic prostatectomy is often associated with significant operative blood loss.
      (5) Laparoscopic prostatectomy with pelvic lymph node dissection requires a steep (>30 degrees) Trendelenburg position for surgical exposure and has the potential for increased carbon dioxide absorption from the retroperitoneum.
    ii) **Preoperative considerations**
      (1) Patients presenting for prostatectomy are usually elderly males. Preoperative evaluation should focus on comorbid disease processes that are prevalent in this patient population (2).

Radical retropubic prostatectomy is often associated with significant surgical blood loss.

iii) **Positioning**

(1) Hyperextended supine position to facilitate exposure of the pelvis.

(2) The operating room table is tilted head-down to make the operative field horizontal.

(3) A steep Trendelenburg position is required for laparoscopic/robotic prostatectomy.

iv) **Monitoring**

(1) ASA standard monitors, temperature monitoring, and an arterial line for continuous blood pressure monitoring are required.

(2) Central venous pressure monitoring might be required to assess the volume status (2).

v) **Access**

(1) Consider large-bore IVs (significant blood loss may occur) and an arterial line ± central venous access (depending on comorbidities) as significant blood loss and large volume shifts occur.

vi) **Anesthetic technique**

(1) Regional, general, or a combined regional/general technique can adequately provide anesthesia for radical retropubic prostatectomy.

(2) General anesthesia with muscle relaxation is preferred for radical perineal prostatectomy because the patient is placed in the exaggerated lithotomy position, which interferes with respiratory function.

vii) **Complications**

(1) Include blood loss, hypothermia, anemia, coagulopathy, venous air embolism, and peroneal nerve injury due to positioning

b) **Transurethral resection of the prostate**

i) **Indications**

(1) Transurethral resection of the prostate (TURP) is the second most common surgical procedure in men over age 65.

(2) The most common indication for TURP is symptomatic benign prostatic hypertrophy. This patient population has a greater anesthetic risk because of a greater prevalence of coexisting cardiovascular and pulmonary problems.

Large amounts of irrigation solution are absorbed during TURP and can cause a syndrome of pulmonary edema, cerebral edema, and hyponatremia.

(3) This procedure is performed using a modified cystoscope (resectoscope) with a wire loop connected to an electrocautery unit for resection of tissue and coagulation of bleeding vessels.

(4) During the procedure, large amounts of irrigation solution are absorbed into the circulation and the periprostatic and retroperitoneal spaces (3).

(a) Normally, about 20 mL/min of irrigation fluid is absorbed (4). In clinical practice, it is almost impossible to assess accurately the volume absorbed.

(b) Absorption of irrigating fluid depends on

(i) Pressure, volume, and type of irrigating fluid

(ii) Intravesical pressure

(iii) Duration, amount, and quality of resection

(iv) Degree of bleeding

(c) Absorption of irrigating fluid will cause hypervolemia, dilutional hyponatremia, hemolysis, and toxicity of solutes in the irrigating fluid.

(d) The ideal irrigating fluid should be

(i) Isotonic

(ii) Nonelectrolytic

(iii) Transparent

(iv) Nonmetabolized, nontoxic, and rapidly excreted.

(e) Irrigation solutions used and their potential side effects during TURP include:
  (i) Glycine: hyperammonemia (coma) and possible visual disturbances (transient postoperative visual syndrome)
  (ii) Distilled water: hemolysis and hyponatremia/ hypo-osmolality
  (iii) Mannitol: osmotic diuresis
  (iv) Sorbitol: hyperglycemia and possible lactic acidosis
  (v) Lactated Ringer is isotonic and does not cause hemolysis upon intravascular absorption.

ii) **Positioning**
  (1) Lithotomy
  (2) Functional residual capacity decreases, predisposing patients to atelectasis and hypoxia.
  (3) Rapid lowering of the legs at the end of the operation acutely decreases venous return and can result in severe hypotension.
  (4) Peroneal nerve compression at fibular head can cause loss of dorsiflexion of the foot if pressure points padding is not adequate (5).

iii) **Monitoring**
  (1) Standard ASA monitors including temperature monitoring

iv) **Anesthetic technique**

Spinal anesthesia may be preferable in TURP because it may reduce the risk of pulmonary edema and permits early detection of mental status changes associated with TURP syndrome.

  (1) Regional or general anesthetic techniques are possible. There is no evidence of a difference in mortality or morbidity between regional and general anesthesia (7).
  (2) Regional anesthesia may be preferred, since an awake patient can be helpful for an early diagnosis of
    (a) TURP syndrome: neurological manifestations
    (b) Bladder perforation: abdominal and/or shoulder pain
  (3) Spinal anesthesia is considered the anesthetic technique of choice for patients undergoing TURP.
    (a) Spinal anesthesia is reported to reduce the risk of pulmonary edema and permits early detection of mental status changes because increased absorption of irrigating fluid during the procedure produces a number of problems with cardiovascular and neurologic implications (6,8).
    (b) For a satisfactory anesthesia, a sensory block up to T10 is required to prevent the discomfort of bladder distention.
    (c) Adequate anesthesia with minimal hemodynamic effects can be achieved with a hyperbaric solution of local anesthetic with or without an opioid.
    (d) Regional anesthesia does not abolish the obturator reflex (external rotation and adduction of the thigh secondary to stimulation of the obturator nerve by electrocautery current through the lateral bladder wall). The reflex is reliably blocked only by muscle paralysis during general anesthesia.

v) **Complications**
  (1) Complications associated with TURP occur in approximately 7% of patients (7) (Tables 134-1 and 134-2).
  (2) Include TURP syndrome (2%), hemorrhage, bladder perforation (1%), hypothermia, septicemia (6%), disseminated intravascular coagulation.

vi) **TURP syndrome**
  (1) Manifestations are primarily of circulatory fluid overload, water intoxication, and, occasionally, toxicity from the solute in the irrigation fluid.

Table 134-1

Signs and Symptoms Attributed to Transurethral Resection of the Prostate (TURP) Syndrome

Neurological Manifestations	Restlessness Disorientation Confusion Depressed consciousness Blurring of vision transient Blindness (glycine neurotoxicity) Convulsions
Cardiovascular Manifestations	Hypertension Chest pain Bradycardia Dysrhythmia ECG changes (wide QRS, S-T changes) In severe and late cases, hypotension, CHF and pulmonary edema may occur
Pulmonary Manifestations	Respiratory distress Hypoxemia Pulmonary edema
Metabolic Changes	Hyponatremia Hyperglycemia Hyperammonemia Hypo-osmolarity

The most important physiologic derangement of CNS function in TURP syndrome is acute hypo-osmolality.

The risk of TURP syndrome can be reduced by limiting surgical time <1 h and suspending irrigation fluid no more than 30 cm above the OR table.

(2) **Clinical signs and symptoms**

    (a)   Early clinical signs and symptoms of TURP syndrome include restlessness, headache, and tachypnea.

    (b)   It may progress to respiratory distress, hypoxia, pulmonary edema, nausea, vomiting, confusion, and coma.

    (c)   TURP syndrome consists of pulmonary edema, cerebral edema, and hyponatremia due to absorption of large amounts of hypotonic irrigation fluids.

        (i)   The most important physiological derangement of CNS function is not hyponatremia, but acute hypo-osmolality because the blood-brain barrier is essentially impermeable to sodium but freely permeable to water.

        (ii)   Cerebral edema caused by acute hypo-osmolality can increase intracranial pressure with bradycardia, hypertension, and neurologic symptoms.

        (iii)   When serum sodium level falls to <120 mEq/L, signs of cardiovascular depression can occur.

        (iv)   Levels <115 mEq/L will cause bradycardia, widening of the QRS complex, ST-segment elevation, ventricular ectopic beats, and T-wave inversion. A serum sodium level <110 mEq/L can cause respiratory and cardiac arrest (8,9).

    (d)   The risk of TURP syndrome can be reduced by limiting the time of surgery to <1 hour, and by maintaining the irrigating fluid suspended no more than 30 cm above the operating room table during the resection (10).

Table 134-2

Other Potential Complications of TURP

Blood Loss	• Blood loss is difficult to quantify, particularly in prolonged cases. • Visual estimation of hemorrhage may be difficult due to dilution of blood with irrigant solution. • Usual warning signs (tachycardia and hypotension) may be overshadowed by overhydration due to irrigant absorption.
Coagulopathy	• Disseminated intravascular coagulation (DIC) is responsible for severe postoperative bleeding after TURP in <1% of the cases. • Caused by release of a plasminogen activator from the prostate into the circulation during surgery. • Treatment may include administration of aminocaproic acid.
Bladder Perforation	• The incidence of bladder perforation during TURP is about 1%. • Can be difficult to recognize in the presence of a high spinal block (may mask abdominal pain) or general anesthesia. • *Extraperitoneal perforation* presents with pain in the periumbilical, inguinal, or suprapubic regions. • *Intraperitoneal perforations* may present with generalized pain in the upper abdomen or referred pain from the diaphragm to the precordial region or the shoulder associated with abdominal rigidity, nausea, vomiting, and hypotension (1).
Bacteremia and Septicemia	• TURP facilitates the entry of bacteria into the bloodstream via open prostatic venous sinuses. • Bacteremia following TURP is usually asymptomatic and transient. • Septicemia may occur and is treated with antibiotics and cardiovascular support is warranted (1).
Hypothermia	• Elderly patients have a reduced thermoregulatory capacity. • Appropriate measures to reduce heat loss are warming blankets (Bear Hugger), heated irrigating solution, and warm intravenous fluids. • Associated with a significantly higher incidence of postoperative myocardial ischemia.

(3) Treatment

    (a) Treatment of TURP syndrome depends on early recognition and should be based on the severity of symptoms. The syndrome has a significant mortality unless it is recognized and treated promptly.

        (i) Signs will be detected earlier in the awake patient.

        (ii) In the anaesthetized patient, the only clue may be tachycardia and hypertension.

        (iii) Diagnosis can be confirmed by finding a low serum sodium. An acute fall to <120 mEq/L is always symptomatic.

    (b) Surgery should be terminated as soon as possible and IV fluid should be stopped.

        (i) Check arterial blood gas, serum sodium, and hemoglobin.

        (ii) Support respiration with oxygen or intubation and ventilation if required.

        (iii) Most patients can be managed with fluid restriction and a loop diuretic.

CONCERNS IN SUBSPECIALTY ANESTHESIA

(iv) If pulmonary edema or hypotension develops, invasive hemodynamic monitoring is recommended as a guide for pharmacologic support and fluid management.

(v) Symptomatic hyponatremia resulting in seizures or coma should be treated with hypertonic saline (NaCl 3%) until symptoms resolve.

Central pontine myelinolysis may occur if hyponatremia is corrected too rapidly.

1. The rate of correction of the serum sodium should not be more than 12 mEq/L in the first 24 hours—rapid administration of hypertonic saline has been associated with an increased risk of central pontine myelinolysis (CPM, a.k.a osmotic demyelination syndrome).

2. CPM has been reported after both rapid and slow correction of serum sodium concentration in TURP patients (9).

3. Endotracheal intubation is advisable to prevent aspiration until the patient's mental status normalizes.

c) **Cystoscopy**
   i) The most commonly performed urological procedure
   ii) Performed to diagnose and treat lesions of the lower (urethra, prostate, bladder) and upper (ureter, kidney) urinary tracts
   iii) **Positioning**
       (1) Lithotomy
   iv) **Monitors**
       (1) Standard ASA monitors
   v) **Access**
       (1) Generally one peripheral IV is all that is required
   vi) **Anesthetic management**
       (1) Varies with the age and gender of the patient and the purpose of the procedure.
       (2) Most cystoscopies are performed as an outpatient procedure and the duration is usually short (15 to 20 minutes) so a general anesthetic is usually used.
       (3) If a regional anesthetic (spinal or epidural) is used, a sensory level to T10 provides good anesthesia for nearly all cystoscopic procedures.
       (4) The obturator reflex that can occur during the procedure is reliably blocked only by muscle paralysis during general anesthesia.
   vii) **Complications**
       (1) Complications are related to lithotomy position and bladder perforation (see TURP).

d) **Cystectomy**
   i) **Indications**
       (1) Radical cystectomy is recommended for invasive bladder tumors (usually transitional cell) and simple cystectomy for interstitial/hemorrhagic/radiation cystitis.
       (2) A procedure to divert the urinary tract is also needed, usually a piece of small bowel brought out as a stoma (ileal conduit). It can also be a pouch constructed out of the bowel and reattached to the urethra (neobladder).
       (3) Extensive lymph node dissection is typical in radical procedures (1).
   ii) **Preoperative evaluation**
       (1) Smoking is a major risk factor for bladder cancer, so patients have high coincidence of CAD and COPD.
       (2) Patients with interstitial cystitis often have chronic pain, and opioid tolerance is common.
   iii) **Positioning**
       (1) Lithotomy or supine

Significant surgical blood loss can occur during radical cystectomy and large-bore IVs and arterial pressure monitoring should be considered.

(2) Good medial padding is needed in lithotomy, as injuries have been described with leg adduction as a result of obturator reflex from use of cautery near obturator nerve during pelvic node dissection.

(3) Robot-assisted procedures are often done with exaggerated Trendelenburg (i.e., 45 degrees or more) (2).

iv) **Access**

(1) Consider large-bore IVs (significant blood loss may occur) and an arterial line ± central venous access (depending on comorbidities) as significant blood loss and large volume shifts occur.

v) **Monitoring**

(1) ASA standard monitors and temperature monitoring

(2) Urine output may not be measurable when bladder is open.

vi) **Anesthetic technique**

(1) General endotracheal anesthesia with a muscle relaxant provides good operating conditions.

(2) A low-thoracic epidural (usually T10-12) should be considered for intraop use and/or postop pain control.

(3) An upper body forced-air warming blanket should be used to prevent hypothermia.

vii) **Complications**

(1) Significant blood loss and fluid shifts are common.

(2) Colonic or ileal conduits, performed immediately following radical cystectomy, are associated with hyperchloremic metabolic acidosis.

e) **Retroperitoneal lymph node dissection**

i) **Indications**

(1) Advanced or recurrent testicular tumors

ii) **Preoperative evaluation**

(1) Patients who have had chemotherapy may have had bleomycin. Pulmonary function should be evaluated. These patients may be at greater risk of pulmonary complications, including oxygen toxicity.

iii) **Positioning**

(1) Usually supine

iv) **Monitoring**

(1) ASA standard monitors and temperature monitoring

v) **Access**

(1) Consider large-bore IVs and an arterial line ± central venous access (depending on patient's comorbidities).

vi) **Anesthetic technique**

(1) General anesthesia; also consider low-thoracic epidural for intraop use and/or postop pain control.

(2) If an epidural is used, it should cover the T6-7 dermatome, depending on the incision (sometimes thoracoabdominal is used).

vii) **Complications**

(1) Plan for possible significant blood loss.

(2) Depending on epidural use, sympathetic discharge might be noticed (e.g., tachycardia) during dissection near sympathetic chain.

Smoking is a risk factor for renal cell carcinoma. Patients may have coincident risk of CAD and COPD.

f) **Nephrectomy**

i) **Indication**

(1) Radical nephrectomy (includes ureter, often adrenal gland) is performed for neoplasms, usually renal cell carcinoma.

(2) Partial nephrectomy is sometimes done for smaller tumors, which spares nephron mass but often results in greater intraoperative blood loss.

CONCERNS IN SUBSPECIALTY ANESTHESIA

(3) Simple nephrectomy is performed for chronic infection, large stones, or transplant donors (1).

ii) **Preoperative evaluation**

(1) Smoking is a risk factor for renal cell carcinoma, so patients have high coincidence of CAD and COPD.

(2) Preoperative anemia and renal insufficiency are common. Renal cell carcinoma patients require preoperative staging.

(3) If the tumor extends into the inferior vena cava (IVC) or right atrium, partially or fully occlude the IVC; poor venous return and hypotension may occur.

iii) **Positioning**

(1) Lateral decubitus or supine position

iv) **Approach**

(1) Retroperitoneal or transperitoneal

(2) Open or laparoscopic

(3) If done laparoscopically with retroperitoneal approach, insufflation of CO_2 into retroperitoneum can track up above diaphragm.

v) **Monitoring and access**

(1) ASA standard monitors and temperature monitoring.

(2) Consider large-bore IVs and an arterial line as significant blood loss and large volume shifts occur.

(3) Central venous access may be necessary for central pressure monitoring as well as for rapid transfusion when necessary.

(4) Intraoperative transesophageal echocardiogram can be used for monitoring patients at risk for having tumor fragments embolize to the pulmonary circulation.

There is a risk of pneumothorax from diaphragmatic injury during nephrectomy.

vi) **Anesthetic technique**

(1) General anesthesia with muscle relaxation plus a thoracic epidural (usually T7-8 level) for intraop use and/or postop pain control should be used.

(2) In case the tumor extends intracardiac and occupies more than 40% of the right atrium, cardiopulmonary bypass may be used intraoperatively (1).

vii) **Complications**

(1) There is a risk of pneumothorax because of diaphragm injury (near superior pole of kidney).

(2) In renal cell carcinoma that involves IVC or right atrium, prepare for significant blood loss, impairment in venous return, possible need to clamp the IVC intraop, venous air embolism, pulmonary embolism of tumor or associated thrombus (2).

g) **Nephroureterectomy**

i) **Indication**

(1) For upper tract transitional cell tumors (e.g., ureter).

(2) Similar considerations as nephrectomy; however, this surgery also involves open component to resect ureteral insertion into bladder with a margin of bladder tissue.

ii) **Monitoring**

(1) ASA standard monitors and temperature monitoring

(2) Urine output may not be measurable when bladder is open.

iii) **Access**

(1) Consider large-bore IVs and an arterial line.

iv) **Anesthetic technique**

(1) General anesthesia with muscle relaxation plus a thoracic epidural (usually T7-8 level) for intraop use and/or postop pain control should be used.

h) **Orchiectomy**
    i) **Indication**
        (1) Testicular tumors most commonly diagnosed in men between the ages of 15 and 34.
    ii) **Preoperative evaluation**
        (1) Patients who have had neoadjuvant chemotherapy may have had bleomycin. Pulmonary function should be evaluated.
    iii) **Positioning**
        (1) Supine or lithotomy
        (2) The incision is usually similar to that for inguinal hernia repair.
    iv) **Anesthetic technique**
        (1) Spinal/epidural (a T9 sensory level is required) or general anesthesia is an acceptable anesthetic technique.
    v) **Complications**
        (1) Patients treated with bleomycin may be at greater risk of pulmonary complications, including oxygen toxicity (11).
        (2) Reflex bradycardia or nausea may occur from traction on the spermatic cord

i) **Laparoscopic surgery in urology**

READ MORE
Anesthesia for laparoscopic surgery, Chapter 133, page 927

    i) Laparoscopic surgery is used to perform traditionally open procedures like pelvic lymph node dissection radical prostatectomy, nephrectomy (radical or partial), cystectomy, pyeloplasty, and stone extraction.
    ii) Laparoscopic surgery reduces perioperative morbidity compared with similar open approaches and allows for better visualization of the operative site (12).
    iii) **Anesthetic considerations**
        (1) Similar to those for laparoscopic procedures in general surgery or gynecology
        (2) General anesthesia with endotracheal intubation and muscle relaxation is required to control ventilation in setting of pneumoperitoneum (13).

Subcutaneous emphysema can occur during laparoscopic surgery due to insufflation of CO_2 gas to create the pneumoperitoneum.

    iv) **Monitoring and access**
        (1) ASA standard monitors and temperature monitoring
        (2) Consider large-bore IVs and an arterial line as significant blood loss can occur during some of these procedures.
        (3) Central venous access is dependent on patient-related comorbidities.
    v) **Complications**
        (1) Related to pneumoperitoneum required during the procedure
        (2) Subcutaneous emphysema may extend all the way up to the head and neck, compromising the upper airway in the most severe cases (14).
        (3) Because of the prolonged duration of these procedures, a significant amount of carbon dioxide can be absorbed, causing marked acidosis (13).

j) **Extracorporeal shock wave lithotripsy (ESWL)**
    i) ESWL is the treatment of choice for disintegration of urinary stones in the kidney and upper part of the ureters.
    ii) Shock wave–induced cardiac arrhythmias previously reported in 10% to 14% of patients undergoing lithotripsy are now extremely rare (15).

 iii) Patients with a pacemaker or an internal cardiac defibrillator (ICD) are at risk for developing arrhythmias induced by shock waves during ESWL.

 iv) The internal components of pacemaker and ICD devices can be damaged during ESWL.

 v) Pregnancy and untreated bleeding disorders are contraindications to ESWL.

 vi) **Immersion** in a heated water bath may produce significant changes in the cardiovascular and respiratory systems.

  (1) Cardiovascular changes include hypotension (caused by vasodilation) and increase in central venous pressure and central venous volume (16).

  (2) Respiratory changes include a reduction in functional residual capacity, tidal volume, and vital capacity (17).

 vii) **Monitoring**

  (1) Electrocardiograph pads should be attached securely with waterproof dressing prior to immersion.

  (2) Synchronization of the shock waves to the R wave from the electrocardiogram (ECG) decreases the incidence of arrhythmias during ESWL. The shock waves are usually timed to be 20 ms after the R wave to correspond to the ventricular refractory period.

 viii) **Anesthetic technique**

  (1) General anesthesia and regional anesthesia (spinal, epidural, or flank infiltration with or without intercostal blocks)

 ix) **Complications**

  (1) Cardiac dysrhythmias, hematuria, ureteral colic, renal (subcapsular) hematoma, and severe pulmonary or intestinal damage

Chapter Summary for Anesthesia for Urologic Surgery

	Overview of Anesthetic Considerations
Radical Prostatectomy	Used for resection of large prostatic masses or tumors. Consider large-bore IV and arterial pressure monitoring in anticipation of blood loss for retropubic approach.
Transurethral Resection of the Prostate	Used for symptomatic benign prostatic hypertrophy. During the procedure, large amounts of irrigation solution are absorbed into the circulation and the periprostatic and the retroperitoneal spaces. Beware of TURP syndrome.
Cytoscopy	The most commonly performed urological procedure, used to diagnose and treat lesions of the lower (urethra, prostate, bladder) and upper (ureter, kidney) urinary tracts. Most cystoscopies are performed as an outpatient procedure.
Cystectomy	Radical cystectomy recommended for invasive bladder tumors (usually transitional cell). A procedure to divert the urinary tract is also needed. Consider large-bore IV and arterial pressure monitoring in anticipation of blood loss for retropubic approach.
Retroperitoneal Lymph Node Dissection	Used for advanced or recurrent testicular tumors. Prepare for significant blood loss.

(continued)

Chapter Summary for Anesthesia for Urologic Surgery (*Continued*)

	Overview of Anesthetic Considerations
Nephrectomy	Radical nephrectomy (includes ureter, often adrenal gland) is performed for neoplasms, usually renal cell carcinoma. Diaphragmatic injury during surgery may result in pneumothorax.
Nephroureterectomy	For upper tract transitional cell tumors (e.g., ureter). Involves open component to resect ureteral insertion into bladder with a margin of bladder tissue.
Orchiectomy	Used for testicular tumors most commonly diagnosed in men between the ages of 15 and 34. Risk of reflex bradycardia from traction on the spermatic cord.
Laparoscopic Surgery in Urology	Used to perform traditionally open procedures like pelvic lymph node dissection radical prostatectomy, nephrectomy (radical or partial), cystectomy, pyeloplasty, and stone extraction. Reduces perioperative morbidity compared with similar open approaches; allows for better visualization of the operative site.
Extracorporeal Shock Wave Lithotripsy	For disintegration of urinary stones in the kidney and upper part of the ureters. Patients with a pacemaker or an internal cardiac defibrillator (ICD) are at risk for developing arrhythmias induced by shock waves during ESWL. Immersion in a heated water bath produces significant changes in the cardiovascular and respiratory systems.

References

1. Whalley DG. Anesthesia for radical prostatectomy, cystectomy, nephrectomy, pheochromocytoma, and laparoscopic procedures. *Anesthesiol Clin North Am* 2000;18(4):899–917.
2. Jaffe R, Samuels SI. *Anesthesiologist's Manual of Surgical Procedures.* 4th ed. Philadelphia, PA: Lippincott Williams & Wilkins; 2009:857–902.
3. Malhotra V. Transurethral resection of the prostate. *Anesthesiol Clin N Am* 2000;18(4):883–897.
4. Hahn RG. Fluid absorption in endoscopic surgery. *Br J Anaesth* 2006;96(1):8–20.
5. Warner MA, Martin JT, Schroeder DR, et al. Lower-extremity motor neuropathy associated with surgery performed on patients in a lithotomy position. *Anesthesiology* 1994;81:6.
6. Hosking MP, Lobdell CM, Warner MA, et al. Anaesthesia for patients over 90 years of age. Outcomes after regional and general anaesthetic techniques for two common surgical procedures. *Anaesthesia* 1989;44:142.
7. Azar I. Transurethral prostatectomy syndrome and other complications of urological procedures. In: McLeskey CH, ed. *Geriatric Anaesthesiology.* Baltimore, MD: Williams & Wilkins; 1997:595–607.
8. Gravenstein D. Transuretheral resection of the prostate: a review of the pathophysiology and management. *Anesth Analg* 1997;84:438.
9. Balzarro M, Ficarra V, Bartoloni A, et al. The pathophysiology, diagnosis and therapy of the transurethral resection of the prostate syndrome. *Urol Int* 2001;66:121–126.
10. Brunner JE, Redmond JM, Haggar AM, et al. Central pontine myelinolysis and pontine lesions after rapid correction of hyponatremia: a prospective magnetic resonance imaging study. *Ann Neurol* 1990;27:61–66.
11. Mathes DD. Bleomycin and hyperoxia exposure in the operating room. *Anesth Analg* 1995;81:624.
12. Guillonneau B, Rozet F, Barret E, et al. Laparoscopic radical prostatectomy: assessment after 240 procedures. *Urol Clin North Am* 2001;28:189–202.
13. Weingram J, Sosa RE, Stein B, Poppas D. Subcutaneous emphysema (SCE) during laparoscopic pelvic lymph node dissection (LPLND). *Anesth Analg* 1993;76:S460.
14. Conacher ID, Soomro NA, Rix D. Anaesthesia for laparoscopic urological surgery. *Br J Anaesth* 2004;93(6):859–864.
15. Walts LF, Atlee JL. Supraventricular tachycardia associated with extracorporeal shock wave lithotripsy. *Anesthesiology* 1986;65:521–523.
16. Behnia R, Shanks CA, Ovassapian A, et al. Hemodynamic responses associated with lithotripsy. *Anesth Analg* 1987;66:354–356.
17. Bromage PR, Bonsu AK, El-Fagih SR, et al. Influence of Dornier HM3 system on respiration during ESWL. *Anesth Analg* 1989;68:363–367.

CONCERNS IN SUBSPECIALTY ANESTHESIA

135 Anesthesia for Orthopedic Surgery

Christie M. Sasso, MD • Danielle B. Ludwin, MD

Orthopedic surgical procedures range from short outpatient procedures (e.g., carpal tunnel) to long, complex cases with the potential for significant blood loss (e.g., revision total hip arthroplasty). Orthopedic procedures are often painful, so it is important to provide both surgical anesthesia and postoperative analgesia. This chapter discusses anesthetic considerations for orthopedic surgical procedures, including potential complications and postoperative rehabilitation.

1) **Overview**

a) Orthopedics is a branch of surgery involving conditions affecting the musculoskeletal system.

  i) A wide range of surgical procedures encompass orthopedic practice, from carpal tunnel release surgeries to complex spinal fusion and laminectomy surgeries.

b) The goals of anesthesia for orthopedic surgery include:

  i) **Surgical anesthesia.** Anesthetic techniques must be adequate to provide optimal surgical operating conditions (see Table 135-1).

    (1) Appropriate depth of anesthesia

    (2) Adequate pain control

    (3) General anesthesia, neuraxial anesthesia, peripheral nerve blocks, or a combination can be used.

The goals of orthopedic surgery are to provide surgical anesthesia, postoperative analgesia, optimize surgical exposure, and prevent stretch or compression nerve injuries.

  ii) **Postoperative analgesia.** Many patients will have significant pain after orthopedic surgeries and a plan for postoperative analgesia should be carefully considered.

    (1) Peripheral nerve blockade with or without catheter

    (2) Opioids for breakthrough pain

    (3) NSAIDs and adjuvant analgesic medications

  iii) **Optimize surgical exposure.** Neuromuscular blockade or neuraxial anesthesia or peripheral nerve block is often required to facilitate optimal surgical exposure for orthopedic surgeries because they involve manipulation of the musculoskeletal system.

  iv) **Prevent stretch/compression nerve injuries.** Orthopedic surgeries can require the lateral, prone, or beach chair position; therefore, careful patient positioning is important to prevent injuries.

READ MORE

Local anesthetics, Chapter 37, page 282

Overview of peripheral nerve blocks, Chapter 34, page 256

2) **Local anesthetics in regional anesthesia**

a) Short- (chloroprocaine, lidocaine), intermediate- (mepivacaine), or long-acting (ropivacaine, bupivacaine) local anesthetics can be used for peripheral nerve blockade or neuraxial blockade depending on the duration of the procedure and the anticipated postoperative pain.

b) Most peripheral nerve blocks are done with 20 to 40 mL of local anesthetic.

c) The ideal spinal anesthetic for ambulatory surgery is controversial.

i)   Lidocaine has a 20% to 30% incidence of transient neurologic syndrome (TNS) especially when used for cases in the lithotomy position.

ii) Mepivacaine has approximately a 6% TNS incidence (4).

iii) Chloroprocaine has been used off-label for spinal anesthesia (5).

d) Care should be taken for patients receiving a combination of anesthetic techniques in regard to local anesthetic toxicity (Table 135-1).

3) **Upper extremity surgery**—Shoulder, elbow, hand surgery (see Table 135-2)

a) Anesthetic considerations: Upper extremity surgery: peripheral nerve block with or without general anesthesia is often used.

i)   Surgery to the proximal arm may limit access to the airway. If the patient has received a regional anesthetic and airway obstruction is a concern, securing the airway with an LMA or an ETT at the beginning of the case may be prudent.

ii) Placement of an IV line and NIBP on the nonoperative arm may interfere with infusions or fluid administration; therefore, consideration should be given to placement of a lower extremity IV.

iii) For patients with comorbidities such as morbid obesity and significant coronary artery disease, invasive BP monitoring may be beneficial.

b) Shoulder surgery

i)   Positioning—"Beach chair" or lateral position is often used. The patient's neck should be maintained in a neutral position.

(1) Bezold-Jarish reflex—Profound hypotension and bradycardia can present in the beach chair position after interscalene block or with general anesthesia.

(a) Pretreatment with β-adrenergic antagonists and vagolytics has been shown to prevent this reflex (6).

(b) Treat with small doses of epinephrine (10 to 100 μg).

(2) Maintenance of cerebral perfusion pressure (CPP) in the beach chair position is critical. CPP is the net perfusion pressure causing blood to flow to the brain (CPP = MAP – ICP or CVP), whichever is greater). There have been case reports of cerebral ischemia in this position (7) as the brain

---

For upper extremity surgery, if the patient has received a regional anesthetic and airway obstruction is a concern, securing the airway with an LMA or an ETT at the beginning of the case may be prudent.

READ MORE

Invasive arterial blood pressure monitoring, Chapter 11, page 70

Anesthesia for intracranial and neurovascular procedures, Chapter 139, page 979

Table 135-1

Benefits/Risks/Considerations for Regional Anesthesia (1,2,3)

Benefits	• ↓Risk of deep venous thrombosis; pulmonary embolism; transfusion; pneumonia; myocardial infarction; renal failure; ileus • May improve postoperative cognitive function
Risks	• Nerve damage • Bleeding risk • Infection risk • Partial/failed block
Additional considerations	• Site for nerve blockade should be assessed preoperatively. • A thorough history and physical exam should be documented. • If there are pre-existing neurologic deficits, risk-benefit ratio should be carefully considered. • Postsurgical therapy goals

CONCERNS IN SUBSPECIALTY ANESTHESIA

Table 135-2

Regional Anesthetic Techniques for Upper Extremity Surgery

Brachial Plexus Technique	Level of Blockade	Peripheral Nerves Blocked	Surgical Applications	Comments
Axillary	Peripheral nerve	Radial, ulnar, median; musculocutaneous unreliably blocked	Surgery to forearm and hand, less used for procedures about the elbow	Unsuitable for proximal humerus or shoulder surgery; patient must be able to abduct the arm to perform
Infraclavicular	Cords	Radial, ulnar, median, musculocutaneous, axillary	Surgery to elbow, forearm, and hand	Catheter site (near coracoid process) easy to maintain; no risk of hemo-, pneumothorax
Supraclavicular	Distal trunk-proximal cord	Radial, ulnar, median, musculocutaneous, axillary	Surgery to mid-humerus, elbow, forearm, and hand	Risk of pneumothorax, unsuitable for outpatient procedures; phrenic nerve paresis in 30% of cases
Interscalene	Upper and middle trunks	Entire brachial plexus, although inferior trunk (ulnar nerve) not blocked in 15%–20% of cases	Surgery to shoulder, proximal/middle humerus	Phrenic nerve paresis in 100% of patients for block duration; unsuitable for patients unable to tolerate 25% reduction in pulmonary function

Duration of block performed with long-acting local anesthetic (bupivacaine or ropivacaine) is 12 to 20 hours; intermediate-acting agents (lidocaine or mepivacaine) will resolve after 4 to 6 hours.

Reproduced from Horlocker TT, Wedel DJ. Anesthesia for orthopaedic surgery. In: Barash PG, Cullen BF, Stoelting RK, et al., eds. *Clinical Anesthesia.* 6th ed. Philadelphia, PA: Lippincott Williams & Wilkins; 2009:1375–1392, with permission.

Maintenance of cerebral perfusion pressure in the beach chair position is critical.

is 20 to 30 cm higher than at the site of BP measurement; thus, the blood pressure is lower in the brain than in the arm. CPP can be maintained with fluids and vasopressors as needed.

c) Hand and elbow surgery

   i) Positioning—Typically, the supine position is used. Occasionally, the patient may be lateral or prone.

   ii) See Table 135-2 for commonly placed peripheral nerve blocks.

   iii) Digital blocks—For distal extremity surgery, digital blocks that block the terminal branch of a nerve can be done by the surgeon or the anesthesiologist.

   iv) Bier block—This is an intravenous regional technique that provides complete anesthesia to an extremity distal to the tourniquet site. It is used in cases of <1.5 to 2 hours (8).

     (1) An IV is inserted into the operative extremity. Another IV on the nonoperative side should also be placed for routine fluid and drug administration.

     (2) A proximal and distal pneumatic tourniquet with alarms is placed on the operative extremity.

     (3) The operative extremity is raised for at least 1 minute to allow for passive exsanguination.

Bupivacaine is contraindicated in a Bier Block due to its cardiotoxic properties if it were inadvertently released systemically.

Do not use epinephrine in a Bier Block because of risk of IV injection; it is contraindicated in distal extremities due to risk of vasoconstriction causing nerve ischemia.

(4) An Esmarch bandage is then wrapped from the distal part of the extremity until the tourniquet site to further exsanguinate the extremity.

(5) The proximal tourniquet is then inflated typically to 100 mm Hg greater than the systolic blood pressure.

(6) Once the tourniquet is adequately inflated, the Esmarch is released.

(7) Local anesthetic, typically lidocaine, is injected into the IV of the operative extremity.

(8) The local anesthetic will diffuse from the bloodstream to anesthetize the surrounding nerves.

(9) If the patient begins to complain of tourniquet pain, inflate the distal tourniquet and then deflate the proximal tourniquet.

(10) The tourniquets cannot be deflated until at least 30 minutes after injection of the local anesthetic for risk of local anesthetic toxicity.

(11) A 2-stage deflation of the cuff can be done by deflating for 10 seconds and then reinflating for 1 minute to slow the washout of the local anesthetic from the extremity.

4) Lower extremity surgery—hip, knee, ankle, and foot surgery (Table 135-3).

   a) **Hip surgery**

Table 135-3
Lumbosacral Techniques for Major Lower Extremity Surgery

Peripheral Technique	Area of Blockade	Duration of Blockade	Perioperative Outcomes
Lumbar plexus femoral	Femoral, partial lateral femoral cutaneous, and obturator	12–18 h	Improved analgesia and joint range of motion, decreased hospital stay compared with PCA; fewer technical problems, less urinary retention, and hypotension than epidural analgesia (TKA)
Fascia iliaca	Femoral, partial lateral femoral cutaneous, obturator, and sciatic (S1)		Improved analgesia and joint range of motion compared with PCA (TKA)
Psoas compartment	Complete lumbar plexus; occasional spread to sacral plexus or neuraxis		Reduced morphine consumption, pain at rest compared with PCA (TKA, THA); reduced blood loss (THA); analgesia equivalent to continuous femoral block (TKA)
Sciatic	Posterior thigh and leg (except saphenous area)	18–30 h	Supplemental sciatic required (TKA); proximal approaches allow block of posterior femoral cutaneous nerve (TKA)

PCA, patient-controlled analgesia; TKA, total knee arthroplasty; THA, total hip arthroplasty.
Duration of block performed with long-acting local anesthetic (bupivacaine or ropivacaine); intermediate-acting agents (lidocaine or mepivacaine) will resolve after 4 to 6 hours.
Outcomes most marked in patients who receive a continuous lumbar plexus catheter with infusion of 0.1% to 0.2% bupivacaine or ropivacaine at 6 to 12 mL/h for 48 to 72 h.
Reproduced from Horlocker TT. Anesthesia and pain management, Revision Hip and Knee Arthroplasty. Edited by Berry DJ, Trousdale RT, Dennis D, et al. 2008 Philadelphia, Lippincott Williams & Wilkins, with permission.

CONCERNS IN SUBSPECIALTY ANESTHESIA

i) **Hip fracture**

(1) Preoperative considerations

Patients undergoing lower extremity surgery often have functional limitations secondary to pain that can make assessing their exercise tolerance difficult and may require further cardiac workup prior to surgical interventions.

   (a) Consider the etiology of the fracture/fall and associated risks and comorbidities, for example, mechanical fall versus cardiac or neurologic cause that may require further workup (i.e., carotid duplex ultrasound, echocardiogram).

   (b) Delaying surgery for cardiac evaluation is an independent risk factor of postoperative complication, irrespective of the patient's medical status (9).

   (c) Patients are often elderly.
      (i) They may have extensive comorbidities such as severe coronary artery disease, pulmonary disease, and renal disease.
      (ii) They can be hypovolemic from prolonged NPO status or diuretic use that may require aggressive fluid resuscitation and slow titration of anesthetics.
      (iii) Fluid administration should be done cautiously in patients with impaired left ventricular function.

(2) Intraoperative considerations/anesthetic techniques

   (a) Supine or lateral position.

   (b) Neuraxial anesthesia, lumbar plexus block, or general anesthesia.
      (i) Neuraxial anesthesia is typically preferred in patients with concomitant cardiopulmonary disease (see Table 135-1).
      (ii) General anesthesia is often preferable for patients unable to cooperate for neuraxial anesthesia and anticoagulated patients who require emergent surgery.

Hip fracture patients are at high risk for perioperative thromboembolic events.

   (c) A preoperative femoral nerve or a fascia iliaca compartment block can be helpful in decreasing perioperative opioid requirements as well as for positioning for a neuraxial anesthetic (10,11).

   (d) Invasive blood pressure monitoring will depend on patient comorbidities such as extensive coronary artery disease or need for frequent blood sampling.

(3) Postoperative considerations

   (a) Patients are at high risk for thromboembolic complications

   (b) Patients often receive compression stocking and thromboprophylaxis medications (e.g., LMWH, Coumadin).

ii) **Total hip arthroplasty**

(1) Intraoperative considerations

   (a) Commonly performed in the lateral position.

   (b) Anesthetic options include neuraxial or general anesthesia with/without a lumbar plexus block for postoperative analgesia.

   (c) Deliberate hypotension may be requested by the surgeon to decrease blood loss and improve surgical exposure.
      (i) Deliberate hypotension is a technique using neuraxial anesthesia, general anesthesia, or IV agents (antihypertensives such as labetalol, nicardipine, or IV sedatives like propofol) to intentionally decrease BP to a MAP of 50 to 65 mm Hg.
      (ii) The acceptable decrease in BP is controversial due to concerns of hypoperfusion and ischemia to vital organs. Benefits and risks must be weighed for each patient and patients with chronic hypertension may be at higher risk for ischemia (12,13).

The acceptable decrease in BP using deliberate hypotension is controversial due to concerns of hypoperfusion and ischemia to vital organs.

b) **Knee surgery**
   i) **Total knee arthoplasty**
      (1) Intraoperative considerations
         (a) Supine position
         (b) Anesthetic options: Neuraxial anesthesia, femoral and sciatic nerve block, general anesthesia, or a combination of the above
      (2) Postoperative analgesia
         (a) Epidural, spinal opioids, femoral block/catheter, sciatic block/catheter
   ii) **Knee arthroscopy/ACL reconstruction**
      (1) Intraoperative considerations
         (a) Anesthetic options: Spinal, femoral and sciatic nerve block, general anesthesia, local and MAC
      (2) Postoperative analgesia
         (a) Spinal opioids, femoral block/catheter, intra-articular opioids, local anesthetic infiltration
c) **Foot and ankle surgery** (Table 135-4)
   i) Intraoperative considerations
      (1) Anesthetic options: Neuraxial anesthesia versus general anesthesia.
   ii) Postoperative analgesia
      (1) Femoral with/without saphenous nerve block, popliteal nerve block, or ankle block.
5) **Complications**
   a) **Fat embolus syndrome**
      i) Definition: The triad of pulmonary distress, mental status changes, and petechial rash 24 to 48 hours after a pelvic or a long-bone fracture.

Table 135-4

Anesthetic Techniques for Common Foot and Ankle Operations

	Surgical Procedure	Regional Technique	Comments
Forefoot	Hallux valgus	Metatarsal, ankle, popliteal blockade	Sural nerve block not necessary for surgery.
	Amputations	Ankle, popliteal blockade	Popliteal blockade is the technique of choice in the presence of infection or swelling
Midfoot	Transmetatarsal amputations	Popliteal, ankle blockade	
Hindfoot	Ankle arthroscopy	Spinal, epidural, or general anesthesia	Operation typically requires good muscle relaxation for manipulation; thigh tourniquet
	Achilles tendon repair	Spinal, epidural, or popliteal blockade	Spinal or epidural anesthesia whenever thigh tourniquet is required
	Triple arthrodesis	Spinal or epidural	Neuraxial technique preferred for bone graft harvesting; popliteal blockade for postoperative analgesia

Femoral or saphenous block required if the incision extends to the medial aspect of the foot or ankle.
Reproduced from Horlocker TT, Wedel DJ. Anesthesia for orthopaedic surgery. In: Barash PG, Cullen BF, Stoelting RK, et al., eds. *Clinical Anesthesia*. 6th ed. Philadelphia, PA: Lippincott Williams & Wilkins; 2009:1375–1392, with permission.

     ii) Signs and symptoms fall into major and minor criteria and are summarized in Table 135-5.

     iii) Treatment is supportive. Fluids and vasopressors should be used as needed to maintain hemodynamics.

   b) **Bone cement implantation syndrome**

     i) Definition: This syndrome is characterized by hypoxia, hypotension, and/or unexpected loss of consciousness occurring around the time of cementation, prosthesis insertion, reduction of the joint or, occasionally, during limb tourniquet deflation in a patient who has received cement.

     ii) Bone cement is used for arthroplasty (joint replacement surgery).

     iii) This can cause sudden hypotension, hypoxemia.

     iv) Treatment includes hydration, vasopressors, 100% FiO_2 (stop N_2O before methylmethacrylate is inserted) (14)

   c) **Thromboembolic events**—Orthopedic patients are at high risk of thromboembolic events such as deep vein thrombosis and pulmonary embolism.

READ MORE

Deep-Vein thrombosis and pulmonary embolism, Chapter 65, page 470

     i) **DVT prophylaxis** should be initiated in every patient.

       (1) Prophylaxis can range from encouraging ambulation, to compression stockings to pharmacological thromboprophylaxis.

     ii) The decision to perform neuraxial anesthesia in patients on anticoagulants should be based on the risks and benefits for each individual patient.

   d) Importantly, regional anesthesia techniques have been shown to decrease the risk of DVT and PE in patients who were not receiving pharmacologic prophylaxis (15).

   e) **Tourniquets** are often used in distal extremity surgery.

     i) A tourniquet is a pressure cuff that is inflated on the operative limb, proximal to the surgical site. Inflation of a tourniquet prevents blood flow to the limb and enables the surgeons to work in a bloodless field.

Tourniquet release leads to a transient metabolic acidosis often with an increase in $ETCO_2$, hypotension, and tachycardia.

     ii) Prolonged tourniquet times typically are defined as >2 hours for the lower extremity and 90 minutes for the upper extremity and may result in permanent injury to muscles, vessels, and nerves.

     iii) Tourniquet pain is believed to involve type C pain fibers (16).

     iv) Tourniquet release leads to a transient metabolic acidosis often with an increase in $ETCO_2$, hypotension, and tachycardia.

Table 135-5

Signs and Symptoms of Fat Embolus Syndrome (17)

Major Criteria	Hypoxemia CNS depression Pulmonary edema Subconjunctival/axillary petechiae
Minor Criteria	Tachycardia Hypothermia Retinal fat emboli Urinary fat globules Anemia Thrombocytopenia Increased erythrocyte sedimentation rate Sputum fat globules

The ideal postoperative regional technique would provide prolonged sensory blockade with intact motor function.

v) Tourniquet pain is best treated with release of the tourniquet. If it is not surgically possible to release the tourniquet, the anesthetic can be deepened.

f) **Peripheral nerve injury** can occur due to a peripheral nerve block or the surgical procedure or be a complication from improper patient positioning.

g) **Comorbid conditions**

i) Patients with rheumatoid arthritis may have associated musculoskeletal, pulmonary, and cardiac complications in addition to cricoarytenoid arthritis and cervical spine instability requiring extra precautions.

6) **Postoperative considerations**

a) Early mobilization is advantageous to improve rehabilitation.

b) Lower extremity peripheral nerve blockade can allow patients to participate more fully in physical therapy.

c) This benefit must be weighed against the possibility of fall risk in a patient with a dense block.

Chapter Summary for Anesthesia for Orthopedic Surgery

Definition	Orthopedics is a branch of surgery involving conditions affecting the musculoskeletal system. A wide range of surgical procedures encompass orthopedic practice, from carpal tunnel release surgeries to complex spinal fusion and laminectomy surgeries.
Preoperative Considerations	In patients with pre-existing neurologic deficits, the risk-benefit ratio of peripheral or central neuraxial blockade must be considered.
Intraoperative Considerations	Since orthopedic procedures are frequently painful, orthopedic anesthesia should provide surgical anesthesia and postoperative analgesia. Regional anesthesia is often used to attain these goals. Patient positioning should optimize surgical exposure and prevent stretch/compression nerve injuries.
Postoperative Considerations	Orthopedic patients are at high risk for thromboembolic events. DVT prophylaxis should be initiated in every patient.

References

1. Wu CL, Fleisher LA. Outcomes research in regional anesthesia and analgesia. *Anesth Analg* 2000;91:1232–1242.
2. Hebl, JR. Ultrasound guided regional anesthesia and the prevention of neurologic injury: fact or fiction. *Anesthesiology* 2008;108:186–188.
3. Neal JM, Bernards CM, Hadzic A, et al. ASRA practice advisory on neurologic complications in regional anesthesia and pain medicine. *Reg Anes Pain Med* 2008;33:404–415.
4. YaDeau JT, Liguori GA, Zayas VM, et al. The incidence of transient neurologic symptoms after spinal anesthesia with mepivacaine. *Anesth Analg* 2005;101:661–665.
5. Yoos JR, Kopacz DJ. Spinal 2-chloroprocaine for surgery: an initial 10-month experience. *Anesth Analg* 2005;100:553–558.
6. Liguori GA, Kahn RL, Gordon J, et al. The use of metoprolol and glycopyrrolate to prevent hypotensive/bradycardic events during shoulder arthroscopy in the sitting position under interscalene block. *Anesth Analg* 1998;87:1320–1325.
7. Cullen DJ, Kirby RR. Beach chair position may decrease cerebral perfusion: catastrophic outcomes have occurred. *APSF Newsletter* 2007;22(2):25–27.
8. Van Zundert A, Hemstadter A, Goerig M, et al. Centennial of intravenous regional anesthesia. Bier's Block (1908–2008). *Reg Anesth Pain Med* 2008;33:483–489.
9. Cluett J, Caplan J, Yu W. Preoperative cardiac evaluation of patients with acute hip fracture. *Am J Orthop* 2008;37(1):32–36.

CONCERNS IN SUBSPECIALTY ANESTHESIA

10. Pedersen SJ, Borgbjerg FM, Schousboe B, et al. A comprehensive hip fracture program reduces complication rates and mortality. *J Am Geriatr Soc* 2008;56:1831–1838.

11. Parker MJ, Griffiths R, Appadu B. Nerve blocks for hip fractures (review). *Cochrane Datab Syst Rev* 2002;1.

12. Sharrock NE, Bading B, Mineo R, et al. Deliberate hypotensive epidural anesthesia for patients with normal and low cardiac output. *Anesth Analg* 1994;79:899–904.

13. Williams-Russo P, Sharrock NE, Mattis S, et al. Randomized trial of hypotensive epidural anesthesia in older adults. *Anesth* 1999;91:926–935.

14. Donaldson AJ, Thomson HE, Harper NJ, et al. Bone cement implantation syndrome. *Br J Anaesth* 2009;102(1):12–22.

15. Modig J, Borg T, Karlstrom G, et al. Thromboembolism after total hip replacement. *Anesth Analg* 1983;62:174–180.

16. Concepcion, MA, Lambert DH, Welch KH, et al. Tourniquet pain during spinal anesthesia. *Anesth Analg* 1988;67:828–832.

17. Horlocker TT, Wedel DJ. Anesthesia for orthopaedic surgery. In: Barash PG, Cullen BF, Stoelting RK, et al., eds. *Clinical Anesthesia*. 6th ed. Philadelphia, PA: Lippincott Williams & Wilkins; 2009:1375–1392.

Suggested Readings

Horlocker TT, Wedel DJ. Anesthesia for orthopaedic surgery. In: Barash PG, Cullen BF, Stoelting RK, et al., eds. *Clinical Anesthesia*. 6th ed. Philadelphia, PA: Lippincott Williams & Wilkins; 2009:1375–1392.

Neal JM, Gerancher JC, Hebl JR, et al. Upper extremity regional anesthesia: essentials of our current understanding. *Reg Anes Pain Med* 2008;34(2):134–170.

Enneking KF, Chan V, Greger J, et al. Lower extremity peripheral nerve blockade: essentials of our current understanding. *Reg Anes Pain Med* 2005;30(1):4–35.

136 Anesthesia for Eye Surgery

Brian M. Davidson, MD

Surgery involving the eyes is common and presents unique challenges for the anesthesiologist. Avoiding anesthesia-related increases in **intraocular pressure (IOP)**, management of systemic side effects of **ophthalmic medications**, and mitigating the **oculocardiac reflex (OCR)** are important anesthesia concepts for eye surgery. Patients will experience improved surgical outcomes when the anesthesiologist recognizes and properly manages the challenges unique to eye surgery (1).

1) Ocular physiology
   a) **IOP** is the pressure within the rigid globe of the eye.
   b) **Increases in IOP**
      i) Increased IOP may result in extrusion of vitreous humor in the situations such as an open globe during a surgical procedure or trauma.
      ii) Increased IOP may result from increases in arterial BP, central or local venous pressure, and local external pressure increases on the eye (1).
   c) **Anesthesia events/procedures that may increase IOP**
      i) Direct laryngoscopy and intubation
      ii) High ventilation pressures—both endotracheal and mask
      iii) Trendelenburg position
2) **Anesthetics and IOP**
   a) Most anesthetic agents (volatiles, opiates, induction agents, benzodiazepines) **reduce IOP.**
      i) Mechanism
         (1) A combination of decreases in systemic vascular pressures, muscle relaxation (extraocular), and pupillary constriction ($\uparrow$ aqueous outflow).
   b) **Ketamine**
      i) **May increase IOP** due to its sympathomimetic effects and tendency to raise BP
      ii) Lacks muscle relaxation properties
   c) **Succinylcholine**
      i) **May increase IOP** via depolarization of extraocular muscles
      ii) The effect may last up to 10 minutes
      iii) Relatively contraindicated for induction in open globe trauma or in patients with known increases in IOP.
      iv) Anesthesia providers must use clinical judgment when weighing the risk of increased IOP versus the risk of aspiration and hypoxia in patients requiring rapid sequence induction (RSI) or with known or potential difficult airways (2).
   d) **Nondepolarizing muscle relaxants do not increase IOP**

3) **Anticholinergic medications**
   a) Topical anticholinergics cause pupil dilation (mydriasis) and may precipitate closed-angle glaucoma.
   b) Systemic atropine and glycopyrolate are not associated with ↑IOP (1).

4) **Oculocardiac reflex**
   a) Results from **traction** on the eye or **extraocular muscles.**
   b) **Signs and symptoms**
      i) **Bradycardia**, junctional rhythm, ventricular ectopy, or asystole
      ii) Awake patients may experience nausea or somnolence.
   c) OCR involves the ophthalmic **trigeminal (V')** **afferent** and **vagal (X)** **efferent** pathway (1).
   d) More common in pediatric patients undergoing **strabismus surgery.**
   e) **Prevention and treatment (Table 136-1)**
      i) Administer anticholinergic drugs such as **atropine (10 μg/kg)** or **glycopyrolate (4 μg/kg).**
         (1) Use with caution in patients with coronary artery disease.
         (2) Care should also be taken when using atropine in elderly patients due to CNS effects.
         (3) The rapid onset of atropine may make it the medication of choice in dire clinical situations (1).

5) **Systemic effects of ophthalmic medications**
   a) Topical medications
      i) Used frequently and absorbed into the body through blood vessels in the eye.
      ii) Rate of absorption is slower than IV but faster than subcutaneous route of administration.
         (1) **Echothiophate:** Irreversible cholinesterase inhibitor for treatment of glaucoma.
            (a) Side effects may include blurred vision, headache, eye erythema, and local or systemic allergic reaction.
         (2) **Epinephrine:** Topical drops used to reduce bleeding in topical ophthalmic procedures
            (a) May cause tachycardia, hypertension, and dysrhythmias in patients with and without a previous cardiac history.
         (3) **Timolol:** β-Adrenergic antagonist used to lower IOP by reducing aqueous humor production
            (a) Rare reports of hypotension, bradycardia, and bronchospasm

The OCR pathway may be easily remembered as the "five and dime" reflex because it involves cranial nerves (CNs) V and X.

Nitrous oxide administration during retinal surgery can cause **gas bubble expansion and ↑IOP** secondary to the agent's increased blood solubility.

Table 136-1

Management of the Oculocardiac Reflex (OCR)

Immediate management of cardiac symptoms resulting from OCR
1. **Cease** surgical traction or stimulation.
2. **Evaluate** vital signs and depth of anesthesia.
3. **Give** atropine 10 mg/kg IV if patient is unstable or reflex persists.
4. **Recurring** reflex symptoms may be managed with further anticholinergic doses or local anesthesia injection into the extraocular muscles by surgeon.

6) Intraocular gas expansion
   a) Gas bubble may be placed by ophthalmologist into posterior chamber to **aid repair of a detached retina.**
      i) **Avoid nitrous oxide** for the entire case or within 10 minutes of any gas bubble insertion.
   b) Sulfur hexafluoride (SF6) may be used for the bubble owing to its lower solubility and prolonged therapeutic effect (1).
      i) SF6 bubble will increase in size naturally and stay in place up to 10 days.
7) **Anesthesia for eye surgery. General, regional, and topical anesthesia approaches are available for ophthalmic surgery patients.**
   a) **Preoperative considerations**
      i) Patient undergoing many eye procedures may be older and have significant systemic medical conditions.
      ii) The ophthalmic surgery patient is more likely to have cardiac, respiratory, endocrine, and orthopedic pathology.
      iii) Appropriate preoperative testing and evaluation should occur in these patients even though the inherent risk of most ophthalmic procedures is low.
      iv) The patients' ability to cooperate and remain still in the supine position must be confirmed before sedation is considered for the anesthetic plan.

When considering sedation for eye surgery, carefully assess the patient's ability to lie still while supine.

   b) **Intraoperative considerations**
      i) Airway access may be limited as the patient's head is usually 90 to 180 degrees from the anesthesiologist
      ii) Standard ASA monitoring requirements apply. Consider special monitors based on the patient's medical history and condition.
      iii) **General anesthesia**
         (1) Indicated for more invasive procedures and uncooperative patients
         (2) Choice of induction technique is based on patient's general medical condition.
            (a) Trauma patients may require RSI without the use of succinylcholine (2).
            (b) Succinylcholine avoidance with open globe injuries has been suggested as it may increase IOP and result in extravasation of ocular contents. Although clinical evidence supporting such avoidance is very limited, succinylcholine has been used successfully in open globe injuries in patients requiring RSI (2).
            (c) Hypoxia and hypercarbia also greatly increase IOP, making a failed airway an equally problematic situation.
         (3) **Patients with traumatic rupture (an open globe) require special care**
            (a) IOP must be controlled during induction and maintenance of anesthesia in order to prevent extrusion of vitreous.
            (b) Deep anesthesia should be maintained to prevent increases in IOP.
            (c) Paralysis to prevent movement should be strongly considered.
            (d) Hemodynamic control is essential
            (e) Smooth extubation plan is necessary to avoid valsalva from coughing.

Oral RAE tubes are useful for eye cases requiring general anesthesia by providing greater surgical field access and less likelihood of tube obstruction/kinking.

CONCERNS IN SUBSPECIALTY ANESTHESIA

(i) Consider extubating the patient under deep anesthesia (contraindicated with difficult airway or full stomach).

(ii) Lidocaine 1.5 mg/kg 2 minutes prior to extubation may reduce laryngeal responsiveness and facilitate extubation.

(iii) Remifentanil (0.025 to 0.1 µg/kg/min) infusion may also be used to provide a smooth emergence with reduced coughing.

PONV after eye surgery is common and can be dangerous due to potential increases in IOP.

iv) **Regional and topical anesthesia** (see below for techniques)

(1) Most common technique for nontraumatic eye surgeries

(2) Sedation must be kept to a minimum for ophthalmic surgery because **patient cooperation and stillness** are necessary for most of the intraoperative period (1).

(a) Short periods of heavier sedation are appropriate for placement of regional blocks (3).

c) **Postoperative considerations**

i) Postoperative nausea and vomiting (PONV)

(1) Valsalva with vomiting can ↑IOP

(2) Adequate antiemetic medication should be given.

(3) PONV is very common after strabismus surgery.

ii) Adequate pain control

(1) Important because increased pain can lead to increased BP and ↑IOP

8) **Regional and local techniques for eye surgery (Fig. 136-1)**

a) **Retrobulbar block**

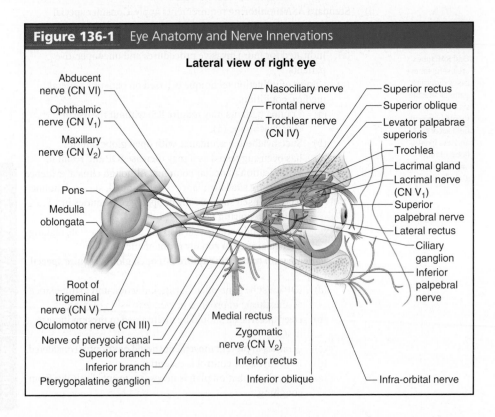

Figure 136-1   Eye Anatomy and Nerve Innervations

Lateral view of right eye

Abducent nerve (CN VI)
Ophthalmic nerve (CN V₁)
Maxillary nerve (CN V₂)
Pons
Medulla oblongata
Root of trigeminal nerve (CN V)
Oculomotor nerve (CN III)
Nerve of pterygoid canal
Superior branch
Inferior branch
Pterygopalatine ganglion

Nasociliary nerve
Frontal nerve
Trochlear nerve (CN IV)
Medial rectus
Zygomatic nerve (CN V₂)
Inferior rectus
Inferior oblique

Superior rectus
Superior oblique
Levator palpabrae superioris
Trochlea
Lacrimal gland
Lacrimal nerve (CN V₁)
Superior palpebral nerve
Lateral rectus
Ciliary ganglion
Inferior palpebral nerve
Infra-orbital nerve

Inadvertent CNS injection during retrobulbar block may cause seizures, apnea, and cardiovascular collapse.

    i)   Local anesthetic is injected behind the operative eye via the lateral third of the lower eyelid.

    ii) A **3.5-cm, 25-gauge needle** is advanced along the floor of the orbit toward the cone formed by the convergence of the extraocular muscles.

    iii) 2.5 mL of local anesthetic (lidocaine or bupivicaine common) *without* epinephrine is injected after **negative aspiration to avoid intravascular or intracranial injection.**

    iv) A successful block provides anesthesia, akinesia, and blockage of the OCR.

    v) Hyaluronidase is added to improve block spread by increasing connective tissue permeability of local anesthetic.

    vi) Complications
- (1) Retrobulbar hemorrhage, globe trauma, optic nerve damage, and systemic/CNS injection of local anesthetics
- (2) **Systemic/CNS injection of local anesthetic may induce seizure, obtundation, apnea, or cardiovascular collapse due to the anatomic continuity between the optic nerve and the CNS (1).**
  - (a) Prompt and aggressive supportive care is necessary for the duration of the local anesthetic.

b) **Peribulbar block (sub-tenon block)**

    i)   Less invasive and more common than retrobulbar block.

    ii) Injection of 0.5 mL of local anesthetic into superior quadrant of subconjunctiva along the sub-Tenon space.

    iii) Not appropriate for anterior chamber surgery.

    iv) Complications include localized bleeding, infection, and eyelid droop.

c) **Topical anesthesia**

    i)   Anesthetic eye drops, such as oxybuprocaine and tetracaine, are applied preoperatively at 5-minute intervals for five applications.

    ii) Anesthetic gel is later applied with a swab to upper and lower conjunctival sacs.

    iii) Common for cataract and other minor **anterior chamber surgery**

    iv) Complications include corneal abrasion and toxic keratopathy.

d) **Facial nerve block**

    i)   It prevents eyelid squinting during surgery and allows placement of lid speculums.

    ii) Multiple techniques are utilized depending on the location and requirements of the surgical procedure (4).
- (1) Examples include lacrimal, zygomatic, supraorbital, supratrochlear, infratrochlear, and infraorbital nerve blocks.

    iii) Complications include local hemorrhage and block failure.

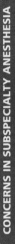

CONCERNS IN SUBSPECIALTY ANESTHESIA

Chapter Summary for Eye Surgery

Management Considerations	Control of IOP, Eye medications, OCR, Patient comorbidities
Effects of Anesthesia on IOP	↑ = intubation, mask ventilation, ketamine, succinylcholine, N_2O with gas bubble for retinal surgery ↓ = volatiles/benzos/opiates ↔ = Nondepolarizing NMBAs
OCR	Caused by traction on eye muscles Mediated by cranial nerves V and X Symptoms: ↓HR, bradyarrhythmias, asystole, nausea Treatment: Cease, Evaluate, Atropine!
Operative Considerations	Sedation, regional, vs. general Prolonged supine position requires patient cooperation/stillness Minimal airway access, RSI has a risk of increasing IOP
Regional Anesthesia	Local/topical, peribulbar, retrobulbar, facial blocks
Open Globe	General: RSI with succinylcholine may ↑IOP, avoid valsalva, smooth emergence

IOP, intraocular pressure; RSI, rapid sequence induction; OCR, oculocardiac reflex; NMBAs, nondepolarizing neuromuscular blocking agents; HR, heart rate.

References

1. McGoldrick K, Gayer S. Anesthesia and the eye. In: Barash P, Cullen B, Stoelting R, et al., eds. *Clinical Anesthesia*. 6th ed. Philadelphia, PA: Lippincott Williams & Wilkins.
2. Vinik, H R. Intraocular pressure changes during rapid sequence induction and intubation: a comparison of rocuronium, atracurium, and succinylcholine. *J Clin Anesth* 1999;11:95.
3. Ripart J, Mehrige K, Della Rocca R. Local and Regional Anesthesia for Eye Surgery 2009. New York School of Regional Anesthesia. *Anesthesiology* 2001;94:56–62.
4. Cousins MJ, Bridenbaugh PO. *Neural Blockade in Clinical Anesthesia and Pain Management*. Philadelphia, PA: JB Lippincott; 1987:1069–1072.

Spine Surgery

Barbara Wilkey, MD

Spine surgery can be very challenging for an anesthesiologist. Perioperative issues potentially include difficult airway management, positioning injury, ventilation challenges, large volume shifts, coagulopathy, and postoperative visual loss. This chapter provides a brief overview of spinal anatomy, pathophysiology, procedures, and fundamental perioperative considerations.

1) Anatomy of the spine (1)
   a) Composed of vertebrae, intervertebral discs, the spinal cord, and vascular structures with support by ligaments.
   b) There are 33 vertebrae
      i) 7 cervical, 12 thoracic, 5 lumbar, 5 sacral, and 4 coccygeal
      ii) The sacral and the coccygeal vertebrae are fused.
   c) Intervertebral discs
      i) Between the vertebral bodies of C2-S1
      ii) They absorb force exerted on the spine, and allow movement between vertebrae (2).
   d) Spinal cord (1)
      i) Located in the vertebral canal.
      ii) Spinal cord ends around L2 in most adults, L3 in newborns.
   e) Spinal nerves
      i) Exist as pairs, with 8 in the cervical region, 12 in the thoracic region, 5 in the lumbar and sacral regions, and one pair in the coccygeal region.
      ii) Most exit through intervertebral foramina.
   f) Cervical spine (Fig. 137-1)
      i) Anatomically divided into the upper and lower cervical spines.
      ii) Upper cervical spine
         (1) It contains the occipitoatlantal articulation between the atlas (C1) and the axis (C2).
         (2) There is no vertebral body associated with the atlas.
         (3) The axis has a small vertebral body that gives rise to the odontoid process.
         (4) The atlas rotates around the odontoid process.
         (5) The axis and atlas are devoid of intervertebral foramina.
         (6) Flexion and extension are greatest at C1–2.
      iii) Lower cervical spine (C3–7)
         (1) More conventional vertebral anatomy.
         (2) Has a lordotic curvature.
         (3) In the lower cervical spine, flexion and extension are greatest at C5–7 (3).
         (4) The cervical enlargement of the spinal cord starts at C3 and traverses the cervical spinal canal down to T2 (2).

Figure 137-1   Anatomy of the lower cervical spine

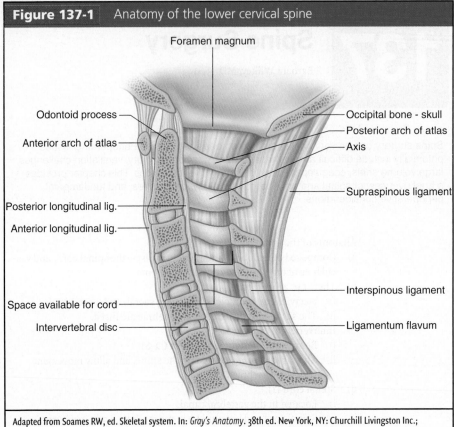

Adapted from Soames RW, ed. Skeletal system. In: *Gray's Anatomy*. 38th ed. New York, NY: Churchill Livingston Inc.; 1995:425–736.

g) Thoracic spine (1)
   i) Upper thoracic vertebrae resemble cervical vertebrae.
   ii) Lower thoracic vertebrae resemble the lumbar vertebrae.
   iii) The thoracic spine has a natural kyphotic curvature.
   iv) The spinous processes slant downward.
   v) The lumbar enlargement of the spinal cord begins at the T9 vertebral body and ends at T12.
h) Lumbar spine
   i) Has a lordotic curvature.
   ii) Spinous processes are nearly horizontal.
2) Spine pathology
   a) **Osteoarthritis (OA) (4)**
      i) Can be idiopathic (primary) or secondary to factors such as injury, congenital anomalies, or metabolic disorders.
      ii) Pathophysiology
         (1) Loss of articular cartilage, which may eventually result in pain and decreased range of motion.
         (2) Spinal OA can involve the facet joints, the uncovertebral joints in the cervical spine (joints of Luschka), and the intervertebral discs.
         (3) Pain can be localized, referred, or radicular.

(a) Radicular pain is due to compression of the spinal nerves and may be accompanied by sensory and/or motor deficits.

    (4) Spinal cord compression can result from osteophytes or ligamentous hypertrophy.

b) **Rheumatoid arthritis**

  i) Pathophysiology

    (1) Inflammatory disease process that, in its natural course, results in proliferation of the synovium (5).

READ MORE

Arthritis, Chapter 92, page 663

      (a) May result in cervical spine instability and spinal cord compression (4)

        (i) Flexion-extension radiographs may be helpful to determine the degree of atlantoaxial instability.

      (b) May be associated with myelopathy.

    (2) Other comorbidities (5)

      (a) Cardiopulmonary sequelae, keratoconjuctivitis sicca, cricoarytenoid arthritis and dislocation, synovitis of the tempomandibular joint.

      (b) Patients are often on chronic steroid therapy.

c) **Ankylosing spondylitis (5)**

  i) Pathophysiology

    (1) Inflammatory arthropathy with localized or systemic findings.

    (2) The entire spine may be involved resulting in the characteristic "bamboo spine."

    (3) Cervical mobility may be significantly limited.

      (a) Fiberoptic intubation may be required.

    (4) **Patients can develop bone fractures with minimal to no trauma.** Even hyperextension can lead to C-spine fracture. Be gentle with initial positioning and subsequent movement. Support kyphosis, if present (6).

    (5) Other comorbidities may include pulmonary fibrosis, decreased chest wall compliance, aortic insufficiency, cardiomegaly, and conduction abnormalities (5).

d) **Spinal cord compression**

  i) Due to multiple etiologies.

  ii) May be acute, subacute, or chronic.

  iii) Spinal cord compression due to arthritis

    (1) Spinal cord compression can occur with OA due to posteriorly directed osteophyte formation (4).

    (2) Spondylosis (7)

      (a) OA involving the intervertebral disks, which may result in osteophyte formation on the disc, inflammation of the disc, and subluxation of the facet joints.

      (b) May be associated with myelopathy if a large posterior osteophyte forms on the disc.

  iv) Herniated nucleus pulposus (7,8)

    (1) Most herniations of intervertebral discs occur posterolaterally, primarily resulting in radicular symptoms.

    (2) If herniation is median or paramedian, spinal cord compression may occur.

    (3) May present as cauda equina syndrome when herniation occurs in the lumbar spine.

  v) Spinal stenosis (7)

    (1) Narrowing of the spinal canal, which may be congenital or acquired.

    (2) Acquired spinal stenosis is generally due to multiple factors, such as disc degeneration, facet joint arthritis, and/or subluxation.

  vi) Tumors (9)

    (1) Cause spinal cord compression by mass effect or by bone destruction resulting in vertebral collapse.

READ MORE

Trauma
Chapter 142,
page 1029

Polytrauma
patients may
require a halo
for spinal
stability, which
can compli-
cate airway
management
and positioning.

Even cleared
plain films
of the cervi-
cal spine in a
trauma patient
do not rule out
ligamentous
injury.

Patients with
acute spinal
cord lesions
above T4 may
not generate a
compensatory
tachycardia
in the face of
hypovolemia.

(2) Pain is usually localized.

(3) Most often occur in the thoracic spine.

vii) **Trauma (10)**

  (1) There is controversy related to the timing of surgery for patients who have suffered trauma to the spine, even when there is cord compression.

  (2) In the polytrauma patient, the spine injury may not be the primary injury requiring surgery

    (a) Patients may have spine instability requiring special management.

      (i) Consultation with a neurosurgeon for guidance on proper positioning and management is recommended

  (3) **Use of succinylcholine in patients with spinal cord injury**

    (a) Polytrauma patients may have crush injuries, which increases their risk of hyperkalemia.

    (b) The amount of time since the spinal cord injury must be considered when choosing a muscle relaxant.

      (i) Succinylcholine is likely safe in the first few hours following injury.

      (ii) Extrajunctional receptors begin to proliferate and place the patient at risk for life-threatening hyperkalemia after 24 to 48 hours (11).

    (c) The risks and benefits of succinylcholine use in the 24 to 48 hours after spinal cord injury should be considered, and **after this time period it should be avoided (11).**

  (4) Hypotension in the trauma patient is often due to hypovolemia.

    (a) With persistent hypotension despite adequate volume resuscitation and surgical hemostasis, consider occult bleeding or spinal shock.

e) **Spinal cord transection**

  i) Acute (12)

    (1) Associated with flaccid paralysis and sympathetic nervous system dysfunction.

    (2) Spinal shock

      (a) Presents as hypotension, often with associated bradycardia.

      (b) Etiology

        (i) Spinal cord injury at the level of T6 or above can result in spinal shock due to a temporary sympathectomy.

        (ii) Lesions at T4 and above can also result in bradycardia.

        (iii) Hemodynamic instability may last for several weeks and will improve when spinal cord reflexes begin to improve.

        (iv) Risk factors for chronic respiratory failure (13)

          1. Age >50

          2. Lesion near C3

          3. Pre-existing pulmonary disease

      (c) Symptomatic treatment of spinal shock (13)

        (i) Hypotension

          1. Treat with volume resuscitation, vasopressors, and inotropes as necessary.

          2. Consider minimizing or avoiding PEEP if hypotension persists.

          3. Be aware that if the patient is placed in reverse Trendelenburg position, there will be significant dependent pooling of intravascular volume.

(ii) Bradycardia should be treated with antimuscarinics and/or b-adrenergic agonists

(iii) Nasogastric tube may be necessary due to risk of paralytic ileus.

(iv) Consider arterial line placement for close monitoring of BP.

(v) Other invasive monitors may be necessary to monitor hemodynamics, especially in patients with injuries above T6.

A common stimulus for autonomic hyperreflexia is bladder or gastrointestinal distention.

ii) **Chronic spinal cord transection**

   (1) Characterized by hyperreflexia, paralysis, and possible spasticity.

   (2) **Autonomic hyperreflexia** (12,14)

      (a) An autonomic dysregulation syndrome caused by lack of sympathetic inhibition due to spinal cord damage.

         (i) When spinal reflexes return, the patient is at risk for autonomic hyperreflexia.

      (b) Patients with lesions at T10 or above are at risk. Highest-risk patients have lesions above T6.

      (c) Stimulation leading to hyperreflexia can be cutaneous or visceral, and must be below the level of the lesion.

Autonomic hyperreflexia may occur in recovery after the anesthetic has worn off.

         (i) May cause severe hypertension and a baroreceptor mediated bradycardia.

         (ii) Other dysrhythmias may also be observed.

         (iii) Above the level of spinal cord injury, vasodilatation occurs.

      (d) Autonomic dysreflexia is a serious situation and may progress to seizures, intracranial hemorrhage, or myocardial infarction if untreated.

Recognize that even if the surgical area is insensate, stimulation of areas below the level of the lesion can result in autonomic hyperreflexia.

      (e) Treatment

         (i) Have quick-onset, relatively short-acting vasodilators and heart rate control agents available.

         (ii) Consider regional or neuraxial anesthesia prior to surgical stimulation. A drawback of this technique is lack of ability to monitor therapy.

         (iii) If signs occur intraoperatively, deepening the anesthetic may help.

         (iv) Consider arterial line placement.

3) **Spinal surgery procedures**

   a) **Spinal fusion** (15)

     i) Indications

       (1) Spinal instability, fracture, stenosis, degenerative disease, tumor removal, disc herniation (post discectomy), vertebral osteomyelitis, tuberculosis, scoliosis, and failed previous fusion.

     ii) Procedure

       (1) Spinal fusion has a wide range of indications; thus, there are many methods used to fuse the spine.

       (2) In general, fusion restores stability and/or relieves deformity.

       (3) Techniques may involve bone grafting, pedicle screws, plates and/or rods at one or more levels.

     iii) Approaches

       (1) Cervical spine

         (a) Anterior approach

CONCERNS IN SUBSPECIALTY ANESTHESIA

        (i)   For upper cervical spine, approach may be transoral or anterior retropharyngeal.

        (ii)   The patient will be supine.

    (b)   Posterior approach requires the patient to be prone and in pins or traction.

        (i)   Patient may possibly be in the sitting position for midcervical spine.

  (2)   Cervical-thoracic junction

    (a)   With a trans-sternal or transclavicular approach, the patient will be supine.

    (b)   If the area is reached via thoracotomy, the patient will be lateral and one-lung ventilation may be required.

  (3)   Thoracic

    (a)   Anterior approach

        (i)   Positioning will be lateral decubitus and may require one-lung ventilation.

    (b)   Transdiaphragmatic approach

        (i)   Used for T11-L1 surgery.

        (ii)   Lateral decubitus position.

        (iii)   One-lung ventilation is generally not required.

    (c)   Posterior approach requires prone positioning.

  (4)   Lumbar

    (a)   Approach may be anterior, posterior, or lateral decubitus.

  (5)   Combined anterior/posterior approaches may require a table that rotates.

b)   **Microdiscectomy** (15)

  i)   Indications

    (1)   Chronic pain from herniated disc.

  ii)   Procedure

    (1)   Performed through a small posterior incision with the appropriate level confirmed radiographically.

    (2)   The ligamentum flavum is exposed and then an operating microscope is used to remove the ligamentum flavum and the disc.

  iii)   Position may be prone, kneeling, or lateral decubitus.

c)   **Laminectomy** (15)

  i)   Indications

    (1)   Spinal element decompression and exposure for removal of intraspinal masses.

  ii)   Procedure

    (1)   Performed through a midline posterior incision with the appropriate level confirmed radiographically.

    (2)   The lamina (and possibly disc) is exposed and removed in pieces.

    (3)   Be aware that there is risk for epidural and retroperitoneal bleeding.

  iii)   Position is prone.

d)   **Kyphoplasty** (16)

  i)   Indication

    (1)   Pain from vertebral compression fracture, either osteoporotic or osteolytic.

  ii)   Procedure

    (1)   The fractured vertebral body is entered percutaneously, and a bone tamp (balloon type device) is inflated, which restores vertebral height.

    (2)   The tamp is then removed, and a filler is placed in the created space to maintain the newly created architecture.

    (3)   Fluoroscopy is used extensively.

  iii)   Position is prone.

4) **Perioperative approach to the patient undergoing spinal surgery (15)**
   a) **Preoperative considerations**
      i) Preoperative Evaluation
         (1) Neurologic
            (a) Perform a preoperative neurologic exam and document any pre-existing sensory or motor deficits or symptomatology.
            (b) Discuss seizure history, current pain issues, and pain medication regimen.
            (c) Discuss postoperative visual loss when the patient is prone, and have wake-up exam (if applicable), and postoperative neurologic reassessment.
      ii) Pulmonary/Airway
         (1) Evaluate for respiratory insufficiency from neuromuscular weakness or diaphragmatic insufficiency. If the patient has scoliosis, determine severity as this could impair pulmonary function.
         (2) In the airway exam, skip neck flexion/extension if patient has an unstable cervical spine or neurologic symptoms with movement. Review cervical spine imaging studies if available. If the surgery is being performed for correction of cervical instability or if it is a trauma patient, the surgeon may be an invaluable reference for determination of stability.
      iii) Cardiovascular
         (1) Evaluate for history of spinal shock or autonomic hyperreflexia.
         (2) For trauma patients, evaluate volume status.
         (3) Consider invasive monitoring if there is concern about extensive blood loss, history of autonomic hyperreflexia, and/or coexisting cardiovascular disease.
      iv) Hematologic
         (1) Over-the-counter, prescription, and herbal medications may impair hemostasis.
         (2) Discuss any history of coagulopathy, transfusion history, and current willingness to accept blood products.
         (3) Discuss cell recovery and normovolemic hemodilution if applicable.
         (4) Consider sending blood for type and cross.
      v) Positioning
         (1) Ask if any position causes significant pain or provokes neurologic symptoms. Some conditions, such as spinal stenosis, may cause dynamic symptoms.
         (2) Prior to placing the patient in the prone position, it is important to evaluate his/her ability to raise the arms above the head.
   b) **Intraoperative considerations**
      i) Airway management
         (1) Cervical spine instability (3)
            (a) Spinal movement should be minimized during management of the airway.
            (b) Blade elevation during laryngoscopy can cause superior rotation at the occiput-C1, and inferior rotation at C2–5. With tracheal intubation, there is superior rotation at the occiput-C1 (3).
            (c) Cervical collars
               (i) The patient may come to the operating room with a cervical collar in place.
               (ii) Cervical collars probably do not decrease cervical spine movement during airway manipulation and may make intubation more difficult due to decreased mouth opening.
               (iii) Some advocate removing the anterior portion of the collar after manual inline immobilization (MILI), prior to laryngoscopy.

(2) Manual inline immobilization (3)

    (a) May be performed either at the head of the bed, or at the side of the bed.

    (b) If performed at the head of the bed, one holds the mastoid processes with the fingertips and the occiput rests in the palms.

    (c) If performed from the side of the bed, the mastoids are held in the palms and the occiput is grasped with the fingertips.

    (d) When laryngoscopy is performed, the individual providing MILI applies pressures equal and opposite to maintain a neutral position.

(3) Techniques (3)

    (a) Mask ventilation

        (i) May cause more cervical spine movement than nasal or oral tracheal intubation.

    (b) Laryngeal mask airway

Awake fiberoptic intubation should be considered in patients with unstable spine injuries.

        (i) May exert pressure on the upper cervical vertebrae, but the clinical significance of this finding is unclear.

    (c) Laryngoscopy versus fiberoptic intubation

        (i) There are no clear data as to which results in better outcomes.

        (ii) Most North American anesthesiologists favor an awake fiberoptic intubation in the setting of unstable cervical spine.

        (iii) However, skill level with fiberoptic intubation should be considered, as failed attempts have been associated with morbidity and mortality.

The benefit of rapid onset with succinylcholine should be weighed against the risk of hyperkalemia due to proliferation of extrajunctional receptors when the injury is <48 hours old (11,14).

ii) Induction

  (1) Hemodynamically stable patient

    (a) Induction agent of choice

  (2) Hemodynamically unstable patient

    (a) Consider ketamine or etomidate if hypotension is present (17).

    (b) If spinal shock is present, anticholinergics and vasopressors should be available.

    (c) Consider maintenance of mean arterial blood pressure at 80 to 85 mm Hg or higher to avoid further spinal cord injury (13).

  (3) Choice of muscle relaxant

    (a) Acutely, succinylcholine is likely safe but should be avoided after the first 24 to 48 hours (11).

iii) Positioning

  (1) Avoid positions that exacerbate pre-existing neuropathies. Consider positioning prior to sedation.

READ MORE

Positioning of the surgical patient, Chapter 5, page 34

Neurophysiologic monitoring and anesthetic management, Chapter 16, page 100

iv) Maintenance

  (1) Prepare for the possibility of autonomic hyperreflexia or spinal shock.

  (2) In the trauma patient, consider that hypotension could be caused by things other than spinal shock (e.g., hypovolemia, myocardial ischemia, tension pneumothorax, etc.)

  (3) Consider invasive monitoring.

  (4) If significant blood loss is anticipated, consider baseline and serial thromboelastograms or arterial blood gases.

(5) Intraoperative Neuromonitoring
- (a) Prior to induction, discuss neuromonitoring with the surgeon.
- (b) Place a bite block between the molars if motor monitoring is to be performed.
- (c) In general, IV anesthetics will have less effect on SSEPs and MEPs than inhaled agents (18).
- (d) Anesthetic technique does not affect EMG but paralytics should be avoided for motor monitoring (18).
- (e) Notify the neuromonitoring team about any changes in hemodynamics or anesthetic technique.
- (f) Wake-up test (12)
    - (i) Involves waking the patient during the operation, and evaluating movement of extremities.
    - (ii) Requires a cooperative patient.
    - (iii) Coordinate timing with the surgeon, so muscle relaxation is not inadvertently given close to the wake-up time.
    - (iv) Generally, anesthetic agents and muscle relaxants are allowed to wear off.
    - (v) Only limited movement of hands and feet is required.

c) **Postoperative considerations**
- i) Neurologic exam
    - (1) A neurologic exam should be performed in the PACU, with a follow-up exam on your postoperative check.
        - (a) Abnormalities should be discussed immediately with the surgeon.
- ii) Pain control
    - (1) Patients undergoing elective spine surgery may be taking a significant amount of narcotics preoperatively, making traditional dosing of narcotics less effective.
    - (2) Multimodal therapy (19)
        - (a) Multimodal therapy including i) preoperative and postoperative gabapentin, acetaminophen, and controlled release oxycodone, ii) intraoperative dolasetron, and iii) postoperative supplemental oxycodone may be more effective than standard IV PCA.
    - (3) Local anesthetic (20)
        - (a) Peri-incisional subfascial local anesthetic infusion may decrease narcotic analgesic requirements postoperatively.
    - (4) Epidural (12)
        - (a) The surgeon can place an epidural catheter intraoperatively through which opioids and/or local anesthetics can be infused. If you plan to use local anesthetic in the epidural infusion, discuss timing with the surgeon, as it may interfere with the postoperative neurologic exam.
    - (5) Ketamine (21)
        - (a) Perioperative ketamine can decrease postoperative opioid use.
    - (6) Intrathecal morphine (12)
        - (a) Preservative-free morphine placed in the intrathecal space by the surgeon has been shown to provide better pain relief than intravenous opioids in patients undergoing lumbar spine surgery.

Chapter Summary for Spine Surgery

Pre-operative Evaluation	Focus on the indication for surgery, pre-existing neurologic deficits, spine stability, hemodynamic stability, need for and type of blood products, and required access. Incorporate neuromonitoring needs into your anesthetic plan.
Intraoperative Management	Consider hemodynamic stability at induction. Succinylcholine should be avoided in patients with spinal cord injuries after the first 24-48 hours. Have an airway plan based on spine stability. Prepare for spinal shock or autonomic hyperreflexia if the clinical situation is appropriate.
Postoperative Pain Control	Consider nontraditional measures such as Ketamine, subfascial local anesthetic infusions, intrathecal preservative-free morphine, or epidural infusion.
Postoperative Neurologic Exam	Notify the surgeon if abnormalities are found.

References

1. Soames RW, ed. Skeletal system. In: *Gray's Anatomy*. 38th ed. New York, NY: Churchill Livingston Inc.; 1995:425–736.
2. Bonica JJ, Cailliet R, Loeser J. General considerations of pain in the neck and upper limb. In: Loesser JD, ed. *Bonica's Management of Pain*. 3rd ed. Philadelphia, PA: Lippincott Williams & Wilkins; 2001:970–1002.
3. Crosby ET. Airway management in adults after cervical spine trauma 2006. *Anesthesiology* 2006;104:1293–1318.
4. Gardner GC, Gilliland BC. Arthritis and periarthritic disorders. In: Loesser JD, ed. *Bonica's Management of Pain*. 3rd ed. Philadelphia, PA: Lippincott Williams & Wilkins; 2001:503–521.
5. Schwartz JJ. Skin and musculoskeletal diseases. In: Hines RL, Marschall KE, ed. *Stoelting's Anesthesia and Co-Existing Disease*. 6th ed. Philadelphia, PA: Churchill Livingston Inc.; 2008:437–467.
6. Woodward LJ, Kam PCA. Ankylosing spondylitis: recent developments and anaesthetic implications. *Anaesthesia* 2009;64:540–548.
7. Mercier LR. *Practical Orthopedics*. 4th ed. St. Louis, MO: Mosby-Year Book Inc.; 1995.
8. Yamazaki S, Kokubun S, Yushin I, et al. Courses of cervical disc herniation causing myelopathy or radiculopaathy: an analysis based on computed tomographic discograms. *Spine* 2003;28:1171–1175.
9. Fitzgibbon DR, Chapman CR. Cancer pain: assessment and diagnosis. In: Loesser JD, ed. *Bonica's Management of Pain*. 3rd ed. Philadelphia, PA: Lippincott Williams & Wilkins; 2001:623–658.
10. Harris M, Sethi R. The initial assessment and management of the multiple-trauma patient with an associated spine injury. *Spine* 2006;31(Suppl):S59–S15.
11. Horlocker TT, Wedel DJ. Anesthesia for orthopedic surgery. In: Barash PG, Cullen BF, Stoelting RK, Cahalan MK, Stock MC, eds. *Clinical Anesthesia*. 6th ed. Philadelphia, PA: Lippincott Williams & Wilkins; 2009:1375–1392.
12. Mahla ME, Horlocker TT. Vertebral column and spinal cord surgery. In: Cucchiara RF, Black S, Michenfelder JD, ed. *Clinical Neuroanesthesia*. 2nd ed. New York, NY: Churchill Livingstone Inc.; 1998:403–448.
13. Miko I, Gould R, Wolf S, et al. Acute spinal cord injury. *Int Anesthesiol Clin* 2009;47:37–54.
14. Pasternak JJ, Lanier WL Jr. Spinal cord disorders. In: Hines RL, Marschall KE, ed. *Stoelting's Anesthesia and Co-Existing Disease*. 6th ed. Philadelphia, PA: Churchill Livingston Inc.; 2008:239–247.
15. Jaffe RA, Samuels SI, eds. *Anesthesiologist's Manual of Surgical Procedures*. 3rd ed. Philadelphia, PA: Lippincott Williams & Wilkins; 2004.
16. Phillips FM. Minimally invasive treatments of osteoporotic vertebral compression fractures. *Spine* 2003;28:S45–S53.
17. Dutton RP, McCunn M. Anesthesia for trauma. In: Miller RD, ed. *Miller's Anesthesia*. 7th ed. Philadelphia, PA: Elsevier Churchill Livingstone; 2005:2451–2495.
18. Mahla ME, Black S, Cucchiara RF. Neurologic monitoring. In: Miller RD, ed. *Miller's Anesthesia*. 7th ed. Philadelphia, PA: Elsevier Churchill Livingstone; 1511–1550.
19. Rajpal S, Gordon D, Pellino T, et al. Comparison of perioperative oral multimodal analgesia versus IV PCA for spine surgery. *J Spinal Disord Tech* 2010;23:139–145.
20. Elder JB, Hoh D, Liu CY, et al. Postoperative continuous paravertebral anesthetic infusion for pain control in posterior cervical spine surgery: a case control study. *Oper Neurosurg* 2010;66:ons99–ons107.
21. Bell RF, Dahl JB, Moore RA, et al. Perioperative ketamine for acute postoperative pain (review). The Cochrane Collaboration 2009.

138 ENT and Laser Surgery

Kevin Malott, MD

Otolaryngologic, or Ear, Nose, and Throat (ENT) surgery can be challenging to the anesthesiologist since the patient often is at risk for airway compromise. Many patients have coexisting illnesses that can complicate anesthetic management. Lasers can be advantageous for airway surgery but require advanced knowledge and preparation to prevent complications.

1) Surgical considerations for ENT procedures
   a) Otolaryngologic procedures constitute a large share of all surgical procedures.
   b) With the population aging, demand will undoubtedly increase, especially for resections of head-and-neck neoplasms and for increasingly sophisticated otological interventions for hearing loss.
   c) Common operations include various ear, nose, sinus, throat, and laryngeal procedures, trachestomy, definitive oncologic resections, surgery to relieve obstructive sleep apnea (OSA), reconstructive procedures, and panendoscopy to aid in the diagnosis of disorders of the aerodigestive tract.

2) Preoperative assessment
   a) Patients are often elderly and may have significant comorbidities
      i) HTN, COPD, and CAD are the most common.
   b) Preoperative assessment of the major organ systems and optimization of pre-existing disorders is warranted.
   c) **Oncologic patients.** These patients not only tend to present at an older age, and with important cancer related comorbidities, but they usually require longer, more invasive, and more complex surgeries.
      i) Tobacco exposure is the most significant risk factor for cancers of the head and neck.
         (1) Patients presenting for oncologic surgery have a high prevalence of COPD.
      ii) May be malnourished secondary to dysphagia and further debilitated from concomitant chemoradiation therapy
      iii) Often present with anemia, coagulopathy, electrolyte imbalances, and occasionally, aspiration pneumonia
   d) **A thorough airway exam is critical (Table 138-1)**
      i) Close attention to the ease of air movement, noting the presence and timing of stridor, wheezing, or other adventitious breath sounds, is helpful in making a plan for airway management.
      ii) If your patient, while wide awake and with intact airway reflexes, is having difficulty breathing, he/she may be impossible or exceedingly difficult to mask ventilate when anesthetized.

For ENT procedures, remember that your surgeon is an airway expert. Preoperative discussion with the surgeon about the patient's airway exam will yield essential information.

iii) Likewise, if supraglottic or glottic anatomy is overly obscured by profuse bleeding, edema, or tumor, direct visualization of the glottis and endotracheal intubation may be impossible, and using a technique to secure the airway with the patient spontaneously ventilating or awake should be considered.

e) Patients with chronic airway obstruction may have chronic hypoventilation with hypoxemia

i) This often can result in increased risk of pulmonary hypertension and right-sided heart failure

ii) Clinical signs

(1) Cyanosis, jugular venous distension, a loud P2, clubbing, right axis deviation and RVH on ECG, poor exercise capability, polycythemia

(2) If present further cardiologic evaluation is recommended (1)

3) **General principles**

a) Airway management

If deliberate hypotension is requested, ALWAYS consider the patient's coexisting diseases when determining a lower limit for hypotension and clearly communicate with the surgeon. In some cases, it may not be safe.

i) For ENT procedures in general, and airway procedures in particular, close communication with the surgeon is paramount.

ii) Discussion about preoperative assessments, such as radiology studies, nasal endoscopies, and your joint physical exam findings, is important in creating a safe plan for managing the airway.

iii) Your surgeon will likely have preferences regarding type of endotracheal tube (ETT) (nasal vs. oral, standard vs. RAE, laser vs. plastic, etc.), the feasibility of using an laryngeal mask airway (LMA), how best to secure the tube, and head positioning.

b) Deliberate hypotension. Except for very superficial procedures, the use of deliberate relative hypotension to limit blood loss and improve surgical visibility may be requested by surgeons for ENT procedures.

i) It is important to accurately assess your patient's ability to tolerate induced hypotension without end-organ dysfunction or injury

(1) Care MUST be taken to maintain a safe minimum BP to assure adequate renal, coronary, and cerebral perfusion.

ii) Achieving deliberate hypotension

(1) In anticipation of a smooth emergence, it is less problematic to achieve deliberate hypotension with antihypertensive agents as opposed to merely deepening anesthetic levels.

If a difficult airway is anticipated, the surgeon should be present to assist during anesthesia induction, as an additional pair of knowledgeable and experienced hands can provide invaluable help in implementing advanced airway techniques and rescue maneuvers, including, establishing a surgical airway.

(2) If hypotension is induced with anesthetic agents, use very short-acting drugs.

c) **Teamwork**

i) A team approach toward airway management is critical.

ii) The surgeon can give an excellent appraisal of the difficulty in managing the airway.

iii) ENT surgeons are also experts at securing an airway, so their abilities and assistance can be invaluable.

(1) Surgeons should be present and ready to assist, as necessary, during anesthetic induction and all crucial steps of airway management.

iv)   It is important to discuss the timing and use of muscle relaxants, use of corticosteroids to reduce airway edema, and postop airway and pain management.

4)   Difficult airway management

READ MORE

Difficult airway management, Chapter 21, page 150

a)   **Awake versus asleep.** If you are confident you can ventilate your patient with a mask, it is reasonable to proceed with induction of general anesthesia.

i)   If difficulty is anticipated with mask ventilation and intubation, the patient's airway should be secured while awake, either after instituting topical anesthesia to the airway, or by tracheostomy.

b)   **Fiberoptic endotracheal intubation**

i)   A complete description of fiberoptic intubation is covered in the "Fiberoptic Intubation" chapter.

ii)   Please also see "Fiberoptic Intubation" cognitive aid.

c)   Special airway management options

Regardless of the airway management plan, it is important to have backup plans should the primary plan fail.

i)   In addition to the standard assortment of straight and curved laryngoscope blades, LMAs, bougies, stylets, and nasal and oral airways, many other options exist for the establishment of a secure or at least manageable patent airway.

(1)   **If the airway is not expected to be fragile or prone to injury**

(a)   A "blind" technique such as a lighted stylet, LMA Fastrak, or bind nasal approach is reasonable.

ii)   **If a tumor is encroaching on the airway**

(1)   Visualization of the passageway to the glottis may be preferable.

(a)   Techniques such as direct laryngoscopy, use of an Airtrak, Glidescope, Bullard scope, or fiberoptic scope, particularly if the tumor may be friable.

If difficult mask ventilation is anticipated, strongly consider securing the patient's airway while awake and/or spontaneously ventilating.

iii)   **LMA use for ENT procedures** (Table 138-2)

(1)   The LMA can be an excellent choice for ENT surgeries as its use avoids the stress of tracheal stimulation and offers a smooth emergence.

(2)   LMAs have been used successfully for a variety of ENT procedures including tonsillectomies.

(3)   Risk/benefit assessment

Table 138-1
Predicting Difficult Airway Management

Previous history of difficult mask ventilation or intubation.

Hoarseness

Congenital defects

Airway obstruction manifested by tachypnea, stridor, or wheezing (stridor at rest suggests severe airway narrowing and the timing suggests the location of obstruction with an inspiratory stridor suggesting a supraglottic process, and an expiratory stridor suggesting a subglottic obstruction)

Decreased C-spine mobility

Poor Mallampati class, large tongue, retrognathia, or poor mouth opening

Prior history of surgery or radiation to head or neck (may also make establishment of a surgical airway difficult)

Acute or chronic oropharyngeal or laryngeal swelling secondary to infection, epiglottitis, allergic reaction, neoplasm, vascular anomaly, or bleeding

CONCERNS IN SUBSPECIALTY ANESTHESIA

READ
MORE
Laryngeal mask
airway,
Chapter 23,
page 173

(a) It may seem against conventional wisdom not to protect the airway from blood and secretions with an ETT during ENT procedures, particularly when the operative table is turned away from the anesthesia machine.

(b) However, blood and secretions will typically pool above the LMA where they can readily be seen and suctioned by the surgeon

(c) Advantages gained by a smoother emergence can be well worth the mild decrease in control of the airway with the LMA as compared to an ETT.

(4) The flexible LMA is aptly suited for ENT cases

    (a) Has a smaller outer diameter per given cuff size

    (b) Less prone to kinking

    (c) Less likely to become dislodged

    (d) More pliable, so manipulation of the LMA shaft does not transmit movement to the cuff as easily as the standard LMA

5) **Anesthetic emergence considerations for ENT procedures**

  a) **Intraoperative considerations**

    i) A smooth controlled emergence is desirable to avoid increased bleeding from excessive hypertension, or damage to freshly sutured tissues from postextubation airway manipulation.

    ii) Upon awakening, blood, secretions, and the inherent irritation from operating on this highly reflexogenic area of the body may predispose to coughing, straining, and laryngospasm.

    iii) Finding a balance between suppression of airway irritation with good analgesia while avoiding oversedation is an important challenge.

      (1) If the case warrants, use of an LMA may decrease the likelihood of a turbulent emergence, with a reduced incidence of coughing on emergence, SaO_2 desaturations, laryngospasm, sore throat, and laryngeal trauma (2).

      (2) Judicious use of local anesthesia and cranial nerve blocks can enhance patient comfort and decrease postoperative narcotic requirements.

      (3) Consider using less typical pharmacologic agents, such as dexmedetomidine and ketamine, as part of a safe and balanced anesthetic plan.

      (4) Measures to prevent PONV should be followed vigorously.

      (5) Consider administering corticosteroids to help reduce airway edema.

    iv) If little postop pain is expected

      (1) Short-acting IV agents such as remifentanil may be advantageous in facilitating a pleasant and cooperative emergence.

6) Postoperative considerations
   a) If doubts remain about the ability to maintain an airway
      i) A leak test or extubation over a tube exchanger should be attempted prior to committing to full extubation.
      ii) Conversely, the patient may be left intubated and sedated until extubation is appropriate.
   b) Airway obstruction secondary to edema
      i) Manifested by stridor, tachypnea, and an increased work of breathing
      ii) Must be treated aggressively.
         (1) Administer steroids, nebulized racemic epinephrine, and humidified O_2.
7) Specific situations
   a) **Otologic and neurotologic surgery**
      I) **Preoperative considerations**
         (1) General concerns, with patients presenting from all age groups
      ii) **Intraoperative considerations**
         (1) Avoidance of muscle paralysis during facial nerve monitoring
         (2) May need to avoid nitrous oxide with tympanoplasty
         (3) Resections of acoustic neuromas and skull-based lesions
            (a) Usually performed in collaboration with neurosurgery
            (b) May require relative hypotension, neuromonitoring, and a smooth emergence.
         (4) If surgery was intradural
            (a) Coughing and straining on emergence may increase ICP and predispose to a dural leak.
      iii) **Postoperative considerations**
         (1) Cranial nerve palsies causing dysphagia and predisposing to pulmonary aspiration possible
   b) **Panendoscopy**
      i) Indications
         (1) Assessment of aerodigestive tract, foreign body removal, removal of superficial lesions
         (2) Procedures include esophagoscopy, laryngoscopy, and bronchoscopy
      ii) **Preoperative considerations**
         (1) Patients may have head-and-neck cancers, so the aforementioned concerns for oncologic patients apply.
      iii) **Intraoperative considerations**
         (1) These procedures are profoundly stimulating, but of brief duration and entail little postoperative pain.
         (2) They often require an open anesthesia circuit to ambient air for surgical access to the airway.
         (3) TIVA with short-acting agents is an excellent choice.
         (4) Use caution when intubating the patient to avoid traumatizing tongue base tumors.
         (5) Flexible bronchoscopy may be performed through a Patil-Syracuse mask during mask ventilation, or a large-diameter ETT.
            (a) See airway management under ventilation strategies below.
         (6) Muscle relaxation
            (a) Suggested to avoid patient injury from movement
            (b) Recommendations include succinylcholine infusion, or short-acting nondepolarizing neuromuscular blocking agents.
      iv) **Postoperative considerations**

(1)   Complications include esophageal perforation and barotrauma

c)   **Tracheostomy**

    i)   Indications

        (1)   Elective tracheostomy

            (a)   Useful for intubated patients requiring prolonged respiratory support

                (i)   Increases comfort level

                (ii)   Decreases potential for laryngeal injury

                (iii)   Enhances airway access for clearance of secretions

                (iv)   Improves airway protection from pulmonary aspiration

            (b)   May be performed for severe OSA

            (c)   Occasionally performed as part of a larger ENT procedure such as total laryngectomy

        (2)   Emergent tracheostomy

            (i)   Patients with impending or progressing airway obstruction in whom other techniques are unsafe.

    ii)   **Preoperative considerations**

        (1)   Intubated patients will have significant comorbidities and may be critically ill.

            (a)   Patients should be reasonably hemodynamically stable, and any significant metabolic or coagulopathic derangements should be corrected.

            (b)   Make an honest assessment of whether the patient can tolerate not only brief periods of apnea inherent to the procedure, but also transport to and from the operating room.

        (2)   Accurate assessment of the airway is important.

            (a)   If safety in inducing unconsciousness and managing the airway is not assured, use a technique to secure the airway with the patient awake, or place the tracheostomy under local anesthesia.

During tracheostomy, it is possible for the surgeon to pass the new tracheal tube into a false passage created by a mucosal separation. Keep the original ETT in the trachea until the new airway is assured.

    iii)   **Intraoperative considerations**

        (1)   Risk of airway fire if electrosurgical techniques are used (see preventing airway fire algorithm)

            (a)   The trachea should not be opened with an electrosurgical device.

        (2)   When the surgeon is ready to open the trachea, increase FiO_2 to 100% and keep the ETT cuff below the level of incision.

        (3)   When the surgeon requests removal of the ETT, only withdraw as much as needed to allow placement of the tracheal tube, but keep the original ETT in the trachea. Placing an airway exchange catheter prior to the exchange can provide another layer of safety.

        (4)   It is possible (even after initial visualization of the ETT/tracheal lumen) for the surgeon to pass the new tracheal tube into a false passage created by a mucosal separation.

            (a)   Patients with tracheal edema or fragile tissues are presumably at highest risk.

        (5)   **Only after the presence of $ETCO_2$ is confirmed through the new airway should the original ETT be removed.**

READ MORE

Epiglottitis, Chapter 122, page 856

d)   **Acute upper airway obstruction**

    i)   **Indications**

        (1)   Oropharyngeal abscess (OA), tumor, trauma, epiglottitis, or angioedema

ii) **Preoperative considerations**
(1) Patients may have stridor at rest, cyanosis, or worsening hypercarbia.
  (a) These patients are in danger of imminent airway loss.
(2) OA may be deceivingly large and result in significant airway obstruction during airway management.
  (a) Manipulation of the airway can lead to disruption of abscess with the potential for copious drainage and aspiration of its contents.
(3) Epiglottitis
  (a) With the widespread use of the *Haemophilus influenza* vaccine, epiglottitis is rarely seen in children and now is most commonly encountered in adults (1).
  (b) Patients are at risk for respiratory failure and may be intubated under general anesthesia in the operating room.

iii) **Intraoperative considerations**
(1) Seriously consider and be prepared for the placement of a surgical airway under local anesthesia.
(2) Induction and airway management
  (a) Anesthesia may be slowly induced with inhalational agents in 100% O_2, while maintaining spontaneous ventilation.
  (b) Once a deep plane of anesthesia is reached, direct visualization of the glottis and endotracheal intubation can be attempted.
  (c) Use smaller-than-normal ETTs (5.0 to 6.0 mm).
  (d) Proceed very cautiously in caring for patients with airway tumors.
    (i) Tumors near the base of the tongue are often fragile and not only may physically block the route to the glottis, but may bleed or become dislodged and further obstruct the airway.

e) **Sinus/maxillofacial/nasal surgery**
  i) Indications
    (1) Chronic sinus disease, nasal polyps, and aesthetic concerns
    (2) Functional endoscopic sinus surgery done for the resection of inflamed bone and tissue to restore normal mucociliary clearance
  ii) **Preoperative considerations**
    (1) May be associated with triad of nasal polyposis, NSAID hypersensitivity, and reactive airway disease
  iii) **Intraoperative considerations**

READ MORE
Obstructive sleep apnea, Chapter 74, page 524

    (1) A LMA may be especially useful, given the importance of a smooth emergence with the avoidance of postoperative mask ventilation.
    (2) The reinforced laryngeal mask airway protects the airway from blood and surgical debris by forming a reliable seal across the oropharyngeal inlet, so any bleeding will typically pool above the LMA and can be readily seen and suctioned by the surgeon (3).
    (3) Expect periods of highly stimulating surgical manipulation with little postoperative pain.
    (4) Safe deliberate hypotension may be preferred to minimize blood loss as hemorrhage can be copious and will diminish surgical visibility.
  iv) **Postoperative considerations**
    (1) Complications include possibility of dural, nasolacrimal, ocular, or carotid injury.
  f) **Surgery to relieve OSA**
    i) **Preoperative considerations**
      (1) See preoperative assessment for chronic airway obstruction.

CONCERNS IN SUBSPECIALTY ANESTHESIA

    ii) **Intraoperative considerations**
        (1) Patients frequently are morbidly obese and may be difficult to mask ventilate.
            (a) Consider awake FOI
        (2) Patients are at risk for airway obstruction after extubation secondary to glossopharyngeal obstruction or bleeding from uncontrolled HTN.
            (a) Avoid overhydration, in order to lessen the incidence of postoperative HTN, airway edema, and pulmonary edema in this potentially susceptible patient population.
        (3) **Postoperative considerations**
            (a) Patients are especially prone to oversedation with narcotic analgesics, and may warrant more vigorous monitoring and longer hospital stays.
            (b) Close BP control may decrease risk of airway hemorrhage and edema.

  g) **Emergent surgical airway**
    i) Indications

↱ READ MORE

Wire Crichothy-roidotomy cognitive aid, Chapter 157, page 1110

        (1) Part of difficult airway algorithm when attempts at endotracheal intubation, and LMA or facemask ventilation have been unsuccessful
        (2) If experienced surgeon not present, should be placed by the anesthetist
        (3) Most expeditious method is an emergent cricothyroidotomy, with a needle inserted or a stab incision made just above the cricoid cartilage
        (4) Jet ventilation or insufflation of O_2 with permissive hypercapnia may be used initially until the airway can be dilated sufficiently to allow adequate tidal ventilation. Convert to definitive tracheostomy early.

8) **Laser surgery**
  a) **Indications**
    i) Ablation or debulking of various tumors of the head, throat, and airway
    ii) Lasers are notably helpful in the precise excision of tumors located on or near critical structures, such as the vocal cords, while causing minimal collateral tissue damage.

  b) **Safety precautions**
    i) Lasers are high-energy focused beams of light that may easily ignite combustible material, particularly in the presence of supplemental O_2.
    ii) Care must be taken to eliminate any readily combustible material from the surgical field.
        (1) Surgical drapes around the patient should be nonflammable and wet towels can be placed over the patient's eyes and face for added safety.
    iii) Eyes are especially prone to damage. Everyone present in the operating room must wear appropriate, laser-specific, eye protection.
    iv) Smoke should be properly scavenged.
    v) If excised lesions are thought to be from an infectious process, such as human papilloma virus, OR personnel should wear fitted masks to filter aerosolized viral particles (4).

  c) **Airway management**
    i) The airway will be shared, so close communication with the surgeon is critical.

  d) **Minimizing risk of airway fire (Tables 138-3 and 138-4)**
    i) FiO_2 should be kept to a minimum, preferably <30%.
    ii) N_2O supports combustion and should not be used.
    iii) Avoid introducing any combustible material into the airway, including oil-based lubricants or dry cottonoids.
    iv) Using PEEP lowers the risk of ETT ignition (5).

9) **Ventilation strategies for laser surgery**
  a) **Endotracheal intubation**
    i) Laser-resistant metal ETTs, or tubes wrapped with metal tape, are safest.
    ii) Double-cuffed ETTs

(1) Provide additional protection because if the proximal cuff is punctured, the distal cuff will prevent airway gases from leaking and supporting combustion.

(2) It is beneficial to fill the cuffs with saline colored with dye (e.g., methylene blue), so the surgeon will notice if one is punctured.

b) **Intermittent apnea**

i) May be utilized if ETT is not used due to the nature of the surgery and the patient can tolerate periods of apnea

(1) Intermittently ventilating by mask, LMA, or ETT and then extubating each time the surgeon works, is a viable option.

(a) The surgeon will have an unimpeded field of view and the problem of potentially combustible airway adjuncts will be avoided (6).

Every anesthesia provider should know the location of the OR's fire extinguisher.

c) **Venturi technique**

i) A small unobtrusive catheter is positioned just above the glottic opening and short bursts of high-pressure ventilation entrain room air to achieve adequate tidal volumes.

ii) Close observation of chest expansion with confirmation of complete exhalation is critical to avoid severe barotraumas, such as pneumothorax, pneumomediastinum, or severe gastric distention and/or rupture.

All unprotected nonmetal tubes are prone to laser induced ignition.

d) **Jet insufflations**

i) Similar to venturi technique, but catheter is placed at or below the level of the vocal cords either by transglottal or transtracheal route.

ii) Should be avoided in patients with obstructive lung disease or severe obesity, as their passive lung deflation is impaired.

iii) Advantages and concerns are similar to the venturi technique, but with higher risk of barotrauma (7).

e) **Manual ventilation through sideport of bronchoscope**

i) Often difficult to achieve effective ventilation secondary to the bronchoscope impeding airflow, but may be acceptable if procedure is of short duration.

Table 138-3
Preventing Fires in ENT During Laser or Electrosurgery

1. Minimize FiO_2, avoid N_2O, use O_2–N_2, O_2–air, or O_2–helium mixtures, use PEEP.
2. If using MAC, meticulous care must be taken to avoid the accumulation of O_2 within the surgical drapes or bedding. At the most, use low-flow supplemental O_2. If higher flows are needed for patient safety, then general anesthesia should be used with an LMA or ETT to isolate airway gases from the surgical field.
3. All flammable prep solutions must be allowed time to completely dry.
4. For laser surgery: the surgeon should use the lowest laser intensity necessary and short intermittent laser bursts. Use metal ETT or wrap ETT with metal tape. Fill ETT cuff with blue dye and keep cuff out of surgical field.
5. Avoid electrosurgery within the airway if patient requires high FiO_2.
6. Saline should be ready and available to extinguish an airway fire.

Table 138-4
Treating an Airway Fire

1. Immediately remove burning material and stop ventilation
2. Disconnect/replace circuit and extinguish fire with saline.
2. Re-establish airway and ventilation.
3. Perform bronchoscopy to assess injury; consider lavage.
4. Supportive care: mechanical ventilation, PEEP, corticosteroids, CXR, ABG, reassessment later if extent of injury unclear. Consider low tracheostomy.

Chapter Summary for ENT and Laser Surgery

Patient Assessment	Emphasis on thorough airway exam and consideration of coexisting disease.
Airway Management	Coordinate plan with surgeon; maintain spontaneous ventilation or secure the airway with the patient awake if necessary.
Fire Prevention	Use caution with laser or electrosurgery within the airway, avoid N_2O, minimize FiO_2, and have a plan to quickly extinguish any fire.
Laser Surgery	Pay meticulous attention to protecting the patient and OR personnel from thermal injury.
Emergence	Strive to avoid coughing, mask ventilation, or loss of the airway on patient awakening.
Postoperative Concerns	Avoid PONV, airway edema, oversedation, or hypertension to help minimize bleeding or airway compromise.

References

1. Nekhendzy V, Guta C, Champeau MW. Otolaryngology-head and neck surgery. In: Jaffe RA, Samuels SI, eds. *Anesthesiologist's Manual of Surgical Procedures*. 4th ed. Philadelphia, PA: Lippincott Williams & Wilkins; 2009:173–258.
2. Webster AC, Morley-Foster PK, Janzen V, et al. Anesthesia for intranasal surgery: a comparison between tracheal intubation and the flexible reinforced laryngeal mask airway. *Anesth Analg* 1999;88:421–425.
3. Ahmed MZ, Vohra A. The reinforced laryngeal mask airway (RLMA) protects the airway in patients undergoing nasal surgery-an observation of 200 patients. *Can J Anesth* 2002;49:863–866.
4. Ferrari LR, Gotta AW. Anesthesia for otolaryngological surgery. In: Barash PG, ed. *Clinical Anesthesia*. 5th ed. Philadelphia, PA: Lippincott Williams & Wilkins; 2006:1006–1007.
5. Pashayan AG, SanGiovanni C, Davis LE. Positive end-expiratory pressure lowers the risk of laser-induced polyvinylchloride tracheal-tube fires. *Anesthesiology* 1993;79:83–87.
6. Werkhaven JA. Microlaryngoscopy-airway management with anaesthetic techniques for CO_2 laser. *Pediatr Anesth* 2004;14:90–94.
7. Jaquet Y, Monnier P, Van Melle G, et al. Complications of different ventilation strategies in endoscopic laryngeal surgery. *Anesthesiology* 2006;104:52–59.

139

Anesthesia for Intracranial and Neurovascular Procedures

Leslie C. Andes, MD

Neuroanesthesia is the provision of anesthesia for intracranial and spine operations. Neurosurgical cases can be quite long, and preoperative planning and meticulous attention to detail intraoperatively will aid in the attainment of a favorable anesthetic and surgical outcome. This chapter gives an overview of the physiology of the central nervous system (CNS), surgical procedures, and perioperative issues to be considered. For a discussion of anesthesia for spinal surgery (see Chapter 137).

The goal of anesthesia for neurosurgical procedures is maintenance of the normal balance between ICP, CPP, and CMRO$_2$.

READ MORE

Increased ICP, Chapter 75, page 528

1) **Intracranial physiology**
   a) **Intracranial pressure (ICP)** (Fig. 139-1)
      i) Normal ICP is <10 mm Hg.
      ii) When growth of an intracranial lesion is slow, ICP will remain stable for a while because of shunting of cerebrospinal fluid (CSF) into spinal reservoirs and blood into the central vascular system.
      iii) When an increase in volume can no longer be accommodated, a small change in volume can cause a large and rapid increase in ICP, which can quickly lead to herniation and death.
   b) **Cerebral perfusion pressure (CPP) and cerebral blood flow (CBF)**
      i) CPP is the net perfusion pressure causing blood to flow to the brain (CBF). This can be expressed as: **CPP = MAP (mean arterial pressure) – ICP (or central venous pressure (CVP), whichever is greater)**
      ii) Autoregulation of CBF (Fig. 139-2A)
         (1) Autoregulation is the ability of the cerebral vasculature to maintain relatively constant CBF despite large changes in blood pressure.
         (2) Effected via dilation or constriction of the cerebral blood vessels, with some matching (or "coupling") of flow to metabolism of glucose and cerebral metabolism of oxygen (CMRO$_2$)
         (3) Range for autoregulation
            (a) Historically thought to be between 50 and 150 mm Hg.
            (b) **Recent expert opinion is that the MAP for the lower limit of autoregulation (LLA) may be ≥70 mm Hg.**
         (4) Once the limits of autoregulation are exceeded, flow is dependent on perfusion pressure.
            (a) Areas of the brain that are chronically underperfused may be maximally vasodilated and blood flow will be dependent on MAP.
            (b) Acceptable intra- and postoperative BP must be individualized for each patient based on usual BP readings (1).

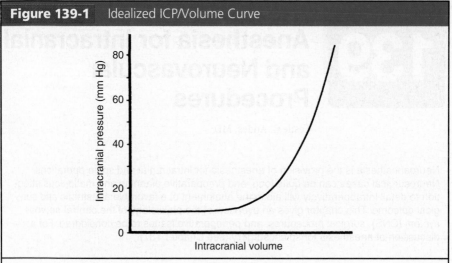

Figure 139-1   Idealized ICP/Volume Curve

Reproduced from Newfield P, Cottrell JE, ed. *Handbook of Neuroanesthesia*. 4th ed. Philadelphia, PA: Lippincott Williams & Wilkins; 2007:21, with permission.

(5)   Cerebral autoregulation is impaired by the following
   (a) Vascular disease
   (b) Anesthesia
   (c) Tumors
   (d) Disruption in the blood-brain barrier (BBB)
   (e) Medications

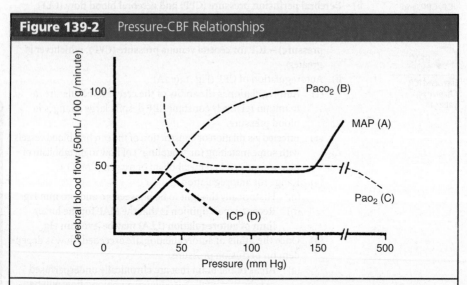

Figure 139-2   Pressure-CBF Relationships

A: The traditional view of CBF autoregulation between MAP 50 to 150 mm Hg. The LLA is more likely ≥70 mm Hg. **B:** Linear relationship between partial pressure of arterial carbon dioxide (PaCO$_2$) and CBF for PaCO$_2$ = 20 to 80 mm Hg. **C:** PaO$_2$ and CBF. **D:** ICP and CBF. Adapted from: Newfield P, Cottrell JE, ed. *Handbook of Neuroanesthesia*. 4th ed. Philadelphia, PA: Lippincott Williams & Wilkins; 2007:113.

(f)   Cerebral Edema

(g)   Trauma

iii)   CBF is directly proportional to $PaCO_2$ between 20 and 80 mm Hg, and tightly coupled regionally (Fig. 139-2B).

> The cerebral autoregulation curve is shifted to the right in patients with chronic HTN, and these patients require higher MAP to maintain CBF.

(1)   **Blood vessels in ischemic regions do not react normally to changes in CO_2 levels.**

(2)   Hypoventilation with hypercarbia may result in a steal phenomenon with increased CBF to normal areas.

(3)   Hyperventilation may result in an inverse steal effect with improved CBF to damaged brain areas.

iv)   CBF is inversely affected by PaO_2 (Fig. 139-2C)

v) CaO_2 and viscosity changes caused by changes in hematocrit will also affect CBF (2).

c)   **Cerebral metabolism of oxygen ($CMRO_2$)**

i)   The cerebral metabolic rate for oxygen ($CMRO_2$) is the brain's oxygen consumption requirement to maintain normal function and viability.

ii)   Normal coupling between $CMRO_2$ and CBF is maintained under anesthesia.

iii)   A decrease in $CMRO_2$ is the basis for most current neuroprotection therapies.

(1)   Burst suppression can decrease $CMRO_2$ by up to 60% from baseline, which is the maximum achievable as the remaining 40% is used for cellular maintenance. Sodium thiopental (STP) has been used for burst suppression in the past, but because it will not be available in the foreseeable future, propofol is the current preferred agent.

(2)   Lowering the patient's temperature will decrease $CMRO_2$ by 5% to 7% per°C (3).

d)   **Blood-brain barrier (BBB)**

i)   A barrier between the vascular system and brain tissue that protects the CNS.

ii)   Tight junctions in capillary endothelial cells prevent passage of large, water-soluble, or charged substances between the blood and brain cells.

iii)   Can be disrupted by hypertension (HTN), tumors, drugs, traumatic brain injury (TBI), and disease (e.g., encephalopathies, meningitis, multiple sclerosis)

e)   **Cerebral edema**

i)   Vasogenic edema

> Location, size, and type of lesion are important determinants of positioning, monitoring, and anesthetic induction and maintenance.

(1)   Results from disruption of the BBB that causes protein leakage into extracellular areas

(2)   Seen with tumors

(3)   Responds to steroids and diuretics

ii)   Cytotoxic edema

(1)   BBB is not disrupted, so there is no protein leak.

(2)   Not improved with steroid use

iii)   Ischemic edema

(1)   Blend of vasogenic and cytotoxic

(2)   May have a delayed onset

2)   **Neuroanesthesia considerations**

a)   **Preoperative assessment and planning**

i)   Recommend discussion with surgeon to assess neurosurgical issues impacting planned anesthetic.

(1) Films should be reviewed for signs of increased ICP or compression or invasion of other structures. Examples include:

    (a) Compression of brain stem by tumor (e.g., large acoustic neuroma) or vascular malformation.

    (b) Large pituitary tumor invading the cavernous sinus, with proximity to the carotid artery (Fig. 139-3)

(2) Underlying structures that may be entered with the chosen surgical approach, especially venous sinuses.

(3) Positioning for best surgical exposure should be discussed with the surgeon.

ii) **Blood should be available** in the OR for neurovascular surgeries and others where rapid and extensive blood loss may be likely.

iii) **Preoperative airway management planning is an important aspect of neuroanesthesia.**

    (1) Difficult airway issues are common in neurosurgical patients, due to concerns such as spinal pathology, presence of a halo fixation device, facial trauma, congenital deformities.

    (2) A wide variety of airway devices should be available.

    (3) Proceed with rapid sequence induction and intubation if full stomach is expected.

    (4) Minimal or no preoperative sedation is best for a patient with increased ICP due to possibility of inducing hypoventilation and intracranial HTN.

iv) Preoperative discussion with patient.

    (1) Prepare patient for frequent serial neurologic exams after the surgery until postoperative stability is assured.

    (2) Instruct pituitary surgery patients that if nasal packing is placed at the conclusion of surgery, they must breathe through the mouth.

Figure 139-3 Structures Within or Near the Cavernous Sinus

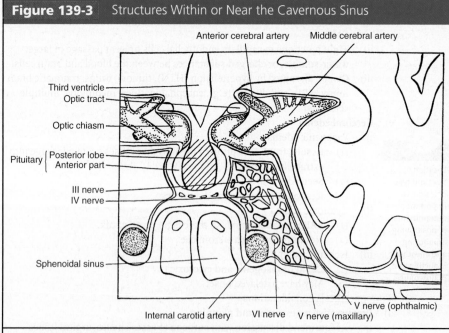

Reproduced from Newfield P, Cottrell JE, ed. *Handbook of Neuroanesthesia*. 4th ed. Philadelphia, PA: Lippincott Williams & Wilkins; 2007:188, with permission.

b) **Intraoperative considerations**

　　i)　Monitoring: In addition to standard ASA monitors, special monitors may be considered for neurosurgical procedures.

　　　　(1)　Intravascular monitors

　　　　　　(a)　Arterial line monitors are useful for continuous monitoring of blood pressure and to obtain arterial blood for analysis.

　　　　　　　　(i)　Helpful when large changes in arterial blood pressure are expected and/or undesirable

　　　　　　　　(ii)　An arterial line may be placed preinduction for patients in whom aggressive BP control is necessary (e.g., ruptured aneurysm).

　　　　　　　　(iii)　Insert an arterial line for all craniotomies, or if indicated for medical condition of patient.

　　　　　　(b)　Central venous access is useful for monitoring central venous pressures and infusing medications quickly to the central circulation.

　　　　　　　　(i)　A central venous pressure (CVP) catheter is placed for larger craniotomies, or may be inserted to improve ease of care in ICU postoperatively.

　　　　　　　　(ii)　Pulmonary artery catheter is used occasionally in patients receiving therapy for vasospasm (to monitor for adverse cardiac effects of hypervolemic hemodilution therapy used in vasospasm), in some sitting craniotomies, or if medically indicated based on patient status.

　　　　(2)　Neurologic monitors

　　　　　　(a)　The use of BIS monitoring to prevent awareness is controversial. The BIS is not reliable for detection of ischemia in carotid endarterectomy (CEA) (4,5).

　　　　　　(b)　Neurophysiologic monitoring

　　　　　　　　(i)　Used to ensure the patient's neurologic status does not change during positioning or surgical approach to the lesion, or if the lesion is in an eloquent brain area

　　　　　　　　(ii)　If the somatosensory evoked potentials (SSEPs) decrease within a short time after positioning, check the extremity involved for pressure issues.

　　　　　　　　(iii)　If SSEPs change after a clamp is applied to a vessel, the clamp must be released and the BP may be increased to high normal levels.

　　　　　　　　(iv)　Increased doses of anesthetic agents will decrease all SSEPs equally; causes should be sought for unilateral changes in SSEPs.

　　　　(3)　Neuroimaging navigation system (aka wand guidance)

　　　　　　(a)　Correlates the topographic anatomy of the patient's head to the preoperative MRI or CT scan

　　　　　　(b)　Used to optimize surgical approach and help the surgeon avoid critical structures

　　　　　　(c)　Once frame is attached to the head holder and calibrated, the frame and the system should not be moved. ICP if monitor or CSF drain is already in situ

　　　　(4)　A urinary catheter is placed for any case longer than 2 to 3 hours, and in all patients with spinal cord injury.

　　　　　　(a)　Positioning

　　　　　　　　(i)　General considerations (6)

READ
MORE

Neuromonitoring, Chapter 16, page 100

Intracranial pressure, Chapter 75, page 528

Positioning of the surgical patient, Chapter 5, page 34

Correct and safe positioning of the neurosurgical patient requires preoperative consultation with the surgeon, and although the ultimate responsibility rests with the surgeon, anesthesiologists are frequently called on to assist.

CONCERNS IN SUBSPECIALTY ANESTHESIA

For a craniotomy, the head will be positioned so that a plane through the craniotomy will be roughly parallel to the floor.

(a) Surgical approach will be chosen by the surgeon to maximize view while minimizing retraction of brain tissue.

(b) The patient must be protected during what could unexpectedly become a very lengthy case.

(c) If table rotation is planned, the patient may be taped to the table across the chest and thighs.

(d) **The position should be as anatomically correct as possible.**

(e) All pressure points should be well padded.

(f) Ensure there are no restrictive elements on the patient (armbands, rings, and so on).

(g) **Patient access will be limited once the case has started.**

    (i) The table will frequently be turned 90 to 180 degrees placing the anesthesiologist at the side or foot of the bed.

    (ii) Secure all lines and tubes completely before draping.

    (iii) The ETT must be well secured to the patient.

(2) **Head positioning**

If BP control is critical, the arterial line should be placed prior to pin application.

  (a) Application of the head holder ("pins")

    (i) Can cause intense adrenergic stimulation, bradycardia, or even asystole (more likely in children or patients with high vagal tone).

    (ii) Pretreat the patient with narcotic, propofol, esmolol, and/or an increase in gas concentration.

    (iii) Pins may also be used in short cases if wand guidance is planned (e.g., VP shunts, brain biopsy).

    (iv) The horseshoe head holder is not used in cases expected to last longer than 2 hours, due to potential effects of pressure on the scalp.

  (b) Limiting rotation of the head to 45 degrees or less is preferred. If more rotation is required, the shoulder opposite from the direction of the head turn can be "bumped up" with a sandbag, and the table can be rotated after the patient is secured to it.

  (c) Disastrous consequences have been reported from overextension or overflexion of the head and/or neck with resultant inadequate arterial flow to the brain stem and spinal cord. Avoid venous outflow obstruction as well.

(3) Prone position

  (a) For high posterior cervical and occipital surgeries, the head will usually be in pins with arms tucked at the sides.

  (b) In cases where the head is quite flexed, a soft bite block or an oral airway will ensure that the patient does not bite the tongue or occlude the ETT.

    (i) Chin position should be checked and padded as needed; at least two fingerbreadths thyromental distance should be maintained.

    (ii) If peak inspiratory pressures increase after positioning, check for ETT obstruction; surgeon to reposition the head as necessary.

(4) Sitting position

  (a) Used infrequently

  (b) Patients with carotid stenosis may have insufficient CBF in the sitting position

  (c) The arterial pressure transducer should be placed at the level of the Circle of Willis (ear level), as it is possible to for CPP to be undesirably low if BP is adjusted based on the pressure transduced at heart level (every 1" is ~ 2 mm difference) (1).

iii) Induction and maintenance

  (1) Choice of anesthesia

    (a) GA is used for most intracranial (IC) cases; no difference in outcome has been shown between use of volatile agents vs. total intravenous anesthetic (TIVA) in intracranial cases.

    (b) Awake craniotomies are used for seizure focus resection (lesion in eloquent area), thermal rhizotomy, and deep brain–stimulating electrode (DBS) placement where the patient will be awake intermittently to facilitate placement of the probe.

(2) **Anesthetic agents and other medications**

    (a) Induction agents

        (i) Intravenous

            1. Propofol (1 to 2 mg/kg) and sodium thiopental (STP, 3 to 5 mg/kg) are acceptable induction agents as both decrease CBF (via vasoconstriction) and ICP and preserve autoregulation.

            2. Etomidate (0.1 to 0.4 mg/kg) decreases CBF and $CMRO_2$ and may be a reasonable induction agent for patients with unstable cardiovascular status.

            3. Ketamine, long thought to increase ICP, is still generally not used in IC surgery but may be acceptable under certain conditions (7).

        (ii) Inhalation agents are rarely used for induction due to potential increase in CBF and ICP

        (iii) Neuromuscular blockade (NMB)

            1. Usually accomplished with an intubating dose of rocuronium (0.5 to 0.6 mg/kg), vecuronium (0.1 to 0.2 mg/kg), or cisatracurium (0.15 to 0.20 mg/kg).

            2. Succinylcholine may transiently increase ICP; it is contraindicated in some chronic neuromuscular and CNS diseases and in trauma with crush injury which has occurred more than 24 hours earlier.

            3. For most neurosurgeries, repeat dosing of NMB is not necessary after intubation as long as anesthetic depth is maintained; they especially should not be redosed in cases where EMGs or motor evoked potentials (MEPs) are monitored.

    (b) Maintenance

        (i) Intravenous agents

            1. Dexmedetomidine, an α_2 agonist, can be useful in BP control and may decrease the dose of narcotics required.

            2. TIVA is popular for cases requiring MEP monitoring; the use of a volatile agent at ≤1 MAC with a small amount of narcotic will be as effective.

            3. Narcotics do not have clinically important direct effects on $CMRO_2$, CBF, or ICP

                a. Fentanyl, sufentanil, alfentanil, remifentanil, morphine, meperidine and hydromorphone are all acceptable choices in neurosurgery.

                b. Ventilation must be adequate to prevent hypercarbia.

        (ii) Inhalation agents

            1. Volatile agents

                  a. At >1 MAC may increase CBF due to vasodilation.

                  b. Sevoflurane is least problematic in terms of effects on CBF; isoflurane would be the next best choice (5,8).

                  c. Desflurane may increase CBF and cause loss of autoregulation, and can also increase ICP through increased CSF production.

CONCERNS IN SUBSPECIALTY ANESTHESIA

Chronic therapy with medications that induce hepatic enzyme production (e.g., antiepileptics) may necessitate increased dose of anesthetic agents.

2. Nitrous oxide (N_2O)
   a. Use of N_2O in intracranial neurosurgery is controversial.
   b. N_2O has been shown to increase CPP (9).
   c. However, a recent study shows no difference in outcomes with use of N_2O in aneurysm surgery in patients with subarachnoid hemorrhage (SAH) (10).
   d. The increase in CBF from N_2O can usually be overcome by hyperventilation.
   e. **N_2O will interfere with MEPs and should not be used in cases when they are monitored.**
   f. N_2O will increase volume of an intracranial air space and if used it may be desirable to turn off near the end of the case before the dura is closed.
   g. Endotracheal tube cuff pressures may increase during a long case if N_2O is used.

(c) Adjuvant agents include
   (i) Mannitol 0.25 to 1 mg/kg
   (ii) Dexamethasone 4 to 10 mg
   (iii) Vasoactive agents
       1. Phenylephrine increases MAP and may cause reflex decrease in HR; it is often used during neuroradiologic procedures, and during STP administration.
       2. Currently, β-adrenergic antagonists or nicardipine are the most frequently used agents to decrease MAP intra- or postoperatively for neurosurgical patients.
       3. Sodium nitroprusside causes vasodilation and impairs autoregulation.
       4. Adenosine is occasionally used in aneurysm surgeries to facilitate clip placement in technically challenging cases by causing short-duration hypotension and possibly asystole. If use is planned, consider application of defibrillator leads to the patient before draping. A 2010 report recommends a dose of 0.3 to 0.4 mg/kg ideal body weight to achieve 45 seconds of profound hypotension.
   (iv) Antibiotics
   (v) Anticonvulsants (phenytoin or fosphenytoin)
   (vi) Desmopressin, vasopressin
   (vii) Hypertonic saline (HS) may rarely be necessary for severe hyponatremia (e.g., SIADH) or cerebral edema.

iv) **Fluid and electrolyte management**
   (1) Goal is euvolemia (normal CVP), while maintaining normal glucose and electrolyte levels.
   (2) Management of intraoperative glucose levels
       (a) Avoid dextrose-containing fluids
           (i) Hyperglycemia worsens outcome in both global and focal ischemia (11,12).
           (ii) Aneurysm patients with SAH who underwent clipping with blood glucose levels >152 mg/dL were more likely to experience postoperative deficits in gross neurologic function (13).
       (b) Current practice is to treat glucose levels >150 to 200; best intraoperative control may be obtained with use of insulin infusion protocols.

v) Cerebral protection

    (1) Neuroprotection entails the use of certain pharmacologic agents or hypothermia to protect the CNS from injury during periods of low blood flow, via decrease in $CMRO_2$.

    (2) The maximum achievable decrease in $CMRO_2$ has occurred when burst suppression is seen on EEG; however, an isoelectric EEG may not be required for cerebral protection (14).

    (3) During a focal ischemic event, STP and propofol may be used to decrease $CMRO_2$ and afford a measure of neuroprotection; these drugs have not been proven to be effective in global ischemia at clinically useful doses.

    (4) Other agents may also decrease $CMRO_2$ but should not be assumed to be neuroprotective.

    (5) Volatile inhalation agents will also decrease cerebral metabolism until the EEG becomes isoelectric, but the dose required to do so (>1.5 to 2 MAC) may increase CBF.

    (6) Moderate hypothermia has also been shown to be neuroprotective, at least in global ischemia (15).

READ MORE

Intracranial pressure, Chapter 75, page 528

        (a) If used during neurovascular cases, the patient may be rewarmed once the lesion has been treated.

        (b) Though hypothermia decreases $CMRO_2$, a recent large prospective study showed that mild intraoperative hypothermia (33°C) did not improve outcome during hospitalization or at 3 months in good-grade (WFNS score I, II, or III) SAH patients (16,17).

    (7) Intraoperatively, begin STP or propofol administration once the risk of an ischemic event is present.

        (a) During aneurysm surgery, this is usually when the aneurysm is visualized but before the surgeon is closely dissecting. If an aneurysm has ruptured preoperatively, a neuroprotective agent may be started on induction.

        (b) Arteriovenous malformations (AVMs) and cavernous malformations are often larger and more complicated lesions, requiring higher total dose.

It is often desirable for the patient to be awake upon completion of surgery in order to assess neurologic status.

        (c) Doses of STP over 6 to 10 mg/kg (depending on age, condition, and tolerance) decrease the probability of successful extubation at the end of the case. The relatively short action of propofol means that most patients can be extubated if indicated.

        (d) Once the lesion has been resected or treated, burst suppression can be discontinued if ICP is not grossly elevated.

vi) **ICP management**

    (1) **Can be critical in the perioperative period**

    (2) Treatment of increased ICP

        (a) Raise head of bed

        (b) Hyperventilation (may sometimes need very high minute ventilation)

        (c) Mannitol; rarely, 3% saline.

        (d) Neuroprotective agents

        (e) Drainage of small amount of CSF if drain is in situ.

vii) High venous pressures:

    (1) May cause excessive intraoperative venous bleeding and obscure surgical field

    (2) Treatment

        (a) Ensure no venous compression or restriction of venous drainage in the neck.

        (b) Raise head of bed up to 30 degrees

      (c) Change respiratory parameters (decrease tidal volume, increase respiratory rate).

      (d) Low-dose venodilators (NTG, morphine) can be administered if increased CBF is not a concern, or if deliberate hypotension may be useful.

      (e) Redose neuromuscular blocking agents.

  c) **Emergence**

    i) **Wakeup must be smooth to avoid increase in ICP or CBF.**

    ii) Extubation

      (1) Most desirable would be to have patient awake at end of case

      (2) Extubation under deep anesthesia, when appropriate, may help prevent coughing.

      (3) If the ability to maintain an airway could be compromised, it may be prudent to keep the patient intubated until awake.

        (a) Use of larger doses of neuroprotective agents

        (b) Posterior fossa surgeries where CNs 9, 10, and 12 might be injured or edematous

        (c) Cases in which brain stem swelling might be expected (tumor, hemorrhage)

        (d) Lengthy prone cases where dependent edema of the airway is possible

    iii) **Watch for BP spikes during emergence and extubation. Treat promptly.**

    iv) If a postoperative MRI is planned, remove all metal from the patient (SaO_2 probe, esophageal stethoscope, wires from neurophysiologic monitoring), and replace EMG-wired ETT with plain ETT if patient is to remain intubated.

  d) **Postoperative care**

    i) Frequent serial neurologic exams should be performed; any postoperative decrement in the exam should prompt immediate investigation as to cause.

    ii) **Continue meticulous BP control (systolic < 160)** so that recently coagulated blood vessels on and within the brain do not bleed. Keep BP even lower (<120) in AVM patients.

    iii) Nausea and vomiting are especially common after posterior fossa cases; consider prophylactic therapy with antiemetics before emergence.

    iv) Intubated patients may be returned directly to the ICU.

    v) Carry vasoactive agents and/or sedation (propofol) during transport in case of hypo- or hypertension.

    vi) Postoperative neurologic assessment

      (1) Assess level of consciousness and mental status.

      (2) Check pupillary response.

      (3) Perform basic cranial nerve function.

        (a) Eyes follow finger

        (b) Smile

        (c) Gag

        (d) Tongue function

      (4) Flexion/extension of all four extremities.

  e) **Potential complications**

    i) Vasospasm

      (1) Usually treated medically with "triple H" therapy (hypertension, hypervolemia, and hemodilution), although a recent study shows that autoregulation may be impaired with hypervolemic hemodilution (18).

      (2) Other options include direct intra-arterial administration of calcium channel blockers (injected by the surgeon, or via radiologic catheter), bathing the artery in papaverine solution, or angioplasty.

Angioplasty is the most medically effective treatment for cerebral vasospasm.

ii) Bleeding
   (1) Because the posterior fossa is a small space, even a small amount of bleeding can cause serious problems, including compression and herniation.
   (2) Watch for somnolence, decreased CN signs such as loss of gag reflex, altered respiratory patterns.

iii) **Venous air embolus (VAE)**
   (1) Sitting craniotomies and any other case where the operative site is higher than the right atrium carry a clinically significant risk of VAE.
   (2) Watch for VAE particularly during turning of flap and bone work, when entry into venous sinuses is most likely.
   (3) Preparation for cases with higher risk of occurrence
      (a) Evaluate patients for patent foramen ovale preoperatively.
      (b) Intraoperative monitoring should include precordial Doppler, as well as multiorifice CVC; TEE may be used if available.
      (c) Sensitivity for detection of VAE: transesophageal echo (TEE) > Doppler > PAP and $ETCO_2$ > CVC > BP > ECG
      (d) It may be preferable to use air instead of N_2O.
   (4) Signs and symptoms
      (a) Consider VAE if severe hypotension is accompanied by decrease in $ETCO_2$.
      (b) Pulmonary HTN and right-sided heart failure secondary to rapid entrainment of 100 to 300 cc of air may be lethal (19).
      (c) Right cardiac inflow/outflow obstruction may also be implicated in the mortality from VAE.
   (5) Treatment
      (a) Immediate treatment of VAE
         (i) Notify surgeons.
         (ii) Call for help.
         (iii) Surgeons flood operative field with saline.
         (iv) Ensure 100% O_2 with controlled ventilation.
         (v) Attempt to aspirate air from CVC.
         (vi) Change position to have operative site lower than right atrium.
         (vii) Consider application of jugular venous compression.
         (viii) Support blood pressure.
         (ix) Prepare for cardiac arrest.
      (b) Rapid administration of fluids through the central line to increase CVP.
         (i) May help prevent further air entry and force the air into the pulmonary circulation where it can be absorbed (20).
         (ii) Must be weighed against the potential increased risk of paradoxical (arterial) air embolism and the possibility of worsening pulmonary HTN.

iv) Syndrome of Inappropriate ADH (SIADH)
   (1) Seen with many malignancies as well as intracranial processes.
   (2) Be suspicious if urine output (UOP) is low relative to IV fluids given, Na + <124, serum Osm < 280, and high urine Osm.
   (3) Treat with restriction of fluids, administration of furosemide, and possibly HS if severe.

v) Diabetes insipidus
   (1) Rarely seen intraoperatively but may develop during surgeries of the pituitary or hypothalamus.

CONCERNS IN SUBSPECIALTY ANESTHESIA

    (2) Large quantity of dilute urine (<200 mOsm, SG 1.001 to 1.005) with normal or elevated serum Osm and Na+.

    (3) Treat with vigorous rehydration with 0.5 NS to match UOP, and 5 to 10 U vasopressin or 1 to 4 μg desmopressin IV.

vi) Neurogenic pulmonary edema (NPE)

    (1) May be due to massive sympathetic activation caused by acute spike in ICP

    (2) Prevented by α blockade

    (3) Frequently accompanied by pulmonary hemorrhage, probably due to increased pulmonary pressures during the sympathetic release

    (4) Incidence of NPE is 50% in patients with severe TBI, and it may also be seen in subarachnoid and intraparenchymal hemorrhage (IPH), as well as status epilepticus.

    (5) HPE develops rapidly within hours of initial injury, and often resolves just as quickly, though may have relapsing course.

    (6) Treatment is symptomatic; use smaller tidal volumes with increased RR.

vii) Eye injury

    (1) Risk with any surgery on the head and neck

    (2) Initial discussion of anesthetic risks may include the potential for postoperative ischemic optic neuropathy especially in patients who will be placed prone.

        (a) Risk may be highest in patients who have substantial blood loss and/or undergo prolonged procedures (>6.5 hours) (20).

        (b) Patients who are diabetic, obese, hypertensive, and smoke may have an incidence as high as 1:100 (21).

        (c) Avoid pressure on the globe, increased venous pressure (a slight head-up position may assist), and overhydration (22).

    (3) Ophthalmic ointment may protect against corneal abrasions.

3) **Intracranial procedures**

  a) **Intracranial neuroendovascular procedures**

    i) Indications

      (1) Diagnostic

        (a) Delineation of size and location of lesions to plan further therapy

      (2) Therapeutic

        (a) Detection and treatment of vasospasm

          (i) Transluminal balloon angioplasty is the most effective treatment for vasospasm, whether it is the reason for the angiogram (e.g., post-SAH) or occurs unexpectedly during an angiogram.

          (ii) Treatment occasionally includes intra-arterial injection of vasodilators (papaverine or calcium channel blockers).

        (b) Coiling and embolization procedures

          (i) May be definitive therapy for vascular lesions such as arteriovenous malformation (AVM) or aneurysm.

          (ii) Often used as a staging procedure to decrease size, minimize blood loss and possibility of rupture during a planned resection to follow

        (c) Placement of stents for stenotic lesions, across ruptured vessels, or to direct flow away from a lesion

    ii) General considerations

      (1) Patient immobility is critical.

      (2) Minimal blood loss is expected.

      (3) **Monitor I/O: Patients may receive several liters of heparinized flush solution.**

      (4) An arterial line is needed if treatment is planned.

      (5) **Do not hyperventilate as this may predispose to vasospasm.**

    (6) Vasopressor and vasodilator therapy should be immediately available.

    (7) Give heparin (70 U/kg) to maintain ACT > 250 if treatment of a lesion is planned; check ACT every hour and redose with partial heparin dose as needed.

    (8) It is desirable to have a rapid but smooth awakening at the end of these procedures.

    (9) Postoperative pain is minimal.

  iii) **Procedures**

    (1) Diagnostic angiograms

      (a) Consider placing an arterial line and a foley catheter prior to beginning the procedure if treatment of lesion might become possible or necessary.

      (b) Have vasopressor ready to administer, as extremely rapid systemic vasodilatory effect may be seen with intra-arterial vasodilator injection by surgeons.

    (2) Aneurysm coiling

      (a) The catheter travels from the femoral artery to the intracranial circulation.

      (b) A pusher wire is threaded through the catheter and numerous platinum coils inserted into the aneurysm where they remain after being disengaged.

    (3) Arteriovenous malformations and dural AV fistulas

      (a) Feeding arteries of large vascular malformations and tumors may be embolized preoperatively to decrease bleeding during subsequent resection.

      (b) Neuroembolic agents include particulates and polymer glues, and the newer nonpolymerizing liquid agents.

  iv) Potential complications

    (1) Vasospasm

    (2) Vessel perforation or rupture with hemorrhage

      (a) Decrease BP and reverse heparin immediately.

      (b) Emergency craniotomy may be required if a stent cannot be placed.

    (3) Vessel occlusion

      (a) Treatment is to increase BP to high normal.

    (4) Contrast-induced nephropathy

      (a) N-acetylcysteine, 600 to 1200 mg before and after the procedure may be effective in reducing the incidence in patients at risk (23).

b) **Carotid endarterectomy**

  i) Indications

    (1) CEA is performed to remove a stenotic plaque from the carotid artery and improve blood flow to the brain.

  ii) Surgical Procedure

    (1) After the carotid artery is exposed, vessel loops are passed around the carotid divisions (common, external or ECA, internal or ICA).

    (2) The common carotid artery is clamped below the lesion; next the ECA and ICA are clamped.

    (3) Before clamping the ICA, the surgeon may elect to measure perfusion pressure ("stump pressure") transmitted to the ICA via the Circle of Willis (Fig.139-4).

      (a) Needle placed into the ICA after clamping the ECA and common carotid

      (b) A (saline-flushed) sterile high-pressure line is attached to the needle, and the distal end passed to the anesthesiologist to be attached to a stopcock in the arterial line monitoring system.

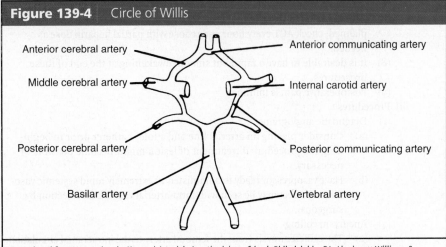

Figure 139-4 Circle of Willis

Anterior cerebral artery

Anterior communicating artery

Middle cerebral artery

Internal carotid artery

Posterior cerebral artery

Posterior communicating artery

Basilar artery

Vertebral artery

Reproduced from Yao et al., eds. *Yao and Artusio's Anesthesiology*. 6th ed. Philadelphia, PA: Lippincott Williams & Wilkins; 2008:553, with permission.

Bradycardia may be observed during dissection in region of carotid body, which may be ameliorated by the surgeon injecting 1 to 2 mL of lidocaine.

(c) If the pressure is <20 to 40 mm Hg (actual number is controversial) or if other monitors (e.g., EEG) indicate ischemia when the ICA clamp is applied, the surgeon may elect to insert a shunt from the common carotid to the ICA to ensure perfusion pressures are adequate.

(4) The common carotid artery is opened, and plaque is stripped off the endothelium at the bifurcation of the common carotid artery into the external and internal branches.

(5) The arterotomy is partially sutured, backflow is allowed in order to flush the artery of air and particulate matter, and the final sutures placed.

(6) The external and internal carotids are unclamped, then the common carotid; the incision is closed.

iii) Preoperative considerations

(1) Studies support early operation in symptomatic patients, but probably not for asymptomatic patients (5,24).

(2) Preoperative BP should be optimized, as preoperative systolic BP > 180 may be associated with postoperative CVA or death, although no study has yet shown a decrease in operative risk if the BP is controlled preoperatively (25).

(3) It is probably appropriate to proceed in patients with severe bilateral stenosis or frequent symptoms (TIAs) even if HTN is not controlled.

iv) Intraoperative anesthetic considerations

(1) Choice of anesthesia

(a) A recent multicenter study found no difference in outcome between general and local anesthesia for CEA (26).

(2) BP Control

(a) Maintain BP high normal (MAP 20% over baseline, especially if a shunt is used) with phenylephrine infusion.

(b) Patient should be hydrated to avoid labile BP.

(3) Maintain normocarbia

(4) Clamping of the carotid artery

        (a) Give heparin 70 U/kg just before clamping; reversal of heparin is not usually necessary but choice can be based on ACT results.

        (b) A neuroprotective agent may be infused for burst suppression before clamping if the surgeon requests.

    (5) The EEG reflects only cortical events and not ischemia of deeper structures.

  v) Postoperative considerations

    (1) Patients with carotid artery disease are often hypertensive preoperatively; higher than normal perfusion pressures may be desirable.

        (a) Postoperative BP control can be difficult; aim for a postoperative systolic pressure of 140 to 160 if appropriate.

        (b) Nicardipine infusion started just before emergence may help prevent BP swings.

    (2) Coughing should be treated with small doses of lidocaine or narcotics.

Wound hematoma after CEA has the potential to rapidly deteriorate into an airway disaster.

  vi) Potential complications

    (1) CVA

    (2) MI

    (3) Nerve injuries (most commonly hypoglossal, sublingual, or recurrent laryngeal)

    (4) Wound hematoma

        (a) If there is any stridor or tracheal deviation, the best course of action may be to bring airway cart into OR, prep the neck and evacuate the hematoma with the patient awake, then perform rapid sequence induction and intubation.

  c) **Craniotomy**

    i) Tumors

      (1) Limit preoperative sedation if ICP is high, there is midline shift, or the patient has signs of impending herniation, and take care to not increase ICP during induction (do not hypoventilate).

      (2) Mannitol (0.25 to 1 gm/kg) infused slowly prior to opening the dura.

      (3) Moderate hyperventilation ($PaCO_2$ 25 to 28) will decrease brain swelling in supratentorial tumors (27). Normalize CO_2 once dura is closed to minimize space available for accumulation of blood, fluid, or air.

      (4) Acoustic neuromas and tumors of the cerebellopontine angle may compress the brain stem and affect cardiovascular status.

      (5) During orbitozygomatic approach the surgeon may exert pressure on the globe, activating the oculocardiac reflex. Treat with anticholinergic agent.

      (6) Anticipate extensive blood loss in the resection of large, highly vascular tumors (e.g., hemangiomas, some glioblastomas).

    ii) Vascular lesions

      (1) Aneurysm

        (a) Use moderate hyperventilation ($ETCO_2$) (28–30) until aneurysm is clipped or wrapped.

        (b) **Keep BP lower than normal to prevent intraoperative rupture or rerupture.**

        (c) A temporary clip may be applied proximally to stop blood flow through the aneurysm, thus easing placement of the permanent titanium clip.

For all craniotomies, it is important to ask the surgeon about size and location of lesion (which will determine site and size of craniotomy as well as position of patient), potential problems (crossing a sinus on opening, etc.), need for dexamethasone, mannitol, and neuroprotection.

Aneurysm cases are an emergency if ruptured.

CONCERNS IN SUBSPECIALTY ANESTHESIA

(i) A temporary clip may be on a vessel that supplies a larger area, which will be at risk for ischemia until the clip is removed.

(d) Once the permanent clip has been applied, minimize potential for vasospasm.

   (i) Resume normal $ETCO_2$.

   (ii) Allow BP to rise to normal-to-increased levels (MAP of 90 to 100); maintain this higher BP postoperatively.

(e) Adenosine administration to cause hypotension or even momentary asystole acts as a "pharmacologic temporary clip."

Nonspecific ST changes mimicking ischemia are common EKG findings in patients with intracranial aneurysm rupture.

   (i) May be used if temporary clip placement is not practicable in large or difficult-to-isolate aneurysms.

   (ii) Defibrillator pads should be placed on the patient during positioning if adenosine may be used.

   (iii) Most commonly recommended initial dose is 12–18 mg followed by up to two more doses.

(f) If clip location causes occlusion of a perforator artery to the brain stem, thalamus, or other structures, cardiovascular instability or loss of neurologic function may follow.

   (i) An intraoperative angiogram may be performed to confirm exclusion of the aneurysm.

(g) **If intraoperative aneurysm rupture occurs, ensure burst suppression and immediately control BP at MAP 40 to 60 until the surgeon regains control of the vessel.** Use shorter-acting agents such as esmolol, nicardipine, sevoflurane, thiopental, and propofol.

(2) Arteriovenous malformation

   (a) Mass of thin-walled blood vessels with direct arterial-to-venous connection without intervening capillaries

      (i) Acts as low resistance circuit (shunt), causing chronic vasodilation with loss of autoregulation in surrounding normal tissue (in order to maintain flow)

      (ii) Up to 10% have an associated aneurysm

   (b) The arterial inflow vessels will be resected first, venous outflow after.

   (c) After AVM resection, the surrounding area that may have been hypoperfused due to the shunt is now exposed to higher CBF.

      (i) This higher CBF in normal tissue may lead to edema or hemorrhage, a situation called normal pressure perfusion breakthrough (NPPB), which can occur intra- or postoperatively.

↳ READ
  MORE

Trauma,
Chapter 142,
page 1029

      (ii) Preoperative embolization decreases the chance of intraoperative hemorrhage and NPPB, and potentially shortens the duration of resection.

      (iii) Treatment of NPPB includes scrupulous control of BP to keep systolic under 110 mm Hg (dexmedetomidine may be a good choice), hyperventilation, increased depth of anesthesia or sedation, mannitol, and diuretics.

   (d) **Slow, calm wakeup of these patients will be helpful** but must be balanced against the surgeon's desire for neurologic exam at end of case.

iii) Traumatic brain injury (TBI)

   (1) Can behave like a mass lesion, 20% mortality.

   (2) Glasgow Coma Scale score of 13 or higher correlates with mild brain injury, 9 to 12 is moderate injury, 8 or less is severe injury; if <8, patient needs immediate intubation.

(3) Consider awake FOI; Patients with trauma above the level of the clavicles have a 15% incidence of cervical spine injury (28).

(4) Cautious induction if hypotensive.

(5) **Maintain BP preferentially over ICP concerns.**

(6) **Do not hyperventilate unless needed for operating conditions:** decreased perfusion of ischemic tissue may follow hyperventilation that causes vasoconstriction (15). Autoregulation may be disrupted and there is not yet consensus on CPP management.

(7) Vasospasm is seen in >30%.

(8) The SAFE-TBI study found a higher mortality level at 24 months in severe TBI patients resuscitated with 4% albumin versus with saline (29).

(9) If acute, use full stomach precautions and RSI for induction.

(10) Changes in ECG morphology and rhythm are common after head trauma and not necessarily due to cardiac issues.

iv) Craniotomy for IPH, aka "strokectomy":

(1) **Risk of rehemorrhage is high, making surgery urgent.**

(2) Volume of clot is a determining factor in outcome (30).

(3) Surgical removal of the clot can decrease pressures and improve prognosis.

(4) Outcome in patients without upper brain stem reflexes is poor (50% die, only 20% recover to be independent).

(5) The posterior fossa is smaller and less compliant than the supratentorial compartment.

  (a) ICP will increase more for a smaller change in volume due to hemorrhage.

  (b) Increased infratentorial pressure is more life threatening due to the possibility of early herniation of the brain stem.

(6) Any coagulopathy must be reversed before surgery.

(7) Maintain systolic BP < 160 (higher in chronically hypertensive patients).

(8) Treat for HTN and risk of vasospasm with nicardipine.

v) Other procedures

(1) Pituitary tumor

  (a) Usually removed via transnasal transsphenoidal approach using endoscope or microscope, or via craniotomy if tumor quite large or invasive.

READ MORE
Pituitary disease, Chapter 84, page 615

  (b) Location is just medial to the cavernous sinuses, which is very vascular and if entered the bleeding will be quite difficult to stop.

  (c) Place arterial line and additional large-bore IV. Consider CVC.

  (d) Have oral airway adjuncts ready at end of case in case patient obstructs, as nares may be packed by surgeon.

(2) Ventriculoperitoneal (VP) shunt

(3) Subdural hematoma (SDH) evacuation

  (a) SDH is due to venous bleeding.

  (b) Acute SDH has high mortality (50% to 80%).

  (c) Surgery will be via burr hole if acute (liquid), craniotomy if chronic (organized clot).

  (d) Insert arterial line and consider CVC for craniotomy.

(4) Epidural hematoma (EDH) evacuation

  (a) EDH is almost always caused by skull fracture above middle meningeal artery.

  (b) Surgery is usually urgent or emergent. Craniotomy often fairly large due to urgency and uncertainty as to exact location of bleeding.

  (c) Vital signs may be quite unstable if hematoma is large.

  (d) Place arterial line and consider CVC.

    (5) Brain biopsy
- (a) Usually a short, low-risk procedure done via either burr hole with a needle, or a minicraniotomy
- (b) Can be done with local or general anesthetic

    (6) Chiari malformation
- (a) In adults, there is disruption of CSF flow through the foramen magnum (FM) and possible herniation of the cerebellar tonsils below the FM. Medullary and cervical cord compression can also occur. Presenting symptoms include headache and weakness.
- (b) Procedure is posterior fossa decompression and dural patch via midline suboccipital incision, with possible concurrent C1-2 laminectomy.
- (c) Place arterial line and extra IV.
- (d) As in any posterior craniotomy, venous sinus entry is possible during opening, with sudden extensive blood loss.
- (e) Watch for postoperative respiratory depression and increased risk of aspiration.

    (7) Intracerebral abscess or empyema
- (a) Similar to SDH and EDH
- (b) Consider arterial line; consider CVC for postoperative ATBs. Surgeon may request delay in antibiotic administration until cultures have been obtained.

    (8) Resection of seizure focus
- (a) Demonstrable discrete focus may be resected (e.g., temporal lobectomy, amygdalo-hippocampectomy).
- (b) If awake surgery is planned (lesion in eloquent area), patient must be able to communicate and cooperate.
  - (i) Oversedation, with resultant respiratory depression, must be avoided.
  - (ii) $ETCO_2$ can be monitored via nasal cannula CO_2 channel.
- (c) Remifentanil, propofol, and/or dexmedetomidine infusions may be useful.
- (d) Hyperventilation can decrease seizure threshold, while methohexital and etomidate can increase activity of seizure focus.

    (9) Surgeries for trigeminal (CN 5) neuralgia
- (a) Suboccipital craniotomy for microvascular decompression requires GA; surgeon will place Gore-tex or Teflon patch between nerve and artery.
- (b) Rhizotomy (thermal or radiofrequency), percutaneous balloon compression, or glycerol or alcohol injection may all be accomplished with the patient intermittently awake but sedated during placement of probe or needle.
- (c) Nerve stimulation during treatment can cause extreme adrenergic response with severe HTN if not treated expectantly. Consider arterial line.
- (d) Potential intraoperative complications include impaling nearby vascular structures including carotid artery.

    (10) Hemifacial spasm (CN 7)
- (a) Microvascular decompression similar to that for CN 5.
- (b) Recommend arterial line placement; other monitoring will include facial nerve and BAERs.

    (11) Stereotactic radiosurgery

      (a) Delivery of radiation to a lesion (tumor, trigeminal neuralgia) via cyber knife or gamma knife.

      (b) Frame placement (used as the guide) requires sedation or "light" general anesthesia for 5 to 20 minutes, during which the patient will be sitting upright with spontaneous ventilation maintained.

(12) Ommaya reservoir

      (a) Short procedure in which a chemotherapy reservoir is implanted under scalp, with distal end inserted into lateral ventricle via burr hole similar to shunt.

(13) Endoscopic procedures

      (a) Current uses are fenestration of third ventricular and other arachnoid cysts, transsphenoidal resection of pituitary tumors, and in some cranial base surgeries.

      (b) Becoming more common in neurosurgery, and can greatly increase visualization of the surgical site with minimal retraction in tight spaces

      (c) Watch patient carefully for signs of herniation, as fluid inflow may be greater than outflow.

      (d) Recommend arterial line.

(14) DBS electrode placement

      (a) Placement of an electrode into deep brain structures (e.g., hypothalamus) to treat various medical disorders, the most common being Parkinson disease.

      (b) Patient will be awake but sedated (propofol infusion works well). The patient must be cooperative for testing during certain parts of the procedure.

Chapter Summary for the Patient for Intracranial Surgery

Definition	
General Considerations	Intracranial surgery cases span a wide variety of problems and can be very challenging. The anesthesiologist must be meticulous in preparing the patient for what may be a multihour procedure.
Preoperative	Consult with the surgeons on planning for any special issues that may exist with the airway, location of lesion, positioning, and monitoring.
Intraoperative	Blood should be immediately available for patients with vascular lesions.
Postoperative	Meticulous attention to BP control is critical. Follow serial neurologic exams in the recovery room and immediately investigate any change. Craniotomy patients usually do not have severe postoperative pain.

CONCERNS IN SUBSPECIALTY ANESTHESIA

References

1. Drummond JC, The lower limit of autoregulation: time to revise our thinking? *Anesthesiology* 1997;86(6):1431–1433.
2. Tomiyama Y, Jansen K, Brian J, et al. Hemodilution, cerebral O$_2$ delivery, and cerebral blood flow: a study using hyperbaric oxygenation. *Am J Physiol* 1999;276(4 Pt 2):H1190–H1196.
3. Cottrell JE, Smith DS, ed. *Anesthesia and Neurosurgery*. 4th ed. St. Louis, MO: Mosby; 2001.
4. Deogaonkar A, Vivar R, Bullock R, et al. Bispectral index monitoring may not reliably indicate cerebral ischaemia during awake carotid endarterectomy. *Br J Anaesth* 2005;94(6):800–804.
5. Howell SJ. Carotid endarterectomy. *Br J Anaesth* 2007;99(1):119–131.

6. Rozet I, Vavilala MS. Risks and benefits of patient positioning during neurosurgical care. *Anesthesiol Clin* 2007;25(3):631–53, x.

7. Himmelseher S, Durieux ME. Revising a dogma: ketamine for patients with neurological injury? *Anesth Analg*, 2005;101(2):524–534.

8. Dinsmore J. Anaesthesia for elective neurosurgery. *Br J Anaesth* 2007;99(1):68–74.

9. Hancock SM, Eastwood JR, Mahajan RP. Effects of inhaled nitrous oxide 50% on estimated cerebral perfusion pressure and zero flow pressure in healthy volunteers. *Anaesthesia*, 2005;60(2):129–132.

10. McGregor DG, Lanier W, Pasternak, J, et al. Effect of nitrous oxide on neurologic and neuropsychological function after intracranial aneurysm surgery. *Anesthesiology* 2008;108(4):568–579.

11. Kushner M, Nencini P, Reivich M, et al. Relation of hyperglycemia early in ischemic brain infarction to cerebral anatomy, metabolism, and clinical outcome. *Ann Neurol* 1990;28(2):129–135.

12. Els T, Klisch J, Orszagh M, et al. Hyperglycemia in patients with focal cerebral ischemia after intravenous thrombolysis: influence on clinical outcome and infarct size. *Cerebrovasc Dis* 2002;13(2):89–94.

13. Pasternak JJ, McGregor D, Schroeder D, et al. Hyperglycemia in patients undergoing cerebral aneurysm surgery: its association with long-term gross neurologic and neuropsychological function. *Mayo Clin Proc* 2008;83(4):406–417.

14. Warner DS, Takaoka S, Wu B, et al. Electroencephalographic burst suppression is not required to elicit maximal neuroprotection from pento-barbital in a rat model of focal cerebral ischemia. *Anesthesiology* 1996;84(6):1475–1484.

15. Fukuda S, Warner DS. Cerebral protection. *Br J Anaesth* 2007;99(1):10–17.

16. Todd MM, Hindman B, Clarke W, et al. Mild intraoperative hypothermia during surgery for intracranial aneurysm. *N Engl J Med* 2005;352(2):135–145.

17. Anderson SW, Todd M, Hindman B, et al. Effects of intraoperative hypothermia on neuropsychological outcomes after intracranial aneurysm surgery. *Ann Neurol* 2006;60(5):518–527.

18. Ogawa Y, Iwataki K, Aoki K, et al. Central hypervolemia with hemodilution impairs dynamic cerebral autoregulation. *Anesth Analg* 2007;105(5):1389–1396.

19. Geissler HJ, Allen S, Mehlhorn U, et al. Effect of body repositioning after venous air embolism. An echocardiographic study. *Anesthesiology* 1997;86(3):710–717.

20. Practice advisory for perioperative visual loss associated with spine surgery: a report by the American Society of Anesthesiologists Task Force on Perioperative Blindness. *Anesthesiology* 2006;104(6):1319–1328.

21. Gill B, Heavner JE. Postoperative visual loss associated with spine surgery. *Eur Spine J*, 2006;15(4):479–84.

22. Williams EL, Hart WM Jr, Tempelhoff R. Postoperative ischemic optic neuropathy. *Anesth Analg* 1995;80(5):1018–1029.

23. Varma MK, Price K, Jayakrishnan V, et al. Anaesthetic considerations for interventional neuroradiology. *Br J Anaesth* 2007;99(1):75–85.

24. Chambers BR, Donnan GA. Carotid endarterectomy for asymptomatic carotid stenosis. *Cochrane Database Syst Rev* 2005(4):CD001923.

25. Rothwell PM, Howard SC, Spence JD. Relationship between blood pressure and stroke risk in patients with symptomatic carotid occlusive disease. *Stroke* 2003;34(11):2583–2590.

26. Lewis SC, Warlow C, Bodenham A, et al. General anaesthesia versus local anaesthesia for carotid surgery (GALA): a multicentre, randomised controlled trial. *Lancet* 2008;372(9656):2132–2142.

27. Gelb AW, Craen R, Rao G, et al. Does hyperventilation improve operating condition during supratentorial craniotomy? A multicenter random-ized crossover trial. *Anesth Analg*, 2008;106(2):585–594.

28. Newfield P, Cottrell JE, ed. *Handbook of Neuroanesthesia*. 4th ed. Philadelphia, PA: Lippincott Williams & Wilkins; 2007.

29. Myburgh J, Cooper J, Finfer S, et al. Saline or albumin for fluid resuscitation in patients with traumatic brain injury. *N Engl J Med* 2007;357(9):874–884.

30. Broderick JP, Brott T, Duldner J, et al. Volume of intracerebral hemorrhage. A powerful and easy-to-use predictor of 30-day mortality. *Stroke* 1993;24(7):987–993.

31. Bebawy J, Gupta D, Bendok B, et al. Adenosine-Induced flow arrest to facilitate intracranial aneurysm clip ligation: Dose-Response data and safety profile. *Anesth Analg* 2010;110(5):1406–1411.

Thoracic anesthesia is one of the most challenging areas of practice in anesthesia. Operations range from lung biopsies or small segmental resections, to complete pneumonectomies, tracheal resections, or esophageal surgery. Surgery involving the airway or lung requires lung isolation, often by different techniques based on the patient's unique anatomy. The anesthesiologist should be prepared to manage airway abnormalities, difficult or unusual ventilation strategies, along with postoperative pain control strategies for open thoracotomy procedures.

1) **Respiratory physiology**
   a) **Lung volumes and capacities (Fig. 140-1)**
      i) An understanding of basic respiratory physiology is important in all aspects of anesthesia care and of paramount importance in thoracic surgery.
      ii) **Tidal volume (TV)** is the volume of gas exchanged during normal breathing.
      iii) **Vital capacity** is the volume of gas expired when one takes a maximal inspiration and maximal expiration.
      iv) **Residual volume (RV)** is the amount of gas remaining in the lung after maximal expiration.
      v) **Functional residual capacity (FRC)** is the amount of gas remaining in the lung after normal expiration.
   b) **Pulmonary ventilation and perfusion (Fig. 140-2)**
      i) Regardless of body position, gravitationally dependent regions of the lung (bases in the upright position, dorsal regions in the supine position) receive greater ventilation (V) and perfusion (Q).
      ii) Although the overall V/Q ratio of the lung is 0.8, gravitationally nondependent alveolar units have greater regional V/Q ratios than the dependent ones.
      iii) Since gas exchange efficiency is directly related to the regional V/Q ratios, and zone 1 is reduced significantly in the supine position, overall V/Q (and oxygenation) decreases when a patient moves from the upright to the supine position.
   c) **Mechanisms of hypoxemia**
      i) **Reduced inspired oxygen (P_iO_2)**
         (1) Occurs with lower atmospheric pressure (i.e., high altitude) or oxygen fraction <0.21 (i.e., toxic fumes in closed environment)
         (2) Alveolar hypoventilation, ventilation/perfusion (V/Q) mismatch, right-to-left (intra/extra-pulmonary) shunt, and diffusion impairment

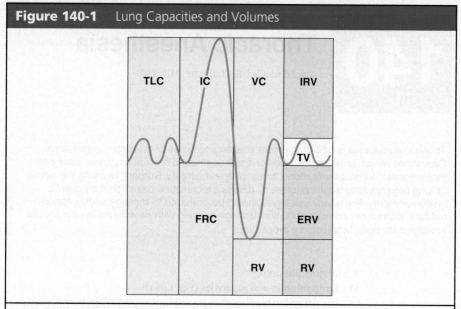

Figure 140-1 Lung Capacities and Volumes

Reproduced from Ault ML, Stock MC. Respiratory Function. In: Barash PG, Cullen BF, Stoelting RK, et al., Eds. *Clinical Anesthesia*. 6th ed. Philadelphia, PA: Lippincott Williams & Wilkins; 2008:247, with permission.

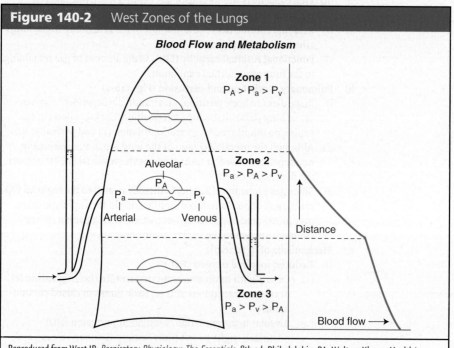

Figure 140-2 West Zones of the Lungs

Reproduced from West JB. *Respiratory Physiology: The Essentials*. 8th ed. Philadelphia, PA: Wolters Kluwer Health/ Lippincott Williams & Wilkins; 2008, with permission.

ii) **Alveolar hypoventilation**
   (1) Impairment in the respiratory drive that reduces inspired volume and/or respiratory rate (i.e., neuromuscular diseases, chest trauma, sedatives)

iii) **V/Q mismatch**
   (1) One of the most frequent and resistant-to-O_2-treatment hypoxemic mechanisms, derives from a dissociation between the degree of ventilation and perfusion in alveolar units.
   (2) These units receive proportionally less ventilation than perfusion (i.e., secretions, edema, etc.).
   (3) Shunt effect (an extreme V/Q mismatch) occurs in perfused alveoli that are unventilated and therefore do not contribute to gas exchange.
      (a) Examples include pulmonary arteriovenous malformations, hepatopulmonary syndrome, alveolar consolidation.
   (4) General anesthesia increases V/Q mismatch because of increased airway closure and inhibition of hypoxic pulmonary vasoconstriction, and shunt effect due to atelectasis. Lateral position and one-lung ventilation (OLV) enhance this V/Q mismatch.

iv) **Impairment of O_2 diffusion through the alveolar-capillary barrier**
   (1) Rarely a main mechanism of hypoxemia, but may contribute in cases of pulmonary fibrosis and advanced Acute Respiratory Distress Syndrome

v) **Physiological dead space**
   (1) Physiological dead space (V_D) refers to the fraction of inspired volume that does not contribute to gas exchange.
   (2) Includes the air that remains in the respiratory tree excluding the alveolar spaces (anatomical V_D, ~2 mL/kg) and the volume that reaches poorly/not ventilated alveoli (functional V_D, variable volume that increases with age, COPD, etc.).
   (3) In a healthy adult, $V_D/V_T < 30\%$.
   (4) Physiological V_D is reflected by the expired-to-arterial PCO_2 ratio $[(PaCO_2 - P_{ET}CO_2)/PaCO_2]$.

vi) **Compliance**
   (1) The ability of the respiratory system (chest wall, lung, or both) to change in volume with a change in distending pressure.
   (2) Respiratory compliance is usually measured as:

$$C = \Delta\text{Volume}/\Delta\text{Pressure} = V_T/(P_{plateau} - \text{Positive End Expiratory Pressure})$$

   (3) In a spontaneously breathing healthy adult, the compliance of the respiratory system or total compliance (lung + chest wall) is around 100 mL/cm H_2O, but it decreases significantly in the supine position, under anesthesia and with respiratory diseases (i.e., pulmonary fibrosis, inflammation, or edema)
   (4) **Airway resistance**
      (a) Resistance to airflow is inversely related to lung volume and airway diameter.
      (b) Determines whether this airflow is laminar or turbulent
      (c) Airway resistance is usually measured as:

$$R = \Delta\text{pressure}/\Delta\text{flow} = (P_{peak} - P_{plateau})/\text{flow}$$

The lateral position and the OLV enhance the V/Q mismatch that occurs during general anesthesia.

vii) **Work of breathing (WOB)**

(1) Reflects the effort performed by respiratory muscles to overcome the resistance and elastance recoil of chest and lung, and is usually estimated as a product of mean airway pressure (Paw) times tidal volume: $WOB = Paw \times V_T$.

2) **Preoperative assessment and management**

a) **General considerations**

i) **A thorough preoperative evaluation should be performed with a focus on the cardiac and respiratory function.**

ii) Pulmonary function must be optimized before surgery

General anesthesia reduces respiratory compliance and increases airway resistance and work of breathing.

(1) **Pulmonary rehabilitation, treatment of underlying infections, and palliative relief of airway obstruction if needed should be carried out.**

(2) Scheduled treatments (including inhalation therapy) should be continued.

iii) **Preoperative** interview is a critical time for discussing the postoperative management including emergence and extubation, risk of postoperative mechanical ventilation, critical role of Patient Controlled Analgesia (PCA) analgesia, etc.

The lower the lung compliance, the stiffer the lung.

iv) Ideally, an epidural thoracic catheter should be placed and tested before proceeding to the operating room.

b) **Pulmonary function tests (PFTs) should be reviewed**

i) **Table 140-1** shows normal and pathological results of the PFTs.

ii) **Pressure-flow curves** for different respiratory conditions are described in **Figure 140-3**.

iii) Preoperative findings described in **Table 140-2** indicate a high risk for postoperative complications after a pneumonectomy.

iv) Postoperative respiratory complications are rare if the preoperative FEV_1 is ≥2 L or ≥50% of predicted value.

Table 140-1
Pulmonary Function Test (PFT) PFT Results

Description	Normal[a]	Obstructive Disease	Restrictive Disease
TLC	5.5 L	↑	↓
FVC	4 L	N/↓	↓
FEV$_1$	3.2 L	↓	N/↓
FEV$_1$/FVC	80%	↓	↑
FRC	2.5 L	↑	↓
RV	1.5 L	↑	↓
FEF$_{25-75}$	>65%	↓	N/↓

[a]Normal PFT values for a healthy 70-kg adult. N, normal.

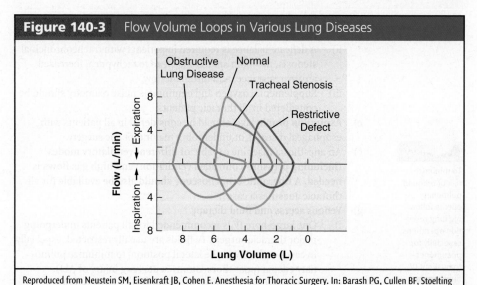

Figure 140-3   Flow Volume Loops in Various Lung Diseases

Reproduced from Neustein SM, Eisenkraft JB, Cohen E. Anesthesia for Thoracic Surgery. In: Barash PG, Cullen BF, Stoelting RK, et al., Eds. *Clinical Anesthesia*. 6th ed. Philadelphia, PA: Lippincott Williams & Wilkins; 2008:1035, with permission.

v) Conversely, an estimated postoperative $FEV_1 < 0.8$ L (postoperative FEV_1 = preoperative FEV_1 × perfusion % of remaining lung after resection, estimated by ^{133}Xe or ^{99}Tc scanning) is indicative of high risk of postoperative respiratory failure.

c) **Other tests**
   i) **Arterial blood gases** are not routinely indicated but may be helpful in particular cases for assessing the severity of the pulmonary condition.
   CT imaging may be required in tracheobronchial stenosis in order to evaluate the size and length of the endotracheal tube (ETT) or to modify the airway management plan.

d) **Preoperative sedation**

Table 140-2

High-risk Preoperative Test Results for Pneumonectomy

Test	High-risk Results
Arterial blood gas (room air)	$PaO_2 < 50$ mm Hg $PaCO_2 > 45$ mm Hg
Preoperative FEV_1	<2 L
Predicted postoperative FEV_1	<0.8 L or <40% of predicted
FEV_1/FVC	<50% of predicted
Maximum breathing capacity	<50% of predicted
Maximum VO_2 during exercise	<10 mL/kg/min

FEV_1, forced expiratory volume in 1 second; FVC, forced vital capacity; VO_2, oxygen consumption.

        i) Sedation should be individually customized to avoid respiratory depression, hypoxemia, and loss of airway protection.

        ii) A delicate balance is required in patients with tracheobronchial stenosis, in whom anxiety may lead to tachypnea, increased airway resistance, and turbulent flow.

        iii) Supplemental oxygen and continuous pulse oximetry should be considered in all thoracic patients.

   e) **Aspiration prophylaxis** should be considered in all patients with esophageal diseases or undergoing major thoracic surgery.

   f) An anesthesia machine capable of **different ventilatory modes (including pressure-controlled ventilation) and high gas flows is needed. A fiberoptic bronchoscope should also be available** for all thoracic anesthesia cases.

   g) **Venous access and fluid therapy.**

        i) One large-bore IV is recommended for all patients undergoing major thoracic surgery. IV fluids are usually restricted, especially in cases with OLV in the lateral position, to minimize pulmonary edema (post-thoracotomy acute lung injury or ALI).

To minimize risk of rebound pulmonary edema following lung resection operations, especially for pneumonectomy, limit IV fluids aggressively (<1 L).

        ii) Consider invasive arterial BP monitoring for open thoracic procedures or as needed based on cardiac risk.

3) Intraoperative management will be discussed in following sections.

4) Postoperative management

   a) **General considerations**

        i) Despite an older population undergoing elective thoracic surgery with their concurrent comorbidities, operative mortality after thoracic surgery remains unchanged from historic controls (<2% for lobectomy, <6% for pneumonectomy) (2).

   b) **Independent risk factors of perioperative mortality**

        i) Increased age, male sex, dyspnea score, functional performance status, the American Society of Anesthesiologists (ASA) score, and the extent of surgical resection (3,4)

   c) **Complications**

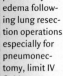

Ideally, an epidural catheter should be checked for efficacy before induction of general anesthesia, and dosed during the case and at thoracotomy closure for a smoother emergence.

        i) The most common postoperative fatal complications are infections and ALI/ARDS.

        ii) Nonfatal complications are more frequent: inadequate analgesia, atelectasis, pneumothorax, bleeding (>200 mL/h through chest tube), hemoptysis, supraventricular tachyarrythmias, and neural injury (i.e., left recurrent laryngeal, vagus, or phrenic nerve injury after mediastinal surgery).

   d) **Postoperative Management**

Epidural medications will not blunt vagal-related airway manipulation, lung re-expansion reflexes, or referred shoulder pain from diaphragmatic irritation.

        i) Patients should be in a semiupright (>30 degrees) position and receive close ECG and hemodynamic monitoring, supplemental O_2 as needed, incentive spirometry, a postoperative chest x-ray, and aggressive pain treatment.

5) Anesthetic management of Specific procedures

   a) **Pulmonary resection via open thoracotomy**

        i) **Regional analgesia**

           (1) Patients undergoing a thoracotomy benefit from a thoracic epidural catheter (T4-7) due to better postoperative pain control and decreased narcotic secondary effects.

           (2) A local anesthetic-opioid mixture is most commonly selected (i.e., bupivacaine 0.06% with fentanyl 2 μg/mL, usually at 5 to 8 mL/h).

(3) **Intercostal nerve blocks** may be used when epidural analgesia is not an option or not effective.

Paravertebral blocks, Chapter 184, page 1247

   (a) Under sterile conditions, a 22-gauge needle is inserted perpendicular to the skin at the posterior axillary line on the inferior edge of the rib. The needle is advanced until it is touching the rib, then slid downward to slip off the rib. After confirmation of no blood or air upon aspiration, 4 to 5 mL of local anesthetic (i.e., bupivacaine 0.5% with epinephrine 1:200,000) is injected. The process is repeated at each intercostal space involved in innervation of the thoracotomy site.

(4) **Paravertebral block**

   (a) Paravertebral blockade can be accomplished either preoperatively or postoperatively. This block can provide supplemental pain control for 12 to 24 hours.

ii) **General anesthesia**

   (1) **Monitoring**

      (a) Standard ASA monitoring plus invasive arterial monitoring are recommended in all patients undergoing major thoracic surgery.

      (b) Blood flow to the dependent arm in a lateral-positioned patient, and to the right arm during mediastinal surgery, should be monitored with either the arterial line or pulseoximeter. Further invasive monitoring will depend on the patient's condition.

   (2) **Induction**

      (a) Can be achieved using various induction agent/muscle relaxant combinations as guided by the preoperative evaluation.

   (3) **Maintenance**

      (a) Can be achieved with a volatile agent or a propofol infusion

      (b) Muscle relaxation is needed during the procedure.

      (c) Nitrous oxide is typically not used due to possible increased atelectasis, as well as increased pulmonary vascular pressures.

   (4) **Emergence**

Vagal-mediated bradycardia may occur with airway surgical manipulation, so atropine should always be available.

      (a) Smooth emergence is ideal to avoid stressing anastomosis lines following pulmonary resection.

      (b) Verify double-lung ventilation with manual recruitment of the lungs (inspiratory pressure < 30 cm H_2O maintained for 2 to 3 seconds).

      (c) Use FiO_2 1.0 and verify patency of chest tubes.

      (d) A supine position with head raised 45 degrees is helpful.

      (e) If postoperative mechanical ventilation is needed, the double lumen tube (DLT) must be exchanged for a conventional ETT prior to emergence.

      (f) Chest tubes are connected to water seal alone after a pneumonectomy, or with 20 cm H_2O suction in all other resections.

iii) **Positioning**

   (1) Pulmonary resection is usually performed with the patient in the lateral position (operative, or nondependent side, up), and the bed sharply flexed.

   (2) Extreme care should be taken to assure a good positioning with enough pressure-relieving padding below head and neck (neutral position of neck, dependent ear, eye), shoulders (brachial plexus), arms (radial, ulnar nerves), legs, and scrotum in males.

   (3) Vital signs and oxygenation should be monitored during positioning.

   (4) After positioning and before preparation of the surgical field, reassessment of vitals, oxygenation, patency of IV catheters, epidural catheter, and position of endobronchial tube or bronchial blocker is mandatory.

iv) **One-lung ventilation**

(1) **Physiological implications**

(a) General anesthesia, mechanical ventilation, lateral position, open chest, and OLV alter ventilation and perfusion (V/Q matching).

(b) Oxygenation will mostly depend on the blood flow directed to the nonventilated lung (intrapulmonary shunt).

(c) The shunt fraction is reduced in the lateral position due to gravity effects along with hypoxic pulmonary vasoconstriction, which reduces perfusion to nonventilated areas.

(d) Additionally, chronically diseased lungs have diminished perfusion overall, which is beneficial if the operative side is the most severely injured lung.

(2) **Multiple devices** are available for lung isolation, including double-lumen tubes, bronchial blockers, and Univent tubes.

(3) **Management**

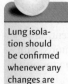
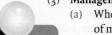

Lung isolation should be confirmed whenever any changes are made in patient position.

(a) When switching from double-lung to OLV or vice versa, a brief period of manual ventilation is recommended for assessing compliance and recruiting collapsed alveoli.

(b) Minute ventilation is ideally maintained, with lower TVs recommended (5 to 7 mL/kg instead of 6 to 9 mL/kg) and higher respiratory rates (5).

(c) Neuromuscular relaxation and controlled ventilation are mandatory during OLV, with the goal of maintaining adequate oxygenation and a CO_2 partial pressure similar to double-lung ventilation. The latter will depend largely on the dependent lung compliance.

(4) Should oxygenation/ventilation difficulties occur during OLV, one should:

(a) **Ensure FiO$_2$ of 1.0.**

(b) **Confirm adequate tube position** by fiberoptic bronchoscopy (**Figs. 140-3 and 140-4**)

(c) **Suction secretions** if needed.

(d) **Apply continuous positive airway pressure (CPAP) to the nonventilated lung** (in open thoracotomy cases) and **notify the surgeon.** Under direct visualization, the nonventilated lung is inflated through a separate circuit and then allowed to deflate and maintained at a volume that does not interfere with the surgical procedure, usually 2 to 5 cm H$_2$O CPAP. This may not be possible in video-assisted thoracic surgery (VATS) cases due to interference with the surgeon's view.

(e) **Add PEEP to the ventilated lung** trying to recruit atelectasic areas. This measure may not be effective if the high airway pressures decrease perfusion to ventilated areas increasing shunted blood to nonventilated ones, so small increases of PEEP are recommended to select the minimum effective PEEP.

(f) **Apneic oxygenation of the nonventilated lung.** The nonventilated lung is periodically inflated with FiO$_2$ 1.0 and then isolated capping the exhalation valve, so that it stays motionless and slowly collapses absorbing the oxygen.

(g) **Periodic manual double-lung ventilation** may be required for adequate oxygenation.

(h) If hypoxemia persists, the surgeon may **clamp the pulmonary artery** perfusing the operative field to improve the V/Q matching.

(i) **Cardiopulmonary bypass** can be established in extreme situations (Table 140-3).

b) **Video-assisted thoracic surgery (VATS)**

i) The number of cases performed with thoracoscopic assistance is rapidly increasing.

ii) Usually performed in the lateral decubitus position with OLV and three or four small incisions

Figure 140-4 Fiberoptic View of the Distal Trachea and Carina

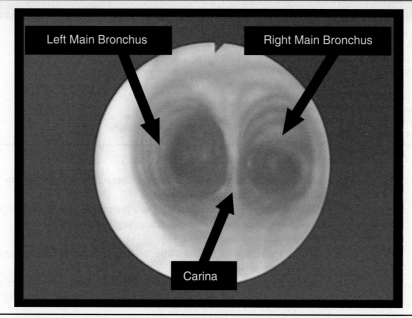

Fiberoptic view of carina anatomy is labelled. It is common practice to identify the right upper lobe in the right mainstem bronchus (usually 2–3 cm past carina) to verify the right from left bronchus. (Image by N. Weitzel MD.)

Figure 140-5 Fiberoptic View of Appropriately Placed Double Lumen ETT

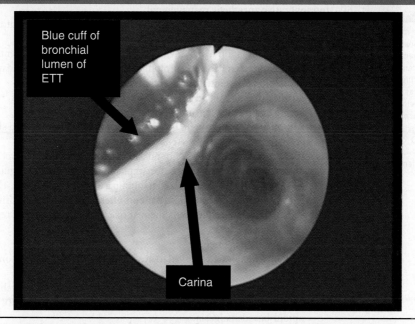

The bronchial lumen is in the left bronchus—with the edge of the bronchial cuff (*blue*) just visible at the carina when viewed from the tracheal lumen. (Image by N. Weitzel MD.)

Table 140-3

Steps to Take When Oxygenation or Ventilation Difficulties Occur During OLV

Ensure FiO_2 of 1.0.
Confirm adequate tube position
Suction secretions if needed
Apply CPAP to the nonventilated lung (open thoracotomy) and notify the surgeon.
Add PEEP to the ventilated lung
Apneic oxygenation of the nonventilated lung
Periodic manual double-lung ventilation
Pulmonary artery clamp
Cardiopulmonary bypass (extreme situations)

iii)   Anesthetic management is similar to open procedures except that no epidural analgesia is usually required.

iv)   CPAP often disrupts the surgical field to a greater degree than with open thoracotomy, and may prevent adequate surgical exposure.

c)   Lung volume reduction surgery (LVRS)

i)   LVRS aims at removing the most affected lung areas in selected patients with severe emphysema.

ii)   The major clinical trial that compared medical + surgical treatment *versus* medical only treatment (National Emphysema Treatment Trial, or NETT trial) showed controversial results (6).

   (1)   LVRS may improve the quality of life of patients without high operative risk who have predominantly apical disease, and a poor baseline exercise tolerance, although it does not alter their overall disease-related mortality. Postoperative mortality is increased in poorly selected patients.

iii)   Intraoperative anesthetic management

   (1)   The risk of hypoxemia and pneumothorax should guide ventilator management.

   (2)   Careful ventilation with individualized FiO_2, pressure limited ventilation below 30 cm H_2O and prolonged expiratory times are mandatory.

   (3)   Extubation is essential at the end of the procedure; therefore, extreme care should be paid to optimize extubation conditions before emergence: maximize SaO_2, ensure adequate analgesia, administer IV steroids and bronchodilator nebulizations, avoid shivering from hypothermia, etc.

   (4)   If immediate extubation is not possible, assure an adequate level of anesthesia of the patient before replacing the DLT with a regular ETT. FiO_2 should be minimized to obtain a SpO_2 ≥88% to 90%. The chronic hypoxic state of these patients alters their respiratory drive such that increased FiO_2 puts them at risk for hypercapnia and respiratory acidosis (7).

iv)   Postoperative management

   (1)   Adequate analgesia is critical to avoid hypoventilation and its consequences.

   (2)   Thoracic epidural analgesia is ideal, but intercostal or paravertebral regional blocks should be considered before opting for a total IV opioid-based analgesia.

   (3)   BiPAP should be considered in patients with $PaCO_2$ ≥70 mm Hg.

Due to chronic hypoxia in extreme COPD, patients breathing high FiO_2 are at risk for developing hypercapnia; thus, aim for SpO_2 of 88% to 90% in these patients.

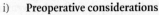

d) **Tracheal resection and reconstruction**
   i) **Preoperative considerations**

For tracheal surgeries, equipment and personnel for an emergency airway loss should be immediately available before induction.

(1) The major anesthetic challenge during these procedures is airway management at induction and during the case. Individualized and detailed communication with the surgical team before the procedure is critical: level and severity of airway lesion and initial airway management (oral vs. tracheostomy, size of device), surgical implications on airway control (change of airway device, need of jet ventilation), postoperative plan.

   ii) **General anesthesia**

(1) **Induction**

   (a) IV agents can be used in patients with a pre-existing tracheostomy or those without critical airway stenosis.

   (b) In patients with critical stenosis, induction can be performed with sevoflurane and spontaneous ventilation.

   (c) Neuromuscular relaxation should be delayed until the airway is instrumented under a deep plane of anesthesia and/or the use of local anesthetic squirted at the vocal cords. Total Intravenous Anesthesia (TIVA) (i.e., propofol and remifentanil) is a convenient method for maintenance of anesthesia because of the changes in ventilatory approaches (with its intermittent loss of ventilatory circuit seal) and the smooth emergence.

(2) **Surgical specifics**

   (a) Rigid bronchoscopy may be performed prior to intubation and the findings may guide the intubation approach: routine oral intubation, tracheostomy, resection of intraluminal tracheal lesion, Laryngeal Mask Airway (LMA) and spontaneous ventilation, jet ventilation from above the lesion, etc. In lower tracheal or carinal stenosis, a long cuffed ETT or jet ventilation through a catheter may be used.

(3) **Tracheal division**

   (a) When the trachea is surgically divided, the ETT or jet catheter is retracted and a sterile armored ETT is placed by the surgeon in the distal airway. If the distal airway is too small to accommodate a tube (i.e., carinal or mainstem bronchial resections), a jet catheter (see below) may be used.

   (b) The airway resection is performed along with the posterior anastomosis around this distal tube/catheter. The anterior sutures are often placed under intermittent apnea before advancing the original ETT.

   (c) The patient's neck is then flexed (extra blankets will be needed to support the head), the anastomosis finished, and skin closed. A suture may be left from the chin to the chest to remove tension at the tracheal anastomosis.

(4) **Emergence and extubation**

   (a) Spontaneous ventilation and extubation is usually the goal to decrease strain on fresh anastomosis, but in certain cases postoperative sedation with mechanical ventilation and a flexed neck may be preferred.

   (b) A small tracheostomy may be placed below the anastomosis for safety reasons (multiple secretions, difficult anatomy).

CONCERNS IN SUBSPECIALTY ANESTHESIA

    (c) Extubation should be performed when patient is awake enough to avoid aspiration but without excessive head movement or coughing (use of mild sedation may be considered).

    (d) Flexible bronchoscopies may be needed postoperatively to clear secretions.

    (e) A small uncuffed tube (5.0 or 6.0 ETT) and a flexible bronchoscope should be easily available for a potential reintubation.

e) **Endoscopic procedures**

  i) **Bronchoscopy**

    (1) **Flexible bronchoscopy**

      (a) Usually performed under local anesthesia (pharynx and airways) with sedation.

      (b) General anesthesia may be needed in certain patients and will require an LMA or ETT big enough to pass the bronchoscope.

Coordination between the surgical and anesthesia teams is critical during rigid bronchoscopy, since ventilation (and surgery) may need to be interrupted for instrumentation or ventilation.

      (c) Premedication with an antisialogogue, local anesthesia of the airways, and short-acting anesthetics and neuromuscular relaxants if needed is recommended.

    (2) **Rigid bronchoscopy**

      (a) Allows visualization of the larynx, trachea, and mainstem bronchi.

      (b) It requires a deep level of general anesthesia or neuromuscular relaxation to prevent movement or coughing.

      (c) Ventilation is accomplished through the working channel of the rigid bronchoscope, attaching the respiratory circuit to the lateral port of the rigid bronchoscope. Jet ventilation may be used (see below).

      (d) In cases of severe stenosis, maintenance of spontaneous ventilation is recommended.

Jet ventilation requires being familiar with the jet equipment and the administration of ventilation with small TV/ high rate in an open respiratory system.

      (e) Due to the potential large air leaks, capnography may not be accurate; TIVA is a convenient option for maintenance.

      (f) **Jet ventilation**

        (i) The major benefits are a continuous ventilation and a lack of movement of the surgical field.

        (ii) May be applied through a thin catheter inserted through the main lumen of the rigid bronchoscope or through a small lateral lumen of a specially designed rigid bronchoscope, with a Sanders' manual jet injector or a specially designed jet ventilator.

        (iii) Jet ventilation consists of administration of very small tidal volumes (close to the pulmonary dead space) at a high frequency or respiratory rate. Air comes into the airways at a very fast speed, dragging more air than is "programmed" (entrapment).

        (iv) Therefore, exact TV or inspired oxygen fraction is not known.

        (v) Make sure that exhaled air escapes into the atmosphere (open respiratory system); if not (closed system), the risk of tension pneumothorax is high.

Check visually thoracic movements to assure air comes in... and OUT!

        (vi) FiO_2 must be reduced below 0.4 during laser surgery.

    (3) **Complications** of bronchoscopy include injuries to eyes, lips, teeth, or larynx, airway rupture, pneumothorax, bleeding, and airway obstruction because of bleeding, dislodged stent.

ii) Mediastinoscopy and mediastinal surgery.
   (1) Usually performed for staging tumoral conditions, allowing for planning of surgical resection, but sometimes is coupled with a VATS or open resection
   (2) **Preoperative evaluation** of the trachea is mandatory to rule out a fixed, deviated, or compressed trachea.
      (a) A large bore (16-gauge at least) venous access is highly recommended because of the risk of bleeding during mediastinal surgery from damage to the large vessels, and the difficulty of controlling it.
   (3) **Monitoring**
      (a) The pulseoximeter or arterial line (if needed) should be placed in the right arm to monitor flow through the innominate artery and detect a potential compression.
      (b) Mediastinoscopy alone is a short procedure and short-acting hypnotics and neuromuscular relaxants should be used.

Chapter Summary for Thoracic Anesthesia

General Population	Wide range of patients and procedures often requiring advanced airway management or OLV
Assessment	Based on extent of procedure, but consider full laboratory workup, Pulmonary Function testing $\pm$ VQ scanning for lung resections, $\pm$ABG, CT scans. Coronary workup based on comorbidity. Aggressive pulmonary therapy preoperatively helps reduce risk of respiratory complications.
Risks	Patients are intermediate risk surgical candidates. May have secondary elevations in PAP leading to right-heart dysfunction—increasing risk level.
Monitoring	Arterial line for open thoracic procedures. Consider central line based on IV access/surgical risk. TEE/PAC typically not indicated unless severe cardiac disease present. Fiberoptic bronchoscope recommended for ETT placement.
Anesthetic Management	General Anesthesia usually employed due to considerations for OLV. Regional analgesia should be considered for open thoracic procedures.

References

1. Barash PG. *Clinical Anesthesia*. 6th ed. Philadelphia, PA: Wolters Kluwer/Lippincott Williams & Wilkins; 2009.
2. West JB. *Respiratory Physiology: The Essentials*. 8th ed. Philadelphia, PA: Wolters Kluwer Health/Lippincott Williams & Wilkins; 2008.
3. Boffa DJ, Allen MS, Grab JD, et al. Data from The Society of Thoracic Surgeons General Thoracic Surgery database: the surgical management of primary lung tumors. *J Thorac Cardiovasc Surg* 2008;135(2):247–254.
4. Licker M, Fauconnet P, Villiger Y, et al. Acute lung injury and outcomes after thoracic surgery. *Curr Opin Anaesthesiol* 2009;22(1):61–67.
5. Schultz MJ, Haitsma JJ, Slutsky AS, et al. What tidal volumes should be used in patients without acute lung injury? *Anesthesiology* 2007;106(6):1226–1231.
6. Fishman A, Martinez F, Naunheim K, et al. A randomized trial comparing lung-volume-reduction surgery with medical therapy for severe emphysema. *N Engl J Med* 2003;348(21):2059–2073.
7. Murphy R, Driscoll P, O'Driscoll R. Emergency oxygen therapy for the COPD patient. *Emerg Med J* 2001;18(5):333–339.

Adult Cardiac Surgery

Christopher Cornelissen, DO

Adults presenting for cardiac surgery make up a diverse population with pathology not limited to coronary artery disease and valve repair or replacement. Increasing numbers of adults with a history of repaired congenital heart disease are presenting for cardiac and noncardiac operations. The surgical spectrum also includes trauma, major aortic repair or reconstruction, heart and lung transplantation, surgical interventions for malignancy/tumor and the placement of intracardiac devices.

Baseline exercise tolerance can give invaluable information about the extent of a patient's coronary artery disease.

I) **Preoperative assessment**
   a) It is important to know the extent of the patient's primary cardiac disease and comorbidities.
      (i) This is especially important in patients with an ongoing or past history of unstable coronary syndromes, decompensated heart failure (HF), significant arrhythmias, or severe valvular disease.
   b) **Myocardial ischemia/infarction**
      i) The key items for evaluation include determination of the amount of myocardium at risk or involved, the angina or ischemic threshold, ejection fraction, stability of symptoms, and medical therapy.
      ii) Baseline exercise tolerance can give invaluable information about extent of coronary disease.
         (1) Resting and stress echocardiography may reveal the extent of damaged or potentially viable myocardium, with stress imaging more indicative.
      iii) Coronary catheterization provides the most optimal means of determining the exact coronary vessels involved as well as a determination of overall coronary anatomy.
      iv) High-resolution CT may provide imaging of the pericardium, chambers, and great vessels.
         (1) Cardiac MRI is emerging as a tool to assess native vessels in addition to prior arterial and venous coronary bypass grafts.
      v) Ongoing heparinization, use of antiplatelet agents (clopidogrel, integrilin) or warfarin may require discontinuation immediately prior to surgery (heparin) or within 6 to 8 hours of surgery (Integrilin®).
         (1) These patients are at higher risk for platelet and fresh frozen plasma transfusion to control bleeding upon separation from cardiopulmonary bypass CPB.
   c) **Heart failure (HF)**
      i) The presence of systolic or diastolic HF has significant implications for the cardiac surgery patient.
      ii) Paroxysmal nocturnal dyspnea and orthopnea may impact the patient's ability to lie supine on induction.

Patients with preoperative congestive HF have a two- to threefold increased risk of postoperative morbidity and mortality.

READ MORE

Cardiac arrhythmias and pacemakers, Chapter 57, page 412

iii) The presence of significant pericardial disease should be determined to guide the induction plan, especially if constrictive physiology is present.

iv) Many patients will remain on ACE inhibitors, angiotensin II receptor blockers, or diuretics until the time of surgery.

v) Preoperative HF may lead to a two- to threefold increase in postoperative morbidity or mortality **(1)**.

d) **Dysrhythmias**

i) Patients presenting with pacemakers or automatic implantable cardioverter defibrillators (AICD) should have their devices interrogated prior to cardiac surgery.

(1) The antitachycardia feature of the AICD should be suspended.

ii) Pacemaker-dependent patients may benefit from their device being placed in an asynchronous mode for continuous pacing.

iii) Defibrillation pads should be considered in patients with critical left main coronary artery disease (or left main equivalency), unstable arrhythmias, critical valvular stenosis, and patients predisposed to ventricular tachycardia.

e) **Coexisting organ dysfunction**

i) **Central nervous system (CNS)**

(1) Patients with a history of transient ischemic attack or cerebrovascular accident (CVA) may have an increased risk of a new CNS event following cardiac surgery.

(2) Brain imaging and carotid duplex ultrasound may establish a baseline of disease preoperatively.

(3) A history of CNS events necessitates maintaining higher mean arterial pressures and hemoglobin levels intraoperatively and during CPB.

(4) Combined carotid endarterectomy/coronary artery bypass grafting (CABG) remains a possibility for patients with critical carotid stenosis and unstable coronary disease.

(a) CABG can present a 9% to 17% risk of stroke to patients with known carotid disease (1).

ii) **Pulmonary**

(1) Chronic lung disease may necessitate further workup with pulmonary function tests and arterial blood gas analysis.

(2) Response to bronchodilator therapy may help guide intraoperative treatment in the event of exacerbations of chronic obstructive pulmonary disease or reactive airway disease.

(3) Purulent secretions and acute respiratory infections may delay extubation postoperatively and negatively impact surgical morbidity.

iii) **GI/hepatic**

(1) Deficiencies of clotting factors may occur in patients with acute or chronic hepatic dysfunction.

(2) Serum albumin <3 g/dL may have a negative impact on patient outcome.

(3) Baseline liver-associated enzymes should be obtained if preoperative dysfunction exists.

iv) **Endocrine**

(1) Perioperative hyperglycemia may place the cardiac surgery patient at an increased risk for wound infection and delayed wound healing in addition to impacting overall patient morbidity and mortality.

READ
MORE

Diabetes mellitus, Chapter 81, page 592

(2) A preoperative insulin infusion ± dextrose should be considered for insulin-dependent diabetics.

    (a) Insulin infusions started during surgery to maintain blood glucose below 140 mg/dL should be continued into the intensive care unit postoperatively.

  v) **Hematologic**

    (1) It is essential to determine a history of bleeding disorders.

      (a) A personal or family history of abnormal bleeding may uncover factor deficiencies or significant platelet dysfunction.

    (2) Coagulation screening tests such as PT (prothrombin time), PTT (partial thromboplastin time), and INR (international normalized ratio) in addition to a complete blood count may reveal important information prior to CPB.

READ
MORE

Coagulopathies, Chapter 89, page 643

      (a) Thromboelastography (TEG) studies and fibrinogen levels may be helpful in coagulopathic or debilitated patients, or those receiving chronic anticoagulation or antiplatelet agents prior to surgery.

    (3) Variables that increase the risk of postoperative blood transfusion include advanced age, preoperative anemia or small body size, preoperative antiplatelet or antithrombotic drugs, redo or complex procedures, emergency operations, and noncardiac patient comorbidities (2).

  vi) **Renal**

    (1) A preoperative creatinine of >2.0 mg/dL has been identified as an independent risk factor for postoperative complications (1).

    (2) Factors associated with the need for postoperative renal dialysis include preoperative serum creatinine, age, race, type of surgery (CABG plus valve or valve only vs. CABG only), diabetes, shock, NYHA class, lung disease, recent MI, and prior cardiovascular surgery (3).

 f) **Special considerations**

  i) Several patient conditions such as pregnancy, the Jehovah Witness, procedures requiring deep hypothermic circulatory arrest, and the potential for complex or combined surgical procedures (e.g., combined carotid endarterectomy/CABG) can create special dilemmas with regard to intraoperative monitoring, blood conservation strategies, and overall potential morbidity and mortality.

2) **Multidisciplinary decision making**

 a) Communication between the anesthesia team, cardiac surgeon, perfusionist, and nursing staff is essential for optimal patient management.

  i) Essential elements of discussion include:

    (1) Surgical approach (median sternotomy vs. thoracotomy in cases of prior IMA grafting)

    (2) Specific surgical objectives (valve repair vs. replacement), on-CPB or off-pump (OPCAB)

    (3) Cannulation strategy

    (4) Potential for circulatory arrest in cases of ascending aortic or aortic arch repairs.

    (5) Preferences for antifibrinolytics or requirements for other intraoperative medications (e.g., inhaled nitric oxide)

    (6) Blood product utilization and availability

    (7) Placement of lines for infusions or monitoring by the anesthesia team.

3) **Perioperative monitoring**

 a) Optimal monitoring of the cardiac patient should begin preoperatively and continue until the patient is received in the cardiac intensive care unit.

  i) **Standard ASA Monitors should be used along with invasive blood pressure monitoring.**

(1) The clinical situation (e.g., emergency surgery, aortic dissection, cardiac tamponade) and patient instability (low CO, presence of intra-aortic balloon pump [IABP], requirement for preoperative inotropes or vasopressors) may determine whether or not further invasive monitors such as central venous pressure (CVP) or pulmonary artery (PA) catheter monitoring is required prior to induction.

ii) **Blood pressure monitoring**

(1) Should include invasive measurements given the potential for nonpulsatile flow present during CBP as well as the need for arterial blood sample measurements

(2) The noninvasive monitor serves as a backup in the event of a nonfunctioning invasive monitor.

(3) Preinduction placement of an arterial line should be guided by the patient's propensity to develop hemodynamic swings on induction of anesthesia in addition to the patient's ability to tolerate the fluctuations given their underlying disease state.

(a) Baseline exercise tolerance is a good indicator in many cases.

(4) Cannulation site should be discussed with surgical team in complex cases such as arch repairs, or CABG with radial grafting.

(5) A femoral arterial line is an acceptable alternative in patients with severe vascular or coronary disease, and provides an avenue for aortic balloon placement in severely dysfunctional patients.

iii) **ECG monitoring**

(1) ECG monitoring is essential given the patient's underlying history of ischemia or dysrhythmias.

(2) A five-lead system utilizing the V5 lead is best for diagnosing myocardial ischemia.

(3) Over 90% of ischemic episodes will be detected if lead II is also utilized (1).

(4) Monitoring of the cardiac patient should occur as soon as the patient arrives in the preoperative area.

b) **CVP monitoring**

i) Can be effective in managing patients with normal left ventricular/valvular function, and in these patients is a reasonable predictor of ventricular filling.

c) **PA catheter placement**

i) Provides the ability to determine left atrial filling pressures via the pulmonary capillary wedge pressure, pulmonary and systemic vascular resistance, cardiac output via thermodilution, and measurement of mixed venous oxygen saturation in addition to CVP and assessments of RV performance.

ii) PA use is recommended in patients with severe valvular disease, shunts, or below-normal ventricular function.

READ MORE

Pulmonary Artery Catheter, Chapter 13, page 82

Transesophageal echocardiography: Indications as a monitoring tool, Chapter 14, page 90

d) **Transesophageal echocardiography (TEE)**

i) TEE is now used for nearly all cardiac surgeries.

ii) TEE can provide an assessment of global cardiac function and specific structural and valvular anomalies (4).

e) **Neurologic monitoring**

i) Neurologic monitoring has become more prevalent in cardiac surgery to prevent and reduce the incidence of brain injury.

    ii) Cerebral near-infrared spectroscopy noninvasively monitors brain oxygenation by measuring regional cerebral venous oxygen saturation, correlating with measures of global brain metabolism even in the absence of flow (5).

    iii) Processed EEG signals such as compressed spectral array or bispectral index monitors may provide a useful indication of anesthetic depth during cardiac anesthesia.

f) Urine output monitoring

    i) Urine output monitoring is crucial during cardiac surgery as renal failure may complicate up to one third of CPB cases.

    ii) Urinary catheter output should be monitored at least hourly and quantified for the duration of CPB.

    iii) Adequacy of urine output while on CPB depends on several factors including volume status, cardiac output, hemoglobin concentration, and amount of surgical bleeding (1).

g) Temperature monitoring

READ MORE

Aortic valvular disease, Chapter 54, page 383

Ventricular assist devices, Chapter 56, page 404

Cardiac arrhythmias and pacemakers, Chapter 57, page 412

    i) Temperature monitoring is essential to ensure the even cooling and rewarming of the myocardium and brain.

    ii) Core (PA catheter, nasopharyngeal, or esophageal) and shell (rectal or bladder) temperatures are commonly measured during procedures involving CPB.

    iii) A myocardial temperature probe is also placed by the surgeons.

    iv) While hypothermia can suppress cerebral metabolism (6% to 7% decline per 1°C), hyperthermia and aggressive rewarming may cause injurious effects.

    v) Myocardial oxygen consumption drops 50% for every 10°C decrease in myocardial temperature (6).

4) Principles of intraoperative management

a) Induction

    i) Hemodynamic goals for induction should consider the patient's cardiac pathology. Several considerations must be made when planning induction.

      (1) Patients with normal LV function may reveal a strong sympathetic response to surgical stimulation requiring the use of vasodilators, beta blockers, and higher doses of opioids and benzodiazepines in addition to the primary induction agent.

      (2) Depressed LV function dictates minimizing cardiodepressant induction and maintenance agents.

        (a) Patients who present for surgery on inotropic therapy such as dopamine or dobutamine should remain on these drugs throughout the induction period.

          (i) These patients may not be able to produce a strong hemodynamic response to sympathetic stimulation.

      (3) Significant valvular lesions such as critical aortic stenosis require maintenance of preload and a higher afterload state.

        (a) Hemodynamic goals for each valvular lesion should be followed

      (4) Ischemic cardiac disease requires minimizing myocardial oxygen consumption and maximizing myocardial oxygen supply.

      (5) In general, a slower heart rate, reduced wall tension, and adequate coronary perfusion pressure (elevated diastolic pressure) represent ideal hemodynamic goals.

      (6) Planning for early extubation requires avoiding high-dose opioids and long-acting neuromuscular blockers.

In general, a slower heart rate, reduced wall tension, and adequate coronary perfusion pressure (elevated diastolic pressure) represent ideal hemodynamic goals for patients with ischemic cardiac disease.

    (a)   Patient factors that may prevent extubation within 4 to 6 hours from ICU admission include impaired LV function, redo operation, extracardiac arteriopathy, preoperative IABP, elevated serum creatinine, and nonelective and complex surgery (7).

b) **Preinduction preparation**
   i)   All anesthesia equipment should be checked and equipment for the unanticipated difficult airway should be available as many cardiac patients will have little physiologic reserve if ventilation and oxygenation are not maintained.
   ii)   Emergent surgeries and the most compromised cardiac patients warrant the presence of the cardiac surgeon during the induction period in the event the patient decompensates acutely or arrests requiring urgent institution of CPB.
   iii)   Benzodiazepines such as midazolam (0.5 to 1 mg titrated increments) or lorazepam while the patient is monitored and receiving supplemental oxygen can be used for anxiolysis.
   iv)   **Medications** to be available on induction for all cardiac surgery cases include:
      (1)   Inotropes such as epinephrine (10 and 100 µg/mL) for bolus and inotropic infusion such as epinephrine, dopamine, or dobutamine.
      (2)   Vasopressors
          (a)   phenylephrine (for bolus) and vasopressin
      (3)   Vasodilators
          (a)   nitroglycerine and nitroprusside
      (4)   Anticholinergics
          (a)   atropine
      (5)   Ephedrine and calcium chloride
      (6)   Antiarrhythmics and rate-control agents such as:
          (a)   esmolol
          (b)   labetolol or metoprolol
          (c)   amiodarone
          (d)   lidocaine
          (e)   adenosine
          (f)   diltiazem or verapamil
      (7)   Heparin should always be immediately available in the event emergent transition to CPB is required.

c) **Induction medications**
   i)   Most induction agents can be used safely for almost all cardiac surgery patients as long as they are titrated slowly and carefully.
   ii)   Each intravenous anesthetic has benefits and drawbacks that should be weighed for each patient.
      (1)   Hypovolemia, depressed cardiac function, and arrhythmias may potentiate the myocardial depressant effects of the intravenous anesthetic agents resulting in hypotension or bradycardia.
   iii)   **Opioids** allow for a blunting of the hemodynamic response to intubation while maintaining stability throughout induction.
      (1)   Fentanyl doses of 3 to 10 µg/kg or sufentanil 0.1 to 1 µg/kg are acceptable induction doses.
   iv)   **Benzodiazepines** titrated during the induction period will be additive to the depressant effects possible with intravenous opioids.
   v)   **Etomidate** (0.15 to 0.3 mg/kg) is useful in maintaining myocardial contractility with only mild decreases in MAP and SVR.
      (1)   When paired with an opioid, it can provide for a very stable induction.
   vi)   **Propofol** (1 to 2 mg/kg) can be utilized in small increments (0.5 mg/kg) but can produce significant hypotension.

(1) It should be used very judiciously in the cardiac surgery patient.

vii) **Ketamine** may cause a stimulation of the cardiovascular system or hypotension in the catecholamine-depleted patient.

(1) Though such stimulation may be undesirable in patients prone to myocardial ischemia, it may be the agent of choice in constrictive pericarditis, tamponade, and major trauma.

viii) **Neuromuscular blocking** agents should be utilized early in the induction period.

(1) Succinylcholine is acceptable in the event a rapid-sequence induction is selected bearing in mind the need to control the sympathetic response to intubation.

(2) Vecuronium (70 to 100 μg/kg), rocuronium (0.3 to 1.2 mg/kg), and cisatracurium (70 to 100 μg/kg) are acceptable neuromuscular blockers.

(3) Pancuronium is an option when vagolysis is desired in the setting of low baseline heart rates and severe valvular regurgitation (1).

d) **Maintenance of anesthesia**

i) Inhalational agents may produce dose-dependent myocardial depression, vasodilation, and reflex tachycardia.

ii) Isoflurane, sevoflurane, and desflurane are commonly used as a balanced anesthetic maintenance strategy along with opioids and benzodiazepines and may exhibit cardioprotective properties (anesthetic preconditioning) that may protect against ongoing myocardial ischemia.

iii) The postinduction period is marked by a lack of surgical stimulation leading up to extremely high stimulation upon sternal retraction.

iv) Appropriate anesthetic depth should be balanced by the need to maintain stable hemodynamics.

v) See Tables 141-1 and 141-2 for a brief overview of the causes and treatment of pre-CPB hypotension and hypertension.

e) **Postinduction tasks**

i) The endotracheal tube, central venous, peripheral and arterial lines should be secured.

Table 141-1
Pre-bypass Hypotension

Prebypass hypotension

Assess for hypovolemia— utilize TEE
  Fluid bolus
Assess anesthetic depth—Is there too much anesthetic?
Assess Venous return
  Mechanical compression due to surgeons, cannulas, etc.
  Elevated airway pressures
Reduced myocardial contractility— utilize TEE
  Consider Inotropic agent such as epinephrine/dopamine
Ischemia—assess ECG/TEE.
  Increase O_2, decrease heart rate (esmolol), increase diastolic blood pressure.
  Alert surgeon of ischemia—consider initiation of CPB if needed.
Low SVR—diagnose with PAC, treat with vasopressor agents (vasopressin or epinephrine)
Dysrhythmia: Loss of atrial contraction can be detrimental
  Consider cardioversion, pharmacologic therapy with amiodarone (150 mg), initiation of CPB if severe

Adapted from Hensley FA, Martin DE, Gravlee GP, eds. A Practical Approach to Cardiac Anesthesia. 4th ed. Philadelphia, PA: Lippincott Williams & Wilkins, 2008:188.

Table 141-2

Pre-Bypass Hypertension

Pre-Bypass Hypertension: (1)
  Manipulation of Sympathetic nerves during aortic cannulation **
  Hypoxia
  Hypercapnia
  Hypervolemia
Rare   Withdrawal from HTN therapy – what outpatient medications were held?
       Thyroid Storm
       Pheochromocytoma
  Light Anesthesia – Most common and easy to fix. **
  Increase anesthetic depth (inhaled agent, opioids)
** Most common causes

Adapted from Hensley FA, Martin DE, Gravlee GP, eds. A Practical Approach to Cardiac Anesthesia. 4th ed. Philadelphia: Lippincott Williams & Wilkins, 2008:189.

(1) Intravenous and arterial line function are confirmed again after patient positioning.
ii) The TEE probe (if utilized) is placed after suctioning with an orogastric tube.
  (1) Atraumatic probe placement should be documented and a mouth guard should be utilized when possible.
iii) Prolonged surgery, surgical positioning, and sternal retraction place the patient at risk for positioning injuries.
  (1) The entire OR team should participate in positioning to ensure proper padding and positioning is achieved.
iv) Antibiotics are administered preincision in accordance with hospital policies.
v) Baseline arterial blood gas and activated clotting time (ACT) samples are obtained.
vi) Antifibrinolytics are generally administered prior to incision.
  (1) These agents inhibit fibrinolysis through inhibition of plasminogen inhibitors and antiplasmin activity.
    (a) **Aminocaproic acid** (epsilon aminocaproic acid, EACA) is a lysine analogue that attaches to the lysine-binding site on the plasminogen molecule.
      (i) EACA dosing is 100 to 150 mg/kg bolus followed by 10 to 15 mg/kg/h (or 1 g/h infusion).
      (ii) EACA is also added to the CPB prime.
    (b) **Tranexemic acid** (TA) is similar in action to aminocaproic acid but is ten times more potent and has higher plasminogen affinity.
      (i) TA dosing is 10 to 20 mg/kg bolus followed by 1 to 2 mg/kg/h infusion.
    (c) **Aprotinin** is a bovine protein that inhibits serine proteases inhibiting trypsin, plasmin, and kallikrein.
      (i) Aprotinin may also attenuate the inflammatory response to CPB but has been unavailable after marketing was suspended by the FDA in 2007.
      (ii) Aprotinin has been associated with an increased risk of postoperative renal dysfunction and overall mortality.

CONCERNS IN SUBSPECIALTY ANESTHESIA

Figure 141-1 Schematic of CBP Circuit

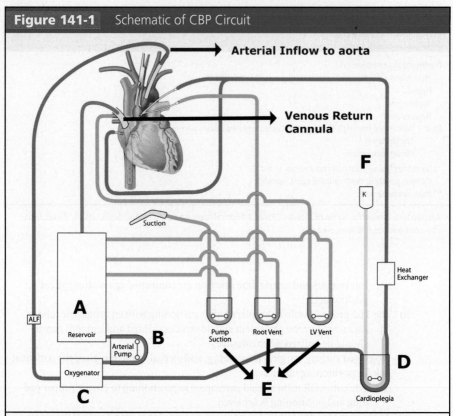

Basic/key components of the CPB circuit are shown here. *A:* Venous reservoir collecting venous return from the venous return cannula (see *arrow* above) thus bypassing the heart. Blood is then routed through the arterial pump *(B)* and oxygenator *(C)* (different configurations depending on CPB machine) prior to being returned to the body via the aortic inflow cannula (labeled above). Accessory components include the heat exchanger (labeled) that can be in different configurations depending on the model. The cardioplegia pump *(D)* allows for administration of cardioplegia (high potassium solution) to the cardioplegia cannula (Fig. 141-2). Additional pumps *(E)* allow for surgical suction, aortic root venting, and LV venting depending on surgeon's needs at various points of the procedure. (Image Courtesy of Bruce Searles, Suny Upstate Medical University, Department of Cardiovascular Perfusion.)

---

5) **Cardiopulmonary bypass (Figs. 141-1 and 141-2)**
   a) CPB allows for systemic perfusion and oxygenation during a period of cardiac inactivity (arrest) to allow for an optimal surgical field.
   b) Through a series of cannulas surgically placed into the heart and great vessels, venous blood is drained by gravity, bypasses the heart, and is oxygenated externally before it is returned via the arterial cannula.
   c) Elements of the CPB pump include the reservoir, oxygenator, heat exchanger, main pump, arterial filter, suction, and vents.
   d) **Overview of CBP process**
      i) A certified clinical perfusionist will ensure all tubing connected to the CPB pump is free from air to prevent a venous air lock or a gas embolus. The pump will also be primed with an electrolyte solution with or without additional blood depending on the patient's initial hemoglobin concentration.

Figure 141-2   Cannulation Diagram

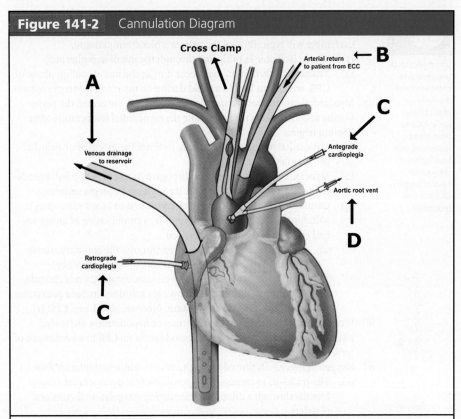

This schematic depicts the cannula insertions into the heart for a typical CPB procedure. venous drainage occurs at (A) with a two-stage venous cannula depicted (note the cannula enters the right atrium, but the distal tip is in the inferior vena cava). Arterial inflow cannula is depicted at (B). Typically, both antegrade and retrograde cardioplegia cannula are placed (C). The cross clamp is depicted and labeled above. Finally, the aortic root vent allows venting of air/blood/cardioplegia as needed (D). If additional venting of the ventricle is required, an LV vent can also be placed (Bot shown in diagram). (Image Courtesy of Bruce Searles, SUNY Upstate Medical University, Department of Cardiovascular Perfusion.)

ii) After adequate anticoagulation (see Pre-CPB period below) and depth of anesthesia, an aortic cannula will be positioned by the surgeon within the aorta. Subsequent venous cannulation will occur through the venae cavae.

iii) Upon initiation of CPB, blood will drain by gravity from the venous circulation through the venous cannulae into a venous reservoir.

iv) After routing through an arterial pump, blood will pass through a membrane oxygenator exchanging oxygen and carbon dioxide. Blood temperature can also be modified at this time.

v) Before passing through a final arterial pump, blood will be filtered to prevent microembolization of air or particles and delivered into the aorta or the other central artery that has been cannulated.

vi) The perfusionist will monitor pressure in the pump's arterial line and can also continuously monitor hematocrit, temperature, and mixed venous oxygen saturation.

e) **Physiology:** A unique set of physiologic variables must be considered during the course of CPB.

Low myocardial temperatures combined with the delivery of cardioplegia solutions produces a quiescent, non-beating heart optimal for cardiac surgery, which is also protective.

    i) Systemic hypothermia has a direct effect on the metabolic rate for oxygen consumption in the myocardium and brain. During CPB, the heat exchanger will typically cool the patient's blood temperature.

      (1) Tissue ischemia is mitigated through the use of hypothermia.

      (2) Ventricular fibrillation may occur during the initial cooling phase of CPB, which can lead to a rapid decline in myocardial energy reserves.

    ii) Myocardial protection: During the course of CPB, surgeons, the perfusionist and anesthesia team will note the myocardial temperature after cooling begins.

      (1) Myocardial temperature can help indicate the extent of myocardial protection while arrested.

      (2) Myocardial protection occurs through hypothermia applied directly to the heart (topical cooling) or through cardioplegia solutions.

      (3) Cardioplegia may be delivered as crystalloid or blood cardioplegia solutions (most commonly). Typically, a combination of antegrade and retrograde cardioplegia is used

        (a) Antegrade cardioplegia is given through the coronary arteries (except in the setting of significant aortic insufficiency).

        (b) Retrograde cardioplegia is given via a coronary sinus cannula.

        (c) Common additives to cardioplegia solutions include potassium, mannitol, THAM, magnesium, glucose, blood, and CPD (1).

    iii) Blood viscosity is increased in the setting of hypothermia. Increased viscosity is counteracted through hemodilution on CPB to a hematocrit of 20%–30%.

    iv) Oxygen delivery is improved through enhanced microcirculatory flow (1).

      (1) The trade-off to increased oxygen delivery is perioperative coagulopathy through a dilution of circulating coagulation factors and platelets.

      (2) Hemodilution to a level of 6 to 7 g/dL may provide adequate oxygen delivery during CPB (2).

    v) Activation of inflammatory mediators, tissue factor, altered platelet function, and combined coagulation and fibrinolysis occur during CPB.

    vi) Nonpulsatile flow may lead to periods of relative hypoperfusion followed by reperfusion as well as the production of microemboli.

  f) **CPB initiation period (Table 141-3)**

Table 141-3
Checklist for Initiation of CBP

O	Observe patient (face and head), surgical field, bypass circuit and lines, appropriate cannulation
N	No ventilation (upon initiating full CPB)
P	PA catheter pulled back 3–5 cm, pumps inspected (vasoactive infusions off)
U	Urine output (recorded)
M	Maintain anesthesia, muscle relaxation (confirm delivery of volatile agent by perfusionist, if utilized)
P	Perioperative TEE exam

   i) Heparinization must be assured prior to arterial cannulation and CPB.

      (1) Heparin bolus dose is 300 to 350 units/kg delivered into a central vein with patency confirmed with blood aspiration.

      (2) ACT monitors the effect of heparin on coagulation.

      (3) 400 seconds is the lowest ACT allowable to initiate CPB.

      (4) Inadequate ACT may occur through technical causes (inadequate dose or low activity) or heparin resistance.

READ
MORE
Coagulopathies,
Chapter 89,
page 643

         (a) Recall that heparin binding to antithrombin III (ATIII) allows heparin to inhibit thrombin and factor Xa.

         (b) Some causes of heparin resistance include ATIII deficiency, previous heparin exposure, hemodilution, shock, endocarditis, or advanced age (1).

      (5) Heparin resistance can commonly be overcome by administering more heparin.

         (a) Alternatively, ATIII deficiency can be overcome through the administration of fresh frozen plasma providing additional ATIII (generally 2 to 4 units must be given) or administration of concentrated AT III supplementation.

  ii) **Surgical factors/concerns**

      (1) Cannulation of the aorta occurs first at a systolic pressure of <100 mm Hg.

      (2) The visible portions of the ascending aorta, aortic arch, and proximal descending thoracic aorta should be inspected with TEE to identify atherosclerotic area that could preclude safe cannulation.

         (a) Epiaortic ultrasound is encouraged prior to cannulation.

         (b) TEE is used to visualize the aortic cannula in the aortic arch.

         (c) The CPB circuit transduced pressure should show a pulsatile waveform after the aorta has been cannulated. The pulsatile waveform should correlate with the patient's radial arterial pressure ensuring that the cannula has not been placed into a false passage within the vessel (e.g., aortic dissection).

         (d) Venous cannulation provides the gravity drainage of blood to the CPB reservoir. For closed heart procedures, a single, two-stage cannula is placed in the right atrium/IVC providing complete venous drainage to the heart. For open heart procedures, bicaval cannulation is used with an individual cannula in the IVC and SVC.

g) **CPB period (Table 141-1 to 141-3)**

   i) Initiation of CPB should take place with an ACT >400 seconds. The following steps are then taken:

      (1) Inspection of flow through the bypass circuit with venous blood draining to gravity and arterial blood returning via the arterial cannula.

      (2) **Inspection of patient**

         (a) The patient's face and head should be inspected for blanching, engorgement, or a harlequin pattern signifying improper cannulation.

      (3) **Anesthetic maintenance**

         (a) Ventilation is suspended once "full flow" on CPB is established.

         (b) Additional muscle relaxant and benzodiazepine can be administered.

         (c) Ensure volatile anesthetic delivery via CPB circuit.

h) **CPB maintenance**

   i) The onset of CPB is a critical time during cardiac surgery. Communication with the perfusionist is crucial.

ii) Though it may be tempting for the anesthesiologist to leave the room for a short period of time during the CPB period, it is imperative that he or she remain with the patient. The anesthesiologist must still remain vigilant.

  (1) Elevated thresholds for perfusion pressure and target mean arterial pressures should be maintained especially in patients with a history of cerebrovascular disease, diabetes, and hypertension.

  (2) Perfusionists will typically deliver a low concentration of volatile anesthetic (~0.5 MAC isoflurane or sevoflurane) directly through the CPB pump. Additional opioid and/or benzodiazepine dosing may be required while on CPB.

iii) Temperature and urine output monitoring should be monitored while on CPB.

  (1) There is debate regarding optimal temperature management during CPB with current practices ranging from "warm" bypass at 35°C to 36°C, to relatively hypothermic CBP at 28°C or lower.

iv) Decreased urine output should be approached by first troubleshooting the urinary catheter for kinking and ensuring adequate systemic perfusion pressures.

v) ACT and ABG monitoring with specific attention to glucose control should occur while on CPB.

vi) Declining hemoglobin values may require transfusion of PRBC while on CPB.

vii) During CPB with moderate hypothermia, transfusion of packed red blood cells for hemoglobin levels <6 g/dL is reasonable except in patients at risk for decreased cerebral oxygen delivery (e.g., CVA, DM, carotid stenosis) in which case higher hemoglobin levels may be required (2).

i) **CPB catastrophes** occur infrequently but may include:

  (i) Misdirected arterial cannula

  (ii) Reversed arterial and venous cannulae

  (iii) Oxygenator failure

  (iv) Inappropriate protamine administration

  (v) Air embolus

j) **CPB-separation** (Table 141-4)

  i) Separation from CBP is a critical time for the cardiothoracic surgical team including the anesthesiologist and perfusionist.

  ii) During this time, the CPB pump flows that provided the patient's full cardiac output will be reduced, the patient's intrinsic cardiac rhythm regained (through the help of defibrillation and possibly internal cardiac pacing), and mechanical ventilation of the patient's lungs must be resumed.

Table 141-4
Mnemonic for Separation from CPB

C	V	P
Cold	Ventilation	Predictors
Conduction	Vaporizer	Protamine
Calcium	Volume expanders	Pressure
Cardiac output	Visualization	Pressors
Cells		Pacemaker
Coagulation		Potassium

Adapted from Hensley, et al. *A Practical Approach to Cardiac Anesthesia*. 4th ed. Philadelphia, PA: Lippincott Williams & Wilkins; 2008:231.

iii) A period of rewarming signals upcoming separation from CPB
    (1) Core temperature should be >36°C and shell temperature should be at least 35°C to 36°C (1).

iv) During CPB separation, the anesthesiologist must be in constant communication with the surgeon and perfusionist as the following steps occur:
    (1) Venous flow to the CPB pump is reduced
        (a) The perfusionist will slowly apply a clamp to the venous return line. This process will fill the right atrium and right ventricle allowing for direct oxygenation and ventilation by the pulmonary circuit. Full mechanical ventilation should occur at this point.
        (b) The perfusionist will be able to adjust RV preload by altering the amount of blood flow that is allowed to remain in the heart rather than drain back to the pump.
        (c) PA and CVPs, TEE, and direct surgical inspection are all important variables at this time.
    (2) Forward flow of oxygenated blood through the aortic cannula is reduced
        (a) Blood flow that is moving forward through the pulmonary circulation is now contributing to the patient's intrinsic cardiac output.
        (b) The perfusionist will continue to reduce pump flow as preload and contractility are optimized.
    (3) CPB is stopped
        (a) Once adequate filling pressures are attained, the pump flow is terminated and no flow is present through the cannulae. Systolic pressures will generally be >85 to 90 mm Hg at this time.

v) Adequate cardiac rate and rhythm will improve the chances for successful separation from CPB.
    (1) Heart rate is ideally 80 to 100 as slight increase in rate compensates for a "stiff ventricle" following CPB.
    (2) Rhythm may be controlled through epicardial pacing wires.
    (3) Arrhythmias can be treated via pharmacologic means, electric cardioversion, or epicardial pacing.

vi) Metabolic status and electrolytes should be optimized prior to separation.
    (1) Calcium chloride should be readily available.

vii) Inotropic agents and vasodilators should be ready for infusion and pumps should be programmed.
    (1) Inodilators (milrinone, amrinone), inhaled nitric oxide, and epoprostenol may be considered in the setting of significant RV dysfunction or rising PA pressures.

viii) Blood products should be available for separation from CPB and intravenous lines should be confirmed to be patent.

ix) Deairing maneuvers are very important if the cardiac chambers were entered. Small microbubbles may have entered the heart through the cannulation process or during the placement of coronary grafts (rarely) or valve repairs or replacements (more commonly).
    (1) The presence of air bubbles in the arterial circulation may contribute to the patient's risk of developing embolic neurologic events.
    (2) TEE may help the anesthesiologist advise the surgeons of the quantity of air detected in the cardiac chambers (if any).
    (3) An aortic root vent (a small cannula placed within the aortic root just proximal to the aortic valve) can be aspirated to mitigate the risk of air bubbles traveling through the systemic circulation.

Predictors of difficult separation from CPB include global decompensation or reduced EF, RV failure, renal disease, emergency surgery, inadequate myocardial preservation, and inadequate surgical repair (1).

CONCERNS IN SUBSPECIALTY ANESTHESIA

  (4) Multiple table position changes and manual recruitment breaths may enable air bubbles to be pushed forward through the aortic root and disposed through the aortic root vent.

 x) Failure to separate may require the use of an intraaortic balloon pump (IABP), ventricular assist device, or continuation of extracorporeal membrane oxygenation

k) **Post-CPB period**

 i) Hemodynamic, metabolic, oxygenation, and surgical concerns must all be addressed in the post-CPB period.

 ii) Hemodynamic considerations include the post-CPB evaluation of hypotension, hypertension, low CO/high CO states, and low/high SVR states. (Table 141-5)

  (1) PA catheter data and TEE may help clarify the etiologies of the hemodynamic conditions.

 iii) Protamine 1 mg for each 100 units of heparin given is a useful starting point for heparin reversal.

  (1) A test dose of Protamine (1 mL or 10 mg) is generally given peripherally. Protamine administration may be associated with:

   (a) Hypotension with rapid administration

   (b) Potential for anaphylactoid reactions

   (c) Pulmonary vasoconstriction/RV failure

  (2) The surgeon, anesthesiologist, and perfusionist must all be aware that protamine is being given and notified when half the dose is administered so that pump suction can be stopped.

   (a) Administration of protamine should be no faster than 20 mg to 40 mg every 60 seconds. Protamine administration can cause complement-mediated reactions of varying severity ranging from mild hypotension requiring coadministration of a vasoconstrictor such as phenylephrine to profound cardiovascular collapse due to anaphylaxis, severe pulmonary vasoconstriction, and RV failure.

Always notify surgeon and perfusionist that protamine is being given. Rapid administration of protamine is associated with hypotension and should be avoided.

Table 141-5
Outline to Maintain Hemodynamic Stability on Termination of CPB

Termination of CPB

1. Adjust rate/rhythm; consider epicardial pacing if needed
2. Partially occlude venous line; observe cardiac filling
3. Decrease arterial flow from pump; ejection begins (partial CPB)
4. Measure arterial blood pressure

BP	High	Low
	1. Completely occlude venous line	1. Maintain partial CPB
	2. Stop pump after ventricle fills	2. Carefully adjust ventricular volume
	3. Estimate or measure preload and SV (contractility)	3. Vasoactive drugs: inotropes, vasocontrictors
		4. Reduce pump flow; readjust volume and infusion dose

Adapted from Thomas. *Manual of Cardiac Anesthesia*, 2nd ed. New York, NY: Churchill Livingstone, 1993.

  (b) Rapid administration is associated with more severe protamine reactions.

6) **Special post-CPB considerations**
   a) Identification and management of post-CPB coagulopathy
      i) Identification of preoperative coagulopathy or platelet dysfunction will help guide therapy.
         (1) TEG can be invaluable in complex coagulation cases.
         (2) Standard coagulation studies post bypass, including platelet count and fibrinogen, can also guide therapy.
   b) **Coronary Artery Spasm**
      i) Evidence of wall motion abnormalities or ST segment elevations may occur in the event of intracoronary air or a "kinked" graft
   c) **Chest closure**
      i) Elevations in CVP, PA pressure, or airway pressures may occur. Persistent instability in the setting of a low CO may require the chest to be left open.
   d) **Dysrhythmias**
      i) Metabolic and electrolyte status should be monitored following separation from CPB.
      ii) Continued dysrhythmias may indicate the need for epicardial pacemaker placement or dependence.

7) **Transition to the cardiac intensive care unit**
   a) The patient should remain completely monitored throughout each transition phase from the operating room table to transport gurney or bed and to the ICU since wide hemodynamic swings can occur during this time.
   b) Direct access to a large bore peripheral or preferably central infusion lines should be maintained in the event inotropes, vasopressors, or fluids need to be administered.
   c) The anesthesia team should be prepared to deal with unanticipated extubation, the need for emergent defibrillation or cardioversion, disruption of cardiac pacing or intracardiac devices (IABP), or the need to emergently reopen the chest.

Chapter Summary for Adult Cardiac Surgery

Indications	Coronary Artery Disease, valvular disease, adult congenital heart disease, HF, major trauma, aortic disease, heart or lung transplant, ventricular assist device placement
Risks	High-risk surgery in high-risk patients. Extreme care must be taken at every aspect of these cases
Monitors	Typically full invasive monitoring, TEE, ± neurologic monitoring
Equipment	CBP circuit, TEE, invasive monitors, pacing equipment, defibrillator, ± rapid transfusion device.
Considerations	Anesthesiologist must prepare for these cases carefully, with specific medications and equipment needed that are outside the scope of most typical OR cases.

CONCERNS IN SUBSPECIALTY ANESTHESIA

References

1. Hensley FA, Martin DE, Gravlee GP, eds. *A Practical Approach to Cardiac Anesthesia*. 4th ed. Philadelphia, PA: Lippincott Williams & Wilkins; 2008.

2. STS/SCA Task Force. Perioperative blood transfusion and blood conservation in cardiac surgery: The Society of Thoracic Surgeons and The Society of Cardiovascular Anesthesiologists Clinical Practice Guideline. *Ann Thorac Surg* 2007;83:S27–S86.

3. Mehta R, Grab J, O'Brien S, et al. Bedside tool for predicting the risk of postoperative dialysis in patients undergoing cardiac surgery. *Circulation* 2006;114:2208–2216.

4. Shanewise, et al. Comprehensive and abbreviated intraoperative TEE examination. In: *Comprehensive Textbook of Intraoperative Transesophageal Echocardiography*. Philadelphia, PA: Lippincott Williams & Wilkins; 2005:81–93.

5. Guarracino F. Cerebral monitoring during cardiovascular surgery. *Curr Opin Anaesthesiol* 2008;21:50–54.

6. Kaplan JA, Reich DL, Lake CL, et al. eds. *Kaplan's Cardiac Anesthesia*. 5th ed. Philadelphia, PA: Saunders Elsevier; 2006.

7. Constantinides V, Tekkis P, Fazil A, et al. Fast-track failure after cardiac surgery: development of a prediction model. *Crit Care Med* 2006;34:2875–2882.

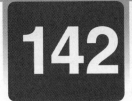

Trauma

James Duke, MD, MBA

Few patients offer greater challenge to the anesthesiologist than the acutely injured patient. The urgency of the situation and uncertainty as to the extent of injury requires the anesthesiologist to be methodical and vigilant. This chapter provides a systematic approach to such patients, including airway management, anesthetic technique, and concerns for injury to specific body regions.

1) **Initial assessment:** There is often little time for a standard preoperative evaluation, but all severely injured patients should be considered at risk for aspiration, cervical spine and closed-head injury, hypovolemia, substance abuse, and multisystem injury (1,2).

   a) Assume the patient is hypovolemic. Vital signs are insensitive for detecting moderate degrees of blood loss (Table 142-1).

   b) A cursory neurologic examination should be performed, noting level of consciousness (Glasgow Coma Scale, Table 142-2), cervical spine tenderness, and lateralizing defects.

Table 142-1

Estimated Blood Loss Based on Patient Presentation

	Class I	Class II	Class III	Class IV
Blood loss (mL)	<750	750–1,500	1,500–2,000	>2,000
Blood loss (%)	<15	15–30	30–40	>40
Blood pressure	Normal	Normal	Decreased	Markedly decreased
Pulse pressure	Normal or ↑	↓	↓	↓
Heart rate	≤100	>100	>120	>140
Respiratory rate	14–20	20–30	30–40	>35
UOP cc/h	>30	20–30	5–20	0–5
Mental status	Slightly anxious	Mildly anxious	Confused	Confused, lethargic

Adapted from American College of Surgeons. *Advanced trauma life support, student course manual.* 7th ed. Chicago, IL: American College of Surgeons; 2004.

Table 142-2
Glasgow Coma Scale Criteria

	1	2	3	4	5	6
Eyes	Does not open eyes	Opens eyes in response to painful stimuli	Opens eyes in response to voice	Opens eyes spontaneously	N/A	N/A
Verebal	Makes no sounds	Incomprehensible sounds	Utters inappropriate words	Confused, disoriented	Oriented, converses normally	N/A
Motor	Makes no movements	Extension to painful stimuli	Abnormal flexion to painful stimuli	Flexion/Withdrawal to painful stimuli	Localizes painful stimuli	Obeys commands

Teasdale G, Jennett B. Assessment of coma and impaired consciousness. A practical scale. *Lancet* 1974;2:81–84.

Trauma patients require a methodical systematic approach to insure proper care.

The triad of coagulopaty, metabolic acidosis, and hypothermia is lethal and should therefore be managed agressively.

c) Gastroparesis and the likelihood of a full stomach predisposing to pulmonary aspiration are assumed.

d) Respiratory drive may be impaired due to head injury or intoxicants, and the mechanical aspects of ventilation may be compromised due to spinal cord, chest wall, or diaphragmatic injury, as well abdominal distention, pulmonary contusion, hemothorax, pneumothorax, etc.

    i) An attempt to oxygenate a hypoxic patient prior to establishing definitive airway control through endotracheal intubation is always advisable.

2) **Airway management:** Establishing airway patency is an essential feature in early trauma care. The injured patient is at risk for a compromised airway for multiple reasons.

a) The tongue is the most common cause of an obstructed airway and is readily treated by anterior displacement of the mandible with a jaw thrust and oral airway.

b) Direct trauma to the face may distort or obstruct the airway through disruption of the supporting bony architecture. Bilateral fractures of the mandible are particularly likely to result in loss of airway patency. Blunt trauma to the anterior neck may fracture the larynx or trachea and precipitate subcutaneous emphysema and soft tissue swelling. Penetrating neck injuries may produce hematomas sufficient to obstruct airflow (3).

    i) Indications for definitive airway control include the need for airway protection, the need for ventilation and oxygenation, and as part of an ongoing massive resuscitation. These problems may be due to

        (1) Loss of consciousness

        (2) Severe brain injury (GCS < 8)

        (3) Severe maxillofacial injury

        (4) Airway obstruction

        (5) Risk of pulmonary aspiration

        (6) Apnea

    (7)   Chest trauma, including pneumothorax

    (8)   Severe brain injury

  ii) Hoarseness, stridor, use of accessory respiratory musculature, and paradoxical motions of the chest or abdominal wall suggest some degree of airway obstruction and impending total airway collapse.

  iii) Cyanosis, pallor, declining pulse oximetry values, and apnea are signs mandating immediate airway intervention.

c) **Cervical spine stabilization.** All forms of airway control, including chin lift, jaw thrust, and oral and nasopharyngeal airway insertion, result in some cervical spine motion, though immobilization may mitigate this somewhat (4).

  i) Airway immobilization precautions include an appropriately sized Philadelphia collar, sand bags placed on each side of the head and neck, and the patient resting on a hard board with the forehead taped and secured to the board.

  ii) Direct laryngoscopy, even with in-line spine stabilization, results in cervical motion, especially at atlanto-occipital and atlantoaxial levels. Straight and curved laryngoscope blades do not differ substantially in the motion they produce, though the Bullard laryngoscope causes less head and cervical spine extension than conventional laryngoscopy (4).

d) Difficult intubations require the use of such airway adjuncts as gum elastic bougies, light wands, LMA, and fiberoptic bronchoscopes.

e) The Bullard laryngoscope facilitates intubation while maintaining the neck in a neutral position, and now there are laryngoscope handles that transmit the viewed image to an attached screen and reduce (but not eliminate) the amount of cervical motion associated with intubation (Glidescope, Saturn Biomedical, Burnaby, BC, Canada).

f) The intubating LMA (Fastrach, LMA North America, San Diego, CA) has led to successful intubations in patients with maxillofacial injuries and where there is difficult tracheal intubation along with difficult mask ventilation.

g) Fiberoptic bronchoscopy is considered by some to be the preferred method of securing the airway in patients with potential cervical spine injuries. However, the overall experience using a standard laryngoscope is satisfactory and no particular recommendation can be made based on outcome data.

h) Failure to establish a definitive airway by intubation necessitates a surgical airway. Cricothyroid puncture with jet ventilation is a useful temporizing measure prior to cricothyrotomy. Often performing a cricothyrotomy will be a bridging maneuver before formal tracheostomy unless oral intubation can be achieved under less stressful circumstances.

3) **Fluid resuscitation**

a) Intravenous (IV) access. Numerous large-gauge IV lines should be inserted (14- and 16-gauge peripheral cannulae and 9 French central introducers are ideal). Placement of IV lines above and below the diaphragm is recommended if physical findings suggest major thoracic or upper extremity vascular injury.

b) Laboratory evaluations. Blood should be drawn for type and cross-match, as well as hematology, chemistry (including lactate), ABG, and coagulation profiles (including thromboelastography)

c) IV infusions should be warmed, isotonic, and compatible with blood products.

d) Blood products are administered predicated upon hemodynamic indicators and serial laboratory examinations. **Failure to respond to crystalloid indicates a need for blood.**

  i) If cross-matched blood is unavailable, transfuse O-negative or type-specific red blood cells. If more than 10 units of O negative red bloods cells are given, consider continuing to administer O-negative blood.

4) **Monitoring**

READ MORE

Massive transfusion and resuscitation, Chapter 29, page 220

a) Depending on patient and surgical factors, invasive monitoring, such as intra-arterial and CVP monitoring, offer additional diagnostic information not provided by standard monitors. Patients with closed head injuries may require ICP monitoring. Urine output should also be followed.

b) Capnography. Measuring expired CO_2 not only verifies endotracheal intubation but may assist in diagnosis of other important events.

c) Trauma patients will have increased gradients between alveolar and end-tidal CO_2 due to increased dead space. This may be due to hypovolemia, atelectasis, pulmonary contusion, pulmonary aspiration, etc.

   i) Acute, exponential increases in the CO_2 gradient are ominous and may be due to air embolism or acute decreases in CO, such as might occur with myocardial ischemia, cardiac tamponade, or tension pneumothorax.

d) Temperature monitoring. Trauma patients usually arrive to the OR hypothermic. The anesthetized state and the OR environment potentiates this problem. Core temperature monitoring is ideal and esophageal monitoring is the norm.

   i) Hypothermia impairs wound healing, increases the likelihood of sepsis, slows drug metabolism and impairs coagulation. The triad of hypothermia, coagulopathy and acidosis is a lethal combination.

   ii) The OR should be warmed, convective air warming devices employed, and all fluids should be warmed. Wrapping the head or extremities in plastic sheeting may also be helpful.

5) **Anesthetic agents:** Anesthetic agents should be titrated to effect, expecting that lower than normal doses may suffice where the patient is hypovolemic.

READ MORE

Intravenous induction agents, Chapter 43, page 306

a) **Induction agents:** While some agents are preferred for trauma patients, any agent, improperly used, can be deleterious. Two induction agents are preferable in this set-ting-ketamine and etomidate.

   i) Etomidate has relatively less effect on decreasing CO and SVR, though it causes adrenal depression and the impact of even a single dose in a critically injured patient remains unclear.

      (I) It is the preferred agent in a patient who may have an evolving head injury as it decreases cerebral metabolic activity and is a cerebral vasoconstrictor.

   ii) Ketamine stimulates the sympathetic nervous system and often used in the hypovolemic patient. It does have some direct myocardial depressant effects but these are noted mostly in catechol-depleted patients.

      (I) Ketamine is a bronchodilator and a cerebral vasodilator and increases cerebral metabolic activity, contraindicating its use where head injury is suspected.

   iii) **Intraoperative awareness:** Trauma patients are at risk for intraoperative awareness. Benzodiazepines and scopolamine should be administered, recognizing the latter has less impact on BP.

   iv) **Nitrous oxide:** Is contraindicated in trauma patients as it can rapidly diffuse into closed gas spaces, increasing the risk of tension pneumothorax, and can also expand any pneumocephalus or air embolism.

   v) **Opioids.** Opioids are cardiostable though they may potentiate the hypotensive effects of induction agents, volatile anesthetics, and benzodiazepines.

vi) **Muscle relaxants:** Succinylcholine is routinely used to facilitate intubation and intermediate or long-acting nondepolarizing relaxants maintain good surgical conditions. Many patients are not extubated at case conclusion.

6) **Trauma-related concerns for specific body regions**

a) **Brain injury**

i) Secondary CNS injury: Little can be done to reverse the primary, direct CNS effects of acute injury. However, it is absolutely clear that without attention to maintaining intravascular volume, cerebral perfusion pressure and oxygenation, CNS injuries can be worsened. Agents that decrease cerebral metabolic activity are preferred. In the short-term, hyperventilation decreases ICP but over time, secondary changes in CSF pH decrease its benefit. Elevation of the head when tolerated and perhaps loosening slightly a cervical collar (facilitating jugular venous drainage) are also useful techniques. At times changing from a volatile anesthetic to an IV anesthetic technique may decrease ICP as volatile anesthetics do have cerebral vasodilator effects. Once a neurologic exam has been performed (looking in particular for lateralizing defects or posturing), use of muscle relaxants is common.

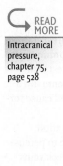

READ MORE

Intracranical pressure, chapter 75, page 528

(a) Coagulopathy: Patients with brain injuries have a high risk of impaired hemostasis. Serial measures of coagulation function should be performed and defects treated appropriately.

b) **Spinal cord injury**

i) All injured patients should be considered to have cervical spine injuries until disproven definitively. Cervical cord injuries can impair the patient's ventilation and result in hypotension due to the inability to produce distal vasoconstriction (neurogenic shock). Like CNS injuries, spinal cord injuries can be worsened by hypotension and hypoxemia. Many of these patients will also receive 24 hours of IV steroids, though this therapy is controversial.

c) **Thoracic injury**

i) Thoracic injuries may be penetrating or blunt in etiology, and include injuries to the heart and pericardium; lung, pleural space, or bronchus; diaphragm.

ii) Blunt cardiac injury

(1) Also called myocardial contusion, blunt cardiac injury is a clinical diagnosis. Associated injuries include sternal fractures, rib fractures, and pulmonary contusion.

iii) **Dysrhythmias:** Sinus tachycardia with nonspecific ST segment changes is most common. Conduction blocks and ventricular rhythms may also be observed.

iv) **Myocardial ischemia:** Patients may sustain injury to valves or papillary muscles. Coronary artery thrombosis is possible and most commonly occurs in the right coronary artery (presenting with ischemic changes in inferior ECG leads). Pump failure is an ominous finding. Cardiac enzymes add little to the evaluation of a patient suspected of having a contusion. Echocardiography is very useful and may reveal segmental wall motion defects.

v) **Cardiac tamponade:** May arise from either blunt or penetrating trauma.

(1) Signs and symptoms. Bleeding into the pericardial space increases pericardial pressures and impairs cardiac filling. Positive-pressure ventilation further decreases venous return and may greatly exacerbate the reduction in CO. Stroke volume decreases, and tachycardia compensates for a time to increase CO.

(2) The classic signs associated with cardiac tamponade (Beck's triad) are: hypotension, distant heart sounds, and distended neck veins. Neck vein distention may not be observed because of hypovolemia.

(3) Electrical alternans, where the major ECG axis is constantly changing, may be noted. This is due to the heart floating freely in the expanded pericardium.

(4) A patient with tamponade is at risk for cardiovascular collapse with anesthetic induction. Consider draining the pericardium using local anesthesia at the operative site (a subxiphoid pericardial window) prior to general anesthetic induction.

vi) **Tension pneumothorax and hemothorax**

   (1) Patients may sustain a pneumothorax in association with rib fractures, stab wounds and central line placement. If the pleural cavity does not communicate with the ambient environment, air may accumulate between the chest wall and lung and expand quickly with positive-pressure ventilation. Eventually, a tension pneumothorax will decrease venous return to the thorax and cause torsion of mediastinal vessels, leading to cardiovascular collapse.

     (a) **Signs and symptoms:** The chest may rise unevenly with inspiration, breath sounds become unequal, the hemothorax is tympanitic to percussion, and the trachea may shift away from the affected side. Neck veins may become distended if the patient is normovolemic. Airway pressures rise.

The needle used to treat a tension pneumothorax should be left in place until a tube thoracostomy is performed.

      (i) **Treatment:** Tension pneumothorax is a clinical diagnosis; do not delay treatment for radiologic confirmation of this life-threatening condition. The immediate treatment is the placement of a large-bore needle through the chest wall in the second intercostal space in the midclavicular line. A rush of air confirms the diagnosis. The needle should be left in place until a tube thoracostomy is performed. Nitrous oxide should not be used in trauma patients because it quickly diffuses into any air-filled cavity, such as a pneumothorax.

vii) **Air embolism.** Penetrating lung injuries may result in systemic air entrainment via bronchovenous or alveolocapillary fistulas.

   (1) **Signs and symptoms:** Air embolism should be suspected whenever unexpected signs of CNS or myocardial ischemia and precipitous cardiovascular collapse occur in the appropriate clinical context. When treating patients at risk, minimize inspiratory airway pressure, avoid PEEP, and administer small tidal volumes.

viii) **Abdominal compartment syndrome (ACS).** The ACS is regularly encountered and challenges the anesthesiologist.

   (1) Signs and symptoms. A victim of polytrauma with hypotension, oliguria, and respiratory failure manifesting as increasing airway pressures and decreasing oxygenation may have ACS. Diagnosis is by clinical suspicion and confirmed by measuring bladder pressure (>25 cm H_2O is diagnostic).

   (2) Prompt recognition is important as the treatment, surgical decompression, is usually straightforward. However, low CO may be associated with elevated pulmonary arterial occlusion pressure, somewhat similar to what might be seen in cardiac failure, calling into question optimal fluid management. A trial of volume expansion is usually indicated when a pathologic increase in abdominal pressure is suspected despite seemingly normal intravascular status as assessed by invasive hemodynamic monitors.

7) **Damage control:** Damage control is the principle of performing the minimum necessary interventions to save life and limb, leaving further procedures for a later time, after the patient has obtained hemodynamic stability. Abbreviating the initial procedure has the advantage decreasing the incidence of metabolic acidosis, hypothermia, and coagulopathy, a triad known to have a high incidence of mortality.

Chapter Summary: Trauma

Trauma	Patients require a systematic, methodical approach
Initial Assessment	Assume hypovolemia, full stomach, perform history and physical exam, assign GCS score
Airway Management	Evaluate need for intubation. In-line cervical spine stabilization may be required. Have emergency airway devices ready
Fluid Resuscitation	Establish large bore IV access, send laboratory studies (T&C, CBC, coagulation studies, electrolytes, ABG), blood transfusion may be required
Monitoring	Invasive monitors may be required, temperature monitoring essential
Anesthetic Management	All induction drugs can potentially cause hemodynamic compromise, etomidate and ketamine most often recommended, consider high risk of awareness, nitrous oxide contraindicated with certain injuries, neuromuscular blockade commonly used

ABG, arterial blood gas; CBC, complete blood count; GCS, glasgow coma scale; T&C, type and cross.

References

1. Bonatti H, Calland JF. Trauma. *Emerg Med Clin N Am* 2008;26:625–648.
2. Cereda M, Weiss YG, Deutschman CS. The critically ill injured patient. *Anesthesiol Clin* 2007;25:13–21.
3. Pierre EJ, McNeer RR, Shamir MY. Early management of the traumatized airway. *Anesthesiol Clin* 2007;25:1–11.
4. Crosby ET. Airway management in adults after cervical spine trauma. *Anesthesiology* 2006;104:1293–1318.
5. Holcomb JB, Jenkins D, Rhee P, et al. Damage control resuscitation: Directly addressing the early coagulopathy of trauma. *J Trauma* 2007;62:307–310.

143

Liver and Kidney Transplantation

Sara Cheng, MD, PhD

Patients with end-stage liver and kidney disease requiring transplantation may enter the operating room with derangements of multiple organ systems. The anesthesiologist must be prepared to handle the presenting pathophysiology as well as the demands of the operative procedure.

READ MORE

Diseases of the liver and biliary tract, Chapter 77, page 551

Donor characteristics can significantly affect liver transplantation outcomes.

1) **Liver transplantation**
   a) **General considerations**
      i) Intraoperative problems often include massive hemorrhage and severe hemodynamic derangements. Aggressive management of coagulopathy and hemodynamic instability is mandatory (1).
   b) **Preoperative considerations**
      i) **Graft allocation**
         (1) **MELD (Model for End-Stage Liver Disease)**
            (a) The MELD is a scoring system originally developed for assessing perioperative risk in cirrhotic patients. It is a disease severity score that is used in the United States to prioritize patients for liver transplantation (2).
               (i) **All liver transplant candidates aged 12 and older are prioritized by the MELD system**
               (ii) Patients under age 12 are prioritized by the PELD system (Pediatric End-stage Liver Disease).
            (b) Liver grafts are allocated to patients in a geographic region with the highest MELD/PELD scores.
            (c) MELD score is calculated based on the serum bilirubin, INR, and creatinine.
            (d) A MELD calculator can be accessed at www.UNOS.org. This score should be calculated and recorded on the anesthetic record.
         (2) **Status 1**
            (a) **Patients with acute (sudden and severe onset) liver failure and a life expectancy of hours to days without transplant**
            (b) Status 1 is the only priority exception to MELD
            (c) Comprises <1% of liver transplant candidates
      ii) **Donor risk index**
         (1) **Strong predictors of graft failure include donor age >40 years, donation after cardiac death, cold ischemia time >12 hours, and split/partial grafts. African-American donor**

race, less height, other causes of brain death, and prolonged ischemia time are also significantly associated (3).

    (2) Liver grafts harvested from donors with a high-risk index (one or more risk factors) are termed *extended criteria* organs.

    (3) Anesthesiologists should be aware of the donor risk index, as recipients receiving extended criteria grafts are at higher risk for poor immediate graft function and coagulopathic blood loss in the operating room.

c) **Preoperative evaluation of the patient**

  i) Patients should have a complete set of laboratory studies available for review, including complete blood counts, electrolytes, coagulation indices, and EKG. Stress echocardiography and pulmonary function tests (PFTs) may also be indicated.

  ii) The patient should be carefully assessed for

    (1) **Severity of liver disease**

      (a) Including the presence of encephalopathy, signs of portal hypertension (ascites, esophageal varices, thrombocytopenia), electrolyte abnormalities, and deficits in hepatic synthetic function (INR, albumin)

    (2) **Comorbidities**

      (a) **Hepatopulmonary syndrome, portopulmonary HTN, renal insufficiency, and cirrhotic cardiomyopathy may all be present.**

      (b) Significant coronary artery disease, cardiac dysfunction, and moderate-to-severe pulmonary HTN are generally considered contraindications to liver transplantation.

      (c) Patients with moderate-to-severe renal insufficiency (hepatorenal syndrome or other renal disease) may require intraoperative hemodialysis.

    (3) **Bleeding risk**

      (a) **Patients with elevated INR, thrombocytopenia, portal HTN, uremia, history of upper abdominal surgery, and intra-abdominal infection are at increased risk of large-volume blood loss in the operating room.**

      (b) **The number of risk factors should dictate the number of blood products that are immediately available for transfusion in the operating room.**

d) **Preoperative checklist for preparation of the operating room (Table 143-1)**

  i) **Blood product availability**

    (1) A predetermined number of blood products based on the patient's bleeding risk should be immediately available in the operating room at the beginning of the surgical procedure.

  ii) **Rapid laboratory analysis**

    (1) **Frequent monitoring of arterial blood gases, hematocrit, coagulation parameters, electrolytes, and glucose must be easily accessible.**

    (2) Thromboelastography is often very helpful and should be used if available.

CONCERNS IN SUBSPECIALTY ANESTHESIA

Table 143-1

Perioperative Checklist for Liver Transplantation

Item	Consider	Notes

Monitoring
Standard ASA monitors
    Arterial line
    Central venous line
	TEE
	PA catheter
		Use varies with institution and patient comorbidities

Intravenous access	14 g IV × 2 *or* 9 F central venous introducer *or* 8.5 F rapid infusion catheter	Large-bore and redundant venous access is essential
Warming system for intravenous solutions	Rapid infusion systems such as Level 1™ or Belmont™	Systems vary in heating capacity and max flow rate
Blood product availability	In a patient with several bleeding risk factors—consider 10 units of PRBCs, 5 units of FFP, and 1 plasmapheresis unit of platelets in room to start.	Amount of blood products will vary with the patient's risk factors and institutional requirements
Rapid laboratory analysis	Thromboelastography may be helpful if available.	

Resuscitation meds
    Amiodarone
    Atropine
    Calcium chloride Epinephrine
    Nitroglycerine Phenylephrine
    Sodium bicarbonate
	Other meds
	    Aminocaproic acid
	    Furosemide
	    Methylprednisolone
	    Propranolol	

Anesthesia induction meds	Minimize benzodiazepine use. Avoid succinylcholine if hyperkalemia present. Avoid rocuronium secondary to heavy hepatic metabolism.	Rapid sequence induction should be used in the presence of ascites, full stomach

iii) **Resuscitation and transplant medications**
    (1) In addition to the standard drugs for induction and maintenance of anesthesia, the following drugs should be readily available
        (a) Epinephrine, calcium chloride, sodium bicarbonate, phenylephrine, atropine, amiodarone, nitroglycerine, furosemide, methylprednisolone, aminocaproic acid, and propranolol
iv) **Intraoperative dialysis may be necessary in the case of hepatorenal syndrome.**
  e) **Intraoperative considerations (Table 143-2)**
    i) **Surgical procedure overview**
      (1) Orthotopic liver transplantation

Table 143-2

Surgical Stages of Orthotopic Liver Transplantation

Stage	Surgical Goals
Preanhepatic	Vascular isolation and removal of the in situ diseased liver. Usually achieved by placing vascular clamps across the superior and inferior vena cava, portal vein, and hepatic artery, followed by *en bloc* removal the diseased liver attached to a segment of the vena cava.
Anhepatic	Formation of the portal vein, inferior vena cava, and hepatic artery anastamoses.
Neohepatic	**Begins with release of all vascular clamps, allowing reperfusion of new liver graft. Followed by biliary reconstruction, surgical hemostasis, and closure of abdomen.**

The surgical procedure for liver transplant involves three distinct stages.

(a) The majority of liver transplantations are performed in an orthotopic manner, in which a whole diseased liver is replaced with a healthy donor liver.

(b) Whole liver grafts are obtained from cadaveric donors.

(c) Split liver grafts are primarily used in the case of child recipients or living donors.

(2) Heterotopic liver transplantation

(a) Donor liver is placed at a different location from the existing diseased liver.

(b) Rare procedure used for bridging recipients to orthotopic transplantation

ii) Anesthetic management of preanhepatic phase

(1) Infectious concerns

(a) Due to the high prevalence of blood-borne pathogens in liver transplant recipients, especially hepatitis C, all medical personnel should use universal precautions.

(b) Patients will require immunosuppression, so every effort must be made to avoid infectious complications.

(i) Use of aseptic technique for all invasive line placement

(ii) Administer appropriate perioperative antibiotics.

(iii) If blood loss is massive or the procedure long, redosing of antibiotics should be considered.

(2) Monitoring

(a) In addition to standard ASA monitors, an arterial catheter should be placed for serial laboratory measurements and real-time BP monitoring during times of rapid hemodynamic change.

(b) A central venous catheter should be used for infusion of drugs into the central compartment and transduction of central venous pressure (CVP).

(c) The use of pulmonary artery catheters and transesophageal echocardiography (TEE) during liver transplantation varies widely between institutions.

CONCERNS IN SUBSPECIALTY ANESTHESIA

(d) In general, the ability to monitor cardiac output should be available to aid in the differential diagnosis of refractory hypotension, especially in high MELD patients.

(3) **Intravenous therapy**

(a) Infusions should be chosen with the intent of reducing portal HTN, maintaining normal cardiac contractility, and counteracting renal retention of sodium and water.

(b) High MELD patients with cirrhotic cardiomyopathy may require the use of ionotropes (Table 143-3).

(4) **Induction and maintenance**

(a) Preoxygenation with 100% oxygen is essential.

(i) All liver failure patients are considered full stomachs, necessitating the use of a rapid-sequence induction.

(b) Thiopental or propofol are appropriate induction agents if the patient has adequate BP; otherwise, etomidate can be used.

(c) Succinylcholine is the preferred neuromuscular blocker if the patient is normokalemic.

(i) Rocuronium is not recommended due to the heavy reliance of this drug on hepatic metabolism.

(d) Anesthesia should be maintained with volatile anesthetics with low blood-gas partition coefficients (desflurane) to allow rapid changes in the anesthetic depth.

(5) **Anesthetic goals**

(a) Maintenance of normothermia

(i) Use of fluid warmers, bed warmers, forced heated air devices, and control of ambient temperature are all appropriate.

(b) Electrolyte management of sodium, potassium, and calcium

Table 143-3

Suggested Dosing of Infusions Commonly Used During Liver Transplantation

Drug	Desired Effect	Suggested Dosing
Octreotide	Portal vasoconstriction	50–75 µg/h
Vasopressin	Portal vasoconstriction	0.04 U/min
Dopamine	Natriuresis	2 µg/kg/min
Mannitol	Osmotic diuresis	5–10 g/h
25% albumin	Normal serum osmolarity	10–15 cc/h
Epinephrine	Maintain cardiac contractility and SVR	0.01–0.1 µg/kg/min
Norepinephrine	Maintain cardiac contractility and SVR	0.05–0.2 µg/kg/min
Phenylephrine	Maintenance of SVR	0.1–5 µg/kg/min

(i) Maintain at as close to normal levels as possible, because derangements can lead to more severe hemodynamic instability at graft reperfusion.

(c) Monitor blood loss

(i) Surgical dissection can cause brisk bleeding during this period. Indicators of volume status include BP, visible blood loss, CVP, and area under the arterial BP tracing.

(d) Monitor coagulation

(i) **Consider partial correction of severe coagulopathy and thrombocytopenia prior to line placement.**

(ii) **Impaired intraoperative hemostasis is usually multifactorial, resulting from a combination of dilutional coagulopathy, thrombocytopenia, platelet dysfunction, hyperfibrinolysis, and poor graft function.**

(e) Administer blood products if necessary

(i) **An intraoperative transfusion ratio close to 1:1 of PRBC:FFP should be considered to avoid dilutional coagulopathy.**

(ii) Reasonable goals for transfusion are a hematocrit of 30% to 35% and platelets >50,000/mL.

(iii) Drugs such as α-aminocaproic acid, DDAVP (arginine vasopressin), and recombinant fVIIa are not given routinely but should be considered on a case-by-case basis.

iii) Anesthetic management of anhepatic phase

(1) This phase begins with surgical occlusion of the hepatic artery, portal vein, and the inferior vena cava above and below the liver.

(2) In addition to continuing attention to the concerns associated with the pre-anhepatic phase, this phase has additional hemodynamic issues related to caval occlusion.

(3) Acute hypotension is common secondary to poor venous return above the cross clamp.

(a) Venous congestion below the cross clamp can cause a decrease in renal blood flow, leading to oliguria or anuria.

(4) Arterial BP can be maintained with use of an arterial vasoconstrictor such as phenylephrine.

(5) Judicious use of volume during this phase is recommended, as overzealous resuscitation during this period can worsen venous congestion and the risk of subsequent volume overload after caval unclamping.

(6) Venovenous bypass

(a) **Used by some centers to maintain cardiac preload during the anhepatic phase**

(b) This may decrease hemodynamic instability.

(c) When used, pump flow rates must be kept above 800 ml/min to avoid pump thrombosis.

(d) **A low threshold of suspicion should be maintained for complications including vascular injury from bypass catheters, catheter kinking, pump thrombosis, hypothermia, and venous air embolus.**

(7) Electrolyte abnormalities

(a) Common electrolyte abnormalities during the anhepatic stage include metabolic acidosis, hyperkalemia, and hypocalcemia.

(b) Must be aggressively corrected since the anhepatic patient has no means of physiologic compensation

READ MORE

Blood component therapy, Chapter 27, page 209

The major issues during the anhepatic phase of liver transplant are due to occlusion of the inferior vena cava.

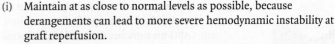
CONCERNS IN SUBSPECIALTY ANESTHESIA

Close communication with the surgeon is necessary to allow adequate preparation for the hemodynamic consequences of unclamping.

Reperfusion syndrome occurs in up to 30% of liver transplants.

(c) Serum potassium should be lowered to below 3.5 mEq/L to lessen the risk of reperfusion syndrome (see below).

(d) ABG measurements should be conducted at least every 30 minutes.

(8) IV steroid should be administered prior to reperfusion as part of induction therapy (short-term immunosuppression given at the time of transplant).

(a) Methylprednisolone 500 to 1,000 mg is commonly used, as this dose has been shown to cause lymphocyte apoptosis and decreased subsequent graft rejection.

iv) **Anesthetic management of neohepatic phase**

(1) Starts with removal of vascular clamps, resulting in reperfusion of the donor graft. It encompasses surgical reconstruction of the biliary tree and the conclusion of the surgery.

(2) **Caval unclamping**

(a) **Typically results in marked** increases in cardiac preload and BP.

   (i) **Pressors should be turned off just prior to unclamping.**

   (ii) **Small doses of nitroglycerin (10 to 20 μg) may be used for extreme HTN (SBP > 180), although higher pressures are preferable in preparation for the next phase of portal vein unclamping.**

(b) **Portal vein unclamping**

   (i) **Allows recipient blood to enter the donor graft.**

   (ii) **Reperfusion syndrome**

   1. Hemodynamic instability manifesting within 1 to 5 minutes after portal vein unclamping

   2. Caused by characteristics of the graft effluent (cold, acidic, hyperkalemic, vasoactive mediators)

   3. Symptoms include severe bradyarrhythmias, hypotension, decreased contractility, and vasodilation

   4. Severity of symptoms is related to the extent that patient parameters are normalized prior to reperfusion.

   5. **Prompt and repeated administration of atropine, epinephrine, phenylephrine, calcium, and bicarbonate may be required.**

   (iii) Hepatic artery unclamping

   1. Does not usually have any noticeable hemodynamic consequences.

   (iv) Assessment of graft function

Markers of good liver graft function include citrate metabolism, adequate urine output, maintenance of normothermia, and visible bile production.

f) **Postoperative management**

i) **Extubation**

(1) Patients who meet certain criteria may be safely extubated at the end of the operation and discharged to the surgical ward.

(a) **The decision to extubate should be based on individual patient criteria and adequacy of hospital infrastructure (Table 143-4).**

(2) Laboratory monitoring

(a) **Postoperative serial measurement of hematocrit, platelets, and coagulation indices should be available.**

(3) Pain control

(a) **Extubated patients are candidates for patient-controlled analgesia.**

Table 143-4

Patient Criteria Associated with Safe Extubation after Liver Transplant (4)

• Awake patient	• Not a Status 1 recipient
• Intact cranial nerve reflexes	• Not a repeat liver transplant recipient
• TV > 8 cc/kg	• Cadaveric donor graft
• RR < 20 breaths/min	• Anesthetic technique allowing resumption of spontaneous
• Normocarbia	respiration (judicious use of narcotics and neuromuscular
• Neuromuscular reversal	blockade)
• Normothermia	
• Hemodynamic stability with minimal drug support	

2) **Kidney transplantation (5)**
  a) **Overview**
    i) Offered to end-stage renal disease (ESRD) patients to allow them freedom from dialysis.
    ii) Classified as deceased-donor or living-donor transplantation.
      (1) Living-donor renal transplants are further characterized as genetically related (living-related) or nonrelated (living-unrelated) transplants.
  b) **Preoperative considerations**
    i) Patients presenting for renal transplantation have ESRD and typically fall into two categories: the young and relatively healthy (on dialysis), or older and more chronically ill
    ii) Preoperative evaluation
      (1) Most patients should have a complete set of laboratory studies available for review, including complete blood counts, electrolytes, coagulation indices, CXR, and ECG. PFTs should be obtained if indicated by comorbidities.

For kidney transplant patients, preoperative evaluation for coexisting cardiac disease and cardiac function is of primary importance.

      (2) Dialysis status
        (a) Patients should be queried about how often they are dialyzed, the date/time of their last dialysis, and whether they make any urine.
        (b) If dialysis has not been performed within 6 to 8 hours of presenting to the operating room, serum potassium should be checked and volume status carefully assessed.
      (3) Comorbidities
        (a) As many as 50% of ESRD patients have comorbidities associated with increased cardiac risk, including severe diabetes, HTN, and atherosclerosis.
        (b) Low-risk patients may proceed directly to the operating room, while intermediate- and high-risk patients should probably undergo perfusion studies and/or invasive studies such as cardiac catheterization.
      (4) Preoperative preparation of the operating room
        (a) Standard preparations for general anesthesia should be made.
        (b) Fluid warmers and pressure transducers for arterial and CVP measurements may be considered.
  c) **Intraoperative considerations**
    i) Surgical procedure
      (1) Kidney transplantation is a fairly short procedure (<3 hours) usually associated with minimal blood loss.

(2) Generally performed in a heterotopic fashion, with the donor graft being placed in a nonanatomic location such as the iliac fossa.

    (a) The diseased recipient kidneys are left in situ.

(3) The renal artery of the donor kidney is often connected to the external iliac artery in the recipient.

(4) The renal vein of the new kidney is often connected to the external iliac vein in the recipient.

ii) **Intraoperative management**

    (1) Monitoring

        (a) Standard ASA monitors are required.

        (b) Arterial BP monitoring and CVP monitoring may be considered based on patient comorbidities and institutional practice, but are generally not demanded by the procedure itself.

    (2) **Induction and maintenance**

        (a) General endotracheal anesthesia is usually used although in selected patients combined spinal epidural or LMA general anesthesia may be appropriate.

        (b) Induction

            (i) There is no preferred IV induction agents provided hemodynamic stability is maintained.

            (ii) Any paralytic agent can be used judiciously. Succinylcholine should be avoided if serum potassium is elevated. Vecuronium, rocuronium, and cisatracurium are all appropriate choices. Drugs with heavy reliance on renal metabolism, such as pancuronium, are best avoided.

        (c) Maintenance

            (i) Can be achieved by a combination of opioid and volatile agents

            (ii) Paralytics, opioids, and volatile anesthetics should all be titrated with the goal of successful extubation at the conclusion of the procedure.

            (iii) Avoid use of ketorolac (possible renal toxicity) and morphine (due to renal clearance of morphine 6-glucuronide).

    (3) **Intraoperative goals**

        (a) The major goal in perioperative management of kidney transplant patients is correction and maintenance of adequate renal perfusion pressure to facilitate immediate graft function.

            (i) Both intraoperative fluid management and pharmacological treatment have been studied in this regard, although there is a no clear consensus on the optimum strategy.

                1. Crystalloid therapy is generally sufficient for volume resuscitation, with little need for colloid therapy due to short duration of the surgery and minimal associated blood loss.

                    a. Lactated Ringers, normal saline, and plasmalyte are all generally safe for use during kidney transplantation.

                2. Euvolemia should be the goal of fluid administration.

                3. Mannitol, loop diuretics, dopamine, and occasionally fenoldapam can all be used to increase urine output and improve graft function.

            (ii) An induction dose of IV steroid such as methylprednisolone should be administered.

iii) **Postoperative considerations**

(1) Most patients meet standard criteria for extubation at the conclusion of the procedure.

(2) Urine output should be closely monitored.

(a) Immediate urine production is seen in over 90% of living donor transplants and between 40% to 70% of deceased-donor transplants.

Chapter Summary for Liver Transplantation

Preoperative Evaluation	Assess severity of liver disease and common comorbidities Assess bleeding risk Warm room Prepare rapid infusion system Blood products immediately available Intraoperative dialysis if needed
Induction of Anesthesia	RSI with succinylcholine unless contraindicated, avoid rocuronium due to heavy hepatic excretion, expect desaturation due to decreased FRC from ascites, minimize preoperative benzodiazepines, use etomidate if BP low.
Maintenance of Anesthesia	Atracurium and cisatracurium are NMBs of choice. Consider desflurane for rapid titration of anesthetic depth. Use short-acting opioids. Invasive monitoring necessary for management of major hemodynamic derangements. Plan for management of IVC occlusion (venovenous bypass vs. pressors). Optimize patient physiology prior to reperfusion. Aggressively manage acid base, electrolyte status, and hemodynamics tailored to phase of surgery (preanhepatic, anhepatic, reperfusion, neohepatic). Steroid administration prior to graft reperfusion.
Postoperative Concerns	Consider extubation if patient characteristics are favorable. Serial monitoring of hemacrit, platelets, INR, transaminases, and clinical signs of bleeding are mandatory.

Chapter Summary for Renal Transplantation

Preoperative Evaluation	Assess severity of kidney disease and comorbidities
Induction of Anesthesia	Short-acting induction agents due to short duration of case Avoid succinylcholine if hyperkalemia present.
Maintenance of Anesthesia	General anesthesia is typically used. Avoid NMBs that rely mainly on renal clearance Balanced anesthetic technique of opioid/volatile Avoid ketorolac (renal toxic) and morphine (renal clearance of morphine 6-glucuronide). Maintain adequate renal perfusion pressure to facilitate immediate graft function. Steroid administration prior to graft reperfusion.
Postoperative Concerns	Most patients can be extubated using standard criteria. Urine output should be closely monitored.

CONCERNS IN SUBSPECIALTY ANESTHESIA

References

1. Niemann CU, Eilers H. Abdominal organ transplantation. *Minerva Anestesiol* 2010 Apr;76(4):266–75.
2. Lake JR. MELD—an imperfect, but thus far the best, solution to the problem of organ allocation. *J Gastrointestin Liver Dis* 2008;17(1):5–7.
3. Feng S, Goodrich NP, Merion RM. Characteristics associated with liver graft failure: the concept of a donor risk index. *Am J Transplant* 2006;6(4):783–790.
4. Mandell MS, Lockrem J, Kelley SD. Immediate tracheal extubation after liver transplantation: experience of two transplant centers. *Anesth Analg* 1997;84(2):249–253.
5. Lemmens HJ. Kidney transplantation: recent developments and recommendations for anesthetic management. *Anesthesiol Clin North Am* 2004;22(4):651–662.

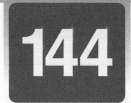

Obstetrical Anesthesia

Andrea J. Fuller, MD

Obstetrical anesthesia is a rewarding and dynamic specialty requiring **constant communication** among nurses, obstetricians, and anesthesiologists. Although some patients prefer to not have medications as part of their birth plan, all patients admitted to the labor ward could potentially require anesthetic intervention. This requires the anesthesia provider be cognizant of all patients on the ward but treat each as an individual, remaining sympathetic to patient's wishes and clearly explaining all procedures necessity, risks, and benefits.

1) **Common obstetrical nomenclature**
   a) The description of a patient by the obstetric and nursing staff will often include abbreviations, the knowledge of which is important to understanding a patient's obstetric history.
   b) **G refers to Gravida**, which is the number of times the patient has been pregnant.
   c) **P refers to Parity** and is often subclassified with the mnemonic TPAL
      i) T is the number of full-term births.
      ii) P is the number of preterm births.
      iii) A is the number of abortions, whether spontaneous or induced.
      iv) L is the number of living children.
   d) For example, a G3P1112 patient has been pregnant three times, with one full term birth, one preterm birth, one abortion, and two living children.
2) **Physiologic changes of pregnancy** (Table 144-1)
   a) Pregnancy significantly alters physiology, which dramatically affects the perioperative management of these patients
3) **Normal Labor**
   a) **First stage:** Onset of labor to complete cervical dilation.
      i) Pain arises in peripheral nociceptors in the lower uterine segment and cervix and travels in **visceral** afferent neurons, which enter the neuraxis at **T10-L1**.
   b) **Second stage:** Pushing and delivery of baby.
      i) Pain is predominantly from the perineum and travels in **somatic** afferent fibers in the pudendal nerve that enter the neuraxis at **S2-4**
   c) **Third stage:** Placental delivery
4) **Analgesia for a laboring patient anticipating a vaginal delivery**
   a) **Nonpharmacologic methods for relieving childbirth pain**
      i) Success varies with the individual and her labor pattern.
      ii) Include Lamaze, transcutaneous electrical stimulation, relaxation training, massage, water baths, and emotional support.

Table 144-1

Physiologic Changes of Pregnancy

System	Physiologic Change	Anesthetic Implication
CNS	MAC ↓ by up to 40% ↑ sensitivity to local anesthetics ↓ CSF volume, distention of epidural veins, ↑ pressure in epidural space	↓ anesthetic requirement ↓ doses required, ↑ risk of toxicity ↑ risk of intravascular catheter placement with attempted epidural
Airway	Capillary engorgement and edema	↑ potential for difficult airway ↓ endotracheal tube size required (6–6.5 mm)
Respiratory	↑ oxygen consumption, ↓ FRC ↑ minute ventilation	Very rapid desaturation with apnea or induction of GA ↓ $PaCO_2$ to approximately 33 mmHg by 3rd trimester
Cardiovascular	↑ cardiac output by 40% by end of 1st trimester and to > 80% above prelabor values after delivery ↓ SVR Aortocaval compression due to uterine enlargement	Potential for decompensation in patients with pre-existing cardiac disease, especially immediately following delivery ↓ arterial BP; considered elevated when > 140/90 Hypotension with supine position; never position patients > 18–20 weeks' supine without displacement of the uterus
Hematologic	↑ blood volume; ↑ red cell mass (not in proportion to blood volume) ↑ coagulability	Able to tolerate blood loss at delivery; "physiologic" anemia of pregnancy Hypercoagulability places patients at risk for DVT/PE and other clotting problems.
Gastrointestinal	↓ gastric emptying ↓ lower esophageal sphincter tone	↑ risk for pulmonary aspiration of gastric contents
Musculoskeletal	↑ lumbar lordosis Widened pelvis	↓ interspinous spaces possibly making neuraxial procedures more difficult Head down tilt when assuming the lateral position
Genitourinary	↑ glomerular filtration rate	↓ creatinine (0.4–0.6 mg/dL)

BP, blood pressure; CSF, cerebrospinal fluid; DVT, deep venous thrombosis; FRC, functional residual capacity; MAC, minimum alveolar concentration; PE, pulmonary embolism; SVR, systemic vascular resistance.

b) **Systemic pain medications**

i)   Do not require a procedure or carry the risk of lower extremity motor block

ii) Opioid medications are the most widely used.

iii) Commonly used where neuraxial analgesia is unavailable or impossible due to contraindications.

iv) **Intravenous (IV) is the preferred route of administration due to the rapid, predictable onset.**

v)   Higher doses of IV opioids are usually required as labor progresses.

Opioid medications are a viable option for labor analgesia but do not completely relieve labor pain in safe doses.

vi) Side effects of opioids include maternal or neonatal respiratory depression, postural hypotension, urinary retention, constipation, nausea, vomiting, and decreased fetal heart rate (FHR) variability (1,2).

vii) Choice of agent is determined by maternal and neonatal effects.

   (1) **Fentanyl**

     (a) **Rapid onset of effective analgesia**

     (b) **Preferred agent for labor and delivery**

     (c) The IV dose is **50 to 75 μg**, with a peak effect of 3 to 5 minutes and duration of 30 to 60 minutes.

     (d) Fentanyl crosses the placenta and can cause neonatal respiratory depression, but the duration of effect on the neonate appears small, especially if it is avoided within 2 hours of delivery (1).

     (e) Fentanyl patient-controlled analgesia (PCA) is an effective option for patients who cannot have neuraxial analgesia.

       (i) PCA doses range from 10 to 50 μg with a lockout period of 8 to 20 minutes.

   (2) **Meperidine** has been widely used in obstetrics.

     (a) The dosage is 25 to 50 mg IV with a peak effect 5 to 10 minutes and duration of 3 to 4 hours.

     (b) Rapidly crosses the placenta

     (c) **Both meperidine and its active metabolite, normeperidine, are present in the neonate for long periods (up to 3 to 6 days),** causing respiratory depression and neurobehavioral changes.

   (3) **Morphine**

     (a) **Causes more neonatal depression than other agents and is a less effective analgesic at clinically safe doses.**

     (b) Not a recommended agent

c) **Neuraxial analgesia for vaginal delivery**

i) Provides the best pain relief and patient satisfaction of all the options for pain management during labor (Table 144-3)

ii) The goal is to provide excellent analgesia and minimize lower extremity motor block (3).

iii) If cesarean delivery becomes necessary, the presence of a properly functioning epidural catheter allows rapid and simple conversion to surgical anesthesia.

iv) Continuous epidural infusion is used with or without an intrathecal injection administered via the combined spinal epidural (CSE) technique.

   (1) The choice of technique depends on many factors, including provider preference and expertise, potential for difficult airway, and progress of the patient's labor.

v) Combined spinal epidural

   (1) Advantages

     (a) Rapid onset of analgesia

     (b) Minimal motor block

   (2) Patients likely to benefit from CSE

     (a) Late in labor, especially multiparous women

     (b) Those with a history of short labor

   (3) Disadvantages

     (a) When the CSE technique is used, the epidural catheter is untested and may be unpredictable if needed for cesarean delivery.

       (i) Therefore, patients with a known or an anticipated difficult airway may not be good candidates for CSE.

Every epidural catheter in a laboring patient should be evaluated for its potential to be used for cesarean delivery if necessary

READ MORE

Combined spinal epidural technique, Chapter 33, page 252

A CSE is an excellent option for labor analgesia, especially in multiparous women late in labor or those with a history of short labor.

CONCERNS IN SUBSPECIALTY ANESTHESIA

READ MORE

Obstetrical emergencies, Chapter 100, page 727

If an instrumented vaginal delivery is not successful, the patient may require immediate cesarean delivery.

4) **Instrumented vaginal delivery**
   a) Accomplished with vacuum extraction or forceps
   b) Requires excellent **perineal anesthesia**
   c) Frequently requires concentrated local anesthetic (Table 144-3)
      i) If an epidural catheter is not present, a spinal injection (preferably via the CSE technique) can be performed and dosed according to Table 144-3.
   d) The anesthesia provider should **remain present (or immediately available) during delivery** in the event of an emergent cesarean delivery, additional medication requirements, neonatal resuscitation, or bleeding.

5) **Anesthesia for cesarean delivery (Table 144-2)**
   a) Regardless of anesthetic technique, the procedure for cesarean delivery can be thought of as having three phases
      i) Phase I: Administration of anesthesia, surgical incision, and dissection
      ii) Phase II: Uterine incision and delivery of the fetus
      iii) Phase III: Hemostasis and closure

6) **Regional anesthesia (RA) for cesarean delivery**
   a) RA is the preferred method of anesthesia for cesarean delivery for the following reasons
      i) Due to the physiologic changes of pregnancy, all parturients are considered a full stomach and are at risk for aspiration of gastric contents.
      ii) The incidence of difficult airway is eight times higher during pregnancy than in the general population.
      iii) Anesthetic mortality with GA was previously reported to be 16 times higher than with RA (4,5).

Table 144-2
Considerations for Cesarean Delivery

Surgical Phase	Events	Anesthetic Considerations
Phase I	Administration of anesthesia, surgical incision and dissection to uterus	Choice of RA or GA based on clinical situation (RA preferred); Hemodynamic stability and adequacy of anesthetic are primary concerns Communication with patient and support person is essential
Phase II	Uterine incision and delivery of fetus	If RA, notify patient of imminent delivery; carefully observe uterine incision and delivery time; observe placental extraction and the surgical field for adequacy of uterine tone and signs of bleeding
Phase III	Hemostasis and closure	Administer uterotonic agents; vigilantly observe and communicate with surgeon about adequacy of uterine tone and bleeding concerns; Patient may spend time bonding with baby; Consider postoperative pain management plans

Table 144-3
Suggested Analgesic/Anesthetic Regimens for Obstetrics (1,2)

Clinical Scenario	Anesthetic Regimen	Comments/Side Effects
Labor epidural[a]	**Initiation:** 10–15 mL Bupivacaine 0.125%–0.25% + fentanyl 50–100 µg or sufentanil 5–10 µg **Maintenance infusion:** 10–15 mL/h Bupivacaine 0.0625%–0.125% Ropivacaine 0.1%–0.2% + fentanyl 2 µg/mL or sufentanil 0.3–0.4 µg/mL **PCEA:** any above infusion with boluses of 4–10 mL every 10–20 min with maximum hourly dose of 12–30 mL.	Lower concentrations and higher volumes of local anesthetics preferred. Side effects include motor block, urinary retention, nausea/vomiting, hypotension, pruritus, and respiratory depression (if narcotics are added)
Labor CSE	Fentanyl 15–25 µg or sufenta 2.5–5 µg ±bupivacaine 1.5–2.5 mg	Narcotic-only techniques do not have motor block ("walking epidural"); Side effects are the same as epidural; Higher doses associated with fetal bradycardia via unclear mechanism, probably uterine hypertonus
Instrumented vaginal delivery[a]	**Epidural:** 5–15 mL lidocaine 1%–2% or 2%–3% 2-choloroprocaine **Spinal:** 2.5–5 mg bupivacaine plus 15–25 µg fentanyl	Cesarean delivery may be necessary if instrumented delivery fails
Cesarean delivery in a patient with functioning labor epidural[a]	20 mL 2% lidocaine with 1 mEq/10 mL HCO_3 and 1:200,000 epinephrine; 20 mL 3% 2-choloroprocaine	For postoperative analgesia, add epidural morphine 3–4 mg
Spinal anesthesia for cesarean delivery (no labor epidural)	Bupivacaine 12 mg (use 0.5% isobaric or 0.75% hyperbaric) + fentanyl 10–25 µg	For postoperative analgesia, add intrathecal morphine 100–200 µg
Epidural anesthesia for cesarean delivery (no labor epidural)[a]	20–25 mL 2% lidocaine with 1 mEq/10 mL HCO_3 and 1:200,000 epinephrine; or 0.5% bupivacaine; 0.5% ropivacaine; 3% 2-cholorprocaine + fentanyl 75–100 µg or sufentanil 10–25 µg	For postoperative analgesia, add epidural morphine 3–4 mg

The majority of elective cesarean deliveries in the United States are performed with spinal anesthesia

(1) Maternal mortality has significantly improved with the overall use of RA and improvements in airway management.

(2) Currently, the prevalence of morbidity and mortality with GA remains higher than with RA, but the overall number of claims is higher with RA because of the widespread use of RA for obstetrics (6).

iv) Maternal satisfaction is higher with RA because the woman is awake for delivery and able to bond with her baby immediately.

v) Postoperative pain management is improved with the use of neuraxial opioids

CONCERNS IN SUBSPECIALTY ANESTHESIA

READ MORE

Spinal anesthesia, Chapter 30, page 225 and Spinal anesthesia, Chapter 160, page 1116

b) If RA is used, a **T4 sensory level is required for adequate anesthesia.** Table 144-3 contains suggested medications and dosage.

c) **Always ensure adequate surgical anesthesia prior to surgical incision.**

d) **Spinal anesthesia**
   i) Advantages
      (1) **Rapid onset** of dense surgical anesthesia
      (2) Usually quick to perform and can be used for urgent delivery
      (3) Low doses of medication are required, which have minimal fetal effects
   ii) Disadvantages
      (1) Hypotension
         (a) Can be minimized by rapid administration of at least 1 L of balanced salt solution with or without 500 mL hetastarch prior to or immediately following block placement (7)
      (2) Inability to add medications if anesthesia is inadequate

READ MORE

Epidural anesthesia, Chapter 31, page 237 and Atlas of anesthesia procedures: Lumbar epidural placement, Chapter 161, page 1118

e) **Epidural anesthesia**
   i) **Advantages**
      (1) Catheter is in place for the duration of surgery
      (2) May be used for postoperative pain management.
      (3) If analgesia is inadequate, the epidural catheter can be redosed and/or manipulated to improve anesthesia.
      (4) Hemodynamic changes may be slower to take effect, which may be preferred in patients who may not tolerate acute hypotension
   ii) **Disadvantages**
      (1) Slower onset
      (2) Possibly less dense block
      (3) Placement can be more time consuming.

f) **CSE anesthesia**
   i) Combines the advantages and the disadvantages of both spinal and epidural techniques
   ii) Examples of situations where CSE may be indicated include
      (1) Patients who would benefit from the rapid onset of spinal medication but in whom the best dose is unclear (i.e., extreme short stature, morbid obesity)
      (2) Patients at risk for long duration of surgery at the time of cesarean delivery (e.g., a patient undergoing her fourth cesarean delivery)

READ MORE

Combined spinal-epidural technique, Chapter 33, page 252

g) **Hypotension during RA** for cesarean delivery is common and should be treated aggressively
   i) May first manifest as **nausea and vomiting**
   ii) **Treatment**
      (1) **Ensure adequate left uterine displacement.**
      (2) Ensure adequate intravascular volume.
      (3) Pharmacologic treatment includes **phenylephrine (50 to 100 μg IV) as a first-line medication if the heart rate is adequate,** or ephedrine (5 to 10 mg IV).
         (a) Due to concerns about neonatal metabolic acidosis with large doses of ephedrine, **phenylephrine may be the preferred agent** (3).
         (b) Reflex bradycardia can occur with phenylephrine administration and can be successfully treated with **glycopyrolate (0.2 to 0.4 mg IV)** or atropine **(0.5 mg IV).**

In a parturient who has a spinal anesthetic for cesarean delivery, a complaint of nausea is a manifestation of hypotension until proven otherwise.

iii) Rarely, severe bradycardia and even cardiac arrest can occur after spinal anesthesia.

(1) In order to maximize the chance of successful outcome, this must be treated **rapidly** with **atropine** starting at 0.2 to 0.3 mg for severe bradycardia up to 1 mg IV for cardiac arrest and/or **epinephrine 0.2 to 0.3 mg** escalating to full resuscitation doses if necessary (8).

READ MORE

Transversus abdominis plane blocks, Chapter 183, page 1242

7) **General anesthesia (GA) for cesarean delivery (Fig. 144-1)**

a) GA in obstetrics can be anxiety provoking and complication prone, but may be required when RA is not possible due to emergency conditions or contraindications. Occasionally GA may be required due to failure of regional technique.

b) **Maintenance of communication among members of the care team is imperative.**

c) Aspiration precautions (Fig. 144-2) should be taken.

d) It is important to remember that all volatile anesthetics decrease uterine tone and can increase bleeding so uterine tone must be carefully monitored.

e) MAC is decreased in pregnancy, so volatile anesthetic requirements may be reduced.

f) Postoperative pain is often severe. IV opioid medications will be required, usually by PCA if neuraxial opioids are not given.

i) Also consider multimodal therapy with NSAIDs, Acetaminophen, and/or transversus abdominal plane blocks.

For optimal airway management in the parturient, consider building a "ramp" to elevate the head and shoulders so that the external auditory meatus is at the level of the sternal notch.

8) **Other pregnancy-related procedures**

a) **Cervical cerclage** is performed for cervical incompetence, often with prior pregnancy loss.

i) Due to the physiologic changes of pregnancy, RA is preferred.

ii) There are situations such as a patient with a dilated cervix and bulging membranes **who cannot assume the upright or the lateral position** for whom GA (with aspiration precautions) may be the best choice.

When performing GA for cesarean delivery, it is important to notify the surgeons in very clear terms when the airway is secure to avoid skin incision while the patient is awake.

iii) It is important to consult the patient's obstetrician prior to determining anesthetic technique.

iv) If RA is used, the sensory level should be **T8-10.**

(1) For spinal anesthesia, 40 mg lidocaine or 7.5 mg of bupivacaine with 20 µg fentanyl is recommended (1).

(2) If an epidural is used, approximately 12 to 15 mL of 2% lidocaine with 50 to 75 µg fentanyl is typically adequate (1).

CONCERNS IN SUBSPECIALTY ANESTHESIA

Figure 144-1	Aspiration Precautions

- Nonparticulate antacid (such as 30 ml sodium bicitrate PO)
- Histamine$_2$ (H$_2$) receptor antagonist (ranitidine 50 mg or famotidine 20 mg IV) preferably given at least 30 minutes prior to procedure
- Gastric motility agent (metoclopramide 10 mg IV)
- Rapid sequence induction
- Cricoid pressure
- Endotracheal intubation
- Awake extubation with airway reflexes intact

Appropriate for all Patients after 12 weeks' gestation and immediately postpartum. (1,2).

Figure 144-2	Suggested Procedure for General Anesthesia for Cesarean Delivery

Ensure well functioning **IV line**

Administer non-particulate antacid and H2-receptor antagonist

Place patient in the supine position with **left uterine displacement**

Apply standard ASA **monitors**

Have surgeons prepped, draped and ready for surgery

Preoxygenate, ideally for 3–5 minutes

Have an assistant apply **cricoid pressure**

Administer induction agent (propofol 2 mg/kg, thiopental 4 mg/kg, etomidate 0.2–0.3 mg/kg) followed by succinylcholine (1–1.5 mg/kg) with **rapid sequence induction**

Intubate the trachea with a cuffed endotracheal tube

Confirm placement of the endotracheal tube with ETCO2 and/or bilateral breath sounds.

Inform the surgeons that the airway is secure and that they may begin surgery

Administer 100% oxygen plus 0.5–1 MAC of halogenated agent

Once baby is delivered, administer 50% nitrous oxide and 50% oxygen, **decrease volatile agent to <0.5 MAC, and consider adding opioids and/or muscle relaxants as necessary**

Administer **uterine contractile agent** (usually oxytocin infusion).

Closely monitor uterine tone and bleeding. Additional uterotonic agents may be necessary.

Administer antibiotics as requested by the surgeon (may be done prior to incision)

Extubate the patient fully awake

v) Regardless of technique, coughing and vomiting must be avoided because it causes increased intra-abdominal pressure, which can be detrimental in this situation.

Oxytocin, especially in large doses, should never be administered via IV bolus as hemodynamically significant hypotension, tachycardia, and flushing may occur.

b) **Emergent Hysterectomy:** In the event of postpartum hemorrhage, hysterectomy may be required. Rarely, a hysterectomy may be done electively at cesarean delivery for medical or other reasons.

 i) **RA is still preferred over GA in the absence of extreme hemodynamic instability and/or coagulation abnormalities (9).**

 ii) If massive hemorrhage occurs and resuscitation is required, **airway difficulty could arise due to edema.** Early intubation in the face of an ongoing resuscitation is preferable (10).

c) **Postpartum tubal ligation:** Tubal ligation may be easily performed in the first several days postpartum.

 i) It is unknown when the risk of gastric aspiration reaches prepartum levels.

  (1) These patients remain at risk for aspiration and difficult airway.

   (a) If GA is performed, appropriate aspiration precautions should be taken (Fig. 144-2)

READ MORE

Hemorrhage in the parturient, Chapter 101, page 740

   (2) **Volatile agents can cause uterine atony and precipitate postpartum hemorrhage;** high doses should be avoided (1).

 ii) A spinal or an epidural anesthetic is the preferred method for this surgery. If an epidural is in place from delivery, it can be used.

  (1) The **failure rate for catheters left in place >24 hours is up to 20%, and it may be faster to remove the catheter and administer spinal anesthesia (11).**

9) Nonobstetric surgery during pregnancy

a) **Incidence:** Approximately 0.75% to 2% of pregnant patients require nonobstetric surgery (12).

b) **Timing**

When determining whether an in situ epidural catheter may function for postpartum tubal ligation, check to see if the catheter has dislodged and ask the patient if it functioned well for her delivery.

 i) Elective surgery should not be performed during pregnancy.

 ii) Surgical procedures during the 1st trimester are associated with **increased risk of spontaneous abortion.**

 iii) Surgery in the third trimester is associated with **preterm labor.**

 iv) If surgery must be done, **the second trimester is preferred** as these risks are minimized.

 v) A procedure should not be postponed until the second trimester if a mother's life is in danger.

c) **Fetal Monitoring:** Intraoperative fetal monitoring should be discussed with the patient's obstetrician.

 i) Prior to 24 weeks' gestation

  (1) FHR should be documented pre- and postoperatively.

 ii) After 24 weeks' gestation, the fetus is viable.

  (1) **Continuous monitoring should be considered,** especially for patients undergoing high-risk procedures (i.e., intra-abdominal, intracranial, or intrathoracic operations) (13).

  (2) **When fetal monitoring is performed, a clear plan for treatment of FHR abnormalities should be determined prior to starting the procedure.**

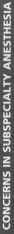

CONCERNS IN SUBSPECIALTY ANESTHESIA

iii) **Anesthetic technique**

(1) No specific technique has been associated with any improved fetal outcome (1).

(2) Fetal oxygenation depends on maternal oxygenation and uterine perfusion.

  (a) The goals of anesthesia during pregnancy are to maintain maternal oxygen tension and to avoid hypotension and acidosis.

  (b) Blood pressure should be vigilantly monitored (by invasive means if necessary) and hypotension promptly treated.

  (c) Hypoxia should be avoided and PCO_2 maintained in the normal range for pregnancy (~33 mm Hg).

(3) RA should be strongly considered if appropriate for the surgical procedure.

iv) Aspiration precautions should be taken and the airway should be protected with endotracheal intubation in most patients >12 weeks' gestation or those with a history significant for gastroesophageal reflux (Fig. 144-2).

v) **After 18 to 20 weeks' uterine size, the patient should always be positioned with left uterine displacement.**

vi) Some evidence supports the avoidance of N_2O very early in the first trimester (6 weeks' gestation or less) or during long cases.

(1) **Complete avoidance of N2O may necessitate large doses of volatile agent, with resulting maternal hypotension.**

(2) Concentrations of N2O of 50% or less appear safe, especially when used to avoid maternal hypotension (1).

vii) **All volatile agents and opiates cause decreased FHR variability**

(1) Probably due to fetal anesthesia

(2) Every effort should be made intraoperatively to ensure fetal oxygenation and uterine perfusion (1).

d) **Postoperative recovery**

i) Pregnant patients are often best recovered on a unit with FHR and uterine tocodynamic monitoring capability.

ii) Postoperative disposition should be a collaborative decision involving the patient's obstetrician and the physician performing the nonobstetric procedure.

Chapter Summary for Obstetrical Anesthesia

Procedure	Overview of Anesthetic Considerations
Labor Analgesia for Vaginal Delivery	Epidural infusion or CSE most commonly used; Aim for maximal pain relief with minimal motor block
RA for Cesarean Delivery	Preferred anesthetic technique; Patient must be positioned with left uterine displacement; Hypotension must be aggressively treated; Block must be tested and adequate anesthesia confirmed prior to surgical incision; Constant communication with patient and surgeon is essential
GA for Cesarean Delivery	May be necessary due to contraindications to RA or emergency; Aspiration precautions should be taken and preparations for difficult airway made; Vigilantly observe blood loss and decrease volatile agents if necessary; PCA analgesia will be necessary for postoperative pain control
Cervical Cerclage	Performed for cervical incompetence; RA preferred; avoid coughing or straining; outpatient procedure for many patients
Postpartum Tubal Ligation	Performed 24–48 h postpartum while uterine size enables smaller surgical incision; RA preferred
Anesthesia for Pregnant Patients Requiring Nonobstetric Surgery	Done for variety of indications; Elective procedures should be delayed until postpartum; 2nd trimester is preferred if surgery is necessary; Strive to optimize maternal hemodynamics; Ensure left uterine displacement; Monitor FHR at beginning/end of procedure and intraoperatively only after consultation with obstetrician regarding clear plan of action based on results

References

1. Chestnut DH, Polley LS, Tsen LC, et al., eds. *Chestnut's Obstetric Anesthesia: Principles and Practice*. Philadelphia, PA: Mosby Elsevier; 2009.
2. Hughes SC, Levinson G, Rosen MA, eds. *Shnider and Levinson's Anesthesia for Obstetrics*. Philadelphia, PA: Lippincott Williams & Wilkins; 2002.
3. Practice Guidelines for Obstetric Anesthesia: An updated report by the American Society of Anesthesiologists Task Force on Obstetric Anesthesia. *Anesthesiology* 2007;106:1–21.
4. Hawkins JL, Koonin LM, Palmer SK, et al. Anesthesia-related deaths during obstetric delivery in the United States, 1979–1990. *Anesthesiology* 1997;86:277–284.
5. Lyons G. Failed intubation: six year's experience in a teaching maternity unit. *Anaesthesia* 1985;40:759–762.
6. Davies JM, Posner KL, Lee LA, et al. Liability associated with obstetric anesthesia: a closed claims analysis. *Anesthesiology* 2009;110:131–139.
7. Riley ET, Cohen SE, Rubenstein AJ, et al. Prevention of hypotension after spinal anesthesia for cesarean section: six percent hetastarch versus lactated Ringer's solution. *Anesth Analg* 1995;81:838–842.
8. Pollard JB. Cardiac arrest during spinal anesthesia: common mechanisms and strategies for prevention. *Anesth Analg* 2001;92:252–256.
9. Chestnut DH, Dewan DM, Redick LF, et al. Anesthetic management for obstetric hysterectomy: a multi-institutional study. *Anesthesiology* 1989;70:607–610.
10. Bhavani-Shankar K, Lynch, EP, Datta, S. Airway changes during Cesarean hysterectomy. *Can J Anaesth* 2000;47:338–341.
11. Goodman EJ, Dumas SD. The rate of reactivation of labor epidural catheters for postpartum tubal ligation surgery. *Reg Anesth Pain Med* 1998;23:258–261.
12. Mazze RI, Kallen B. Reproductive outcome after anesthesia and operation during pregnancy: A registry study of 5405 cases. *Am J Obstet Gynecol* 1989;161:1178–1185.
13. ACOG Committee on Obstetric Practice. ACOG committee opinion No. 284. Nonobstetric surgery in pregnancy. *Int J Gynaecol Obstet* 2003;83(1):135.

145 Out of OR Anesthesia and Transport

Carlee Clark, MD

Each year, the number of anesthetics delivered at sites outside of the operating room (OR) has been steadily increasing. As procedures continue to move toward the minimally invasive, there will be a continued need for anesthesiologists to provide the quality of anesthesia expected in the OR at remote locations. With each out of OR location, there are unique challenges for the anesthesia team. The goal is to hold these sites to the standards of the OR. *An easy way to prepare is to think about each case in terms of how the anesthetic is influenced by the patient, the procedure (Table 145-1), and the environment.*

1) **Overview**
   a) All patients should have a thorough preoperative anesthesia evaluation.
   b) An anesthetic plan should be formulated by determining the unique needs of the patient.
      i) Take into consideration the anticipated procedure and environment.
      ii) Special equipment should be anticipated and ordered in advance.
   c) Patients requiring the presence of an anesthesiologist are frequently **high-risk, difficult to sedate,** or may have a **movement disorder.**
      i) A high-risk patient can have comorbidities. Some examples include:
         (1) A morbidly obese patient with obstructive sleep apnea (OSA).
         (2) An elderly patient with aortic stenosis or significant coronary artery disease (CAD).
         (3) A patient who is not a candidate for invasive surgery due to the extent of their disease and presents for a less invasive procedure.
      ii) Difficult-to-sedate patients may have:
         (1) High levels of anxiety
         (2) Psychiatric disorders
         (3) Chronic opioid use
         (4) Mental status changes
         (5) Dementia
      iii) Patients with movement disorders may require an anesthesiologist to help provide patient immobility.
2) **Procedures** (Table 145-1)
   a) Most out of OR procedures are radiographic (magnetic resonance imaging [MRI]/computed tomography [CT]), percutaneous, endoscopic, or electroconvulsive in nature.
   b) These procedures usually do not involve major surgical interventions, but can involve manipulation of large blood vessels (e.g., transjugular intrahepatic portosystemic shunt (TIPPS)).
   c) Some examples of procedures frequently performed out of the OR are summarized in Table 145-1.

For out of OR anesthesia, prepare for each case by thinking about how the anesthetic is influenced by the patient, the procedure, and the environment.

READ MORE

Anesthetic plan and induction of anesthesia, Chapter 1, page 1

Table 145-1

Procedures Frequently Requiring Out of OR Anesthesia

Neuroradiology	Cerebral angiography Cerebral stenting Cerebral coiling
Radiology	MRI CT Interventional radiology TIPPS
Cardiology Cath Lab	Cardioversion Radiofrequency ablations/EP studies AICD testing Coronary angiography/angioplasty/stenting
PACU or Monitored Ward	Electroconvulsive therapy
Endoscopy	Upper endoscopy Esophageal dilatation/stenting ERCP Colonoscopy/sigmoidoscopy
Intensive Care Unit	Tracheostomy Endoscopic procedures
Infertility Clinic	Oocyte retrieval

3) **Environment**
   a) Out of OR locations range from a crowded intensive care unit (ICU) room to state-of-the-art endoscopy and fluoroscopy suites.
   b) Not all sites were developed with the anesthesiologist in mind.
      i) Adaptability and having a plan are very important.
   c) The goal is to provide a safe anesthetic for the patient.
   d) There are ASA guidelines for anesthesiologists to apply to each new environment before administering anesthesia (Table 145-2).

4) **Anesthetic considerations for specific procedures**
   a) Magnetic resonance imaging
      i) **Indications**
         (1) Pediatric patients and in adult patients with movement disorders, psychiatric disorders, claustrophobia, or obstructive sleep apnea.
      ii) **Technique**

For adequate MRI imaging, the patient often needs to be immobile.

         (1) MRIs can be several hours in duration and it can be critical for adequate imaging that the patient be immobile.
            (a) Can require sedation or a general anesthetic.
         (2) Most patients receive propofol for sedation, with a total intravenous anesthesia technique for general anesthesia.
      iii) **Anesthetic considerations**
         (1) Patients are far away, and must be viewed at all times via a window or a video screen or the provider can remain next to the MRI scanner.
         (2) Patient monitors must be visible.

Table 145-2

ASA Guidelines for Nonoperating Room Anesthetizing Locations (1)

Oxygen	• Reliable source and quantity • Backup cylinder—full
Suction	• Adequate and reliable
Scavenging	• Adequate and reliable when administering anesthetic gases
Anesthetic Equipment	• Self-inflating bag for PPV providing at least 90% oxygen • Drugs, supplies, and equipment for intended level of anesthetic • Monitoring equipment to allow adherence to Standards for Basic Anesthetic Monitoring (3) • Administration of inhaled anesthetics requires an anesthesia machine equivalent to those in the OR and maintained with the same standards
Electrical Outlets	• Sufficient for machine and monitors • Isolated electrical power or ground fault circuit interrupters if "wet location"
Adequate Lighting	• Requires illumination of the patient, monitors, and equipment • Battery-powered backup available
Sufficient Space	• Space for personnel and equipment • Easy access to patient, machine, and monitors
Resuscitation Equipment	• Emergency drugs • Defibrillator • Cardiopulmonary resuscitation equipment
Staff	• Adequately trained staff for support • Reliable means of two-way communication to request assistance
Building and Safety Codes	• All should be observed
Postanesthesia Care Facilities	• Appropriate postanesthesia management • Adequately trained staff • Appropriate equipment for safe transport

(3) Airway equipment, medication pumps, poles, monitors, and the anesthesia machine must be MRI compatible.
   (a) MRI compatible equipment is MRI safe, works correctly in the presence of the magnet, and does not interfere with the correct operation of the MRI equipment.
   (b) Using non-MRI compatible equipment can have devastating consequences including the projectile effect, burns, and equipment malfunction.
   (c) If using non-MRI compatible equipment, extensions for tubing, breathing circuits, or monitoring cables must be immediately available as non-MRI compatible equipment must remain in the scanner control room (4).
(4) Organization of lines and cables is important, so they are not dislodged while moving the patient through the MRI.

(5) **Airway management and maintenance are critical when working in the MRI suite.**

b) **Computed tomography**

   i) **Anesthetic Considerations**

     (1) Similar to MRI but CT is typically a shorter procedure.

     (2) Risk of radiation exposure.

c) **Neuroradiology**

   i) **Indications**

     (1) Cerebral angiography, stenting, or coiling of cerebral aneurysms.

   ii) **Technique**

     (1) Most healthy patients can tolerate cerebral angiography with nurse-administered sedation.

     (2) **Stenting or coiling of cerebral aneurysms or unstable, emergent procedures require a general anesthetic or deep sedation to provide patient immobility and close hemodynamic monitoring.**

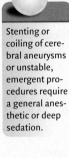

Stenting or coiling of cerebral aneurysms or unstable, emergent procedures require a general anesthetic or deep sedation.

   iii) **Anesthetic considerations**

     (1) Typically, the anesthesiologist does not have close proximity to the patient or the airway.

       (a) All breathing circuits, IVs, and arterial line tubing must have extensions.

     (2) Arterial lines are commonly used for hemodynamic monitoring.

       (a) May be from the percutaneous sheath placed by the interventionalist.

     (3) Radiation exposure

       (a) Stay behind the provided shield and wear lead.

     (4) **Complications include intracranial bleeding with resulting intracranial hypertension and hemodynamic instability.**

d) **Cardiac catheterization laboratory**

   i) **Cardioversion**

     (1) **Indications**

       (a) Conversion of aberrant rhythm patterns.

         (i) Atrial fibrillation

         (ii) Atrial flutter to sinus rhythm

     (2) **Technique**

       (a) Cardioversion is painful, so patients need to be unconscious for the procedure.

       (b) The procedure only lasts a few seconds.

         (i) The key is to provide deep short-acting sedation.

         (ii) Low doses of propofol are an option and allow for quick recovery (5).

       (c) The patient should wear a nonrebreather oxygen mask with high-flow oxygen.

       (d) Phenylephrine and IV fluids should be administered to treat hypotension.

       (e) Patients with or without OSA may develop brief airway obstruction.

       (f) A chin lift, jaw thrust, or nasal airway may be helpful.

     (3) **Anesthetic considerations**

       (a) These patients often have an extensive history of cardiac disease.

         (i) Ideally are nothing per os (NPO) for at least 8 hours.

    ii) **Radiofrequency ablations**
      (1) **Indications**
        (a) These procedures typically last many hours depending on the difficulty of the atrial mapping.
      (2) **Technique**
        (a) Many of these procedures can begin and end with the patient receiving low-dose IV sedation and nurse monitoring.
          (i) However, the ablation requires induction and maintenance of a general anesthetic.
      (3) **Anesthetic considerations**
        (a) There is radiation exposure.
        (b) Emergence and extubation of a patient with a femoral sheath warrants special attention because the patient needs to remain still to avoid dislodging the sheath and bleeding.
   iii) **Coronary angiography**
      (1) **Indications**
        (a) Angiography can be done to evaluate the patency and flow patterns of coronary arteries.
      (2) **Technique**
        (a) Most elective procedures are performed with nurse-administered sedation.
        (b) Many pediatric patients require an anesthesiologist depending on the age of the patient and the cardiac lesion.
        (c) An adult for emergent catheterization may require a general anesthetic if the patient is in respiratory failure or has hemodynamic compromise.
      (3) **Anesthetic considerations**
        (a) Pediatric patients with congenital lesions require understanding of their cardiac anatomy.
        (b) Adults needing general anesthesia can be unstable and have a full stomach.
        (c) In emergency cases, the patient may be in a location without an anesthesia machine or a ventilator.
        (d) Ask the support staff in the procedure room to obtain any additional equipment needed and call for anesthesia backup if necessary.
        (e) Be prepared for the worst-case scenario and a potential transport directly to the OR or ICU.
        (f) There is a risk of radiation exposure.
 e) **Intensive care unit**
   i) **Indications**
      (1) ICUs may need anesthesia staffing for bedside procedures.
      (2) Percutaneous, open tracheostomies, and endoscopic procedures are frequently performed at the bedside to minimize patient complications from transport.
      (3) Bedside endoscopy for GI bleeding frequently requires airway protection and sedation and continuous hemodynamic monitoring.
   ii) **Technique**
      (1) Procedure and patient specific.
   iii) **Anesthetic considerations**
      (1) Usually, this is a tight workspace.
        (a) Plan ahead and have emergency medications and airway equipment at the head of the bed.

(2) Always confirm that the tracheostomy is in the trachea with direct visualization via a fiberoptic scope or $ETCO_2$ before removing the endotracheal tube (ETT).

(3) Patients with GI bleeds can become hemodynamically unstable with intubation and sedation, so be prepared to fully support the patient.

(4) Other complications to be concerned about are loss of the airway, bleeding, and/or viscous perforation.

f) **Endoscopy suite**

i) **Indications**

(1) Many patients requiring monitored anesthesia care for endoscopic procedures are healthy, but have requested to be "asleep."

(2) Other patients have chronic GI disorders or comorbidities that warrant close hemodynamic or airway monitoring.

(3) Invasive procedures such as ERCP, stenting, or dilatations require a deeper level of sedation or a general anesthetic.

(4) The procedure length is operator and patient dependent.

ii) **Technique**

(1) Deep sedation and patient position can lead to airway obstruction in any patient, so monitoring $ETCO_2$ is helpful.

(2) Having access to the patient's airway is important because patients may need a chin lift or a jaw thrust to relieve airway obstruction.

(3) Have fluids and phenylephrine available to treat hypotension.

iii) **Anesthetic considerations**

(1) Workspace varies, so organization is very important.

(2) Patients often are dehydrated due to their bowel preparation and NPO status.

(3) There is also a chance of bleeding and viscous perforation during the procedure.

Patient's undergoing endoscopy procedures may be prone to hypotension due to dehydration from bowel preparation and fasting.

g) **Transport**

i) There are many situations in which a member of the anesthesia team will find themselves transporting a patient: from the OR to the postanesthesia care unit (PACU) to the ICU, or in reverse.

ii) During any patient transport, a member of the anesthesia team ideally should be with the patient to continually monitor, evaluate, and treat the patient.

iii) Transporting patients requires preparation.

(1) Obtain the following items for transport:

(a) A transport monitor capable of displaying pulse oximetry, invasive or noninvasive blood pressure, and telemetry.

(b) Emergency airway equipment (including a mask, laryngoscope, and ETT)

(c) Resuscitation medications (including sedatives, pain medications, vasopressors, and antihypertensives) must be obtained before transport.

(2) Some patients may need to be transported with a ventilator, but most intubated patients can be transported with a self-inflating bag with a person dedicated to ventilating the patient and a full oxygen tank.

(3) Patients coming to and from ICUs often have several invasive catheters and monitors with multiple intravenous infusions.

(4) All lines and monitors should be well organized.

(5) If the patient's condition warrants it, a defibrillator should be obtained for transport.

(6) In order to ease the transition, report can be called to the PACU or ICU prior to leaving the procedure site to give the receiving team time to prepare.

(7) To facilitate a safe and expedient transport, someone from the surgical or the medical service should help transport and supporting staff should aid in retrieving elevators or opening doors.

h) **Postoperative care**

i) Some offsite facilities have their own recovery unit.

ii) The standards for postanesthesia care should be the same as the PACU in the main OR environment.

iii) A verbal signout should be given to whoever is assuming care of the patient.

iv) A member of the anesthesia team should stay with the patient until the effects of the anesthetic has worn off allowing the patient to be extubated, spontaneously ventilating and supporting their airway, hemodynamically stable with adequate pain control (2).

v) The offsite staff should have contact information in case of any postoperative issues relating to the anesthetic.

Chapter Summary for Out of OR Anesthesia and Transport

Definition	Out of OR anesthesia refers to anesthesia services provided in areas that may not frequently support the anesthesiologist, such as diagnostic radiology facilities. The same standards for OR anesthetic care should be applied to anesthesia practices outside of the OR.
General Considerations	For out of OR anesthetics, consider the patient, the procedure, and the environment. Difficult-to-sedate patients may have high levels of anxiety, psychiatric disorders, chronic opioid use, mental status changes, or dementia. Patients with movement disorders may require an anesthesiologist to help provide patient immobility.
Preoperative Considerations	All patients should have a thorough preoperative anesthesia evaluation. The anesthetic plan should be tailored to the patient's individual needs and the available facilities in the practice environment.
Intraoperative Considerations	The ASA Guidelines for Nonoperating Room Anesthetizing Locations (1) make recommendations about availability of equipment including oxygen, suction, and resuscitative medications.
Postoperative Considerations	The standards of postoperative care should be the same as those implemented in the OR perioperative environment.

References

1. Statement on Nonoperating Room Anesthetizing Locations. Committee of Origin: Standards and Practice Parameters (Approved by the ASA House of Delegates on October 15, 2003 and amended on October 22, 2008).

2. Standards for postanesthesia care. Committee of Origin: Standards and Practice Parameters (Approved by the ASA House of Delegates on October 12, 1988, and last amended on October 27, 2004).

3. Standards for Basic Anesthetic Monitoring. Committee of Origin: Standards and Practice Parameters (Approved by the ASA House of Delegates on October 21, 1986, and last amended on October 25, 2005).

4. Provision of Anaesthetic Services in Magnetic Resonance Units. The Association of Anaesthetists of Great Britain and Ireland, May 2002. http://www.aagbi.org/publications/guidelines/docs/mri02.pdf

5. Herregods LL, Bossuyt GP, De Baerdemaeker LE, et al. Ambulatory Electrical External Cardioversion with Propofol or Etomidate. *J Clin Anesth* 2003;15(2):91–96.

146

Challenges in Anesthesia: The Patient with Chronic Low Back Pain Presenting for Total Knee Replacement Surgery

Raymond Gaeta, MD

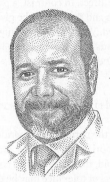

Clinical Vignette

A 68-year-old woman presents to the preop clinic scheduled for knee replacement surgery the following day. She remains quite active despite a history of chronic low back pain for which she is maintained on methadone and gabapentin. She appears anxious and is particularly concerned about postoperative pain control as she feels that she was undermedicated for a previous surgery leading to a horrible experience. She in fact has delayed this surgery out of such concerns.

Introduction

The role of the anesthesiologist as a perioperative physician is paramount when considering the continuum of patient experiences when undergoing surgery. The patient's experience in fact encompasses the preoperative period and the postoperative period, while the appropriate delivery of anesthesia generally makes the patient oblivious to the actual surgery. The appropriate consideration of preoperative factors for the conduct of the anesthetic is always important but no more so when the opioid-tolerant patient presents for surgery. Not only does the use of chronic opioids impact the conduct of the intraoperative phase of anesthesia, it also impacts their emergence from anesthesia and subsequent postoperative pain management. Obviously, patients are concerned with the outcome of the surgery, but the horror stories of uncontrolled pain either as a personal experience or that of friends and family weighs on them considerably. Thus, the anesthesiologist of today must be well versed in the continuum of care in order to provide the best experience for the patient.

Preoperative Concerns

The patient presents with chronic low back pain as the most significant past feature. She is status post L5-S1 discectomy and laminectomy at L5 without fusion experiencing chronic unrelenting pain. After the institution of methadone and gabapentin, the patient became much more active, bringing to light the pain from her knee. Her current medications include methadone 15 mg bid and gabapentin 600 mg tid. As an additional point of interest, a preoperative EKG should be checked for evidence of QT prolongation that can be seen on higher doses of methadone.

Opioid Tolerance

The definitions of opioid tolerance are easy to recite. Whether one discusses the decreased effect of medications over time or the requirement of more medication over time to achieve the same result, the clinical scenario is easily recognized based upon the types of medications the patient is taking. What is more difficult, however, is to determine the level of tolerance the patient will exhibit as even the exposure to a small amount of opioid preoperatively can predispose some patients to analgesic tolerance.

This wide distribution of patient response after opioid exposure follows the bell distribution curves commonly found in biological systems. It is the spread, however, that makes it difficult to apply uniform dosing instructions for this population. In the extremes, a patient exposed to a small amount of opioid may be horribly opiate tolerant and require many multiples of the usual dose to achieve the desired opiate affect. In contrast, a patient on significant doses of opioid may still retain some responsiveness and thus would be given a massive overdose if multiples of the usual doses were administered. With such variability, an anesthetic plan and a postoperative pain plan relying solely on opioids are likely to have a less-than-satisfactory affect with displeasure voiced by surgeon, patient, and family alike.

Preoperative Instructions to Patient

On the morning of surgery, the patient was instructed to take her regular dose of the long-acting opioid, in this case methadone.

Fentanyl patches should be continued in the perioperative period noting the site of placement so that subsequent caregivers may appropriately plan for its administration. If the patient is taking multiple doses of a short-acting opioid, then they should continue taking them as well.

Even though the determination of the level of tolerance may be difficult, it is clear that patients denied their usual chronic opioid will undergo withdrawal symptoms if their chronic medications are withheld. As the patients have taken this level of medication on a chronic basis, its presence will not interfere with the conduct of the anesthetic and in fact may allow for a less problematic anesthetic because the patients will not have to "catch up" as they might if the long-acting opioid were withheld.

Perioperative Pain Management Strategy and Postoperative Pain Plan

In the opioid-tolerant patient, particularly, the coadministration of the regional anesthetic technique provides not only appropriate analgesia but in fact may decrease the need for massive doses of opioids to achieve the desired effect. In this circumstance, conduction blockade of the nociceptive pathways is preferable to the modulation of pain signals that occurs with the administration of opioids.

Various techniques of local anesthetic administration can be utilized from local infiltration, peripheral nerve blockade, plexus block, or even neuroaxial anesthesia. Each has its benefits with less or more expertise required for implementation. The duration of analgesia provided by regional blockade is also variable; thus, the installation of local anesthetic through an indwelling catheter will more reliably provide analgesia over a longer period of time.

In the case of this patient's knee replacement, the use of an indwelling femoral catheter delivering local anesthetic provided a suitable region of anesthesia over the anterior knee. As the incision generally is over the anterior portion of the knee and the patella, this region is easily in the distribution of the femoral nerve. Placement of the catheter was facilitated by the use of ultrasound guidance (neurostimulation can also be used) that may improve the efficacy of these blocks postoperatively.

Unfortunately, some of the surgical technique will occur in areas outside the femoral nerve distribution including branches of the sciatic nerve posteriorly. While the patient may have an entirely anesthetic anterior knee, the patient may still complain bitterly about pain in the posterior knee. The anesthesiologist should be prepared for this and provide appropriate postoperative pain care to be discussed subsequently as some surgeons prefer no sciatic block so as to assess distal sciatic nerve function. Should the surgeon have no preference, then a single shot sciatic block via a posterior approach may provide several hours of relief in the transition from the surgical theater to the hospital ward.

Intraoperative Concerns

Generally speaking, the delivery of the preoperative oral dose of opioid makes many different intraoperative anesthetic techniques possible. It is critical to remember that the oral dose of opioids preoperatively replaces the patients' regular requirement; thus, additional intraoperative opioids may be required based on usual clinical grounds to provide for a smooth emergence. The titration of short-acting opioids intravenously during the case fits the bill nicely.

The use of intravenous anesthetics such as propofol or inhalation agents such as desflurane and sevoflurane can be utilized at the discretion of the anesthesiologist. Again, the need for additional opioid intraoperatively and immediately postoperatively should be anticipated despite the fact that the patient has already received a dose of opioid preoperatively. In the case of methadone, the dose can be given intravenously as well should the patient forget to take it on the morning of surgery. An interesting option for intraoperative management is the use of a low-dose ketamine infusion during the case. In addition to providing excellent anesthesia, it may also reduce the postoperative opioid requirement.

Postoperative Pain Management

With the planning as previously discussed, the postoperative pain management would likely consist of a local anesthetic through a femoral catheter along with the continuation of the patients' chronic opioid. In addition to this, because of posterior knee pain uncovered by the femoral nerve block, patient-controlled analgesia intravenously should be utilized. Because the patients are maintained on their chronic oral opioid, the doses of PCA are likely to be relatively similar or slightly higher than the opiate-naive patient.

Appropriate monitoring of the patient should be afforded as variability of opiate response is the norm and this will assure that a patient is neither undermedicated nor overmedicated with this regimen. While short-acting oral medications such as hydrocodone preparations can be utilized instead of the intravenous PCA, the lack of patient control and more difficult titration is less desirable especially in the first 24 hours.

After discussion with the surgeon and coordination with the acute pain management team, the patient's femoral catheter remained in place until the second postoperative day, providing excellent postsurgical analgesia. On the second postoperative day, the catheter was removed and the patient was titrated off the PCA and onto a fully oral regimen consisting of the long-term oral opioid and short-acting medications for breakthrough pain. Maintenance of the gabapentin was continued perioperatively and also likely reduced the patient's opioid requirement and may minimize postoperative wound hyperalgesia.

Special Considerations

Occasionally, despite these appropriate considerations and implementations, the patient may still have pain that is less well controlled owing to extreme levels of tolerance, lack of consent for regional anesthesia, or other unforeseen circumstances. While escalation to an epidural catheter is possible, the loss of motor function and monitoring of sensory function is generally considered undesirable. Adjunctive medications such as acetaminophen while appropriate in the multimodal approach to analgesia may still leave the patient with significant pain complaints.

The NMDA-receptor antagonist ketamine is an important consideration in opiate tolerant patients. The analgesic and anesthetic properties are profound and do not demonstrate cross-tolerance with the opioids. In those patients where the pain is uncontrolled, analgesia may be quickly recovered with the institution of ketamine if the following precautions are observed.

Ketamine is a potent analgesic-anesthetic and should not be used in an unmonitored setting. The psychomimetic effects of ketamine may often require the use of concomitant benzodiazepines to avoid the bad dreams that patients may experience. The combination of these medications and the complicated regimen thus require the level of monitoring often seen in intensive care units or highly staffed intermediate care units. Nursing experience with the use of these medications is paramount as they are the first line of defense against overdosage in these patients.

The use of ketamine 10 to 20 mg/hr intravenously titrated to effect may allow the difficult patient to get through the first 24 hours when some of the pain stimulus has subsided. While it appears the placement of the patient in an intensive care unit is an escalation of care, the difficulties of managing these patients on the regular wards readily supersede bed control issues. The use of intense monitoring in this situation provides appropriate analgesia in a safe environment producing the desired outcome for physicians and patients alike.

The patient was subsequently discharged home on a regimen of methadone, gabapentin, and a prescription of oxycodone for any episodes of acute breakthrough pain. Her perioperative course was unremarkable owing to a carefully orchestrated pain management strategy.

The opioid-tolerant patient can be quite a challenge to manage perioperatively. This case illustrates some of the basic concepts including tolerance and the need to plan for it in the anesthetic and subsequent care. Maintenance of chronic opioid medications through the perioperative period allows for a smooth transition through the operation and into the postoperative period. Regional local anesthetic techniques provide conduction blockade unaffected by the use of chronic opioids. When patients still experience unmitigated pain, the use of special agents such as ketamine with appropriate monitoring may yet save the day. With the maintenance of the preoperative medications, the prescription of a short-acting opioid as with any other patient should suffice. Oxycodone 5 to 10 mg q4–6h should be sufficient.

Selected Readings

1. Himmelseher S, Durieux ME. Ketamine for perioperative pain management. *Anesthesiology* 2005;102:211–220.
2. Subramaniam K, Subramaniam B, Steinbrook RA. Ketamine as adjuvant analgesic to opioids: a quantitative and qualitative systematic review. *Anesth Analg* 2004;99:482–495.
3. Mitra S, Sinatra RS. Perioperative management of acute pain in the opioid-dependent patient. *Anesthesiology* 2004;101:212–227.
4. Morin AM, Kratz CD, Eberhart LH, et al. Postoperative analgesia and functional recovery after total-knee replacement: comparison of a continuous posterior lumbar plexus (psoas compartment) block, a continuous femoral nerve block, and the combination of a continuous femoral and sciatic nerve block. *Reg Anesth Pain Med* 2005;30(5):434–445.
5. Hogan MV, Grant RE, Lee L Jr. Analgesia for total hip and knee arthroplasty: a review of lumbar plexus, femoral, and sciatic nerve blocks. *Am J Orthop (Belle Mead NJ)* 2009;38(8):E129–E133.
6. Tiippana EM, Hamunen K, Kontinen VK, et al. Do surgical patients benefit from perioperative gabapentin/pregabalin? a systematic review of efficacy and safety. *Anesth Analg* 2007;104:1545–1556.

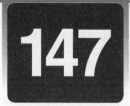

Post Anesthesia Care Unit

Wesley Liao, MD • Jamie Murphy, MD • Danielle B. Ludwin, MD

The post anesthesia care unit (PACU) provides close monitoring of patients immediately following anesthesia. It facilitates the transition between the operating room and discharge home or transfer to a hospital ward. Common PACU issues include hypotension, hypertension, dysrhythmias, airway obstruction, hypoxemia, hypercarbia, delayed emergence, and oliguria. Equipment and medications should be readily available for routine and critical care situations.

I) Overview
  a) The PACU is a high-level facility that provides expert postoperative care of patients immediately following surgery.
  b) Staffing models
    i) Nurses
      (1) Highly trained nurses with experience in caring for patients who have had general anesthesia and sedation.
      (2) Many nurses have advanced certifications in critical care (CCRN) and/or postoperative care (CPAN or CAPA).
    ii) Nurse staffing
      (1) The American Society of Perianesthesia Nurses have a position statement on minimum nursing staffing requirements for Phase I PACU stating that two registered nurses, one competent in Phase I postanesthesia nursing, will be in the same room where the patient is receiving Phase I level of care (1).
    iii) Physicians
      (1) According to the ASA standards and practice guidelines for postoperative care, an anesthesiologist should be responsible for general medical supervision and coordination of patient care in the PACU (2,3).
  c) **ASA Standards for postoperative care** (2)
    i) Standard I: All patients who have received general anesthesia, regional anesthesia or monitored anesthesia care shall receive appropriate postanesthesia management.
      (1) The setting should be a PACU or ICU or equivalent unless waived by the anesthesiologist responsible for the patient's care.
      (2) The care provided in this area should follow the policies and procedures reviewed by the Anesthesiology Department.
      (3) The PACU design, equipment and staffing should meet expectations of facility's accrediting and licensing bodies.

ii) **Standard II:** A patient transported to the PACU shall be accompanied by a member of the anesthesia care team who is knowledgeable about the patient's condition. The patient shall be continually evaluated and treated during transport with monitoring and support appropriate to the patient's condition.

iii) **Standard III:** Upon arrival in the PACU, the patient shall be re-evaluated and a verbal report provided to the responsible PACU nurse by the member of the anesthesia care team who accompanies the patient.

    (1) The patient's preoperative history and perioperative history should be relayed to the PACU nurse.

    (2) A member of the anesthesia care team should stay in the PACU until the PACU nurse accepts responsibility for the patient.

iv) **Standard IV:** The patient's condition shall be evaluated continually in the PACU.

    (1) Observation and monitoring should include oxygenation, ventilation, circulation, level of consciousness and temperature.

    (2) Documentation should be done to record the patient's vital signs and notable events while in the PACU.

v) **Standard V:** A physician is responsible for the discharge of the patient from the PACU.

    (1) In the absence of the physician responsible for the discharge, the PACU nurse shall determine that the patient meets the discharge criteria. The name of the physician accepting responsibility for discharge shall be noted on the record.

> When transferring a patient to the PACU, a member of the anesthesia care team should stay in the PACU until the PACU nurse is ready and able to accept responsibility for the patient.

> The patient's condition shall be evaluated continually in the PACU.

2) **Phases of postoperative care (1)**

  a) **Phase 1**

    i) Nursing is focused on providing care in the immediate postoperative period and transitions the patient to either Phase 2 recovery, the inpatient general floors or step-down or ICU settings.

      (1) Vital signs are typically recorded every 5 to 15 minutes but frequency should depend on the patient's condition.

      (2) Nursing is typically staffed one nurse to two patients.

  b) **Phase 2**

    i) Nursing is focused on preparing the patient/family/significant others for care at home, extended observation level of care or the extended care environment.

      (1) Nursing is typically staffed one nurse to three patients.

      (2) "Fast-tracking"—this concept is applied to patients who bypass Phase 1 recovery and go directly to Phase 2 recovery.

        (a) Fast-tracking may assist in cost reduction and reduce recovery room time. It is important to appropriately select patients for fast-tracking. ASA 1 or 2 patients undergoing local or monitored anesthesia care (MAC) anesthesia are potentially good candidates.

  c) **Phase 3/Extended care**

    i) Nursing is focused on ongoing care after transfer or discharge from Phase 1 and Phase 2.

      (1) Nursing is typically staffed one nurse to three to five patients.

3) **Admission and monitoring (4–7)**

  a) Role of the anesthesia team

    i) The anesthesia team typically transports the patient from the operating room to the PACU and is responsible for patient care until the PACU team receives signout.

ii) Most patients are transported with supplemental O_2. Transport monitoring, for example, pulse oximetry, ECG, and BP, may be used.

iii) Upon PACU arrival, a complete report is given consisting of:

PACU signout should include a pertinent summary of the patient's history and perioperative events.

(1) Background information (name, age, procedure performed, diagnosis, past medical history, medications, allergies, preoperative vital signs, pertinent labs)

(2) Perioperative course

(a) Type of anesthetic

(b) Drugs given (premedication, induction, maintenance, opioids, muscle relaxants and reversal agents, antiemetics, vasoactive agents, antibiotics)

(c) Anesthetic course (complications, difficult IV access, difficult airway management, hemodynamic instability)

(d) Presence of lines, tubes, or drains (location, sizes, specific instructions on use or care)

(e) Fluid input and output (estimated blood and fluid losses, urine output, and fluids administered), and any other specific needs or instructions.

Hypotension in the PACU can be due to hypovolemia, impaired venous return, vasodilation, and/or decreased cardiac output.

b) PACU monitoring

i) Vital signs measured in the PACU include BP, respiratory rate, continuous ECG, pulse oximetry, and temperature.

ii) Typically, vital signs are recorded at intervals no greater than every fifteen minutes.

iii) Level of consciousness, airway patency, breathing patterns, and peripheral perfusion should also be routinely assessed.

c) Common PACU issues include cardiac, respiratory and renal complications (Table 147-1)

Table 147-1
Common Problems Observed in the PACU

Problem	Differential Diagnosis
Hypotension	Hypovolemia, ↓venous return, vasodilation, ↓CO, medications
Hypertension	Pre-existing HTN, pain, fluid overload, hypercarbia, hypoxemia, hypothermia, ↑ICP, bladder distention, medications
Dysrhythmias	Hypercarbia, hypoxemia, acidosis, residual anesthetics, myocardial ischemia, ↑sympathetic discharge, metabolic abnormalities, pre-existing cardiac/respiratory disease, medications
Airway Obstruction	Mechanical, ↑secretions, vomitus/blood, glottic swelling, external compression
Hypoxemia	Atelectasis, hypoventilation, diffusion hypoxia, obstruction, bronchospasm, aspiration, pulmonary edema, pneumothorax, pulmonary embolus, medications
Hypercarbia	Respiratory depression from anesthetics/opioids, hypothermia, inadequate reversal of neuromuscular blockade, pain, splinting, abdominal distention
Delayed Awakening	Residual anesthetics, ↓cerebral perfusion, stroke, hypoglycemia, sepsis, encephalopathy, metabolic abnormalities
Oliguria	Prerenal—hypovolemia; intrarenal—kidney injury; postrenal—obstruction

4) **Cardiac complications in the PACU**
   a) **Hypotension**—Causes include hypovolemia, impaired venous return, vasodilation, and decreased cardiac output.
      i) **Hypovolemia**
         (1) Causes include inadequate intraoperative fluid resuscitation, third-space loss, osmotic polyuria, or ongoing surgical bleeding.
         (2) Consider fluid boluses followed by reassessment of hemodynamics.
         (3) Potential sources of ongoing bleeding should be further evaluated and surgical colleagues consulted.
         (4) Persistent hypotension despite fluid resuscitation should prompt further investigation and consideration of urinary catheter placement and invasive monitoring.
      ii) **Impaired venous return**
         (1) Causes include positive end-expiratory pressure (PEEP), pneumothorax, and pericardial tamponade.
         (2) Clinically, impaired venous return may present as increased jugular venous distention, elevated CVP, and decreased breath or heart sounds.
         (3) Treatment involves addressing the underlying cause.
      iii) **Vasodilation**
         (1) Causes include residual inhalational anesthetic agents, adrenal insufficiency, neuraxial anesthesia, rewarming, anaphylaxis, transfusion reactions, drug effects, liver failure, systemic inflammation, and sepsis.
         (2) Treatment addresses the underlying cause.
         (3) Consider administration of α-adrenergic drugs (phenylephrine, norepinephrine, epinephrine).
      iv) **Decreased cardiac output**
         (1) Causes include congestive heart failure, arrhythmias, myocardial ischemia or infarction, negative inotropic drugs, sepsis, hypothyroidism, malignant hyperthermia.
         (2) Labs (Basic Metabolic Profile, complete blood count (CBC)), 12 lead electrocardiogram (ECG), and CXR should be considered in the initial workup.
         (3) Consider treatment with diuresis, antiarrhythmic agents, afterload reducers, inotropic agents, and cardioversion.
   b) **Hypertension**—Causes include pain, fluid overload, pre-existing hypertension, medications, hypercarbia, hypoxemia, hypothermia, increased intracranial pressure (ICP), and bladder distention.
      i) Although patients are usually asymptomatic, physical manifestations of hypertension may include visual changes, headache, restlessness, or dyspnea.
      ii) The goal of management is to identify the underlying cause and, in most cases, to restore the BP to the patient's baseline.
      iii) Postoperative hypertension (HTN) can be more pronounced if patients have held antihypertensive medications pre-operatively.
      iv) β-adrenergic antagonists, calcium-channel antagonists, hydralazine, and nitrates can be used as antihypertensives.
      v) If pain is the etiology of the hypertension, opioids as well as non-steroidal anti-inflammatory agents should be used.
   c) **Dysrhythmias**—Causes include hypercarbia, hypoxemia, acidosis, residual anesthetic effects, increased sympathetic discharge from surgical procedures, metabolic derangements, and preexisting cardiac and respiratory disease (Table 147-2).
      i) **Bradycardia** can be a residual effect of cholinesterase inhibitors, β-blockers, or opioids.
      ii) **Tachycardia** can be due to anticholinergic agents, vagolytic drugs and β-receptor agonists, in addition to fever, pain, hypovolemia, and anemia.

Table 147-2
Common Dysrhythmias (8–10)

READ MORE

Crisis management: ventricular tachycardia & ventricular fibrillation, Chapter 206, page 1321

READ MORE

Crisis management: myocardial ischemia, Chapter 213, page 1332

Common Supraventricular Dysrhythmias
  Sinus Bradycardia, Sinus Tachycardia
Paroxysmal Supraventricular Tachydysrhythmias
  Consider synchronized cardioversion, adenosine, verapamil, amiodarone, β-blockers, digoxin, ibutilide, procainamide
Stable Ventricular Dysrhythmias
  Premature ventricular contractions (PVCs), stable nonsustained ventricular tachycardia
  Usually do not require further intervention
  Assess for reversible causes (hypoxemia, hypercarbia, acidosis, hypotension, electrolyte imbalances, mechanical irritation, hypothermia, adrenergic stimulation, proarrhythmic drugs, micro/macro shock, cardiac ischemia)
Unstable Ventricular Dysrhythmias
  Ventricular tachycardia, ventricular fibrillation
Myocardial Ischemia and Infarction
  T-wave changes (such as inversions, flattening), ST-segment changes (elevation or depression)
  In patients at high risk for cardiac events, perioperative β-blockade has been shown to decrease risk
  Consider cardiology consultation, 12-lead EKG, cardiac enzymes (CK, CK-MB, troponins), supplemental O_2, β-blockade, nitrates, opioids, aspirin been shown to decrease risk

5) **Respiratory complications in the PACU (4–7)**

   a) **Airway obstruction**—Causes include mechanical obstruction, increased secretions, vomitus or blood in the airway, glottic swelling, or from external compression (e.g., expanding neck hematoma).

      i) In **partial airway obstruction**, stridor occurs due to limited air movement.

      ii) In **complete airway obstruction**, there may be paradoxical chest wall movement with lack of associated respiratory sounds.

Treat laryngospasm with CPAP. Refractory cases can be treated with succinylcholine (10 to 20 mg IV for normal adult patients without contraindications) and 100% O_2 via positive pressure ventilation.

      iii) Any patient with a suspected airway obstruction should immediately receive supplemental O_2 and a jaw-thrust, head-tilt, chin-lift, oral/nasal airways and suctioning, to relieve the obstruction.

      iv) If these maneuvers are still ineffective, **laryngospasm** should be considered as a cause of airway obstruction.

        (1) **Laryngospasm can be treated with continuous positive airway pressure (CPAP). Succinylcholine (10 to 20 mg in normal adult patients) and continuation of 100% O_2 delivery via positive pressure ventilation should be considered for refractory cases.** In the most severe cases, re-intubation may be required.

      v) For cases of glottic edema, intravenous corticosteroids or aerosolized racemic epinephrine should be considered (4–7).

      vi) For head and neck cases, the surgical site should be carefully inspected for signs of bleeding.

      vii) Expanding hematomas can lead to airway compression and the incision site may have to be reopened to relieve the compression (4–7).

   b) **Hypoxemia**—Causes include atelectasis, hypoventilation, diffusion hypoxia, upper airway obstruction, bronchospasm, aspiration, pulmonary edema, pneumothorax, and pulmonary embolism.

      i) Hypoxemia is commonly encountered in the PACU as patients recover from general anesthesia.

Progression of hypoxemia can lead to acidosis, bradycardia, hypotension, neurologic obtundation and cardiac arrest.

ii) Transient mild to moderate hypoxemia (PaO_2 50 to 60 mm Hg) is generally tolerated well by otherwise healthy individuals.

iii) Signs and symptoms of hypoxemia include tachycardia, cyanosis, restlessness, and cardiac irritability.

iv) As hypoxemia progresses, acidosis, bradycardia, hypotension, neurologic obtundation, and cardiac arrest may occur.

v) Early detection of hypoxemia in the PACU is critical in identifying potential oxygenation and ventilation abnormalities (11).

vi) **Decreased functional residual capacity** (FRC) is common following surgery especially after upper abdominal and thoracic procedures.

    (1) Decreased FRC can lead to increased intrapulmonary shunting resulting in hypoxemia.

    (2) Other causes of right to left intra-pulmonary shunting include prolonged intraoperative low tidal volume ventilation, airway obstruction, pulmonary aspiration and pulmonary edema.

        (a) Pulmonary edema usually presents as wheezing within the first hour after surgery.

        (b) It can be from cardiogenic causes, acute respiratory distress syndrome (ARDS), or a sudden relief of a prolonged airway obstruction, unintentional endobronchial intubation, and lobar collapse.

vii) **Pneumothorax** may occur in patients who have central venous catheters, intercostal nerve blocks, history of rib fractures or lung disease (blebs, bullae), neck dissection, tracheostomy, retroperitoneal procedures, or other cases involving potential diaphragmatic penetration.

viii) **Treatment**—O_2 therapy is the mainstay treatment for hypoxemia.

    (1) Treatment with 30% to 60% O_2 is sufficient to prevent hypoxemia in patients with mild to moderate hypoventilation and hypercapnea.

    (2) Pulse oximetry (SpO_2) and arterial blood gas measurements can be used to guide O_2 treatment.

    (3) Consider 100% O_2 via nonrebreather mask, positive pressure ventilation, and intubation and mechanical ventilation for patients having severe or persistent hypoxemia.

    (4) A chest radiograph (CXR) (ideally upright) can help assess for pneumothorax, infiltrates, and heart and lung volume and size.

    (5) In cases of suspected atelectasis, a semi-upright position can facilitate maintaining and improving FRC.

    (6) Therapeutic bronchoscopy can help re-expand areas of atelectasis, and remove debris or mucous plugs.

    (7) Persistent hypoxemia requiring >50% O_2 supplementation is an indication for the use of PEEP or CPAP (5,6).

c) **Hypoventilation/Hypercarbia**—Causes include respiratory depression from residual anesthetic agents or opioids, medication overdose, hypothermia, inadequate reversal of neuromuscular blockade, pharmacologic interaction (e.g., mycins, magnesium), alterations in pharmacokinetics or metabolism, discomfort or splinting from pain, diaphragmatic dysfunction, abdominal distention, and restrictive abdominal dressings or surgical closures.

i) **Definition:** Hypoventilation is defined as $PaCO_2$ >45 mm Hg.

    (1) Mild hypoventilation occurs commonly in postoperative patients after general anesthesia.

    (2) Significant hypoventilation is usually only clinically appreciated when $PaCO_2$ is >60 or pH is <7.25.

(3) Signs and symptoms of hypoventilation may include labored respirations, depressed respiratory rate, rapid and shallow breathing, excessive or prolonged somnolence, or airway obstruction.

(4) Progression of respiratory acidosis can increase sympathetic stimulation resulting in tachycardia and hypertension.

(5) Severe acidosis can lead to circulatory depression.

(6) Shivering, hyperthermia, and sepsis, can worsen the clinical changes associated with hypoventilation by contributing to increased CO_2 production.

Progression of respiratory acidosis can increase sympathetic stimulation resulting in tachycardia and hypertension.

ii) **Treatment:** The underlying cause must be addressed.

(1) Patients with obtunded mental status, circulatory depression, and severe acidosis (pH < 7.15) should for considered for emergent intubation and controlled ventilation.

(2) Consider diuretics for cases of circulatory fluid overload, aerosolized bronchodilators for bronchospasm, naloxone for cases of opioid-induced respiratory depression, and additional cholinesterase inhibitor for suspected residual muscle paralysis.

(3) With persistent residual respiratory depression despite a full dose of neuromuscular paralytic reversal, controlled ventilation should be maintained until spontaneous recovery occurs.

6) Neurological problems in the PACU include delayed awakening, neurologic damage, emergence delirium, peripheral neurologic lesions, and awareness/recall. **Presence of residual anesthetics is the most common cause of delayed awakening (5,6).**

a) **Stroke**

i) The perioperative incidence of stroke ranges from 0.08% to 2.9%. (4)

ii) The incidence of stroke is higher following intracranial surgery, carotid endarterectomy, cardiac surgery, and patients with multiple traumas (7).

iii) Initial signs and symptoms of stroke, such as slurred speech, visual disturbances, dizziness, agitation, confusion, numbness, muscular weakness, paralysis, and psychosis, can be nonspecific making early diagnosis challenging.

iv) Prompt neurologic consultation and imaging should be performed in all cases of suspected stroke.

READ
MORE

Crisis management: delayed emergence, Chapter 223, page 1345

b) **Emergence delirium** (4,7)

i) May present as agitation alternating with disorientation, lethargy, and inappropriate behavior.

ii) It occurs more often in patients with history of drug dependency, dementia, psychiatric disorders, and the elderly. (4,7)

iii) Drugs used in the perioperative period (especially benzodiazepines, ketamine, anticholinergics, opioids, droperidol, and large doses of metoclopromide) may contribute to emergence delirium.

iv) Other causes of delirium include hypoglycemia, metabolic derangements, hypoxemia, hypothermia, electrolyte and acid–base disorders, intracranial injury, pre-existing encephalopathies, sepsis, pain, and drug withdrawal.

v) Treatment for emergence delirium includes supplemental O_2, pain control, fluid and electrolyte repletion, and supportive care.

vi) The use of antipsychotics (haloperidol), benzodiazepines, and physostigmine (to reverse delirium from anticholinergics) may also be considered.

Prompt neurologic consultation and imaging should be performed in all cases of suspected stroke.

c) **Awareness/recall** (4,12)

i) Risk factors include ASA III-V, light anesthesia, substance abuse history, young age, and use of intraoperative muscle relaxants.

        ii)   The long-term sequelae of these experiences range from mild anxiety to severe posttraumatic stress disorder.

        iii)   Patients who note having these experiences should be provided with reassurance and additional support resources, including a referral for counseling.

7) **Renal issues in the PACU** (4–7)

  a) **Oliguria**

     i)   Is typically defined as urine output less than 0.5 mL/kg/h.

     ii)   It may be attributed to prerenal, intrarenal, or postrenal causes. **In the PACU, the prerenal (via hypovolemia) cause is most common.**

        (1)   In prerenal states, urine electrolytes show low urine Na concentration (<10 mEq/L).

        (2)   A fluid bolus trial (e.g., 250 to 500 mL crystalloid) should be considered and urine output reevaluated.

     iii) Persistent oliguria warrants further diagnostic workup.

     iv) The prognosis of acute renal failure is not improved with medication-induced diuresis to temporarily sustain urine output.

     v)   Intrarenal causes of oliguria may stem from acute tubular necrosis secondary to renal hypoperfusion, toxin exposure, or trauma. Granular casts may be present on urinalysis.

     vi) Post-renal oliguria is commonly related to mechanical causes, such as urinary catheter obstruction, trauma, or iatrogenic injuries.

  b) **Polyuria**

     i)   Is a disproportionately high urine output for a given fluid intake.

     ii)   The differential diagnosis includes large intraoperative volume administration, postobstructive diuresis, nonoliguric renal failure, osmotic diuresis, and diabetes insipidus.

     iii) Symptomatic treatment typically involves volume replacement to maintain hemodynamic stability. Electrolytes and acid–base status should be followed.

  c) Renal insufficiency or failure can make a patient susceptible to electrolyte imbalances.

     i)   Hyperkalemia, hypokalemia, hypomagnesemia, and acidemia can lead to cardiac arrhythmias.

⤷ READ MORE

Acute pain management, Chapter 149, page 1085

Postoperative nausea and vomiting, Chapter 7, page 47

Outpatient anesthesia, Chapter 130, page 909

8) **Postoperative pain**

  a) When treating postoperative pain in the PACU setting important considerations include whether the patient is an inpatient or outpatient in terms of choosing a short or long acting medication and its associated safety profile.

  b) IV or oral medications can be given depending on the patient's ability to tolerate medications by mouth.

  c) Multimodal therapy can be a useful option utilizing opioids, nonsteroid anti-inflammatories, acetaminophen and peripheral nerve blocks in select patients.

9) **Postoperative nausea/vomiting**

  a) Can be a significant factor in delayed PACU discharge.

  b) Treatment is a low-dose 5HT3 antagonist.

  c) It PONV persists, consider other agents such as dexamethasone, droperidol, or low-dose propofol.

10) **Discharge criteria** (3–7)
  a) According to the ASA Practice Guidelines for Postanesthetic Care, PACU discharge criteria should be based upon evaluating many factors.
    i) Factors include neurologic status, vital signs, respiratory status, control of nausea/vomiting, and pain.
    ii) Patients should be arousable and oriented or at their baseline pre-operative neurologic status.
    iii) Vital signs should be stable and within normal parameters or within the patient's pre-operative baseline for at least 30 minutes.
    iv) Patients should be free from any obvious surgical complications or active bleeding, and should be comfortable, without nausea and emesis, and with pain well controlled.
    v) Peripheral nerve function should be assessed and signs of returning sensory and motor function should be documented.
    vi) Patients can go home with an insensate limb if they receive appropriate counseling and support (e.g., knee brace if received a femoral nerve block).
    vii) Patients that receive respiratory depressant drugs should be observed for at least 30 minutes prior to discharge.
    viii) Patients receiving supplemental O_2 in the PACU should be observed for at least 15 minutes on room air to ensure that hypoxemia does not develop (10).
    ix) Use of discharge scoring systems may help in determining readiness for discharge.
    x) Outpatients should be discharged to a responsible adult who will accompany them home and be provided with written instructions including diet, medications, activities and an emergency phone number.

Chapter Summary for PACU

Definition	The PACU facilitates the transition between the operating room and discharge home or transfer to a hospital ward.
ASA Standards	All patients shall receive appropriate postanesthesia management. Patients transported to the PACU will be accompanied by a member of the anesthesia care team. On arrival to the PACU, the patient will be reevaluated and a verbal report given to the PACU nurse. Patients will be evaluated continuously in the PACU. A physician is responsible for PACU patient discharge.
Admission and Monitoring	PACU signout should include a pertinent summary of the patient's history and perioperative events. Monitoring typically includes pulse oximetry, telemetry, and blood pressure.
Common Problems	Common PACU issues include hypotension, hypertension, dysrhythmias, airway obstruction, hypoxemia, hypercarbia, delayed emergence, and oliguria. Hypoxemia can lead to acidosis, bradycardia, hypotension, neurologic obtundation, and cardiac arrest. Respiratory acidosis can cause sympathetic stimulation resulting in tachycardia and hypertension.
Discharge Criteria	Patients should be arousable, oriented or at their baseline pre-operative neurologic status. Vital signs should be stable or within the patient's baseline for at least 30 min. Patients should be free from any obvious surgical complications. Patients' pain should be well controlled. Patients that have received respiratory depressant drugs should be observed for at least 30 min before discharge. Outpatients should be discharged to a responsible adult and should be provided with written instructions on outpatient care.

References

1. http://www.aspan.org/Portals/6/docs/ClinicalPractice/PositionStatement/4-Min_Staffing.pdf.
2. http://www.asahq.org/publicationsAndServices/standards/36.pdf.
3. American Society of Anesthesiologists Task Force on Postanesthetic Care. Practice Guidelines for Postanesthestic Care. *Anesthesiology* 2002:96:742–752.
4. Diaconescu, D, Grecu L. The postanesthesia care unit. In: Dunn PF, ed. *Clinical Anesthesia Procedures of the Massachusetts General Hospital.* 7th ed. Philadelphia, PA: Lippincott Williams & Wilkins; 2007:623–644.
5. Feeley TW, Macario A. *Miller's Anesthesia.* 6th ed. 2005;2703–2723.
6. Nicholau D. The postanesthesia care unit. In: Miller RD, ed. *Miller's Anesthesia.* 7th ed. Philadelphia, PA: Churchill Livingstone Elsevier; 2009:2707–2728.
7. Fowler MA, Spiess BD. PostAnesthesia recovery. In: Barash PG, Cullen BF, Stoelting RK, et al., eds. *Clinical Anesthesia.* 6th ed. Philadelphia, PA: Lippincott Williams & Wilkins; 2009:1421–1443.
8. Lindenauer PK, Pekow P, Wang K, et al. Perioperative beta-blocker therapy and mortality after major noncardiac surgery. *N Engl J Med* 2005;353:349–361.
9. Priebe HJ. Perioperative myocardial infarction—aetiology and prevention. *Br J Anaesth* 2005;95(1):3–19.
10. Thompson A, Balser JR. Perioperative cardiac arrhythmias. *Br J Anaesth* 2004;93:86–94.
11. Fu ES, Downs JB, Schweiger JW, et al. Supplemental oxygen impairs detection of hypoventilation by pulse oximetry. *Chest* 2004;126:1552–1558.
12. Sebel PS, Bowdle TA, Ghoneim MM, et al. The incidence of awareness during anesthesia: a multicenter United States Study. *Anesth Analg* 2004;99:833–839.

148 Post-op Ventilation of the Surgical Patient

Matthew Coleman, MD

Respiratory management of the postoperative patient has unique considerations. Up to 5% of patients will fail extubation following a surgical procedure (1,2). This population typically endures relatively short duration intubation and rapid weaning from mechanical ventilatory support. These patients are emerging from anesthesia, which includes drugs that alter respiratory efforts and require adequate pharmacologic reversal. The decision to extubate the trachea and discontinue mechanical ventilation is sometimes difficult, but the underlying pathophysiology, duration of surgery, and site of surgery must be considered. Considerations for extubation are addressed in this chapter in an effort to address when it is appropriate to discontinue mechanical ventilation, prevent failed extubation, and treat patients who fail extubation.

Successful extubation after mechanical ventilation depends on a variety of parameters, including the patient's ability to protect the airway, maintain adequate ventilation, and maintain adequate oxygenation.

1) Discontinuation of mechanical ventilation
   a) **General considerations**
      i) Weaning a patient from mechanical ventilation in the operating room is a rapid process.
      ii) The decision to extubate the trachea is often based on practitioner experience; however, subjective and objective data should be used.
      iii) In order to facilitate successful extubation, the patient must have the following: **a patent airway, return of muscle strength, the ability to cough and protect the airway, spontaneous respiratory drive, and adequate blood oxygenation.**
   b) **Extubation criteria (Table 148-1)**
      i) When evaluating a patient for discontinuation of mechanical ventilation and extubation in the operating room, it is helpful to use a systems approach.
      ii) Failure to meet these criteria will often preclude extubation and lead to intensive care unit (ICU) admission for a more gradual weaning process.

Strongly consider the use of noninvasive positive-pressure ventilation patients with emphysema undergoing thoracotomy to avoid reintubation.

2) Surgery specific extubation considerations (Table 148-2)
   a) **Cardiac**
      i) 8.5% of adult patients undergoing cardiac surgery will have postoperative respiratory complications (8).
      ii) **Fast tracking**
         (1) The practice of **"fast tracking"** involves rapid weaning within a few hours after transfer to the ICU, as opposed to the traditional 24 hours or more of mechanical ventilation.
         (2) Postoperative respiratory complications are a significant cause of morbidity and mortality, and earlier extubation is clinically and economically favored over prolonged intubation (5,8,9).

Table 148-1

Criteria to Assess Whether a Patient Should be Extubated

Extubation Criteria/Assessment		Example
General	The acute disease process is addressed or resolved	Open wounds Impending sepsis
	Chronic systemic disease does not preclude extubation	Acute or chronic lung disease Cardiovascular disease Musculoskeletal disease
	Acceptable surgical duration	Usually <8 h
	No major surgical involvement of the chest, lungs, or muscles of respiration	
Neurologic	Arousable patient	GCS > 13 Follows commands
	Adequate pain control	Postoperative epidural or regional analgesia RR < 35
Respiratory	Sufficient respiratory drive	pCO_2 < 60 mm Hg Minute ventilation > 4 L/min
	Normal mechanics of ventilation	Tidal volume 4–6 mL/kg RR < 35 Negative inspiratory force <–20 to –30 cm H_2O
	Normal oxygenation	SpO_2 > 95% on FiO_2 1.0 PaO_2 > 60 mm Hg with FiO_2 <0.4 PEEP < 5–10 cm H_2O PaO_2/FiO_2 > 200–300 mm Hg
	Airway protection intact	Muscle relaxants reversed Cough to eliminate secretions No upper airway edema No hemorrhage
Cardiovascular	Hemodynamic stability	Vasopressors not required for BP stability HR < 120 bpm
	No active bleeding	Hemoglobin > 8 mg/dL and stable Drain output stable
Infection, Fluids, and Metabolic	No metabolic abnormalities	Sodium, phosphate, magnesium, and blood glucose in the normal range
	Normal pH	Range 7.35–7.45
	Normal temperature	Range 35.5°C–38°C
	No evidence of fluid overload	Absence of obvious facial or extremity edema Normal cuff leak test

Table 148-2

Special Considerations with Subspecialty Surgery (3–7)

Special Patient Population	Extubation and Ventilation Considerations
Otolaryngology	Tumors may compress airway Airway stenosis may be present Caution should be taken following surgery in the neck, pharynx, mandible, maxilla, or adjacent structures.
Thoracic Surgery	Many patients have severe lung disease, which makes extubation challenging Up to 30% of patients with severe emphysema undergoing thoracotomy will have postoperative respiratory complications Patients undergoing lung volume reduction surgery, pneumonectomy, and lung transplant benefit from early discontinuation from mechanical ventilation due effects of positive pressure on suture lines and prevention of reintubation.
Cardiac Surgery	Respiratory complications are usually due to cardiac dysfunction Consider rapid weaning of ventilation in patients with no sign of cardiac dysfunction, excess bleeding, or neurologic injury.
Neurosurgery	GCS >8 is a strong predictor of extubation success in the ICU Possibility of ICP manipulation Prolonged mechanical ventilation may be necessary
Trauma	Consider the possibility of undiagnosed head injury

GCS, glascow coma scale; ICP, intracranial pressure; ICU, intensive care unit.

Great caution should be taken when extubating patients following surgery on the neck, pharynx, maxilla, mandible, and adjacent structures.

READ MORE

Asthma and reactive airway disease, Chapter 72, page 512

(3) Rapid weaning should be reserved for patients with no sign of cardiac dysfunction, excess bleeding, or neurologic injury.

3) **Treatment methods for acute respiratory distress following surgery**

a) **O_2 therapy (Table 148-3)**

i) The delivery of O_2 via low flow systems is dependent on the minute ventilation of the patient and the reservoir volume obtained by the O_2 delivery device.

b) **Medications**

i) Multiple medications may be used in the post anesthesia care unit (PACU) to prevent or treat respiratory distress.

ii) Pain medications, sedatives, opioid antagonists, GABA antagonists, β-adrenergic antagonists, vasodilators, vasopressors, or anticonvulsants may be needed depending on the underlying problem.

iii) **Acute bronchospasm**

(1) May be effectively treated with β_2-adrenergic agonists, antimuscarinics, racemic epinephrine, H_2 receptor antagonists, or a combination.

iv) **Postoperative stridor**

(1) Racemic epinephrine or helium/O_2 mixture (Heliox) may be useful treatments.

Table 148-3

The Reservoir Volume and Fraction of Attainable O_2 with Various O_2 Delivery Devices (10)

Device	Reservoir Volume (mL)	Oxygen Flow (L/min)	FiO_2
Nasal cannula	50	1–6	0.21–0.46
Simple face mask	150–250	5–10	0.4–0.6
Partial rebreather mask with reservoir bag	750–1,250	5–7	0.35–0.75
Nonrebreather mask with reservoir bag	750–1,250	5–10	0.4–1.0

Adapted from Marino PL. Oxygen inhalation therapy. In: *The ICU Book*. 3rd ed. Philadelphia, PA: Lippincott Williams & Wilkins; 2007:403–418.

   v) **Upper airway obstruction**
      (1) **Sitting the patient up in bed, oral and/or nasal airway may be useful.**
   c) **Respiratory therapy**
      i) Multiple therapy modalities are used to treat postoperative respiratory distress.
      ii) Aggressive coughing, suctioning, sitting the patient up in bed, and incentive spirometry may improve a patient's oxygenation, ventilation, and mental status.
      iii) Regional anesthesia techniques (epidural, paravertebral blockade) can reduce pain associated with coughing and/or incentive spirometry for patients with large abdominal incisions (especially upper abdomen) or open thoracotomy.
      iv) Noninvasive positive-pressure ventilation (NIPPV) (see below) is also a useful method to treat selected postoperative patients, including those with COPD, cardiogenic pulmonary edema, and various forms of hypoxemic respiratory failure (11–13).
4) **Noninvasive ventilation (NIV)**
   a) NIPPV, noninvasive mechanical ventilation (NIMV), and NIV, describe ventilatory support delivered to a patient in the absence of an endotracheal tube or tracheostomy (11).
      i) Support is delivered through a full mask or nasal mask strapped snugly to the face to avoid leaks.
      ii) The delivery of NIV can be from a specifically designed machine, ventilator (in the ICU or operating room), or less precisely by hand mask ventilation.
   b) **NIV criteria**
      i) There are several criteria that patients must meet in order to use NIV (11)
      ii) A patient who does not meet these criteria and is in acute respiratory failure would require endotracheal intubation or tracheostomy.
      iii) Conscious and cooperative
         (1) COPD patients may be an exception (11)
            (a) Randomized trials suggest that NIV is beneficial for hypercapnic patients with acute respiratory distress in the setting of chronic disease.
            (b) NIV can reduce ICU stay, length of ventilator dependence, and mortality
      iv) Hemodynamic and cardiac rhythm stability
      v) Adequately fitted face mask

vi) Contraindications to NIV

   (1) Acute facial trauma

   (2) Recent gastroesophageal surgery

   (3) Active gastrointestinal bleeding

   (4) Impaired swallowing

   (5) Copious respiratory secretions necessitating endotracheal suctioning

c) **Bilevel positive airway pressure (BiPAP)**

   i) BiPAP refers to provision of inspiratory positive airway pressure (IPAP) along with expiratory positive airway pressure.

   ii) In adjusting BiPAP, an IPAP level and a positive expiratory airway pressure (PEEP) are set.

   iii) The patient's spontaneous breaths trigger the machine to deliver the IPAP.

   iv) During expiration, the PEEP is maintained.

   v) As with invasive ventilation, settings on the BiPAP may require multiple adjustments.

      (1) For example, an initial PEEP can be set to 0 cm H_2O and slowly titrated to 3–5 cm H_2O, or 8–10 cm H_2O if the patient is hypoxemic.

      (2) The initial IPAP can be set to 10 cm H_2O and titrated to achieve a tidal volume of >7 mL/kg and a respiratory rate of <25 breaths/min. The FiO_2 can then be titrated to achieve an oxygen saturation of >90%.

d) **Continuous positive airway pressure (CPAP)**

   i) CPAP is the provision of a constant positive airway pressure, which acts to maintain positive pressure in the airway; CPAP does not offer pressure support ventilation.

CPAP is commonly used in patients for home treatment of obstructive sleep apnea.

   ii) Adjusted by changing the level of positive pressure to the patient, typically 4 to 6 cm H_2O.

   iii) Useful modality to increase the functional reserve capacity and improve oxygenation.

   iv) Not useful in patients who lack respiratory drive, such as those patients overdosed with narcotics.

Chapter Summary: Postoperative Ventilation of the Surgical Patient

Extubation Criteria	Patient should be awake, with a patent airway, have return of muscle strength, be able to cough and protect the airway, have the drive to breathe spontaneously, and be able to oxygenate the blood.
Surgical Considerations	1) Surgical procedure may determine ability to extubate. Take great caution with patients following ENT, **thoracic, cardiac, trauma, and neurological surgeries.** 2) Reintubation of patients with emphysema significantly elevates risk of barotraumas.
NIV	Multiple modalities are available that may avoid reintubation in patients at risk of respiratory failure, including CPAP and BiPAP. **Avoid NIV with significant airway swelling, severe GERD/airway secretions/blood, altered consciousness, and acute facial trauma.**

References

1. MacIntyre NR, Cook DJ, Ely EW Jr, et al. Evidence-based guidelines for weaning and discontinuing ventilatory support: a collective task force facilitated by the American College of Chest Physicians, the American Association for Respiratory Care, and the American College of Critical Care Medicine. *Chest* 2001;120:375S.
2. Demling RH, Read T, Lind LJ, et al. Incidence and morbidity of extubation failure in surgical intensive care patients. *Crit Care Med* 1988;16:573–577.
3. Sharafkhaneh A, Falk JA, Minai OA, et al. Overview of the perioperative management of lung volume reduction surgery patients. *Proc Am Thorac Soc* 2008;5(4):438–441.
4. Seigne PW, Hartigan PM, Body SC. Anesthetic considerations for patients with severe emphysematous lung disease. *Int Anesthesiol Clin* 2000;38(1):1–23.
5. Cohen A, Katz M, Katz R, et al. Chronic obstructive pulmonary disease in patients undergoing coronary artery bypass grafting. *J Thorac Cardiovasc Surg* 1995;109:574–581.
6. Namen AM, Ely EW, Tatter SB, et al. Predictors of successful extubation in neurosurgical patients. *Am J Respir Crit Care Med* 2001;163:658–664.
7. Daley B, Garcia-Perez F, Ross S. Reintubation as an outcome predictor in trauma patients. *Chest* 1996;110:1577–1580.
8. Rady MY, Ryan T. Perioperative predictors of extubation failure and the effect on clinical outcome after cardiac surgery. *Crit Care Med* 1999;27:340–347.
9. Weissman C. Pulmonary complications after cardiac surgery. *Semin Cardiothorac Vasc Anesth* 2004;8(3):185–211.
10. Marino PL. Oxygen inhalation therapy. In: *The ICU Book.* 3rd ed. Philadelphia, PA: Lippincott Williams & Wilkins; 2007:403–418.
11. Antonelli M, Conti G. Noninvasive positive pressure ventilation as treatment for acute respiratory failure in critically ill patients. *Crit Care* 2000;4:15–22.
12. Hill NS, Brennan J, Garpestad E, et al. Noninvasive ventilation in acute respiratory failure. *Crit Care Med* 2007;35(10):2402–2407.
13. Esteban A, Frutos-Vivar F, Ferguson ND, et al. A Noninvasive Positive-Pressure Ventilation for Respiratory Failure after Extubation. *N Engl J Med* 2004;350(24):2452–2460.

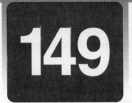

149 Acute Pain Management

Jason G. Ramirez, MD

Pain control is a very important aspect of modern medical care. The American Society of Anesthesiologists (ASA) Task Force on Acute Pain Management currently recommends a choice of three modalities forming the cornerstone of acute pain management. The focus of this chapter will be to address these recommendations from the perspective of an Acute Pain Service. Pharmacologic treatment of acute post operative surgical pain will be the focus. Neuraxial and peripheral regional techniques are discussed at length elsewhere in this text. Complex chronic pain states including cancer pain, complex regional pain syndrome (CRPS) I, CRPS II, and neuropathic pain syndromes are beyond the scope of this chapter and should be addressed under the directive of Chronic Pain Management.

1) **Overview of acute pain management.** Pharmacologic advancements have placed the goal of effective pain control within reach for the patient. Unfortunately, many patients continue to suffer when their pain is not responsive to the most basic of interventions.

Inadequately controlled acute pain has many adverse effects on cardiovascular, pulmonary, gastrointestinal, immune, renal and hematologic systems.

   a) **Poor pain management in the acute postsurgical setting remains a problem.**
      i) Inadequately controlled acute pain has adverse effects on many physiologic systems including the cardiovascular, pulmonary, gastrointestinal, immunologic, renal, and hematologic systems (1).
      ii) Most agree regarding the ethical mandate to provide adequate pain control.
         (1) Growing evidence suggests that inadequate pain control may lead to increases in morbidity, mortality and the development of chronic pain syndromes (1–3).
   b) **The ASA Task Force on Acute Pain Management currently recommends a choice of three modalities** forming the cornerstone of acute pain management. These cornerstone modalities include:
      i) **Systemic opioid therapy** via patient controlled analgesia (PCA),
      ii) **Neuraxial techniques,** such as spinal or epidural anesthesia, and
      iii) **Regional anesthesia** in the form of peripheral nerve blocks (PNBs) (4).
   c) The Task Force also recommends the use of multimodal analgesia and specifically discusses the use of scheduled NSAIDs, COX-2 inhibitors, or acetaminophen (4). Furthermore, others advocate for the use of a nonopioid as part of any analgesic regimen (5). These types of interventions can be described as **adjuvant therapy.**
2) **Pathophysiology and Neurobiology of Pain Transmission.** Formulating an effective pain control plan requires an understanding of pain transmission. Pain perception is a complex interaction involving neural, biochemical, and emotional inputs. However, a reasonable model of acute pain can be described at the most basic level.

1085

A-delta noci-
ceptors are
responsible
for fast pain
response and
sharp sensation
of acute pain. C
nociceptors are
responsible for
dull throbbing
pain.

a) **Acute tissue damage leads to activation of specialized neurons termed nociceptors.** Two types of nociceptors, A-delta and C, have been described.

    i) **A-delta nociceptors** respond to thermal and mechanical stimuli.

        (1) They are responsible for the fast pain response to tissue injury and the sharp sensation of acute pain.

    ii) **C nociceptors** respond to thermal, mechanical and chemical stimuli.

        (1) C nociceptors are involved with a slower response to tissue injury and the release of chemical mediators of pain.

        (2) They are also responsible for the dull, throbbing aspect of acute pain and may play a role in chronic pain development.

b) Afferent **nerve signals** travel from these nociceptors via peripheral nerves to the spinal cord where they synapse on second order neurons.

    i) The nerve signal travels up spinal tracts where it is processed in higher brain centers.

    ii) The efferent nerve response travels down descending spinal tracts when it can interact and modulate further ascending pain signals or it can travel and terminate at peripheral motor neurons.

c) In addition, the initial tissue injury leads to the **release of chemical mediators** including leukotrienes, bradykinins, serotonin, histamine, potassium, substance P, thromboxanes, and prostaglandin. These mediators serve to activate or modulate further nociceptive afferent signals (6).

3) **Receptor targets—Understanding this neurobiological pathway involved in pain signal processing provides the clinician with various cellular targets for pharmacologic intervention in an effort to control pain.**

    a) Examples include **opioids** which bind to opioid receptors located primarily in the spinal cord.

    b) **Local anesthetics** bind and inhibit nerve signal transmission at the peripheral nerve (PNBs) or at the spinal roots (neuraxial block.)

    c) **NSAIDs and acetaminophen** interact with various chemical mediators mentioned above involved in pain transmission.

    d) **Ketamine** binds to the N-Methyl-D-aspartate (NMDA) receptor located in the brain.

4) **Medication classes—the clinician should develop familiarity with some of the basic medications used in the treatment of acute postoperative pain.**

    a) **Opioids**

        i) **Mechanism of action**—Opioids bind and activate opioid receptors.

            (1) Opioid receptors are mostly located in lamina I and the substantia gelatinosa of the spinal cord.

            (2) However, they have also been identified in the brain and in the periphery.

                (a) Peripheral opioid receptors are activated in the presence of inflammation (7).

        ii) **Adverse effects**—The general side effects of opioids include respiratory depression, impaired gastric motility, nausea, vomiting, sedation, pruritis, and urinary retention.

        iii) **Dosing**—It is important to note that opioids should be dosed for each patient's individual needs. Unlike other medication classes, opioids do not have a "maximum dose."

            (1) The proper dose is the dose that produces the desired effect without significant adverse side effects (2,7).

        iv) Specific agents

            (1) **Morphine**

Morphine may be a poor choice in patients with renal failure due to accumulation of morphine-6-glucuronide metabolites.

    (a) Morphine is the most commonly used and most commonly studied opioid in the United States.

    (b) Morphine is a good initial choice for somatic pain but is has low efficacy in the treatment of neuropathic pain (8).

    (c) Morphine is metabolized in the liver

        (i) Principal metabolites include morphine-3-glucuronide and morphine-6-glucuronide.

        (ii) These metabolites are excreted by the kidneys. Morphine 6-glucuronide is an active metabolite possessing sedating and analgesic properties (7,9).

        (iii) Therefore, morphine may be a poor choice for a patient with renal failure.

    (d) Appropriate initial intravenous PCA settings for morphine in the opioid naive patient should be 1 to 2 mg every 8 to 10 minutes.

(2) **Hydromorphone**

    (a) Hydromorphone is a commonly used opioid that has been described as anywhere from **three to eight times more potent than morphine** (7,9,10).

    (b) If the potency of hydromorphone is considered as being five times more potent than morphine, conversions between the two medications can be easily accomplished.

        (i) For example, 1 mg of morphine would be equalanalgesic to 0.2 mg of hydromorphone.

        (ii) Hydromorphone is **metabolized in the liver to inactive metabolites** (9,10). Therefore hydromorphone may be a better choice in patients with renal insufficiency.

    (c) Initial intravenous PCA settings for hydromorphone should be 0.2 to 0.4 mg every 8 to 10 minutes.

(3) **Fentanyl**

    (a) Fentanyl is a synthetic opioid and anywhere from 80 to 125 times more potent than morphine (9,10).

    (b) It is metabolized in the liver to inactive metabolites which are excreted in the urine (7).

    (c) Fentanyl is administered in **micrograms**. If the potency of fentanyl is considered to be 100 times greater than morphine, conversions become easy to accomplish.

        (i) For example, 10 mcg of fentanyl would equal 1,000 mcg (1 mg) of morphine.

    (d) Appropriate initial intravenous PCA settings for fentanyl should be 10 to 20 mcg every 6 to 8 minutes.

(4) **Meperidine**

    (a) Meperidine is seven to ten times less potent as compared morphine (7,9,10).

    (b) Meperidine's mechanism of action is at opioid receptors but it also possesses some antagonist activity at NMDA receptors (7).

    (c) It addition, meperidine inhibits norephinephrine (NE) and serotonin reuptake (7).

    (d) Meperidine is metabolized in the liver (7).

        (i) An active metabolite, normeperidine is formed which relies on renal excretion (9).

        (ii) Normeperidine lowers the seizure threshold.

Meperidine should be used with caution in patients with renal failure or seizure disorders or in those who are taking monoamine oxidase inhibitors.

Methadone is associated with risk of QT interval prolongation and Torsade de pointes.

(iii) Caution should be used with patients who have seizure disorders or with renal failure. Concomitant use with monoamine oxidase inhibitors has been associated with malignant hyperpyrexia. (9)

(e) Meperidine is not recommended for use in PCA. Morphine, fentanyl or hydromorphone represent better alternatives.

(5) **Methadone**

    (a) Methadone has been described as being anywhere from equipotent or up to seven times more potent than morphine (7,11).

    (b) It is metabolized in the liver by the Cytochrome P-450 system to primarily inactive metabolites (8,11).

        (i) Methadone metabolites are **excreted in the urine and bile** (fecal route) (11).

    (c) Methadone is unique in that is has an extremely long half life.

        (i) The $t_{1/2}$ alpha is 2 to 12 hours while the $t_{1/2}$ beta is anywhere between 15 and 60 hours (8,11).

    (d) **Primary action is at opioid receptors.**

        (i) However, methadone exhibits some antagonism at NMDA receptors (7,8,11).

        (ii) Methadone also inhibits NE and serotonin reuptake (7,8,11).

        (iii) Therefore, methadone is a useful agent for patients with both somatic and neuropathic pain components.

    (e) Methadone is associated with the risk of **QT interval prolongation** and **Torsade de pointes** (11).

b) **Nonsteroidal antiinflammatory drugs (NSAIDs)**

  i) NSAIDs can be used solely for the treatment of mild to moderate pain (2,12).

  ii) Additive and/or synergistic effects have been shown when used with other agents (12).

  iii) Therefore, NSAIDs represent a useful component of a multimodal analgesic plan for severe post operative pain. The use of NSAIDS is specifically mentioned by the ASA Task Force on Acute Pain Management.

  iv) **Mechanism of action** NSAIDs inhibit prostaglandin synthesis through the arachadonic acid pathway.

    (1) Prostaglandins are important mediators of pain, inflammation and fever.

    (2) Specifically, NSAIDs reversibly inhibit the enzyme cyclooxygenase (COX) that converts arachidonic acid to prostaglandins (2,5,12–14).

    (3) There are two major isoforms of the COX enzyme, COX-1 and COX-2.

      (a) COX-1 is constitutively expressed and is involved platelet aggregation.

      (b) COX-1 also exerts protective effects within the kidneys and gastrointestinal tract.

      (c) The COX-2 isoform is inducible and is involved in pain and inflammatory states (2,12,13).

    (4) Traditional NSAIDs inhibit both isoforms of the COX enzyme and are termed nonselective NSAIDs.

    (5) Newer COX-2 specific agents, termed Coxibs, were developed in an effort to minimize side effects associated with COX-1 inhibition (5,15).

  v) Adverse effects

    (1) Side effects attributed to NSAIDs are associated with inhibition of the COX enzymes.

    (2) Patients utilizing nonselective **NSAIDs are at risk from bleeding, gastroduodenal ulceration and renal failure** (5,14).

      (3) COX-2 selective agents have a lower risk of bleeding and ulceration (5).

         (a) However, the risk of renal failure is unchanged with these agents (5). Information suggests that the COX-2 enzyme may play a role in cardiovascular protection (12).

         (b) **COX-2 inhibitors have been associated with an increased risk of myocardial infarction and stroke** (5).

   vi) Specific agents

      (1) **Ketorolac**

         (a) Ketorolac is a potent nonselective NSAID and should be considered part of a multimodal analgesic plan.

         (b) Ketorolac is very effective in managing pain associated with recovery following thoracotomy.

         (c) Dosing is 30 mg IV followed by 15 mg IV every 6 hours for 3 days (5).

         (d) Ketorolac can be associated with renal failure and should be used with caution in the elderly (5).

      (2) **Celecoxib**

         (a) Celecoxib is a COX-2 specific inhibitor used for mild to moderate pain control or as an adjuvant as part of a multimodal analgesic plan. Celecoxib is administered orally.

         (b) Dosing is 200 mg orally every 12 hours with a maximum dose of 400 mg/d (5).

         (c) Celecoxib is metabolized in the liver to inactive metabolites (12). The $t_{1/2}$ beta is approximately 11 hours (12).

         (d) Celecoxib is contraindicated in those with an allergy to sulfa containing medications (12).

         (e) As mentioned previously, Coxibs have been associated with an increased risk of myocardial infarction and stroke.

           (i) The other two COX-2 specific medications, rofecoxib and valdecoxib, were initially approved and later withdrawn from the United States market (5).

           (ii) However, the use of celecoxib is considered appropriate in those without a significant cardiovascular history who may derive benefit from its COX-2 specificity.

  c) **Acetaminophen**

    i) Acetaminophen is often overlooked as part of an effective post operative pain management plan.

    ii) Synergistic and/or additive effects have been suggested when it has been used in combination with opioids, NSAIDs, and tramadol (15).

      (1) Therefore, this agent may be considered as an adjuvant in the setting of multimodal analgesia.

    iii) **Mechanism of action**

      (1) Acetaminophen's mechanism of action is unclear but research suggests that it acts as a central inhibitor of prostaglandin synthesis through COX inhibition.

      (2) In addition, it has been demonstrated to inhibit spinal transmission of nociception in the dorsal horn via serotonergic interactions (15,16).

      (3) Some evidence points to inhibition of a third isoform of the COX enzyme (COX-3) (5,14).

    iv) **Adverse effects**

      (1) Acetaminophen has been associated with hepatic necrosis during an acute overdose (5).

Acetaminophen has been associated with hepatic necrosis during acute overdose.

The daily dose of acetaminophen should be limited to 4,000 g/d for healthy individuals.

Ketamine can be associated with psychomimetic side effects including hallucinations, bad dreams and delirium.

(2) Risk factors include those with known liver disease, excessive alcohol consumption and those with decreased glutathione stores (malnutrition, starvation) (5,14).

(3) Acetaminophen has no adverse effects on platelets or upon the gastrointestinal mucosa (5).

v) **Dosing**

(1) Current dosing is focused on the total amount of acetaminophen ingested per day.

(2) 4,000 mg orally per day has been traditionally considered safe for healthy individuals.

(3) A maximum dose of 3,000 mg orally per day should be utilized in those with mild liver impairment and in the elderly (5).

d) **Ketamine**

i) Ketamine is used as an intravenous general anesthetic. Ketamine is also a potent analgesic and can be used at subanesthetic doses for the treatment of acute pain.

(1) It is useful as an adjuvant to opioid therapy and should be considered when severe pain is resistant to opioid therapy (3,17).

(2) In addition, ketamine is effective for the treatment of neuropathic pain states (8).

ii) **Mechanism of action**

(1) Ketamine is an NMDA receptor antagonist (3,8,17).

  (a) Ketamine also may have some effects at opioid receptors (3).

iii) **Adverse effects**

(1) Ketamine can be associated with psychomimetic side effects including hallucinations, dreams and delirium (3,8,17).

(2) Ketamine is a potent sialagogue.

iv) **Dosing**

(1) Low dose ketamine is defined as intravenous dosing of <1 mg/kg (3).

(2) Doses of 12.5 mg intravenously can be administered at the bedside with proper hemodynamic and respiratory monitoring (blood pressure cuff, pulse oximetery).

(3) Do not exceed a dose of 1 mg/kg total.

(4) Ketamine is metabolized in the liver to norketamine (8).

e) **Tramadol**

i) Tramadol is useful in the treatment of mild to moderate pain or as an adjuvant.

ii) **Mechanism of action**

(1) Tramadol possesses opioid agonist properties although it is not classified as an opioid.

(2) Tramadol also acts as an inhibitor of serotonin and NE reuptake (7).

iii) **Metabolism** occurs in the liver with renal elimination of metabolites.

(1) The $t_{1/2}$ beta is approximately 6 hours.

(2) Unlike traditional opioid receptor agonist, Tramadol has no effects on respiration and a low incidence of constipation (7,18).

5) **Clinical management.** When formulating a specific analgesic plan there are several key concepts to consider.
   a) **History.** A detailed patient history must be obtained.
      i) **Classify**—Classify the pain as acute or chronic. Remember, it is possible to have acute post operative pain while also having an ongoing chronic pain syndrome.
      ii) **Qualify**—Qualify the pain as being somatic, visceral or neuropathic in nature. Again, it is possible for multiple types of pain to exist in the same patient at the same time.
      iii) **Quantify**—Quantify the level of baseline pain. It is unreasonable to expect a pain free postoperative recovery period for the chronic pain patient who experiences 7/10 pain on a daily basis. On the other hand, a healthy patient can probably expect to have postoperative surgical pain kept to a minimum during his/her recovery period.
      iv) **Medication intake**—It is important to note the types of pain medications the patient requires to maintain baseline functioning prior to surgery. This will help in choosing appropriate initial PCA settings. An opioid naive patient will respond differently than the patient taking chronic opioid therapy at home.
   b) **Cornerstone therapy.** Patients should be placed on at least one of the cornerstone therapies outlined by the ASA Task Force on Acute Pain Management. Some patients will be candidates for two of the cornerstone therapies.
      i) **Opioids**
         (1) Consider opioid therapy for all patients with moderate to severe pain.
         (2) Morphine, hydromorphone or fentanyl should be considered for most patients.
         (3) Methadone should be reserved for those with coexisting chronic pain syndromes and those with significant neuropathic components to their pain.
      ii) **Peripheral nerve blocks**
         (1) Local anesthetic single injection or continuous block techniques should be considered for all procedures involving the upper and lower extremities.
         (2) PNBs are considered standard of care at many institutions for hand, elbow, hip, knee, ankle, and foot procedures.
      iii) **Neuraxial techniques**
         (1) Epidural catheter placement with a continuous infusion of local anesthetic is the modality of choice for thoracotomy, upper and lower abdominal and gynecologic procedures.
         (2) Along with local anesthetics, opioids can be administered directly through a properly functioning epidural catheter resulting in improved pain control at lower medication doses.
   c) **Adjuvant medications**
      i) Following the initiation of appropriate cornerstone therapy, adjuvant medications should be considered for most patients expected to experience moderate to severe postoperative pain.
      ii) **NSAIDs**
         (1) Scheduled ibuprofen, 200 mg orally three times per day, can be an effective adjuvant for healthy patients.
         (2) A short course of IV ketorolac is very helpful for the management of severe pain particularly those recovering after a thoracotomy.
         (3) Celecoxib is effective for those with a history of gastrointestinal ulceration.
      iii) **Acetaminophen**
         (1) Scheduled acetaminophen is also an effective adjuvant when used at the appropriate strength.
         (2) Remember to limit the daily dose under 4,000 mg/d for healthy adult patients.

iv) **Ketamine**
- (1) Ketamine should be reserved to help with severe pain that has been unresponsive to opioid therapy.
- (2) Ketamine is particularly helpful in those with coexisting neuropathic and chronic pain syndromes.

v) **Tramadol**
- (1) Tramadol can also be helpful for the acute pain patient with coexisting neuropathic and chronic pain syndromes.
- (2) It should be considered for the patient with mild to moderate pain complaints despite opioid and other adjuvant therapy use.

Chapter Summary for Acute Pain Management

Overview	Effective treatment of acute pain requires an understanding of the pathophysiology and receptor targets involved with pain transmission.
Acute Pain Management Approach	A thorough history should be taken and physical exam performed. Pain should be classified, qualified and quantified. Current pain medications should be noted. Together, these factors should be considered when implementing cornerstone therapies.
Cornerstone Therapies	The ASA Task Force on acute pain recommends that patients be given at least one cornerstone therapy: systemic opioids, neuraxial anesthesia or PNB. Some patients may qualify for more than one therapy.
Adjuvant Therapies	Adjuvant therapy should be considered and added as necessary. Adjuvant therapies include: NSAIDs, acetaminophen, ketamine, tramadol

References

1. Joshi GP, Ogunnaike BO. Consequences of inadequate post operative pain relief and chronic persistent post operative pain. *Anesthesiol Clin North America* 2005;23:21–36.
2. Brown AK, Christo PJ, Wu CL. Strategies for postoperative pain management. *Best Pract Res Clin Anesthesiol* 2004;318:703–717.
3. De Kock MF, Lavand'homme PM. The clinical role of NMDA receptor antagonist for the treatment of postoperative pain. *Best Pract Res Clin Anaesthesiology* 2007;21:85–98.
4. American Society of Anesthesiologists Task Force on Acute Pain Management Practice, Guidelines for Acute Pain Management in the Perioperative Setting An Updated report by the American Society of Anesthesiologists Task Force on Acute Pain Management. *Anesthesiology* 2004;100:1573–1581.
5. Munir MA, Enany N, Zhang J-M. Nonopioid analgesics. *Anesthesiol Clin* 2007;25:761–774.
6. Walter AF. The pathophysiology of acute pain. *Emerg Clin North America* 2005;23:277–284.
7. Berger JM. Opioids in anesthesia. *Semin Anesth Periop Med Pain* 2005;24:108–119.
8. De Pinto M, Dunbar PJ, Edwards TW. Pain management. *Anesthesiol Clin North America*. 2006;24:19–37.
9. Grass JA. Patient-controlled analgesia. *Anesth Analg* 2005;101:S44–S61.
10. Fugere F. Patient controlled analgesia (PCA): additions or alternatives to morphine. *Anesthesiol Rounds* 2003;2(8).
11. Peng PWH, Tumber PS, Gourlay D. Review article: perioperative management of patients on methadone therapy. *Can J Anesth* 2005;52:513–523.
12. Gajraj NM, Joshi GP. Role of cyclooxygenase-2 inhibitors in postoperative pain management. *Anesthesiol Clin North America* 2005;23:49–72.
13. Kayne AD, Baluch A, Kaye AJ, et al. Pharmacology of cyclooxygenase-2 inhibitors and preemptive analgesia in acute pain management. *Curr Opin Anaesthesiol* 2008;21:439–445.
14. Schug SA, Manopas A. Update on the role of non-opioids for postoperative pain treatment. *Best Pract Res Clin Anaesthesiol* 2007;21:15–30.
15. Remy C, Marret E, Bonnet F. State of the art of paracetamol in *Acute Pain Therapy*. *Curr Opin Anaesthesiol* 2006;19:562–565.
16. Pickering G, Esteve V, Loriot M-A, et al. Acetaminophen reinforces descending inhibitory pain pathways. *Clin Pharmacol Therapeut* 2008;84:47–51.
17. Knotkova H, Pappagallo M. Adjuvant analgesics. *Anesthesiol Clin* 2007;25:775–786.
18. Grond S, Sablotzki A. Clinical pharmacology of tramadol. *Clin Pharmacokine* 2004;43:879–923.

150 Insertion of Peripheral IV

By Larry F. Chu, MD, MS

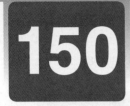

Equipment: Alcohol pad, tourniquet, gauze, 2% lidocaine with 30-g needle, IV catheter, clear dressing, adhesive tape.

Identify anatomy. Hand veins are usually easily visualized, and bifurcation sites on veins can be easier to cannulate. Antecubital veins are usually large and easy to palpate. Explain the procedure to the patient. Always wear gloves and use universal precautions.

A Apply a tourniquet tightly to the arm. Sterile prep with alcohol.

B Place a small local anesthetic wheal proximal to the IV site.

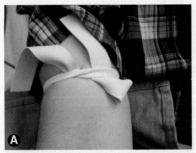
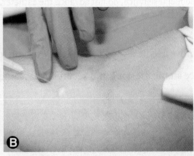

A. A tourniquet is applied tightly to the proximal arm. Loosen the tourniquet if the patient complains of excessive pain. **B.** Insert the 30-gauge needle intradermally and inject a small (0.1 to 0.2 mL) volume of 1% to 2% lidocaine proximal to the planned IV insertion site. It is important not obscure the IV site with the wheal.

C Palpate the vein with one hand and direct the IV with the other.

D Stop when a flash of blood is seen. Advance IV 1 to 2 mm further.*

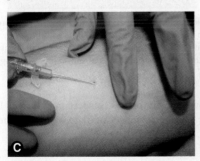
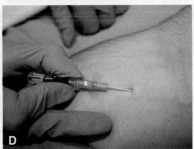

C. Gently palpate the vein with the non-dominant hand. Puncture the skin wheal and advance toward vein. **D.** Stop advancing the catheter when a flash of blood is seen. The needle extends 1 to 2 mm past the catheter tip, so the assembly should be advanced 1 to 2 mm further to ensure the catheter is in the vein.

---

*The needle assembly should be advanced further for large bore IVs.

ANESTHESIA PROCEDURES

E Hold the needle assembly with your dominant hand and advance the catheter into the vein in one smooth motion.

F Release the tourniquet and prepare to connect the catheter to the IV tubing.

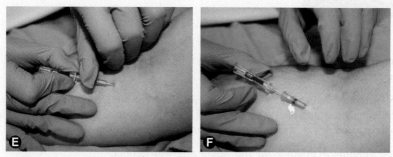

E. Stabilize the needle assembly with your dominant hand and advance the catheter in one smooth motion. A flash of red blood between the catheter and the needle as you advance the catheter into the vein is reassuring. If you feel resistance, do not advance the catheter. **F.** Release the arm tourniquet to minimize bleeding through the catheter when you remove the needle assembly in order to connect the catheter to the IV tubing.

G Remove needle assembly. Attach IV tubing to catheter.

H Place sterile dressing and secure the IV catheter to the skin with adhesive tape.

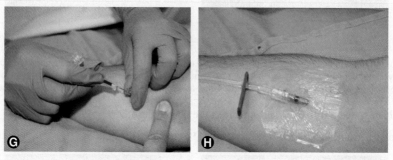

G. Remove the needle assembly from the catheter while stabilizing the catheter site. Applying pressure at the end of the catheter can help prevent bleeding from the catheter when the needle is withdrawn.
H. Attach IV tubing to the catheter and secure the IV with adhesive tape and/or clear adhesive dressing. Additional adhesive tape should be applied to secure the IV to the arm, but is not shown in the photograph so that the IV site can be clearly shown.

Open the IV fluid flow valve to check that free flow to gravity occurs. Suspect an infiltrated IV if the patient complains of pain, fluid does not freely flow to gravity, or if the IV site becomes indurated or swollen.

151

Standard Induction of General Anesthesia

By Larry F. Chu, MD, MS • T. Kyle Harrison, MD

M (**M**achine checked, High flow O₂).
S (**S**uction on, Yankauer catheter at patient's head).
M (**M**onitors on, NIBP every minute, baseline measurement).
A (**A**irway equipment ready and available).
I (**I**V access and free flow IV with adequate fluid in bag).
D (**D**rugs for induction of anesthesia ready and available).
S (**S**pecial—extra equipment for case).

A Re-check anesthesia machine and OR setup (see MSMAIDS).

B Place ASA standard monitors on patient.

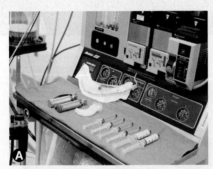
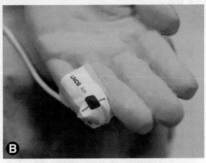

A. Check the anesthesia machine, verify high-flow O₂, suction, airway equipment, drugs according to the MSMAIDS meumonic above. **B.** ASA standard monitors should be used and placement of pulse oximeter probe (avoid index finger as patients can scratch their eyes inadvertently), EKG, NIPB cuff.

C Reassure patient and explain induction. Preoxygenate.

D Confirm vital signs every minute. **Titrate** induction agent.

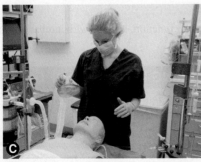
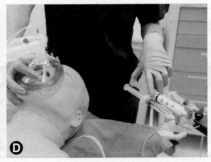

C. Reassure patient and explain induction. Preoxygenate with 100% O₂ 3 minutes or 8 deep breaths over 60 seconds. **D.** Obtain baseline vitals, and check every 1 minute. Titrate IV induction agent to effect.

ANESTHESIA PROCEDURES

1095

E Confirm induction of anesthesia by testing eyelash reflex. Tape eyelids with eye tape.

F Confirm ability to mask ventilate patient. Consider insertion of oral or nasal airways to improve mask ventilation.

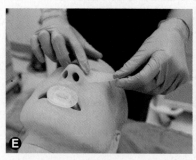 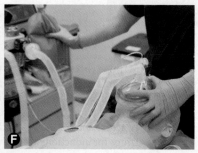

E. Test eyelash reflex to confirm patient is unconscious. Tape eyelids shut to protect eyes from corneal abrasion during airway manipulation and surgery. **F.** Confirm ability to mask ventilate patient.

 If mask ventilation is not possible, call for help! Implement ASA Difficult Airway Algorithm.

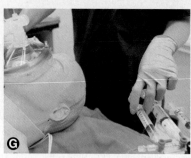 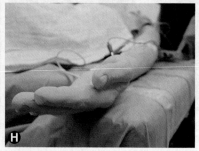

G. Administer neuromuscular blocking agent through the IV. **H.** Attach nerve simulator leads to ulnar aspect of the patient's arm and monitor twitches continuously. Mask ventilate patient while awaiting full neuromuscular blockade in order to produce ideal intubation conditions.

G Administer neuromuscular blocking agent.

H Mask ventilate patient and monitor neuromuscular function. Proceed with intubation when neuromuscular blockade is adequate.

PATIENT CONSIDERATIONS DURING INDUCTION OF GA

1. **Make patient comfortable** (warm room temperature, apply warm blankets when moved to OR table, introduce OR staff).
2. **Reassure patient** during this anxious period of time. Maintain patient modesty by draping body while positioning and applying monitors.

152 Mask Ventilation

By Larry F. Chu, MD, MS • T. Kyle Harrison, MD

Equipment: Anesthesia machine, airway supplies including oral and or nasal airways, face mask, ventilation system.

Mask ventilation of a patient is a vital skill for anesthesiologists

Mask ventilation allows the anesthesiologist time to safely manage and instrument the airway. **Confirm MSMAIDS mnemonic** (see Induction of Anesthesia cognitive aid).

A Preoxygenate patient and induce general anesthesia.

B Place nasal part of mask on nose and lever mask down on face.

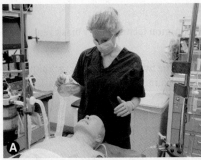 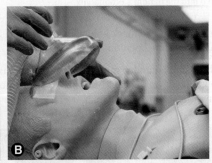

A. Preoxygenation and induction of anesthesia should proceed as previously described (see Induction of anesthesia cognitive aid) **B.** The nasal aspect of mask is placed on the bridge of the nose and the body of the mask is levered down onto the face, covering the nose and mouth.

C The non-dominant hand thumb and index finger hold the mask.

D The remaining fingers pull mandible into mask to open airway.

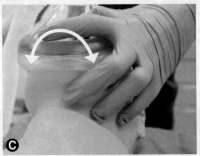 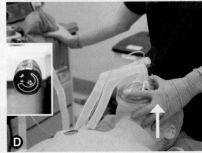

C. The non-dominant thumb and index finger hold the mask, and can rock gently side to side to achieve the best mask seal. **D.** The remaining fingers pull upward on the mandible to open the airway and ease bag ventilation. The machine pop-off valve (inset) can be rotated to adjust airway pressures if needed.

ANESTHESIA PROCEDURES

E An oral airway can be inserted to facilitate mask ventilation. Insert the curved tip toward patient's face.

F Rotate the airway 180 degrees as it is inserted into the oropharynx.

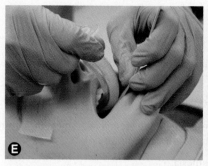
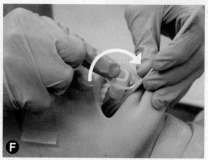

E. An oral airway can be inserted to open airway structures and ease mask ventilation. The airway is inserted with the curved tip pointing toward the patient's face **F.** The airway is rotated 180 degrees as it is fully inserted into the patient's oropharynx.

G A single-handed mask hold with oral airway is a common technique for mask ventilation of patients in the operating room.

H If the single-handed method is inadequate, institute the two-handed mask technique. Place both hands on the mask, thumbs opposite the mask connector. Create firm mask seal with jaw-thrust and chin-lift maneuvers.

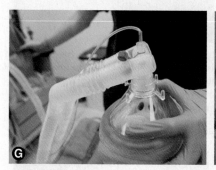
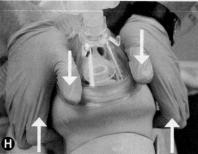

G. Single-handed mask hold with oral airway. **H.** A two-handed mask technique can be employed if difficult mask ventilation is encountered using the single-handed mask hold technique. The metacarpophalangeal (MCP) joints of both thumbs are placed opposite the mask connector. This allows four fingers to create a firm mask seal, while maintaining jaw-thrust and chin-lift maneuvers. This position can be maintained comfortably for prolonged ventilation.

 If mask ventilation is not possible, call for help! Implement ASA Difficult Airway Algorithm.

153

Laryngeal Mask Airway Insertion

By Larry F. Chu, MD, MS • T. Kyle Harrison, MD

Equipment: Laryngeal mask airway, 30 cc air syringe, lubricant, adhesive tape, airway management equipment including face mask, and oral airways.

Confirm MSMAIDS mnemonic (see Induction of Anesthesia cognitive aid).

A Assemble equipment, deflate LMA cuff with air syringe.

B Lubricate LMA cuff.

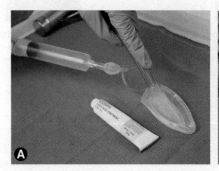
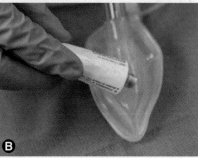

A. Assemble the components necessary for LMA insertion. Deflate the LMA cuff according to the manufacturer's guidelines so that the leading edge is smooth **B.** Lubricate the LMA with lubricant, such as lidocaine ointment.

C Explain the procedure and reassure patient. Induce general anesthesia (see Induction of anesthesia cognitive aid). Place patient in "sniffing" position.

D Open mouth with "scissor" technique using non-dominant hand.

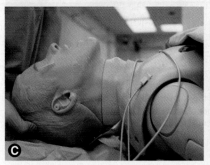
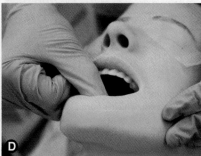

C. Explain procedure and induce general anesthesia. Neuromuscular blockade is usually unnecessary for LMA insertion. Place patient in proper "sniffing" position. **D.** Tilt the patient's head backward (caution in patients with uncleared c-spine injuries) or open mouth with "scissor" technique.

ANESTHESIA PROCEDURES

E Grasp LMA in dominant hand. Flat side of the cuff should face patient's head. Place first finger in space between tube and cuff.

F The leading edge of the cuff should be flat and pressed upward against the hard palate during insertion. Guide LMA above tongue and down oropharynx in a smooth continuous motion.

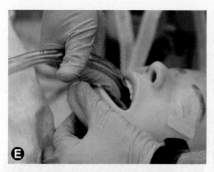
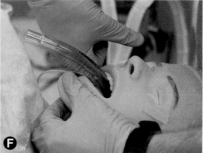

E. Grasp the LMA in your dominant hand with the curved tube and flat side of cuff facing the patient. Place your index finger in the space between the tube and the LMA cuff. F. Insert the LMA into the mouth and press the cuff upward against the hard palate. Guide the cuff above the tongue and down the oropharynx in a smooth motion. Inadequate anesthesia may cause difficulty with insertion of the LMA.

G Stop when resistance is met (7 to 10 cm of LMA should protrude).

H Inflate cuff with approximately 30 cc air. The LMA may slide out of the mouth 1 to 2 cm during inflation. This is normal.

Confirm proper placement of the LMA with bilateral auscultation of breath sounds and capnography. The neck should be auscultated and air leakage should not be heard below 20 cm H_2O, indicating proper positioning of the device. Secure the LMA with adhesive tape.

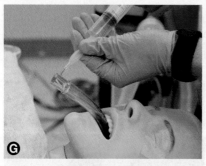
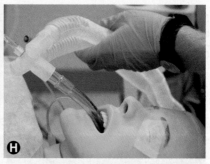

G. Stop advancing LMA when resistance is met. Inflate the cuff with about 30 cc air. The LMA my slide out of the mouth 1 to 2 cm, which is normal. **H.** Confirm proper placement by auscultation and capnography. A leak pressure should be assessed by insuflatting 20 cm H_2O of air pressure through LMA. No air leakage at the patient's neck should be observed.

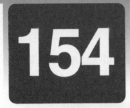

154

Endotracheal Intubation

By Larry F. Chu, MD, MS • T. Kyle Harrison, MD

Equipment: Endotracheal tube (ETT), stylet, air syringe, stethoscope, bag mask ventilation device, adhesive tape.

Confirm MSMAIDS mnemonic (see Induction of Anesthesia cognitive aid).

A Assemble equipment for airway manipulation and intubation.

B Explain procedure and reassure patient. Induce general anesthesia (see Induction of anesthesia cognitive aid). Place patient in "sniffing" position.

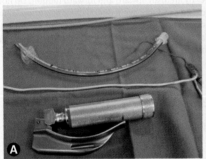
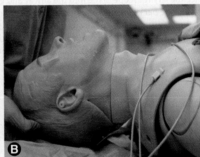

A. Assemble the airway equipment needed for endotracheal intubation, including an ETT, stylet, laryngoscope and Macintosh 3 blade. **B.** Place the patient in the "sniffing" position after induction of anesthesia and establishing optimal neuromuscular blockade and intubating conditions.

C Use right thumb and third finger to "scissor" open mouth widely.

D Insert laryngoscope sweeping tongue aside from right to left.

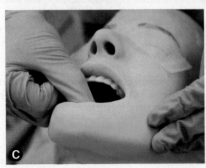
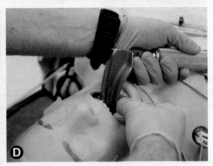

C. Use the right hand to scissor open the mouth with thumb and third finger **D.** Insert the Macintosh laryngoscope blade into the mouth, sweeping the tongue to the side (right to left).

E Advance laryngoscope blade into the airway. Lift in an upward and forward motion toward the corner of the room.

F Once VCs are visualized, advance ETT through glottic opening. Stop advancing when ETT cuff is past the VCs.

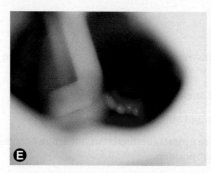 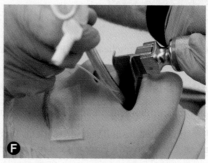

E. Advance the laryngoscope blade into the airway and gently lift in an upward and forward motion. Do not tilt the laryngoscope backward and do not use excessive force. Be careful to avoid dental damage during laryngoscopy. Beginners often do not advance the blade far enough into the Vallecula. Cricoid pressure can assist airway visualization **F.** Once the vocal cords (VC) are visualized, do not take your eyes off glottic opening–have an assistant hand you the ETT. Advance ETT through glottic opening. Stop when cuff is past VCs.

G Inflate the ETT with 2 to 6 cc air to achieve 20 cm H_2O pressure.

H Attach anesthesia circuit to airway connector at end of ETT.

Proper placement should be confirmed by capnography and bilateral auscultation of breath sounds on lung examination.
Secure the ETT with adhesive tape.

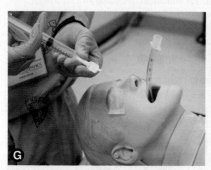 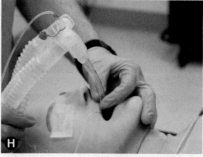

G. Remove ETT stylet. Inflate the ETT cuff with 2 to 6 cc air (cuff pressure can be measured and adjusted to a minimum 20 cm H_2O) **H.** Attach anesthesia circuit to the airway connector at the end of the ETT. Confirm proper placement of the ETT by capnography and auscultation of bilateral breath sounds.

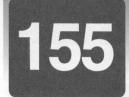
155

Awake Fiber Optic Intubation

By Larry F. Chu, MD, MS • T. Kyle Harrison, MD

Equipment: Airway topicalization supplies, including 4% lidocaine solution. Fiberoptic bronchoscope (FOB), endotracheal tube (ETT), air syringe, and McGill forceps.

Confirm MSMAIDS mnemonic (see Induction of Anesthesia cognitive aid). An assistant should be available throughout procedure.

Ⓐ Assemble equipment for airway anesthesia and intubation.

Ⓑ Explain procedure and reassure patient. Sedate as appropriate. Administer nebulized lidocaine. Consider antisialogogue.

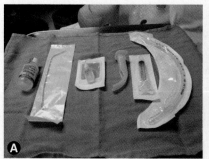
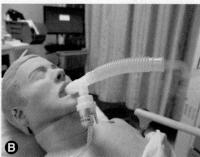

A. Assemble equipment including 4% lidocaine solution, topicalization devices such as spray wand or nebulizer, oral airway, ETT and air syringe. **B.** Nebulized lidocaine is an effective method for topical anesthesia of the airway to tolerate awake fiberoptic intubation (FOI). Ensure total topical lidocaine does not exceed maximum dose of 5 mg/kg. Consider 0.2 mg IV glycopyrrolate antisialogogue.

Ⓒ Lidocaine should also be applied directly to the airway.

Ⓓ Insert an oral airway. The patient should not react or "gag."

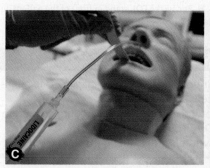
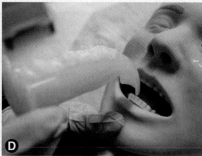

C. Lidocaine should also directly to the airway with a spray wand. **D.** Test adequate airway topicalization by placing oral airway with lidocaine ointment. The patient should not react or "gag."

ANESTHESIA PROCEDURES

E Test the fiberoptic broncho scope (FOB) to ensure that it is functioning properly.

F Remove the airway connector from the end of an ETT and apply lidocaine ointment for lubrication.

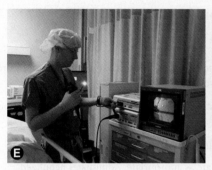 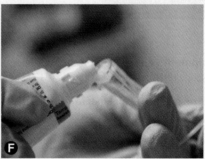

E. Assemble and test the FOB according to the manufacturer's instructions. **F.** Remove the airway connector from the end of an ETT and apply a small amount of lidocaine ointment for lubrication so the ETT will glide smoothly over the FOB.

G Slide lubricated ETT over the FOB. Remove any excess ointment from the FOB. Consider applying anti-fog spray to FOB.

H Elevate the head of the bed. Adjust bed height for easy positioning.

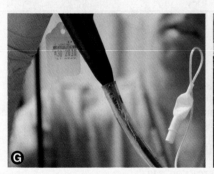 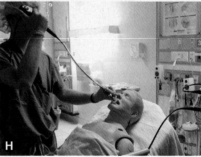

G. Slide the lubricated ETT over the FOB. Remove any excess ointment from the end of the FOB. Consider applying anti-fog spray or liquid to the end of the FOB. **H.** For awake FOI, stand in front of the patient and place video monitor within easy viewing distance. Elevate the head of the patient's bed 45 degrees.

IMPORTANT TASKS DURING FOI

1. An assistant should be present to **continuously monitor** the patient's vital signs during FOI. **Help should be immediately available.**
2. An assistant can titrate sedation, as appropriate during the procedure, under the direction of an anesthesiologist. **AVOID APNEA.**
3. Patient should **breathe spontaneously at all times** during the awake FOI procedure.

I Insert the tip of the FOB through the airway into the mouth.

J Look through the eyepiece or video monitor of the FOB.

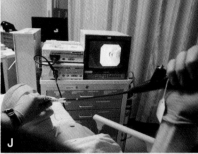

I. Insert tip of the FOB through the airway. **J.** Once the FOB is inserted, focus your attention on the video monitor (or FOB eyepiece) to visualize the airway structures as you advance the FOB.

K Tip of airway and patient's soft palate will come into view as the FOB is advanced into the airway.

L Anteflex (or flex) the tip of the FOB and advance until epiglottis and vocal cords (VCs) come into view.

M Advance through cords.

N Advance the scope past the vocal cords.

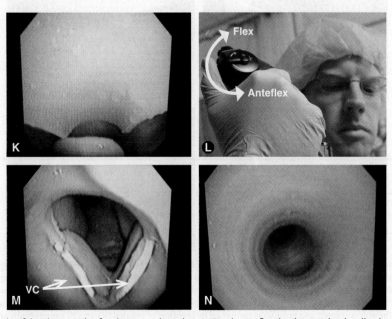

K. The tip of the airway and soft palate come into view. **L.** Gently anteflex the tip to assist visualization of the glottis or epiglottis. You may occasionally need to flex (thumb up) to assist visualization **M.** Advance the FOB under the epiglottis, rotating the scope or flexing the tip to keep the VCs in the middle of the screen. **N.** Advance the scope past the VCs.

O Advance to mid-trachea.

P Advance ETT over FOB into airway in a smooth motion.

Q Confirm placement as FOB is withdrawn from airway.

R Remove FOB from the airway

S Secure ETT with McGill forceps while oral airway is removed over the ETT.

T Reattach airway connector to ETT. Inflate the ETT cuff and re-confirm position by auscultation and capnography.

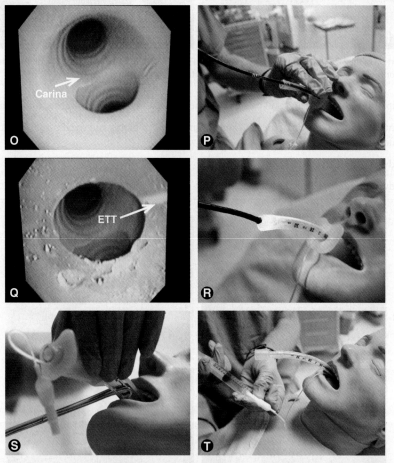

O. Advance FOB until the carina is visualized and stop. **P.** Advance the ETT over the FOB into the airway. If difficulty is encountered, grasp the ETT and rotate 90 degrees counter clockwise to minimize impingement behind arytenoid. **Q.** Confirm proper ETT placement above carina as FOB is withdrawn **R.** Remove FOB from ETT. **S.** Grasp ETT with McGill forceps as the oral airway is removed. **T.** Reattach airway connector to ETT The cuff is inflated and position is confirmed by presence of exhaled CO_2 gas by capnography and auscultation of bilateral breath sounds.

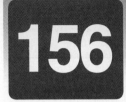

Insertion of Left-Sided Double Lumen Tube

By Larry F. Chu, MD, MS • Vivek Kulkarni, MD • T. Kyle Harrison, MD

Equipment: Appropriately sized double lumen tube (DLT), clamp, fiberoptic bronchoscope, laryngoscope, stethoscope, and standard airway management equipment (see Intubation and Mask Ventilation cognitive aids).

Confirm MSMAIDS mnemonic (see Induction of Anesthesia cognitive aid).

A Assemble equipment for airway instrumentation and intubation.

B Explain procedure and reassure patient. Induce general anesthesia (see Induction cognitive aid). Place patient in "sniffing" position.

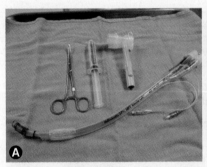
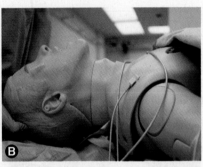

A. Assemble equipment including appropriately sized DLT (Table 156-1) **B.** Explain the procedure to the patient. Confirm MSMAIDS mnemonic. After confirming normal stable vital signs, proceed with induction (see Induction of Anesthesia cognitive aid). Place the patient in the proper "sniffing position."

ANESTHESIA PROCEDURES

Table 156-1

Guidelines for Left-Double Lumen Tube Selection

Tracheal Width (mm)	Recommended Size
>18	41 Fr (M,R,S,P)
>17	41 Fr (M,S) 39 Fr (R,P)
>16	39 Fr (MS) 37 Fr (R,P)
>15.5	37 Fr (MS) 35 Fr (R,P)
>15	35 Fr (M,RS,P)
>14	32 Fr (M)
>13	32 Fr (M)
>12	28 Fr (M)
>11	26 Fr (R)

Manufacturer: M, Mallinckrodt (St. Louis, MO); P, Portex (Keene, NH); R, Rusch (Duluth, GA); S, Sheridan (Argyle, NY).

C Perform direct laryngoscopy under ideal intubating conditions.

D Advance DLT into the airway. Stop when blue cuff passes vocal cords.

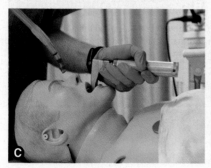
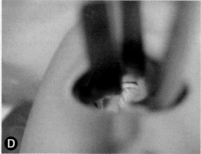

C. Perform direct laryngoscopy to visualize the glottic opening under optimized intubating conditions.
D. Advance the DLT under direct visualization into the airway and stop advancing the DLT when the blue bronchial cuff passes the vocal cords. The tracheal (clear) cuff should be above the vocal cords.

E Remove stylet from the DLT. Rotate DLT 90 degrees counterclockwise and advance with a smooth motion into the airway.

F Attach connectors to end of bronchial (blue) and tracheal (clear) lumens.

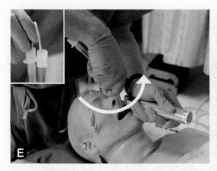
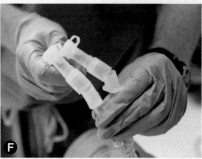

E. Remove stylet from DLT. Rotate DLT 90 degrees counterclockwise as you advance the tracheal cuff through the DLT. This will help direct the end of the DLT with the bronchial cuff into the left mainstem bronchus. **F.** When the tube is inserted to a depth of 29 cm at the lips, attach the tracheal and bronchial lumens to the airway connectors.

G Confirm proper placement by auscultation.

H Confirm proper placement by fiberoptic bronchoscope (FOB) through tracheal lumen.

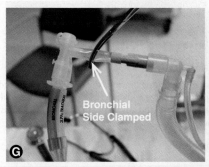
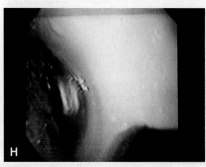

Bronchial
Side Clamped

G. Inflate both tracheal and bronchial cuffs and auscultate bilateral breath sounds. Occlude bronchial lumen and auscultate right-side only breath sounds. Occlude tracheal lumen and auscultate left-side only breath sounds, confirming placement. **H.** Insert FOB through tracheal lumen and visualize only the rim of the blue cuff in the left main bronchus, just beyond the carina, confirming proper placement. If the blue cuff herniates across the carina it is shallow and needs to be advanced until only the blue rim is visible

ANESTHESIA PROCEDURES

Wire Crichothyroidotomy

By Larry F. Chu, MD · Pedro Tanaka, MD

Equipment: Crichothyroidotomy kit including aspiration needle and syringe, wire, scalpel, dilator, and cannula.

Call for help: Call for surgeon capable of performing emergency tracheotomy and have tracheotomy tray immediately available.

Sterile prep the patient's neck. Wear sterile gown, face mask and sterile gloves (*photographs do not show gloves but they should be worn*).

Ⓐ Puncture cricothyroid membrane (CTM) with a needle attached to a 5 mL syringe.

Ⓑ Confirm tracheal entry by aspirating air into the syringe.

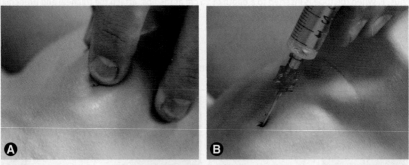

A. The cricothyroid membrane is identified by palpation and is located between the thyroid cartilage and cricoid cartilage. **B.** Insert the aspiration needle through the cartilage and direct 45 degrees caudad while aspirating the saline-filled syringe for the presence of air bubbles. Stop advancing the needle when air is aspirated in the syringe. The needle is now in the trachea.

Ⓒ Insert wire through the needle and remove the needle.

Ⓓ Make a stab incision caudally with a scalpel.

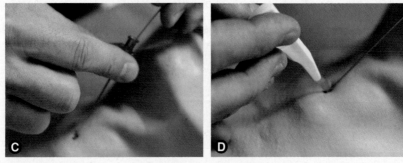

C. Insert the soft (pliable) end of the wire through the needle 3 to 5 cm. **D.** Make a small incision in the skin/cricothyroid membrane holding the scalpel in the caudal direction.

E Assemble the dilator/cannula.

F Pass the assembly device over the wire into the trachea in a smooth motion.

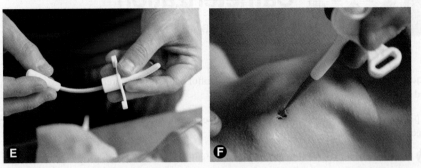

E. Assemble the dilator/cannula by placing the pointed introducer into the cannula. F. Pass the wire through the introducer and advance the assembly into the airway over the wire in a smooth motion.

Ensure the dilator is fully and completely seated inside the airway. Advance the assembly with moderate force over wire through the skin and into the airway.

G Remove the wire and introducer.

H Attach self inflating bag or circuit and ventilate the patient.

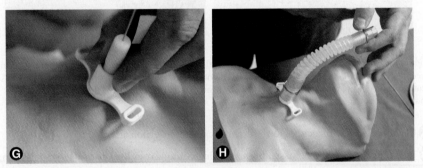

G. Ensure the introducer/assembly is completely seated inside the airway. Remove the dilator and the wire from the airway. H. Attach a self-inflating bag or circuit to the airway device and ventilate the patient.

Confirm ventilation with auscultation of the lung fields and change of color on a CO_2 indicator device.
Secure the airway device to the patient's neck.

158 Radial Artery Catheterization

By Larry F. Chu, MD, MS • T. Kyle Harrison, MD

Equipment: Radial artery catheter, gauze, alcohol pad, suture material, adhesive dressing, and tape.

Explain the procedure to the patient and obtain consent. **Always wear gloves and use universal precautions.**

A Place the wrist in extension as shown. Wrist splints can assist with proper positioning.

B Palpate the radial artery pulse using the fingertips of your non-dominant hand.

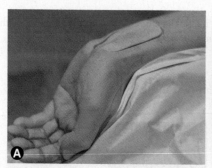
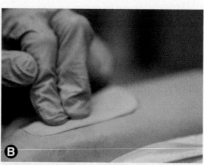

A. Place the wrist in extension as shown. The use of wrist splints can assist with proper positioning during placement. The splint may be removed after placement is accomplished **B.** Palpate the radial artery pulse located 1 to 2 cm from the wrist, between the bony head of the distal radius and the flexor carpi radialis tendon.

C Clean the wrist with alcohol to sterilize the catheter insertion site.

D Insert the needle/catheter assembly at a 45 degree angle over the site of arterial pulsation.

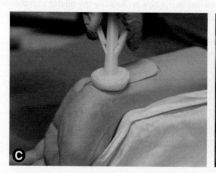
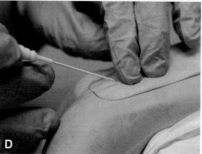

C. Clean the insertion site with alcohol prep. **D.** Insert the needle/catheter assembly into the wrist at the site of arterial pulsation.

E Advance the needle/catheter assembly slowly toward arterial pulse. Stop once arterial blood is observed in the assembly barrel.

F Advance the guide wire by sliding the black tab on the barrel down toward the catheter. Stop if resistance is encountered.

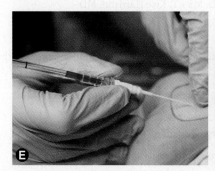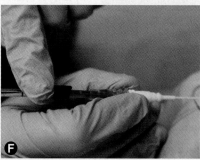

E. Advance the needle/catheter assembly slowly toward the arterial pulsations until a flash of blood is visualized. Stop advancing assembly. **F.** Free flow of arterial blood indicates proper needle placement. Advance guide wire into artery by sliding the black tab down the barrel of the assembly. Do not advance wire if resistance is encountered. Smooth and easy guide wire advancement is reassuring.

G Apply downward pressure on the radial artery at the catheter tip. Remove the needle/wire assembly.

H Attach arterial pressure transducer tubing to the catheter and secure the catheter with sutures to the patient's wrist. Alternatively transparent adhesive dressing and tape can be used.

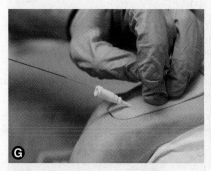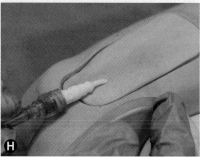

G. Apply pressure to the artery at the catheter tip and remove the needle/wire assembly. **H.** Attach arterial pressure transducer tubing to the catheter and secure with sutures or an adhesive dressing. Confirm proper placement by evaluating arterial pressure waveform on the patient monitors.

Confirm proper placement by evaluating the arterial pressure waveform on the patient monitors.

ANESTHESIA PROCEDURES

1113

159

Central Venous Catheterization

By Larry F. Chu, MD, MS • T. Kyle Harrison, MD

Equipment: Central line kit and full body sterile drape. Ultrasound machine and probe with sterile transducer sheath.

Wear sterile gown, face mask, and sterile gloves. Explain procedure to patient. **Always wear gloves and use universal precautions.**

A Sterile prep the patient's neck. Trendelenberg if possible.

B Place gel on ultrasound (US) probe. Place probe into sterile sheath.

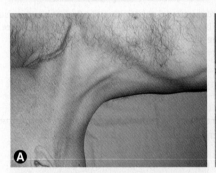
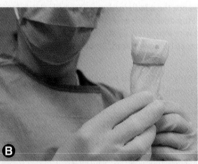

A. If needed and appropriate, Trendelenberg position (head down) can be used to increase venous return to the heart and facilitate central venous cannulation. The neck should be sterile prepped with alcohol.
B. Ultrasound gel should be placed on the probe and covered with a sterile sheath by an assistant.

C Sterile drape neck (not shown). Place the US probe parallel and cephalad to the clavicle between the two heads of the sternocleidomastoid muscle. The internal jugular vein is visualized.

D Puncture the skin at a 45 degree angle and aspirate until the needle is seen on US and a flash of blood is aspirated into syringe.

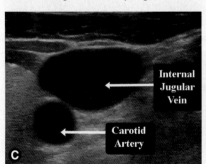
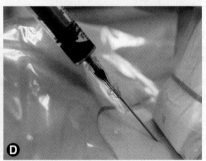

C. The internal jugular vein is easily compressible while the common carotid artery is pulsatile and not compressible. **D.** Advance needle at a 45 degree angle and aspirate needle until blood is aspirated. Stop.

E Prepare wire by retracting the soft tip into the holder.

F Confirm free flow blood and advance the wire through the needle. Monitor EKG. If ventricular ectopy is observed, stop and retract wire.

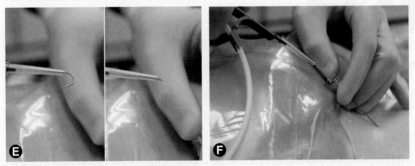

E. Retract wire into the holder. **F.** Confirm free flow venous blood and pass the wire through the needle in a smooth motion. Monitor EKG. If ventricular ectopy is observed, stop and retract wire.

G Advance dilator over wire.

H Nick skin and advance dilator.

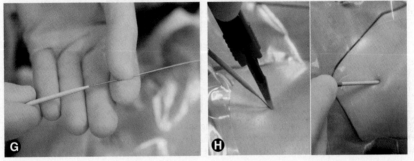

G. Advance dilator over wire, retaining control of wire at all times. **H.** Create a small skin incision at insertion site and advance dilator in a smooth motion. Remove dilator, retaining control of wire.

I Remove dilator, advance catheter over wire.

J Suture catheter.

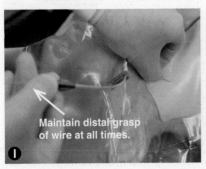
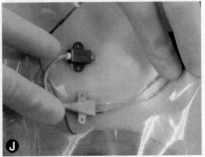

Maintain distal grasp of wire at all times.

I. Advance catheter over wire, grasp wire as it exits catheter. Retract wire from catheter. **J.** Flush lumens of catheter with saline. Secure the catheter with sutures and a dressing.

ANESTHESIA PROCEDURES

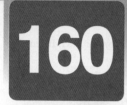

Spinal Anesthesia

Larry F. Chu, MD • Andrea J. Fuller MD • T. Kyle Harrison, MD

Equipment: Spinal anesthesia kit, sterile gloves, mask, and hat.

ASA Standard Monitors should be placed prior to spinal placement. An assistant should be available throughout procedure.

Ⓐ Assemble equipment for spinal placement.

Ⓑ Explain procedure and reassure patient. Sedation as appropriate. Patient positioning is critical for successful placement. Instruct the patient to round his/her back to facilitate spinal placement.

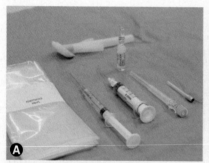
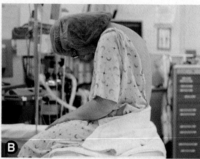

A. Assemble equipment for spinal anesthesia including spinal medications and local anesthetic for skin wheal. **B.** The patient should be instructed to sit with his/her back rounded in order to open the spaces between the spinous processes to facilitate placement of spinal anesthesia.

Ⓒ Examine surface anatomy of the patient's back. Identify the spinous processes on the top of the iliac crests (L4 spinous process).

Ⓓ Sterile prepare the back widely around the L4-5 interspace.

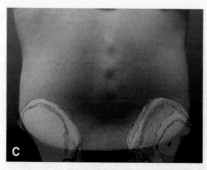
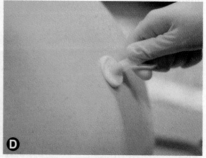

C. The surface anatomy of the back can be examined for spinous process landmarks. The superior margin of the iliac crests can be palpated and represent the approximate level of the L4 spinous process. **D.** Sterile prep the back with sterile prep solution widely around the L3-4 or L4-5 interspace.

E Drape patient. With sterile technique, reconfirm landmarks for lumbar interspace.

F Place a skin wheal of local anesthetic. Infiltrate deeper.

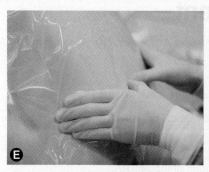 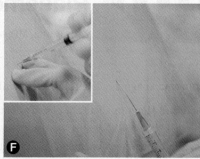

E. Drape the patient and reconfirm L3-4 or L4-5 level. **F.** Inject local anesthetic skin wheal and then redirect the needle through the wheal to infiltrate deeper tissues along the intended spinal needle path.

G Insert introducer needle perpendicular to back, midline.

H Insert spinal needle through introducer until "pop" is felt.

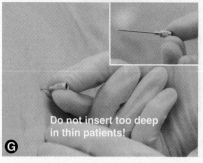 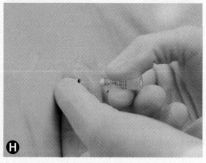

Do not insert too deep in thin patients!

G. Place the introducer perpendicular to the back, midline at L3-4 or L4-5. **H.** Advance the spinal needle until a "pop" is felt, indicating dural puncture. Stop advancing the needle immediately.

I Remove stylet. Observe free flow cerebrospinal fluid (CSF).

J Slowly inject spinal medication.

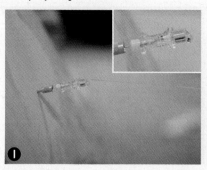 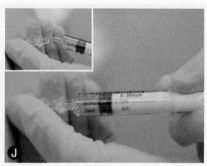

I. Remove the stylet from the spinal needle. Observe free flow CSF fluid, noting absence of blood. **J.** Attach syringe with spinal medications. Aspirate slightly to reconfirm CSF flow, then inject medication while stabilizing needle at the introducer. Aspirate at the end to reconfirm the full dose was administered.

ANESTHESIA PROCEDURES

161

Lumbar Epidural Placement

Larry F. Chu, MD, MS • Andrea J. Fuller, MD • T. Kyle Harrison, MD

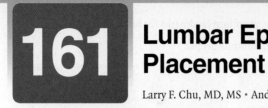

Equipment: Epidural catheterization kit, sterile gloves, mask, and hat.

ASA Standard Monitors should be placed prior to epidural placement. An assistant should be available throughout procedure.

A Assemble equipment for epidural placement.
Explain procedure and reassure patient. Sedation as appropriate.

B Patient positioning is critical for successful placement. Instruct the patient to round his/her back to facilitate epidural placement.

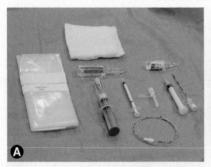
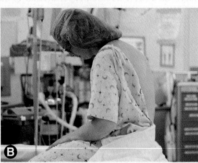

A. Assemble equipment for epidural including saline for loss of resistance syringe and local anesthetic for skin wheal. **B.** The patient should be instructed to sit with his/her back rounded in order to open the spaces between the spinous processes to facilitate epidural catheter placement.

C The back should be sterile prepped widely around L4-5 interspace.

D Place sterile drape. With sterile technique, palpate L4 spinous process (level of iliac crests). Inject local anesthetic wheal in the interspace.

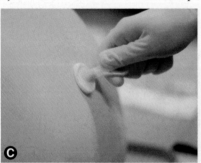
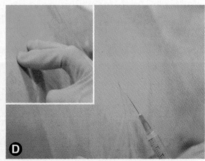

C. The back should be widely sterile prepped with sterile prep solution. **D.** The L4 spinous process should be palpated (level with the top of the iliac crests) and a small local anesthetic wheal injected in the L4-5 interspace. Local anesthetic can be infiltrated deeper through the skin wheal. 2% lidocaine can be used.

E The Tuohy epidural needle should be inserted midline.

F Once the Tuohy is seated into interspinous ligament (1 to 2 cm), remove stylet.

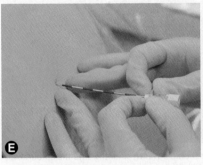
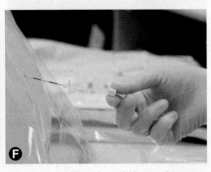

E. The Tuohy needle should be inserted perpendicular to the back, midline, through the L4-5 interspace.
F. Once the Tuohy needle has passed subcutaneous tissues and is firmly seated in ligament (a "crunching" sensation is felt), the stylet can be removed.

G A saline-filled loss of resistance (LOR) syringe should be attached to the Tuohy needle. Apply gentle constant pressure to the plunger as the Tuohy needle is advanced through ligament by the non-dominant hand.

H As ligamentum flavum is encountered an increase in resistance may be felt, followed by a sudden LOR. Stop.

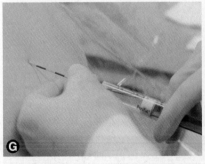
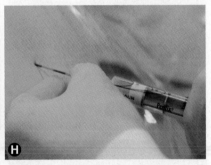

G. A saline-filled loss of resistance syringe should be attached to the Tuohy and slowly advanced while constant gentle pressure is applied to the plunger. H. Resistance to the plunger will suddenly decrease when the epidural space is entered (loss of resistance, LOR). Stop. Note the depth of LOR.

PATIENT CONSIDERATIONS DURING EPIDURAL PLACEMENT

1. **Make patient comfortable** (warm room temperature, apply warm blankets when moved to OR table, introduce OR staff).
2. **Reassure patient** during this anxious period of time. Maintain patient modesty by draping body while positioning and applying monitors.

ANESTHESIA PROCEDURES

1119

I Place catheter into Tuohy needle. (For CSE, first do Steps **O** to **T**.)

J The catheter should advance smoothly into the epidural space.

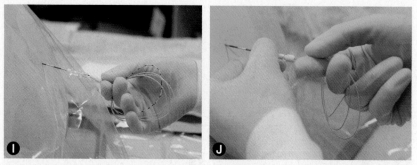

I. Epidural catheter is placed into Tuohy. **J.** The catheter should advance smoothly into the epidural space. If resistance is felt, consider dilating the epidural space with saline or repeating LOR technique.

K The needle can be removed after 15 to 20 cm has been threaded into the epidural space. Provide counter-traction on catheter.

L Once needle has been removed, pull the catheter out until 5 cm remains in the epidural space.

M Aspirate the catheter.

N Cap/label catheter.

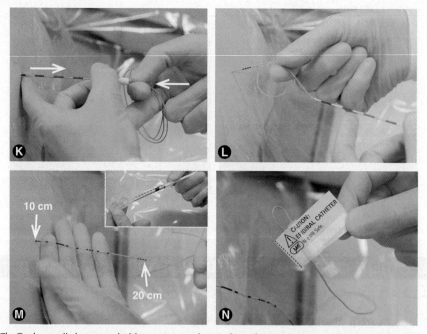

K. The Tuohy needle is removed with counter-traction on the catheter to prevent catheter migration during needle removal. **L.** Once the needle is removed, pull the catheter out until 5 cm remains in the epidural space. **M.** Aspirate the catheter with a 1 cc syringe to confirm absence of cerebrospinal fluid (CSF) (intrathecal) or blood (intravascular). **N.** Place a cap and label on the end of the catheter.

E Place a Tuohy needle into the epidural space (Steps **A-E**).

O Prepare spinal needle (SN).

P Insert SN through Tuohy needle until a "pop" is felt

Q Remove stylet.

R Observe CSF flow.

S Aspirate CSF, then slowly inject spinal medication.

T Remove SN.

G Go to Steps **K–N**.

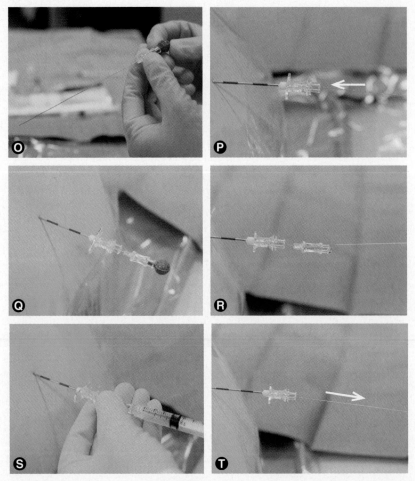

O. Prepare a 26-27 pencil point spinal needle (SN) by loosening the stylet. **P.** Advance the SN through the Tuohy from Step **E. Q.** Continue to advance the SN until a "pop" is felt, at which point stop advancing the needle. **R.** Remove the stylet from the SN and observe free flow CSF to gravity. **S.** Stabilize Tuohy needle and attach a syringe containing spinal medications (Luer lock preferable), being careful not to inadvertently reposition the SN. Gently inject the spinal medication through the SN. **T.** Remove SN from the Tuohy needle.

ANESTHESIA PROCEDURES

162 Transesophageal Echocardiography Basic Views

Prairie Neeley Robinson, MD • Nathaen Weitzel, MD

Intraoperative transesophageal echocardiography (TEE) is widely used in modern operating rooms as it provides valuable real time information to the surgical team. The TEE allows intraoperative decisions to be made based on data collected throughout the procedure instead of waiting until after the case to evaluate surgical outcomes. Outcomes have been shown to improve secondary to intraoperative TEE evaluation specifically in cardiac valvular surgery (1), which has promoted the routine use in most cardiac cases today. The anesthesiologist performs the TEE at most institutions intraoperatively and may perform exams in emergency situations in noncardiac operating rooms or locations such as the intensive care unit. Therefore, it is useful for all anesthesiologists to have basic knowledge of the TEE and the intraoperative exam.

READ MORE

ASE/SCA 20 view exam overview, Chapter 168, page 1161

1) **TEE exam basics:** A TEE exam is performed by placing the TEE probe into the esophagus.

    a) Placement: Consider placing an orogastric tube first to suction the gastric contents; then use a lubricant jelly and a mouth/bite guard when placing the probe.

    b) **Relative contraindications:** Patient history of: mediastinal radiation, dysphagia, recent upper gastrointestinal surgery or bleeding. Known esophageal pathology is also a relative contraindication including stricture, varices, tumor, diverticulum, or esophagitis.

2) **TEE views**

The basic TEE exam consists of 20 views adapted from Shanewise et al. (2) **(Fig. 162-1).** These are the basic views used by anesthesiologists to evaluate the heart in the operating room. Not every view is utilized in every patient, but it is useful to know the structures present and how to obtain each view. Each of the 20 views is described in this chapter as well as how to obtain the view. The views are discussed as they are found cephalad to caudad in the esophagus. There are markings of the depth in centimeters on the TEE probe. The depth is usually measured at the patient's incisors.

| **Figure 162-1** | Twenty Views of the Recommended Comprehensive TEE Exam |

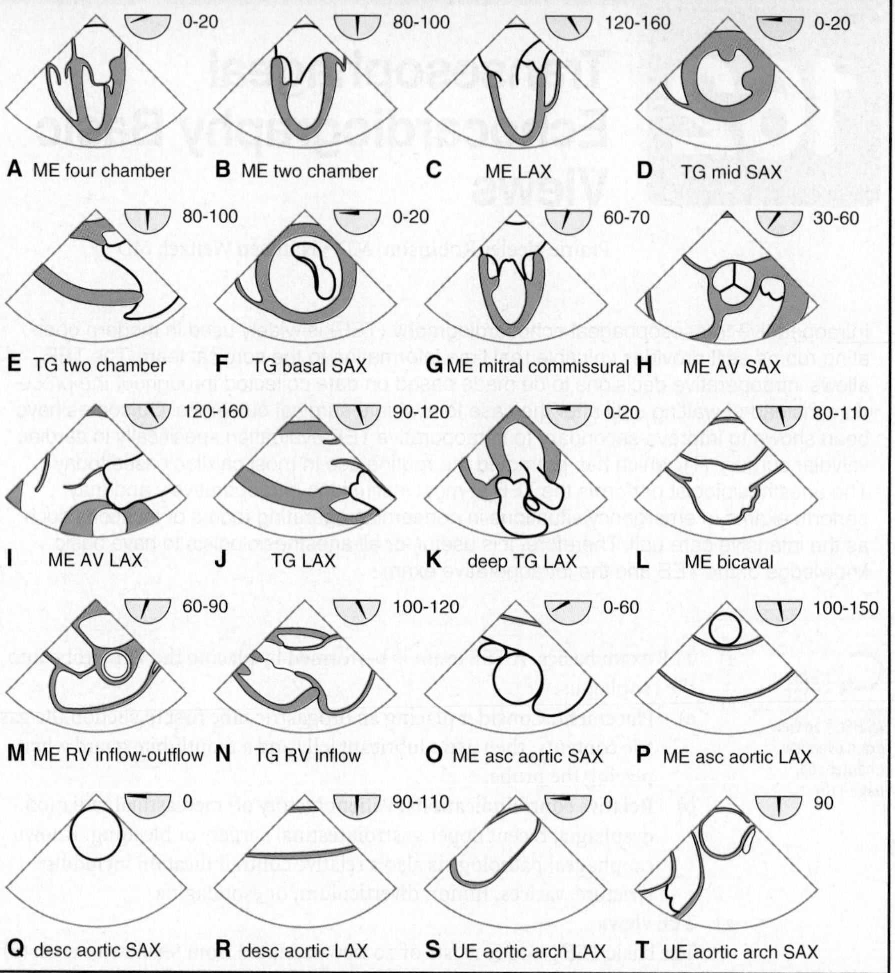

A ME four chamber 0-20
B ME two chamber 80-100
C ME LAX 120-160
D TG mid SAX 0-20

E TG two chamber 80-100
F TG basal SAX 0-20
G ME mitral commissural 60-70
H ME AV SAX 30-60

I ME AV LAX 120-160
J TG LAX 90-120
K deep TG LAX 0-20
L ME bicaval 80-110

M ME RV inflow-outflow 60-90
N TG RV inflow 100-120
O ME asc aortic SAX 0-60
P ME asc aortic LAX 100-150

Q desc aortic SAX 0
R desc aortic LAX 90-110
S UE aortic arch LAX 0
T UE aortic arch SAX 90

Reproduced from Shanewise js, Cheung at, Aronson S, et al. Ase/Sca guidelines for performing a comprehensive intraoperative multiplane transesophageal echocardiography examination. *Anesth Analg* 1999;89:870–884, with permission.

Upper Esophageal 20 to 25 cm

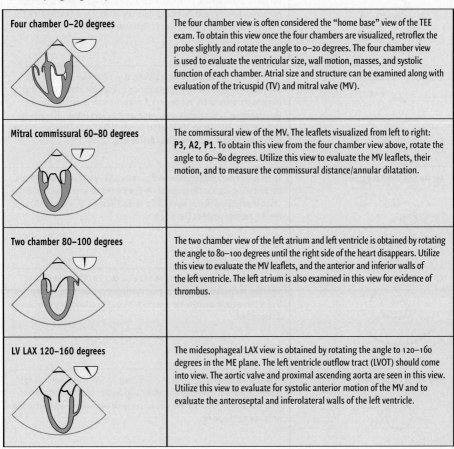

Aortic arch LAX 0 degree	The long axis (LAX) view of the aortic arch. It is typically found after imaging the descending thoracic aorta. The probe is withdrawn and the thoracic aorta is followed superiorly until the arch is in view. This view is useful to look for aortic pathology including atherosclerotic plaques, mobile plaques, calcification and dissections.
Aortic arch SAX 90 degrees	The short axis (SAX) view of the aortic arch. It is found similarly to the above view of the arch in LAX. Once the LAX is in view, rotate the angle to 90 degrees to obtain the SAX view. The aortic arch is seen along with the subclavian artery. The pulmonary valve and main pulmonary artery are seen in LAX. The aorta is evaluated for pathology in this view similarly to the LAX aortic arch view above.

Mid Esophageal 30 to 40 cm

Four chamber 0–20 degrees	The four chamber view is often considered the "home base" view of the TEE exam. To obtain this view once the four chambers are visualized, retroflex the probe slightly and rotate the angle to 0–20 degrees. The four chamber view is used to evaluate the ventricular size, wall motion, masses, and systolic function of each chamber. Atrial size and structure can be examined along with evaluation of the tricuspid (TV) and mitral valve (MV).
Mitral commissural 60–80 degrees	The commissural view of the MV. The leaflets visualized from left to right: **P3, A2, P1.** To obtain this view from the four chamber view above, rotate the angle to 60–80 degrees. Utilize this view to evaluate the MV leaflets, their motion, and to measure the commissural distance/annular dilatation.
Two chamber 80–100 degrees	The two chamber view of the left atrium and left ventricle is obtained by rotating the angle to 80–100 degrees until the right side of the heart disappears. Utilize this view to evaluate the MV leaflets, and the anterior and inferior walls of the left ventricle. The left atrium is also examined in this view for evidence of thrombus.
LV LAX 120–160 degrees	The midesophageal LAX view is obtained by rotating the angle to 120–160 degrees in the ME plane. The left ventricle outflow tract (LVOT) should come into view. The aortic valve and proximal ascending aorta are seen in this view. Utilize this view to evaluate for systolic anterior motion of the MV and to evaluate the anteroseptal and inferolateral walls of the left ventricle.

(continued)

Mid Esophageal 30 to 40 cm (Continued)

AV SAX 30–50 degrees	The aortic valve SAX view (AV SAX) is obtained in the ME plane usually at 30–50 degrees. Adjust the probe depth until the AV is centered in screen. In this view, all three cusps of the AV can be visualized. The noncoronary cusp is adjacent to the interatrial septum, the right coronary cusp is anterior, and the remaining cusp is left. The right and left coronary arteries can often be visualized superior to their corresponding cusp. Utilize this view to evaluate the aortic valve cusps for prolapse, calcification, restriction, and for aortic insufficiency.
AV LAX 120–150 degrees	The aortic valve LAX view (AV LAX) can be obtained by starting from the AV SAX view and rotating the angle to 120–150 degrees. Utilize this view to examine the aortic valve movement, prolapse, restriction, calcification, and for aortic insufficiency using color flow Doppler. In addition, this view is used to measure the annulus, sinus, and ascending aorta.
RV Inflow–Outflow 60–90 degrees	This is the right ventricle (RV) inflow-outflow view. To obtain this view, start at the four chamber view and rotate the probe to the right until the TV is in the center of the screen. Then rotate the angle to 60–90 degrees to see the pulmonic valve (PV) and the main pulmonary artery. The RV outflow tract is well visualized. Utilize this view to evaluate the TV and PV.
Bicaval 80–110 degrees	To obtain the midesophageal bicaval view, start at the four chamber view and **rotate** the probe to the right, centering on the right atrium (RA). Then increase the angle to 80–110 degrees. Utilize this view to evaluate the RA, the inferior vena cava (left) and the superior vena cava (right). This view is also useful to evaluate for atrial septal defects (ASDs). A bubble study can be performed while in this view to look for the ASD.
Asc Ao SAX 0–60 degrees	To obtain the midesophageal ascending aortic SAX view (Asc Ao SAX), locate the ascending aorta in the center of the screen, and advance or withdraw the probe to examine different levels of the aorta. The main PA and right PA and the SVC are also visualized here.
Asc Ao LAX 100–150 degrees	The midesophageal ascending aortic LAX view (Asc Ao LAX) is obtained by adjusting the multiplane angle to 100–150 degrees from the Asc Ao SAX view. Utilize this view to examine the aorta in LAX as well as the right pulmonary artery in SAX.
Desc Ao SAX 0 degrees	To obtain the descending aortic SAX view (Desc Ao SAX), begin with the four chamber view and turn the probe left by ~90 degrees until the aorta comes into view. The length of the thoracic aorta can be examined by advancing and withdrawing the probe.

Desc Ao LAX 90 degrees 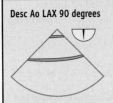	To obtain the descending aortic LAX view (Desc Ao LAX), start with the Desc Ao SAX view and adjust the multiplane angle to 90 degrees. Utilize this view to complement the SAX evaluation of the descending aorta.

Transgastric 40 to 45 cm

TG basal MV SAX 0–20 degrees	The transgastric views are obtained by advancing the probe into the stomach and strongly anteflexing the tip. The basal MV SAX view (Basal MV SAX) is located superior/proximal to the Mid SAX view and corresponds to the basal segments of the left ventricle. Utilize this view to evaluate the MV.
TG Mid SAX 0–20 degrees	The transgastric mid SAX view (TG Mid SAX) is obtained by advancing the probe from the ME plane or TG Basal view until the papillary muscles are visualized. Anteflexion is typically required. Utilize this view to evaluate global ventricular function, monitor regional wall motion abnormalities, and assess volume status (preload) of the LV.
TG two chamber 80–100 degrees	This is the transgastric two chamber view. To obtain this view from the TG Mid SAX view, adjust the multiplane angle to between 80–100 degrees. Utilize this view to evaluate the MV, chordae tendinae, MV leaflets, along with the anterior (bottom) and inferior (top) left ventricular walls.
LV LAX 90–120 degrees	This is the transgastric left ventricular LAX view. To obtain this view from the above image, further advance the multiplane angle to 120 degrees. Utilize this view to evaluate the AV and LVOT, especially to take measure gradients through the AV.
RV inflow 100–120 degrees	This is the RV inflow view. To obtain this view, rotate the probe to the right from the mid SAX view. Utilize this view to examine the RA, RV, TV, and papillary muscle.

Deep Transgastric 45 to 50 cm

Deep TG LAX 0–20 degrees 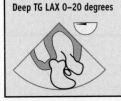	This is the deep transgastric LAX (TG LAX) view. To obtain this view, advance the probe in the neutral position deep into the stomach and maximally ante-flex the probe. Then slowly withdraw the probe until it contacts the stomach wall. Utilize this view to interrogate the aortic valve and LVOT, again like the **LV LAX**, a useful view for the measurement of aortic valve gradients.

TRANSESOPHAGEAL ECHOCARDIOGRAPHY

The 20 views above are important for every anesthesiologist to understand and be able to recognize cardiac structures. TEE is an excellent tool to evaluate cardiac function and pathology in the OR as well outside the OR.

References

1. Marymont J, Murphy GS. Intraoperative monitoring with transesophageal echocardiography: indications, risks, and training. *Anesthesiol Clin* 2006;24:737–753.
2. Shanewise JS, Cheung AT, Aronson S, et al. ASE/SCA guidelines for performing a comprehensive intraoperative multiplane transesophageal echocardiography examination: recommendations of the American Society of Echocardiography Council for Intraoperative Echocardiography and the Society of Cardiovascular Anesthesiologists Task Force for Certification in Perioperative Transesophageal Echocardiography. *Anesth Analg* 1999;89:870–884.

TEE Evaluation of the Aortic Valve

Prairie Neeley Robinson, MD • Nathaen Weitzel, MD

Aortic valve (AV) replacement is a common surgical procedure in the cardiac operating room. A complete transesophageal echocardiographic (TEE) exam is important to determine etiology of AV disease as well as severity. An overview of the basic TEE evaluation techniques for both regurgitant and stenotic lesions is presented.

READ MORE

Evaluation of aortic valve, Chapter 171, page 1170

1) **TEE evaluation of the AV:** The real time evaluation of the heart prior to and following bypass is an invaluable tool in the operating room both to the surgeon and the anesthesiologist.

a) **Basic anatomy:** The AV is a semilunar valve with three cusps. The cusps are named for the coronary artery that exits superior to them. Therefore, there is a right coronary cusp that sits anteriorly, a noncoronary cusp (NCC) which is closest to the interatrial septum and a left coronary cusp. Key anatomic features associated with the AV are the left ventricular outflow tract (LVOT) and the aortic root.

   i) The **LVOT** is the outflow region of the left ventricle (LV) immediately inferior to the valve.

   ii) The **aortic root** refers to the AV annulus, cusps, sinuses of Valsalva, coronary artery ostia, sinotubular junction, and proximal ascending aorta (**Fig. 163-1**).

2) **TEE views of the AV**

   The TEE exam for the AV uses the following four views from the ASE/SCA 20 TEE views (1)

a) **Mid esophageal AV short axis view**—This cross-section view of the AV allows the echocardiographer to view all three cusps of the valve at one time. In this view, the cusp adjacent to the atrial septum is the NCC, the most anterior cusp is the right coronary cusp, and the remaining cusp is the left coronary cusp. This view can be used to measure the area of the AV using planimetry. Color Doppler can be used here to evaluate aortic insufficiency, or prosthetic ring abnormalities following AV replacement.

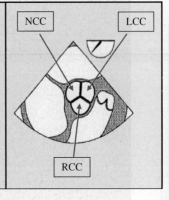

TRANSESOPHAGEAL ECHOCARDIOGRAPHY

b) **Mid esophageal AV long axis view**—This view is useful to assess aortic regurgitation (AR) using color flow Doppler, along with evidence of turbulent flow seen in aortic stenosis. It is also used to assess the aortic root measuring the diameters of the AV annulus, sinuses of Valsalva, sinotubular junction, and the proximal ascending aorta.

c) **Transgastric long axis view**—Utilize this view to obtain Doppler quantification of blood flow through the LVOT and AV.

d) **Deep transgastric view**—Like the transgastric LAX view, this image is used to obtain Doppler quantification of flow velocities in the LVOT, AV, and can be useful in measuring elevated gradients for patients with LVOT obstruction, (HOCM patients, or patients with systolic anterior motion of the mitral valve). Also, a good view for measuring pressure half-time of the AR Doppler tracing. Finally, this view can provide good imaging in patients with prosthetic AV or MV where there are significant artifacts at the ME levels, but the deep transgastric approach avoids this.

Figure 163-1 Long Axis View of LVOT

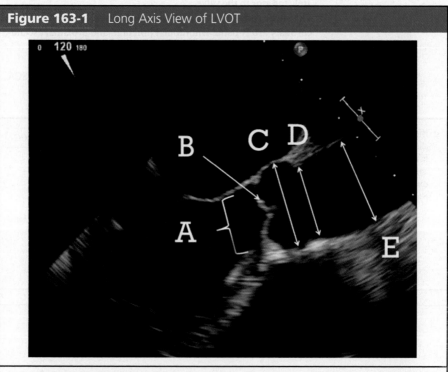

ME LAX view showing the LVOT (**A**), aortic valve (**B**), sinus of valsalva (**C**), sinotubular junction (**D**), and ascending aorta (**E**).

Table 163-1
Aortic Regurgitation (3)

	Mild	Moderate	Severe
Qualitative			
Angiographic data	1+	2+	3–4+
Color Doppler jet width	Central jet, width <25% of LVOT	Greater than mild, but no signs of severe AR	Central jet, width >65% LVOT
Doppler vena contracta width (cm)	<0.3	0.3–0.6	>0.6
Quantitative (cath or echo)			
Regurgitant volume (mL/beat)	<30	30–59	≥60
RF (%)	<30	30–49	≥50
ROA (cm²)	<0.1	0.1–0.29	≥0.3
Pressure half-time (ms)	>500	200–500	<200
Additional Criteria			
LV size			Increased
Aortic diastolic flow reversal			Holodiastolic flow reversal

Source: Adapted from Bonow RO, Carabello BA, Chatterjee K, et al. ACC/AHA 2006 Guidelines for the management of patients with valvular heart disease: executive summary. *Circulation* 2006;114.

3) **Aortic regurgitation**

AR describes an AV that is incompetent and allows reversal of blood flow into the LV during diastole. For assessment and quantification of AR, see Table 163-1.

a) **Qualitative measures**: The Color Doppler jet width and vena contracta represent the main tools in assessing the severity of AI.

b) **Quantitative assessment**: A quantitative assessment of the valve is undertaken by calculating the regurgitant volume, regurgitant fraction (RF), and regurgitant orifice area (ROA).

Quantitative echocardiography, Chapter 165, page 1143

i) The **regurgitant volume** is the difference between the LV stroke volume and the right ventricular (RV) stroke volume.

$$RV_{AV} = SV_{LV} - SV_{RV}$$

The LV stroke volume is calculated by multiplying the cross-sectional area of the LVOT by the velocity time integral (VTI) of LVOT flow. The LVOT VTI can be obtained using pulsed wave Doppler at the LVOT (**Fig. 163-2**).

Calculate the RV stroke volume similarly by multiplying the cross-sectional area of the pulmonary out flow tract by the VTI measured in the proximal pulmonary artery. This technique is time consuming and requires multiple measurements leading to possible error and thus is used infrequently.

ii) The **RF** is the regurgitant volume divided by the forward flow or cardiac output. **Cardiac output = HR × SV.**

iii) The **pressure half-time** is defined as the time interval between the maximal regurgitant pressure gradient and the time when the gradient is half of the maximum (**Fig. 163-3**). To obtain this measurement, use either the

Figure 163-2	Pulsed Wave Doppler Evaluation of AV

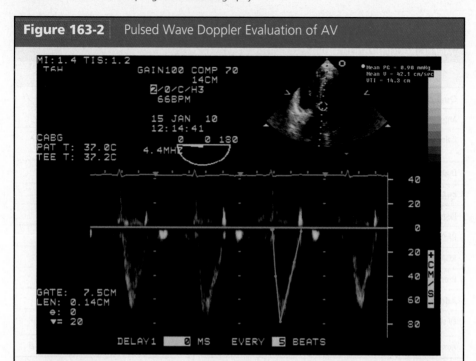

This is the deep transgastric view with pulse wave Doppler across the AV. A VTI can be measured in this view by outlining the Doppler flow. The VTI is used to calcuate the stroke volume by multiplying it by the LVOT area.

Figure 163-3	Continuous Wave Doppler Evaluation of AV

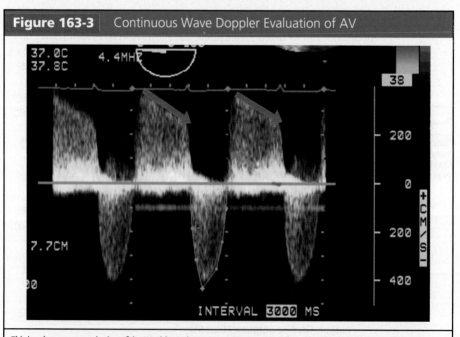

This is a deep transgastric view of the AV with continuous wave Doppler across the valve. There is AR in the patient as seen by the reversal of flow during diastole. The arrows represent the pressure half-time measurement, with an average value of 375 milliseconds, indicating moderate aortic insufficiency.

Table 163-2
Aortic Stenosis

Indicator	Mild	Moderate	Severe
Peak Jet velocity (m/s)	<3.0	3.0–4.0	>4.0
Mean gradient (mm Hg)	<25	25–40	>40
Valve area (cm²)	>1.5	1.0–1.5	<1.0
Valve area index (cm²/m²)			<0.6

Sources: Adapted from Bonow RO, Carabello BA, Chatterjee K, et al. ACC/AHA 2006 guidelines for the management of patients with valvular heart disease: executive summary. Circulation 2006;114; Perrino A, Reeves S. *Transesophageal Echocardiography*. Philadelphia, PA: Lippincott Williams & Wilkins; 2008.

transgastric long axis view or the deep transgastric view. A pressure half-time <200 milliseconds indicates severe AR.

iv) **Aortic flow reversal:** Measurement of aortic flow in the descending aorta is an adjunct measure of AR severity. Presence of holodiastolic flow reversal in the descending aorta confirms severe AR.

4) **Aortic valve stenosis (AS)**

AS is the narrowing of the AV orifice, typically due to calcification/sclerosis of the valve leaflets. The normal area of an AV in an adult is 2.6 to 3.5 cm². **Severe AS is defined as a valve area <1.0 cm² or a mean gradient >40 mm Hg.** Table 163-2 describes the criteria for grading aortic stenosis (2).

a) **Quantitative measures**

i) **Bernoulli equation:** To calculate the above values and estimate the severity of aortic stenosis, use the modified Bernoulli equation to measure the gradient across the valve and the continuity equation to measure the AV area. To obtain the peak velocity, place the continuous wave Doppler beam parallel to the flow of blood across the AV in the deep transgastric view **(Fig. 163-4)**. With this velocity, use the modified Bernoulli equation to calculate the mean gradient.

READ MORE

Quantitative echocardiography, Chapter 165, page 1143

Peak gradient (mm Hg) = 4 (aortic peak velocity)²

Mean gradient (mm Hg) = 4 (mean velocity)²

$$= 2.4 \ (V_{max})^2$$

ii) **The continuity equation**

LVOT stroke volume = AV Stroke volume

Stroke volume = CSA × VTI

The equation rearranges to:

$$VTI_{LVOT} \times area_{LVOT} = VTI_{AV} \times area_{AV}$$
$$Area_{AV} = VTI_{LVOT} \times area_{LVOT} \div VTI_{AV}$$

The LVOT velocity is obtained from the deep transgastric view; however, use the pulsed wave Doppler placed directly in the LVOT to obtain this Doppler tracing.

iii) **Planimetry**

The area of the valve can also be measured using planimetry in systole by measuring the narrowest orifice of the valve. Planimetric techniques are not considered as accurate as the continuity equation in severely calcified and sclerotic valves as significant shadowing can result in errors in measurement. Despite this, planimetry can provide a rapid estimate of valve area **(Fig. 163-5)**.

Figure 163-4 Deep Transgastric View of the AV Using Continuous Wave Doppler

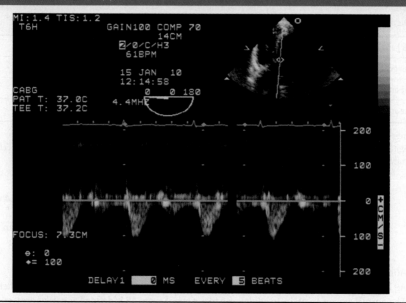

This CW Doppler across the AV is used to measure a peak velocity. The peak velocity measurement is then used to calculate a peak pressure by the equation:

Peak gradient (mm Hg) = 4 (peak velocity)²

A high gradient indicates a stenotic valve.

Figure 163-5 Planimetry of AV in the Short Axis

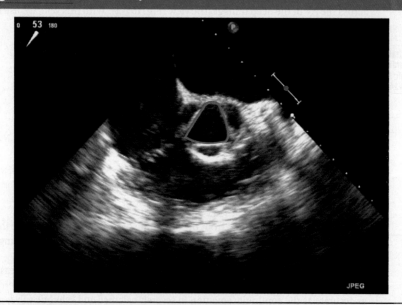

The short axis view of the AV is used to estimate valve area using planimetry. The valve area is outlined using software on the tee machine. This is a quick estimate of area most useful in normal valves. Calcified and stenotic valve area is difficult to measure with this method.

References

1. Shanewise JS, Cheung AT, Aronson S, et al. ASE/SCA Guidelines for performing a comprehensive intraoperative multiplane transesophageal echocardiography examination. *Anesth Analg* 1999;89:870–884.
2. Bonow RO, Carabello BA, Chatterjee K, et al. ACC/AHA 2006 Guidelines for the management of patients with valvular heart disease: executive summary: a report of the American College of Cardiology/American Heart Association Task Force on Practice Guidelines. *Circulation* 2006; 114 (5):e84-231.
3. Perrino A, Reeves S. *Transesophageal Echocardiography*. Philadelphia, PA: Lippincott Williams & Wilkins; 2008.

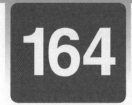

164

TEE Evaluation of the Mitral Valve

Prairie Neeley Robinson, MD • Nathaen Weitzel, MD

Mitral valve surgery remains a mainstay in the cardiothoracic surgical arena. New interventional approaches are also in practice and development for mitral valve repair. These procedures require the anesthesiologist to have a solid understanding of the mitral valve anatomy both for physiologic management as well as TEE interpretation.

READ
MORE

Evaluation of the mitral valve, Chapter 170, page 1168

1) **Anatomy**

The mitral valve separates the left atrium from the left ventricle. Two leaflets make up the mitral valve—the anterior and posterior leaflets. The anterior leaflet makes up approximately 55% of the surface area of the valve, while the posterior leaflet makes up approximately 45%. The leaflets meet at the anterolateral and posteromedial commissures. The valve is surrounded by a fibromuscular ring called the mitral annulus (Fig. 164-1).

Figure 164-1 Schematic of the Mitral Valve Illustrating the Anterior and Posterior Leaflets

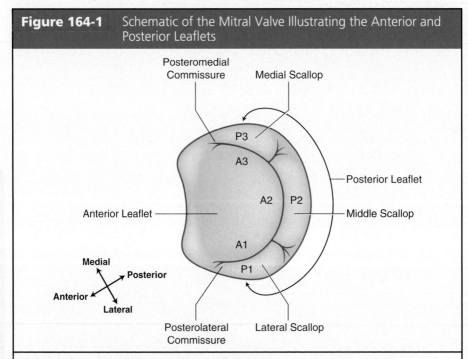

This illustration uses the widely accepted carpentier classification system.
Adapted from Shanewise JS, Cheung AT, Aronson S, et al. ASE/SCA guidelines for performing a comprehensive intraoperative multiplane transesophageal echocardiography examination. Anesth Analg 1999;89:870–884.

---

2) **Nomenclature:** The Carpentier system used to describe the mitral anatomy (2)
   a) The **posterior** leaflet is comprised of three scallops: P1, P2, and P3. P1 is closest to the atrial appendage (Fig. 164-2).
   b) The **anterior** leaflet is not scalloped but is named with a corresponding numerical system for easy identification: A1, A2, and A3.
3) **TEE views of mitral valve**
   To image the mitral valve, use the following 6 of the 20 standard TEE views (1).

ME four chamber—Utilize this view to evaluate MV with and without color flow Doppler. In this view, P2 is on the right and A2 is on the left.	
ME mitral commissural—Utilize this view to evaluate MV annular size. This is a good view to evaluate restriction, calcification, and specific leaflet motion. In this view, A2 is in the middle, P1 is on the right, and P3 is on the left.	
ME Two chamber—Utilize this view to evaluate MV with and without color flow Doppler. In this view, P3 is on the left and A3/A2 are on the right.	
ME long axis—Utilize this view to evaluate the MV, and look for systolic anterior leaflet of the motion of the valve. In this view, P2 is on the left and A2 is on the right.	
TG Basal short axis—Utilize this view to evaluate the MV. This view can be used to calculate the MV area. In this view, the posteromedial commissure is in the upper left of the display, and the anterolateral commissure is in the lower right. The posterior leaflet is on the right side, and the anterior leaflet is to the left.	
TG two chamber—Utilize this view to evaluate the mitral valve attachments to the papillary muscles and chordae tendinae.	

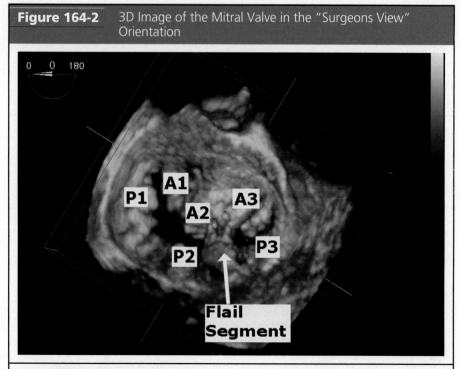

Figure 164-2 3D Image of the Mitral Valve in the "Surgeons View" Orientation

3D Magnified image of the mitral valve looking down on the atrial surface of the mitral valve. Note that in this image, there is a flail segment at the P2/P3 junction.

4) **Mitral valve regurgitation (MR)**

MR is a condition where blood can flow back into the left atrium during systole due to coaptation defects in the mitral apparatus.

a) **Classification**—A classification system by Carpentier describes the leaflet motion in relation to the regurgitation (2).

  i) **Type 1 lesion**: MR is present—with normal leaflet motion. The most common cause for this is annular dilatation. Other causes include mitral valve clefts, perforations or aneurysms. In this type of lesion, the jet is often centrally directed.

  ii) **Type 2 lesion**: MR with excessive leaflet motion. The jet in these cases is often directed away from the involved leaflet. Examples of this include:

   (1) **Billowing**—Part of the mitral leaflet projects above the annulus in systole.

   (2) **Prolapse**—The leaflet tip is above the level of the mitral annulus.

   (3) **Flail**—The leaflet tip is free flowing in the left atrium in systole, usually with chordal rupture.

  iii) **Type 3 lesion**: MR with restricted leaflet motion.

   (1) **Type 3a**—Structural restriction—leaflet motion affected in systole and diastole.

   (2) **Type 3b**—Functional restriction—leaflet motion affected in systole.

5) **Evaluation**

a) **Qualitative**

  i) Color flow Doppler allows a visual estimation of the severity of regurgitation based on the size of the regurgitant jet. (See **Table 164-1** for the severity grading in MV disease.)

Table 164-1

MR Classification

Indicator	Mild	Moderate	Severe
Qualitative			
Angiographic grade	1+	2+	3–4+
Color Doppler jet area	Small, central jet, <4 cm², <20% LA area	Signs of MR greater than mild but not severe criteria	Jet area > 8 cm², >40% LA area, wall hugging jet
Doppler vena contracta width (cm)	<0.3	0.3–0.69	≥0.7
Quantitative (cath or echo)			
Regurgitant volume (mL/beat)	<30	30–59	≥60
RF (%)	<30	30–49	≥50
ROA (cm²)	<0.10	0.2–0.39	≥0.4
Additional Essential Criteria			
Left atrial size			Enlarged
Left ventricular size			Enlarged

Reproduced from Bonow RO, Carabello BA, Chatterjee, K, et al. ACC/AHA 2006 guidelines for the management of patients with valvular heart disease: executive summary: a report of the American College of Cardiology/American Heart Association Task Force on Practice Guidelines. *Circulation* 2006;114(5):e84–231, with permission.

ii) The vena contracta is measured at the narrowest portion of the regurgitant jet (**Fig. 164-3**).

b) **Quantitative:** A quantitative assessment of the mitral valve is undertaken by calculating the regurgitant volume, regurgitant fraction (RF) and regurgitant orifice area (ROA).

i) To calculate the **regurgitant volume**, first calculate the stroke volume across the left ventricular outflow tract (LVOT).

$$\text{LVOT SV} = (\text{VTI}_{LVOT} \times \text{area}_{LVOT})$$

Subtract this value from the stroke volume measured at either the mitral valve in diastole ($\text{VTI}_{MV} \times \text{Area}_{MV}$) or the pulmonary artery.

ii) The **RF** is the percentage of left ventricular volume that flows back in to the left atrium in systole. To calculate this percentage, the regurgitant volume is divided by the overall stroke volume.

iii) Calculation of the effective regurgitant orifice area (EROA) is done using the **PISA method**. This method is explained in detail in Quantitative Echocardiography, Chapter 165. The equation is:

$$\text{EROA} = \frac{2\pi r^2 \times \text{Nyquist limit}}{\text{MR velocity}}$$

TRANSESOPHAGEAL ECHOCARDIOGRAPHY

Figure 164-3 Measurement of Vena Contracta

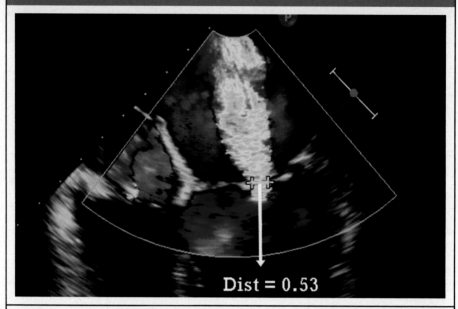

Dist = 0.53

Measurement of vena contracta utilizing the ME 4 chamber view. The diameter of the regurgitant jet is measured using the caliper function of the TEE machine. The diameter here (0.53 cm) is consistent with severe mitral regurgitation.

6) **Mitral valve stenosis**—describes the condition of a narrowed mitral valve orifice. The normal MV area is 4 to 6 cm². A valve area <2 cm² causes an increase in transvalvular pressure; however, the clinical presentation of MS and significant increase in the transvalvular pressure is not seen until the valve area is <1.4 cm² **(Table 164-2).**

   a) **Gradient—calculate the mean pressure gradient across the mitral valve with the modified Bernoulli equation**

↪ READ MORE

Quantitative echocardiography, Chapter 165, page 1143

$$\text{Pressure gradient (mm Hg)} = 4V^2$$

$$V = \text{instantaneous velocity}$$

Table 164-2

Mitral Stenosis

Indicator	Mild	Moderate	Severe
Mean gradient (mm Hg)	<5	5–10	>10
Pulmonary artery systolic pressure (mm Hg)	<30	30–50	>50
Valve Area (cm²)	>1.5	1.0–1.5	<1.0

Reproduced from Bonow RO, Carabello BA, Chatterjee, K, et al. ACC/AHA 2006 guidelines for the management of patients with valvular heart disease: executive summary: a report of the American College of Cardiology/American Heart Association Task Force on Practice Guidelines. *Circulation* 2006;114(5):e84–231, with permission.

Figure 164-4 Planimetry Measurement of MV Area

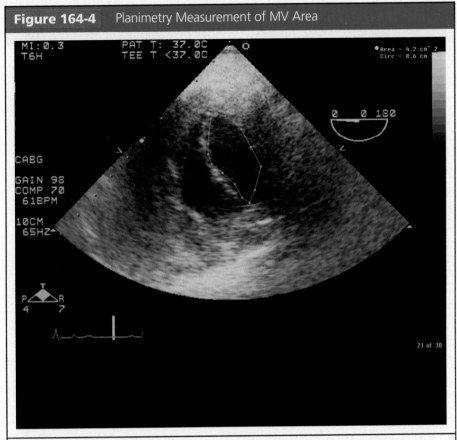

Planimetry measurement of the mitral valve area is accomplised with the transgastric basal view. The valve opening is traced using the measurement software embedded in the TEE machine.

The velocity measurement is obtained using continuous wave Doppler across the mitral valve.

b) **Valve area:** The valve area is obtained by either measuring the valve opening in diastole using planimetry or by the pressure half-time technique.

i) **Planimetry** involves tracing the valve opening in the TG basal view during diastole—giving an estimate of the open valve area. Image quality is the main limitation with this technique **(Fig. 164-4).**

ii) **Pressure half-time:** To use the pressure half-time technique, the transmitral flow velocity is measured using continuous wave Doppler **(Fig. 164-5).** The time it takes to decrease by a factor of the square root of 2 is calculated. A normal value for pressure half-time is <60 milliseconds. Severe mitral stenosis will have a pressure half-time >220 milliseconds. To calculate the valve area from the pressure half-time, use the following formula:

$$\text{MV area (cm}^2) = 220/\text{pressure half-time (ms)}$$

TRANSESOPHAGEAL ECHOCARDIOGRAPHY

Figure 164-5 Midesophageal four Chamber View with Continuous Wave Doppler to Measure Pressure Half-Time

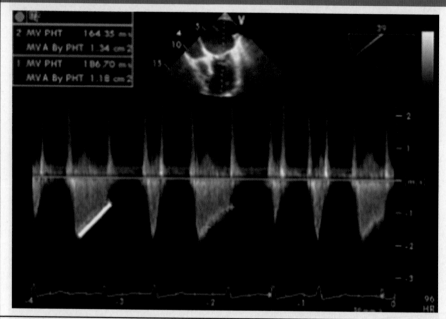

The pressure half-time is measured using continuous wave doppler through the valve. The white line is the slope of the decrese of the velocity in diastole. The pressure half-time is calculated by the TEE machine and can be used to calculate the valve area using the formula:

MV area (cm²) = 220/pressure half-time (ms).

iii) **Alternatives:** The continuity equation and PISA method can also be used to calculate the valve area. These are explained in detail in chapter "Post-op Ventilation of the Surgical Patient." The basic equations are below.

$$\text{Continuity equation: } \text{MVA} = \frac{(\text{LVOT}_{\text{AREA}} \times \text{LVOT}_{\text{VTI}})}{\text{MV}_{\text{VTI}}}$$

$$\text{PISA: } \text{MVA} = 2\pi r^2 \times \frac{\alpha}{180} \times \frac{V_a}{V_p}$$

References

1. Shanewise JS, Cheung AT, Aronson S, et al. ASE/SCA Guidelines for performing a comprehensive intraoperative multiplane transesophageal echocardiography examination: recommendations of the American Society of Echocardiography Council for Intraoperative Echocardiography and the Society of Cardiovascular Anesthesiologists task Force for Certification in Perioperative Transesophageal Echocardiography. *Anesth Analg* 1999;89:870–884.
2. Carpentier AF, Lessana A, Relland JY, et al. The Physio Ring: an advanced concept in mitral valve annuloplasty. *Ann Thorac Surg* 1995;60:1177–1185.
3. Bonow RO, Carabello BA, Chatterjee, K, et al. ACC/AHA 2006 Guidelines for the management of patients with valvular heart disease: executive summary: a report of the American College of Cardiology/American Heart Association Task Force on Practice Guidelines. *Circulation* 2006;114(5):e84–231.

165 Quantitative Echocardiography

Tamas Seres, MD, PhD

Transesophageal echocardiography (TEE) is an important monitoring and diagnostic modality in the field of cardiac anesthesia. Due the reliability and safety of TEE, its application is extending into other areas of anesthesiology as well. This chapter provides an overview of TEE evaluation of systolic and diastolic function along with tools to evaluate pressure gradients (PGs) and valve areas in patients with stenotic or regurgitant valves.

1) **General concepts—myocardial function**
One of the most common indications for a TEE exam in the regular OR is to evaluate left ventricular (LV) systolic function. It is the most important part of the intraoperative exam in cardiac anesthesia before and after cardiopulmonary bypass. The TEE measurements provide parameters to evaluate the LV systolic function in patients with chronic or acute heart failure (HF).

   a) **Myocardial remodeling**: Myocardial remodeling is manifested clinically by changes in cardiac size, shape, and function in response to increased load or myocardial injury. The cause of pathologic myocardial remodeling can be

   i) **Pressure overload** (e.g., aortic stenosis (AS), hypertension)
   (1) Concentric myocardial hypertrophy—normal heart volumes and ejection fraction (EF)

   ii) **Volume overload** (e.g., valvular regurgitation)
   (1) Eccentric myocardial hypertrophy—large LV end diastolic volume (LVEDV), LV end systolic volume (LVESV), ↓ EF, along with normal or altered stroke volume (SV) and cardiac output (CO)

   iii) **Altered myocardial contractility**
   (1) Myocardial infarction, inflammatory myocardial disease, idiopathic dilated cardiomyopathy
   (2) Characterized by ↓ SV, ↑ LVESV and LVEDV and ↓ EF. The SV may be normal depending on the stage of the remodeling process and the treatment of the heart disease (1).

2) **Systolic function of the left ventricle**
Principle: A heart with normal systolic function generates appropriate CO with low filling pressures for appropriate oxygen delivery to the body to cover the oxygen consumption at rest or during exercise (2).

   a) **TEE Image planes:** For the evaluation of the LV volumes and systolic function, the following TEE image planes are considered (3,4):
   i) ME 4-chamber view, ME 2-chamber view, ME long axis (LAX) view
   ii) Transgastric (TG) views are used for diameter, area change, and direct Doppler measurements
   iii) TG mid short axis (SAX) view, deep TG view, TG LAX

READ MORE

Heart failure, Chapter 60, page 436

b) **Evaluation of systolic function includes the measurement of**
   i)   LVEDV/LVESV

Principle: As the LV contracts, it shortens in the LAX/SAX, and there is a twisting effect where the base and the apex rotate around the LAX of the left ventricle. Based on the complex pattern of the LV systolic contraction, the ME LV views are the most appropriate (5). LVEDV and LVESV are measured by using the method of discs (MOD) or Simpson's method by using two ME views. The Simpson's method slices the LV into several discs and measures the volume of each disc. Aberrations in LV shape will not introduce as much error into the result compared to other standard measurements (6).

Image planes: ME 4-chamber and 2-chamber views.

Measurement: The measurement is performed by tracing the endocardial border of the LV in 4-chamber and 2-chamber views in end-diastole and end-systole. After tracing the endocardial border under the option of MOD, the computer automatically calculates the volumes (**Fig. 165-1, Panel A**).

Normal values can be seen in **Table 165-1**.

   ii)   LVEDV and LVESV measurement by using M-mode images

Principle: The measurement of LV internal diameter at end-diastole (LVIDd) and end-systole (LVIDs) can be used for mathematical assumption of the LV volume using the Teichholz method.

Image planes: TG SAX mid-papillary view.

Figure 165-1   Examples for Systolic Function Determined by Simpson's Method and M-mode

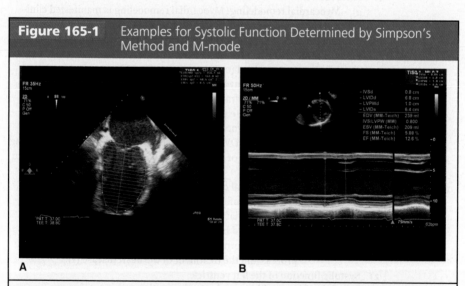

A   **B**

A: LVEDV and LVESV were measured in 4- and 2-chamber views by tracing the endocardial border. The LV was divided to discs and the volume was calculated by the summation of the volumes of each disc. **B:** The LVIDd and LVIDs were measured in the same patient. Fractional shortening (FS) can be calculated: (LVIDd-LVIDs)/LVIDd x 100 (%). The EDV and ESV were computed by the Teichholz method. This patient has a dilated heart with severe systolic dysfunction.

Table 165-1

LV Systolic Function

	Men	Women
LVEDV (mL)	62–170	55–101
LVESV (mL)	14–76	13–60
LVIDd (cm)	4.2–5.9	3.9–5.3
LVIDs (cm)	2.6–4.0	2.3–3.5
SV (mL)		70–100
CO (L/min)		4–8
CI (L/min/m²)		2.5–4.2
EF (%)		55–70
FS (%)		28–44
FAC (%)		40–75
Wall thickness		
Posterior wall (cm)		0.6–1.1
Septum (cm)		0.6–1.1
Contractilty (dP/dt) (mm Hg):		>1,200 (normal)
		<1,000 (abnormal)

Measurement: The diameter can be measured by caliper under the M-mode measurement option, and the volume will be calculated by the computer of the echo machine using the Teichholz method:

$$V = [7/(2.4 + LVID)] \times LVID^3$$

Comment: The measurement of LVEDV, LVESV, and EF with the Teichholz method requires absence of regional wall motion abnormalities and normal shape of the LV (see **Fig. 165-1**) (7).

iii) Ejection fraction
Principle: EF can be calculated quantitatively by using the volumes measured by the Simpson's or Teichholz methods (see **Fig. 165-1, Panel B**).

$$EF = (EDV - ESV)/EDV \times 100$$

Normal values: 55% to 75%
Comment: The advantage of EF is the uniformity among patients. While the patient's size, body habitus, and sex may be different, EF represents systolic function that is comparable between patients and comparable in a single patient under different conditions. Preload, afterload, and contractility can affect the EF. An increase in preload or contractility as well as a decrease in afterload will increase the EF.

iv) **SV, CO, cardiac index (CI)**
  (1) Volumetric measurement
    Principle: SV can be measured by using the volume data of the Simpson's or Teichholz methods (see **Fig. 165-1**). SV = EDV – ESV
    Normal values: 70 to 100 mL
  (2) Doppler measurement
    Principle: There is a direct way to measure SV by using pulsed wave Doppler (PWD) in LV outflow track (LVOT). The SV measurement is based on the concept that the blood is flowing through the LVOT cross-sectional area (CSA_{LVOT})

TRANSESOPHAGEAL ECHOCARDIOGRAPHY

Figure 165-2 Typical Views for CSA$_{LVOT}$ and Doppler Measurement

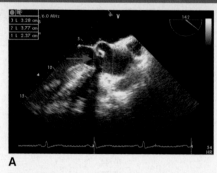 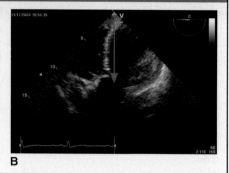

A **B**

A: The LVOT diameter is measured on the LV LAX view and the CSA is calculated using the equation for area of circle.
LVOT diameter = 2.37 cm
CSA$_{LVOT}$ = 2.37² x 0.785 = 4.4 cm²
B: The deep TG view is seen for Doppler measurements. The arrow shows the site of the LVOT diameter. The arrow localizes the cursor of the pulse wave Doppler at the level where the diameter was measured.

---

with changing velocity during systole. The time integral of the velocity curve (VTI) or the area under the curve is the distance that the blood travels during systole through the CSA$_{LVOT}$. The SV is the product of the CSA$_{LVOT}$ × VTI$_{LVOT}$. The velocity curve should be obtained at the level of the measurement of the CSA to get exact result.

Image plane: ME LAX view, deep TG view or TG LAX view **(Fig. 165-2, Panel A and B)**

Measurement: The calculation of CSA$_{LVOT}$ is based on the measurement of the diameter (D) of the LVOT in the ME LAX view **(Fig. 165-2, Panel A).**

Assuming that the LVOT area is a circle, the area is:

$$CSA_{LVOT} = r^2 \times \pi = (D/2)^2 \times \pi = D^2 \times \pi/4 = D^2 \times 0.785$$

The SV is calculated as follows:

$$SV = CSA_{LVOT} \times VTI_{LVOT} \text{ (Fig. 165-3, Panel A) (8)}.$$

Comment: The SV derived from volumetric measurements can be different from Doppler SV measurement in the LVOT. For example, in a patient with mitral regurgitation (MR) or ventricular septal defect, the volumetric SV is bigger than the Doppler SV. The difference is the regurgitant or the shunt volume, respectively.

(3) **CO and CI**

Principle: The measured SV is multiplied with the heart rate (HR) to obtain the CO:

$$CO = SV \times HR$$

CI: CO/body surface area

Normal values: 2.5 to 4.2 L/min/m²

Figure 165-3   Evaluation of AS with Using the Continuity Equation

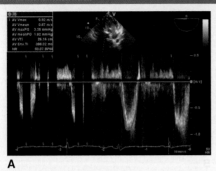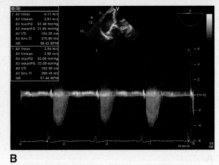

A   **B**

A: PWD is used to measure the flow and SV in the LVOT. The CSA_{LVOT} = 4.4 cm² from Fig. 165-2. V_{LVOT} = 92 cm/s, VTI_{LVOT} = 26 cm

$Flow_{LVOT} = CSA_{LVOT} \times V_{LVOT}$ = 405 mL/s

$SV = CSA_{LVOT} \times VTI_{LVOT}$ = 4.4 × 26 = 114 mL.

B: CWD is used to measure the flow and SV at the AS. The AS cross-sectional area (CSA_{AS}) can be calculated by the flow or SV continuity equations. V_{AS} = 402 cm/s, VTI_{AS} = 104 cm

Calculation of the AS area (CSA_{AS}) with flow continuity: $CSA_{LVOT} \times V_{LVOT} = CSA_{AS} \times V_{AS}$

$CSA_{AS} = CSA_{LVOT} \times V_{LVOT} / V_{AS}$ = 405/402 = 1 cm²

Calculation of the AS area with SV continuity: $CSA_{LVOT} \times VTI_{LVOT} = CSA_{AS} \times VTI_{AS}$

$CSA_{AS} = CSA_{LVOT} \times VTI_{LVOT} / VTI_{AS}$ = 114/104 = 1.1 cm²

The severity of AS can be evaluated by the peak and mean PG measured by CWD.

PG_{peak} = 64 mmHg and PG_{mean} = 32 mm Hg represent moderate AS.

v)   **Evaluation of regional wall motion abnormality (RWMA)**

Principle: The LV is divided to 16 segments to describe the wall motion of different areas supplied by different coronary arteries. There are basal, mid, and apical segments. There are six segments in the basal and mid level (anterior, anteroseptal, septal, inferior, posterior, lateral) and four segments at apical level (anterior, septal, inferior, lateral).

Image planes: To evaluate the different segments, multiple views should be used: ME 4-chamber, ME 2-chamber, ME LAX views. TG SAX views are frequently used to evaluate the SAX movement of the segments.

Measurement of wall motion: During systole, the myocardial wall thickens and the endocardial wall moves toward the center of the heart (wall motion). In current clinical practice, analysis of LV segmental function is based on a qualitative visual assessment of the motion and thickening of a segment during systole. The recommended qualitative grading scale for wall motion is

(1)   Normal (>30% movement of the endocardium to the center of the LV)

(2)   Mildly hypokinetic (10% to 30% movement of the endocardium)

(3)   Severely hypokinetic (<10% movement of the endocardium)

(4)   Akinetic (no movement of the endocardium)

(5)   Dyskinetic (moves paradoxically during systole).

Figure 165-4   LV SAX Area Measurement

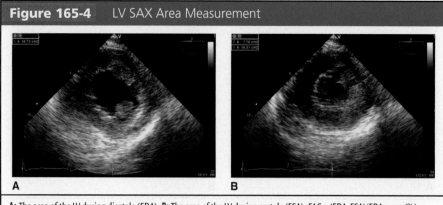

A: The area of the LV during diastole (EDA). **B:** The area of the LV during systole (ESA). FAC = (EDA-ESA)/EDA x 100 (%).

Comments: RWMA represents segmental systolic dysfunction and alters long-term morbidity and mortality in ischemic heart disease (9). The causes of RWMA include ischemia, infarction, hibernation, stunning, bundle branch block, pacemaker, or artifact. Myocardial ischemia can be detected early by monitoring wall motion in intraoperative setting (3).

vi) **Additional measurements**

(1) **LV SAX area measurement**

Principle: More than 80% of the SV is due to the shortening of the SAX. Therefore, the change in area during systole in LV SAX view at mid papillary level may represent the systolic volume change of the LV.

Image planes: TG mid SAX

Measurement: The LV areas are measured by manual planimetry of the area of the LV at end-diastole (EDA) and end-systole (ESA) excluding the papillary muscles (**Fig. 165-4, Panel A and B**).

Normal values: EDA: 9.5–22 cm², ESA: 4–11.6 cm²

Comments: Changes of ESA may reflect the changes in contractility (increased contractility decreases ESA) or afterload (increased afterload increases ESA). Qualitatively, if the papillary muscles are seen "kissing" or making contact during systole, then hypovolemia (most frequent), low peripheral resistance, or increased contractility can be present (10).

(2) Fractional area change (FAC)

Principle: The area change during systole compared to the EDA is the FAC, which correlates well with EF (see **Fig. 165-4**).

$$FAC = (EDA - ESA)/EDA \times 100$$

Normal values: 40% to 75%

Comment: Although the value of FAC is generally used for off-line quantitative analysis, a qualitative assessment of ESA, EDA, and FAC is important in evaluating the etiology of hemodynamic instability (3).

(3) **LV internal diameter measurement with M-mode and fractional shortening (FS)**

Principle: LVIDd and LVIDs can be measured in either 2D or M-mode images. Internal diameters can be obtained easily, and they are characteristic in different remodeling conditions.

Image planes: TG mid SAX view

Measurement: Fractional shortening

After obtaining the TG mid SAX view the diameter of the LV can be measured in diastole (LVIDd) or in systole (LVIDs) by using a caliper in the M-mode option of the echo software (see **Fig. 165-1, Panel B**). The percentage change in the LVID during systole compared to end-diastole can be used to evaluate LV systolic function.

$$FS = (LVIDd - LVIDs)/LVIDd \times 100$$

Normal values: Table 165-1.

Comments: The papillary muscles should be excluded from the measurement. The LVIDd and LVIDs can be used to evaluate eccentric remodeling in mitral or aortic valve regurgitation (11) (see **Fig. 165-1, Panel B**). FS has limited value in evaluating systolic function because it measures changes only in a narrow segment of the LV in one dimension (3).

3) Diastolic function
   a) **Principle:** The optimal performance of the left ventricle depends on its ability to cycle between two states:
      i) A compliant chamber in diastole that allows the left ventricle to fill with low left atrial (LA) pressure
      ii) A stiff chamber with rapidly rising pressure in systole that ejects the SV at arterial pressures

      Furthermore, the SV must increase in response to demand, such as exercise, without much increase in LA pressure. Elevated filling pressures are the main physiologic consequence of diastolic dysfunction. Filling pressures are considered elevated when the mean pulmonary capillary wedge pressure (PCWP) is >12 mm Hg or when the LVEDP is >16 mm Hg.

      Impaired LV relaxation and/or poor LV compliance may lead to elevated filling pressures with or without the clinical symptoms of HF. Diastolic HF represents patients with abnormal diastolic function and normal EF. The staging and functional classes of diastolic HF are the same as it was described for systolic HF (2).

   b) **The phases of diastole**
      i) **Isovolumic relaxation time (IVRT):** The time from the aortic valve closure to mitral valve opening. During isovolumic relaxation, the volume of the left ventricle is constant but the pressure falls. The period of IVRT is an active, ATP burning phase. The mitral valve will open when the LAP exceeds the LV pressure. If the LA pressure is elevated, the IVRT will be shortened. Conversely, if the relaxation of the left ventricle is decreased, then the IVRT will be increased.
      ii) **Rapid filling phase:** The rapid filling phase accounts for most of the filling of the left ventricle (80%). The factors that account for the amount of filling during this phase are the LV suction, pressure difference between the left atrium and the left ventricle, the LV compliance, and the left atrial volume.
      iii) **Diastasis:** During diastasis, the LA-LV pressure difference is small. Filling of the left ventricle (5%) is mostly due to pulmonary venous flow with the LA acting as a conduit. LV compliance is the main determinant of filling during diastasis.
      iv) **Atrial contraction:** Factors determining the filling of the left ventricle (15% to 20%) from an atrial contraction are ventricular compliance, pericardial restraint, atrial contractility, and electrical synchrony (PR interval) (2,12).

   c) **Evaluation of diastolic function with TEE**
      i) Mitral Doppler inflow velocity

Figure 165-5 Evaluation of Diastolic Function with PWD at the MV and Pulmonary Vein

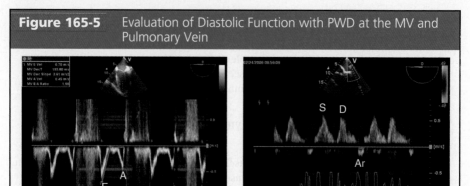

A: Mitral valve inflow was obtained with PWD. The early diastolic wave (E) and the atrial kick (A) can be differentiated. The red lines represent DT measurement at the E wave and A duration at the A wave. **B:** Pulmonary vein flow was obtained with PWD. The S wave represents the flow during systole, the D wave is the early diastolic flow and the Ar is a backflow into the pulmonary veins during the atrial contraction. The red line represents the duration of Ar.

Principle: Pulsed wave Doppler is used to visualize the flow through the mitral valve. The early diastolic wave of the mitral inflow is the E wave. In normal patients, the LV relaxation and untwisting generate negative pressure in the LV at the time of the opening of the MV—generating the E wave. The second wave or A wave is generated by the atrial contraction.

The velocity of E and A, their ratio, deceleration time (DT) of E, and duration of A are used to characterize the diastolic function (**Fig. 165-5, Panel A**).

Image plane: ME 4-chamber view

Measurements: The PWD cursor is positioned at the tip of the mitral leaflets to gain the best possible velocity curve. Maximum velocity of the E and A wave is measured by using the velocity scale. DT of the E wave can be measured by using the slope measurement tool, which calculates the time from the maximum velocity to zero velocity. The duration of the A wave can be measured by time measurement options (see **Fig. 165-5, Panel A**).

Comments: Decreased relaxation accompanies decreased E wave, E/A ratio and increased A wave. Increased LA pressure increases the PG during early diastole resulting in high E wave and E/A ratio. Increased LV end diastolic pressure causes decreased A wave velocity and duration (**Table 165-2**).

ii) **Pulmonary vein flow**

Principle: Pulsed wave Doppler is used to measure the velocity of the flow through the pulmonary vein. The wave during LV systole is the S wave, which has two components. The S1 wave represents the relaxation of the LA after atrial contraction. The S2 wave is more prominent than S1 and represents the flow from the pulmonary vein into the LA during LV systole due to the movement of the closed MV toward the LV apex. The D wave represents the flow from the pulmonary vein into the LA during early diastole after the opening of the MV. The A reversal (Ar) is a flow from the LA into the pulmonary vein during the atrial contraction (see **Fig. 165-5 , Panel B**).

Image plane: ME 2-chamber view focusing on the area of left atrial appendage and the left upper pulmonary vein running close to it.

Table 165-2
LV Diastolic Function

	Normal	Grade I	Grade II	Grade III
Decreased Relaxation		+	+	+
Increased LV-EDP			+	++
Decreased compliance			+	++
NYHA functional class	I	I-II	II-III	III-IV
Mitral inflow				
E/A ratio	1–2	<0.8	0.8–1.5	≥2
DT (ms)	160–200	>200	160–200	<160
IVRT (ms)	60–100	>100	60–100	<60
Pulmonary vein flow				
S/D	≥1	>1	<1	≪1
Ar (m/s)	<0.38	<0.35	≥0.35	≥0.35
Ar–A (ms)	<0	<0	≥30	≥30
Tissue Doppler velocity of the MV annulus				
E′ (cm/s)	>10	<8	<8	<8
E′/A′ ratio	1–2	<1	<1	<1
E/E′ average ratio	≤8	≤8	9–12	≥13
Flow propagation velocity				
Vp (cm/s)	>50	<50	<50	<50

Measurement: The PWD cursor is placed into the pulmonary vein, and the velocity curve is registered. The velocities of S2, D, and Ar waves; the S/D ratio; as well as the duration of the Ar wave are measured and used to characterize the diastolic function in addition to the parameters of the mitral inflow.

Comments: Increased LA pressure decreases the S wave velocity. Relaxation abnormality decreases the velocity of the D wave. Increased LV end-diastolic pressure may increase the velocity and duration of Ar (see **Table 165-2, Panel B**).

iii) **Tissue Doppler velocity measurement**

Principle: By eliminating high velocity/low amplitude signals in color Doppler, the low velocity high amplitude movements of the myocardium during systole and diastole can be visualized and measured. The MV annulus moves toward the apex during systole (S wave) and away from the apex during early and late diastole. The early diastolic annular velocity is expressed as E′ and the late diastolic velocity as A′. The peak velocity of these diastolic movements and their ratio are measured for characterization of the diastolic function parallel with the flow evaluation through the MV and pulmonary vein. For the assessment of global LV diastolic function, it is recommended to acquire and measure tissue Doppler signals at least at the septal and lateral sides of the mitral annulus and their average (E′average), given the influence of regional function on these velocities and time intervals (**Fig. 165-6, Panel A**).

Image plane: ME 4-chamber view using tissue Doppler image

TRANSESOPHAGEAL ECHOCARDIOGRAPHY

Figure 165-6	Evaluation of Diastolic Function with Tissue Doppler and Color M-Mode Method

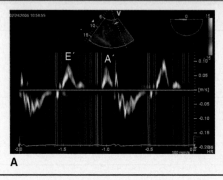

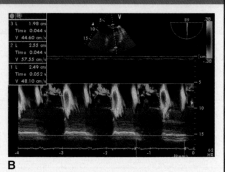

A | **B**

A: Tissue Doppler modality was used and the PWD cursor was placed on the lateral part of the mitral valve annulus. The annulus is moving toward the apex during systole (first negative wave) and away from the apex during early diastole (E') and late diastole or atrial kick (A'). The E/E' ratio is depending on the LA pressure. B: Color Doppler on the MVA and M-mode is directed through the color flow. The red line is at the flow propagation during early diastole. The measurement is performed at the yellow-blue transition line using the slope measurement option on the computer.

Measurement: For obtaining the velocity curve of the MV annulus, the PWD cursor is placed on the septal or lateral edge of the MV annulus in tissue Doppler mode.
Comments: Tissue Doppler parameters are important for full evaluation of diastolic function and LV filling pressures. Low E' (<8 cm/s) represents impaired relaxation. The MV inflow E/tissue Doppler E'average ratio < 8 is usually associated with normal LV filling pressures, whereas a ratio > 13 is associated with increased filling pressures (see **Table 165-2**).

iv) **Color M-mode flow propagation velocity**
Principle: The most widely used approach for measuring mitral-to-apical flow propagation is the slope method. Acquisition is performed in the apical 4-chamber view, using color flow imaging. The M-mode scan line is placed through the center of the LV color inflow from the mitral valve to the apex. Flow propagation velocity (V_p) is expressed as the slope (cm/s) of the first aliasing velocity during early filling, measured from the mitral valve plane to 4 cm distally into the LV cavity. V_p >50 cm/s is considered normal.
Image plane: ME 4-chamber view with optimal MV opening
Measurement. The edge of the aliasing velocity, as it described above, is traced by the slope function and the V_p can be obtained (see **Fig. 165-6, Panel B**).
Comment: In patients with depressed EF V_p can provide useful information for the prediction of LV filling pressures. The E/V_p ratio ≥ 2.5 predicts PCWP > 15 mm Hg with reasonable accuracy.

d) **Evaluation of the severity of LV diastolic dysfunction:** Three grades of diastolic dysfunction are identified by Doppler echocardiography:

i) **Grade I—impaired relaxation**
(1) In patients with mild diastolic dysfunction, the mitral E/A ratio is <0.8, DT is >200 milliseconds, IVRT is ≥ 100 milliseconds, predominant systolic flow is seen in pulmonary venous flow (S/D ≥ 1), annular E'septal is <8 cm/s and E' lateral is <10 cm/s, and the E/E' average ratio is <8 (see **Table 165-2**). Importantly, even in asymptomatic patients, grade I diastolic dysfunction was associated with a fivefold higher 3- to 5-year mortality in comparison with subjects with normal diastolic function.

(2) Because the majority of subjects aged >60 years without a history of cardiovascular disease have E/A ratios <1 and DTs >200 milliseconds, such values in the absence of further indicators of cardiovascular disease (e.g., LV hypertrophy) can be considered normal for age.

(3) Reduced mitral E/A ratio in the presence of normal annular tissue Doppler velocities can be seen in volume-depleted normal subjects, so an E/A ratio <0.8 should not be universally used to infer the presence of grade I diastolic dysfunction.

ii) **Grade II—pseudonormal**

(1) In patients with moderate diastolic dysfunction (**pseudonormal pattern**), the mitral E/A ratio is 0.8 to 1.5 (pseudonormal) and decreases by >50% during the Valsalva maneuver. DT is 160 to 200 milliseconds and IVRT is 60 to 100 milliseconds. E' septal is <8 cm/s and E' lateral is <10 cm, and the E/E' average ratio is 9 to 12. Other supporting data include an Ar velocity >30 cm/s and an S/D ratio <1 (see **Table 165-2**).

(2) **Grade II** diastolic dysfunction represents impaired myocardial relaxation with mild to moderate elevation of LV filling pressures due to moderately decreased LV compliance. These patients may have symptoms of HF with NYHA II–III functional status.

iii) **Grade III—restrictive**

(1) Severe diastolic dysfunction or restrictive LV filling occurs with an E/A ratio >2, DT <160 milliseconds, IVRT <60 milliseconds, E/E' average ratio >13, S/D << 1, Ar duration – A duration (Ar–A) >30 milliseconds (see **Table 165-2**).

(2) LV filling may revert to pseudonormal or impaired relaxation pattern with successful therapy in some patients (grade IIIa), whereas in others, LV filling remains restrictive (grade IIIb). The later predicts a high risk for cardiac morbidity and mortality. Patients with grade III diastolic function may have symptoms of HF with NYHA III–IV functional status.

(3) Grade IIIb dysfunction should not be determined by a single examination and requires serial studies after treatment is optimized. LA volume is increased in grades II and III of diastolic dysfunction but can be within normal limits in grade I.

e) **Hemodynamic measurements using the diastolic parameters**

Elevated LV filling pressures are important characteristics of clinically significant systolic and diastolic dysfunction. The increased filling pressures represent elevated preload. A clinical scenario of elevated preload with small SV and EF suggests significant systolic dysfunction. However, elevated preload with normal SV and EF may represent significant diastolic dysfunction. Elevated LV filling pressures in the OR might suggest high risk for pulmonary edema in cases with significant fluid shifts and volume changes (**Table 165-3**) (12).

4) **Doppler measurements of pressure gradients (PG) and valve areas**

a) **Measurement of PGs**

Principle: The PG through a stenotic valve needs to be evaluated to determine the severity of the valve disease. Based on the physical principle of flow continuity in a closed system, wherever the area of the flow is decreased the velocity is increased. The velocity is highest at the point where the area is the smallest. In the case of AS or mitral stenosis (MS), the velocity of the flow is highest at the site of the stenosis. Measurement of the peak velocity allows calculating the peak PG at the site of the stenosis by using the simplified Bernoulli equation.

$$\text{Peak PG} = 4 \times V^2$$

V = the peak velocity of the flow through the stenotic valve

Table 165-3
Increased Filling Pressures Suggested by Diastolic Parameters

Patient with Depressed EF and LA Pressure > 12 mm Hg
1. E/A ratio $\geq$ 2 and DT <160 ms
2. E/A ratio 1–2: E/E' average >15
   E/V_p ratio $\geq$ 2.5
   S/D < 1
   Ar–A $\geq$ 30 ms

Patient with Normal EF and LA Pressure > 12 mm Hg
1. E/E' average >13
2. E/E' average 9–13: Ar–A $\geq$ 30 ms

Image planes: Deep TG or TG LAX view for AS and ME 4-chamber view for MS (8)

Measurement: Continuous wave Doppler (CWD) aligned to the blood flow through the stenotic valve is used to measure the highest velocity in the direction of the flow. After obtaining the velocity curve, the curve is traced and the peak and mean PG are determined by the computer of the echo machine. In clinical practice, the mean PG gradient is used to determine the severity of the stenosis (see **Fig. 165-3, Panel B**).

b) **Evaluation of LV contractility by measuring PGs in MR**

Principle: Contractility is described as the change of pressure in the LV over time (dP/dt). The highest dP/dt can be measured during the isovolumic contraction. The isovolumic contraction becomes visible for TEE measurement in patients with MR. The MR jet can be used for the measurement of contractility using CWD.

Image plane: ME 4-chamber view

Measurement: A velocity measurement, early in the flow acceleration phase of systolic ejection, is used to calculate an early pressure, using the Simplified Bernoulli Equation (PG = $4 \times V^2$). Another velocity, later in the flow acceleration phase is used to calculate another pressure. The difference in pressures is the dP part of the dP/dt value. The difference in time between the last and first velocity measurements make the dt part of the formula. The typical values used are the time difference, in seconds, between the velocity values of 3 and 1 m/s. The pressures are $4 \times 3^2 = 36$ mm Hg and $4 \times 1^2 = 4$ mm Hg with a difference of 32 mm Hg divided by the seconds between the velocity measurements (**Fig. 165-7**).

Normal value: 1,200 mm Hg/s, abnormal value is <1,000 mm Hg/s

Comment: One study found that dP/dt <600 mm Hg/s identified a high-risk group with a reduced event-free survival after myocardial infarction (13).

c) **Measurement of MS area with pressure half-time (PHT)**

Principle: PHT is the time required for the gradient between the left atrium and the left ventricle to fall to one half of its initial value. Based on catheterization data, a PHT of 220 milliseconds is equivalent to a mitral valve area (MVA) of 1 cm². MVA can be calculated by obtaining PHT from the MS velocity curve:

MVA = 220/PHT

Image planes: ME 4-chamber view

Measurement: CWD aligned trough the MS. The PHT is measured on the slope between the E and A wave with the PHT option (**Fig. 165-8**).

Comments. In case of MS and MR, the MVA will be overestimated because of the increased flow and decreased PHT during the diastole (8).

d) **Measurement of the AS area with the continuity equation**

| **Figure 165-7** | Measurement of LV Contractility Using CWD Image of the MR Jet |

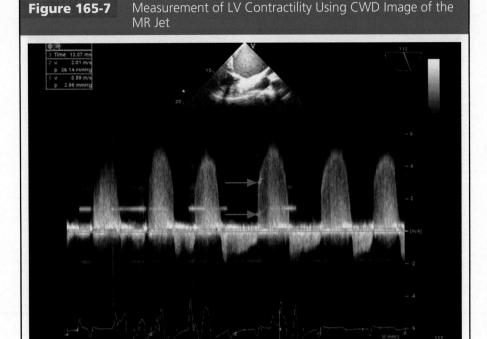

CWD measures the velocity change through the MR orifice. The PG at 1 and 3 m/s was calculated by using the simplified Bernoulli equation (4 x V²). The pressure difference and the time difference were determined between the two points (red arrows) and the contractility was computed by using the dP/dt formula. Contractilty = 32 mmHg/0.13 s = 2461 mmHg/s.

Principle: Continuity equation is an important tool to evaluate areas with unknown size such as areas of AS, MS or regurgitant areas of aortic insufficiency or MR. The severity of the AS can be graded by the mean PG and area of the stenosis. The area measurement is especially important when the patient has low CO because the PG generated through the aortic valve is low in this situation and underestimates the severity of the AS.

The continuity equation is based on assuming a constant flow of fluid through a conduit. Flow (cm³/s) in a conduit is the product of CSA of the conduit (cm²) and the velocity (V) of the fluid (cm/s). If there is a stenosis in the conduit, the velocity of fluid will increase at the site of stenosis to keep the continuity of flow. In case of AS, the flow in the LVOT is the same as the flow at the AS. The flow in the LVOT can be calculated by determining CSA_{LVOT} and multiplying it wit the V_{LVOT} (see **Figs. 165-2 and 165-3**). The flow at the AS cannot be calculated because the CSA_{AS} is unknown. V_{AS} can be measured by CWD as the highest velocity in the direction of the flow through the CSA_{AS} (see **Fig. 165-3, Panel B**). From the flow continuity, CSA_{AS} can be calculated (8):

$$CSA_{LVOT} \times V_{LVOT} = CSA_{AS} \times V_{AS}$$
$$CSA_{AS} = CSA_{LVOT} \times V_{LVOT}/V_{AS}$$

The SV continuity states that the SV is the same in the LVOT as at the AS. SV is defined as the product of CSA and VTI. The VTI values in the LVOT and at the AS can be used to express CSA_{AS}:

$$CSA_{AS} = CSA_{LVOT} \times VTI_{LVOT}/VTI_{AS}$$

TRANSESOPHAGEAL ECHOCARDIOGRAPHY

Figure 165-8

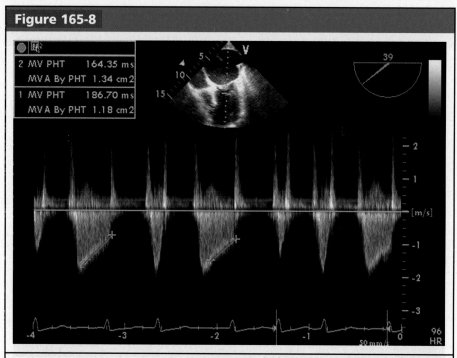

2 MV PHT	164.35 ms
MV A By PHT	1.34 cm2
1 MV PHT	186.70 ms
MV A By PHT	1.18 cm2

The flow through MS was visualized by CWD. The red line represents the slope of the decrease of velocity during diastole. The PHT is calculated by the computer of the echo machine. MVA = 220/PHT–220/186.7 = 1.2 cm².

Comments: Although the method is mostly used for AS area measurement, the MS area can also be measured by this method. In this case, the LVOT flow will be compared to the flow through MS. The peak velocity of MS can be measured by CWD. The MVA can be calculated as follows:

$$CSA_{LVOT} \times V_{LVOT} = MVA \times V_{MS}$$
$$MVA = CSA_{LVOT} \times V_{LVOT}/V_{MS}$$

e) **Proximal isovelocity surface area (PISA) technique**
   Principle: The area of MR, called effective regurgitant orifice area (EROA), can be calculated as a reliable parameter for grading the severity of the MR. The measurement is based on the fact that as blood flows toward a regurgitant orifice, the blood flow velocity increases with the formation of multiple concentric isovelocity shells. Using color Doppler, the isovelocity shell with the aliasing velocity can be identified. The aliasing velocity is the peak velocity on the color Doppler velocity scale.

   In MR, using the 4-chamber view the regurgitant flow is toward the transducer (red color). Close to the regurgitant orifice the velocity of the flow is high (yellow color). At the shell surface where the velocity is higher than the maximum velocity on the color scale, the color turns blue from the yellow. This shell surface represents the PISA where the velocity equals to the maximum velocity on the color scale or aliasing velocity. This shell is a hemisphere and its area can be calculated from the radius (r), which is the distance between the PISA and the orifice (**Fig. 165-9, Panel A**).

$$PISA = 2 \times r^2 \times \pi$$

Figure 165-9 | Calculation of the EROA in MR

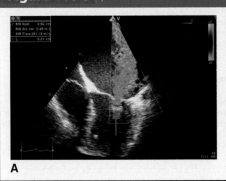 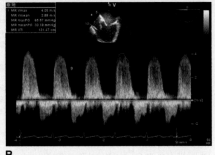

A   **B**

A: Color Doppler image of the MR. The tip of the arrow is positioned at the transition of color from yellow to blue (PISA). The area of PISA = $2 \times \pi \times r^2$. The velocity at PISA is 49 cm/s, which is the peak velocity on the color scale ($V_{aliasing}$). The flow at PISA = $2 \times \pi \times 0.96^2 \times 49 = 284$ ml/s. **B:** The velocity curve of the MR obtained by CWD. The peak velocity of MR ant the VTI of the MR can be measured. $V_{MR} = 405$ cm/s, $VTI_{MR} = 131$ cm

The $Flow_{MR} = EROA \times V_{MR} = Flow_{PISA}$

$EROA = Flow_{PISA} / V_{MR} = 284/405 = 0.7$ cm^2

$RV = EROA \times VTI_{MR} = 0.7 \times 131 = 92$ mL

The flow through the PISA can be calculated because the aliasing velocity can be identified as the maximum velocity on the color scale.

$$Flow_{PISA} = PISA \times V_{aliasing}$$

Using the continuity equation, the flow through the PISA should be the same as the flow through the EROA. The flow through the EROA can be derived from the product of EROA and the maximum velocity of the MR (V_{MR}) (see **Fig. 165-9, Panel B**):

$$Flow_{EROA} = EROA \times V_{MR}$$
$$Flow_{PISA} = Flow_{EROA}$$
$$PISA \times V_{aliasing} = EROA \times V_{MR}$$
$$EROA = PISA \times V_{aliasing}/V_{MR} \quad (8)$$

Image plane: ME 4-chamber view

Measurement: At first, the PISA radius is measured. The aliasing velocity is determined from the color scale. The second step is the measurement of the maximum velocity of MR using CWD. The MR velocity curve is traced, and the maximum velocity (V_{MR}) as well as the VTI_{MR} is measured (see **Fig. 165-9, Panel A and B**).

EROA is calculated as it was described above. Knowing the EROA and the VTI_{MR} of the regurgitant flow, the regurgitant volume (RV) can be calculated:

$$RV = EROA \times VTI_{MR}$$

Regurgitant fraction (RF) expresses the percentage of the RV of the volumetric SV. Volumetric SV can be calculated with the Simpson's or the Teichholz method.

$$RF = RV/SV \times 100$$

PISA measurement value in severe MR: EROA > 0.4 cm^2

$$RV > 60 \text{ mL}$$
$$RF > 60\%$$

Comment: Measurement of EROA is a relatively volume independent measurement of the severity of MR.

References

1. Cohn JN, Ferrari R, Sharpe N. Cardiac remodeling—concepts and clinical implications: a consensus paper from an international forum on cardiac remodeling. Behalf of an International Forum on Cardiac Remodeling. *J Am Coll Cardiol* 2000;35:569–582.
2. Hunt SA, Abraham WT, Chin MH, et al. ACC/AHA 2005 Guideline Update for the Diagnosis and Management of Chronic Heart Failure in the Adult: a report of the American College of Cardiology/American Heart Association Task Force on Practice Guidelines (Writing Committee to Update the 2001 Guidelines for the Evaluation and Management of Heart Failure): developed in collaboration with the American College of Chest Physicians and the International Society for Heart and Lung Transplantation: endorsed by the Heart Rhythm Society. *Circulation* 2005;112:e154–e235.
3. Odell DH, Cahalan MK. Assessment of left ventricular global and segmental systolic function with transesophageal echocardiography. *Anesthesiol Clin* 2006;24:755–762.
4. Shanewise JS, Cheung AT, Aronson S, et al. ASE/SCA guidelines for performing a comprehensive intraoperative multiplane transesophageal echocardiography examination: recommendations of the American Society of Echocardiography Council for Intraoperative Echocardiography and the Society of Cardiovascular Anesthesiologists Task Force for Certification in Perioperative Transesophageal Echocardiography. *J Am Soc Echocardiogr* 1999;12:884–900.
5. Dorri F, Niederer PF, Lunkenheimer PP, et al. The architecture of the left ventricular myocytes relative to left ventricular systolic function. *Eur J Cardiothorac Surg* 2009.
6. Schiller NB, Shah PM, Crawford M, et al. Recommendations for quantitation of the left ventricle by two-dimensional echocardiography. American Society of Echocardiography Committee on Standards, Subcommittee on Quantitation of Two-Dimensional Echocardiograms. *J Am Soc Echocardiogr* 1989;2:358–367.
7. Teicholz LE, Kreulen T, Herman MV, et al. Problems in echocardiographic volume determinations: echocardiographic-angiographic correlations in the presence or absence of asynergy. *Am J Cardiol* 1976;37:7.
8. Quinones MA, Otto CM, Stoddard M, et al. Recommendations for quantification of Doppler echocardiography: a report from the Doppler Quantification Task Force of the Nomenclature and Standards Committee of the American Society of Echocardiography. *J Am Soc Echocardiogr* 2002;15:167–184.
9. Gustafsson F, Torp-Pedersen C, Brendorp B, et al. Long-term survival in patients hospitalized with congestive heart failure: relation to preserved and reduced left ventricular systolic function. *Eur Heart J* 2003;24:863–870.
10. Leung JM, Levine EH. Left ventricular end-systolic cavity obliteration as an estimate of intraoperative hypovolemia. *Anesthesiology* 1994;81:1102–1109.
11. Bonow RO, Carabello BA, Kanu C et al. ACC/AHA 2006 guidelines for the management of patients with valvular heart disease: a report of the American College of Cardiology/American Heart Association Task Force on Practice Guidelines (writing committee to revise the 1998 Guidelines for the Management of Patients With Valvular Heart Disease): developed in collaboration with the Society of Cardiovascular Anesthesiologists: endorsed by the Society for Cardiovascular Angiography and Interventions and the Society of Thoracic Surgeons. *Circulation* 2006;114:e84–e231.
12. Nagueh SF, Appleton CP, Gillebert TC, et al. Recommendations for the evaluation of left ventricular diastolic function by echocardiography. *J Am Soc Echocardiogr* 2009;22:107–133.
13. Kolias TJ, Aaronson KD, Armstrong WF. Doppler-derived dP/dt and -dP/dt predict survival in congestive heart failure. *J Am Coll Cardiol* 2000;36:1594–1599.

Part A: Atlas of Transesophageal Echocardiography Cognitive Aids
Normal Values

Larry F. Chu, MD, MS • Nathaen Weitzel, MD

NORMAL

Aortic annulus size	1.8–2.3 cm
Mitral annulus size	3.0–3.5 cm
Aortic VTI	18–25 cm
Mitral VTI	10–13 cm

MITRAL VALVE

Normal area	4.0–6.0 cm²
Mild stenosis	1.5–2.5 cm²
Moderate stenosis	1.0–1.5 cm²
Severe stenosis	<1.0 cm²

MITRAL VALVE MEAN GRADIENT

Mild MS	<5 mm Hg
Moderate MS	5–10 mm Hg
Severe MS	>10 mm Hg

MITRAL REGURGITATION (MR)

	Mild	Moderate	Severe[a]
Vena contracta (cm)	<0.3	0.3–0.7	>0.7
Color Doppler jet area (cm²)	<4.0	4–8	>8.0[b]

[a]ERO ≥0.4 cm², radius ≥1.0 cm, color Nyquist = 40 cm/s, MR peak velocity = 500 cm/s
[b]or wall hugging jet.

AORTIC VALVE

Normal area	2.5–4.5 cm²
Mild stenosis	>1.5 cm²
Moderate stenosis	1.0–1.5 cm²
Severe stenosis	<1.0 cm²

AORTIC STENOSIS

	Mild	Moderate	Severe
Peak jet velocity (m/s)	<3.0	3–4	>4.0
Mean gradient (mm Hg)	<25	25–40	>40

AORTIC REGURGITATION

	Mild	Moderate	Severe
Vena contracta (cm)	<0.3	0.3–0.6	>0.6
PHT (ms)	>500	<500–200	<200
Decel rate (m/s²)	<2.0	2.0–3.5	>3.5

CW Doppler evaluation: holosystolic flow reversal in descending aorta

Decel rate, deceleration rate; ERO, effective regurgitant orifice; PHT, pressure half time.

AR JET WIDTH AND LVOT RATIO

Mild AR	<25%
Moderate AR	25%–65%
Severe	>65%

AORTIC AND MITRAL REGURGITANT FRACTION

Mild	<30%
Moderate	30%–50%
Severe	>50%

PULMONARY HYPERTENSION

Mild	30–40 mm Hg
Moderate	40–70 mm Hg
Severe	>70 mm Hg
Severe mean PA pressure	>40 mm Hg
Normal dP/dt	>1,200 mm Hg/s (<27 ms)
Borderline	1,000–1,200 mm Hg/s (27–32 ms)
Abnormal	<1,000 mm Hg/s (>32 ms)

NORMAL LV SYSTOLIC FUNCTION PARAMETERS

Stroke volume	70–100 mL
Cardiac output	4–8 L/min
Fractional shortening	28%–44%
Fractional area change	40%–75%
Ejection fraction	55%–70%
Mild dysfunction	40%–55%
Moderate dysfunction	26%–39%
Severe dysfunction	<25%

LV HYPERTROPHY (TG SAX)

End-diastole	>1.2 cm

LV wall thickness

Patterns of diastolic dysfunction by TEE

TRANSESOPHAGEAL ECHOCARDIOGRAPHY

167 Performing a TEE Examination

Once you have properly set up your TEE according to manufacturer's guidelines, taken care of the four A's (Antibiotics, ACT, ABG, Amicar) you may perform a TEE exam.

1. Place an OG tube and suction air out of the stomach.
2. Place approximately 10 cc of gel into the mouth.
3. Jaw lift and gently intubate the esophagus with the TEE probe, it should pass easily. **If you feel resistance, stop and reevaluate the positioning.** Occasionally direct laryngoscopy with a MAC 3 to visualize the esophagus assists in probe placement.
4. Start by advancing the probe to 35 cm at the incisors and then take a look for the 4 chamber view (0 degree) and evaluate LV/RV size and function. Evaluate the mitral (MV) and tricuspid valves. If desired, a 2 chamber (90 degrees) view can examine the LV apex for pathology.
5. Pull the probe out ever so slightly until the 5 chamber view is visualized (0 degree). Examine the MV and aortic valve (AV) at various angles and in color (see AV and MV pages).
6. Advance the probe to 40 to 45 cm and obtain the transgastric LV mid-papillary short axis view (0 degree) to assess LV filling and function and SWMA (segmental wall motion abnormalities). To obtain the transgastric view you will need to anteflex the probe (push down on the wheel with your thumb so that turns clockwise).

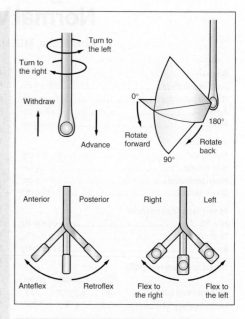

7. The deep transgastric long axis view (see 20 views card) which is useful to assess the AV by Doppler (this view can be challenging to obtain).
8. Evaluate the aorta, beginning with the descending and moving up all the way to the arch. Note abnormalities such as dissection and plaques. The surgeon will occasionally ask you to look for their bypass cannulas in the aorta.

CAVEAT: This is an abbreviated exam. The ASE/SCA guidelines describe a comprehensive 20 view TEE examination. The key is to be systematic so important pathology and information is not missed during the ETT exam.

DID YOU KNOW? The contraindications for TEE include: UGI bleed, perforation, diverticulum, tumor, stricture, varices, and recent gastric or esophageal surgery.

168

ASE/SCA 20 View Exam Overview

Shanthala Keshavacharya, MD

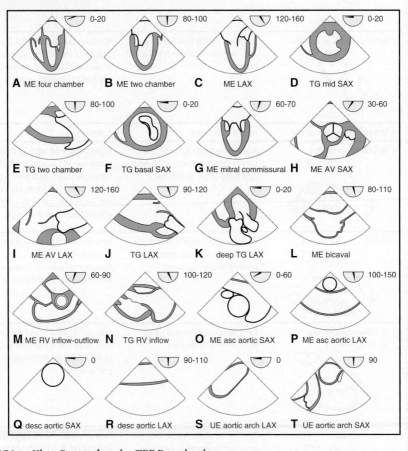

ASE/SCA 20 View Comprehensive TEE Examination

Journal of the American Society of Echocardiography, 12(10):887–900.

20 cross-sectional views composing the recommended comprehensive transesophageal echocardiographic examination. Approximate multiplane angle is indicated by the icon adjacent to each view. ME, mid esophageal (30 to 40 cm at incisors); LAX, long axis, TG, transgastric (40 to 45 cm at incisors); SAX, short axis; AV, aortic value; RV, right ventricle, asc, ascending; desc, descending; UE, upper esophageal (20 to 25 cm at incisors).

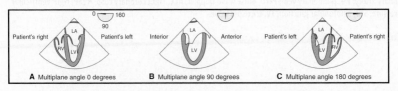

TRANSESOPHAGEAL ECHOCARDIOGRAPHY

ASE/SCA 20 View Exam Card 1/4
Guided ASE/SCA 20 View Comprehensive TEE Examination (1/4)

20	A. Upper Esophageal (20–25 cm)	How to Obtain View	Comments
	1. Aortic arch LAX. 0 degree	Obtained at the highest level. Can also be imaged by withdrawing probe after imaging the descending thoracic aorta evaluation.	Look for evidence of atherosclerosis, calcification, mobile plaques, and dissection flaps. PWD for flow reversal in AI.
	2. Aortic arch SAX. 90 degrees	As above. Slightly retroflex the probe and move side to side to evaluate arch vessels.	As above. Examine PV, MPA. Spectral Doppler of PV, parallel intercept angle. Look for L brachiocephalic vein adjacent to L subclavian artery.
30	B. Mid esophageal (30–40 cm)	How to obtain view	Comments
	3. AV SAX. 30–50 degrees	Advance the probe from the above view to obtain the classic "Mercedes-Benz" sign at 30–50 degrees.	Highest and most anterior valve. RCC is anterior, NCC is adjacent to IAS, the remainder is LCC. Look for R & L coronary arteries. CFD for AI, any calcification, vegetation, prolapse, restriction of leaflet motion or dissection.
	4. AV LAX. 120–150 degrees	Move the probe slightly to open up the Ao and LVOT, with valve cusps opening parallel to Ao wall.	Look for valve thickening, opening motion, prolapse, vegetation, dissection. CFD for AI. Measure annulus, sinus, STJ and ascending Ao.
	5. RV inflow-outflow view. 60–80 degrees	From the aortic valve view rotate forward to 60–80 degrees.	Evaluate TV, PV with and with out CFD. Spectral (CW) Doppler of TR jet for RVSP. Look for PA catheter, pacing wires.
	6. 4 chamber view. 0–20 degrees	Advance the probe slightly from the aortic image. Retroflex and angle 0–20 degrees to minimize LVOT and to open the LV apex to prevent foreshortening.	Evaluate all the chambers for size, wall motion, thrombi (in LAA and LV apex), and thickening. Evaluate TV, MV with and without CFD, mitral inflow spectral Doppler. Evaluate septal motion and thickening.

AI, aortic insufficiency; Ao, aorta; CFD, color flow Doppler; CW, color wave; IAS, interatrial septum; LAA, left atrial appendage; LCC, left coronary cusp; LVOT, left ventricular outflow tract; MPA, main pulmonary artery; NCC, noncoronary cusp; PA, pulmonary artery; PV, pulmonary vein; PWD, pulse wave Doppler; RCC, right coronary cusp; RVSP, right ventricular systolic pressure; STJ, sinotubular junction; TV, tricuspid valve.

ASE/SCA 20 VIEW EXAM CARD 2/4

Guided ASE/SCA 20 View Comprehensive TEE Examination (2/4)

30	B. Mid Esophageal (30–40 cm)	How to Obtain View	Comments
	7. Mitral commissural view. 60–80 degrees	Rotate the angle forward to 60–80 degrees to get "trap door" view.	Measure the commissural distance for annular dilation. Look for restriction, calcification, redundancy of leaflet motion, CFD. See MV card.
	8. 2-chamber view. 80–100 degrees	Increase the angle further to obtain the 2 chamber view.	Evaluate MV, CFD, look for regional wall motion, thickening in anterior and inferior wall, also examine the LAA for evidence of thrombus. PWD: A LAA velocity >0.5 m/s indicates good atrial contractility and less likelihood of thrombus or low flow state. PWD LUPV.
	9. LV long axis view. 120–160 degrees	Increase the angle further from above image.	Examine the LV anteroseptal, posterior wall thickening and wall motion. Look for SAM.
	10. Bicaval view. 80–110 degrees	From 4-chamber view, rotate the probe to the right in order to center the RA. Increase the multiplane angle to 80–110 degrees.	Examine RA, RAA, IAS, SVC, IVC. CFD for ASD, PFO. Perform bubble study, look for lines, aid in femoral cannulation.
	11. ME Asc Ao SAX. 0–60 degrees	From AV SAX pull the probe back to evaluate great vessels.	Can be used to image Asc Ao, MPA, RPA, LPA and SVC. Look for PAC, saddle embolus in MPA and bifurcation, Ao dissection, plaque.
	12. ME Asc Ao LAX. 100–150 degrees	As above, increase the angle 100–150 degrees.	Can be used to view the asc Ao in long axis and can image RPA in SAX.

Ao, aorta; Asc, ascending; ASD, atrial septal defect; CFD, color flow Doppler; IAS, interatrial septum; IVC, inferior vena cava; LAA, left atrial appendage; LUPV, left upper pulmonary vein; MV, mitral valve; MPA, main pulmonary artery; PA, pulmonary artery; PAC, pulmonary artery catheter; PFO, patent foramen ovale; PV, pulmonary vein; PWD, pulse wave Doppler; RA, right atrium; RAA, right atrial appendage; RPA, right pulmonary artery; RVSP, right ventricular systolic pressure; SAM, systolic anterior motion; SAX, short axis; SVC, superior vena cava; TV, tricuspid valve.

TRANSESOPHAGEAL ECHOCARDIOGRAPHY

ASE/SCA 20 View Exam Card 3/4

Guided ASE/SCA 20 View Comprehensive TEE Examination (3/4)

40	C. Trans Gastric Views (40–45 cm)	How to Obtain View	Comments
	13. Basal MV SAX. 0–20 degrees	Advance the probe gently to the stomach and anteflex the tip. Pull the probe back until the MV is seen.	Evaluate the MV, trace the MV area. CFD to localize the leaflet pathology.
	14. Mid papillary SAX. 0–20 degrees	Advance the probe to image at the level of the papillary muscle.	Assess global ventricular function, regional WMA all RCA, LAD, LCX distributions. Evaluate preload. Obtain cine loop for comparison. M Mode for LV dimension.
	15. Trans gastric 2 chamber. 80–100 degrees	Increase the angle to 90 degrees from the above image.	Evaluate the mitral apparatus i.e., papillary muscle, chordae, leaflet, anterior and inferior basal ventricular wall motion. Look for restriction or redundancy of chordae.
	16. LV long axis. 90–130 degrees	Further advance the angle from the above image.	Provides reasonable image for spectral Doppler interrogation of AV and LVOT.
	17. RV inflow. 100–120 degrees	Rotate the probe to right form mid papillary view to center the RV and increase the angle.	Examine right atrium, right ventricle, tricuspid valve and papillary muscle. Further rotation of the angle can sometimes reveal RVOT and PV.
	18. Deep trans gastric view. 0–20 degrees	Advance the probe deep into stomach and maximally anteflex and slowly withdraw the probe. This view is hard to obtain and probe needs manipulation in terms of advance, pull, rotate etc.	This view aligns the probe almost parallel to the heart to facilitate spectral Doppler interrogation of AV and LVOT.

AV, aortic valve; **CFD,** color flow Doppler; **LCA,** left coronary artery; **Lcx,** left circumflex; **LVOT,** left ventricular outflow tract; **MV,** mitral valve; **PV,** pulmonary vein; **RCA,** right coronary artery; **RV,** right ventricle; **RVOT,** right ventricular outflow tract; **WMA,** wall motion abnormality.

ASE/SCA 20 View Exam Card 4/4
Guided ASE/SCA 20 View Comprehensive TEE Examination (4/4)

40	C. Trans Gastric Views (40–45 cm)	How to Obtain View	Comments
	19. Evaluation Of Desc Thoracic. 0 degree **A** 90–130 degrees **B**	For complete examination of the aorta, rotate the probe to the left until the descending thoracic aorta is visualized. Reduce the image depth and increase the transducer frequency. Withdraw the probe slowly to image the entire length up to the aortic arch. Rotate the probe as required to keep the image in the center.	Image in 0 and 90 degrees. Look for dissection, false and true lumen plaques, aneurysm or thrombus. PWD for flow reversal in AI.
	20. Pulmonary veins <small>Courtesy of Kent Garman, MD</small>	Begin with 4-chamber view. LUPV— Adj to LAA at 0 and 90 degrees. LLPV— turn probe further left and advance 1–2 cm. RUPV—turn probe to right from LAA at 90 degrees. RLPV— advance 1–2 cm from above.	Confirm the pulmonary vein with CFD. Do PWD to evaluate diastolic dysfunction and assess the severity of MR. Localize source air during de-airing maneuver.
	21. Coronary sinus 0–20 degrees	Obtain 4-chamber view. Rotate the probe to center TV. Advance 1–2 cm and retroflex.	Assist with placement and confirmation of retrograde cardioplegia catheter. Can also be imaged in SAX 2-chamber view, transgastric basal view and in cross section in bicaval view.

Ao, aorta; **AV,** aortic valve; **CFD,** color flow Doppler; **CWD,** continuous wave Doppler; **IAS,** inter atrial septum; **LAA,** left atrial appendage; **LAX,** long axis view; **LCC,** left coronary cusp; **LVOT,** left ventricular outflow tract; **NCC,** noncoronary cusp; **PV,** pulmonary vein, right, left, upper, lower; **PWD,** pulse wave Doppler; **RCC,** right coronary cusp; **RVOT,** right ventricular outflow tract; **SAX,** short axis view; **WMA,** wall motion abnormality.

TRANSESOPHAGEAL ECHOCARDIOGRAPHY

169

Evaluation of Myocardial Perfusion

Larry F. Chu • Nathaen Weitzel

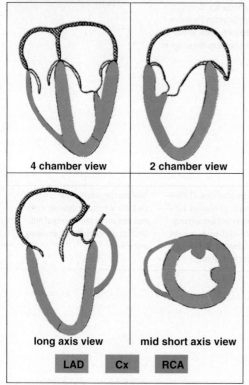

4 chamber view

2 chamber view

long axis view

mid short axis view

| LAD | Cx | RCA |

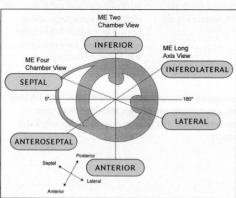

ME Two
Chamber View

INFERIOR

ME Long
Axis View

ME Four
Chamber View

INFEROLATERAL

SEPTAL

0°—

—180°

LATERAL

ANTEROSEPTAL

Posterior

Septal

ANTERIOR

Lateral

Anterior

Once you have mastered obtaining the different TEE views, you can use your skills to assist the surgeon in identifying areas of myocardial ischemia.

This can be done by recording loops during the pre-bypass period and comparing contractility and wall motion abnormalities to the post-bypass heart.

By looking for segmental wall motion abnormalities, you can help localize areas of ischemia to specific vessels.

The mid short axis view (see "20 view overview, D", Chapter 168) may be best to visualize LV function. However, changes that occur in the apex will not be visualized.

You should also familiarize yourself with the orientation of the heart in the mid short axis view. The mnemonic "**SALI**" describes the main four segments-septal, anterior, lateral, and inferior. The remaining two segments are "sandwiched in between—anteroseptal and inferolateral." You should know what these are and how to identify them on your TEE examination.

Qualitative grading of wall motion is:

1 = Normal (>30% thickening)
2 = Mildly hypokinetic (10% to 30%)
3 = Severely hypokinetic (<10%)
4 = Akinetic (does not thicken)
5 = Dyskinetic (paradoxical movement)

DID YOU KNOW? TEE experts divide the left ventricle into 16 segments by examining 5 cross-sectional views (see "Left Ventricle 16 Segment Model").

Left Ventricle 16 Segment Model

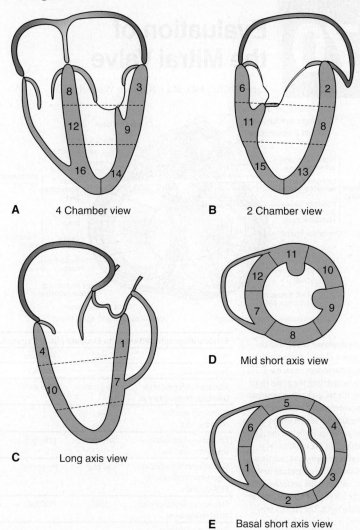

Basal Segments	Mid Segments	Apical Segments
1 = Basal anteroseptal	7 = Mid anteroseptal	13 = Apical anterior
2 = Basal anterior	8 = Mid anterior	14 = Apical lateral
3 = Basal lateral	9 = Mid lateral	15 = Apical inferior
4 = Basal posterior	10 = Mid posterior	16 = Apical septal
5 = Basal inferior	11 = Mid inferior	
6 = Basal septal	12= Mid septal	

Journal of the American Society of Echocardiography 1999;12(10):884–900.

170 Evaluation of the Mitral Valve

Larry F. Chu, MD, MS • Nathaen Weitzel, MD

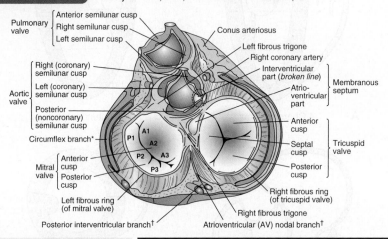

The anatomy displayed above, and on following page will help to orient you to the valve structures seen in each 2-D TEE view. Begin by inserting the probe to 30 to 35 cm for the ME 4-chamber view and identify the anterior and posterior mitral leaflets. The anterior leaflet will be on the left and the posterior leaflet on the right. Move through the 5 ME views to fully evaluate leaflet anatomy and function. As the multiplane angle is increased beyond 90 degrees, note that the posterior leaflet will be to the left of your screen, and the anterior to the right. The ME LAX view (120 degrees) is a key view looking at the coaptation of A2/P2 for most patients.

Once oriented, assess the overall structure and function of the valve. This includes looking for and describing prolapsing or flail segments, stenotic or restricted leaflet motion (CW Doppler through the valve), and degree of annular dilation (try to describe lesion by location—i.e., prolapse at A1). Color Doppler is paramount in evaluation of MR and aids in locating the site of the lesions. Surgeons want to know the degree of MR, whether it is central or eccentric, which segment is affected (i.e., P2 flail), mitral valve dimensions (commissural view, ME LAX view), and degree of annular calcification.

Echocardiographic Methods to Evaluate Mitral Regurgitation

Method	Mild	Moderate	Severe
Vena contracta (cm)	<0.3	0.3–0.7	>0.7
Spatial area mapping of the color Doppler regurgitant jet	1.5–4.0 cm^2	4.0–8.0 cm^2	>8.0 cm
Pulmonary vein flow characteristics	S wave > D wave		Systolic flow reversal
Estimation of the mitral regurgitant fraction	20%–30%	30%–50%	>50%
Estimation mitral effective regurgitant orifice by the PISA method	<20 mm^2	20–39 mm^2	>40 mm
Secondary 2-D changes: left atrial enlargement	Mild	Moderate	Severe
Peak E-wave velocity			>1.2 m/s

Assessment of mitral stenosis severity

	Normal Values	Mild	Moderate	Severe
Valve area (cm^2)	4–6	1.5–2.0	1.0–1.5	<1.0
Mean gradient (mm Hg)	0–4	5	5–10	>10
Pressure half-time (ms)	70–100	100–150	150–220	>220

Calculation of mitral valve area

$$MVA\ (cm^2) = \frac{220}{Pressure\ half\text{-}time} = \frac{760}{Deceleration\ time}$$

LVOT (area) × LVOT (TVI) = MV (area) × MV (TVI) {continuity equation}
PISA (area) × PISA (velocity) = MV (area) × MV (velocity) {PISA method}

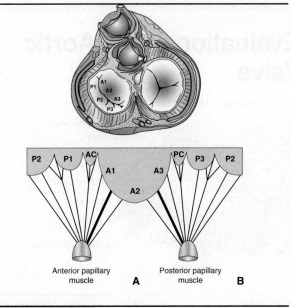

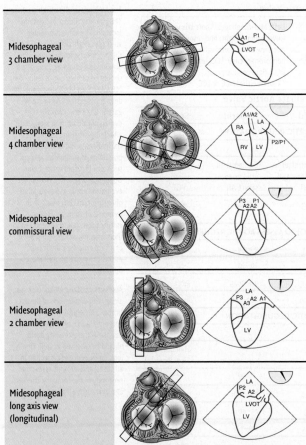

Midesophageal 3 chamber view	A1 P1 / LVOT
Midesophageal 4 chamber view	A1/A2 / RA LA / RV LV / P2/P1
Midesophageal commissural view	P3 P1 / A2 A2
Midesophageal 2 chamber view	LA / P3 A2 A1 / A3 / LV
Midesophageal long axis view (longitudinal)	LA / P2 A2 / LVOT / LV

Mitral Valve ASE/SCA Terminology (per Carpentier)

Chordal relationships: Anterior leaflet divided into A1, A2, A3.

Posterior leaflet divided into P1 (anterolateral scallop), P2 (middle scallop), P3 (posteromedial scallop).

Commissural clefts not named anterior or posterior.

Chordae arising from the anterior papillary muscle attach to A1, AC, P1, and lateral half of P2, A2.

Chordae arising from the posterior papillary muscle attach to A3, PC, P3, and medial half of P2, A2.

Carpentier Terminology

Column A illustrates the cross section the midesophageal views make through the mitral valve leaflets. Anatomical diagram is drawn viewing mitral and tricuspid leaflets from their atrial side. Column B shows schematic of TEE view seen. Section transversed by TEE plane may vary from patient to patient, however general relationship remains.

TRANSESOPHAGEAL ECHOCARDIOGRAPHY

171

Evaluation of the Aortic Valve

Larry F. Chu, MD, MS • Nathaen Weitzel, MD

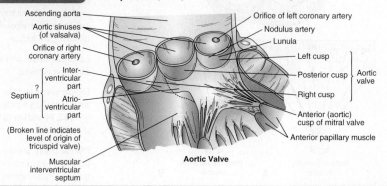

Ascending aorta
Aortic sinuses (of valsalva)
Orifice of right coronary artery
Inter-ventricular part
? Septium
Atrio-ventricular part
(Broken line indicates level of origin of tricuspid valve)
Muscular interventricular septum

Orifice of left coronary artery
Nodulus artery
Lunula
Left cusp
Posterior cusp } Aortic valve
Right cusp
Anterior (aortic) cusp of mitral valve
Anterior papillary muscle

Aortic Valve

Echocardiographic Views of the Aortic Valve

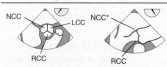

NCC
LCC
RCC

NCC*
RCC

Left: Mid-esophageal short axis view of Aortic valve leaflets. **Right:** Mid- esophageal long axis view of the aortic valve leaflets. NCC, noncoronary cusp; LCC, left coronary cusp; RCC, right coronary cusp.
* Can be either NCC or LCC

Echocardiographic Methods to Evaluate Aortic Valve

Method	Mild	Moderate	Severe
QUALITATIVE METHODS TO ASSESS AORTIC REGURGITATION			
Angiographic data	1+	2+	3–4+
Color Doppler jet width	Central jet width <25% LVOT	Greater than mild no signs severe AR	Central jet width >65% LVOT
Doppler vena contracta width (cm)	<0.3	0.3–0.6	>0.6
QUANTITATIVE METHOD (CATH OR ECHO) TO ASSESS AORTIC REGURGITATION			
Regurgitant volume (mL/beat)	<30	30–59	≥60
Regurgitant fraction (%)	<30	30–49	≥50
Regurgitant orifice area (cm²)	<0.1	0.1–0.29	≥0.3
Pressure half-time (ms)	>500	200–500	<200
ADDITIONAL CRITERIA TO ASSESS AORTIC REGURGITATION			
Left ventricular Size			Increased
Aortic diastolic flow reversal			Holodiastolic Flow Reversal
Assessment of aortic stenosis			
Peak jet velocity (m/s)	<3.0	3.0–4.0	>4.0
Mean gradient (mm Hg)	<25	25–40	>40
Valve area (cm²)	>1.5	1.0–1.5	<1.0
Valve area index (cm²/m²)			<0.6

The AV lends itself to high quality TEE imaging due to its anatomic location. The valve is oriented such that slight anterior flexion of the probe is typically required to obtain ideal imaging. Evaluation should be carried out utilizing the ME AV SAX and LAX views, and the deep transgastric LAX or trans-gastric LAX view. Look for the degree of calcification along with any flail/prolapsing segments of the leaflets. Additionally, look for possibility of congenital lesions such as a bicuspid valve. Color Doppler, along with CW Doppler evaluation are key in evaluation of regurgitant flow along with elements of stenosis. Heavy calcification should be reported to the surgeons, along with degree of mitral annular calcification as this can make an AVR more difficult.

Assessment of the AV annular size, along with dimensions of the aortic root are helpful in aortic valve surgery. Degree of atheromatous disease in the ascending aorta should be assessed as well. Finally, look for evidence of dissection in all cases, and if found assess the proximity to the coronary arteries and aortic valve leaflets.

Regional Anesthesia in the Anticoagulated Patient

Larry F. Chu, MD, MS · Bassam Kadry, MD

WARNING

The following cognitive aid was created using the 2010 Practice Advisory from the American Society of Regional Anesthesia for patients receiving regional anesthesia and antithrombotic therapy and Fleischmann KH, et al. "Practice guidelines often fail to keep pace with the rapid evolution of medicine: a call for clinicians to remain vigilant and revisit their own practice patterns." *Reg Anesth Pain Med* 2010; 35(1):4–7. As noted in their guidelines, "An understanding of the complexity of this issue is essential to patient management; a 'cookbook' approach is not appropriate. Rather, the decision to perform spinal or epidural anesthesia/analgesia and the timing of catheter removal in a patient receiving antithrombotic therapy should be made on an individual basis, weighing the small, although definite risk of spinal hematoma with the benefits of regional anesthesia for a specific patient." Deriving time intervals to minimize risk of hematoma depends on the amount of time it takes the drug to undergo three elimination half-lives. Periodic neurological assessments should be conducted for minimum of 24 hours post intervention if clinical situation is unclear.

Guidelines for Regional Anesthesia in the Anticoagulated Patient (Chu and Kadry)

Anticoagulant	Time Interval for Placement or Removal of Catheter After Last Dose	Time Interval to Restart Anticoagulation After Catheter Removal
Abciximab	48 h	12 h
Argatroban	6 h; check ACT or PTT	2 h
Cilostazol (alone)	None	None
Cilostazol + Aspirin	48 h	1 h
Clopidogrel	7 d	24 h
Dalteparin[a,b] 120 U/kg q 12h	24 h	Indwelling catheters should be removed prior to starting LMWH thromboprophylaxis. After removal: minimum of 2 h. If catheter not removed, wait 24 h.
Dalteparin[a,b] 200 U/kg qd	24 h	Not explicitly specified
Enoxaprin (low dose)[a,b] (0.5 mg/kg/qd)	10–12 h	2 h
Enoxaprin (high dose)[a,b] (1 mg/kg q 12h)	24 h	Indwelling catheters should be removed prior to starting LMWH thromboprophylaxis. After removal: minimum of 2 h. If catheter not removed, wait 24 h.

The recommendations in the following tables were adapted from the 2010 Consensus Conference of the American Society of Regional Anesthesia and Pain Medicine, "Regional Anesthesia in the Patient Receiving Antithrombotic or Thrombolytic Therapy (Third Edition)." *Reg Anesth Pain Med* 2010; 35(1):64–101 and Fleischmann KH, et al. Practice guidelines often fail to keep pace with the rapid evolution of medicine: a call for clinicians to remain vigilant and revisit their own practice patterns. *Reg Anesth Pain Med* 2010; 35(1):4–7. Variances from the recommendations may be acceptable based on the judgment of the responsible anesthesiologist. The recommendations are designed to encourage quality patient care and safety but cannot guarantee a specific outcome. They are subject to revision at any time and updates can be found at http://www.asra.com

[a] Monitoring of anti-Xa level is not predictive of the risk of bleeding and is therefore NOT recommended.

[b] The presence of blood during needle and catheter placement does not necessitate postponing surgery, however LMWH therapy in this setting should be delayed for 24 h.

Guidelines for Regional Anesthesia in the Anticoagulated Patient (Chu and Kadry)

Anticoagulant	Time Interval for Placement or Removal of Catheter After Last Dose	Time Interval to Restart Anticoagulation After Catheter Removal
Enoxaprin (high dose) (1.5 mg/kg qd)	24 h	Indwelling catheters should be removed prior to starting LMWH thromboprophylaxis. After removal: minimum of 2 h. If catheter not removed, wait 24 h.
Eptifibatide Tirofiban	8 h	4 h
Fondaparinux	2.5 mg: 4 d	Suggest 12 h
	5 mg: 7 d	Suggest 24 h
Heparin IV[c]	2–4 h, PTT < 35	1 h
Heparin SC 5000 U BID	None	None
NSAIDS Cox2 Inhibitors Herbal	None	None
Ticlopidine	14 d	Not explicitly specified

[c] Because heparin-induced thrombocytopenia (HIT) may occur during heparin administration, patients receiving heparin > 4d should have a platelet count prior to neuraxial block.

"An understanding of the complexity of this issue is essential to patient management; a "cookbook" approach is not appropriate. Rather, the decision to perform spinal or epidural anesthesia/analgesia and the timing of catheter removal in a patient receiving antithrombotic therapy should be made on an individual basis, weighing the small, although definite risk of spinal hematoma with the benefits of regional anesthesia for a specific patient."

PERIPHERAL NERVE BLOCK PROCEDURES

Guidelines for Regional Anesthesia in the Anticoagulated Patient (Chu and Kadry)

Anticoagulant	Time Interval for Placement or Removal of Catheter After Last Dose	Time Interval to Restart Anticoagulation After Catheter Removal
Tinzaparin [a,b] 175 U/kg qd	24 h	Not explicitly specified
Tirofiban	8 h	4 h
Warfarin [d,e,f] 5 mg/PO (low dose)	Patient on chronic warfarin therapy must stop for 4–5 d. Patients receiving an initial dose 24 h prior to surgery or who have already received a second dose should have PT/INR checked prior to block placement (Goal: INR < 1.5)	An INR > 3 should prompt the physician to withhold or reduce the warfarin dose in patients with indwelling catheters. Neuraxial catheters should be removed when the INR is < 1.5. A neurological assessment is recommended for at least 24 h after catheter removal if in doubt.

[d] Early after discontinuation of warfarin, PT/INR reflect predominately factor VII levels. In spite of acceptable factor VII levels, factors II and X levels may not be adequate for normal hemostasis. Thus, caution should be used when placing blocks in patients recently disconnected from chronic warfarin therapy.

[e] PT/INR should be monitored daily and checked prior to catheter removal if the initial dose was given more than 36 h preoperatively.

[f] Neurologic testing of sensory and motor function should be performed routinely, and continued at least 24 h after catheter removal (and longer if INR was >1.5).

173

Part A:
The Upper Extremity
Interscalene Block

Edward R. Mariano, MD, MAS · Vanessa J. Loland, MD

The interscalene block of the brachial plexus is commonly performed for surgical procedures of the shoulder and the upper arm. It may be performed with the arm in any position and provides excellent anesthesia and postoperative analgesia (1,2). Important surface landmarks to identify include the sternocleidomastoid (SCM), cricoid cartilage, and interscalene muscles. Techniques employing ultrasound (3) or electrical stimulation (4) for localization of the brachial plexus have largely supplanted the historic paresthesia-seeking technique of Winnie (5), although the anatomic considerations remain the same. Continuous interscalene blocks provide prolonged analgesia following shoulder surgery among other benefits.

1) **Indications and contraindications**
   a) Indications
      i) Surgical anesthesia or postoperative analgesia of the shoulder or the upper arm
      ii) Frequent sparing of the C8 and T1 nerve roots makes this block unreliable for hand or wrist procedures unless selective ulnar nerve and/or medial antebrachial cutaneous nerve blocks are performed.

READ MORE
Continuous peripheral nerve blocks, Chapter 35, page 266

   b) Contraindications
      i) Absolute contraindications
        (1) Local infection at the site of planned needle placement
        (2) Pneumonectomy or hemidiaphragmatic paresis on the contralateral side
          (a) A ultrasound study confirmed 100% ipsilateral hemidiaphragmatic paresis due to phrenic nerve blockade following interscalene block (6).
          (b) In patients with normal pulmonary function, phrenic nerve blockade is not clinically significant.

Interscalene block frequently spares C8 and T1 nerve roots.

      ii) Relative contraindications
        (1) Comorbid pulmonary disease, coagulopathy, or preexisting nerve injury

2) **Risks and complications**
   a) General risks involving peripheral nerve blockade are localized bleeding, intravascular injection with local anesthetic toxicity, and infection at the site of needle puncture.
   b) Site-specific side effects from interscalene block
      i) Phrenic nerve blockade
      ii) Ipsilateral Horner syndrome (ptosis, miosis, and anhydrosis)
      iii) Hoarseness due to laryngeal vasodilation or recurrent laryngeal nerve block

The incidence of ipsilateral hemidiaphragmatic paresis with interscalene block is 100%.

      c) Potential complications specific to the interscalene block

          i) Vertebral artery injection

          ii) Epidural or intrathecal injection

          iii) Pneumothorax

3) **Equipment**

    a) Common equipment for all peripheral nerve block techniques includes sterile skin cleansing solution, sterile gloves, a marking pen, and two 20-mL syringes of local anesthetic solution with extension tubing.

    b) A nerve stimulator technique requires an electrical nerve stimulator with a compatible insulated needle and a grounding electrode.

    c) The paresthesia technique only requires a needle attached to syringes of local anesthetic and a cooperative patient.

      i) If using a paresthesia-seeking or stimulation-guided technique, a needle of appropriate length (~2 cm for single injection) may help reduce the likelihood of serious complications.

    d) Ultrasound-guided regional anesthesia requires portable ultrasound equipment and a high-frequency linear transducer for interscalene block.

4) **Technique**

    a) **Monitoring**

      i) Peripheral nerve blocks should be placed in a location where the patient's noninvasive BP, SpO_2, and EKG may be monitored.

      ii) Supplemental O_2 should be provided via face mask or nasal cannulae especially when IV sedation is administered.

    b) **Positioning and preparation**

      i) Position the patient supine with the back slightly elevated. A small shoulder roll may be placed for slight neck extension.

      ii) Apply monitors and supplemental O_2.

      iii) IV sedation should be administered, but the patient must be able to follow commands and volunteer sensory information.

      iv) With the head turned away from the side to be blocked, the patient should lift the head to aid in the identification of the SCM muscle.

    c) **Identification of surface anatomy**

      i) A line should be drawn along the posterior border of the SCM.

      ii) The cricothyroid cartilage should be identified and a line drawn along a skin crease at this level to approximate C6 level.

      iii) Standing next to the head of the bed, the person performing the procedure should palpate quadrant closest to the clavicle posterior to the SCM while the patient takes a forceful inspiration through the nose. This should delineate the interscalene groove and allow marking of the anterior and middle scalene muscles (Cognitive Aid: Panel A).

    d) **Stimulating interscalene block**

      i) Using sterile technique and following injection of a local anesthetic skin wheal, a short insulated block needle should be inserted at a 45 degrees angle to the skin surface in the interscalene groove at the C6 level with the tip directed slightly medial, caudad, and posterior (Fig. 173-1). A perpendicular angle should be avoided as this angle is more likely to lead to intraforaminal needle placement.

      ii) The brachial plexus is superficial at this level and should be contacted within 2 cm of needle insertion in nearly all patients (Fig. 173-2).

A needle angle perpendicular to skin should be avoided as this angle is more likely to lead to infraforaminal needle placement.

Figure 173-1   Needle Position When Performing the Interscalene Block

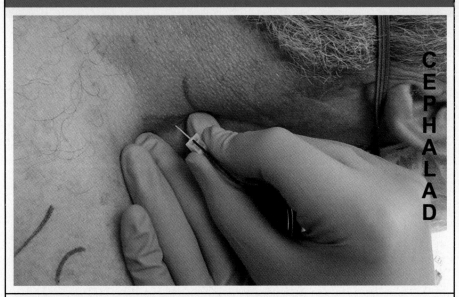

CEPHALAD

Perpendicular to skin with an angle slightly medial, caudad, and posterior.

    iii) Once an appropriate sensory paresthesia or motor response is elicited in the affected limb at a stimulating current <0.5 mA, 30 to 40 mL of local anesthetic should be slowly injected in incremental volumes following careful aspiration. A deltoid response is as effective as a biceps twitch when using a peripheral nerve stimulator (7).

  e) **Ultrasound-guided interscalene block**

    i) With a high-frequency linear transducer positioned perpendicular to skin over the posterior border of the SCM (Cognitive Aid: Panel B), the brachial plexus is visualized in short axis between the anterior and the middle scalene (Cognitive Aid: Panel C).

    ii) After sterile skin preparation, a local anesthetic skin wheal is raised posterior to the edge of the ultrasound transducer.

    iii) The block needle is inserted through the skin wheal and directed anteriorly using in-plane guidance toward the target nerve bundle (3).

    iv) Once the needle tip passes through the middle scalene muscle into the interscalene groove, local anesthetic is injected incrementally after a negative aspiration test for blood until circumferential injectate spread is visually confirmed.

5) **Evaluation of the block**

  a) The quality of nerve blockade must be evaluated prior to surgical incision even if intraoperative general anesthesia is planned.

  b) Motor testing

    i) Strength of elbow flexion against resistance tests the biceps muscle innervated by the musculocutaneous nerve.

    ii) Similarly, strength of elbow extension tests the triceps muscle innervated by the radial nerve.

    iii) Strength of shoulder abduction tests the deltoid muscle innervated by the axillary nerve.

Figure 173-2 The Safe Performance of the Interscalene Block Requires Superficial Needle Placement

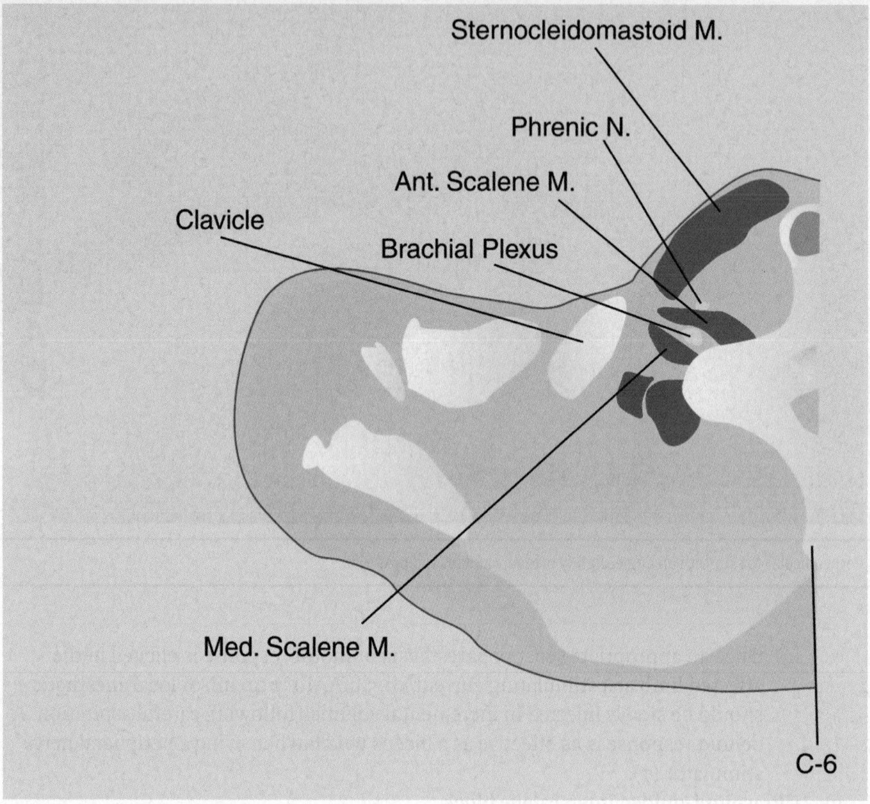

Sternocleidomastoid M.

Phrenic N.

Ant. Scalene M.

Clavicle

Brachial Plexus

Med. Scalene M.

C-6

Reproduced from Brown AR. Interscalene block. In: Chelly JE, ed. *Peripheral nerve blocks: A color atlas*. 3rd ed. Philadelphia: Lippincott Williams & Wilkins, 2009: 59, with permission.

   c) Sensory testing
      i) Pinching the base of the index finger, small finger, and medial aspect of the forearm assesses anesthesia in the distribution of the median, ulnar, and medial antebrachial cutaneous nerves, respectively.
      ii) Pinching over the posterior aspect of the shoulder over the scapula evaluates the block of the suprascapular nerve.
6) **Postoperative management**
   a) All patients who undergo brachial plexus blockade should be discharged with a supportive sling.
   b) Patients with Horner syndrome and uncomfortable anhydrosis of the ipsilateral eye may benefit from artificial tears.
   c) For outpatient procedures, respiratory status should be assessed prior to discharge, but a routine chest radiograph for pneumothorax or hemidiaphragmatic paresis is not recommended in asymptomatic patients.

References

1. Long TR, Wass CT, Burkle CM. Perioperative interscalene blockade: an overview of its history and current clinical use. *J Clin Anesth* 2002;14:546–556.
2. Singelyn FJ, Lhotel L, Fabre B. Pain relief after arthroscopic shoulder surgery: a comparison of intraarticular analgesia, suprascapular nerve block, and interscalene brachial plexus block. *Anesth Analg* 2004;99:589–992.
3. Mariano ER, Loland VJ, Ilfeld BM. Interscalene perineural catheter placement using an ultrasound-guided posterior approach. *Reg Anesth Pain Med* 2009;34:60–63.
4. Klein SM, Grant SA, Greengrass RA, et al. Interscalene brachial plexus block with a continuous catheter insertion system and a disposable infusion pump. *Anesth Analg* 2000;91:1473–1478.
5. Winnie AP. Interscalene brachial plexus block. *Anesth Analg* 1970;49:455–466.
6. Urmey WF, Talts KH, Sharrock NE. One hundred percent incidence of hemidiaphragmatic paresis associated with interscalene brachial plexus anesthesia as diagnosed by ultrasonography. *Anesth Analg* 1991;72:498–503.
7. Silverstein WB, Saiyed MU, Brown AR. Interscalene block with a nerve stimulator: a deltoid motor response is a satisfactory endpoint for successful block. *Reg Anesth Pain Med* 2000;25:356–359.

US-Guided Interscalene Block

By Edward R. Mariano, MD, MAS · Larry F. Chu, MD, MS · Vanessa J. Loland, MD

Patient Position: Position the patient supine with the back slightly elevated. A small shoulder roll may be placed for slight neck extension. With the head turned away from the side to be blocked, the patient should lift the head to aid in the identification of the sternocleido-mastoid (SCM) muscle.

Needle Size: 22 to 17-gauge, 50 to 100-mm block needle

Volume: 20 to 40-mL local anesthetic

Anatomic Landmarks

A A line should be drawn along the posterior border of the SCM. The cricoid cartilage should be identified and a line drawn along a skin crease at this level to approximate C6 level. Standing next to the head of the bed, palpate the quadrant closest to the clavicle posterior to the SCM while the patient takes a forceful inspiration through the nose. This should delineate the interscalene groove and allow marking of the anterior and middle scalene muscles.

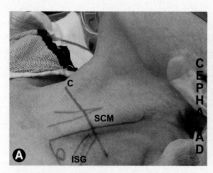 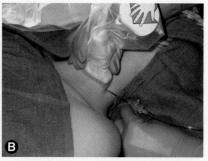

A. Surface anatomy relevant to the interscalene block. SCM, sternocleidomastoid muscle; C, cricoid cartilage; ISG, interscalene groove. **B.** A HF linear transducer is placed perpendicular to skin posterior to the sternocleidomastoid muscle. The block needle is inserted posterior to the transducer and directed antero-medially for in-plane needle guidance.

Approach and Technique

B With a high-frequency (HF) linear transducer positioned perpendicular to skin over the posterior border of the SCM, **C** the brachial plexus is visualized in short-axis between the anterior and middle scalene.

After sterile skin preparation, a local anesthetic skin wheal is raised posterior to the edge of the ultrasound transducer.

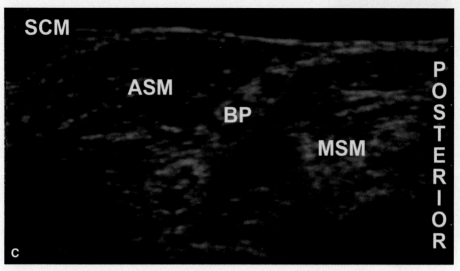

C. Short-axis image of the brachial plexus in the interscalene groove. SCM, sternocleidomastoid muscle; ASM, anterior scalene muscle; MSM, middle scalene muscle; BP, brachial plexus.

The block needle is inserted through the skin wheal and directed anteriorly using in-plane guidance toward the target nerve bundle.

Once the needle tip passes through the middle scalene muscle into the interscalene groove, local anesthetic is injected incrementally after a negative aspiration test for blood until the circumferential injectate spread is visually confirmed.

Evaluation of Block
Motor testing
Strength of elbow flexion against resistance tests the biceps muscle innervated by the musculocutaneous nerve. Strength of elbow extension tests the triceps muscle innervated by the radial nerve. Strength of shoulder abduction tests the deltoid muscle innervated by the axillary nerve.

Sensory testing
Pinching the base of the index finger, small finger, and medial aspect of the forearm assesses anesthesia in the distribution of the median, ulnar, and medial antebrachial cutaneous nerves, respectively. Pinching over the posterior aspect of the shoulder over the scapula evaluates the block of the suprascapular nerve.

174 Supraclavicular Block

Vanessa J. Loland, MD • Edward R. Mariano, MD, MAS

The supraclavicular block anesthetizes the brachial plexus at the level of the distal trunks/divisions as the plexus crosses over the first rib between the insertion sites of the anterior and the middle scalene muscles (1). At this point, the brachial plexus is typically posterolateral and slightly cephalad to the subclavian artery and still within the interscalene groove. An advantage of this block is that it can be performed with the arm in any position. The use of real-time ultrasound guidance may significantly reduce the potential risk of pneumothorax associated with this approach (2,3) and improves the efficacy and speed of onset of this block (4).

1) **Indications and contraindications**
   a) **Indications**
      i) Surgical anesthesia or postoperative analgesia of the upper arm, elbow, forearm, or hand
      ii) If this block is to be used for surgery extending to the shoulder, a superficial cervical plexus block and/or suprascapular nerve block may need to be performed to anesthetize the skin overlying the shoulder.
   b) **Contraindications**
      i) Absolute contraindications
         (1) Local infection at the site of planned needle insertion
         (2) Pneumonectomy or hemidiaphragmatic paresis on the contralateral side due to the risk of ipsilateral phrenic nerve block (5).
      ii) Relative contraindications
         (1) Coagulopathy
         (2) Preexisting nerve injury
         (3) Emphysema or other severe pulmonary disease due to possible phrenic nerve block and the potential risk of pneumothorax

Supraclavicular block should not be performed in a patient with one functional lung for fear of ipsilateral hemidiaphragmatic paresis or possible pneumothorax.

2) **Risks and complications**
   a) General risks involving peripheral nerve blockade are localized bleeding, intravascular injection with local anesthetic toxicity, and infection at the site of needle puncture.
   b) Potential risks specific to the supraclavicular block
      i) The most dreaded complication of the supraclavicular block is pneumothorax with a prevalence of 0.5% to 6.1% (1).
         (1) This quoted risk is higher than with other brachial plexus blocks but is most likely technique dependent with the classic vertical approach carrying a higher risk than the plumb-bob approach (6,7) and ultrasound-guided techniques (2).

Pneumothorax is a known risk of the supraclavicular block, but it occurs less often with this block compared to the interscalene block and may be avoided with ultrasound guidance.

(2) However, the fact that the presentation of pneumothorax may be delayed for many hours makes this technique less appealing for outpatient surgery (1).

ii) In addition, the proximity of the nerves to the subclavian artery introduces the risk of intravascular injection.

c) Site-specific side effects from supraclavicular block include phrenic nerve blockade and ipsilateral Horner syndrome (ptosis, miosis, and anhydrosis) (1).

i) Phrenic nerve blockade is less common following supraclavicular block than interscalene block (5).

ii) Ultrasound guidance with lower injectate volume may further reduce the risk of inadvertent phrenic nerve block (8).

3) **Equipment**

a) Common equipment for all peripheral nerve block techniques include sterile skin cleansing solution, sterile gloves, a marking pen, and two 20-mL syringes of local anesthetic solution with extension tubing.

b) The nerve stimulator technique requires an electrical nerve stimulator with a compatible 1- to 2-inch insulated needle and a grounding electrode.

c) Ultrasound-guided regional anesthesia requires portable ultrasound equipment and a high-frequency linear transducer (preferred) or small curvilinear transducer for supraclavicular block.

4) **Technique**

a) **Monitoring**

i) Peripheral nerve blocks should be placed in a location where the patient's noninvasive BP, SpO_2, and ECG may be monitored.

ii) Supplemental O_2 should be provided via a face mask or nasal cannulae especially when IV sedation is administered.

b) **Positioning and preparation**

i) Position the patient supine with back slightly elevated.

ii) The head should be turned away from the side to be blocked and the arm placed at the side.

iii) Apply monitors and supplemental O_2

iv) IV sedation should be administered, but the patient must be able to follow commands and volunteer sensory information.

v) The anesthesiologist should stand next to the patient's shoulder on the side to be blocked.

c) **Identification of surface anatomy**

i) Important surface landmarks include the sternocleidomastoid (SCM) and clavicle (Cognitive Aid: Panel A).

ii) The SCM may be identified by asking the patient to turn the head away from the affected side and flex the neck.

iii) Palpating the interscalene groove and subclavian artery pulsation posterior to the SCM is also helpful.

d) **Stimulating supraclavicular block (plumb-bob technique)**

i) After sterile skin preparation and injection of a local anesthetic skin wheal, a 1- to 2-inch needle is inserted above the clavicle lateral to the insertion point of the SCM clavicular head and directed perpendicular to the bed or angled slightly cephalad (up to 45 degrees) with the patient supine (6).

    ii) Once the desired motor response is elicited (**hand flexion or extension**) and maintained at <0.5 mA of current, 30 to 40 mL of local anesthetic should be slowly injected in incremental volumes following negative aspiration for blood.

    iii) The needle should not be directed medially toward the cupola of the lung.

    iv) If the subclavian artery is encountered, redirect the needle in a posterolateral direction.

e) **Ultrasound-guided supraclavicular block**

    i) The supraclavicular block may be performed with real-time ultrasound guidance with or without nerve stimulation (2,3).

    ii) With a linear ultrasound transducer positioned cephalad and medial to the midpoint of the clavicle and oriented vertically (Cognitive Aid: Panel B), the brachial plexus is visualized in short axis posterolateral to the subclavian artery (Cognitive Aid: Panel C).

    iii) After sterile skin preparation, a local anesthetic skin wheal is raised lateral to the ultrasound transducer.

    iv) The block needle is inserted through the skin wheal and directed anteromedially toward the subclavian artery.

    v) To ensure blockade of the C8 and T1 divisions for complete upper extremity anesthesia, the needle tip should be directed into the "corner pocket" between the posterolateral portion of the subclavian artery and the first rib (9).

    vi) The total volume of local anesthetic can be injected incrementally after negative aspiration for blood until injectate is visualized surrounding the entire plexus.

5) **Evaluation of the block**

a) The quality of nerve blockade must be evaluated prior to surgical incision even if intraoperative general anesthesia is planned.

b) Motor testing

    i) Strength of elbow flexion against resistance tests the biceps muscle innervated by the **musculocutaneous** nerve.

    ii) Similarly, strength of elbow extension tests the triceps muscle innervated by the **radial** nerve.

    iii) Strength of shoulder abduction tests the deltoid muscle innervated by the **axillary** nerve.

c) Sensory testing

    i) Pinching the base of the index finger, small finger, and medial aspect of the forearm assesses anesthesia in the distribution of the **median, ulnar, and medial antebrachial cutaneous** nerves, respectively.

    ii) Pinching over the medial upper arm and the elbow evaluates the block of the **medial brachial cutaneous** nerve.

6) **Postoperative management**

a) All patients who undergo brachial plexus blockade should be discharged with a supportive sling.

b) Patients with Horner syndrome and uncomfortable anhydrosis of the ipsilateral eye may benefit from artificial tears.

c) For outpatients, respiratory status should be assessed prior to discharge, but a routine chest radiograph for pneumothorax or hemidiaphragmatic paresis is not recommended in asymptomatic patients.

References

1. Neal JM, Gerancher JC, Hebl JR, et al. Upper extremity regional anesthesia: essentials of our current understanding, 2008. *Reg Anesth Pain Med* 2009;34:134–170.

2. Chan VW, Perlas A, Rawson R, et al. Ultrasound-guided supraclavicular brachial plexus block. *Anesth Analg* 2003;97:1514–1517.

3. Kapral S, Krafft P, Eibenberger K, et al. Ultrasound-guided supraclavicular approach for regional anesthesia of the brachial plexus. *Anesth Analg* 1994;78:507–513.

4. Williams SR, Chouinard P, Arcand G, et al. Ultrasound guidance speeds execution and improves the quality of supraclavicular block. *Anesth Analg* 2003;97:1518–1523.
5. Neal JM, Moore JM, Kopacz DJ, et al. Quantitative analysis of respiratory, motor, and sensory function after supraclavicular block. *Anesth Analg* 1998;86:1239–1244.
6. Klaastad O, VadeBoncouer TR, Tillung T, et al. An evaluation of the supraclavicular plumb-bob technique for brachial plexus block by magnetic resonance imaging. *Anesth Analg* 2003;96:862–867.
7. Brown DL, Cahill DR, Bridenbaugh LD. Supraclavicular nerve block: anatomic analysis of a method to prevent pneumothorax. *Anesth Analg* 1993;76:530–534.
8. Renes SH, Spoormans HH, Gielen MJ, et al. Hemidiaphragmatic paresis can be avoided in ultrasound-guided supraclavicular brachial plexus block. *Reg Anesth Pain Med* 2009;34:595–599.
9. Soares LG, Brull R, Lai J, et al. Eight ball, corner pocket: the optimal needle position for ultrasound-guided supraclavicular block. *Reg Anesth Pain Med* 2007;32:94–95.

US-Guided Supraclavicular Block

By Vanessa J. Loland, MD · Larry F. Chu, MD, MS · Edward R. Mariano, MD, MAS

Patient Position: Position the patient supine with back slightly elevated. The head should be turned away from the side to be blocked and the arm placed at the side.

Needle Size: 22 to 17-gauge, 70 to 100-mm block needle

Volume: 20 to 40-mL local anesthetic

Anatomic Landmarks

Ⓐ Important surface landmarks include the sternocleidomastoid (SCM) and clavicle.

The SCM may be identified by asking the patient to turn the head away from the affected side and flex the neck. Palpating the interscalene groove and subclavian artery pulsation posterior to the SCM is also helpful.

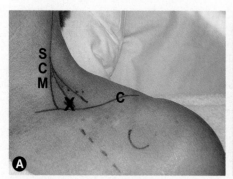
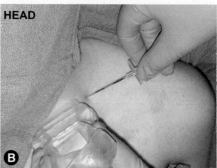

A. Surface anatomy relevant to the supraclavicular block. The "X" marks the suggested site for needle insertion when performing the plumb-bob technique with nerve stimulation. SCM, sternocleidomastoid muscle; C, clavicle. **B.** A high-frequency linear transducer is placed perpendicular to skin medial to the clavicle. The block needle is inserted lateral to the transducer and directed antero-medially for in-plane needle guidance.

Approach and Technique

Ⓑ With a HF linear ultrasound transducer positioned cephalad and medial to the midpoint of the clavicle and oriented vertically, **Ⓒ** the brachial plexus is visualized in short-axis postero-lateral to the subclavian artery.

After sterile skin preparation, a local anesthetic skin wheal is raised lateral to the ultrasound transducer. The block needle is inserted through the skin wheal and directed antero-medially toward the subclavian artery.

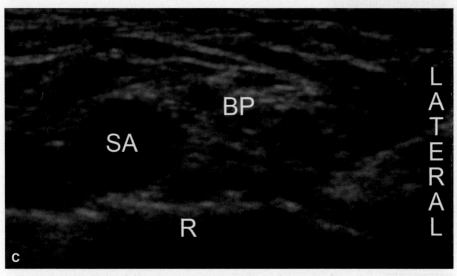

C. Short-axis image of the brachial plexus during supraclavicular block performance. SA, subclavian artery; R, first rib periosteum; BP, brachial plexus.

To ensure blockade of the C8 and T1 divisions for complete upper extremity anesthesia, the needle tip should be directed into the "corner pocket" between the posterolateral portion of the subclavian artery and first rib.

The total volume of local anesthetic can be injected incrementally after negative aspiration for blood until the injectate is visualized surrounding the entire plexus.

Evaluation of Block
Motor testing
Strength of elbow flexion against resistance tests the biceps muscle innervated by the musculocutaneous nerve. Similarly, strength of elbow extension tests the triceps muscle innervated by the radial nerve. Strength of shoulder abduction tests the deltoid muscle innervated by the axillary nerve.

Sensory testing
Pinching the base of the index finger, small finger, and medial aspect of the forearm assesses anesthesia in the distribution of the median, ulnar, and medial antebrachial cutaneous nerves, respectively. Pinching over the medial upper arm and elbow evaluates the block of the medial brachial cutaneous nerve.

175

Infraclavicular Block

Vanessa J. Loland, MD • Edward R. Mariano, MD, MAS

The infraclavicular block may be performed using a variety of techniques to anesthetize the cords of the brachial plexus. This site is often chosen for patients requiring prolonged brachial plexus analgesia via continuous nerve catheters. An approach to this block using the coracoid process as a major landmark may be performed with the arm abducted or at the side, which may be preferable in patients unable to abduct the arm (1,2). A nerve stimulator or an ultrasound guidance is recommended for localization of the brachial plexus at this level.

READ MORE

Continuous peripheral nerve blocks, Chapter 35 , page 266

1) **Indications and contraindications**
   a) **Indications**
      i) Surgical anesthesia or postoperative analgesia for procedures on the elbow, forearm, wrist, or hand
   b) **Contraindications**
      i) Absolute contraindications
         (1) Local infection at the site of planned needle insertion
      ii) Relative contraindications
         (1) Coagulopathy
         (2) Preexisting nerve injury
         (3) Emphysema or other severe pulmonary disease due to the theoretical risk of pneumothorax.

2) **Risks and complications**
   a) General risks involving peripheral nerve blockade are localized bleeding, intravascular injection with local anesthetic toxicity, and infection at the site of needle puncture. The three cords of the brachial plexus (medial, lateral, and posterior) surround the axillary artery at this level.
   b) Potential complications specific to the infraclavicular block
      i) **Pneumothorax**
         (1) Inadvertent pleural puncture with the coracoid approach is less likely when utilizing proper technique.
         (2) Evaluation of the classic technique of Raj using magnetic resonance imaging has demonstrated imprecision and greater potential for pneumothorax (3).
      ii) **Hemothorax**
      iii) **Chylothorax** (for a left-sided block)

3) **Equipment**
   a) Common equipment for all peripheral nerve block techniques include sterile skin cleansing solution, sterile gloves, a marking pen, and two 20-mL syringes of local anesthetic solution with extension tubing.

The medial, lateral, and posterior cords of the brachial plexus surround the axillary artery as it passes caudad to the coracoid process.

b) A nerve stimulator technique requires an electrical nerve stimulator with a compatible insulated needle and a grounding electrode.

c) Ultrasound-guided regional anesthesia requires portable ultrasound equipment and a low-frequency small curvilinear transducer (preferred) or a high-frequency linear transducer for infraclavicular block.

4) Technique

   a) **Monitoring**

      i) Peripheral nerve blocks should be placed in a location where the patient's noninvasive BP, SpO_2, and ECG may be monitored.

      ii) Supplemental O_2 should be provided via a face mask or nasal cannulae, especially when IV sedation is administered.

   b) **Positioning and preparation**

      i) Position the patient supine with the head turned away from the side to be blocked and the arm abducted at 90 degrees (preferred) or at the patient's side.

      ii) Apply monitors and supplemental O_2.

      iii) IV sedation should be administered, but the patient must be able to follow commands and volunteer sensory information.

      iv) The anesthesiologist should stand next to the patient's shoulder on the side to be blocked.

   c) **Identification of surface anatomy**

      i) The coracoid process is the most anterior portion of the scapula and can be palpated at the shoulder between the acromioclavicular joint and the deltopectoral groove.

      ii) If the coracoid process has been correctly identified, forward elevation of the arm should rotate the scapula and displace the coracoid process superiorly and therefore not palpable.

      iii) After identification of this landmark, a point is marked 2 cm medial and 2 cm caudad to the most anterior tip of the coracoid process (Cognitive Aid: Panel A).

   d) **Stimulating infraclavicular block**

      i) After sterile skin preparation and injection of a local anesthetic skin wheal, a 2- to 4-inch insulated needle is inserted at the predetermined point using a plumb-bob approach (perpendicular to the floor), and motor responses of the wrist or hand are sought using a nerve stimulator (Fig. 175-1).

      ii) The average depth from skin to brachial plexus is 4.24 ± 1.49 cm in men and 4.01 ± 1.29 cm in women (1). The brachial plexus and blood vessels are located between the pectoralis minor anteriorly and the subscapularis muscle of the rotator cuff posteriorly.

      iii) If the brachial plexus is not located initially, redirect cephalad-caudad within the same parasagittal plane, and avoid deviation of the needle medially toward the chest wall.

      iv) Once a motor evoked response from the desired nerve(s) is elicited and maintained at <0.5 mA of electrical current, 30 to 40 mL of local anesthetic should be slowly injected in incremental volumes following careful aspiration.

      v) A multiple-injection technique (depositing local anesthetic in divided doses at two or more sites following elicitation of distinct motor responses) has been shown to increase the efficacy of this technique (4–6).

   e) **Ultrasound-guided infraclavicular block**

      i) With a small curvilinear (preferred) or linear transducer positioned medial to the coracoid process and oriented vertically (Cognitive Aid: Panel B),

Avoid deviation of the block needle medially toward the chest wall.

Figure 175-1 Stimulating Infraclavicular Block Technique Employing the Coracoid Approach

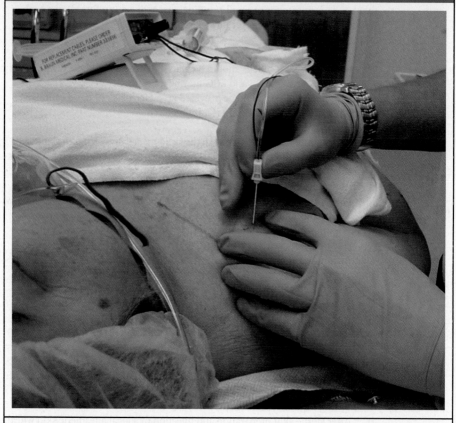

A 4-Inch insulated needle is inserted "Plumb-Bob" at a site 2 cm medial and 2 cm caudad to the coracoid process.

    the brachial plexus cords are visualized in short axis surrounding the axillary artery (Cognitive Aid: Panel C).

ii) After sterile skin preparation, a local anesthetic skin wheal is raised cephalad to the ultrasound transducer.

iii) The block needle is inserted through the skin wheal and directed caudad toward the axillary artery.

iv) Local anesthetic can be injected around each individual cord (7) or incrementally as a single injection posterior to the axillary artery (8) after a negative aspiration for blood until injectate spread surrounding all three cords is visually confirmed.

5) **Evaluation of the block**

  a) The quality of nerve blockade must be evaluated prior to surgical incision even if intra-operative general anesthesia is planned.

  b) Motor testing

    i) Strength of elbow flexion against resistance tests the biceps muscle innervated by the **musculocutaneous** nerve.

    ii) Similarly, strength of elbow extension tests the triceps muscle innervated by the **radial** nerve.

     iii) Strength of shoulder abduction tests the deltoid muscle innervated by the *axillary* nerve.

  c) Sensory testing

     i) Pinching the base of the index finger, small finger, and medial aspect of the forearm assesses anesthesia in the distribution of the **median, ulnar, and medial antebrachial cutaneous** nerves, respectively.

     ii) Pinching over the medial upper arm and the elbow evaluates the block of the **medial brachial cutaneous** nerve.

6) **Postoperative management**

  a) All patients who undergo brachial plexus blockade should be discharged with a supportive sling.

  b) Routine chest radiograph for pneumothorax is not recommended in asymptomatic patients.

References

1. Wilson JL, Brown DL, Wong GY, et al. Infraclavicular brachial plexus block: parasagittal anatomy important to the coracoid technique. *Anesth Analg* 1998;87:870–873.

2. Whiffler K. Coracoid block—a safe and easy technique. *Br J Anaesth* 1981;53:845–848.

3. Klaastad O, Lilleas FG, Rotnes JS, et al. Magnetic resonance imaging demonstrates lack of precision in needle placement by the infraclavicular brachial plexus block described by Raj et al. *Anesth Analg* 1999;88:593–598.

4. Rodriguez J, Barcena M, Lagunilla J, et al. Increased success rate with infraclavicular brachial plexus block using a dual-injection technique. *J Clin Anesth* 2004;16:251–256.

5. Rodriguez J, Barcena M, Taboada-Muniz M, et al. A comparison of single versus multiple injections on the extent of anesthesia with coracoid infraclavicular brachial plexus block. *Anesth Analg* 2004;99:1225–1230.

6. Gaertner E, Estebe JP, Zamfir A, et al. Infraclavicular plexus block: multiple injection versus single injection. *Reg Anesth Pain Med* 2002;27:590–594.

7. Sandhu NS, Capan LM. Ultrasound-guided infraclavicular brachial plexus block. *Br J Anaesth* 2002;89:254–259.

8. Desgagnes MC, Levesque S, Dion N, et al. A comparison of a single or triple injection technique for ultrasound-guided infraclavicular block: a prospective randomized controlled study. *Anesth Analg* 2009;109:668–672.

US-Guided Infraclavicular Block

By Vanessa J. Loland, MD • Larry F. Chu, MD, MS • Edward R. Mariano, MD, MAS

Patient Position: Position the patient supine with the head turned away from the side to be blocked and the arm abducted at 90 degrees (preferred) or at the patient's side.

Needle Size: 22 to 17-gauge, 70 to 100-mm block needle

Volume: 20 to 40-mL local anesthetic

Anatomic Landmarks

The coracoid process is the most anterior portion of the scapula and can be palpated at the shoulder between the acromioclavicular joint and the deltopectoral groove. If the coracoid process has been correctly identified, forward elevation of the arm should rotate the scapula and displace the coracoid process superiorly and therefore not palpable.

A After identification of this landmark, a point is marked 2 cm medial and 2 cm caudad to the most anterior tip of the coracoid process.

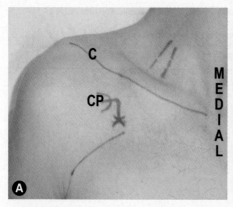
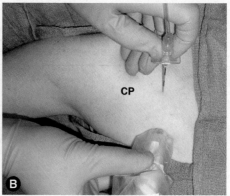

A. View of right shoulder demonstrating surface anatomy relevant to the infraclavicular block. CP, coracoid process of the scapula; C, clavicle. **B.** A small curvilinear transducer is placed medial and caudad to the coracoid process with the arm abducted 90 degrees to optimize the cross-sectional imaging of the neuro-vascular bundle. The block needle is inserted cephalad to the transducer and directed caudad for in-plane needle guidance.

Approach and Technique

B With a small curvilinear (preferred) or linear transducer positioned medial and caudad to the coracoid process and oriented vertically, **C** the brachial plexus cords are visualized in short-axis surrounding the axillary artery.

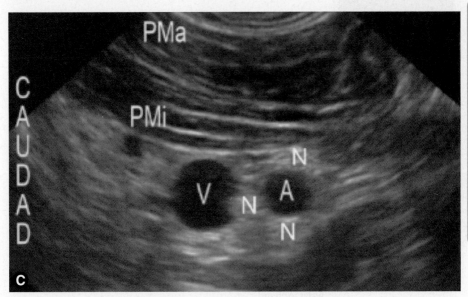

C. Short-axis image of the brachial plexus below the clavicle. PMa, pectoralis major muscle; PMi, pectoralis minor muscle; V, axillary vein; A, axillary artery; N, nerve (cord of the brachial plexus).

After sterile skin preparation, a local anesthetic skin wheal is raised cephalad to the ultrasound transducer. The block needle is inserted through the skin wheal and directed caudad toward the axillary artery. Local anesthetic can be injected around each individual cord or incrementally as a single injection posterior to the axillary artery after a negative aspiration for blood until the injectate spread surrounding all three cords is visually confirmed.

Evaluation of Block
Motor testing
Strength of elbow flexion against resistance tests the biceps muscle innervated by the musculocutaneous nerve. Strength of elbow extension tests the triceps muscle innervated by the radial nerve. Strength of shoulder abduction tests the deltoid muscle innervated by the axillary nerve.

Sensory testing
Pinching the base of the index finger, small finger, and medial aspect of the forearm assesses anesthesia in the distribution of the median, ulnar, and medial antebrachial cutaneous nerves, respectively. Pinching over the medial upper arm and elbow evaluates the block of the medial brachial cutaneous nerve.

Axillary Block

Edward R. Mariano, MD, MAS · Vanessa J. Loland, MD

The axillary block is performed at the level of the terminal branches. The three major nerves that remain in close proximity to the axillary artery at this level are the median, radial, and ulnar nerves. Evaluation of the perineural sheath with magnetic resonance imaging has demonstrated incomplete spread of local anesthetic solution following large-volume single injection resulting in unsatisfactory anesthesia (1). Therefore, a multiple compartment approach to the axillary block is recommended (2). Ultrasound guidance for axillary block may improve onset time and initial success rates (3,4).

1) Indications and contraindications
   a) **Indications**
      i) Surgical anesthesia or postoperative analgesia of the forearm, wrist, or hand
      ii) To provide cutaneous anesthesia for upper arm surgery, the intercostobrachial nerve (from the dorsal ramus of T1) and the medial brachial cutaneous nerve may need to be supplemented with local anesthetic infiltration. The need for this supplemental infiltration for tourniquet analgesia is controversial (5).
   b) **Contraindications**
      i) Absolute contraindications
         (1) Inability to abduct the arm at the shoulder
         (2) Local infection at the site of planned needle insertion
      ii) Relative contraindications
         (1) Preexisting nerve injury
         (2) Coagulopathy (although manual compression and hemostasis may be readily achieved in the event of vascular puncture)
2) Risks and complications
   a) General risks involving peripheral nerve blockade are localized bleeding, intravascular injection with local anesthetic toxicity, and infection at the site of needle puncture.
   b) Site-specific risks
      i) Due to the proximity of the nerves to the axillary artery, there is a **risk of intravascular injection or hematoma from vascular puncture.**
         (1) The risk of intravascular injection can be reduced by a multiple compartment technique, since smaller volumes of local anesthetic are deposited at multiple sites rather than a large volume injected at one site.
         (2) However, there is an increased risk of hematoma formation that can lead to postoperative nerve dysfunction (6).
         (3) Since the nerves are superficial in this location, nerve impalement and intraneural injection are possible (7).

There is no risk of pneumothorax with the axillary block when proper technique is used.

The axillary block may be performed without the aid of nerve stimulation or ultrasound guidance to provide anesthesia or postoperative analgesia following distal upper extremity surgery.

3) Equipment

    a) Common equipment for all peripheral nerve block techniques include sterile skin cleansing solution, sterile gloves, a marking pen, and two 20-mL syringes of local anesthetic solution with extension tubing.

    b) A nerve stimulator technique requires an electrical nerve stimulator with a compatible insulated needle (1 to 2 inches) and a grounding electrode.

    c) The perivascular and transarterial techniques require a 1- to 2-inch 22-gauge B-bevel needle with or without extension tubing attached to syringes of local anesthetic solution.

    d) Ultrasound-guided regional anesthesia requires portable ultrasound equipment and a high-frequency linear transducer for axillary block.

4) Technique

    a) **Monitoring**

       i) Peripheral nerve blocks should be placed in a location where the patient's noninvasive BP, SpO_2, and ECG may be monitored.

       ii) Supplemental O_2 should be provided via a face mask or nasal cannulae especially when IV sedation is administered.

    b) **Positioning and preparation**

       i) Position the patient supine with his/her head turned away from the side to be blocked and the affected arm abducted 90 degrees at the shoulder and flexed 90 degrees at the elbow.

       ii) Extreme abduction of the shoulder may obscure the axillary pulse.

       iii) Apply monitors and supplemental O_2.

       iv) IV sedation should be administered, but the patient must be able to follow commands and volunteer sensory information.

       v) The anesthesiologist should stand or sit at the patient's side facing the patient's axilla.

    c) **Identification of surface anatomy** (Cognitive Aid: Panel A)

       i) The axillary artery should be located below the coracobrachialis muscle with the arm abducted.

       ii) If the pulse is difficult to palpate, Doppler or ultrasound may aid identification.

       iii) The expected location of the median nerve is superficial and lateral to the artery with the radial nerve posterior to the artery and the ulnar nerve medial to the artery (Cognitive Aid: Panel B).

         (1) At this level, the musculocutaneous nerve is located further lateral and away from the axillary artery.

         (2) The precise position of each of these terminal branch nerves is highly variable (5).

    d) **Perivascular axillary block**

       i) After sterile skin preparation and injection of a local anesthetic skin wheal over the axillary artery pulse, a uniform field block of local anesthetic is deposited around the axillary artery using a 1- to 2-inch B-bevel needle and three-ring control syringes of local anesthetic solution (Fig. 176-1).

         (1) If one imagines the artery as the center of a clock face, the four major nerve branches are typically located in each of the four quadrants, and local anesthetic should be injected in each of these locations (8).

Figure 176-1 The Perivascular Axillary Block Technique is Performed by Injecting Local Anesthetic in a Ring Around the Axillary Artery and does not Require Electrical Nerve Stimulation or Ultrasound Guidance

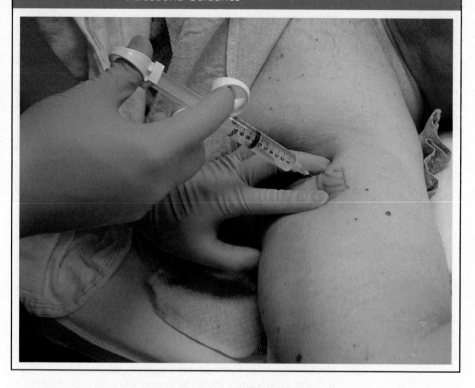

(2) Paresthesias may occur inadvertently during the performance of this block and may help confirm the location of nerves.

(3) Neural puncture and intraneural injection occur frequently when performing techniques that involve deliberate elicitation of paresthesias (7).

ii) The practitioner should perform needle insertion in a steady, controlled manner on each pass to avoid nerve impalement.

e) **Stimulating axillary block**

Nerve impalement occurs frequently when performing deliberate paresthesia-seeking axillary blocks.

i) When using an electrical nerve stimulator, the multiple-injection technique (using a peripheral nerve stimulator to elicit distinct motor responses with subsequent divided local anesthetic injections) has been shown to provide superior anesthesia compared to single injection with lower rates of supplementation (9,10).

ii) After sterile skin preparation, a 1- to 2-inch insulated needle is inserted and directed around the axillary artery in similar fashion to the perivascular technique while seeking motor responses of at least two terminal branch nerves (median, ulnar, or radial).

iii) For each motor response elicited at <0.5 mA of stimulating current, 10 to 20 mL of local anesthetic is injected incrementally after negative aspiration for blood.

f) **Transarterial axillary block**

   i)   After sterile skin preparation and injection of a local anesthetic skin when over the axillary artery pulse, a 1- to 2-inch B-bevel needle connected to extension tubing and syringes containing local anesthetic is intentionally directed toward the axillary artery.

   ii) Deliberate arterial puncture is confirmed by aspiration of blood and then the needle is advanced until it passes through the artery.

      (1) After confirming negative aspiration, half of the volume of local anesthetic is incrementally injected at this location.

      (2) Intermittent aspiration is crucial to ensure that the needle has not migrated back into the vessel.

      (3) The needle is then withdrawn back through the artery as confirmed by aspiration of blood to a position anterior to the artery.

      (4) After confirming negative aspiration for blood in this location, the remaining local anesthetic volume is incrementally injected.

g) **Ultrasound-guided axillary block**

   i)   With a linear transducer positioned perpendicular to skin over the axillary artery (Cognitive Aid: Panel C), the terminal nerves can be visualized at various locations around the axillary artery (Cognitive Aid: Panel D).

      (1) The musculocutaneous nerve is located lateral to the axillary artery between the fascia layers of the biceps brachii and the coracobrachialis muscles.

      (2) The radial nerve is normally posterior to the axillary artery and can be traced distally as it passes into the spiral groove of the humerus.

      (3) The median and ulnar nerves are typically anterior to the axillary vessels, sometimes in close proximity to each other, and may be difficult to differentiate.

   ii) After sterile skin preparation, a local anesthetic skin wheal is raised lateral to the ultrasound transducer.

   iii) The block needle is inserted through the skin wheal and directed medially toward the axillary artery.

      (1) Concurrent use of electrical stimulation may aid in the identification of individual nerve branches.

      (2) Multiple needle insertions may be required to avoid vascular puncture.

   iv) Local anesthetic solution should be injected around each individual nerve to ensure a successful block (4).

5) **Evaluation of the block**

   a) The quality of nerve blockade must be evaluated prior to surgical incision even if intraoperative general anesthesia is planned.

   b) Motor testing

      i)   Strength of elbow flexion against resistance tests the biceps muscle innervated by the **musculocutaneous** nerve.

      ii) Similarly, strength of elbow extension tests the triceps muscle innervated by the **radial** nerve.

   c) Sensory testing

      i)   Pinching the base of the index finger, small finger, and medial aspect of the forearm assesses anesthesia in the distribution of the **median, ulnar, and medial antebrachial cutaneous** nerves, respectively.

      ii) Pinching over the medial upper arm and the elbow evaluates the block of the **medial brachial cutaneous** nerve.

6) **Postoperative management**

   a) All patients who undergo brachial plexus blockade should be discharged with a supportive sling.

References

1. Klaastad O, Smedby O, Thompson GE, et al. Distribution of local anesthetic in axillary brachial plexus block: a clinical and magnetic resonance imaging study. *Anesthesiology* 2002;96:1315–1324.
2. Koscielniak-Nielsen ZJ, Stens-Pedersen HL, et al. Readiness for surgery after axillary block: single or multiple injection techniques. *Eur J Anaesthesiol* 1997;14:164–171.
3. Casati A, Danelli G, Baciarello M, et al. A prospective, randomized comparison between ultrasound and nerve stimulation guidance for multiple injection axillary brachial plexus block. *Anesthesiology* 2007;106:992–996.
4. Chan VW, Perlas A, McCartney CJ, et al. Ultrasound guidance improves success rate of axillary brachial plexus block. *Can J Anaesth* 2007;54:176–182.
5. Neal JM, Gerancher JC, Hebl JR, et al. Upper extremity regional anesthesia: essentials of our current understanding, 2008. *Reg Anesth Pain Med* 2009;34:134–170.
6. Ben-David B, Stahl S. Axillary block complicated by hematoma and radial nerve injury. *Reg Anesth Pain Med* 1999;24:264–266.
7. Bigeleisen PE. Nerve puncture and apparent intraneural injection during ultrasound-guided axillary block does not invariably result in neurologic injury. *Anesthesiology* 2006;105:779–783.
8. Brown DL. *Atlas of Regional Anesthesia.* 2nd ed. Philadelphia, PA: WB Saunders Company; 1999.
9. Inberg P, Annila I, Annila P. Double-injection method using peripheral nerve stimulator is superior to single injection in axillary plexus block. *Reg Anesth Pain Med* 1999;24:509–513.
10. Sia S, Lepri A, Ponzecchi P. Axillary brachial plexus block using peripheral nerve stimulator: a comparison between double- and triple-injection techniques. *Reg Anesth Pain Med* 2001;26:499–503.

US-Guided Axillary Block

Edward R. Mariano, MD, MAS · Larry F. Chu, MD, MS · Vanessa J. Loland, MD

Patient Position: Position the patient supine with the head turned away from the side to be blocked and the affected arm abducted 90 degrees at the shoulder and flexed 90 degrees at the elbow.

Needle Size: 22 to 17-gauge, 50 to 100-mm block needle

Volume: 20 to 40-mL local anesthetic

Anatomic Landmarks

A The course of the axillary artery is palpated and marked in the proximal axilla.

B The expected location of the median nerve is superficial and lateral to the artery with the radial nerve posterior to the artery and the ulnar nerve medial to the artery.

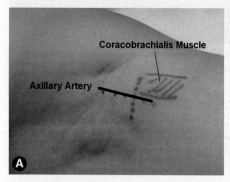

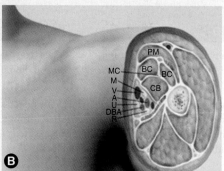

A. Image of the left axilla demonstrating surface anatomy relevant to the axillary block: axillary artery and coracobrachialis muscle. **B.** Illustration of the cross-sectional anatomy through the axillary artery in the proximal axilla demonstrating the expected distribution of the terminal branch nerves in this location. PM, pectoralis major; MC, musculocutaneous; BC, biceps; CB, coracobrachialis; M, median; V, axillary vein; A, axillary vein; U, ulnar; DBA, deep brachial artery; R, radial; H, humerus. Reproduced from Bigeleisen P, Orebaugh S. Ultrasound guided axillary block. In: Chelly JE. Peripheral nerve blocks: a color atlas. 3rd Edition. Philadelphia: Lippincott Williams & Wilkins, 2009: 286, with permission.

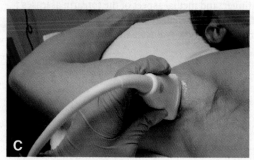

C. A linear ultrasound transducer is placed perpendicular to skin in the proximal axilla to visualize the axillary vessels and terminal branch nerves in cross section.

Approach and Technique

C With a HF linear transducer positioned perpendicular to skin over the axillary artery, **D** the terminal nerves can be visualized at various locations around the axillary artery.

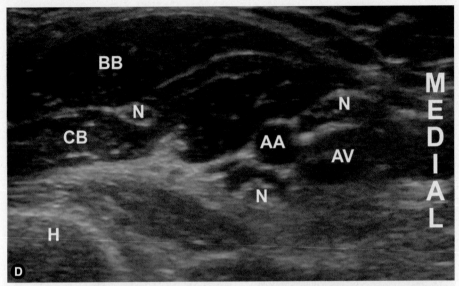

D. Short-axis image of the axillary vessels and terminal branch nerves in the proximal axilla. BB, biceps brachii muscle; CB, coracobrachialis muscle; H, humerus; AA, axillary artery; AV, axillary vein; N, nerve.

After sterile skin preparation, a local anesthetic skin wheal is raised lateral to the ultrasound transducer. The block needle is inserted through the skin wheal and medially directed toward the axillary artery. 5 to 10 mL of local anesthetic solution should be injected around each individual nerve to ensure a successful block.

Evaluation of Block
Motor testing
Strength of elbow flexion against resistance tests the biceps muscle innervated by the musculocutaneous nerve. Similarly, strength of elbow extension tests the triceps muscle innervated by the radial nerve.

Sensory testing
Pinching the base of the index finger, small finger, and medial aspect of the forearm assesses anesthesia in the distribution of the median, ulnar, and medial antebrachial cutaneous nerves, respectively. Pinching over the medial upper arm and elbow evaluates the block of the medial brachial cutaneous nerve.

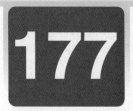

177 Distal Upper Extremity Peripheral Nerve Blocks

Amanda L. Peterson, MD · Edward R. Mariano, MD, MAS

Selective peripheral nerve blocks of the terminal branches of the brachial plexus may be performed distal to the axilla (1). The ulnar, radial, median, medial antebrachial cutaneous, and lateral antebrachial cutaneous nerves may be anesthetized at the elbow. The "wrist block" is composed of individual median, ulnar, and radial nerve blocks (2). The sonoanatomy of these three distal branches in the forearm has been described (3), and ultrasound-guided peripheral nerve blocks at this level are feasible (4).

1) **Indications and contraindications**
   a) Indications
      i) Individual nerve blockade of any or all of the terminal branches may be used to supplement brachial plexus anesthesia or may be used alone to provide surgical anesthesia for procedures of the distal forearm, wrist, or hand.
      ii) The site of the tourniquet should also be considered when planning the most appropriate regional anesthetic plan.
      iii) Although appropriate for postoperative pain management, the use of distal peripheral nerve blocks as a sole anesthetic is typically reserved for procedures limited to the hand or fingers of short duration when a tourniquet is not required or a wrist tourniquet will suffice.
   b) Contraindications
      i) An absolute contraindication is local infection at the site of planned needle insertion.
      ii) Relative contraindications
         (1) Preexisting nerve injury
         (2) Coagulopathy (although nerve blocks distal to the elbow may have advantages over deeper blocks in the patient with bleeding tendencies since compression can be easily applied)

2) **Site-specific risks and complications**
   a) General risks involving peripheral nerve blockade are localized bleeding, intravascular injection with local anesthetic toxicity, and infection at the site of needle puncture.
   b) Site-specific risks
      i) Procedure-induced pain resulting from multiple needle insertions
      ii) Injection of local anesthetic solution into terminal arteries
         (1) Significant IV injection is rare due to division of local anesthetic volume into multiple sites of injection.
         (2) Epinephrine-free local anesthetic solutions are commonly used for distal upper extremity blocks to avoid vasoconstriction of the terminal arteries that supply blood flow to the hand and digits.

Epinephrine-free local anesthetic solutions are used for distal upper extremity blocks to avoid vasoconstriction of the terminal arteries that supply blood flow to the hand.

3) **Equipment**
   a) Common equipment for all peripheral nerve block techniques includes a sterile skin cleansing solution, sterile gloves, a marking pen, and up to 30 mL of local anesthetic solution with extension tubing (or may be divided into 10 mL three-ring control syringes).
   b) When performing elbow and wrist blocks with an infiltration technique, a 25-gauge needle with local anesthetic solution in three-ring control syringes should be used.
   c) A nerve stimulator technique may be employed at the elbow and the wrist, requiring an electrical nerve stimulator, a compatible insulated needle (1 inch), and a grounding electrode.
   d) Ultrasound-guided regional anesthesia requires portable ultrasound equipment and a high-frequency linear transducer for distal upper extremity peripheral nerve blocks.
4) **Technique**
   a) **Monitoring**
      i) Peripheral nerve blocks should be placed in a location where the patient's noninvasive BP, O_2 saturation, and ECG may be monitored.
      ii) Supplemental O_2 should be provided *via* a face mask or nasal cannulae, especially if sedation is to be administered.
   b) **Positioning and preparation**
      i) These blocks are most commonly performed with the patient supine.
      ii) For elbow blocks, the arm should be abducted at 90 degrees with the elbow in extension on a flat surface, except for the ulnar nerve block in which the elbow should be flexed 90 degrees over the patient's chest.
      iii) For wrist blocks, the arm should be abducted at 90 degrees and positioned initially on a flat surface with the wrist supinated, although suspending the wrist with the elbow at 90 degrees of flexion may facilitate blocks of the radial and ulnar nerves.
   c) **Identification of surface anatomy**
      i) Elbow (Cognitive Aid: Panel A)
         (1) With the elbow extended, identify the intercondylar line at the elbow crease between the lateral and the medial epicondyles of the humerus.
         (2) Palpate the brachial artery pulse medially and the tendon of the biceps brachii muscle laterally.
            (a) The median nerve lies medial to the brachial artery.
            (b) The radial nerve is located lateral to the biceps tendon and along the medial border of the brachioradialis muscle.
         (3) Elevate the shoulder 90 degrees and flex the elbow 90 degrees across the patient's chest to palpate the ulnar groove between the olecranon and the medial epicondyle of the humerus where the ulnar nerve is located.
      ii) Wrist (Cognitive Aid: Panel B)
         (1) With the forearm supinated, identify three tendons arranged lateral to medial on the volar surface of the wrist: flexor carpi radialis (FCR), palmaris longus (PL), and flexor carpi ulnaris (FCU).
         (2) The ulnar artery pulse is another helpful landmark since it is reliably located lateral to the ulnar nerve.
         (3) The radial artery runs medial to the radial nerve (Cognitive Aid: Panel B).
         (4) The PL tendon may be congenitally absent in some patients.
   d) **Landmark-based elbow block technique**
      i) After sterile skin preparation, the median nerve block is performed by inserting the needle perpendicular to skin medial to the brachial artery at the elbow crease (Fig. 177-1). When an appropriate motor response is elicited (wrist flexion and pronation with opposition of the thumb) and maintained <0.5 mA, 3 to 5 mL of local anesthetic solution should be injected after negative aspiration for blood.

| **Figure 177-1** | Illustration Showing the Cross-Sectional Anatomy at the Elbow |

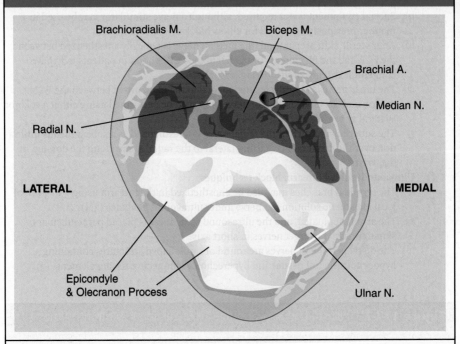

Individual blocks of the median, radial, and ulnar nerves may be performed at or near this level. From Chelly JE. Terminal nerve blocks. C: Blocks at the elbow. In: Chelly JE, ed. Peripheral nerve blocks: A color atlas. 3rd Edition. Philadelphia: Lippincott Williams & Wilkins, 2009: 79, with permission.

ii) The radial nerve is located approximately lateral to the biceps tendon and deep to the medial border of the brachioradialis muscle (see Fig. 177-1).
   (1) A 1-inch needle is inserted perpendicular to skin at this point and advanced toward the lateral epicondyle.
   (2) After eliciting a radial nerve motor response (wrist and/or finger extension), 3 to 5 mL of local anesthetic should be injected after negative aspiration for blood.

iii) Median and radial nerve blockade may also be performed without a nerve stimulator by local anesthetic infiltration using anatomic landmarks.

iv) The lateral antebrachial cutaneous nerve (termination of the musculocutaneous nerve providing innervations of the lateral forearm) may be blocked by infiltration of local anesthetic solution within the sheath of the biceps tendon at the elbow.

v) The medial antebrachial cutaneous nerve may be anesthetized as a field block anterior to the medial epicondyle of the humerus at the elbow.

vi) With the shoulder elevated and the elbow flexed across the patient's chest, the ulnar nerve may be anesthetized posteriorly at a point proximal to the ulnar groove using a nerve stimulator or an infiltration technique (see Fig. 177-1).

Avoid potential ulnar nerve impalement by inserting the block needle proximal to the ulnar groove in the upper arm and not directly into the groove.

e) **Landmark-based wrist block technique**
  i) Wrist blocks are reliably performed as infiltration techniques with 3 to 5 mL of plain local anesthetic solution per nerve.
  ii) Special equipment is not required, although a nerve stimulator may be used in a manner previously described for elbow blocks.
  iii) After sterile skin preparation, the median nerve is typically anesthetized between the FCR and the PL tendons or medial to the FCR tendon in patients who have congenital absence of the PL (Fig. 177-2).
  iv) The ulnar nerve is typically located medial to the ulnar artery between the FCU tendon and the ulna, and ulnar nerve block can be performed using either a volar or a lateral approach (see Fig. 177-2).
  v) The superficial branch of the radial nerve is anesthetized as a subcutaneous infiltration over the distal radius starting lateral to the radial artery along the dorsum of the wrist.

f) **Ultrasound-guided forearm block techniques**
  i) The terminal branches may also be anesthetized in the forearm using 3 to 5 mL of local anesthetic solution per nerve under ultrasound guidance (3,4).
  ii) The arm is supinated, and the ultrasound transducer is placed perpendicular to skin to image the target nerves in short axis.
  iii) The distal peripheral nerves are round or oval-shaped structures containing hypoechoic (neural tissue) and hyperechoics (connective tissue) elements (3).

Figure 177-2   Illustration Showing the Cross-Sectional Anatomy at the Wrist

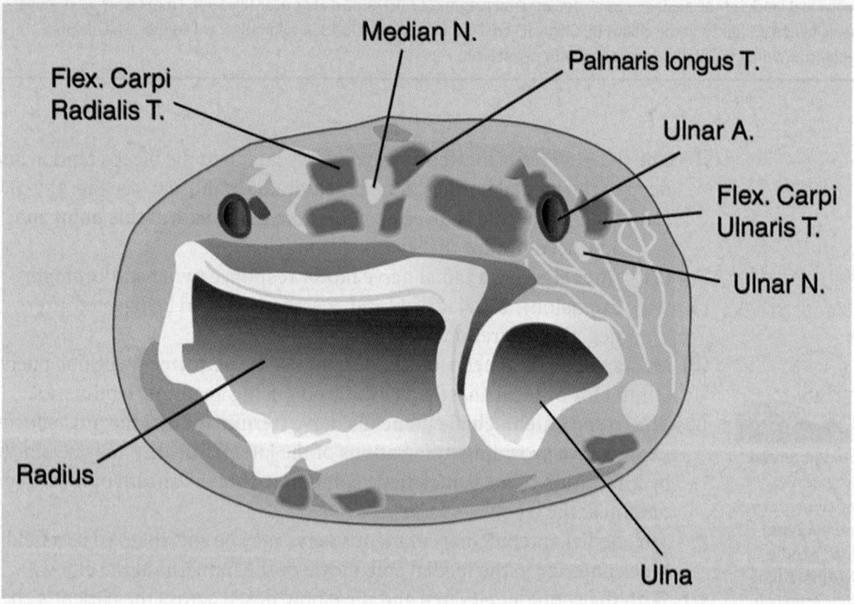

Individual blocks of the median, radial, and ulnar nerves may be performed at this level. From Chelly JE. Terminal nerve blocks. D: Blocks at the wrist. In: Chelly JE. Peripheral nerve blocks: A color atlas. 3rd Edition. Philadelphia: Lippincott Williams & Wilkins, 2009: 83, with permission.

   iv) Scanning from distal at the wrist to the proximal forearm may help to distinguish nerve from tendon.

   v) Median nerve block

     (1) The median nerve is easily visualized in the midforearm medial to the radial artery and between the flexor digitorum superficialis and the flexor digitorum profundus muscles (Cognitive Aid: Panel C).

     (2) After sterile skin preparation and local anesthetic skin infiltration, a 22-gauge B bevel needle is inserted lateral to the transducer and directed medially toward the median nerve (Cognitive Aid: Panel D).

     (3) Note the position of the radial artery to prevent accidental arterial puncture.

   vi) Ulnar nerve block

     (1) The ulnar nerve can be identified in the midforearm deep to the FCU muscle and next to the ulnar artery (Cognitive Aid: Panel E).

     (2) After sterile skin preparation and local anesthetic skin infiltration, a 22-gauge B bevel needle is inserted lateral to the transducer and directed medially toward the ulnar nerve (Cognitive Aid: Panel F).

   vii) Radial nerve block

     (1) The radial nerve is best visualized immediately distal to the elbow crease and deep to the brachioradialis muscle (Cognitive Aid: Panel G).

     (2) After sterile skin preparation and local anesthetic skin infiltration, a 22-gauge B bevel needle is inserted lateral to the transducer and directed medially toward the radial nerve (Cognitive Aid: Panel H).

5) **Evaluation of the block**

   a) Pinching the base of the index finger, small finger, dorsum of the hand, medial aspect of the forearm, and lateral aspect of the forearm assesses anesthesia in the distribution of the median, ulnar, radial, medial antebrachial cutaneous, and lateral antebrachial cutaneous nerves, respectively.

Wrist blocks do not result in significant motor block of the digits.

   b) Patients who receive wrist blocks will most likely not demonstrate significant weakness of finger flexion/extension since the responsible tendons and muscles originate more proximally in the forearm.

6) **Postoperative management**

   a) All patients who undergo upper limb regional anesthesia should be discharged with a supportive sling and a protective wrist splint when indicated.

References

1. Neal JM, Gerancher JC, Hebl JR, et al. Upper extremity regional anesthesia: essentials of our current understanding, 2008. *Reg Anesth Pain Med* 2009;34:134–170.
2. Brown DL. *Atlas of Regional Anesthesia*. 2nd ed. Philadelphia, PA: WB Saunders Company; 1999.
3. McCartney CJ, Xu D, Constantinescu C, et al. Ultrasound examination of peripheral nerves in the forearm. *Reg Anesth Pain Med* 2007;32: 434–439.
4. Gray AT, Schafhalter-Zoppoth I. Ultrasound guidance for ulnar nerve block in the forearm. *Reg Anesth Pain Med* 2003;28:335–339.

US-Guided Distal Upper Extremity

Median, Radial and Ulnar Nerve Blocks

Amanda L. Peterson, MD • Larry F. Chu, MD, MS • Edward R. Mariano, MD, MAS

Patient Position: For elbow blocks, abduct the arm at the shoulder 90 degrees with the elbow in extension on a flat surface; in the ulnar nerve block, flex the elbow 90 degrees over patient's chest. For wrist blocks, abduct the arm at 90 degrees and position on flat surface with the wrist supinated.

Needle Size: 22-gauge, Tuohy-tip or B bevel block needle

Volume: 5 to 10-mL local anesthetic per individual nerve

Anatomic Landmarks

A Elbow: Extend the elbow and identify the intercondylar line. Palpate the brachial artery pulse medially and the tendon of the biceps brachii muscle laterally. Elevate the shoulder 90 degrees and flex the elbow 90 degrees across patient's chest to palpate the ulnar groove between the olecranon and the medial epicondyle of humerus where the ulnar nerve is located.

B Wrist: Supinate the forearm and identify the flexor carpi radialis, palmaris longus, and flexor carpi ulnaris. The radial artery runs medial to the radial nerve.

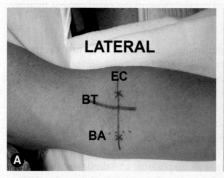 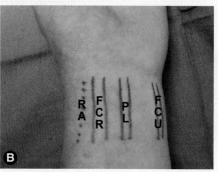

A. Surface anatomy relevant to nerve blocks at the elbow (left arm shown abducted 90 degrees at the shoulder). EC, elbow crease; BT, biceps tendon; BA, brachial artery. **B.** Surface anatomy relevant to nerve blocks at the wrist (left hand and wrist shown). RA, radial artery; FCR, flexor carpi radialis tendon; PL, palmaris longus tendon; FCU, flexor carpi ulnaris tendon.

Median Nerve Block

Approach and Technique

Supinate the arm and place the ultrasound transducer perpendicular to skin.

C Visualize the median nerve in the mid-forearm medial to the radial artery and between flexor digitorum superficialis and flexor digitorum profundus muscles.

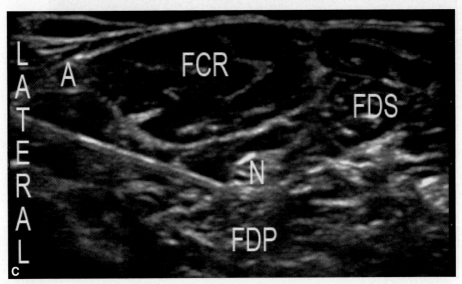

C. Short-axis ultrasound image of the mid-forearm demonstrating sonoanatomy relevant to the median nerve block. A, radial artery; FCR, flexor carpi radialis muscle; FDS, flexor digitorum superficialis muscle; FDP, flexor digitorum profundus muscle; N, median nerve.

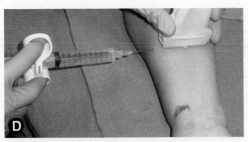

D After sterile skin preparation and local anesthetic skin infiltration, insert the block needle lateral to the transducer and direct it medially toward the median nerve.

D. Ultrasound-guided median nerve block technique employing a high-frequency linear transducer and in-plane needle guidance.

Ulnar Nerve Block

Approach and Technique

Supinate the arm and place the ultrasound transducer perpendicular to skin.

E Identify the ulnar nerve in the mid-forearm deep to the flexor carpi ulnaris muscle and next to the ulnar artery.

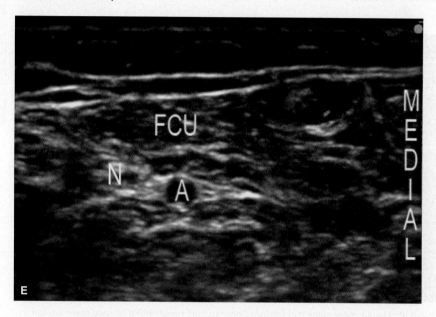

E. Short-axis ultrasound image of the mid-forearm demonstrating sonoanatomy relevant to the ulnar nerve block. A, ulnar artery; FCU, flexor carpi ulnaris muscle; N, ulnar nerve.

F After sterile skin preparation and local anesthetic skin infiltration, insert the block needle lateral to the transducer and direct it medially toward the ulnar nerve.

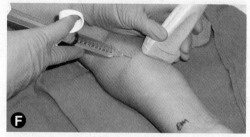

F. Ultrasound-guided ulnar nerve block technique employing a high-frequency linear transducer and in-plane needle guidance.

Radial Nerve Block

Approach and Technique

Supinate the arm and place the ultrasound transducer perpendicular to skin.

G Visualize the radial nerve distal to the elbow crease and deep to the brachioradialis muscle.

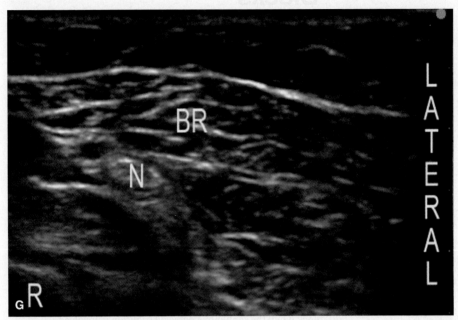

G. Short-axis ultrasound image distal to the elbow demonstrating sonoanatomy relevant to the radial nerve block. BR, brachioradialis muscle; R, radius; N, radial nerve.

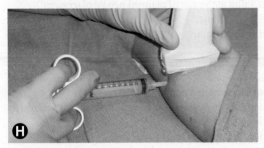

H After sterile skin preparation and local anesthetic skin infiltration, insert the block needle lateral to the transducer and direct it medially toward the radial nerve.

H. Ultrasound-guided radial nerve block technique employing a high-frequency linear transducer and in-plane needle guidance.

Evaluation of Block

Pinch the base of the index finger, small finger, and dorsum to assess anesthesia in the distribution of median, ulnar, and radial nerves, respectively.

Matthew T. Charous, MD • Edward R. Mariano, MD, MAS

The sciatic nerve is formed by the ventral rami of nerve roots L4-S3. The roots exit the pelvis via the greater sciatic foramen and then converge under the piriformis muscle to form the sciatic nerve (Fig. 178-1). The sciatic nerve innervates the posterior aspect of the knee and the entire lower leg and foot except for the distribution of the saphenous nerve (1). The classic transgluteal approach described by Gaston Labat is a proximal sciatic nerve block that may also reliably anesthetize the posterior femoral cutaneous nerve that innervates the posterior thigh (1). The subgluteal approach is performed distal to the gluteal crease where the sciatic nerve is more superficial and requires lower injectate volume (2). Continuous sciatic nerve block catheters can also be readily placed using the subgluteal approach to prolong postoperative analgesia (3).

READ MORE

Lumbar plexus (psoas compartment) block, Chapter 180, page 1223

Femoral nerve block, Chapter 181, page 1229

Patients with proximal tibia or tibial plateau injury should be considered high risk for compartment syndrome postoperatively. A detailed discussion with the patient and trauma team should precede any regional anesthesia technique in these patients.

1) **Indications and contraindications**
   a) Indications
      i) Surgical anesthesia or postoperative analgesia for knee and thigh procedures when combined with lumbar plexus blockade
      ii) Surgical anesthesia for procedures involving the lower leg, ankle, and foot when combined with a femoral or a saphenous nerve block when the saphenous nerve distribution is involved
   b) Contraindications
      i) Absolute contraindications
         (1) Local infection at the site of planned needle placement
      ii) Relative contraindications
         (1) Preexisting nerve injury
         (2) Coagulopathy
         (3) There is theoretical concern that a dense sciatic nerve block may mask pain produced by compartment syndrome in the lower extremity trauma patient.
            (a) Prospectively gathered data supporting this concern are lacking (4).
            (b) A detailed discussion of the potential risks and benefits of regional anesthesia with the patient and trauma team is indicated before performing a peripheral or neuraxial block when compartment syndrome is a concern.

2) **Risks and complications**
   a) General risks
      i) Hematoma formation
         (1) Inferior gluteal artery lies in close proximity to the sciatic nerve when using the transgluteal approach.

Figure 178-1 Illustration Demonstrating the Course of the Sciatic Nerve as it Exits the Greater Sciatic Foramen and Divides Into its Terminal Branches

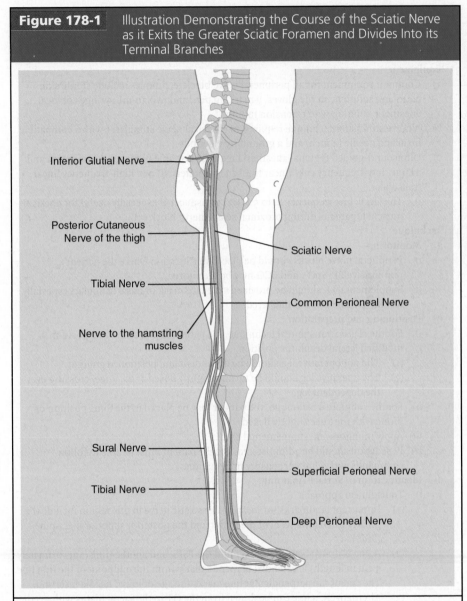

Inferior Glutial Nerve

Posterior Cutaneous Nerve of the thigh

Sciatic Nerve

Tibial Nerve

Common Perioneal Nerve

Nerve to the hamstring muscles

Sural Nerve

Superficial Perioneal Nerve

Tibial Nerve

Deep Perioneal Nerve

Reproduced from Chelly, Jacques E. *Peripheral nerve blocks: a color atlas.* 2nd ed. Philadelphia, PA: Lippincott Williams & Wilkins, 2004. Fig. 10-3, p. 79, with permission.

      (2) Localized bleeding
    ii) Intravascular injection with or without local anesthetic toxicity
    iii) Infection at the site of needle puncture
  b) Site-specific complications
    i) Needle-induced nerve trauma
      (1) The sciatic nerve is widest at this location and may be at risk for needle-nerve contact.
    ii) Patient procedure–related discomfort

(2) Transgluteal sciatic nerve block necessitates that the needle traverse a thick layer of muscle.

(3) Careful titration of sedatives and analgesics helps to attenuate patients' discomfort during block performance.

3) Equipment

a) Common equipment for all peripheral nerve block techniques include sterile skin cleansing solution, sterile gloves, a marking pen, and two 20-mL syringes of local anesthetic solution with extension tubing.

b) A nerve stimulator technique requires an electrical nerve stimulator with a compatible insulated needle (4 inch) and a grounding electrode.

c) Ultrasound-guided regional anesthesia requires portable ultrasound equipment and a large, low-frequency curvilinear transducer (preferred) or a high-frequency linear transducer

i) The large, low-frequency (2 to 5 MHz) transducer is especially useful for obese or muscular patients during proximal sciatic nerve block (5).

4) Technique

a) **Monitoring**

i) Peripheral nerve blocks should be placed in a location where the patient's noninvasive BP, SpO_2, and ECG may be monitored.

ii) Supplemental O_2 should be provided via a face mask or nasal cannulae, especially when IV sedation is administered.

b) **Positioning and preparation**

i) For the classic transgluteal technique, the patient is placed in Sims position, a modified lateral decubitus position.

(1) The nonoperative leg should be dependent and positioned straight.

(2) The operative leg should be up and slightly flexed at the knee, crossing over the dependent leg.

ii) For the subgluteal technique, the patient may be placed in the Sims position or prone with the knee slightly flexed.

iii) Apply monitors and supplemental O_2.

iv) IV sedation should be administered, but the patient must be able to follow commands and volunteer sensory information.

c) **Identification of Surface Anatomy**

i) Transgluteal approach

(1) Important landmarks for locating the sciatic nerve in this region include the greater trochanter (GT) of the femur and the posterior superior iliac spine (PSIS).

(2) A line is drawn between the GT and the PSIS, and another line (approximately 5 cm in length) is extended perpendicularly from the midpoint of the first line. The end of the perpendicular line marks the site of initial needle insertion.

(3) Alternatively, a line can be drawn from the GT to the sacral hiatus with needle insertion at the midpoint of this line.

(4) These two methods can be combined since they identify approximately the same point in most patients.

ii) Subgluteal approach

(1) Surface landmarks for the infragluteal parabiceps approach include the lateral border of the biceps femoris and the lower border of the gluteus maximus muscle.

(2) Caudad to the gluteal crease, the sciatic nerve lies along the lateral border of the long head of the biceps femoris as it crosses medially toward the ischial tuberosity (IT).

(3) When these landmarks are not palpable, alternative landmarks include the GT of the femur and the IT at the level of the inferior gluteal crease (Cognitive Aid: Panel A).

(4) A line is drawn between the GT and the IT, and the midpoint of this line should be marked as the site for needle insertion.

d) **Stimulating classic transgluteal technique**

i) Using sterile skin preparation and technique, a 4-inch insulated needle is inserted at the marked point perpendicular to skin in all planes and advanced while seeking a sciatic nerve motor response.

ii) If bone is contacted, this can represent either the IT or the lesser trochanter of the femur, and the needle should be redirected laterally or medially, respectively, and advanced another 1 to 2 cm.

iii) After an acceptable evoked motor response is elicited (tibial preferred) at a stimulating current < 0.5 mA, 20 to 40 mL of local anesthetic is incrementally injected following careful aspiration.

iv) The "double-injection" technique (identifying each branch of the sciatic nerve using nerve stimulation with separate injections of local anesthetic targeting the tibial and common peroneal contributions) has demonstrated faster onset and increased efficacy compared to the single-injection technique (6).

e) **Stimulating infragluteal parabiceps (subgluteal) technique**

i) Using sterile skin preparation and technique, a 2- to 4-inch insulated needle is inserted at the marked point at the intersection of the inferior border of the gluteus maximus and the lateral border of biceps femoris or at the midpoint of a line drawn between the GT and IT.

ii) The needle is introduced at a 70 to 80 degrees angle aiming cephalad in a parasagittal plane (7).

iii) If bone is contacted, the femur is the most likely source, indicating that the plane of the needle is too far lateral and should be redirected medially.

iv) If direct stimulation of the biceps femoris muscle occurs, this is an indication that the plane of the needle is too far medial and should be redirected more laterally.

v) When performing this block as a single injection technique, injecting local anesthetic after evoking an inversion motor response (from the tibial component of the sciatic nerve) at < 0.5 mA leads to the fastest onset and the greatest likelihood of a complete block (8).

f) **Ultrasound-guided subgluteal technique**

i) With the patient in Sim's position, the ultrasound transducer is placed perpendicular to skin between the IT and the GT of the femur caudad to the gluteal crease and oriented parallel to the crease (Cognitive Aid: Panel B).

ii) The sciatic nerve lies deep to the gluteus maximus muscle between the IT medially and femur laterally (Cognitive Aid: Panel C) (5,9).

iii) A local anesthetic skin wheal is raised lateral to the ultrasound transducer after sterile skin preparation.

iv) The block needle is inserted through this skin wheal using in-plane guidance in a lateral-to-medial direction toward the sciatic nerve.

v) Alternatively, the block needle may be inserted caudad to the center of the ultrasound transducer, aiming cephalad, and directed out-of-plane toward the sciatic nerve.

Blockade of the sciatic nerve distal to the transgluteal approach does not reliably provide anesthesia of the posterior thigh. The posterior cutaneous nerve of the thigh diverges from the sciatic nerve in a more proximal location.

The sciatic nerve will appear flat or oval in the subgluteal region; if the nerve is difficult to identify, trace the course of the nerve cephalad from the popliteal fossa.

5) **Evaluation of the block**

   a) The quality of the nerve blockade must be evaluated prior to surgical incision even if intraoperative general anesthesia is planned.

   b) Motor testing

      i) Testing strength of plantar flexion and dorsiflexion of the foot test blockade of the posterior tibial nerve and the common peroneal nerve, respectively.

      ii) Asking the patient to flex the knee against resistance (by grasping the ankle) allows for assessment of hamstring motor blockade.

   c) Sensory testing

      i) Decreased temperature and pinprick sensation over the lateral calf and the dorsal/plantar surfaces of the foot confirm appropriate sciatic nerve block.

6) **Postoperative management**

   a) Outpatients who undergo sciatic nerve blockade should be discharged with a supportive ankle splint (due to foot drop) and weight-bearing restriction.

      i) The patient is at risk for falling if ambulation is initiated prior to nerve block resolution.

   b) Hospitalized patients with single-injection or continuous sciatic nerve blocks should have similar restrictions but may participate in physical therapy-directed activities (i.e., continuous passive motion or ambulation with assistance).

References

1. Enneking FK, Chan V, Greger J, et al. Lower-extremity peripheral nerve blockade: essentials of our current understanding. *Reg Anesth Pain Med* 2005;30:4–35.
2. Taboada M, Rodriguez J, Valino C, et al. What is the minimum effective volume of local anesthetic required for sciatic nerve blockade? A prospective, randomized comparison between a popliteal and a subgluteal approach. *Anesth Analg* 2006;102:593–597.
3. di Benedetto P, Casati A, Bertini L, et al. Postoperative analgesia with continuous sciatic nerve block after foot surgery: a prospective, randomized comparison between the popliteal and subgluteal approaches. *Anesth Analg* 2002;94:996–1000.
4. Olson SA, Glasgow RR. Acute compartment syndrome in lower extremity musculoskeletal trauma. *J Am Acad Orthop Surg* 2005;13:436–444.
5. Chan VW, Nova H, Abbas S, et al. Ultrasound examination and localization of the sciatic nerve: a volunteer study. *Anesthesiology* 2006;104:309–314.
6. Bailey SL, Parkinson SK, Little WL, et al. Sciatic nerve block. A comparison of single versus double injection technique. *Reg Anesth* 1994;19: 9–13.
7. Sukhani R, Candido KD, Doty R Jr, et al. Infragluteal-parabiceps sciatic nerve block: an evaluation of a novel approach using a single-injection technique. *Anesth Analg* 2003;96:868–873.
8. Sukhani R, Nader A, Candido KD, et al. Nerve stimulator-assisted evoked motor response predicts the latency and success of a single-injection sciatic block. *Anesth Analg* 2004;99:584–588.
9. Karmakar MK, Kwok WH, Ho AM, et al. Ultrasound-guided sciatic nerve block: description of a new approach at the subgluteal space. *Br J Anaesth* 2007;98:390–395.

US-Guided Subgluteal Sciatic Block

Matthew T. Charous, MD • Larry F. Chu, MD, MS • Edward R. Mariano, MD, MAS

Patient Position: For subgluteal technique, the patient can be in Sims position or prone with the knee slightly flexed.

Needle Size: 22 to 17-gauge, 70 to 100-mm block needle

Volume: 20 to 40-mL local anesthetic

Anatomic Landmarks

Ⓐ Landmarks for the ultrasound-guided subgluteal sciatic nerve block include the greater trochanter (GT) laterally and ischial tuberosity (IT) medially.

Caudad to the gluteal crease, the sciatic nerve lies along the lateral border of the long head of biceps femoris and anterior to the gluteus maximus muscle.

Approach and Technique

Ⓑ With the patient in Sim's position, place the ultrasound transducer perpendicular to skin between the ischial tuberosity and the greater trochanter of the femur caudad to the gluteal crease and oriented parallel to the crease.

Ⓒ The sciatic nerve lies deep to the gluteus maximus muscle between the IT medially and the femur laterally.

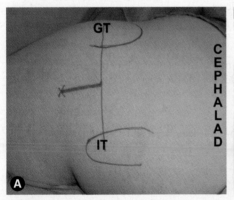 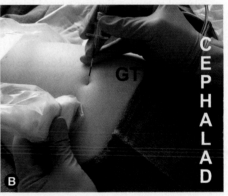

A. Surface anatomic landmarks relevant to the classic subgluteal sciatic nerve block. GT, greater trochanter of the femur; IT, ischial tuberosity. **B.** The ultrasound transducer is placed distal to the gluteal crease between the greater trochanter (GT) of the femur and the ischial tuberosity to image the sciatic nerve in cross section. The block needle is inserted lateral to the transducer and directed medially for in-plane needle guidance (left hip shown).

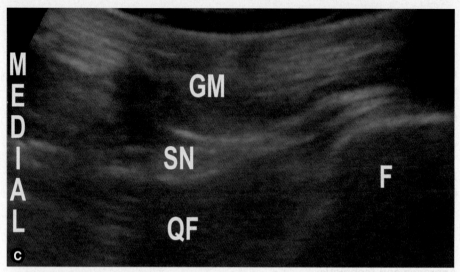

C. Short-axis ultrasound image demonstrating the relevant cross-sectional anatomy for the subgluteal sciatic nerve block approach. GM, gluteus maximus muscle; QF, quadratus femoris muscle; F, femur; SN, sciatic nerve.

A local anesthetic skin wheal is raised lateral to the ultrasound transducer after sterile skin preparation. The block needle is inserted through the skin wheal using in-plane guidance in a lateral-to-medial direction toward sciatic nerve.

Evaluation of Block
Motor testing
Test strength of plantar flexion and dorsiflexion of foot to test blockade of posterior tibial and common peroneal nerve. Asking the patient to flex the knee against resistance allows to assess the hamstring motor blockade.

Sensory testing
Decreased temperature and pinprick sensation over the lateral calf and dorsal/plantar surfaces of the foot confirm the appropriate block.

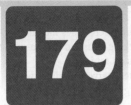

179 Popliteal Fossa Sciatic Nerve Block

Sarah J. Madison, MD · Edward R. Mariano, MD, MAS

The popliteal fossa is bordered laterally by biceps femoris and medially by semimembranosus and semitendinosus (1). Sciatic nerve block at the level of the popliteal fossa is a distal approach that preserves sensation in the posterior femoral cutaneous distribution and the motor innervation of the hamstring muscles, permitting the patient to flex the knee when crutch walking. Ultrasound-guided popliteal block with perineural catheter insertion is safe and effective, which may offer the advantages of faster placement and less patient discomfort compared to stimulating techniques (2).

READ MORE

Femoral nerve block,
Chapter 181,
page 1229

Continuous peripheral nerve blocks,
Chapter 35,
page 266

Ankle block,
Chapter 182,
page 1236

Consider planned surgical site, tourniquet application, patient disposition, and any physical limitations when determining the right regional anesthesia technique for each patient.

1) **Indications and contraindications**
   a) **Indications**
      i) The sciatic nerve may be blocked in the popliteal fossa to provide surgical anesthesia and postoperative analgesia for procedures of the lower leg, ankle, and foot.
         (1) A supplementary block of the femoral or saphenous nerves may be required to provide complete surgical anesthesia if the procedure will involve the medial aspect of the leg or ankle.
         (2) The site of the tourniquet should also be considered when planning the most appropriate regional anesthetic plan.
      ii) A continuous peripheral nerve block catheter may be placed in the popliteal fossa to provide a continuous sciatic perineural local anesthetic infusion for prolonged postoperative analgesia (3,4).
   b) **Contraindications**
      i) Absolute contraindications
         (1) Local infection at the site of planned needle insertion
      ii) Relative contraindications
         (1) Preexisting nerve injury
         (2) Coagulopathy
         (3) Disposition and physical limitations
            (a) Ability to ambulate on crutches should be considered prior to performing lower extremity peripheral nerve blocks in outpatients.
            (b) If a patient is unable to use crutches and has no weight-bearing restriction following foot surgery, an ankle block may be more appropriate.

2) **Risks and complications**
   a) General risks
      i) Localized bleeding
      ii) Infection at the site of needle puncture
   b) Site-specific risks due to the close proximity of the sciatic nerve to the popliteal artery and vein and include:
      i) Hematoma formation

   ii) Intravascular injection

3) **Equipment**

  a) Common equipment for all peripheral nerve block techniques include sterile skin cleansing solution, sterile gloves, a marking pen, and two 20-mL syringes of local anesthetic solution with extension tubing.

  b) A nerve stimulator technique requires an electrical nerve stimulator with a compatible insulated needle (2 to 4 inch) and a grounding electrode.

  c) Ultrasound-guided regional anesthesia requires portable ultrasound equipment and a high-frequency linear transducer or low-frequency curvilinear transducer (obese patients) for sciatic nerve block at the popliteal fossa.

4) **Technique**

  a) **Monitoring**

   i) Peripheral nerve blocks should be placed in a location where the patient's noninvasive BP, SpO_2, and ECG may be monitored.

   ii) Supplemental O_2 should be provided via a face mask or nasal cannulae, especially when IV sedation is administered.

  b) **Positioning and preparation**

   i) This block is most commonly performed with the patient in the prone position although the procedure may be performed from a lateral approach in patients who are unable to maneuver themselves into the prone position.

   ii) Placing a towel roll under the patient's affected ankle permits passive flexion of the knee and can facilitate identification of surface landmarks.

   iii) Apply monitors and supplemental O_2.

   iv) IV sedation should be administered, but the patient must be able to follow commands and volunteer sensory information.

Performing a popliteal sciatic block at least 8 cm proximal to the popliteal crease will increase the likelihood of anesthetizing both major branches of the sciatic nerve with a single injection.

  c) **Identification of surface anatomy**

   i) The popliteal crease is identified and marked while the patient flexes the knee.

   ii) The medial and lateral borders of the popliteal fossa are formed by the semimembranosus and biceps femoris tendons, respectively (Cognitive Aid: Panel A).

   iii) An anatomic study of 28 cadavers demonstrated division of the sciatic nerve into its tibial and common peroneal branches a mean of 60.5 ± 27.0 mm above the popliteal crease (5).

   iv) In order to increase the likelihood of anesthetizing the sciatic nerve prior to division, the site for needle insertion should be marked approximately 8 to 10 cm cephalad to the midpoint of the popliteal crease.

   v) Alternatively, the proximal "junction" of the biceps femoris and semimembranosus tendons may also successfully predict sciatic nerve location (6).

  d) **Stimulating popliteal sciatic nerve block**

   i) After sterile skin preparation, a 2 to 4 inch insulated needle is inserted at a 45 degrees angle to skin aiming cephalad while seeking motor responses from either the tibial or the peroneal nerve branches (Fig. 179-1).

   ii) When a sciatic nerve motor response is elicited and maintained at a stimulating current <0.5 mA, 30 to 40 mL of local anesthetic solution is incrementally injected following careful aspiration for blood.

Figure 179-1 Stimulating Technique for the Posterior Popliteal Fossa Sciatic Nerve Block

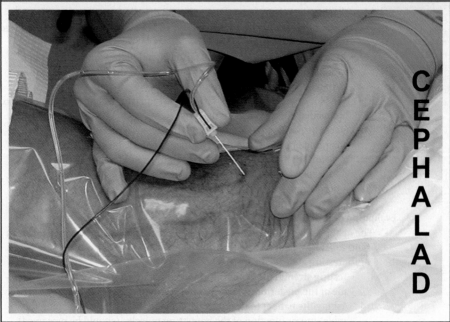

A 2- to 4-inch insulated needle is inserted at a point 8 to 10 cm proximal to the popliteal crease angled 45 degrees cephalad and advanced while seeking a sciatic nerve motor response.

    iii) Given the likelihood of proximal sciatic nerve bifurcation, this block may be performed as a double-injection technique by specifically identifying the motor responses of the tibial nerve (plantar flexion or inversion) and peroneal nerve (dorsiflexion or eversion) individually followed by separate local anesthetic injections.

    iv) For patients who are unable to assume the prone position, the popliteal fossa can be approached laterally with the patient in the supine position to produce effective sciatic nerve blockade, although onset time to complete block is longer when compared to the posterior approach (7).

        (1) With the patient supine, a 10-cm line is drawn cephalad along the lateral thigh from the popliteal crease between the vastus lateralis and the biceps femoris muscles.

        (2) At the top of the line, a 4-inch insulated needle is inserted parallel to the floor and directed medially.

        (3) Upon contact with the femur, the needle is withdrawn and redirected approximately 30 degrees posteriorly while seeking motor responses produced by tibial nerve stimulation.

  e) **Ultrasound-guided popliteal sciatic nerve block**

    i) With the patient in the prone position and a high-frequency linear transducer oriented perpendicular to the long axis of the femur over the intertendinous junction (Cognitive Aid: Panel B), the sciatic nerve can be identified in short axis anterior to the fascia of the biceps femoris muscle, posterior and medial to the femur, and posterior to the popliteal vessels when visible (Cognitive Aid: Panel C).

        (1) The ultrasound-guided technique may also be performed with the patient in the supine position.

(2) The distal leg is elevated on a pillow, and the transducer is applied under the patient's thigh at the level of the intertendinous junction to image the sciatic nerve in short axis.

ii) Tracing the sciatic nerve proximally and distally from this point should reveal bifurcation of the sciatic nerve, and the block should be commenced proximal to this point.

iii) A local anesthetic skin wheal is raised lateral to the transducer on the lateral thigh at a position corresponding to the depth of the sciatic nerve estimated by ultrasound imaging.

iv) The block needle is inserted through this skin wheal using in-plane guidance in a medial direction toward the target nerve.

v) Once the needle tip passes through the biceps femoris fascia and is positioned near the sciatic nerve, incremental aspiration and injection of local anesthetic solution should result in circumferential spread around the target.

vi) A perineural catheter may be placed in proximity to the nerve following local anesthetic injection (2).

5) **Evaluation of the block**

a) The quality of nerve blockade must be evaluated prior to surgical incision even if intraoperative general anesthesia is planned.

b) Motor testing

i) Testing strength of plantar flexion and dorsiflexion of the foot test blockade of the **posterior tibial nerve** and **common peroneal nerve**, respectively.

ii) Asking the patient to flex the knee against resistance (by grasping the ankle) motor function of the hamstring muscles (should be preserved)

c) Sensory testing

i) Decreased temperature and pinprick sensation over the lateral calf and dorsal/plantar surfaces of the foot confirm appropriate **sciatic nerve** block.

6) **Postoperative management**

a) Outpatients who undergo popliteal sciatic nerve blockade should be discharged with a supportive ankle splint (due to foot drop) and weight-bearing restriction.

i) The patient is at risk for falling if ambulation is initiated on the anesthetized extremity prior to nerve block resolution.

b) Hospitalized patients with single-injection or continuous sciatic nerve blocks should have similar restrictions but may participate in physical therapy–directed activities with appropriate assistance.

References

1. Enneking FK, Chan V, Greger J, et al. Lower-extremity peripheral nerve blockade: essentials of our current understanding. *Reg Anesth Pain Med* 2005;30:4–35.

2. Mariano ER, Cheng GS, Choy LP, et al. Electrical stimulation versus ultrasound guidance for popliteal-sciatic perineural catheter insertion: a randomized controlled trial. *Reg Anesth Pain Med* 2009;34:480–485.

3. Ilfeld BM, Morey TE, Wang RD, et al. Continuous popliteal sciatic nerve block for postoperative pain control at home: a randomized, double-blinded, placebo-controlled study. *Anesthesiology* 2002;97:959–965.

4. White PF, Issioui T, Skrivanek GD, et al. The use of a continuous popliteal sciatic nerve block after surgery involving the foot and ankle: does it improve the quality of recovery? *Anesth Analg* 2003;97:1303–1309.

5. Vloka JD, Hadzic A, April E, et al. The division of the sciatic nerve in the popliteal fossa: anatomical implications for popliteal nerve blockade. *Anesth Analg* 2001;92:215–217.

6. Hadzic A, Vloka JD, Singson R, et al. A comparison of intertendinous and classical approaches to popliteal nerve block using magnetic resonance imaging simulation. *Anesth Analg* 2002;94:1321–1324.

7. Hadzic A, Vloka JD. A comparison of the posterior versus lateral approaches to the block of the sciatic nerve in the popliteal fossa. *Anesthesiology* 1998;88:1480–1486.

US-Guided Popliteal Block

By Sarah J. Madison, MD · Larry F. Chu, MD, MS · Edward R. Mariano, MD, MAS

Patient Position: Place patient in prone position. Place a towel roll under patient's affected ankle to permit passive flexion of knee and to facilitate identification of surface landmarks. This block may also be performed in the supine position when necessary.

Needle Size: 22 to 17 gauge, 50 to 100 mm block needle

Volume: 20 to 40 mL local anesthetic

Anatomic Landmarks

Ⓐ The popliteal crease is identified and marked while the patient flexes the knee. The medial and lateral borders of popliteal fossa are formed by semimembranosus and biceps femoris tendons. The sciatic nerve is located between these two muscle groups.

Approach and Technique

Ⓑ With patient in prone position, a high frequency (HF) linear transducer is oriented perpendicular to the long axis of the femur over the intertendinous junction.

Ⓒ Identify the sciatic nerve in short axis anterior and medial to the fascia of biceps femoris muscle, posterior and medial to femur, and posterior to the popliteal vessels when visible.

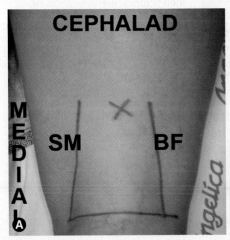
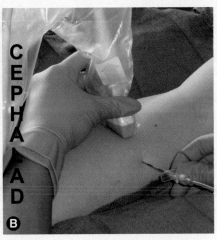

A. The popliteal fossa is bordered laterally by the biceps femoris tendon and medially by the tendons of semimembranosus and semitendinosus (right popliteal fossa shown). The sciatic nerve is reliably located below the intertendinous junction identified by the "X." **B.** The ultrasound transducer is oriented perpendicular to the long axis of the femur across the intertendinous junction to image the sciatic nerve in cross-section. The block needle is inserted lateral to the transducer and directed medially for in-plane needle guidance (left thigh shown).

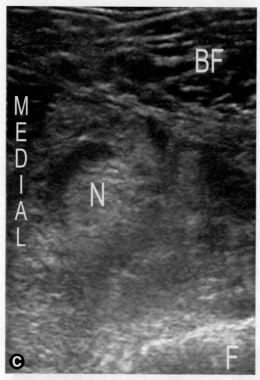

C. Short-axis ultrasound image demonstrating the relevant cross-sectional anatomy for the popliteal sciatic nerve block. RF, biceps femoris muscle; F, femur; N, sciatic nerve.

Trace sciatic nerve proximally and distally from this point to reveal bifurcation of sciatic nerve. Commence block proximal from this point. A local anesthetic skin wheal is raised lateral to the transducer on aterial thigh at a position corresponding to the depth of the sciatic nerve. Insert the block needle through skin wheal using in-plane guidance in a medial direction toward the target nerve. After the needle tip passes through biceps femoris fascia and is positioned near the sciatic nerve, incremental aspiration and injection of local anesthetic solution should result in circumferential spread around the target.

Evaluation of Block
Motor testing
Testing strength of plantar flexion and dorsiflexion of the foot test blockade of the posterior tibial nerve and common peroneal nerve, respectively.

Sensory testing
Decreased temperature and pinprick sensation over lateral calf and dorsal/plantar surfaces of foot confirms appropriate sciatic nerve block.

180 Lumbar Plexus (Psoas Compartment) Block

Jason G. Ramirez, MD · Edward R. Mariano, MD, MAS

The lumbar plexus is formed from the L1-4 spinal nerve roots with inconsistent contributions from T12 (1–3). The plexus ultimately gives rise to the genitofemoral, iliohypogastric, ilioinguinal, femoral, obturator, and lateral femoral cutaneous (LFC) nerves. Of these, the femoral, obturator, and LFC nerves are most important for lower extremity surgery, providing the major innervation of the thigh, hip, and knee (Fig. 180-1) (1). The posterior lumbar plexus block (LPB), also known as the psoas compartment block, can be utilized to provide anesthesia and analgesia for surgical procedures of the hip, thigh, and knee and may be combined with blocks of the sacral plexus to produce anesthesia of the entire lower extremity.

READ MORE

Regional anesthesia in the anticoagulated patient, Chapter 172, page 1171

The LPB is a deep block close to the neuraxis and is not advised for patients at high risk for bleeding.

1) **Indications and contraindications**
   a) Indications
      i) Postoperative analgesia following total hip arthroplasty (1,6,7)
      ii) Postoperative analgesia for major knee and thigh procedures (4)
      iii) May be combined with a parasacral block to provide surgical anesthesia for hip fracture surgery (1,5)
   b) Contraindications
      i) Absolute contraindications
         (1) Patient refusal
         (2) Infection at the planned block site
      ii) Relative contraindications
         (1) Preexisting peripheral neuropathy
         (2) Bacteremia
         (3) Previous spine surgery
         (4) Coagulopathy
            (a) This block is not recommended in patients taking medications affecting hemostasis.
            (b) The lumbar plexus is deep and lies in close proximity to the neuraxis. It is not amenable to compression in the event of vascular puncture (1).

2) **Risks and complications**
   a) General risks include infection, nerve injury, and localized bleeding.
   b) Site-specific risks and side effects
      i) The risk of systemic local anesthetic toxicity, leading to seizures and cardiovascular collapse, is a major concern when injecting large doses of local anesthetic solution into the highly vascular psoas muscle.
      ii) Diffusion or direct injection of large amounts of local anesthetic into the neuraxis may result in various degrees of epidural or subarachnoid block (1,2).
         (1) Epidural spread occurs in up to 16% of LPBs and is attributed to retrograde spread of local anesthetic solution (1,2).

Figure 180-1	Illustration Demonstrating the Main Distal Branches of the Lumbar Plexus that Contribute Significantly to Lower Extremity Innervation

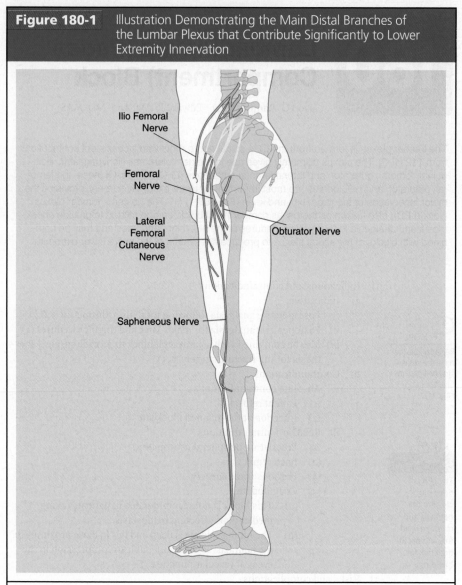

Ilio Femoral Nerve

Femoral Nerve

Lateral Femoral Cutaneous Nerve

Obturator Nerve

Sapheneous Nerve

From Clark L. Anatomy of the lumbar and sacral plexus. In: Chelly JE, ed. *Peripheral nerve blocks: A Color Atlas.* 3rd ed. Philadelphia: Lippincott Williams & Wilkins, 2009: 100, with permission.

  (2) Epidural spread can result in bilateral motor and sensory block and sympathectomy.

  (3) Subarachnoid injection can result in an excessively high spinal block and total spinal anesthesia (1,2).

  iii) Complications associated with deep needle placement may include renal hematoma, retroperitoneal hematoma, and intra-abdominal or intervertebral catheter placement (1,2).

3) **Equipment**
   a) Common equipment for all peripheral nerve block techniques includes a sterile skin cleansing solution, sterile gloves, a marking pen, and two 20-mL syringes of local anesthetic solution with extension tubing (6).
   b) A nerve stimulator technique requires an electrical nerve stimulator with a compatible insulated needle (4 to 6 inch) and a grounding electrode. Using a needle of appropriate length based on the patient's body habitus may help reduce the likelihood of serious complications.

4) **Technique**
   a) **Monitoring**
      i) Peripheral nerve blocks should be performed in a location where the patient's noninvasive BP, SpO$_2$, and ECG may be monitored.
      ii) Supplemental O$_2$ should be provided via a face mask or nasal cannulae, especially when IV sedation is administered.
   b) **Positioning and preparation**
      i) The patient should be placed in the lateral decubitus position with the operative side up.
      ii) The hips should be flexed with the lower back pushed out toward the practitioner.
      iii) Apply monitors and supplemental oxygen.
      iv) IV sedation should be administered, but the patient must be able to follow commands and volunteer sensory information.
   c) **Identification of surface anatomy**
      i) The LPB is routinely performed at the L4 vertebral level (3,5).
      ii) A line marking the midline should be drawn in a caudad-cephalad fashion along the spinous processes of the lumbar vertebrae.
      iii) Draw the intercrestal line between the tops of the iliac crests which intersects the midline at a 90 degree angle.
      iv) A third line parallel to midline is marked through the posterior superior iliac spine in a cephalad direction to intersect the intercrestal line. The distance between the two intersections is divided into thirds, and the site for needle insertion will be 1 cm cephalad from the junction of the middle and lateral thirds, approximating the location of the L4 transverse process (Cognitive Aid: Panel A) (5).
   d) **Stimulating LPB**
      i) After sterile skin preparation and injection of a local anesthetic skin wheal, a 4 to 6 inch stimulating needle is advanced perpendicular to the skin (Cognitive Aid: Panel A).
      ii) The distance from skin to lumbar transverse process is highly variable and dependent on body mass index (BMI) and gender (1,2). However, the distance from transverse process to the lumbar plexus anteriorly is independent of BMI or gender and is fairly constant at approximately 2 to 3 cm (1,2,5).
      iii) Elicitation of a quadriceps contraction signifies correct needle tip placement within the lumbar plexus.
      iv) If bony contact with the L4 transverse process is established, the needle is withdrawn, walked caudally off of the transverse process, and then advanced up to 3 cm seeking an evoked motor response of the quadriceps muscle.
   e) **Ultrasound-guided LPB**
      i) Real-time ultrasound-guided techniques for the LPB have been described but remain challenging (7,8).
      ii) To date, most practitioners continue to rely on electrical nerve stimulation techniques for this procedure in adults, even with ultrasound guidance (3,9,10).
      iii) Prepuncture ultrasound scanning may help practitioners confirm the location and depth of the lumbar transverse processes prior to performing a stimulating LPB (Cognitive Aid Panel C) (11).

5) **Evaluation of the block**

a) The quality of nerve blockade should be evaluated prior to surgical incision even if intraoperative general anesthesia is planned.

b) Sensory and motor testing of the lumbar plexus can be accomplished using the three "P's"—Pull, Pinch, and Punt (1).

i) "Pull" involves abducting the patient's leg and then asking the patient to move the leg voluntarily toward midline to evaluate the strength of the adductor muscles innervated by the *obturator* nerve.

ii) The *lateral femoral cutaneous* nerve is a purely sensory nerve, so a "Pinch" assesses anesthesia in this nerve distribution by pinching the skin over the lateral thigh.

iii) "Punt" involves supporting the patient's leg under the knee and asking the patient to perform a kicking motion against resistance to test the quadriceps muscle innervated by the *femoral* nerve.

6) **Postoperative management**

a) Outpatients who undergo LPB should be discharged with a knee immobilizer and weight-bearing restriction.

b) Hospitalized patients with single-injection or continuous LPBs should have similar restrictions but may participate in physical therapy-directed activities (i.e., continuous passive motion and ambulation with assistance).

i) Quadriceps weakness from a LPB and hip or knee surgery places the patient at high risk for falling if unassisted ambulation is initiated prior to nerve block resolution.

ii) Ambulating patients with LPBs and perineural catheters is possible with the assistance of trained nursing staff and physical therapists (12).

c) Patients experiencing epidural spread of local anesthetic may exhibit signs of sympathectomy and may require temporary supportive treatment including volume resuscitation and/or vasoactive medications.

Patients who have received an LPB should be considered **high fall risk** *and should not ambulate without proper assistance.*

References

1. Enneking FK, Chan V, Greger J, et al. Lower-extremity peripheral nerve blockade: essentials of our current understanding. *Reg Anesth Pain Med* 2005;30:4–35.
2. Capdevila X, Coimbra C, Choquet O. Approaches to the lumbar plexus: success, risks, and outcome. *Reg Anesth Pain Med* 2005;30:150–162.
3. Awad IT, Duggan EM. Posterior LPB: anatomy, approaches, and techniques. *Reg Anesth Pain Med* 2005;30:143–149.
4. Horlocker TT, Hebl JR, Kinney MA, et al. Opioid-free analgesia following total knee arthroplasty—a multimodal approach using continuous lumbar plexus (psoas compartment) block, acetaminophen, and ketorolac. *Reg Anesth Pain Med* 2002;27:105–108.
5. Capdevila X, Macaire P, Dadure C, et al. Continuous psoas compartment block for postoperative analgesia after total hip arthroplasty: new landmarks, technical guidelines, and clinical evaluation. *Anesth Analg* 2002;94:1606–1613.
6. Hebl JR. The importance and implications of aseptic techniques during regional anesthesia. *Reg Anesth Pain Med* 2006;31:311–323.
7. Karmakar MK, Ho AM, Li X, et al. Ultrasound-guided LPB through the acoustic window of the lumbar ultrasound trident. *Br J Anaesth* 2008;100:533–537.
8. Kirchmair L, Entner T, Wissel J, et al. A study of the paravertebral anatomy for ultrasound-guided posterior LPB. *Anesth Analg* 2001;93:477–481.
9. Marhofer P, Greher M, Kapral S. Ultrasound guidance in regional anaesthesia. *Br J Anaesth* 2005;94:7–17.
10. Marhofer P, Chan VW. Ultrasound-guided regional anesthesia: current concepts and future trends. *Anesth Analg* 2007;104:1265–1269.
11. Ilfeld BM, Loland VJ, Mariano ER. Prepuncture ultrasound imaging to predict transverse process and lumbar plexus depth for psoas compartment block and perineural catheter insertion: a prospective, observational study. *Anesth Analg* 2010 Jun 1;110(6):1725–1728.
12. Ilfeld BM, Ball ST, Gearen PF, et al. Ambulatory continuous posterior lumbar plexus nerve blocks after hip arthroplasty: a dual-center, randomized, triple-masked, placebo-controlled trial. *Anesthesiology* 2008;109:491–501.

Lumbar Plexus Block

By Jason G. Ramirez, MD • Larry F. Chu, MD, MS • Edward R. Mariano, MD, MAS

Patient Position: The patient should be placed in the lateral decubitus position with the operative side up. The hips should be flexed with the lower back pushed out towards the practitioner.

Needle Size: 4 to 6 in. insulated needle

Volume: 20 to 40 mL local anesthetic

Anatomic Landmarks

The lumbar plexus block (LPB) is routinely performed at the L4 vertebral level.
A line marking the midline should be drawn in a caudad-cephalad fashion along the spinous processes of the lumbar vertebrae.

A Draw the intercrestal line between the tops of the iliac crests which intersects the midline at a 90 degree angle.

A third line parallel to midline is marked through the posterior superior iliac spine in a cephalad direction to intersect the intercrestal line. The distance between the two intersections is divided into thirds, and the site for needle insertion will be 1 cm cephalad from the junction of the middle and lateral thirds, approximating the location of the L_4 transverse process.

Approach and Technique

B After sterile skin preparation and injection of a local anesthetic skin wheal, a 4 to 6 in stimulating needle is advanced perpendicular to the skin.

C Prepuncture ultrasound scanning may help practitioners confirm the location and depth of the lumbar transverse processes prior to performing LPB.

The distance from skin to lumbar transverse process is highly variable and dependent on body mass index (BMI) and gender.

However, the distance from transverse process to the lumbar plexus anteriorly is independent of BMI or gender and is fairly constant at approximately 2 to 3 cm.

Elicitation of a quadriceps contraction signifies correct needle tip placement within the lumbar plexus.

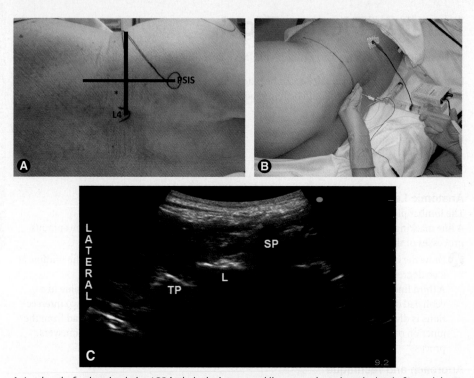

A. Landmarks for the stimulating LPB include the intercrestal line approximately at the level of L4 and the posterior superior iliac spine (PSIS); * marks the recommended site for needle insertion (5). **B.** Stimulating LPB technique: a 4 to 6 in insulated needle is inserted perpendicular to skin at a puncture site predetermined by surface anatomic landmarks. The intersection of the intercrestal line with the parasagittal line determines the site of introduction of the needle. IS, iliac spine, PSIS, postsuperior iliac spine. **C.** Short-axis ultrasound image at the level of the lumbar vertebra; SP, spinous process; L, lamina; TP, transverse process.

If bony contact with the L4 transverse process is established, the needle is withdrawn, walked caudally off of the transverse process, and then advanced up to 3 cm seeking an evoked motor response of the quadriceps muscle.

Evaluation of Block

The quality of nerve blockade should be evaluated prior to surgical incision even if intraoperative general anesthesia is planned.

Sensory and motor testing of the lumbar plexus can be accomplished using the three "P's"— Pull, Pinch, and Punt.

"Pull" involves abducting the patient's leg and then asking the patient to move the leg voluntarily toward midline to evaluate the strength of the adductor muscles innervated by the obturator nerve.

The lateral femoral cutaneous nerve is a purely sensory nerve, so a "Pinch" assesses anesthesia in this nerve distribution by pinching the skin over the lateral thigh.

"Punt" involves supporting the patient's leg under the knee and asking the patient to perform a kicking motion against resistance to test the quadriceps muscle innervated by the femoral nerve.

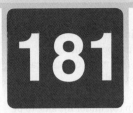

181 Femoral Nerve Block

Matthew T. Charous, MD • Edward R. Mariano, MD, MAS

The femoral nerve supplies the sensory and motor innervation of the anterior thigh and knee and then terminates as the saphenous nerve that innervates the medial aspect of the leg. Techniques employing electrical stimulation, ultrasound guidance, or both have been described. Femoral perineural catheters provide prolonged analgesia following total knee arthroplasty and other major knee surgeries. Other potential benefits of femoral nerve blocks/catheters in total knee arthroplasty include decreased bleeding and need for transfusion (1) and shorter time to achieve hospital discharge criteria (1–3).

READ MORE

Continuous peripheral nerve blocks, Chapter 35, page 266

READ MORE

Proximal sciatic nerve blocks, Chapter 178, page 1210

When the potential benefits outweigh the risks, femoral nerve block may be safely performed in the coagulopathic patient below the inguinal ligament since manual compression of vascular structures may be performed if necessary.

1) **Indications and contraindications**
   a) **Indications**
      i) **Surgical anesthesia or postoperative analgesia of the anterior and medial thigh or the medial aspect of the of the leg below the knee**
      ii) The posterior thigh is supplied by the sacral plexus *via* the posterior cutaneous nerve of the thigh.
      iii) Surgical anesthesia of the entire lower extremity requires blockade of the sciatic nerve in addition to the lumbar plexus branches—femoral, lateral femoral cutaneous (LFC), and obturator nerves
   b) **Contraindications**
      i) Absolute contraindications
         (1) Local infection at the site of planned needle placement
      ii) Relative contraindications
         (1) Coagulopathy
         (2) Preexisting nerve injury

2) **Risks and complications**
   a) General risks involving peripheral nerve blockade are localized bleeding, intravascular injection with or without local anesthetic toxicity, and infection at the site of needle puncture.
   b) Site-specific side effects from femoral nerve block include injury to femoral vessels and subsequent hematoma.

3) **Equipment**
   a) Common equipment for all peripheral nerve block techniques includes a sterile skin cleansing solution, sterile gloves, a marking pen, and two 20-mL syringes of local anesthetic solution with extension tubing.
   b) A nerve stimulation technique requires an electrical nerve stimulator with a compatible insulated needle (1 to 2 in) and a grounding electrode.
   c) The fascia iliaca approach utilizes a Tuohy-tip needle with or without extension tubing attached to syringes of local anesthetic and is performed without nerve stimulation (4).
   d) Ultrasound-guided regional anesthesia requires portable ultrasound equipment and a high-frequency linear transducer for femoral nerve block.

4) **Technique**

   a) **Monitoring**

The fascia iliaca block anesthetizes the femoral and LFC nerves and is performed without nerve stimulation or ultrasound.

   i) Peripheral nerve blocks should be placed in a location where the patient's noninvasive BP, SpO_2, and ECG may be monitored.

   ii) Supplemental O_2 should be provided via a face mask or nasal cannulae, especially when IV sedation is administered.

   b) **Positioning and preparation**

   i) Position the patient supine with a small hip roll under the side to be blocked to flatten the inguinal crease.

      (1) The leg should be straight and not internally or externally rotated.

   ii) Apply monitors and supplemental O_2.

   iii) IV sedation should be administered, but the patient must be able to follow commands and volunteer sensory information.

   c) **Identification of surface anatomy**

The femoral nerve is widest and most superficial at the level of the inguinal crease.

   i) The important landmarks for this block include the inguinal crease and the femoral artery (Cognitive Aid: Panel A).

      (1) An anatomic study has shown the femoral nerve to be widest and most superficial at the level of the inguinal crease (Cognitive Aid: Panel B) where it can be found immediately **lateral** to the artery 71% of the time (5).

      (2) If the femoral pulse is difficult to palpate, Doppler or ultrasound may be helpful.

   ii) After identifying the femoral artery, a point should be marked 1 cm **lateral** to the artery along the inguinal crease.

   d) **Stimulating femoral nerve block**

   i) After sterile skin preparation and injection of a local anesthetic skin wheal, a 1- to 2-in insulated needle should be inserted at a 45 degree angle, aiming cephalad at the point identified above (Fig. 181-1).

   ii) Eliciting an appropriate femoral nerve motor response should involve contraction of the quadriceps muscle and the patellofemoral ligament.

      (1) The ability to maintain the motor response at <0.5 mA of stimulating current confirms proper needle tip placement.

      (2) The total local anesthetic volume (30 to 40 mL) is then injected incrementally after negative aspiration for blood.

READ MORE

Continuous peripheral nerve block, Chapter 35, page 266

      (3) A continuous peripheral nerve block catheter may be placed at this location to administer a postoperative perineural infusion of local anesthetic.

   iii) The classic "3-in-1" block originally described a large-volume single-injection femoral nerve block with firm distal pressure to encourage cephalad spread of the anesthetic to the lumbar plexus to block the LFC and obturator nerves.

      (1) Magnetic resonance imaging has since disproved this theoretical concept by demonstrating local anesthetic spread only in the lateral, caudad, and medial directions (6).

      (2) A clinical study evaluating the "3-in-1" block consistently produced anesthesia in the LFC and femoral nerve distributions but only achieved obturator nerve block in 4% of patients (7).

| **Figure 181-1** | Stimulating Femoral Nerve Block Technique |

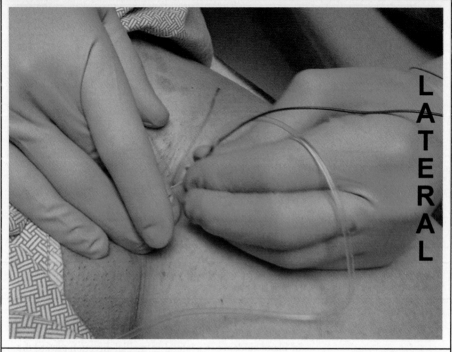

LATERAL

A 1- to 2-in insulated needle is inserted lateral to the femoral artery at a 45-degree angle aiming cephalad at the level of the inguinal crease (left inguinal region shown).

e) **"Fascia Iliaca" block technique**
   i) Performed 1 cm caudad to the junction of the lateral and middle thirds of the inguinal ligament.
      (1) This technique does require nerve stimulation or ultrasound guidance.
      (2) May be useful for "rescue" analgesia following knee or hip surgery or for acute pain management of orthopaedic trauma cases such as hip fractures
   ii) A Tuohy-tip needle is inserted at a 45 degree angle aiming cephalad (Fig. 181-2) until two distinct losses of resistance are palpated as the needle traverses the fascia lata and fascia iliaca, respectively.
   iii) After confirming negative aspiration for blood, the total volume of local anesthetic solution is injected incrementally, producing a very reliable block of the femoral and LFC nerves (4).
f) **Ultrasound guided femoral nerve block**
   i) With a high-frequency linear transducer positioned at the level of the inguinal crease and oriented parallel to the inguinal ligament (Cognitive Aid: Panel C), the femoral artery is identified.
      (1) If both the femoral and profunda femoris arteries are visible, move the transducer more cephalad until the two vessels merge to form the common femoral artery.
      (2) At this level, the femoral nerve lies lateral to the femoral artery between the fascia iliaca and the iliacus muscle (Cognitive Aid: Panel D).
   ii) A local anesthetic skin wheal is raised lateral to the ultrasound transducer after sterile skin preparation.

Figure 181-2   Fascia Iliaca Block Technique

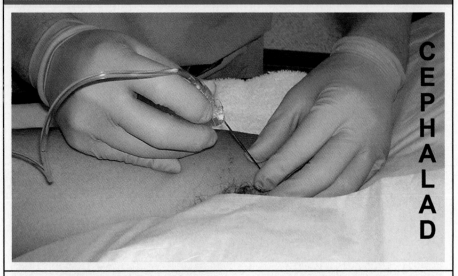

A tuohy-tip epidural needle is inserted 1 cm below the junction of the lateral and middle thirds of the inguinal ligament at a 45 degree angle aiming cephalad until the needle tip traverses the fascia lata and fascia iliaca (right inguinal region shown).

        iii) The block needle is inserted through this skin wheal using in-plane guidance in a lateral-to-medial direction toward the femoral nerve (8).

        iv) Once the needle tip has traversed the fascia iliaca lateral to the femoral nerve, local anesthetic is injected incrementally until visual confirmation of injectate spread surrounding the femoral nerve is achieved.

5) **Evaluation of the block**

    a) The quality of nerve blockade should be evaluated prior to surgical incision even if intraoperative general anesthesia is planned.

    b) Motor testing

        i) Strength of leg extension against resistance or gravity tests the quadriceps muscle innervated by the *femoral* nerve.

    c) Sensory testing

        i) Testing cold temperature and pinprick sensation over the anterior thigh assesses sensory anesthesia in the *femoral* nerve distribution.

        ii) Similar testing over the lateral thigh assesses anesthesia in the LFC nerve distribution.

6) **Postoperative management**

    a) Outpatients who undergo femoral nerve blockade should be discharged with a knee immobilizer and weight-bearing restriction.

    b) Hospitalized patients with single-injection or continuous femoral nerve blocks should have similar restrictions but may participate in physical therapy–directed activities (i.e., continuous passive motion and ambulation with assistance).

Patients who have received a femoral nerve block should be considered **high fall risk** and should not ambulate without proper assistance.

i) Quadriceps weakness from a femoral nerve block and knee surgery places the patient at high risk for falling if unassisted ambulation is initiated prior to nerve block resolution.

ii) Ambulating patients with femoral nerve blocks and perineural catheters is possible with the assistance of trained nursing staff and physical therapists (3).

References

1. Chelly JE, Greger J, Gebhard R, et al. Continuous femoral blocks improve recovery and outcome of patients undergoing total knee arthroplasty. *J Arthroplasty* 2001;16:436–445.
2. Wang H, Boctor B, Verner J. The effect of single-injection femoral nerve block on rehabilitation and length of hospital stay after total knee replacement. *Reg Anesth Pain Med* 2002;27:139–144.
3. Ilfeld BM, Le LT, Meyer RS, et al. Ambulatory continuous femoral nerve blocks decrease time to discharge readiness after tricompartment total knee arthroplasty: a randomized, triple-masked, placebo-controlled study. *Anesthesiology* 2008;108:703–713.
4. Capdevila X, Biboulet P, Bouregba M, et al. Comparison of the three-in-one and fascia iliaca compartment blocks in adults: clinical and radiographic analysis. *Anesth Analg* 1998;86:1039–1044.
5. Vloka JD, Hadzic A, Drobnik L, et al. Anatomical landmarks for femoral nerve block: a comparison of four needle insertion sites. *Anesth Analg* 1999;89:1467–1470.
6. Marhofer P, Nasel C, Sitzwohl C, et al. Magnetic resonance imaging of the distribution of local anesthetic during the three-in-one block. *Anesth Analg* 2000;90:119–124.
7. Lang SA, Yip RW, Chang PC, et al. The femoral 3-in-1 block revisited. *J Clin Anesth* 1993;5:292–296.
8. Mariano ER, Loland VJ, Sandhu NS, et al. Ultrasound guidance versus electrical stimulation for femoral perineural catheter insertion. *J Ultrasound Med* 2009;28:1453–1460.

US-Guided Femoral Nerve Block

By Matthew T. Charous, MD · Larry F. Chu, MD, MS · Edward R. Mariano, MD, MAS

Patient Position: Position the patient supine with a small hip roll under the side to be blocked to flatten the inguinal crease. The leg should be straight and not internally or externally rotated.

Needle Size: 22 to 17 gauge, 50 to 100 mm block needle

Volume: 20 to 40 mL local anesthetic

Anatomic Landmarks

Ⓐ The important landmarks for this block include the inguinal crease and femoral artery (FA).

Ⓑ An anatomic study has shown the femoral nerve (FN) to be widest and most superficial at the level of the inguinal crease where it can be found immediately lateral to the artery 71% of the time.

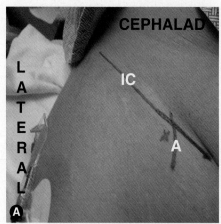
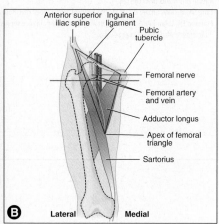

A. Surface anatomic landmarks relevant to the FN block. IC, inguinal crease; A, femoral artery. An "X" is placed lateral to the FA to identify the site for needle insertion (left inguinal region shown). **B.** Illustration of the relationship of the FN, FA, and femoral vein below the inguinal ligament. Reproduced from Perlas A. Ultrasound Guided Femoral Nerve Block. In: Chelly JE, ed. Peripheral Nerve Blocks: A Color Atlas. 3rd ed. Philadelphia: Lippincott Williams & Wilkins, 2009: 295, with permission.

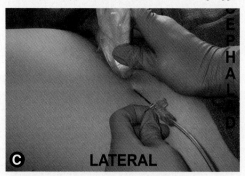

Approach and Technique

Ⓒ With a high frequency linear transducer positioned at the level of the inguinal crease and oriented parallel to the inguinal ligament, the FA is identified.

C. A high frequency linear transducer is placed over the FA pulsation at the level of the inguinal crease. The block needle is inserted lateral to the transducer and directed medially for in-plane needle guidance (left inguinal region shown).

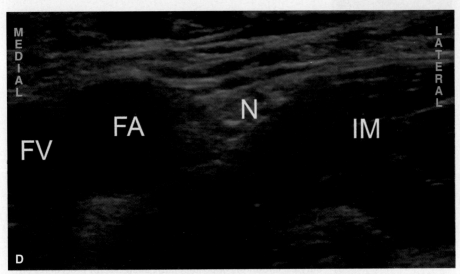

D. Short-axis ultrasound image of the femoral vessels and FN at the inguinal crease; FV, femoral vein; FA, femoral artery; IM, iliacus muscle; N, femoral nerve.

D If the femoral and profunda femoris arteries are both visible, move the transducer more cephalad until the two vessels merge to form the common FA. At this level, the FN lies lateral to the FA between the fascia illiaca and iliacus muscle. The block needle is inserted through the skin wheal using in-plane guidance in a lateral-to-medial direction toward the FN. Once the needle tip has traversed the fascia iliaca lateral to the FN, local anesthetic is injected incrementally until visual confirmation of injectate spread surrounding the FN is achieved.

Evaluation of Block
Motor testing
Strength of leg extension against resistance or gravity tests the quadriceps muscle innervated by the FN.

Sensory testing
Testing cold temperature and pinprick sensation over the anterior thigh assesses sensory anesthesia in the FN distribution. Similar testing over the lateral thigh assesses anesthesia in the lateral femoral cutaneous nerve distribution.

182

Ankle Block

Matthew T. Charous, MD • Edward R. Mariano, MD, MAS

The ankle block anesthetizes the five most distal branches of the lumbosacral plexus: the posterior tibial, sural, deep peroneal, superficial peroneal, and saphenous nerves (1). An advantage of this technique for foot surgery is that motor function is essentially spared since the tendons that are responsible for motor function originate proximal to the site of local anesthetic injection. Therefore, the ankle block is regularly performed for patients undergoing ambulatory foot surgery (2).

1) **Indications and contraindications**
   a) Indications
      i) Surgical anesthesia or postoperative analgesia for procedures on the toes or foot (1)
         (1) Ankle blocks provide adequate surgical anesthesia for foot procedures of limited duration with an ankle tourniquet.
         (2) Prolonged foot surgeries or proximal tourniquet locations (e.g., thigh or calf) will likely require an additional regional or general anesthetic.
      ii) Individual branches may be anesthetized to supplement more proximal nerve blocks of the sciatic or saphenous nerves.
   b) Contraindications
      i) Absolute contraindications
         (1) Local infection at the site of planned needle insertion
         (2) In patients with localized infection of the lower limb, tissue acidosis may limit the amount of nonionized local anesthetic available to cross cell membranes.
      ii) Relative contraindications
         (1) Preexisting nerve injury
         (2) Coagulopathy (although the ankle block may have advantages over deeper blocks in the patient with bleeding tendencies since compression can be easily applied)

2) **Risks and complications**
   a) General risks involving peripheral nerve blockade are localized bleeding, intravascular injection with local anesthetic toxicity, and infection at the site of needle puncture.
   b) Site-specific risks
      i) Procedure-induced pain resulting from multiple needle insertions
      ii) Injection of local anesthetic solution into terminal arteries. However, significant IV injection is rare due to division of local anesthetic volume into multiple sites of injection.
         (1) Even large volumes of local anesthetic solution (up to 30 mL) injected at the ankle result in relatively low serum levels (3).

(2) Epinephrine-free local anesthetic solutions are commonly used for ankle block to avoid vasoconstriction of the terminal arteries that supply blood flow to the foot and digits.

3) **Equipment**

a) Common equipment for all peripheral nerve block techniques include sterile skin cleansing solution, sterile gloves, a marking pen, and up to 30 mL of local anesthetic solution with extension tubing.

b) A nerve stimulator technique may be employed for the tibial nerve block and requires an electrical nerve stimulator with a compatible 1-inch insulated needle and grounding electrode.

c) Ultrasound guidance for tibial nerve block at the ankle requires portable ultrasound equipment and a small high-frequency linear transducer or a small curvilinear transducer.

4) **Technique**

a) **Monitoring**

i) Peripheral nerve blocks should be placed in a location where the patient's noninvasive BP, SpO_2, and ECG may be monitored.

ii) Supplemental O_2 should be provided via a face mask or a nasal cannula especially if sedation is to be administered.

b) **Positioning and preparation**

i) Position the patient supine (preferred) or prone with the foot to be anesthetized elevated on a roll.

ii) Apply monitors and supplemental O_2 prior to administering IV sedation.

c) **Identification of surface anatomy**

i) Important surface landmarks to identify include the most cephalad portions of the medial malleolus (MM), lateral malleolus (LM), and the Achilles tendon posteriorly.

(1) The sural nerve is located in the subcutaneous tissue between the LM and the Achilles tendon (Cognitive Aid: Panel A).

(2) Between the MM and the Achilles tendon, the posterior tibial nerve is located immediately posterior to the tibial artery and is the largest of the five nerves innervating the foot (Cognitive Aid: Panel A).

ii) Next, have the patient dorsiflex the great toe to identify the extensor hallucis longus (EHL) tendon.

(1) The tendon of tibialis anterior (TA) lies medial to the EHL, and the dorsalis pedis artery is typically palpable between these two tendons.

(2) The deep peroneal nerve, which innervates the webspace between the first and the second toes, lies deep to the extensor retinaculum between the two tendons and is closely associated with the dorsalis pedis artery (Cognitive Aid: Panel A).

iii) Superficial branches of the saphenous nerve run anterior to the MM, while the superficial peroneal nerve runs anterior to the LM to innervate the dorsum of the foot (Cognitive Aid: Panel A).

d) **Landmark-based ankle block** (4)

i) After sterile skin preparation, externally rotate the leg.

ii) While palpating the posterior tibial artery behind the MM, insert a 1-inch 22-gauge B-bevel needle posterior to the pulse at a 45 degrees angle toward the MM.

iii) If bone is contacted without eliciting a paresthesia, inject 5 mL of anesthetic while slowly withdrawing the needle to block the posterior tibial nerve.

iv) Alternatively, a 1-inch insulated needle may be used with electrical stimulation to locate the posterior tibial nerve by eliciting plantar flexion of the toes at a stimulating current <0.5 mA.

v) Next, internally rotate the leg to expose the posterior border of the LM and infiltrate 3 to 5 mL of local anesthetic subcutaneously between the LM and the Achilles tendon to anesthetize the sural nerve.

vi)   While palpating the EHL and TA tendons on the dorsum of the foot, insert a 1-inch 22-gauge B-bevel needle between the two tendons and inject 3 to 5 mL of local anesthetic after bony contact.

vii) From this needle insertion site, inject local anesthetic subcutaneously toward the MM and the LM using a 1.5-inch 25- or 27-gauge needle to anesthetize the saphenous and superficial peroneal nerves to complete the ankle block.

The posterior tibial nerve gives rise to three terminal branches: medial plantar, lateral plantar, and calcaneal nerves at the level of the MM. Therefore, complete blockade requires blockade at or proximal to this level.

e)   **Ultrasound-guided tibial nerve block (Cognitive Aid: Pannels B, C, and D)**

i)   Compared to the landmark-based approach, ultrasound guidance for tibial nerve block at the ankle results in a higher success rate (5).

ii)   Place the transducer cephalad to the MM and image the posterior tibial artery in short axis.

iii) The nerve will appear immediately posterior to the artery.

iv)   Injection of 5 mL of local anesthetic around the nerve will result in reliable anesthesia.

f)   **Ultrasound-guided sural nerve block**

i)   The sural nerve travels in close proximity to the lesser saphenous vein posterior to the LM, and ultrasound guidance improves success rates compared to landmark-based sural nerve block techniques (6).

ii)   Using a small linear transducer or a small curvilinear transducer, image the lesser saphenous vein in short axis.

iii) Applying a tourniquet proximally helps to distend the lesser saphenous vein and facilitates its identification.

iv)   Insert a 1 to 1.5 inch 22-gauge B-bevel needle in plane and deposit up to 5 mL of local anesthetic solution circumferentially around the lesser saphenous vein.

g)   **Ultrasound-guided deep peroneal nerve block**

i)   Compared to traditional landmark-based deep peroneal nerve block, ultrasound guidance may speed the onset but does not improve the overall success or quality of the block (7).

Ultrasound guidance has been shown to improve success rates for sural and tibial nerve block at the ankle but not for deep peroneal nerve block (5–7).

ii)   Superficial to the tibial surface, the deep peroneal nerve can be visualized lateral to the anterior tibial artery (continuing as the dorsalis pedis artery distally).

iii) Applying the transducer at the level of the superior margin of the MM, image the deep peroneal nerve and anterior tibial artery in short axis.

iv)   Insert a 1 to 1.5 inch 22-gauge B-bevel needle in plane and deposit up to 5 mL of local anesthetic solution circumferentially around the deep peroneal nerve or lateral to the anterior tibial artery if the nerve cannot be identified.

5)   Evaluation of the block

a)   The quality of the block in each of the five nerve distributions should be evaluated prior to surgical incision.

b)   Blockade of the deep and superficial peroneal nerves may be assessed by testing sensation in the webspace between the first and the second toes and over the dorsum of the foot.

c)   The plantar surface, medial aspect, and lateral aspect of the foot are innervated by the posterior tibial nerve, saphenous nerve, and sural nerve, respectively. The major innervation of the foot is supplied by the posterior tibial nerve.

6) Postoperative management
   a) **All patients who undergo ankle block should be discharged with a hard walking shoe.**
   b) Patients may bear weight as tolerated and may safely ambulate with minimal assistance.

References

1. Enneking FK, Chan V, Greger J, et al. Lower-extremity peripheral nerve blockade: essentials of our current understanding. *Reg Anesth Pain Med* 2005;30:4–35.
2. Klein SM, Pietrobon R, Nielsen KC, et al. Peripheral nerve blockade with long-acting local anesthetics: a survey of the Society for Ambulatory Anesthesia. *Anesth Analg* 2002;94:71–76.
3. Mineo R, Sharrock NE. Venous levels of lidocaine and bupivacaine after midtarsal ankle block. *Reg Anesth* 1992;17:47–49.
4. Brown DL. *Atlas of Regional Anesthesia*. 2nd ed. Philadelphia, PA: WB Saunders Company; 1999.
5. Redborg KE, Antonakakis JG, Beach ML, et al. Ultrasound improves the success rate of a tibial nerve block at the ankle. *Reg Anesth Pain Med* 2009;34:256–260.
6. Redborg KE, Sites BD, Chinn CD, et al. Ultrasound improves the success rate of a sural nerve block at the ankle. *Reg Anesth Pain Med* 2009;34:24–28.
7. Antonakakis JG, Scalzo DC, Jorgenson AS, et al. Ultrasound does not improve the success rate of a deep peroneal nerve block at the ankle. *Reg Anesth Pain Med* 2010;35:217–221.

US-Guided Ankle Block

By Matthew T. Charous, MD • Larry F. Chu, MD, MS • Edward R. Mariano, MD, MAS

Patient Position: Position the patient supine (preferred) or prone with the foot to be anesthetized elevated on a roll.

Needle Size: 22-gauge Tuohy-tip or B-bevel block needle

Volume: 5 mL per nerve

Anatomic Landmarks

Ⓐ Important surface landmarks to identify include the most cephalad portions of the medial malleolus (MM), lateral malleolus (LM), and the Achilles tendon posteriorly. The sural nerve is located in the subcutaneous tissue between the LM and Achilles tendon. Have the patient dorsiflex the great toe to identify the extensor hallucis longus (EHL) tendon. The tendon of tibialis anterior lies medial to the EHL, and the dorsalis pedis artery is typically palpable between these two tendons. The deep peroneal nerve innervates the webspace between the first and second toes. It lies deep to the extensor retinaculum between the two tendons and is closely associated with the dorsalis pedis artery.

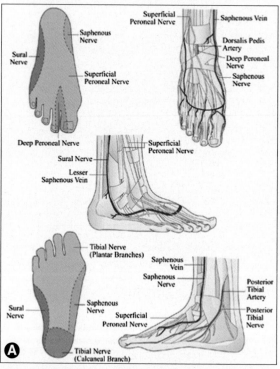

Approach and Technique
US-Guided Tibial Nerve Block

Ⓑ Place the transducer cephalad to the MM and image the posterior tibial artery in short axis. The nerve will appear immediately posterior to the artery.
Injection of 5 mL of local anesthetic around the nerve will result in reliable anesthesia.

A. Anatomic landmarks. From Clanton TO, Loncarich DP. Ankle block. In: Chelly JE. Peripheral nerve blocks: A color atlas. 3rd ed. Philadelphia: Lippincott Williams & Wilkins, 2009: 158, with permission.

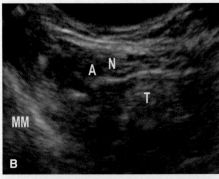

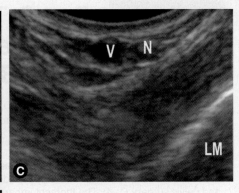

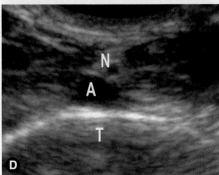

B. Sonoanatomy relevant to the tibial nerve block; MM, medial malleolus; A, posterior tibial artery; N, nerve; T, flexor hallucis longus tendon. **C.** Sonoanatomy relevant to the sural nerve block; LM, lateral malleolus; V, lesser saphenous vein; N, nerve. **D.** Sonoanatomy relevant to the deep peroneal nerve block; T, tibia; A, anterior tibial artery; N, nerve

US-Guided Sural Nerve Block

C Using a small linear transducer or small curvilinear transducer, image the lesser saphenous vein in short-axis.

Applying a tourniquet proximally helps to distend the lesser saphenous vein and facilitates its identification. Insert the block needle in-plane and deposit up to 5 mL of local anesthetic solution circumferentially around the lesser saphenous vein.

US-Guided Deep Peroneal Nerve Block

D Apply the transducer over the anterior tibia at the level of the superior margin of the malleoli. Superficial to the tibial surface, the deep peroneal nerve can be visualized lateral to the anterior tibial artery (continuing as the dorsalis pedis artery distally).

Insert the block needle in-plane and deposit up to 5 mL of local anesthetic solution circumferentially around the deep peroneal nerve or lateral to the anterior tibial artery if the nerve cannot be identified.

Evaluation of Block

Blockade of the deep and superficial peroneal nerves may be assessed by testing sensation in the webspace between the first and second toes and over the dorsum of the foot. Testing sensation along lateral and plantar surfaces of the foot will assess anesthesia in the sural and tibial nerve distributions, respectively.

Part C: Truncal Blocks
Transversus Abdominis Plane Blocks

Justin W. Heil, MD, PhD · Matthew T. Charous, MD · Edward R. Mariano, MD, MAS

Transversus abdominis plane (TAP) blocks anesthetize the somatic nerves that innervate the abdominal wall and may provide postoperative analgesia for abdominal and pelvic surgery (1–4). The thoracolumbar nerves supplying the abdomen arise from spinal nerves T7-L1 and course through the plane between the transversus abdominis (TA) muscle and the internal oblique muscle—the TAP (3). By infiltrating the space between these muscles with local anesthetic solution, distal spinal nerves and peripheral branches of L1 (ilioinguinal and iliohypogastric nerves) may be blocked. However, the distance between the nerves is substantial, and coverage of the entire abdominal wall requires multiple injections (5,6). The TAP block may be performed using surface anatomic landmarks and a "double loss-of-resistance" technique in the triangle of Petit (3) but may also be performed with real-time ultrasound guidance (7,8).

1) Indications and contraindications
   a) **Indications**
      i) TAP blocks anesthetize the somatic nerves innervating the abdominal wall and can provide postoperative analgesia for procedures in the abdominal, pelvic, or inguinal regions.
         (1) A TAP catheter and continuous local anesthetic infusion extend the duration of analgesia and may have other benefits (9).
      ii) The specific distribution of the nerves within this plane requires consideration of the site of surgery.
         (1) A single-injection posterior TAP block reliably anesthetizes the ipsilateral abdominal wall in the dermatomal distributions of T10-L1 (6).
         (2) Subcostal TAP blocks may need to be performed for upper abdominal surgeries.
         (3) Bilateral TAP blocks are necessary for midline surgeries.
         (4) Extensive midline incisions require bilateral multiple-injection techniques (5,6).
   b) **Contraindications**
      i) Absolute contraindications to TAP block include local infection at the site of planned needle placement.
      ii) Relative contraindications
         (1) Coagulopathy
         (2) Previous abdominal wall surgery may distort anatomy and make TAP block more difficult to perform with and without ultrasound guidance.

TAP blocks only anesthetize somatic nerves; therefore, patients may still experience visceral pain following intra-abdominal or pelvic procedures.

The distribution of a single-injection posterior TAP block is T10-L1 ipsilaterally; extensive midline procedures will likely require multiple bilateral injections.

2) **Risks and complications**
   a) General risks involving peripheral nerve blockade are localized bleeding, intravascular injection with local anesthetic toxicity, and infection at the site of needle puncture.
   b) Site-specific side risks for TAP blocks include (10):
      i) Peritoneal puncture
      ii) Bowel or organ perforation
3) **Equipment**
   a) Common equipment for all peripheral nerve block techniques include sterile skin cleansing solution, sterile gloves, a marking pen, and two 20-mL syringes of local anesthetic solution with extension tubing.
   b) Ultrasound-guided regional anesthesia requires portable ultrasound equipment and a high-frequency linear transducer or a large low-frequency curvilinear transducer (obese patients) for TAP block.
4) **Technique**
   a) **Monitoring**
      i) Peripheral nerve blocks should be placed in a location where the patient's noninvasive BP, SpO_2, and ECG may be monitored.
      ii) Supplemental O_2 should be provided via a face mask or nasal cannulae especially when IV sedation is administered.
   b) **Positioning and preparation**
      i) Position the patient supine or lateral decubitus with affected side up to expand the space between the costal margin and the iliac crest.
         (1) The supine position is preferred when performing bilateral TAP block for postoperative pain.
         (2) The lateral decubitus position is helpful when placing a TAP catheter for unilateral inguinal hernia repair preoperatively (displaces the catheter insertion site further away from the planned sterile surgical field).
      ii) Apply monitors and supplemental O_2.
      iii) IV sedation should be administered, but the patient must be able to follow commands and volunteer sensory information.
   c) **Identification of surface anatomy**
      i) The borders of the Triangle of Petit serve as the major surface anatomic landmarks: the iliac crest inferiorly, the external oblique (EO) muscle anteriorly, and the latissimus dorsi muscle posteriorly (Cognitive Aid: Panel A).
      ii) For the ultrasound-guided technique, a line can be drawn along the costal margin cephalad and the iliac crest caudad on the affected side.
   d) **Landmark-based TAP block**
      i) After identifying the Triangle of Petit, a needle suitable for nerve blockade (e.g., 22-gauge Tuohy-tip needle or other blunt bevel needle) is inserted perpendicular to skin.
      ii) The needle will penetrate two layers of fascia; thus, the practitioner should palpate two distinct "pops" or losses to resistance.
         (1) The first loss of resistance denotes penetration of the EO fascia.
         (2) The second loss of resistance indicates that the needle has penetrated the internal oblique (IO) fascia and suggests that the needle tip should be located properly in the TAP.
   e) **Ultrasound-guided TAP block**
      i) The patient may be positioned supine (bilateral and/or single-injection TAP blocks) or in lateral decubitus (preferred for preoperative TAP catheter placement).
      ii) A high-frequency linear transducer is oriented anterior/posteriorly on the lateral abdominal wall, cephalad to the iliac crest, along the midaxillary line (Cognitive Aid: Panel B).

The final location for local anesthetic for TAP block is the plane between IO and TA muscles.

iii) The EO, IO, and TA muscles should be visualized.

iv) For preoperative TAP catheter insertion, a local anesthetic skin wheal is raised posterior to the edge of the ultrasound transducer after sterile skin preparation.

v) The block needle is inserted through this skin wheal using in-plane guidance in an anterior direction through the EO and IO. A "pop" may be felt and observed under ultrasound.

   (1) For single-injection TAP, the patient may be positioned supine.

   (2) The block needle is inserted anterior to the transducer and directed posteriorly in plane toward the TAP.

vi) Once the needle tip passes through into the plane between the IO and TA, local anesthetic is injected incrementally until visual confirmation of a discrete, elliptical fluid deposit is confirmed (Cognitive Aid: Panel C).

   (1) Intramuscular local anesthetic injection results in a more diffuse pattern with less clearly defined boundaries.

   (2) If intramuscular injectate is detected, advance or withdraw the needle until the tip is positioned within the TAP.

5) **Evaluation of the block**

   a) The quality of nerve blockade must be evaluated prior to surgical incision even if intraoperative general anesthesia is planned.

   b) Sensory testing can be performed by loss of sensation to cold or pinprick in the target dermatomes of the planned surgical procedure.

6) **Postoperative management**

   a) Patients may be discharged as outpatients following TAP block.

   b) Since there is no loss of significant motor function or risk of pulmonary compromise, a patient can be discharged when they meet standard discharge criteria.

References

1. Carney J, McDonnell JG, Ochana A, et al. The transversus abdominis plane block provides effective postoperative analgesia in patients undergoing total abdominal hysterectomy. *Anesth Analg* 2008;107:2056–2060.

2. McDonnell JG, Curley G, Carney J, et al. The analgesic efficacy of transversus abdominis plane block after cesarean delivery: a randomized controlled trial. *Anesth Analg* 2008;106:186–191.

3. McDonnell JG, O'Donnell B, Curley G, et al. The analgesic efficacy of transversus abdominis plane block after abdominal surgery: a prospective randomized controlled trial. *Anesth Analg* 2007;104:193–197.

4. O'Donnell BD, McDonnell JG, McShane AJ. The transversus abdominis plane (TAP) block in open retropubic prostatectomy. *Reg Anesth Pain Med* 2006;31:91.

5. Barrington MJ, Ivanusic JJ, Rozen WM, et al. Spread of injectate after ultrasound-guided subcostal transversus abdominis plane block: a cadaveric study. *Anaesthesia* 2009;64:745–750.

6. Tran TM, Ivanusic JJ, Hebbard P, et al. Determination of spread of injectate after ultrasound-guided transversus abdominis plane block: a cadaveric study. *Br J Anaesth* 2009;102:123–127.

7. Belavy D, Cowlishaw PJ, Howes M, et al. Ultrasound-guided transversus abdominis plane block for analgesia after Caesarean delivery. *Br J Anaesth* 2009.

8. El-Dawlatly AA, Turkistani A, Kettner SC, et al. Ultrasound-guided transversus abdominis plane block: description of a new technique and comparison with conventional systemic analgesia during laparoscopic cholecystectomy. *Br J Anaesth* 2009;102:763–767.

9. Gucev G, Yasui GM, Chang TY, et al. Bilateral ultrasound-guided continuous ilioinguinal-iliohypogastric block for pain relief after cesarean delivery. *Anesth Analg* 2008;106:1220–1222.

10. Jankovic Z, Ahmad N, Ravishankar N, et al. Transversus abdominis plane block: how safe is it? *Anesth Analg* 2008;107:1758–1759.

US-Guided TAP Block

By Justin W. Heil, MD, PhD · Larry F. Chu, MD, MS · Matthew T. Charous, MD ·
Edward R. Mariano, MD, MAS

Patient Position: The patient may be positioned supine (bilateral and/or single-injection transversus abdominis plane [TAP] blocks) or in lateral decubitus (preferred for preoperative TAP catheter placement).

Needle Size: 22–17-gauge Tuohy-tip or B-bevel block needle

Volume: 20 mL local anesthetic per side

Anatomic Landmarks

Ⓐ The borders of the Triangle of Petit serve as the major surface anatomic landmarks: the iliac crest inferiorly, the external oblique (EO) muscle anteriorly, and the latissimus dorsi muscle posteriorly.
A line can be drawn along the costal margin cephalad and the iliac crest caudad on the affected side.

Approach and Technique

Ⓑ A high-frequency linear transducer is oriented anterior/posteriorly on the lateral abdominal wall, cephalad to the iliac crest, along the midaxillary line.
The EO, internal oblique (IO), and transversus abdominis (TA) muscles should be visualized.

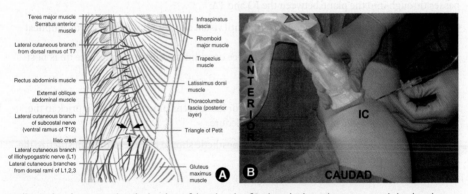

A. Illustration demonstrating the borders of the triangle of Petit and other relevant anatomic landmarks for the TAP block. Figure reproduced from McDonnell JG, et al. RAPM 2007;32:399-404, Fig. 1, pg. 400, with permission. **B.** The ultrasound transducer is positioned cephalad to the iliac crest, oriented anterior-posterior, and slightly anterior to the mid-axillary line to image the abdominal wall layers in short axis. For preoperative ultrasound-guided TAP catheter insertion, the patient is positioned lateral decubitus, and the needle is inserted posterior to the transducer and directed anteriorly toward the target layer.

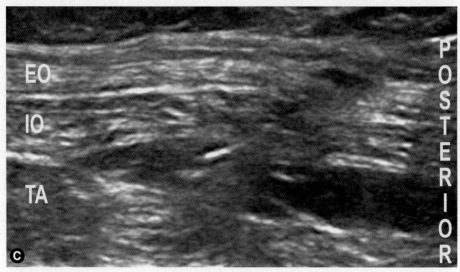

C. Short-axis ultrasound image demonstrating the relevant cross-sectional anatomy for the TAP block. EO, external oblique muscle; IO, internal oblique muscle; TA, transversus abdominis muscle.

A skin wheal with local anesthetic is raised at the site of planned needle insertion.

The block needle is inserted through this skin wheal using in-plane guidance and directed through the EO and IO. A "pop" may be felt and observed under ultrasound as the needle tip passes through into the plane between the IO and TA.

Local anesthetic is injected incrementally until visual confirmation of a discrete, elliptical fluid deposit is confirmed.

If intramuscular injectate is detected, advance or withdraw the needle until the tip is positioned within the TAP.

Evaluation of Block

Sensory testing can be performed by checking for loss of sensation to cold or pinprick in the target dermatomes of the planned surgical procedure.

A single-injection TAP block with 20 mL local anesthetic should be expected to anesthetize the ipsilateral T_{10}-L_1 dermatomes.

184 Paravertebral Blocks

Justin W. Heil, MD, PhD · Edward R. Mariano, MD, MAS

Paravertebral block (PVB) can be performed at the thoracic or lumbar levels to provide anesthesia in specific dermatomal distributions using landmark-based techniques (1–3) or ultrasound guidance (4,5). The wedge-shaped paravertebral space contains spinal and sympathetic nerves as well as segmental vessels. In the thoracic region, it is bounded anteriorly by the parietal pleura, posteriorly by the superior costotransverse ligament, and medially by the posterolateral aspect of the vertebral column (6). In the lumbar region, it is bounded anteriorly by the fascia transversalis over the psoas muscle, posteriorly by the ligaments of the lumbar spine, and medially by the vertebral column (7). Multiple-level injections demonstrate higher efficacy in anesthetizing the desired region over larger volume single injection (3). Paravertebral catheters may be inserted for continuous perineural infusion and can provide prolonged postoperative analgesia.

1) **Indications and contraindications**
   a) **Indications**
      i) Surgical anesthesia or postoperative analgesia for breast surgery, thoracotomy, cholecystectomy, inguinal herniorrhaphy, and other thoracic and abdominal procedures (select levels based on antici-pated dermatomes to be included in the planned surgical site)
      ii) Bilateral PVBs may be performed to provide analgesia for bilateral breast surgery (8) or midline thoracic or abdominal procedures (9).
   b) **Contraindications**
      i) Absolute contraindications to PVBs include local infection at the site of planned needle placement.
      ii) Because of the risk of pneumothorax, care should be taken in selecting patients with emphysema or other significant respiratory compromise.
      iii) Relative contraindications
         (1) Patients receiving anticoagulation therapy
         (2) Preexisting coagulopathy
         (3) Spine deformities that would increase the risk of pleural puncture
         (4) Local tumors
2) **Risks and complications**
   a) General risks involving peripheral nerve blockade are localized bleeding, intravascular injection with local anesthetic toxicity, and infection at the site of needle puncture.
   b) Potential complications specific to PVBs
      i) Pneumothorax
      ii) Hypotension from local anesthetic–induced sympathectomy (may be pronounced for bilateral PVBs)
      iii) Inadvertent intrathecal or epidural injection

3) **Equipment**

    a) Common equipment for all peripheral nerve block techniques include sterile skin cleansing solution, sterile gloves, a marking pen, and two 20-mL syringes of local anesthetic solution with extension tubing.

    b) A nerve stimulator technique requires an electrical nerve stimulator with a compatible insulated needle and a grounding electrode.

    c) Ultrasound-guided regional anesthesia requires portable ultrasound equipment and a low-frequency large curvilinear (preferred) or high-frequency linear transducer for PVB.

4) **Technique**

    a) **Monitoring**

       i) Peripheral nerve blocks should be placed in a location where the patient's noninvasive BP, SpO_2, and ECG may be monitored.

       ii) Supplemental O_2 should be provided via a face mask or nasal cannulae, especially when IV sedation is administered.

    b) **Positioning and preparation**

       i) Position the patient sitting with neck flexed. Placing a bedside table in front of the patient to rest the arms may provide more stability during the procedure.

       ii) The patient may also be placed in the lateral decubitus or prone position if unable to maintain the sitting position. The prone position is preferred during the in-plane ultrasound-guided technique.

       iii) Apply monitors and supplemental O_2.

       iv) IV sedation should be administered, but the patient must be able to follow commands and volunteer sensory information.

Due to the cephalad angulation of the thoracic TPs, the mark 2.5 cm lateral to each SP should overlie the TP of the vertebra one level caudad.

    c) **Identification of surface anatomy**

       i) The spinous processes (SPs) of the vertebrae representing the target dermatomal levels are the most important surface landmarks.

       ii) Start by marking the SP one level above the desired target area and then mark each subsequent SP in the same fashion.

       iii) A point 2.5 cm lateral to each marked SP (toward the affected side) should be marked (Cognitive Aid: Panel A).

         (1) Each of these lateral marks should overlie the transverse process (TP) of the next caudad vertebra in the thoracic region.

         (2) These marks will be the sites for needle insertion when performing landmark-based PVB (Table 184-1).

Despite depth estimates, the exact distance from skin to TP is highly variable. Ultrasound guidance is recommended, if not for real-time needle guidance, then as a "scout" to estimate the distance to the TP prior to employing traditional techniques.

    d) **Landmark-based PVB technique**

       i) Using sterile technique and following injection of a local anesthetic skin wheal at each planned insertion site, a 22-gauge Tuohy-tip needle or a short insulated block needle (nerve stimulation technique) should be inserted perpendicular to the skin at each marked point.

       ii) Advance the needle until it contacts the TP.

         (1) The distance from skin to TP is approximately 2 to 4 cm (thoracic levels) or 4 to 6 cm (lumbar levels).

         (2) This distance is highly variable and is affected by body habitus (12).

         (3) Ultrasound guidance may be very helpful in estimating depth to TP and confirming surface landmarks even if not used for real-time guidance (10,13).

       iii) Withdraw the needle and walk off the cephalad or caudad aspect of the TP (Fig. 184-1).

Table 184-1

Recommended Levels for PVB by Surgical Procedure (7,10,11)

Surgical Procedure	Suggested Levels
Mastectomy with axillary node dissection	T1-6
Breast biopsy or lumpectomy	T2-5 (or planned dermatomes if needle localization performed preoperatively)
Inguinal hernia	T11-L2
Lithotripsy	T8-L1
Thoracotomy or thoracoscopy	Variable depending on involved dermatomes
Cholecystectomy	T8-10

When performing landmark-based PVB, only one of three criteria (loss of resistance, predetermined depth, or evoked motor response) needs to be met before needle advancement is stopped.

Remember that the pleura forms the anterior border of the paravertebral space, so use caution when advancing the needle past the TP to avoid pneumothorax.

    iv) Once the needle clears the TP, advance the needle up to 1 cm (thoracic levels) or 0.5 cm (lumbar levels) maximum (7).

        (1) If a tactile loss of resistance is identified when passing through the superior costotransverse ligament (thoracic levels only), do not advance further.

        (2) If employing a nerve stimulator technique, an intercostal (thoracic levels) or a unilateral abdominal wall (thoracic or lumbar levels) evoked motor response at <0.8 mA serves as the needle endpoint (10).

    v) At each level, inject 4 to 5 mL of local anesthetic solution after negative aspiration for blood.

  e) **Ultrasound-guided PVB technique**

    i) Although varying approaches have been described (4,5), no ultrasound-guided PVB technique is considered standard to date.

    ii) When using a high-frequency linear transducer for out-of-plane needle guidance, position the patient sitting or in lateral decubitus similar to the landmark-based techniques.

        (1) Apply the transducer perpendicular to skin in a parasagittal plane approximately 2 cm lateral to the midline and oriented parallel to the spine.

        (2) Identify the TP of the vertebral bodies cephalad and caudad to the target paravertebral space.

        (3) Visualize the pleura anterior to the paravertebral space and note the depth.

        (4) Insert the block needle perpendicular to skin next to the ultrasound transducer after injecting a local anesthetic skin wheal and advance the needle out-of-plane toward the paravertebral space (Cognitive Aid: Panel B).

          (a) When the desired depth is achieved based on visualization of corresponding tissue movement in the target area or predetermined depth, inject 4 to 5 mL of local anesthetic solution after negative aspiration for blood.

Figure 184-1	Illustrated Sagittal Section Through the Thoracic Paravertebral Region Demonstrating Needle Advancement into the Paravertebral Space and Relevant Anatomy

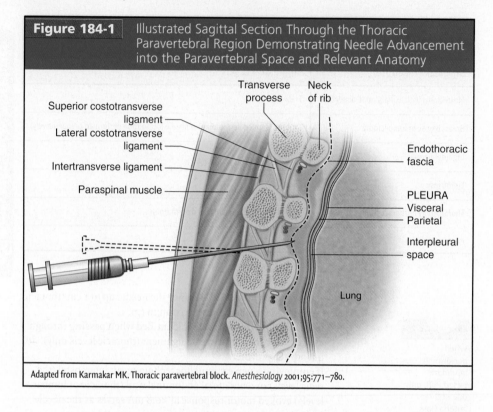

Adapted from Karmakar MK. Thoracic paravertebral block. *Anesthesiology* 2001;95:771–780.

    (b)   Injectate spread should be confirmed within the paravertebral space under ultrasound.

    (c)   Repeat this process for each subsequent level.

  iii) When performing in-plane needle guidance, position the patient prone.

    (1)   The large low-frequency curvilinear transducer is preferred because it enables the practitioner to visualize the needle even at steeper angles.

    (2)   Apply the transducer perpendicular to skin in a parasagittal plane approximately 2 cm lateral to the midline and oriented parallel to the spine (Cognitive Aid: Panel C).

    (3)   Identify the TP of the vertebral bodies cephalad and caudad to the target paravertebral space and the pleura anteriorly (Cognitive Aid: Panel D).

    (4)   With the large curvilinear transducer, often more than one paravertebral space may be visualized. This allows the performance of more than one PVB by simply redirecting the needle cephalad or caudad utilizing one needle insertion.

    (5)   A local anesthetic skin wheal is injected caudad to the ultrasound transducer, and the block needle is inserted through this skin wheal and directed in plane toward the paravertebral space.

        (a)   When the needle tip is visualized within the target paravertebral space, inject 4 to 5 mL of local anesthetic solution after negative aspiration for blood.

        (b)   Injectate spread should be confirmed within the paravertebral space under ultrasound.

        (c)   Repeat this process for each subsequent level; often, more than one PVB may be performed for a single needle insertion.

If a patient presents with shortness of breath after PVB, the diagnosis is pneumothorax until proven otherwise.

5) **Evaluation of the block**
   a) The quality and extent of nerve blockade must be evaluated prior to surgical incision even if intraoperative general anesthesia is planned.
   b) Sensory testing can be performed by loss of sensation to cold or pinprick in the region of the surgical procedure.

6) **Postoperative management**
   a) Patients may be discharged as outpatients following PVB.
   b) Although routine postoperative chest x-ray for pneumothorax is not warranted, the practitioner should have a low index of suspicion should the patient report symptoms of respiratory compromise.

References

1. Eason MJ, Wyatt R. Paravertebral thoracic block-a reappraisal. *Anaesthesia* 1979;34:638–642.
2. Greengrass R, O'Brien F, Lyerly K, et al. Paravertebral block for breast cancer surgery. *Can J Anaesth* 1996;43:858–861.
3. Naja ZM, El-Rajab M, Al-Tannir MA, et al. Thoracic paravertebral block: influence of the number of injections. *Reg Anesth Pain Med* 2006;31:196–201.
4. Ben-Ari A, Moreno M, Chelly JE, et al. Ultrasound-guided paravertebral block using an intercostal approach. *Anesth Analg* 2009;109:1691–1694.
5. Luyet C, Eichenberger U, Greif R, et al. Ultrasound-guided paravertebral puncture and placement of catheters in human cadavers: an imaging study. *Br J Anaesth* 2009;102:534–539.
6. Karmakar MK. Thoracic paravertebral block. *Anesthesiology* 2001;95:771–780.
7. Greengrass R, Buckenmaier CC III. Paravertebral anaesthesia/analgesia for ambulatory surgery. *Best Pract Res Clin Anaesthesiol* 2002;16:271–283.
8. Buckenmaier CC III, Steele SM, Nielsen KC, et al. Bilateral continuous paravertebral catheters for reduction mammoplasty. *Acta Anaesthesiol Scand* 2002;46:1042–1045.
9. Naja Z, Ziade MF, Lonnqvist PA. Bilateral paravertebral somatic nerve block for ventral hernia repair. *Eur J Anaesthesiol* 2002;19:197–202.
10. Jamieson BD, Mariano ER. Thoracic and lumbar paravertebral blocks for outpatient lithotripsy. *J Clin Anesth* 2007;19:149–151.
11. Klein SM, Pietrobon R, Nielsen KC, et al. Paravertebral somatic nerve block compared with peripheral nerve blocks for outpatient inguinal herniorrhaphy. *Reg Anesth Pain Med* 2002;27:476–480.
12. Naja MZ, Gustafsson AC, Ziade MF, et al. Distance between the skin and the thoracic paravertebral space. *Anaesthesia* 2005;60:680–684.
13. Pusch F, Wildling E, Klimscha W, et al. Sonographic measurement of needle insertion depth in paravertebral blocks in women. *Br J Anaesth* 2000;85:841–843.

PERIPHERAL NERVE BLOCK PROCEDURES

US-Guided Paravertebral Block

By Justin W. Heil, MD, PhD · Larry F. Chu, MD, MS · Edward R. Mariano, MD, MAS

Patient Position: Position patient sitting with neck flexed or prone. If unable to place in a sitting position, the prone position is preferred.

Needle Size: 22-gauge, Tuohy-tip block needle

Volume: 5 mL local anesthetic per paravertebral space

Anatomic Landmarks
Ⓐ Mark a 2.5 cm point lateral to each spinous process.

Approach and Technique
Ⓑ Out-of-plane needle guidance: Apply transducer perpendicular to skin in a parasagittal plane 2 cm lateral to the midline and parallel to the spine. Insert the block needle perpendicular to the skin after injecting a local anesthetic skin wheal and advance the needle out-of-plane toward the paravertebral space.

When the needle tip passes the superior costotransverse ligament (thoracic) or the desired depth is achieved (~ 1 cm past the transverse process for thoracic; 0.5 cm past the transverse process for lumbar), inject 5 mL of local anesthetic solution after negative aspiration for blood. Repeat process for each level.

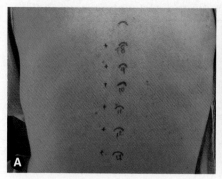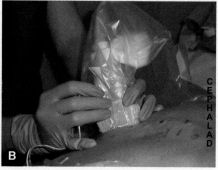

A. When performing out-of-plane thoracic paravertebral block, identify the spinous processes of the vertebrae representing the desired dermatomal levels of anesthesia. Approximate sites for needle insertion are then marked 2.5 cm lateral to each spinous process over the transverse process of the vertebra one level caudad. **B.** Transducer positioning and needle insertion technique during out-of-plane ultrasound-guided paravertebral block.

Ⓒ In-plane needle guidance: Apply the transducer perpendicular to the skin in a parasagittal plane 2 cm lateral to the midline and parallel to the spine.

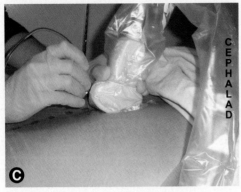

C. Transducer positioning and needle insertion technique during in-plane ultrasound-guided paravertebral block.

D Identify the TP of the vertebral bodies cephalad and caudad to the target paravertebral space and the pleura anteriorly.

Inject a local anesthetic skin wheal caudad to the ultrasound transducer, and insert the block needle through the wheal directed in-plane toward the paravertebral space.

When the needle tip is visualized within the target space, inject 5 mL of local anesthetic solution after negative aspiration for blood. Repeat this process for each level.

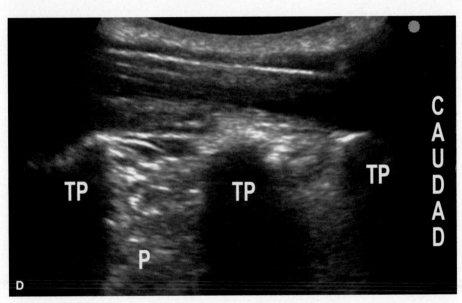

D. Ultrasound image of the paravertebral space. TP, transverse process; P, pleura.

Evaluation of Block

The quality and extent of nerve blockade must be evaluated prior to surgical incision even if intraoperative general anesthesia is planned. Sensory testing can be performed by checking for loss of sensation to cold or pinprick in the distribution of the desired dermatomes.

Anesthesia Phrases in Spanish

By Lynn Ngai • Laura Downey, MD

 Medical translation should always be performed by a professional medical translator. However, there may be instances when a translator is not immediately available in the setting of urgent patient care. The phrases below may be useful in assisting with communication under these circumstances.

 Always document the name and title of the person providing medical translation services in the patient's chart.

Phonetic spellings are provided in italics to assist the anesthesiologist in pronouncing commands necessary for intraoperative care, when a translator or family member may not be present to assist with communication. No phonetic spellings are provided for the remaining phrases; consider showing the patient or family the given translated phrases instead.

Commands	
Open your mouth.	Abra la boca. *(Ah-bra la bow-ka.)*
Take a deep breath in and out.	Respire profundo. Entre y saque el aire. *(Respeer-eh pro-foon-doh. Ahn-tre e sah-ke el ire-eh.)*
Open your eyes.	Abra los ojos. *(Ah-bra los oh-hos.)*
Hold still, please.	Por favor, no se mueva. *(Poor fah-vohr, no say moo-eva.)*
Be calm.	Manténgase tranquilo. *(Man-ten-gas-eh tran-keel-oh.)*
Squeeze your hands.	Apriete las manos. *(Ah-pree-etay las mah-nos.)*
Wiggle your toes.	Mueva los dedos de los pies. *(Moo-eva los day-dose de los pee-ehs.)*
Pre-operative	
Yes/No	Sí/No
Have you had any problems with anesthesia? Surgery?	¿Alguna vez ha tenido problemas con la anestesia o con alguna cirugía?
Has anyone in your family had problems with anesthesia? Surgery?	¿Alguien en su familia ha tenido problemas con la anestesia o con alguna cirugía?
Do you have any allergies to medicines? Tape? Latex?	¿Tiene alergia a alguna medicina, a la cinta adhesiva o al látex?
Do you have any problems with your heart or lungs?	¿Tiene algún problema del corazón o los pulmones?

Can you walk up two flights of stairs?	¿Puede subir dos pisos de escaleras?
Any recent fevers? Colds?	¿Ha tenido fiebre o un resfriado recientemente?
Have you eaten within the last 8 hours? *(Solid, fatty foods are OK if more than 8 hours ago. If the answer is no, see below.)*	¿Ha comido algo en las últimas 8 horas? (no hay problema si comió alimentos sólidos grasosos hace más de 8 horas)
Have you had infant formula, non-human milk, or a light meal in the last 6 hours?	¿Ha tomado fórmula para bebés, leche no materna o alguna comida ligera en las últimas 6 horas?
Have you had breast milk in the past 4 hours?	¿Ha tomado leche materna en las últimas 4 horas?
Have you had clear liquids in the past 2 hours?	¿Ha tomado líquidos claros en las últimas 2 horas?

Anesthesia Consent

I need to start an IV so I can give you medications.	Necesito ponerle un acceso intravenoso para poder darle medicinas.
In the operating room, I will put on monitors and have you breathe oxygen through a mask.	En la sala de operaciones le pondremos monitores y una máscara por la cual va a respirar oxigeno .
When you are asleep, I will put in a breathing tube for surgery.	Cuando esté dormido/a, le colocaremos un tubo para respirar durante la cirugía.
I will take it out before you wake up, but you may have a sore throat for 1-2 days.	Antes de que despierte, sacaremos el tubo, pero es posible que tenga dolor de garganta por 1 o 2 días.
You may have nausea or pain after surgery. I can give you medications for this.	Es posible que tenga náusea o dolor después de la cirugía. Le podemos dar medicina para esto.

Procedures/Explanations

I will give you medicine to help you relax.	Le voy a dar medicina para que se relaje.
I will give you medicine to go to sleep.	Le voy a dar medicina para que se duerma.
This might hurt a little bit.	Esto puede dolerle un poquito.

Epidurals

Have you had an epidural before?	¿Le han puesto una epidural antes?
I will place a catheter in your back so I can give you medicine to control the pain.	Le voy a poner un catéter en la espalda para darle medicina para controlar el dolor
The common risks of an epidural are headaches, backache, bleeding, or infection. I will take precautions to prevent these.	Los riesgos más comunes de una epidural son dolor de cabeza, dolor de espalda, sangrado o infección. Voy a tomar precauciones para prevenir estos riesgos
Please place your chin to your chest, drop your shoulders and push your lower back out.	Ponga su barbilla en el pecho, baje los hombros y mueva la parte baja de la espalda hacia atrás
You might feel a small bee sting and then some pressure.	Es posible que sienta un piquete y luego algo de presión.

Post-operative

Do you have any pain?	¿Tiene dolor?
Where is the pain?	¿Dónde tiene el dolor?
Are you nauseous?	¿Tiene náusea?

Anesthesia Phrases in Russian

By Lynn Ngai • Laura Downey

 Medical translation should always be performed by a professional medical translator. However, there may be instances when a translator is not immediately available in the setting of urgent patient care. The phrases below may be useful in assisting with communication under these circumstances.

Always document the name and title of the person providing medical translation services in the patient's chart.

Phonetic spellings are provided in italics to assist the anesthesiologist in pronouncing commands necessary for intraoperative care, when a translator or family member may not be present to assist with communication. No phonetic spellings are provided for the remaining phrases; consider showing the patient or family the given translated phrases instead.

Commands	
Open your mouth.	Откройте рот. Otkroite rot. *(Aht-CROY-tsay rote.)*
Take a deep breath in and out.	Глубоко вдохните и выдохните. Gluboko vdokhnite I vydokhnite. *(Glue-buck-oh duck-KNEE-tsay ee veeduck-knee-tsay.)*
Open your eyes.	Откройте глаза. Otkroite glaza. *(Aht-CROY-tsay gla-ZA.)*
Hold still, please.	Пожалуйста, не шевелитесь. Pozhaluista, ne shevelites'. *(Pa-SHAWL-sta, nee shey-vel-EE-tays.)*
Be calm.	Успокойтесь. Uspokoites'. *(Ooze-puck-oh-EAT-es.)*
Squeeze your hands.	Сожмите руки в кулаки. Sozhmite pal'tsy v kulaki. *(Suz-MEE-tse RULE-tse cool-la-KEY.)*
Wiggle your toes.	Пошевелите пальцами ног. Poshevelite pal'tsiami nog. *(Push-evel-EE-tse PULL-tsay-mee nohg.)*

Pre-operative	
Yes/No	Да/Нет Da/Net
Have you had any problems with anesthesia? Surgery?	Были ли у Вас проблемы с анестезией? Операцией? Byli li u Vas problemy s anesteziei? Operatsiei?
Has anyone in your family had problems with anesthesia? Surgery?	Были ли проблемы с анестезией у кого-нибудь в Вашей семье? А с операцией? Byli li problemy s anasteziei u kogonibud' v Vashei sem'e? A s operatsiei?
Do you have any allergies to medicines? Tape? Latex?	Есть ли у Вас аллергия к лекарствам? Лейкопластырью? Латексу? Est' li u Vas allergiia k lekarstvam? Leikoplastyriu? Lateksu?
Do you have any problems with your heart or lungs?	Есть ли у Вас проблемы с сердцем или лёгкими? Est' li u Vas problemy s serdtsem ili legkimi?
Can you walk up two flights of stairs?	Можете ли Вы подняться на два лестничных пролёта? Mozhete li Vy podniatsia na dva lestnichnykh proleta?
Any recent fevers? Colds?	Была ли недавно температура? Простуда? Byla li nedavno temperature? Prostuda?
Have you eaten within the last 8 hours? *(Solid, fatty foods are OK if more than 8 hours ago. If the answer is no, see below.)*	Ели ли Вы в течение последних 8 часов? *(твердую, жирную пищу можно было есть, если это было больше 8 часов назад. Если ответ – «Нет», смотрите ниже.)* *Eli li Vy v techenie poslednikh 8 chasov? (tverduiu, zhirnuiu pishchu mozhno bylo est', esli eto bylo bol'she 8 chasov nazad. Esli otvet – "Net", smotrite nizhe.)*
Have you had infant formula, non-human milk, or a light meal in the last 6 hours?	Потребляли ли Вы детскую молочную смесь, молоко (за исключением грудного) или лёгкую закуску в течение последних 6 часов? Potrebliali li Vy detskuiu molochnuiu smes', moloko (za iskliucheniem grudnogo) ili legkuiu zakusku v techenie poslednikh 6 chasov?
Have you had breast milk in the past 4 hours?	Потребляли ли Вы грудное молоко в течение последних 4 часов? Potrebliali li Vy grudnoe moloko v techenie poslednikh 4 chasov?
Have you had clear liquids in the past 2 hours?	Потребляли ли Вы прозрачную жидкость в течение последних 2 часов? Potrebliali li Vy prozrachnuiu zhidkost' v techenie poslednikh 2 chasov?

Anesthesia Consent	
I need to start an IV so I can give you medications.	Я должна поставить капельницу, чтобы вводить Вам лекарства. Ia dolzhna postavit' Vam kapel'nitsu, chtoby vvodit' Vam lekarstva.
In the operating room, I will put on monitors and have you breathe oxygen through a mask.	В операционном зале я подключу Вас к мониторам, и Вы будете дышать кислородом через маску. V operatsionnom zale ia podkliuchu Vas k monitoram, I Vy budete dyshat' kislorodom cherez masku.
When you are asleep, I will put in a breathing tube for surgery.	Когда Вы заснёте, я введу Вам дыхательную трубку на время операции. Kogda Vy zasnete, ia vvedu Vam dykhatel'nuiu trubku na vremia operatsii.
I will take it out before you wake up, but you may have a sore throat for 1-2 days.	Перед тем, как Вы проснётесь, Я выну трубку, но горло ещё может болеть в течение 1 -2х дней. Pered tem, kak Vy prosnetes', ia vynu trubku, no gorlo eshche mozhet bolet' v techenie 1-2kh dnei.
You may have nausea or pain after surgery. I can give you medications for this.	После операции у Вас может быть тошнота или боль. Я дам Вам от этого лекарства. Posle operatsii u Vam mozhet byt' toshnota ili rvota. Ia dam Vam ot etogo lekarstva.
Procedures/Explanations	
I will give you medicine to help you relax.	Я дам Вам лекарство, чтобы помочь. Вам расслабиться. Ia dam Vam lekarstvo, chtoby pomoch Vam rasslabit'sia.
I will give you medicine to go to sleep.	Я дам Вам лекарство, чтобы Вы уснули. Ia dam Vam lekarstvo, chtoby Vy usnuli.
This might hurt a little bit.	Может быть немножко больно. Mozhet byt' nemnozhko bol'no.

Epidurals	
Have you had an epidural before?	Была ли у Вас раньше эпидуральная анестезия? Byla li u Vas ran'she epidural'naia anesteziia?
I will place a catheter in your back so I can give you medicine to control the pain.	Я поставлю Вам катетер в спину, чтобы ввести лекарство от боли. Ia postavliu Vam kateter v spiny, chtoby vvesti lekarstvo ot boli.
The common risks of an epidural are headaches, backache, bleeding, or infection. I will take precautions to prevent these.	Обычные риски эпидуральной анестезии включают в себя головные боли, боли в спине, кровотечение или инфекцию. Я буду принимать все меры, чтобы их предотвратить. Obychnye riski epidural'noi anestezii vkliuchaiut v sebia golovnye boli, boli v spine, krovotechenie ili infektsiiu. Ia budu prinimat' vse mery, chtoby ikh predotvratit'.
Please place your chin to your chest, drop your shoulders and push your lower back out.	Пожалуйста, прижмите подбородок к груди, опустите плечи и выгните назад нижнюю часть спины. Pozhaluista, prizhmite podborodok k grudi, opustite plechi i vygnite nazad nizhniuiu chast' spiny.
You might feel a small bee sting and then some pressure.	Вы почувствуете небольшое жжение, а затем – небольшое давление. Vy pochuvstvuete nebol'shoe zhzhenie, a zatem – nebol'shoe davlenie.
Post-operative	
Do you have any pain?	У Вас что-нибудь болит? U Vas chto-nibud' bolit?
Where is the pain?	Где болит? Gde bolit?
Are you nauseous?	Вас тошнит? Vas toshnit?

Anesthesia Phrases in Traditional Chinese

By Lynn Ngai • Laura Downey

 Medical translation should always be performed by a professional medical translator. However, there may be instances when a translator is not immediately available in the setting of urgent patient care. The phrases below may be useful in assisting with communication under these circumstances.

 Always document the name and title of the person providing medical translation services in the patient's chart.

Phonetic spellings are provided in italics to assist the anesthesiologist in pronouncing commands necessary for intraoperative care, when a translator or family member may not be present to assist with communication. No phonetic spellings are provided for the remaining phrases; consider showing the patient or family the given translated phrases instead.

Commands	
Open your mouth.	張開嘴巴。 Zhāng kāi zuǐba *(Zahng kye zway-ba.)*
Take a deep breath in and out.	深呼吸，吸氣(in)，呼氣(out) Shēnhūxī, xī qì, hu qì. *(Shun who she, she chee, who chee.)*
Open your eyes.	張開眼睛。 Zhāng kāi yǎnjīng *(Zahng kye yen-jing.)*
Hold still, please.	請不要動。 Qǐng bùyào dòng. *(Ching boo-yao dohng.)*
Be calm.	保持冷靜。 Bǎochí lěngjìng. *(Bao-che leng-jeen.)*
Squeeze your hands.	擠壓您的手。 Jǐ yā nín de shǒu. *(Gee yeah neen de show.)*
Wiggle your toes.	擺動您的腳趾。 Bǎidòng nín de jiǎozhǐ. *(Bye-dohng neen de jow-zhe.)*

Pre-operative	
Yes/No	是(有) / 否 (沒有) Shì (yǒu)/fǒu (méiyǒu)
Have you had any problems with anesthesia? Surgery?	您以前在接受麻醉或手術時，有沒有出現任何問題？ Nín yǐqián zài jiēshòu mázuì huò shǒushù shí, yǒu méiyǒu chūxiàn rènhé wèntí?
Has anyone in your family had problems with anesthesia? Surgery?	您的家人以前在接受麻醉或手術時，有沒有出現任何問題？ Nín de jiārén yǐqián zài jiēshòu mázuì huò shǒushù shí, yǒu méiyǒu chūxiàn rènhé wèntí?
Do you have any allergies to medicines? Tape? Latex?	您是否對藥物，膠布，乳膠過敏？ Nín shìfǒu duì yàowù, jiāobù, rǔjiāo guòmǐn?
Do you have any problems with your heart or lungs?	您的心臟或肺部是否有問題？ Nín de xīnzàng huò fèi bù shìfǒu yǒu wèntí?
Can you walk up two flights of stairs?	您能否步行上兩層樓梯嗎？ Nín néng fǒu bùxíng shàng liǎng céng lóutī ma?
Any recent fevers? Colds?	最近有沒有發燒？感冒？ Zuìjìn yǒu méiyǒu fāshāo? Gǎnmào?
Have you eaten within the last 8 hours? *(Solid, fatty foods are OK if more than 8 hours ago. If the answer is no, see below.)*	您在過去的八個小時內有沒有吃東西？(如果您在超過八小時以前曾吃過固體或油膩的食物是可以的。如果您的答案是沒有，請參閱以下問題。) Nín zài guòqù de bā gè xiǎoshí nèi yǒu méiyǒu chī dōngxi? (Rúguǒ nín zài chāoguò bā xiǎoshí yǐqián céng chī guò gùtǐ huò yóunì de shíwù shì kěyǐ de. Rúguǒ nín de dáàn shì méiyǒu, qǐng cānyuè yǐxià wèntí.)
Have you had infant formula, non-human milk, or a light meal in the last 6 hours?	您在過去的六個小時以內有沒有喝嬰兒奶粉，非母乳奶製品，或吃過便餐？ Nín zài guòqù de liù gè xiǎoshí yǐnèi yǒu méiyǒu hē yīngér nǎifěn, fēi mǔrǔ nǎi zhìpǐn, huò chī guò biàncān?
Have you had breast milk in the past 4 hours?	您在過去的四個小時以內有沒有喝母乳？ Nín zài guòqù de sì gè xiǎoshí yǐnèi yǒu méiyǒu hē mǔrǔ?
Have you had clear liquids in the past 2 hours?	您在過去的兩個小時以內有沒有喝清透的流液？ Nín zài guòqù de liǎng gè xiǎoshí yǐnèi yǒu méiyǒu hē qīng tòu de liú yè?

Anesthesia Consent	
I need to start an IV so I can give you medications.	我必須開始進行靜脈注射以便給您輸入藥物。 Wǒ bìxū kāishǐ jìnxíng jìngmài zhùshè yǐbiàn gěi nín shūrù yàowù.
In the operating room, I will put on monitors and have you breathe oxygen through a mask.	在手術室裡，我會使用監察器，和為您戴上呼吸氧氣的面罩。 Zài shǒushù shì lǐ, wǒ huì shǐyòng jiānchá qì, hé wèi nín dài shàng hūxī yǎngqì de miànzhào.
When you are asleep, I will put in a breathing tube for surgery.	您入睡的時候，我會置入手術所需的呼吸插管。 Nín rùshuì de shíhou, wǒ huì zhì rù shǒushù suǒ xū de hūxī chā guǎn.
I will take it out before you wake up, but you may have a sore throat for 1-2 days.	我會在您醒來之前把管子取出，但是您可能在一至兩天內有喉痛的感覺。 Wǒ huì zài nín xǐng lái zhīqián bǎ guǎnzi qǔchū, dànshì nín kěnéng zài yīzhì liǎng tiānnèi yǒu hóu tòng de gǎnjué
You may have nausea or pain after surgery. I can give you medications for this.	手術後您可能會覺得噁心或疼痛。我可以給您藥物來控制這些症狀。 Shǒushù hòu nín kěnéng huì juéde ěxīn huò téngtòng. Wǒ kěyǐ gěi nín yàowù lái kòngzhì zhèxiē zhèngzhuàng.
Procedures/Explanations	
I will give you medicine to help you relax.	我會給您藥物幫助您放鬆。 Wǒ huì gěi nín yàowù bāngzhù nín fàngsōng.
I will give you medicine to go to sleep.	我會給您藥物讓您入睡。 Wǒ huì gěi nín yàowù ràng nín rùshuì.
This might hurt a little bit.	這樣可能會有點痛。 Zhèyàng kěnéng huì yǒudiǎn tòng.
Epidurals	
Have you had an epidural before?	您以前有沒有接受過脊椎硬膜外麻醉？ Nín yǐqián yǒu méiyǒu jiēshòu guò jǐzhuī yìng mó wài mázuì?
I will place a catheter in your back so I can give you medicine to control the pain.	我會在您的背部放置一條導管以便我為您輸入藥物以控制疼痛。 Wǒ huì zài nín de bèibù fàngzhì yītiáo dǎoguǎn yǐbiàn wǒ wèi nín shūrù yàowù yǐ kòngzhì téngtòng.

The common risks of an epidural are headaches, backache, bleeding, or infection. I will take precautions to prevent these.	脊椎硬膜外麻醉的常見風險包括頭痛，背痛，流血或感染。我會採取預防措施以防止這些情況。 Jǐzhuī yìng mó wài mázuì de chángjiàn fēngxiǎn bāokuò tóutòng, bèi tòng, liúxuè huò gǎnrǎn. Wǒ huì cǎiqǔ yùfáng cuòshī yǐ fángzhǐ zhèxiē qíngkuàng.
Please place your chin to your chest, drop your shoulders and push your lower back out.	請把您的下巴貼在胸部，放鬆肩膀，並且把您的腰部往外挪。 Qǐng bǎ nín de xiàba tiē zài xiōngbù, fàngsōng jiānbǎng, bìngqiě bǎ nín de yāobù wǎngwài nuó.
You might feel a small bee sting and then some pressure.	您可能感覺到如被蜜蜂輕微的針刺，然後有一些壓力感。 Nín kěnéng huì yǒurú bèi mìfēng qīngwéi zhēn cì de gǎnjué, ránhòu yǒu yīxiē yālì gǎn.
Post-operative	
Do you have any pain?	您覺得疼痛嗎？ Nín juéde téngtòng ma?
Where is the pain?	那裡痛？ Nàlǐ tòng?
Are you nauseous?	您覺得噁心嗎？ Nín juéde ěxīn ma?

Anesthesia Phrases in Vietnamese

By Lynn Ngai • Laura Downey

Medical translation should always be performed by a professional medical translator. However, there may be instances when a translator is not immediately available in the setting of urgent patient care. The phrases below may be useful in assisting with communication under these circumstances.

Always document the name and title of the person providing medical translation services in the patient's chart.

Phonetic spellings are provided in italics to assist the anesthesiologist in pronouncing commands necessary for intraoperative care, when a translator or family member may not be present to assist with communication. No phonetic spellings are provided for the remaining phrases; consider showing the patient or family the given translated phrases instead.

Commands	
Open your mouth.	Há miệng ra. *(Ha ming ra.)*
Take a deep breath in and out.	Hít vào sâu rồi thở ra dài. *(Hit vow sow, roy tuh ra yai.)*
Open your eyes.	Mở mắt ra. *(Muh maht ra.)*
Hold still, please.	Xin giữ yên đừng động đậy. *(Sin yuh yin dung dom dai.)*
Be calm.	Cứ bình tĩnh. *(Guh ben den.)*
Squeeze your hands.	Nắm tay lại. *(Num tie lie.)*
Wiggle your toes.	Nhúc nhích những ngón chân. *(Nyuck nick nyung nong gin.)*
Pre-operative	
Yes/No	Có/Không
Have you had any problems with anesthesia? Surgery?	Trước đây quý vị đã có vấn đề gì khi được gây mê hay không? Có vấn đề gì khi giải phẫu hay không?
Has anyone in your family had problems with anesthesia? Surgery?	Có ai trong gia đình quý vị đã có vấn đề khi gây mê? Khi giải phẫu?
Do you have any allergies to medicines? Tape? Latex?	Quý vị có bị dị ứng với dược phẩm nào không? Với băng keo dán? Với cao su làm bao tay?

Do you have any problems with your heart or lungs?	Quý vị có vấn đề gì về tim hay phổi không?
Can you walk up two flights of stairs?	Quý vị có thể leo hai tầng cầu thang được không?
Any recent fevers? Colds?	Quý vị mới đây có nóng sốt không? Có cảm cúm không?
Have you eaten within the last 8 hours? *(Solid, fatty foods are OK if more than 8 hours ago. If the answer is no, see below.)*	Quý vị có ăn gì trong tám tiếng đồng hồ vừa qua không? *(Đồ ăn đặc, có mỡ nếu dùng trước 8 tiếng đồng hồ thì được. Nếu trả lời không, xin xem phía dưới.)*
Have you had infant formula, non-human milk, or a light meal in the last 6 hours?	Quý vị có uống sữa theo công thức cho trẻ nhỏ, sữa động vật, hay ăn nhẹ trong 6 tiếng đồng hồ trở lại đây không?
Have you had breast milk in the past 4 hours?	Quý vị có uống sữa từ vú người trong vòng 4 tiếng đồng hồ vừa qua không?
Have you had clear liquids in the past 2 hours?	Quý vị có uống chất lỏng màu trong nội trong 2 tiếng đồng hồ vừa qua không?

Anesthesia Consent	
I need to start an IV so I can give you medications.	Tôi cần đưa ống chích vào tĩnh mạch quý vị để có thể tiêm thuốc cho quý vị.
In the operating room, I will put on monitors and have you breathe oxygen through a mask.	Trong phòng mổ, tôi sẽ đặt các máy kiểm tra và cho quý vị thở dưỡng khí qua mặt nạ.
When you are asleep, I will put in a breathing tube for surgery.	Khi quý vị đã ngủ, tôi sẽ đặt một ống thở cho quý vị để thực hiện cuộc giải phẫu.
I will take it out before you wake up, but you may have a sore throat for 1-2 days.	Tôi sẽ lấy nó ra trước khi quý vị tỉnh dậy, nhưng quý vị có thể thấy đau cổ trong 1 đến 2 ngày sau đó.
You may have nausea or pain after surgery. I can give you medications for this.	Quý vị có thể buồn nôn buồn ói hay đau sau khi giải phẫu.Tôi có thể cho quý vị thuốc để giúp cho việc này.

Procedures/Explanations	
I will give you medicine to help you relax.	Tôi sẽ cho quý vị thuốc để giúp cho thoải mái.
I will give you medicine to go to sleep.	Tôi sẽ cho quý vị thuốc để ngủ.
This might hurt a little bit.	Có thể thấy đau một chút đấy.

Epidurals	
Have you had an epidural before?	Quý vị đã từng được gây mê dây cột sống bao giờ chưa?
I will place a catheter in your back so I can give you medicine to control the pain.	Tôi sẽ đặt một ống thông vào lưng quý vị để có thể cho thuốc làm giảm đau.
The common risks of an epidural are headaches, backache, bleeding, or infection. I will take precautions to prevent these.	Những rủi ro thông thường của thủ thuật gây mê dây cột sống là nhức đầu, đau lưng, chảy máu hay nhiễm trùng. Tôi sẽ thực hiện mọi biện pháp phòng ngừa để ngăn chặn những chuyện này.

Please place your chin to your chest, drop your shoulders and push your lower back out.	Xin ép cằm xuống ngực, xuôi vai và đẩy phía dưới của lưng ra.
You might feel a small bee sting and then some pressure.	Quý vị có thể cảm thấy như ong đốt và sau đó là một chút lực ép.
Post-operative	
Do you have any pain?	Quý vị có đau chỗ nào không?
Where is the pain?	Chỗ đau ở đâu?
Are you nauseous?	Quý vị có buồn nôn buồn ói không?

Anesthesia Phrases in French

By Lynn Ngai • Laura Downey

 Medical translation should always be performed by a professional medical translator. However, there may be instances when a translator is not immediately available in the setting of urgent patient care. The phrases below may be useful in assisting with communication under these circumstances.

 Always document the name and title of the person providing medical translation services in the patient's chart.

Phonetic spellings are provided in italics to assist the anesthesiologist in pronouncing commands necessary for intraoperative care, when a translator or family member may not be present to assist with communication. No phonetic spellings are provided for the remaining phrases; consider showing the patient or family the given translated phrases instead.

Commands	
Open your mouth.	Ouvrez la bouche. *(Oh-fray la boosh.)*
Take a deep breath in and out.	Inspirez et soufflez profondément. *(In-spee-ray eh soo-flay pro-fon-day-mon.)*
Open your eyes.	Ouvrez les yeux. *(Oh-fray leis you.)*
Hold still, please.	Ne bougez pas, s'il vous plaît. *(No boo-shay pa, see voo play.)*
Be calm.	Restez calme. *(Rest-ay calm.)*
Squeeze your hands.	Serrez les mains. *(Ser-ray lei men.)*
Wiggle your toes.	Bougez les orteils. *(Boo-shay leis or-tay.)*
Pre-operative	
Yes/No	Oui/Non
Have you had any problems with anesthesia? Surgery?	Avez-vous déjà eu des problèmes d'anesthésie ? de chirurgie ?
Has anyone in your family had problems with anesthesia? Surgery?	Quelqu'un dans votre famille, a-t-il déjà eu des problèmes d'anesthésie ? de chirurgie ?
Do you have any allergies to medicines? Tape? Latex?	Avez-vous des allergies médicamenteuses ? au ruban adhésif ? au latex ?
Do you have any problems with your heart or lungs?	Avez-vous des problèmes de coeur ou de poumons ?

Can you walk up two flights of stairs?	Pouvez-vous monter deux étages à pieds ?
Any recent fevers? Colds?	Avez-vous eu de la fièvre récemment ? des refroidissements ?
Have you eaten within the last 8 hours? (Solid, fatty foods are OK if more than 8 hours ago. If the answer is no, see below.)	Avez-vous mangé au cours des 8 dernières heures ? *(Des aliments solides, gras, sont autorisés s'ils ont été ingérés il y a plus de 8 heures. En cas de réponse négative, voir cidessous.)*
Have you had infant formula, non-human milk, or a light meal in the last 6 hours?	Avez-vous eu du lait maternisé, non humain, ou un repas léger au cours des 6 dernières heures ?
Have you had breast milk in the past 4 hours?	Avez-vous eu du lait maternel au cours des 4 dernières heures ?
Have you had clear liquids in the past 2 hours?	Avez-vous ingurgité des liquides transparents au cours des 2 dernières heures ?

Anesthesia Consent

I need to start an IV so I can give you medications.	Je dois démarrer une perfusion intraveineuse, afin de vous donner des médicaments.
In the operating room, I will put on monitors and have you breathe oxygen through a mask.	Dans la salle d'opération, je vais allumer des moniteurs et vous ferez respirer de l'oxygène à travers un masque.
When you are asleep, I will put in a breathing tube for surgery.	Une fois que vous serez endormi, j'introduirai un tube de respiration pour l'intervention.
I will take it out before you wake up, but you may have a sore throat for 1-2 days.	Je le retirerai avant votre réveil, mais il se peut que vous ayez des maux de gorge pendant 1 à 2 jours.
You may have nausea or pain after surgery. I can give you medications for this.	Après l'opération, il se peut que vous ayez des nausées ou des douleurs. Je peux vous donner des médicaments pour cela.

Procedures/Explanations

I will give you medicine to help you relax.	Je vais vous donner des médicaments pour vous aider à vous relaxer.
I will give you medicine to go to sleep.	Je vais vous donner des médicaments pour vous endormir.
This might hurt a little bit.	Cela peut faire un peu mal.

Epidurals

Have you had an epidural before?	Avez-vous déjà eu une épidurale auparavant ?

APPENDIX A

I will place a catheter in your back so I can give you medicine to control the pain.	Je vais placer un cathéter dans votre dos, afin de pouvoir vous donner des médicaments pour contrôler la douleur.
The common risks of an epidural are headaches, backache, bleeding, or infection. I will take precautions to prevent these.	Les risques courants d'une épidurale sont des maux de tête, un mal de dos, des saignements ou une infection. Je prendrai toutes les précautions nécessaires pour éviter cela.
Please place your chin to your chest, drop your shoulders and push your lower back out.	Veuillez placer le menton sur votre poitrine, baisser les épaules et faire ressortir le bas du dos.
You might feel a small bee sting and then some pressure.	Il se peut que vous ressentiez une petite piqûre d'abeille, puis une certaine pression.
Post-operative	
Do you have any pain?	Avez-vous des douleurs ?
Where is the pain?	À quel endroit ?
Are you nauseous?	Avez-vous des nausées ?

Note: Phonetic spellings are provided in italics to assist the anesthesiologist in pronouncing commands necessary for intraoperative care where a translator/family member is normally not available.

For the remaining phrases, consider showing the patient or family the given translated phrases to assist with communication. No phonetic spellings are provided.

Local Anesthetics

Jonathan T. Bradley, MD • Tony Cun, BS
Consultant Pharmacist: Anita Y. Chu, BPharm, RPh, PharmD

	Toxic/ Max Adult Dosing WITHOUT Epi	Toxic/ Max Adult Dosing WITH Epi	pK	Onset	Duration After Infiltration	Miscellaneous Facts
ESTERS—Metabolized by Pseudocholinesterase						
Chloro-procaine (Nesacaine)	7 mg/kg	11 mg/kg	9.1	Infiltration/ epidural: 6–12 min	Infiltration/epidural: 30–60 min (prolonged with epinephrine)	Administer over 30 min. Observe for symptoms of toxicity, for example, hypotension, slurred speech, drowsiness, and adjust rate accordingly.
Procaine (Novocain)	10 mg/kg	15 mg/kg	8.9	Infiltration/ spinal: 2–5 min Epidural: 5–25 min	Infiltration: 0.25–0.5 h (w/epi 0.5–1.5 h) Epidural/spinal: 0.5–1.5 h/ prolonged with epi	Metabolized to PABA. Caution if sunblock allergy
Tetracaine (Ponto-caine)	3 mg/kg	3 mg/kg	8.5	Infiltration: 15 min Spinal: <10 min	Infiltration: 2–3 h Spinal: 1.25–3 h	Prolongs the effect of succinylcholine; metabolite (PABA) inhibits the action of sulfonamides and aminosalicylic acid.
AMIDES—Metabolized through Hepatic Metabolism						
Bupi-vacaine (Marcaine)	2.5 mg/kg	2.5–3 mg/kg	8.1	Infiltration: 2–10 min Epidural: 4–17 min Spinal: <1 min	Infiltration/ epidural/spinal: 200–400 min	Most cardiac toxic, levobupivicaine (L-isomer) less cardiotoxic.
Lidocaine (Xylocaine)	4–5 mg/kg	7 mg/kg	7.9	IV: (antiarrhythmic effects) 45–90 s Intratracheal: 1–2 min Infiltration: 0.5–1.0 min Epidural: 5–15 min	IV(antiarrhythmic effects): 10–20 min Intratracheal: 30–50 min Infiltration: 0.5–1.0 h (w/epi 2–6 h) Epidural: 1–3 h	Intrathecal associated with Transient Neurologic Symptoms (TNS) and Cauda Equina Syndrome.

(continued)

	Toxic/ Max Adult Dosing WITHOUT Epi	Toxic/ Max Adult Dosing WITH Epi	pK	Onset	Duration After Infiltration	Miscellaneous Facts
Mepiva-caine (Carbo-caine, Polocaine)	4 mg/kg	7 mg/kg	7.6	**Infiltration:** 3–5 min **Epidural:** 5–15 min	**Infiltration:** 0.75–1.5 h (w/epi 2–6 h) **Epidural:** 3–5 h/ prolonged with epinephrine	
Prilocaine (Citanest)	8 mg/kg	8 mg/kg	7.9	**Infiltration:** 1–2 min **Epidural:** 5–15 min **Peak Effect:** Infiltration/ epidural <30 min IV 15–20 min	**Infiltration:** 0.5–1.5 h (w/epi 2–6 h) **Epidural:** 1–3 h	Can cause methemoglobinemia at high doses (greater than 600 mg (including EMLA-benzocaine/prilocaine). No more than 600 mg prilocaine should be administered within a 2-h period in healthy adults.
Ropi-vacaine (Naropin)	2.5 mg/kg (max 300 mg)	2.5 mg/kg	8.1	**Infiltration:** 1–15 min **Epidural:** 10–20 min **Spinal:** <2 min	**Infiltration/epi-dural:** 20–45 min **Spinal:** 10–13 min	Possibly preferentially blocks sensory fibers over motor fibers. Not to exceed 200 mg for minor nerve block.

Shortcut for deciding if it is an amide or ester: If it has an "i" in the letters before the "–caine" it is an amide. If not it is an ester.

Treatment of Toxicity–LA-induced seizures can be managed by protecting the airway and providing oxygen. Seizures may be terminated with IV thiopental, midazolam, or propofol. If LA intoxication produces cardiac arrest, the ACLS guidelines should be followed, but intralipid should be given and no lidocaine as an antiarrhythmic.

⌐ READ
  MORE

Local anesthetic toxicity, Chapter 218, page 1340

References

Morgan GE, Mikhail MS, Murray MJ. *Clinical Anesthesiology.* New York, NY: McGraw-Hill Medical Publishing Division; 2005.
Omoigui S. *Sota Omoigui's Anesthesia Drugs Handbook.* Hawthorne, CA: State-of-the-Art Technologies, Inc.; 1999.
Stoelting RK, Hillier SC. *Handbook of Pharmacology and Physiology in Anesthetic Practice.* Philadelphia, PA: Lippincott Williams & Wilkins; 2005.

Neuromuscular Blocking Agents

Vikas Shah, MD, PhD • Lynn Ngai, BS
Consultant Pharmacist: Anita Y. Chu, B.Pharm, R.Ph, Pharm.D

	Adult Dosing	Onset	Duration	Elimination Half-life (Normal/ ESRD/ESLD)	Primary Elimination
Atracurium[a,b] (nondepolarizing)	*Intubating*: **IV**: 0.3–0.5 mg/kg *Maintenance*: **IV**: 0.1–0.2 mg/kg *Infusion*: 2–15 μg/ kg/min	<3 min	20–35 min	Normal: 21 min ESRD: 18–25 min ESLD: 20–25 min	90% nonenzymatic degradation in plasma via Hoffman elimination and hydrolysis 10% renal
Cisatracurium[a,b] (nondepolarizing)	*Intubating*: **IV**: 0.15–0.2 mg/kg *Maintenance*: **IV**: 0.02–0.1 mg/kg *Infusion*: 1–2 μg/kg/min	1.5–2 min	20–35 min	Normal: 22–30 min ESRD: 25–34 min ESLD: 21 min	100% nonenzymatic degradation in plasma via Hoffman elimination and hydrolysis
Mivacurium[a,b] (nondepolarizing)	*Intubating*: **IV**: 0.15–0.2 mg/ kg over 15–30 s *Maintenance*: **IV**: 0.01–0.1 mg/kg *Infusion*: 1–15 μg/kg/min	<2 min	6–16 min	Normal: 1–3 min	100% hydrolysis via plasma cholinesterase
Pancuronium[*,a,b] (nondepolarizing) [*]atropine-like drug; may see tachycardia	*Intubating*: **IV**: 0.04–0.1 mg/kg *Maintenance*: **IV**: 0.01–0.05 mg/kg *Infusion*: 1–15 μg/kg/min	1–3 min	40–65 min	Normal: 1.5–2 h ESRD: 4–18 h ESLD: 3–4 h	80% renal 10% hepatic 10% biliary
Rocuronium[a,b] (nondepolarizing)	*Intubating*: **IV**: 0.6–1.2 mg/ kg (higher dose for RSI) *Maintenance*: **IV**: 0.06–0.6 mg/kg *Infusion*: 5–15 μg/kg/min *Rapid sequence*: **IV**: 0.6–1.2 mg/kg	45–90 s	15–150 min	Normal: 90 min ESRD: 1.5–3.5 h ESLD: 2–6 h	10%–25% renal 10%–20% hepatic 50%–70% biliary

(continued)

	Adult Dosing	Onset	Duration	Elimination Half-life (Normal/ ESRD/ESLD)	Primary Elimination
Succinycholine[c] (depolarizing)	*For skeletal muscle relaxation:* **IV:** 0.7–1 mg/kg **Deep IM:** 2.5–4 mg/kg, maximum 150 mg **Infusion:** 10–200 µg/kg/min *To relieve laryngospasms:* **IV:** 0.1–0.5 mg/kg, start at the low end e.g. 10–20 mg for 70 kg adult *Maximum total (to avoid prolonged phase II block):* <5 mg/kg	**IV:** 30–60 s **IM:** 2–3 min	**IV:** 4–6 min **IM:** 10–30 min	N/A	Plasma pseudocholinesterase
Vecuronium[a,b] (nondepolarizing)	*Intubating:* **IV:** 0.08–0.1 mg/kg *Maintenance:* **IV:** 0.01–0.015 mg/kg *Infusion:* 1–2 µg/kg/min	<3 min	25–30 min	Normal: 1–2 h ESRD: 1.5–3 h ESLD: 1–3 h	15%–25% renal 20%–30% hepatic 40%–75% biliary

Adverse effects:

[a]Nondepolarizing agents: Because they have a steroid-like structure, they have been implicated in causing critical illness myopathy. In addition, nondepolarizing drugs may be an underappreciated source of allergic reactions during anesthesia.

[b]Interactions of nondepolarizing agents: A large number of drugs interact with the nondepolarizers, specifically causing prolonged effect. Volatile inhalational anesthetics, aminoglycoside antibiotics, local anesthetics, antiarrhythmics, diuretics, magnesium, lithium, and cyclosporine may all prolong NMB. In addition, myasthenia gravis, hypothermia, female gender and hyperkalemia can potentiate the effects of these drugs. Hypokalemia, burns, and spinal cord injuries can all cause resistance to these agents.

[c]Succinylcholine: Administration of succinylcholine will lead to a 0.5–1 mEq/dL rise in serum potassium concentrations and should not be used in patients who have preexisting elevated serum potassium. This rise can be exaggerated in patients who have altered numbers of ACh receptors at the motor endplate. Though not an exhaustive list, this includes patients with spinal cord injury, burns, and genetic myopathies. It is also a trigger for malignant hyperthermia. Activation of muscarinic ACh receptors may cause bradycardia, an important consideration in the pediatric population that has rate-dependent cardiac output.

IV, intravenous; IM, intramuscular; ESRD, end-stage renal disease; ESLD, end-stage liver disease.

References

Jaffe RA, Samuels SI. *Anesthesiologist's Manual of Surgical Procedures*. 3rd ed. Philadelphia, PA: Lippincott Williams & Wilkins; 2004. Print.

Omoigui S. *Sota Omoigui's Anesthesia Drugs Handbook*. Hawthorne, CA: State-of-the-Art Technologies, Incorporated; 1999.

Stoelting RK, Hillier SC. *Handbook of Pharmacology and Physiology in Anesthetic Practice*. Philadelphia, PA: Lippincott Williams & Wilkins; 2005.

Beers MH, Berkow R. *The Merck Manual of Diagnosis and Therapy*. 17th ed. Philadelphia, PA: John Wiley & Sons; 1999.

Anticholinesterases

Eric Gross, MD, PhD • Tony Cun, BS
Consultant Pharmacist: Anita Y. Chu, BPharm, RPh, PharmD

	Adult Dosing	Duration	Chemical Structure	Site of Action[a]
Edrophonium	*Reverse Neuromuscular blockade or Diagnosis of Myasthenia Gravis:* **IV:** 0.5–1.0 mg/kg. Max dose 40 mg w/atropine 0.015 mg/kg, or glycopyrrolate 0.01 mg/kg	**IV:** 5–20 min **IM:** 10–40 min	Quaternary amine	Neuromuscular junction
Neostigmine	*Reverse Neuromuscular blockade:* **IV:** 0.05 mg/kg, max dose 5 mg, with atropine (**IV** 0.015 mg/kg) or glycopyrrolate (**IV** 0.01 mg/kg)	**IV:** 40–60 min **IM/PO:** 2–4 h	Quaternary amine	
Physostigmine	*Anticholinergic Reversal:* **IV/IM:** 0.5–2.0 mg (10–30 μg/kg) at a rate of ≤1 mg/min	**IV/IM:** 30 min to 5 h	Tertiary amine[b]	
Pyridostigmine	*Reversal of Neuromuscular blockade or Myasthenia Gravis Treatment:* **IV:** 0.25 mg/kg (max dose 30 mg) w/atropine 0.015 mg/kg, or glycopyrrolate 0.01 mg/kg	**IV:** 90 min **PO:** 3–6 h **IM:** 2–4 h	Quaternary amine	

Use: Neuromuscular blockade reversal, myasthenia gravis.
[a]All agents act as competitive inhibitors of acetylcholinesterase.
[b]Tertiary amines penetrate the blood brain barrier.

References

Omoigui S. *Sota Omoigui's Anesthesia Drugs Handbook*. Hawthorne, CA: State-of-the-Art Technologies, Incorporated; 1999:133–136, 316–319, 353–355, 397–400.

Stoelting RK, Hillier SC. *Handbook of Pharmacology and Physiology in Anesthetic Practice*. Philadelphia, PA: Lippincott Williams & Wilkins; 2005:251–265.

Benzodiazepines

Andrew Wall, MD • Tony Cun, BS
Consultant Pharmacist: Anita Y. Chu, BPharm, RPh, PharmD

	Adult Dosing	Peak Effect	Duration	Elimination Half-life*	Pain on Injection	Clinically Active Metabolites
Diazepam	**IV** (sedation/ premedication): 0.05–0.2 mg/kg **IV:** (induction): 0.3–0.5 mg/kg **PO:** (sedation/ premedication): 0.05–0.2 mg/kg	**IV:** 3–4 min **PO:** 60 min	**IV:** 15 min to 1 h **PO:** 2–6 h	30 h	++	Many
Lorazepam	**IV** (sedation/pre-medication): 1–4 mg (0.02–0.08 mg/kg) **PO:** (sedation): 2–3 mg, for elderly 1–2 mg **IM:** 1–4 mg (0.02–0.08 mg/kg) use undiluted injectate solution (max 4 mg)	**IV:** 15–20 min **PO:** 120 min	**IV/IM/PO:** 6–10 h	15 h	++	None
Midazolam	**IV:** (sedation/pre-medication): 0.5–5.0 mg (0.025–0.1 mg/ kg). Typical premedi-cation for surgery dose of 2.0 mg IV for normal healthy adult. **IV:** (induction): 50–350 µg/kg **PO:** (premedication): 20–40 mg **IM:** (premedica-tion): 2.5–10.0 mg (0.05–0.2 mg/kg)	**IV:** 3–5 min **IM:** 15–30 min **PO:** 30 min **Intrana-sal:** 10 min **PR:** 20–30 min	**IV/IM:** 15–80 min **PO/PR:** 2–6 h	2 h	0	Few

(continued)

	Adult Dosing	Peak Effect	Duration	Elimination Half-life[a]	Pain on Injection	Clinically Active Metabolites
Flumazenil (antagonist)	**IV:** for adults 4–20 μg/kg For reversal of sedation and benzodiazepines used during general anesthesia: 0.2 mg IV over 15 s, may be repeated at 1-min intervals (max total dose: 1 mg)	5–10 min	45–90 min	1 h	+	None

[a]Elimination: All the above benzodiazepines are highly protein bound, rely on the liver for initial biotransformation, and are renally cleared. Peak effect, duration, and half-life can vary based on patient characteristics. Consider decreasing dose/frequency in liver or kidney disease. Lorazepam may be preferable for use in renal failure because of inactive metabolites. Synergistic respiratory depression occurs with concomitant narcotic usage, consider decreasing dose in this situation.

0, none.

+, moderate.

++, severe.

References

Omoigui S. *Sota Omoigui's Anesthesia Drugs Handbook*. 3rd ed. Hawthorne, CA: State-of-the-Art Technologies, Incorporated; 1999: 102–105, 183–187, 245–248, 293–299.

Stoelting RK, Hillier SC. *Handbook of Pharmacology and Physiology in Anesthetic Practice*. Philadelphia, PA: Lippincott Williams & Wilkins; 2005: 133–149.

Opioids

Jack Kan, MD • Lynn Ngai, BS
Consultant Pharmacist: Anita Y. Chu, B.Pharm, R.Ph, Pharm.D

	Potency (Relative to Morphine IV)	Adult Dosing	Peak Effect	Duration	Elimination Half-life	Primary Elimination	Interactions/Toxicities
Alfentanil (IV)	15–30	*Analgesia:* IV/IM: 250–500 µg *Induction:* IV bolus: 50–300 µg/kg *Anesthesia supplement:* IV bolus: 10–100 µg/kg Infusion: 0.05–1.25 µg/kg/min *For retrobulbar/peribulbar block:* IV: 50–100 µg/kg	IV: 1–2 min IM: <15 min Epidural: 30 min	IV: 10–15 min IM: 10–60 min	1.4–1.5 h	Hepatic	Chest wall rigidity, bradycardia
Fentanyl (IV)	50–100	*Premedication:* IV/IM: 25–100 µg *Analgesia:* IV/IM: 25–100 µg PCA: 25–100 µg every 5–30 min *Induction:* IV bolus: 1–2 (up to 20) µg/kg *Anesthesia supplement:* IV: 0.5–5 µg/kg Infusion: 0.5–5 µg/kg/h *Epidural* **Bolus:** 50–100 µg **Infusion:** 10–50 µg/h	IV: 5–15 min IM: <15 min Epidural/spinal: <30 min	IV: 30–60 min IM: 1–2 h Epidural/spinal: 1–2 h	IV: 2–4 h	Hepatic, pulmonary	Chest wall rigidity, bradycardia, pruritus, nausea, constipation

(continued)

	Potency (Relative to Morphine IV)	Adult Dosing	Peak Effect	Duration	Elimination Half-life	Primary Elimination	Interactions/Toxicities
Hydromorphone (IV)	5–7	*Analgesia:* **IV:** 0.5–2 mg every 4–6 h **IM/SC/PO:** 2–4 mg every 4–6 h **PCA:** 0.2–1 mg every 10–15 min **Spinal:** 0.1–0.2 mg *Epidural:* **Bolus:** 0.4–2 mg (lower dose for thoracic epidurals) **Infusion:** 0.15–0.3 mg/h	**IV:** 5–20 min **IM/SC/PO:** 30–60 min **Epidural:** 30 min	**IV:** 2–4 h **IM/SC/PO:** 4–6 h **Rectal:** 6–8 h **Epidural:** 10–16 h	For immediate release formulations: 1–3 h	Hepatic	Nausea, constipation, myoclonus
Meperidine (IV)	0.1	*Analgesic:* **PO/IM/SC:** 50–150 mg **IV:** 25–100 mg *Epidural:* **Bolus:** 50–100 mg **Infusion:** 10–20 mg/h *Spinal:* **Bolus:** 10–50 mg **Infusion:** 5–10 mg/h *Shivering/rigors:* **IV:** 12.5–25 mg	**PO:** <1 h **IV:** 5–20 min **IM:** 30–50 min **Epidural/spinal:** 30 min	**PO/IV/IM:** 2–4 h **Epidural/spinal:** 0.5–3 h	2.5–4 h	Hepatic	Normeperidine accumulation may result in seizures (especially in renally insufficient patients); can act as a local anesthetic; can act as anticholinergic, nausea

Morphine (IV)	1	*Analgesic:* **IV:** 2.5–15 mg **Infusion:** 0.5–10 mg/h **IM/SC:** 2.5–20 mg **PO:** 10–30 mg every 4 h **PO, extended release:** 30–60 mg every 8–12 h **Rectal:** 10–20 mg every 4 h *Epidural:* **Bolus:** 2–5 mg **Infusion:** 0.1–1 mg/h *Spinal:* 0.1–1 mg	**IV:** 5–20 min **IM:** 30–60 min **SC:** 50–90 min **PO:** 30–60 min **PO (slow release):** 1–4 h **Rectal:** 20–60 min **Epidural/spinal:** 90 min	**IV/IM/SC/PO:** 4–6 h **PO (slow release):** 6–12 h **Epidural/spinal:** 6–24 h	2–4 h	Hepatic	Histamine release; morphine-6-glucuronide is an active metabolite and can accumulate in renally insufficient patients; morphine-3-glucuronide can lower seizure threshold and can accumulate in renally insufficient patients; pruritus, nausea, constipation, myoclonus
Remifentanil (IV)	50–100	*Anesthesia induction:* **IV bolus:** 1 µg/kg over 30–60 s, then infusion 0.05–0.1 µg/kg/min *Anesthesia maintenance:* **Infusion:** 0.03–0.25 µg/kg/min **Supplemental IV bolus:** 0.5–1 µg/kg *Analgesia/monitored anesthesia care:* **IV bolus:** 0.6–2.0 µg/kg over 30–60 s, then infusion 0.03–0.1 µg/kg/min	**IV:** 1–2 min	**IV:** 5–10 min	3–10 min	Plasma and tissue esterases	Chest wall rigidity, bradycardia; no metabolic interaction with other esterase-hydrolyzed drugs; remifentanil clearance is reduced by approximately 20% during hypothermia

(continued)

APPENDIX B

	Potency (Relative to Morphine IV)	Adult Dosing	Peak Effect	Duration	Elimination Half-life	Primary Elimination	Interactions/Toxicities
Sufentanil (IV)	250–500	*Analgesia* **IV/IM:** 10–30 µg *Induction:* **IV bolus:** 0.5–1 µg/kg *Anesthesia supplement:* **IV bolus:** 0.1–0.5 µg/kg **Infusion:** 0.1–0.5 µg/kg/h *Epidural:* **Bolus:** 10–50 µg **Infusion:** 5–30 µg/h *Spinal:* 1–10 µg	**IV:** 3–5 min **Epidural/spinal:** <30 min	**IV:** 20–45 min **IM:** 2–4 h **Epidural/spinal:** 2–4 h	2.2–4.6 h	Hepatic and small intestine	Chest wall rigidity, bradycardia, constipation
Codeine (PO)	0.25–0.5	**PO:** 15–120 mg every 4–6 h	1–1.5 h	4–6 h	2.5–3.5 h	Hepatic	Pruritus, nausea, constipation
Hydrocodone (PO)	1.5	**PO:** 2.5–10 mg every 4–6 h	1.5 h	4–6 h	3–6 h	Hepatic	Pruritus, nausea, constipation
Methadone (PO)	2–5	**IV/PO:** 2.5–10 mg every 8–12 h	**IV:** 5–20 min **IM:** 30–60 min	**IV/IM:** 4–6 h **PO:** 22–48 h	8–59 h (increased with repeated doses)	Hepatic	Pruritus, nausea, possible severe reaction with MAO inhibitors; slow half-life may lead to overdose when first starting long-term treatment, prolonged QT interval
Oxycodone (PO)	1	**PO:** 5–30 mg every 4 h	0.5–1 h	3–6 h	2–5 h	Hepatic	Pruritus, nausea, constipation
Propoxyphene (PO)	0.1–0.2	**PO:** 65–100 mg every 4 h	2–2.5 h	4–6 h	6–12 h	Hepatic	Pruritus, nausea, constipation

Note: Most opioids will cause respiratory depression.

IV, intravenous; IM, intramuscular; PCA, patient-controlled analgesia; PO, per oral; SC, subcutaneous.

References

Omoigui S. *Sota Omoigui's Anesthesia Drugs Handbook*. Hawthorne, CA: State-of-the-Art Technologies, Incorporated; 1999.
Stoelting RK, Hillier SC. *Handbook of Pharmacology and Physiology in Anesthetic Practice*. Philadelphia, PA: Lippincott Williams & Wilkins; 2005.
Beers MH, Berkow R. *The Merck Manual of Diagnosis and Therapy*. 17th ed. Philadelphia, PA: John Wiley & Sons; 1999.

Opioid Antagonists

Andrew Wall, MD • Tony Cun, BS
Consultant Pharmacist: Anita Y. Chu, BPharm, RPh, Pharm.D

	Route/Adult Dosing	Onset	Duration	Elimination Half-life	Site of Clearance
Naloxone	*Post-op opioid reversal:* **IV:** 0.1–0.2 mg[a] *Intoxication/Respiratory Arrest:* **IV:** 0.4–2 mg **Endotracheal:** 2–2.5× IV dose (less preferred route)	**IV:** 1–2 min **Endotracheal (less preferred):** 2–5 min	30–120 min depending on route	0.5–1.5 h	Hepatic
Naltrexone	*Prophylaxis/treatment of opioid addiction or ethanol abuse:* **PO:** 12.5–50.0 mg daily *Opiate cessation:* **PO:** 12.5–25.0 mg daily initially, then 50 mg daily for maintenance.	**PO:** 15–30 min (Peak ~60 min)	24–72 h (dose dependent)	4 h	Hepatic

Used for complete or partial reversal of opioid drug effects, including respiratory depression and management of known or suspected opioid overdose.
[a]Dose every 2 to 3 minutes until desired response (adequate ventilation/alertness). Repeat dosing may be needed depending on type, dose, and timing of the last opioid administered. Titrate to assure adequate ventilation and minimize withdrawal symptoms.

References

Omoigui S. *Sota Omoigui's Anesthesia Drugs Handbook*. 3rd ed. Hawthorne, CA: State-of-the-Art Technologies, Incorporated; 1999: 310–316.

Stoelting RK, Hillier SC. *Handbook of Pharmacology and Physiology in Anesthetic Practice*. Philadelphia, PA: Lippincott Williams & Wilkins; 2005: 81–117.

Baughman VL, et al. *Anesthesiology and Critical Care Drug Handbook: Including Select Disease States & Perioperative Management*. 9th ed. Hudson: Lexi-Comp, Incorporated; 2009.

NSAIDS

Rohith Piyaratna, MD • Lynn Ngai, BS
Consultant Pharmacist: Anita Y. Chu, B.Pharm, R.Ph, Pharm.D

	Mechanism of Action	Adult Dosing	Peak Effect	Duration	Elimination Half-life	Primary Metabolism
Aspirin	Irreversibly acetylates the COX-1 and COX-2 enzymes, which causes decreased synthesis of prostaglandin precursors	*For analgesic purposes:* 10–15 mg/kg every 4–6 h *For anti-inflammatory purposes:* Initial: 2.4–4 g/d PO in divided doses (typically every 4–6 h) Maintenance: 3.6–5.4 g/d PO in divided doses (typically every 4–6 h) Monitor serum concentration and/or clinical signs of toxicity (tinnitus, nausea, presyncope, etc.)	2 h	4–6 h	Parent drug: 15–20 min Salicylates: 3–10 h (dose dependent)	Hepatic
Celecoxib	Inhibits synthesis of prostaglandins by decreasing mainly COX-2 (and not COX-1) enzyme activity	**PO:** 100–200 mg once or twice daily	3 h	12–24 h	~11 h (fasted)	Hepatic
Ibuprofen	Reversibly inhibits COX-1 and COX-2, with mechanisms including inhibition of chemotaxis, altering lymphocyte activity, inhibiting neutrophil aggregation, or decreasing proinflammatory cytokine levels	*For analgesic purposes:* **IV:** 400–800 mg every 6 h	1–2 h	4–6 h	2–4 h	Hepatic

(continued)

	Mechanism of Action	Adult Dosing	Peak Effect	Duration	Elimination Half-life	Primary Metabolism
Indomethacin	Reversibly inhibits COX-1 and COX-2	*For anti-inflammatory purposes:* **PO:** 25–50 mg 2–3 daily *Maximum total:* 200 mg daily	2 h	4–6 h	4.5 h	Hepatic
Ketorolac[a]	Reversibly inhibits COX-1 and COX-2; may be considered more of a peripherally acting analgesic; useful as a non-narcotic adjunct since ~30 mg of parenteral toradol is equivalent to 10 mg parenteral morphine	*Single-dose:* **IV:** 30 mg **IM:** 60 mg *Multiple-dose:* **IV/IM:** 30 mg every 6 h. Not to exceed 120 mg/d **PO:** Intended to be continuation of parenteral routes only. 10–20 mg initially and then 10 mg every 4–6 h. Not to exceed 40 mg/d. Duration of treatment should not exceed 5 d for combined PO/parenteral routes.	**IV/IM/ PO:** 1–3 h	**IV/IM/PO:** 3.5–8 h	2–6 h	Hepatic
Naproxen	Reversibly inhibits COX-1 and COX-2	*For analgesic purposes:* **PO:** 500 mg initially, followed by 250 mg every 6–8 h. *Maximum total:* 1250 mg/d	1–4 h	*Analgesic:* 7 h *Anti-inflammatory:* 12 h	12–17 h	Hepatic

General NSAID side effects:
May cause fluid retention, kidney or liver failure, antiplatelet aggregation leading to increased risk of bleeding; may cause gastric mucosal damage with ulceration and bleeding. COX-2 specific NSAIDS are believed to cause less damage to gastric mucosa and less antiplatelet effects versus COX-1 agents. However, studies have shown an increased risk for thrombosis, myocardial infarction, and stroke (which led to Rofecoxib being removed from the market in September 2004).
[a]Do not use in patients with bleeding or platelet problems.
IV, intravenous; IM, intramuscular; PO, per oral.

References

Epocrates® Online
Omoigui S. *Sota Omoigui's Anesthesia Drugs Handbook.* Hawthorne, CA: State-of-the-Art Technologies, Incorporated; 1999.
Stoelting RK, Hillier SC. *Handbook of Pharmacology and Physiology in Anesthetic Practice.* Philadelphia, PA: Lippincott Williams & Wilkins; 2005.
Beers MH, Berkow R. *The Merck Manual of Diagnosis and Therapy.* 17th ed. Philadelphia, PA: John Wiley & Sons; 1999.

IV Induction Agents

Christopher Tirce, MD • Lynn Ngai, BS
Consultant Pharmacist: Anita Y. Chu, B.Pharm, R.Ph, Pharm.D

	Mechanism of Action	Adult Dosing	Elimination Half-life	Elimination	Interactions/Toxicities
Etomidate (R-1-ethyl-1-[a-methylbenzyl] imidazole-5-carboxylate)	A carboxylated imidazole. Mechanism is unclear; modulates or activates $GABA_A$ receptors by potentiating GABA-induced chloride currents	*Induction:* IV: 0.2–0.4 mg/kg **Infusion:** 0.25–1 mg/min	2.6 h (terminal)	*Metabolism:* Hepatic *Excretion:* Renal	Cardiovascular and CNS depressant effects potentiated by other sedatives, narcotics, and volatile anesthetics; venous pain and myoclonus on rapid injection. Inhibits the activity of 11-β-hydroxylase, an enzyme necessary for the synthesis of cortisol, aldosterone, 17-hydroxy-progesterone, and corticosterone; adrenal suppression can persists for 5–8 h.
Ketamine	A phencyclidine derivative that acts as a noncompetitive antagonist at the glutamatergic *N*-methyl-D-aspartate (NMDA) receptor	*Sedation/analgesia:* IV: 0.5–1.0 mg/kg IM/PR: 2.5–5 mg/kg PO: 5–6 mg/kg (dilute in 5–10 mL cola-flavored drink) *Induction:* IV: 1.0–2.5 mg/kg IM/PR: 5–10 mg/kg *Infusion:* 15–80 µg/kg/min *Epidural/caudal:* 0.5 mg/kg	Alpha: 10–15 min Beta: 2.5 h	*Metabolism:* Hepatic *Excretion:* Primarily renal	May cause emergence delirium, decreased requirement for volatile anesthetics, hypertension, arrhythmias, or myocardial ischemia with concomitant use of sympathomimetics. Enhancement of depolarizing and nondepolarizing neuromuscular blockers.
Methohexital (1-methyl-5-allyl-5-[1-methyl-2-pent anyl] barbituric acid)	Pharmacodynamic effects are due to allosteric enhancement of the duration of $GABA_A$ receptor opening. At higher doses, may also be GABA-mimetic. Also depresses the transmission of excitatory neurotransmitters in the CNS, including acetylcholine and glutamate	*Sedation:* IV: 0.25–1 mg/kg *Induction:* IV: 1–3 mg/kg IM: 7–10 mg/kg **Infusion:** 50–150 µg/kg/min (0.2% solution) PR: 20–30 mg/kg	4 h	*Metabolism:* Systemic: Hepatic *Excretion:* Systemic: Renal	Circulatory depression, thrombophlebitis (rare), seizure (typically in patients with a history of seizures). Potentiates CNS and circulatory depressant effects of narcotics, sedative hypnotics, alcohol, and volatile anesthetics.

Propofol (2,6-diisopropylphenol)	Allosteric binding to GABA$_A$, increasing the duration of Cl$^-$ channel opening	*Induction:* 1.5–2.5 mg/kg *Maintenance:* 100–200 μg/kg/min *Sedation:* **IV bolus:** 25–50 mg **Infusion:** 25–75 μg/kg/min	Biphasic: Initial: 40 min Terminal: 4–7 h	*Metabolism:* Systemic: Hepatic, extrahepatic (pulmonary) *Excretion:* Systemic: Renal	Circulatory depression, pancreatitis, propofol infusion syndrome (characterized by dysrhythmia, heart failure, hyperkalemia, lipemia, metabolic acidosis, and/or rhabdomyolysis or myoglobinuria with subsequent renal failure). Potentiates CNS and circulatory depressant effects of narcotics, sedative hypnotics, and volatile anesthetics; pulmonary extraction decreased and plasma levels increased with concomitant administration of alfentanil, fentanyl, or halothane; potentiates neuromuscular blockade of nondepolarizing muscle relaxants.
Thiopental (5-ethyl-5-[1-methylbutyl]-2-thio-barbituric acid)	Pharmacodynamic effects are due to allosteric enhancement of the duration of GABA$_A$ receptor opening. At higher doses, may also be GABA-mimetic. Also depresses the transmission of excitatory neurotransmitters in the CNS, including acetylcholine and glutamate	*Induction:* **IV:** 3–5 mg/kg *Anesthesia supplementation:* **IV:** 0.5–1 mg/kg	3–11.5 h	*Metabolism:* Hepatic *Excretion:* Primarily renal	Myocardial dysfunction; thrombosis (intra-arterial injection); hemolytic anemia (rare), radial nerve palsy (rare), renal failure (rare). Potentiates CNS and circulatory depressant effects of narcotics, sedative hypnotics, alcohol, and volatile anesthetics; arterial or extravascular injection can produce necrosis and gangrene; can form precipitates when injected with muscle relaxants. Interferes with porphyrin metabolism: administration of the drug may result in elevated concentrations of porphyrins in serum and/or urine, which may exacerbate acute intermittent porphyria.

APPENDIX B

	Protein Binding	Volume of Distribution	Time to Onset	Peak Effect	Duration of Action
Etomidate	76%	2–4.5 L/kg	15–45 s	1 min	3–12 min
Ketamine	12%	2–3 L/kg	IV: 45–60 s	1 min	5–20 min
Methohexital	85%	1.9–2.2 L/kg	IV: <30 s / PR: 5–15 min	IV: 45 s / PR: 5–10 min	IV: 5–10 min / PR: 30–90 min
Propofol	97%–99%	2–10 L/kg	15–45 s	1 min	5–10 min
Thiopental	72%–86%	1.6–2.5 L/kg	IV: <30 s	IV: 30–40 s	IV: 5–15 min

IV, intravenous; IM, intramuscular; PO, per oral; PR, per rectum.

References

Omoigui S. *Sota Omoigui's Anesthesia Drugs Handbook*. Hawthorne, CA: State-of-the-Art Technologies, Incorporated; 1999.

Stoelting RK, Hillier SC. *Handbook of Pharmacology and Physiology in Anesthetic Practice*. Philadelphia, PA: Lippincott Williams & Wilkins; 2005.

Beers MH, Berkow R. *The Merck Manual of Diagnosis and Therapy*. 17th ed. Philadelphia, PA: John Wiley & Sons; 1999.

Inhaled Anesthetics

Shaun Kunnavatana, MD • Tony Cun, BS
Consultant Pharmacist: Anita Y. Chu, BPharm, RPh, PharmD

	Desflurane	Isoflurane	Nitrous Oxide	Sevoflurane
1 MAC	6.0%	1.2%	105%	2%
Vapor Pressure (mm Hg at 20°C)	681	240	Gas at room temperature	160
Blood/Gas Partition Coefficient	0.42	1.4	0.47	0.65
CNS Effects	↑CBF ↓↓CMRO$_2$ ↑ICP	↑CBF at >1 MAC ↓↓CMRO$_2$ ↑ICP at >1 MAC EEG suppression at >2 MAC	↑CBF ↑CMRO$_2$ ↑ICP	↑CBF ↓↓CMRO$_2$ ↑ICP
Cardiovascular Effects	↓↓BP ↑ or N/C HR ↓↓SVR ↓ or N/C CO Rapid ↑ associated with transient elevations in HR, BP, and catechols	↓↓BP ↑HR ↓↓SVR N/C CO Rapid ↑ associated with transient elevations in HR, BP, and catechols	N/C BP N/C HR N/C SVR N/C CO Increases pulmonary vascular resistance due to constriction of pulmonary smooth muscle	↓BP N/C HR ↓SVR ↓CO May prolong QT interval
Pulmonary Effects	↓TV ↑RR Depresses ventilatory response to ↑PaCO$_2$	↓↓TV ↑RR Depresses ventilatory response to ↑PaCO$_2$ Modest bronchodilation	↓TV ↑RR Depresses hypoxic ventilatory drive	↓TV ↑RR Depresses ventilatory response to ↑PaCO$_2$ Mild bronchodilation
Hepatic Effects	↓Hepatic blood flow	↓Hepatic blood flow	↓Hepatic blood flow	N/C Hepatic blood flow
Renal Effects	↓Renal blood flow ↓GFR ↓UOP	↓↓Renal blood flow ↓↓GFR ↓↓UOP	↓↓Renal blood flow ↓↓GFR ↓↓UOP	↓Renal blood flow ↓GFR ↓UOP

(continued)

	Desflurane	Isoflurane	Nitrous Oxide	Sevoflurane
Metabolism	<0.1% absorbed anesthetic metabolized with pulmonary, hepatic, renal elimination	0.2% absorbed anesthetic metabolized with pulmonary, hepatic, renal elimination	0.004% absorbed anesthetic metabolized with pulmonary, renal, GI elimination	5% absorbed anesthetic metabolized with pulmonary, hepatic, renal elimination
Considerations Against Use	Patients with known or suspected malignant hyperthermia Pungency can cause airway irritation, breath-holding, coughing and laryngospasm	Patients with known or suspected malignant hyperthermia	Tends to diffuse into air-containing cavities. Beware in conditions where air embolism, pneumothorax, acute intestinal obstruction, intracranial air, intraocular air bubbles, tympanic membrane perforation may exist. Avoid use in patients with preexisting pulmonary HTN or Right sided CHF: due to increased pulmonary vascular resistance via vasoconstriction of pulmonary artery	Patients with known or suspected malignant Hyperthermia
Additional Pearls	Ultra-short duration with quick wake-up times Desflurane emergence associated with delirium in some pediatric patients Special vaporizer needed given high vapor pressure	Some evidence of coronary steal via dilation of normal coronary arteries	Avoid in patients with pulmonary HTN or where increased pulmonary vascular resistance is problematic Increased incidence of postoperative nausea, vomiting. Addition of N_2O decreases requirements of other agents for generating same MAC Nitrous oxide has mild analgesic properties Nitrous oxide reduced inspired concentration of inhalational agents: reduction in the cardiovascular and respiratory depressant effects of the volatile agents. N_2O smoothens the anaesthetic.	Accumulation of Compound A seen in low-flow anesthesia, dry barium hydroxide (Baralyme) absorbent, high sevoflurane concentrations Nonpungent features mixed with rapid increase in alveolar concentration make ideal for inhalational induction in pediatric and adult patients when mixed with N_2O

↑, increase; ↓, decrease; ↓↓, large decrease; BP, blood pressure; CBF, cerebral blood flow; CHF, congestive heart failure; $CMRO_2$, cerebral metabolic rate of oxygen; CO, cardiac output; GFR, glomerular filtration rate; GI, gastrointestinal; HR, heart rate; HTN, hypertension; ICP, intracranial pressure; N/C, no change; $PaCO_2$, arterial CO_2 partial pressure; RR, respiratory rate; SVR, systemic vascular resistance; TV, tidal volume; UOP, urine output.

References

Morgan GE, Mikhail MS, Murray MJ. *Clinical Anesthesiology*. New York, NY: McGraw-Hill Medical Publishing Division; 2005.
Omoigui S. *Sota Omoigui's Anesthesia Drugs Handbook*. Hawthorne; CA: State-of-the-Art Technologies, Incorporated; 1999.
Stoelting RK, Hillier SC. *Handbook of Pharmacology and Physiology in Anesthetic Practice*. Philadelphia, PA: Lippincott Williams & Wilkins; 2005.

Adrenergic Agonists

Jonathan T. Bradley, MD • Lynn Ngai, BS
Consultant Pharmacist: Anita Y. Chu, B.Pharm, R.Ph, Pharm.D

	Mechanism of Action	Adult Dosing	Onset	Peak Effect	Duration	Elimination Half-life	Primary Metabolism
Dobutamine	A direct β_1-adrenergic agonist with mild α_1- and β_2-adrenergic receptor agonist effects	**Infusion:** 2–20 µg/kg/min	1–2 min	1–10 min	<10 min	2 min	Hepatic
Dopamine	Both a direct and indirect agonist; stimulates α_1- and β_1-adrenergic receptors	**Infusion:** 1–20 µg/kg/min	2–4 min	2–10 min	<10 min	2 min	Hepatic
Ephedrine	An indirect agonist with some direct agonist effects; stimulates α_1- and β-adrenergic receptors	*For hypotension:* **IV:** 5–20 mg (100–200 µg/kg) **IM/SC:** 25–50 mg	**IV:** almost immediate **IM:** a few minutes	**IV:** 2–5 min **IM:** <10 min	**IV/IM:** 10–60 min	2.5–3.6 h	Hepatic, renal
Epinephrine	Directly activates α- and β-adrenergic receptors; β-adrenergic effects predominate at therapeutic parenteral doses, and α-adrenergic effects predominate at higher doses	*Cardiac arrest:* **IV bolus:** 1 mg or 0.02 mg/kg every 3–5 min, followed by a 20-mL flush of IV fluid *Inotropic support:* **Infusion:** 0.1–1 µg/kg/min *Anaphylaxis:* **IM/SC:** 0.1–5 mg *Test dose in regional anesthesia (a marker for accidental intravascular injection):* 10–15 µg	**IV:** 30–60 seconds **SC:** 6–15 min **Intratracheal:** 5–15 seconds **Inhalation:** 3–5 min	**IV:** within 3 min	**IV:** 5–10 min **Intratracheal:** 15–25 min **Inhalation/SC:** 1–3 h		Enzymatic degradation (hepatic, renal, and GI tract)

	Mechanism	Dose	Onset		Duration		Metabolism
Isoproterenol	Directly activates β_1- and β_2-adrenergic receptors almost exclusively	*Arrhythmias/resuscitation:* **IM/SC:** 0.2 mg **IV push:** 0.02–0.06 mg **Infusion:** 0.02–0.15 µg/kg/min **Sublingual:** 10 mg then 5–50 mg as needed *Bronchospasm:* **Metered dose inhaler:** 120–262 µg every 3–4 h	**IV:** immediate Inhalation: 2–5 min Sublingual/SC: 15–30 min	**IV:** 1 min	**IV:** 1–5 min Inhalation: 0.5–2 h Sublingual/SC: 1–2 h	2.5–5 min	Hepatic
Norepinephrine	Directly activates α- and β_1-adrenergic receptors	**Infusion:** 0.04–0.4 µg/kg/min	<1 min	1–2 min	2–10 min		Enzymatic degradation, pulmonary
Phenylephrine	Directly activates α-adrenergic receptors with minimal β activation	*Hypotension:* **IM/SC:** 2–5 mg **IV:** 50–100 µg **Infusion:** 0.15–4.0 µg/kg/min *Shunt reversal:* **IV:** 1–2 µg/kg	**IV:** <1 min **IM/SC:** 10–15 min	**IV:** <1 min	**IV:** 15–20 min **IM/SC:** 0.5–2 h		Hepatic

IV, intravenous; IM, intramuscular; SC, subcutaneous; PO, per oral.

References

Omoigui S. *Sota Omoigui's Anesthesia Drugs Handbook.* Hawthorne, CA: State-of-the-Art Technologies, Incorporated; 1999.

Beers MH, Berkow R. *The Merck Manual of Diagnosis and Therapy.* 17th ed. Philadelphia, PA: John Wiley & Sons; 1999.

Adrenergic Antagonists

Christopher Tirce, MD • Lynn Ngai, BS
Consultant Pharmacist: Anita Y. Chu, B.Pharm, R.Ph, Pharm.D

	Mechanism of Action	Adult Dosing	Onset	Peak Effect	Duration	Elimination Half-life	Primary Elimination
Atenolol	β₁ selective antagonist	*For antihypertensive/antianginal effects:* **PO:** 50–200 mg once daily *For definite or suspected acute MI:* **IV:** 5 mg over 5 min, followed by another 5 mg intravenous injection 10 min later *For alcohol withdrawal/migraine prophylaxis:* **PO:** 50–100 mg once daily	**IV:** <5 min **PO:** <1 h	**IV:** 5 min **PO:** 2–4 h	**IV:** up to 12 h **PO:** >24 h	6–7 h	Little to no biotransformation; majority is excreted from the kidneys as unchanged drug
Bisoprolol	β₁ selective antagonist	**PO:** 2.5–20 mg once daily	1–2 h	2–4 h	>24 h	9–12 h	Hepatic (significant first-pass effect)
Carvedilol	α₁, β₁, and β₂ antagonist	**PO:** 6.25–25 mg twice daily	1–2 h	1–2 h	12–24 h	7–10 h	Hepatic (significant first-pass effect)
Esmolol	β₁ selective antagonist	*For antihypertensive effects:* **IV:** 0.5–2 mg/kg, repeated every 5 min if necessary **Infusion:** 50–300 μg/kg/min, titrated to blood pressure response *For supraventricular tachyarrhythmias:* **IV:** 500 μg/kg, given over 1 min **Infusion:** 50–200 μg/kg/min—dose is increased to titrate to effect	1–2 min	5 min	10–20 min	10 min	Esterases in the cytosol of red blood cells
Labetalol	Predominant β₁ and β₂ antagonist	**IV bolus:** 0.25 mg/kg slowly over 2 min **Infusion:** 0.5–2 mg/min, maximum 1–4 mg/kg **PO:** 100–400 mg twice daily *Maximum total dose:* 300 mg **IV**	**IV:** 2–5 min **PO:** 20 min to 2 h	**IV:** 5–15 min **PO:** 1–4 h	**IV:** 2–4 h **PO:** 8–24 h	**IV:** 5.5 h **PO:** 6–8 h	Hepatic; urine and feces

(continued)

	Mechanism of Action	Adult Dosing	Onset	Peak Effect	Duration	Elimination Half-life	Primary Elimination
Metoprolol	β₁ selective antagonist, but can inhibit β₂-receptors in high doses	*For antihypertensive effects:* **IV:** 1–5 mg every 2 to 5 min up to 15 mg, with titration to heart rate and blood pressure **PO:** 50–400 mg daily in 1–3 divided doses *For acute myocardial infarction:* **IV:** 15 mg over 6 min in 3 divided doses, **PO:** 50 mg every 6 h, beginning 15 min after the last IV dose for 48 h, and then **PO:** 100 mg twice daily *For migraine prophylaxis:* **PO:** 50–100 mg twice daily	**IV:** <1 min **PO:** <15 min	**IV:** 20 min **PO:** 1.5–4 h	**IV:** 5–8 h **PO:** 10–20 h	3–8 h	Hepatic (significant first-pass effect)
Phenoxybenzamine	An irreversible, nonselective alpha-receptor antagonist	**PO:** 10 mg—dose is increased to titrate to effect	Kinetics are not well known	Kinetics are not well known	14–48 h	**IV:** 24 h **PO:** unknown	Hepatic
Propranolol	Nonselective β blockade	*For antihypertensive effects:* **PO:** 20–40 mg twice daily, usually ≤320 mg daily, but can be up to 640 mg daily **IV:** 10–30 μg/kg every 2 min (maximum 6–10 mg) **IV bolus:** Usual dose is 1–3 mg administered under careful monitoring. Rate of administration should not exceed 1 mg (1 mL)/min. If necessary, a second dose may be given after 2 min. Thereafter, additional drug should not be given for at least 4 h. Additional propranolol hydrochloride should not be given when the desired alteration in rate or rhythm is achieved. *Maximum total dose:* ≤5–10 mg or 0.1 mg/kg	**IV:** <2 min **PO:** <30 min	**IV:** within 1 min **PO:** variable (immediate release: 1–4 h; extended-release formulations: ~6–14 h)	**IV:** 1–6 h **PO:** 6–12 h	3–6 h (for immediate release formulation)	Hepatic, pulmonary

IV, intravenous; PO, per oral.

References

Forssman B, Lindblad CJ, Zbornikova V. Atenolol for migraine prophylaxis. *Headache* 1983;23(4):188–190.

Frischman W, Cheng-Lai A, Nawarskas J. *Current Cardiovascular Drugs*. 4th ed. Philadelphia, PA: Current MedicineLLC; 2005.

Johannsson V, Nilsson LR, Widelius T, et al. Atenolol in migraine prophylaxis a double-blind cross-over multicentre study. *Headache* 1987;27(7): 372–374.

Katzung BG, Masters SB, Trevor A. *Basic and Clinical Pharmacology*. 11th ed. NewYork: McGraw-Hill Medical; 2009.

Kraus ML, Gottlieb LD, Horwitz RI, et al. Randomized clinical trial of atenolol in patients with alcohol withdrawal syndrome. *NEJM* 1985;313(15):905-909.

Miller RD, Eriksson LI, Fleisher LA, et al. *Miller's Anesthesia*. 7th ed. Philadelphia, PA: Churchill Livingstone; 2009.

Omoigui S. *Sota Omoigui's Anesthesia Drugs Handbook*. Hawthorne, CA: State-of-the-Art Technologies, Incorporated; 1999.

Pacak K. Preoperative management of the pheochromocytoma patient. *J Clin Endocrinol Metab* 2007;92(11):4069–4079.

Stoelting RK, Hillier SC. *Handbook of Pharmacology and Physiology in Anesthetic Practice*. Philadelphia, PA: Lippincott Williams & Wilkins; 2005.

Beers MH, Berkow R. *The Merck Manual of Diagnosis and Therapy*. 17th ed. Philadelphia, PA: John Wiley & Sons; 1999.

Wiest D. Esmolol. A review of its therapeutic efficacy and pharmacokinetic characteristics. *Clin Pharmacokinet* 1995;28(3):190–202.

APPENDIX B

Corticosteroids

Rohith Piyaratna, MD • Lynn Ngai, BS
Consultant Pharmacist: Anita Y. Chu, B.Pharm, R.Ph, Pharm.D

Drug Name (Approximate mg of Equivalent Dose)	Mechanism of Action	Adult Dosing	Peak Effect	Duration	Elimination Half-life	Primary Elimination	Glucocorticoid, Mineralcortioid Potency (Relative to Cortisol)
Hydrocortisone (Cortisol) (20)	Has anti-inflammatory and mineralocorticoid activity; binds specific intracellular cytoplasmic receptors in target tissues (a mechanism of all steroidal agents). The receptor-hormone complex then acts as a transcription factor in the nucleus, turning certain genes on or off. Cortisol has rapid onset, but a short duration of action.	*For inflammatory diseases:* **IV/IM:** 20–300 mg every 2–10 h *Steroid replacement:* **IV:** 50–100 mg preoperatively, intraoperatively, and postoperatively	*For anti-inflammatory effects:* **IV/IM:** <1 h	*For anti-inflammatory effects/HPA suppression:* 30–36 h	Biological: 8–12 h	Hepatic	1, 2
Dexamethasone (0.75)	Similar to hydrocortisone; synthetic long-acting glucocorticoid with potent anti-inflammatory effects	*For inflammatory diseases:* Dexamethasone phosphate: **(IA/IT)** 1–16 mg Dexamethasone acetate **(IA/IM/IT):** 4–16 mg Dexamethasone phosphate **(IV/IM):** 0.5–25 mg/d *For cerebral edema or raised ICP:* Dexamethasone phosphate: **IV:** 10–50 mg, then **IV/IM:** 4–20 mg every 6 h or **PO:** 1–15 mg 3 times daily *For airway swelling:* Dexamethasone phosphate **(IV):** 10–25 mg every 6 h in 4–6 doses *For bronchospasm:* Dexamethasone phosphate **(inhalation):** 300 µg (3 inhalations) 3–4 times daily	*For anti-inflammatory effects:* **IV/IM:** 12–24 h	36–54 h	1.8–3.5 h	Hepatic	25–30, 0

(continued)

APPENDIX B

Drug Name (Approximate mg of Equivalent Dose)	Mechanism of Action	Adult Dosing	Peak Effect	Duration	Elimination Half-life	Primary Elimination	Glucocorticoid, Mineralcortioid Potency (Relative to Cortisol)
Fludrocortisone (–)	Similar to hydrocortisone, but has prolonged effect on electrolyte balance and carbohydrate metabolism; produces significant sodium retention, increased potassium excretion from renal distal tubules, and rise in blood pressure	**PO:** 0.05–0.2 mg/d	1.7 h	24 h	Plasma: 30–35 minutes Biological: 18–36 h	Hepatic	10, 125
Prednisone (5)	See hydrocortisone; intermediate acting	**PO:** 5–60 mg/d	1–2 h	12–36 h	~3.5 h	Hepatic	4, 1

General corticosteroid side effects:

Osteoporosis, impaired wound healing and increased risk of infection, increased appetite, hypertension, edema, peptic ulcers, euphoria, and psychoses. Systemic corticosteroids used for <7 d, even at high doses, are not likely to cause adverse side effects, nor are inhaled corticosteroids.

IA, intra-articular; ICP, intracranial pressure; IV, intravenous; IM, intramuscular; IT, intratissue; PO, per oral.

References

Omoigui S. *Sota Omoigui's Anesthesia Drugs Handbook*. Hawthorne: State-of-the-Art Technologies, Incorporated; 1999.

Stoelting RK, Hillier SC. *Handbook of Pharmacology and Physiology in Anesthetic Practice*. Philadelphia, PA: Lippincott Williams & Wilkins; 2005.

Beers MH, Berkow R. *The Merck Manual of Diagnosis and Therapy*. 17th ed. Philadelphia, PA: John Wiley & Sons; 1999.

Antibiotics

Becky Wong, MD • Tony Cun, BS
Consultant Pharmacist: Anita Y. Chu, BPharm, RPh, PharmD

	Surgery Type and Likely Pathogens	Adult Dosing	Administration Dosing	Excretion	Class and Mechanism of Action	Comments
Ampicillin	To treat *Proteus mirabilis*, *E. coli*, and *Streptococcus*. Colorectal, appendectomy procedures.	**IV:** 1–2 g	**Redose:** 4–6 h	Hepatic metabolism; renal excretion	Penicillinase-susceptible with activity against Gram-negative bacilli	Associated with skin rash. Allergic reactions.
Cefazolin	At-risk surgical procedures (cardiac, noncardiac thoracic, colorectal, esophageal and gastroduodenal, biliary tract, appendectomy, pancreatic, vascular, genitourinary, neurosurgery, head and neck, vaginal or abdominal hysterectomy)	**IV:** 1 g (if < 80 kg), 2 g (if > 80 kg)	**Intraop:** Redose every 2–6 h **Post-op:** Redose every 8 h	Renal excretion	1st-generation cephalosporins	Allergic reactions. Toxicity: prolonged thrombin time, neutropenia
Cefoxitin, Cefotetan, Cefuroxime	**Cefoxitin:** colorectal, appendectomy **Cefotetan:** colorectal **Cefuroxime:** cardiac, noncardiac thoracic, pancreatic, vascular	**IV:** 1–2 g (**cefoxitin** and **cefotetan**). **IV:** 1.5 g (**cefuroxime**)	**Redose:** 6–8 h (**cefoxitin**) 12 h (**cefotetan**) 8 h, max 6–9 g/d (**cefuroxime**)	Renal excretion	2nd generation Cephalosporins	Allergic reactions. Toxicity: prolonged thrombin time, neutropenia
Ceftriaxone	Good CNS penetration for neurosurgical procedures. To treat meningtis or epiglottitis (*Haemophilus influenzae*)	**IV:** 1–2 g	**Redose:** 24 h	Renal excretion	3rd-generation cephalosporins	Allergic reactions. Toxicity: prolonged thrombin time, neutropenia
Ciprofloxacin	To treat upper and lower respiratory tract infections, bone and joint infections, and most strains of mycobacterium tuberculosis. Colorectal, esophageal and gastroduodenal, biliary tract, appendectomy, genitourinary	**IV:** 400 mg **PO:** 500 mg	**Redose:** 8–12 h	Hepatic metabolism (active metabolites) Renal excretion	Fluoroquinolones	Allergic reactions. Toxicity: prolongation of QTc interval, tendinitis, photosensitivity, teratogenicity. maternal toxicity: GI irritation

	Indications	Dose	Infusion time / Redose	Metabolism	Class / Mechanism	Toxicity
Clindamycin	Cardiac, noncardiac thoracic, colorectal, esophageal and gastroduodenal surgery, biliary tract, appendectomy, head and neck. Used with gentamycin for urological procedures.	IV: 600–900 mg	**Infusion time:** 60 min **Redose:** 6–8 h	Hepatic metabolism (active metabolites) Renal excretion	Lincomycin	Allergic reactions. Pseudomembranous colitis can be a complication; produces prejunctional and postjunctional effects at the neuromuscular junction; maternal toxicity: alcohol intolerance, peripheral neuropathy
Gentamycin	To treat pseudomonas aeruginosa. Colorectal, esophageal and gastroduodenal, biliary tract, appendectomy, head and neck. Used with clindamycin for urological procedures.	IV: 1–2.5 mg/kg	**Infusion time:** 60 min **Redose:** 8–12 h	Renal excretion	Aminoglycoside	Allergic reactions. Ototoxicity, nephrotoxicity
Metronidazole	Colorectal, appendectomy	IV: 500 mg	**Infusion time:** 60 min **Redose:** 6–8 h	Hepatic metabolism, renal excretion	Antiprotozoal, bactericidal (forms toxic metabolites in the bacterial cell)	Allergic reactions. Toxicity: seizures, peripheral neuropathy, teratogenicity
Piperacillin/ Tazobactam	Broad spectrum for sepsis or skin/soft tissue infections, good for pseudomonas coverage	IV: 3.375 g (4.5 g for antipseudomonas)	**Redose:** 6–8 h	Hepatic metabolism; Renal excretion	Antipseudomonal penicillin, β-lactamase inhibitor	Does not cover MRSA, VRE, atypicals; extended use >1 d may cause neutropenia
Vancomycin	Cardiac and orthopedic surgery. To treat MRSA, staphylococcus epidermidis. Cardiac, noncardiac thoracic, vascular, neurosurgery. Good alternative for Penicillin-allergic patients.	IV: 1 g (patients >70 kg); 500–750 mg (patients <70 kg)	**Infusion time:** 60 min **Redose:** 6–12 h	Renal excretion	Bactericidal glycopeptide that impairs cell wall synthesis of Gram-positive bacteria	Rapid infusion (<30 min) associated with hypotension and cardiac arrest, facial and truncal erythema. Allergic reactions. Toxicity: neutropenia, ototoxicity

APPENDIX B

References

Anderson DJ, Sexton DJ. Control measures to prevent surgical site infection. UpToDate. August 18, 2009. Accessed April 20, 2010. http://www.uptodate.com/online/content/topic.do?topicKey=hosp_inf/6955&view=print

Gilbert DN, Moellering RC, Eliopoulos GM, et al. *The Sanford Guide to Antimicrobial Therapy. Sanford Guide Ser.* Hyde Park, VT: Antimicrobial Therapy, Incorporated; 2009.

Stoelting RK, Hillier SC. *Handbook of Pharmacology and Physiology in Anesthetic Practice*. Philadelphia, PA: Lippincott Williams & Wilkins; 2005.

Antiemetics

Amy Wang, MD • Lynn Ngai, BS
Consultant Pharmacist: Anita Y. Chu, B.Pharm, R.Ph, Pharm.D

	Mechanism of Action	Adult Dosing	Elimination Half-life	Site of Metabolism	Interactions/Toxicities
Dexamethasone	Mechanism of action in regard to antiemesis is currently unknown	*Antiemetic (before incision):* **IV:** 4–8 mg	1.8–3.5 h Biological half-life: 36–54 h	Hepatic	Primary adrenocortical insufficiency. Clearance enhanced by phenytoin, phenobarbital, rifampin, ephedrine; increases requirements of insulin; increases risk of GI bleeding with concomitant NSAID use.
Droperidol	Antiemetic effect is due to dopamine blockade in the chemoreceptor trigger zone	*Antiemetic:* **IV/IM:** 0.625–1.25 mg	2.3 h	Hepatic	Respiratory depression, neuroleptic malignant syndrome. May be sedating. May cause extrapyramidal signs. Can cause anticholinergic effects. May intensify hypotensive effects of vasodilators. **Black box warning:** May cause QT prolongation and torsade de pointes. Use with caution in patients with cardiac disease, electrolyte disturbances.
Metoclopramide	Blocks dopamine D_2 receptors; enhances GI motility and accelerates gastric emptying; increases lower esophageal sphincter tone	**IV/IM:** 10–20 mg every 4–6 h as needed **PO:** 10 mg	5–6 h	Renal	Neuroleptic malignant syndrome. May cause extrapyramidal symptoms; antagonized by anticholinergics and opioids; potentiated by sedatives, opioids, tranquilizers, and hypnotics. **Black box warning:** May cause tardive dyskinesia, which is often irreversible.
Ondansetron	Serotonin $5\text{-}HT_3$ receptor antagonist, targets vagal nerve terminals and chemoreceptor trigger zone of the area postrema	*For postoperative nausea (before end of surgery):* **IV/IM:** 4 mg **PO:** 8–16 mg	3–6 h	Hepatic	Cardiac dysrhythmia, anaphylaxis, bronchospasm. Toxicities potentiated by hepatic disease; use with caution in patients with risk factors for QT prolongation and patients allergic to other $5\text{-}HT_3$ receptor antagonists.

	Mechanism of Action	Dosage	Metabolism	Adverse Effects/Warnings
Prochlorperazine	Antiemetic activity is mediated via dopaminergic blockade in the chemoreceptor trigger zone of the medulla	**IV:** 2.5–10 mg every 3–4 h (maximum 40/d) **IM:** 5–10 mg every 3–4 h (maximum 40 mg/d) **PO:** 5–10 mg 3–4 times/d (maximum 40 mg/d) **PR:** 25 mg twice daily	Hepatic	Prolonged QT interval, torsade de pointes, agranulocytosis, cholestatic jaundice syndrome. May potentiate or increase levels of alcohol, opioid analgesics, anticholinergics, beta-blockers, and CNS depressants; hypersensitivity may result in jaundice and/or extrapyramidal symptoms. **Black box warning:** Increased risk of death seen in elderly patients being treated with antipsychotics for dementia-related psychosis.
Promethazine	Blocks dopaminergic receptors in the brain. Histamine blocking agent at H₁ receptors; antimuscarinic activity may be responsible for antiemetic properties	**IV/IM/PO/PR:** 12.5–25 mg every 4–6 h	9–16 h Hepatic	Injection site reaction, agranulocytosis, jaundice, neuroleptic malignant syndrome. Potentiates CNS, respiratory and circulatory depressant effects of alcohol, volatile anesthetics, and sedative hypnotics. May increase levels/effects of anticholinergics; serotonin modulators. **Black box warning:** Contraindicated in children <2 y.
Propofol	Mechanism of action in regard to antiemesis is currently not well understood	*Antiemetic:* **IV:** 10–20 mg	Biphasic: Initial: 40 min Terminal: 4–7 h Hepatic	May cause sedation, hypotension, respiratory depression, or anaphylaxis; potentiates CNS and circulatory depressant effects of narcotics, sedative hypnotics, and volatile anesthetics.
Scopolamine	Antagonizes action of acetylcholine at cholinergic postganglionic nerve ending; weak peripheral muscarinic cholinergic effect; its tertiary amine structure allows it to readily cross blood–brain barrier, exerting effects on the CNS	*Scopolamine base:* **Transdermal patch:** 1.5 mg, apply to postauricular skin **SC:** 0.6–1 mg	9.5 h Hepatic	Alteration in heart rate, drug-induced psychosis. Central anticholinergic syndrome. Potentiates sedative effects of narcotics, benzodiazepines, anticholinergics, antihistamines, and volatile anesthetics; may cause amnesia, dry mouth, and vertigo; use with caution in patients with narrow-angle glaucoma.

IV, intravenous; IM, intramuscular; PO, per oral; PR, per rectum; SC, subcutaneous.

APPENDIX B

References

Barash PG. *Handbook of Clinical Anesthesia*. 6th ed. Philadelphia, PA: Lippincott Williams & Wilkins; 2009.

Baughman VL, Julie Golembiewski, Jeffrey P. Gonzales, William Jr. Alvarez, et al. *Anesthesiology and Critical Care Drug Handbook*. Hudson, OH: Lexi-Comp, Incorporated; 2009.

Omoigui S. *Sota Omoigui's Anesthesia Drugs Handbook*. Hawthorne, CA: State-of-the-Art Technologies, Incorporated; Jan. 1999.

Miller RD, Stoelting RK. *Basics of Anesthesia*. 5 ed. Philadelphia, PA: Churchill Livingstone; 2006.

Beers MH, Berkow R. *The Merck Manual of Diagnosis and Therapy*. 17th ed. Philadelphia, PA: John Wiley & Sons; 1999.

Stoelting RK, Hillier SC. *Handbook of Pharmacology and Physiology in Anesthetic Practice*. Philadelphia, PA: Lippincott Williams & Wilkins; 2005.

Hematologics

Jack Kan, MD • Tony Cun, BS
Consultant Pharmacist: Anita Y. Chu, B.Pharm, R.Ph, Pharm.D

> Disclaimer: Anticoagulant and antiplatelet medications should not be discontinued without first taking into account the patient's clinical situation. Abrupt discontinuation of these medications may be life threatening or may lead to serious morbidity.

	Effect Site	Adult Dosing	Peak Effect	Half-life	Stop Before Surgery	Metabolism	Adverse Reactions	Usage
			Anticoagulant Drugs					
Argatroban	Thrombin	**IV** (*infusion*): start at 2 μg/kg/min, target PTT 1.5–3 times normal or <100 s	**IV:** steady state 1–3 h	50 min	4–6 h	Hepatic elimination	Hemorrhage	Alternative to heparin in patients that have heparin induced thrombocytopenia
Aspirin[a]	COX, irreversible inhibition of platelet activation and aggregation	81–325 mg daily **ACS:** 325 mg (chewed)	**PO:** 1–2 h	6 h	7 d	Hepatic elimination	Anaphylaxis, angioedema, GI bleed, hemorrhage, anion gap metabolic acidosis, reyes syndrome	ACS, stroke
Clopidigrel	ADP blocking IIb/IIIa activity and inhibition of platelet aggregation	**PO:** 75–150 mg qd	**PO:** 45 min	7 h	7–10 d	Hepatic	Neutropenia, hepatic dysfunction, hemorrhage	CAD, PVD, ischemic stroke, prevention of thrombosis
Eptifibatide	Blocking IIb/IIIa activity and inhibition of platelet aggregation	**IV:** Load with 180 μg/kg then 2 μg/kg/min up to 96 h for **PCI**, stop within 24 h post-procedure	**IV:** 5 min	2.5 h	4 h	Renal	Hemorrhage, anaphylaxis, hypotension	ACS, PCI

Drug	Mechanism	Dose	Onset	Peak	Duration	Elimination	Adverse effects	Indications
Heparin	Binds to antithrombin III to inhibit factor Xa and thrombin	**IV flush:** 10–100 U *Cardiopulmonary bypass:* **IV:** 350–450 U/kg *Low-dose thrombosis prophylaxis:* **SC:** 5,000 U 2 h before surgery then every 8–12 h *Full-dose continuous IV therapy:* **Loading IV:** 5,000 U then infusion 20,000–40,000 U over 24 h	1–3 h	SQ: 2–4 h	4–6 h	Hepatic elimination	Allergy, hemorrhage, thrombocytopenia, decreased antithrombin concentrations	Prophylaxis and treatment against VTE, treatment of ACS, ischemic stroke
Low molecular weight heparin (LMWH) (Enoxaparin)	Binds to antithrombin to inhibit factor Xa only	VTE prophylaxis 30 mg SQ q12 h; treatment for VTE 1–1.5 mg/kg SQ q12 hrs, MI 1 mg/kg SQ q12 h Bridge to warfarin: 1–1.5 mg/kg SQ q12 h until INR in desired range	3 h	SQ: 3 h	12 h if VTE prophylaxis dose, 24 h if full anticoagulation dose	Hepatic elimination	Allergy, hemorrhage, thrombocytopenia	Monitor by factor Xa level, VTE prophylaxis, VTE prophylaxis and treatment, MI
Warfarin	Vitamin K-dependent clotting factors (II, VII, IX, X, C, S)	**Initial:** 10–15 mg **Daily: PO** 2–10 mg	1–5 d	24–60 h	≥5 d	Renal and hepatic elimination	Hemorrhage, skin necrosis	Prophylaxis and treatment of VTE disease including PE, DVT, ischemic stroke, dysrhythmia (a-fib, a-flutter)

Hemostatic Drugs

	Site	Dose	Onset	Duration	Elimination	Adverse Effects	Indications
DDAVP (Desmopressin)	Kidney, endothelium	IV: 0.3 µg/kg over 30 min	IV: 90–120 min	3 h (up to 9 h in renal failure)	Renal	Volume overload, hyponatremia, thrombosis	Hemophilia, vWD[b], diabetes insipidus, platelet dysfunction
FEIBA	Factor II, VII, IX, X	100–200 U/kg/d IV div q6–12h; Max: 200 U/kg/d; Info: dose, frequency, duration varies by site/severity of bleeding, severity of deficiency	10–15 min	Factor dependent	Factor dependent	Anaphylaxis, anaphylactoid, thrombosis, DIC, MI	Pts with factor VIII inhibitors (also hemophilia A or B)
Protamine	Binds to heparin (heparin antagonist)	Slow IV: 1 mg neutralizes 100 U of heparin. Dose is determined by dose of heparin given and time since last dose.	<5 min	(unknown half-life) duration of action: 2 h; dependent on body temperature	Hepatic elimination	Hypo- and hyper-tension, bradycardia, pulmonary HTN, dyspnea, broncho-spasm, anaphylactoid, anaphylaxis, histamine release, thrombocytopenia	Heparin antagonism

| Recombinant Factor VIIa | Activates factor IX and X | IV: 15–90 μg/kg depending on situation (slow IV bolus) | 10–15 min | 2–3 h | Anaphylaxis, thrombosis, hypertension, hemarthrosis, fever, MI, supraventricular tachycardia Blood coagulation disorder, disseminated intravascular coagulation, hemorrhage, acute renal failure, VTE | Bleeding, uncontrolled hemorrhage, long CPB duration, hemophilia A or B FDA-Labeled Indications: Acquired factor VIII deficiency disease-bleeding; bleeding-Factor VII deficiency; Factor VII/VIII deficiency-postoperative hemorrhage; prophylaxis. Bleeding-hemophilia, with inhibitors to Factor VIII or Factor IX. Hemophilia, with inhibitors to Factor VIII or Factor IX—postoperative hemorrhage; prophylaxis |

ACS, acute coronary syndrome; a-fib, atrial fibrillation; CAD, coronary artery disease; COX, cyclooxygenase; CPB, cardiopulmonary bypass; DVT, deep vein thrombosis; HTN, hypertension; INR, international normalized ratio; MI, myocardial infarction; Pt, patient; Pts, patients; PVD, peripheral vascular disease; PCI, percutaneous coronary intervention; PE, pulmonary embolism; qday, daily; VTE, venous thromboembolism; vWD, von Willebrand disease

[a]Aspirin: Half-life elimination: Parent drug: 15–20 min; Salicylates (dose dependent): 3 h at lower doses (300–600 mg), 5–h (after 1 g), 10 h with higher doses.

[b]vWD type I patients are usually responsive, vWD type II patients may have variable responses, vWD type III patients are usually not responsive. Consult a hematologist to address your individual patient needs.

References

Barash PG, et al. *Clinical Anesthesia.* Philadelphia, PA: Lippincott Williams & Wilkins; 2009.

Lloyd Jones M, Wight J, Paisley S, et al. Control of bleeding in patients with haemophilia a with inhibitors: a systematic review. *Haemophilia* 2003;9(4):464–520.

Omoigui S. *Sota Omoigui's Anesthesia Drugs Handbook.* Hawthorne: State-of-the-Art Technologies, Incorporated; 1999.

Stoelting RK, Hillier SC. *Handbook of Pharmacology and Physiology in Anesthetic Practice.* Philadelphia, PA: Lippincott Williams & Wilkins; 2005.

Crisis Management Cognitive Aids

How to Use Cognitive Aids in Crisis Management

The use of cognitive aids to manage crises in anesthesia is controversial. The goal of these cognitive aids is to provide a reference for the management of certain clinical conditions and emergency situations.

The use of cognitive aids should not replace individual clinical judgment and may not be applicable to all clinical situations.

PULSELESS ELECTRICAL ACTIVITY

By Sara Goldhaber-Fiebert, MD • Larry F. Chu, MD • T. Kyle Harrison, MD

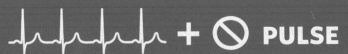 **+** 🚫 **PULSE**

CPR:
1. ≥ **100** compressions/minute
2. Minimize breaks in CPR

CALL FOR HELP **CODE CART**

CHECK

Always Check:
1. Backboard
2. Establish airway
3. IV access (consider IO)
4. Monitor for rhythm changes
5. If shockable rhythm
   (VF/VT), defibrillate

In the OR:
1. Turn **OFF** volatile
2. 100% O_2
3. Check ventilation rate
   (**8 breaths/minute**)
4. Consider: Local Anesthetic
   Toxicity, Malignant
   Hyperthermia, Autopeep,
   Anaphylaxis

TREATMENT

1. **Epinephrine** - 1 mg IV push q 3–5 minutes
2. Consider: **Vasopressin** - 40 units IV (x1, could replace one specific epinephrine dose)

DIAGNOSE

Search for Treatable Causes

H's:
1. Hypovolemia
2. Hypoxia
3. Hydrogen ions - acidosis
4. Hyper- or Hypokalemia
5. Hypo- or Hyperthermia
6. Hypoglycemia or Hypocalcemia

T's:
7. Toxins (overdose)
8. Tamponade - cardiac
9. Tension penumothorax
10. Thrombosis coronary
11. Thrombosis pulmonary

FIND AND TREAT CAUSE: H & T's

FOR ASYSTOLE AND PULSELESS ELECTRICAL ACTIVITY

TREATMENT

1. **Hypovolemia:** Administer rapid bolus of IV fluid and check hemoglobin/hematocrit. Give blood for anemia or massive hemorrhage.

2. **Hypoxia:** 100% FiO_2. Confirm oxygen connections. Check for bilateral breath sounds. Suction ET tube and reconfirm ET tube placement. Consider chest x-ray.

3. **Hydrogen ion (acidosis):** Check blood gas for acidosis. Administer sodium bicarbonate. Consider increasing ventilation rate (this will decrease effectiveness of CPR).

4. **Hyperkalemia:** Check blood gas for electrolyte abnormalities. Give Calcium Chloride 1 g IV; D50 1 Amp IV (25 g Dextrose) + Regular Insulin 10 units IV (monitor glucose). **Hypokalemia:** Rapid but controlled infusion of potassium & magnesium.

5. **Hypothermia:** Active warming by forced air blanket, warm IV. Consider cardiopulmonary bypass. **Hyperthermia:** Cool with axillary ice packs, cold IV. Consider peritoneal lavage. If anesthetic exposure, consider Malignant Hyperthermia. Call for MH Cart. Treat with dantrolene.
MH Hotline: 800-644-9737 (MH-Hyper).

6. **Hypoglycemia or Hypocalcemia:** Check blood gas or finger stick.

7. **Toxins:** Consider overdose of medication. Confirm no infusions are running. Confirm volatile anesthetic off.

8. **Tamponade** (Cardiac): Consider placing transesophageal (TEE) or transthoracic (TTE) echo to rule out. Treat with pericardiocentesis.

9. **Tension Pneumothorax:** Unilateral breath sounds, possibly distended neck veins and deviated trachea (late signs). Perform emergent needle decompression (2nd intercostal space at mid-clavicular line) followed by chest tube placement. Call for chest x-ray, but do not delay treatment.

10. **Thrombosis (Myocardial Infarction):** Consider using TEE to evaluate wall motion of ventricle. Consider emergent coronary revascularization or fibrinolytic agents.

11. **Thrombosis (Pulmonary Embolus):** Consider TEE to evaluate right ventricle. Consider fibrinolytic agents.

VENTRICULAR TACHYCARDIA & VENTRICULAR FIBRILLATION

By Sara Goldhaber-Fiebert, MD • Larry F. Chu, MD • T. Kyle Harrison, MD

V-TACH: **V-FIB:**

CPR:
1. ≥ **100** compressions/minute
2. Minimize breaks in CPR

CALL FOR HELP **CODE CART**

WHEN IT ARRIVES: DEFIBRILLATE!

CHECK

Always Check:
1. Backboard
2. Establish airway
3. IV Access

In the OR:
1. Turn **OFF** volatile
2. 100% O_2
3. Check vent rate (**8 breaths/min**)
4. Do not overventilate

TREATMENT

DEFIBRILLATE: 200 Joules (biphasic)
RESUME CPR IMMEDIATELY
EPINEPHRINE: 1 mg IV push q 3–5 minutes **OR**
VASOPRESSIN: 40 units IV push once

REPEAT CYCLE OF CPR, DEFIB, & MEDS!

CONSIDER

Consider Antiarrhythmics: Amiodarone 300 mg IV
Lidocaine 100 mg IV
If HypoMg or Torsades: Magnesium sulfate 2 grams IV
If HyperK: Calcium, insulin & glucose, sodium bicarbonate

ASYSTOLE

By Sara Goldhaber-Fiebert, MD • Larry F. Chu, MD • T. Kyle Harrison, MD

FLAT LINE:

CPR:
1. ≥ **100** compressions/minute
2. Minimize breaks in CPR

CALL FOR HELP CODE CART

CHECK

Always Check:
1. Backboard
2. Establish airway
3. IV access (consider IO)
4. Monitor for rhythm changes
5. If shockable rhythm (VF/VT), defibrillate

In the OR:
1. Turn **OFF** volatile
2. 100% O_2
3. Check vent rate (**8 breaths/minute**)
4. Consider: Local Anesthetic Toxicity, Malignant Hyperthermia, Autopeep, Anaphylaxis

TREATMENT

1. **Epinephrine** - 1 mg IV push q 3–5 minutes
2. Consider: **Vasopressin** - 40 units IV (x1, could replace one specific epinephrine dose)

DIAGNOSE

Search for Treatable Causes

H's:
1. Hypovolemia
2. Hypoxia
3. Hydrogen ions - acidosis
4. Hyper- or Hypokalemia
5. Hypo- or Hyperthermia
6. Hypoglycemia or Hypocalcemia

T's:
7. Toxins (overdose)
8. Tamponade - cardiac
9. Tension penumothorax
10. Thrombosis coronary
11. Thrombosis pulmonary

FIND AND TREAT CAUSE: H & T's

FOR ASYSTOLE AND PULSELESS ELECTRICAL ACTIVITY

1. **Hypovolemia:** Administer rapid bolus of IV fluid and check hemoglobin/hematocrit. Give blood for anemia or massive hemorrhage.

2. **Hypoxia:** 100% FiO_2. Confirm oxygen connections. Check for bilateral breath sounds. Suction ET tube and reconfirm ET tube placement. Consider chest x-ray.

3. **Hydrogen ion (acidosis):** Check blood gas for acidosis. Administer sodium bicarbonate. Consider increasing ventilation rate (this will decrease effectiveness of CPR).

4. **Hyperkalemia:** Check blood gas for electrolyte abnormalities. Give Calcium Chloride 1 g IV; D50 1 Amp IV (25 g Dextrose) + Regular Insulin 10 units IV (monitor glucose). **Hypokalemia:** Rapid but controlled infusion of potassium & magnesium.

5. **Hypothermia:** Active warming by forced air blanket, warm IV. Consider cardiopulmonary bypass. **Hyperthermia:** Cool with axillary ice packs, cold IV. Consider peritoneal lavage. If anesthetic exposure, consider Malignant Hyperthermia. Call for MH Cart. Treat with dantrolene.
MH Hotline: 800-644-9737 (MH-Hyper).

6. **Hypoglycemia or Hypocalcemia:** Check blood gas or finger stick.

7. **Toxins:** Consider overdose of medication. Confirm no infusions are running. Confirm volatile anesthetic off.

8. **Tamponade** (Cardiac): Consider placing transesophageal (TEE) or transthoracic (TTE) echo to rule out. Treat with pericardiocentesis.

9. **Tension Pneumothorax:** Unilateral breath sounds, possibly distended neck veins and deviated trachea (late signs). Perform emergent needle decompression (2nd intercostal space at mid-clavicular line) followed by chest tube placement. Call for chest x-ray, but do not delay treatment.

10. **Thrombosis (Myocardial Infarction):** Consider using TEE to evaluate wall motion of ventricle. Consider emergent coronary revascularization or fibrinolytic agents.

11. **Thrombosis (Pulmonary Embolus):** Consider TEE to evaluate right ventricle. Consider fibrinolytic agents.

BRADYCARDIA - UNSTABLE

By T. Kyle Harrison, MD • Larry F. Chu, MD • Sara Goldhaber-Fiebert, MD

SIGNS

1. **CHECK FOR PULSE**
   - If NO pulse, go to PEA algorithm.
   - If pulse present but hypotensive, proceed with treatment.

CALL FOR HELP **CODE CART**

INFORM SURGEON

TREATMENT

1. Increase **FiO$_2$ 100%.**
2. Confirm adequate **ventilation** and **oxygenation.**
3. Consider turning down or **OFF** all anesthetics.
4. **Atropine**: 0.4 to 1.0 mg IV, may repeat up to 3 mg. Consider infusions below.
5. Consider trancutaneous **pacing**:
   - Set rate to at least 80 bpm.
   - Increase current until capture achieved.
   - Confirm patient has pulse with capture.

SECONDARY

1. Place **arterial line.**
2. Send **labs**: ABG, hemoglobin, electrolytes.
3. Rule out **ischemia**: Consider EKG, troponins.

Consider Infusions

1. **Dopamine**: 5 to 20 mcg/kg/min.
2. **Epinephrine**: 2 to 10 mcg/min.
3. **Isoproterenol**: 2 to 10 mcg/min.

AMNIOTIC FLUID EMBOLISM

By T. Kyle Harrison, MD • Larry F. Chu, MD • Sara Goldhaber-Fiebert, MD

SIGNS

Consider amniotic fluid embolism if there is the sudden onset of the following in a pregnant or post-partum patient:

1. Respiratory distress, decreased O_2 saturation
2. Cardiovascular collapse: hypotension, tachycardia, arrhythmias, cardiac arrest
3. Coagulopathy
4. Disseminated intravascular coagulation (DIC)
5. Seizures
6. Altered mental status

INFORM SURGEON **CALL FOR HELP**

TREATMENT

1. Administer **100% O_2**.
2. **Consider/prepare for emergent intubation**.
3. Place patient in left uterine displacement (LUD).
4. Establish **IV access** (large volume lines).
5. Consider placing **invasive monitoring** (arterial line).
6. Anticipate possible **cardiopulmonary arrest** and **emergent C-section.**
7. Anticipate the **development of DIC.**
8. Support circulation with **IV fluid, vasopressors, and inotropes.**
9. Consider **circulatory support**: IABP/ECMO/CPB.

RULE OUT

Rule out other causes that might present in a similar fashion:

1. Eclampsia
2. Hemorrhage
3. Air embolism
4. Aspiration
5. Anaphylaxis
6. Pulmonary embolism
7. Anesthetic overdose
8. Sepsis
9. Cardiomyopathy/cardiac valvular abnormality/MI

DIFFICULT AIRWAY

By T. Kyle Harrison, MD • Larry F. Chu, MD • Sara Goldhaber-Fiebert, MD

If unsuccessful after initial attempt at direct laryngoscopy (DL):
1. Attempt to reposition patient's head to improve "sniffing position"
2. Change to a different laryngoscope blade
3. Consider placing towels under the patient's shoulders to align the tragus of the ear with the sternal notch

If grade II or III view attempt to place gum elastic bougie then pass ET tube over bougie, confirm with $ETCO_2$ and bilateral breath sounds.

⬇

Attempt face mask ventilation, maintain cricoid pressure if rapid sequence induction

UNSUCCESSFUL → → → SUCCESSFUL

CALL FOR HELP!
PLACE ORAL, NASAL AIRWAY

SEE NEXT PAGE

UNSUCCESSFUL ⬇

Place LMA — SUCCESSFUL →

CONSIDER:
1. Awakening patient
2. Doing the case with LMA
3. LMA as a conduit for intubation
4. +/- fiber optic guidance

UNSUCCESSFUL ⬇

Emergency Airway Ventilation ← If ventilation becomes inadequate

⬇

CALL FOR HELP
Attempt: Needle cricothyrotomy
Percutaneous cricothyrotomy
Transtracheal Jet Ventilation
Tracheostomy
Confirm successful placement with $ETCO_2$ and bilateral breath sounds.

DIFFICULT AIRWAY

Continued from previous page

IF SUCCESSFUL face mask ventilation, attempt 3rd DL after changing position/blade again if needed. Consider external pressure on the anterior neck/larynx.
- Move left/right, push down and up on larynx.
- Briefly release cricoid pressure may improve view of glottic structure.

UNSUCCESSFUL

Attempt face mask ventilation, maintain cricoid pressure if rapid sequence induction

SUCCESSFUL   UNSUCCESSFUL

CONSIDER:
1. Awakening patient
2. Completing case with LMA or face mask ventilation
3. Fiber optic intubation
4. Intubating LMA
5. Using LMA as a conduit for intubation +/- fiber optic guidance
6. Light wand
7. Retrograde wire intubation
8. Blind nasal intubation

CALL FOR HELP!
PLACE ORAL, NASAL AIRWAY

SEE PREVIOUS PAGE

If ventilation becomes inadequate

Place LMA (see previous page)

Modified from: Practice Guidelines for the Management of Difficult Airway. *Anesthesiology*, 2003.

MALIGNANT HYPERTHERMIA

By T. Kyle Harrison, MD • Larry F. Chu, MD • Sara Goldhaber-Fiebert, MD

SIGNS

EARLY:
1. Increased $ETCO_2$
2. Tachycardia
3. Tachypnea
4. Acidosis
5. Masseter spasm/trismus

LATE:
1. Hyperthermia
2. Trunk/limb rigidity
3. Myoglobinuria

INFORM SURGEON **CALL FOR HELP**

CALL FOR MH CART • START PREPARING DANTROLENE!

RULE OUT

- Light anesthesia
- Hypoventilation
- Over-heating (external)
- Thyroid storm
- Pheochromocytoma
- Hypoxemia

TREATMENT

1. **Discontinue** anesthetic triggers (volatiles and succinylcholine) and **increase** fresh gas flow to 10 L/min. Do NOT change machine or circuit.
2. Convert to TIVA for maintenance.
3. **Hyperventilate**, FiO_2 100%, high flow O_2.
4. Prepare 2.5 mg/kg IV Dantrolene bolus. Dilute each 20 mg Dantrolene vial in 60 mL sterile water.
5. **Rapidly administer dantrolene.** Continue giving until patient stable (may give up to 10 mg/kg).
6. **Administer** sodium bicarbonate 1–2 mEq/kg for metabolic acidosis/hyperkalemia.

MALIGNANT HYPERTHERMIA

Continued from previous page

TREATMENT

7. Actively **cool patient** with ice packs and cold saline lavage.

8. Arrhythmias are usually secondary to hyperkalemia: **treat** with insulin/glucose, sodium bicarbonate and/or calcium chloride. **Avoid calcium channel blockers.**

9. Send labs for ABG, CPK, myoglobin, PT/PTT, and lactic acid.

SECONDARY

Once successfully treated, monitor the patient for 36 hours in the intensive care unit. The patient should continue to receive **1 mg/kg dantrolene every 6 hours for 36 hours**.

Contact the Malignant Hyperthermia Association of the United States (MHAUS) at any time for consultation if MH is suspected: 1-800-986-4287, or online at http://www.mhaus.org/.

ANAPHYLAXIS

By T. Kyle Harrison, MD • Larry F. Chu, MD • Sara Goldhaber-Fiebert, MD

SIGNS

Some signs may be absent in an anesthetized patient:

1. Hypoxemia, difficulty breathing, tachypnea
2. Rash/hives
3. Hypotension (may be severe)
4. Tachycardia
5. Bronchospasm/wheezing/hypoxemia
6. Increase in peak inspiratory pressure (PIP)
7. Angioedema (potential airway swelling)

INFORM SURGEON **CALL FOR HELP**

PREPARE EPINEPHRINE 10 mcg/mL OR 100 mcg/mL

If patient becomes pulseless, start CPR, continue Epinephrine 1 mg IV boluses, large volume IVF, and switch to PEA algorithm

---

RULE OUT

Consider and rule out other causes:

- Pulmonary embolus
- Myocardial infarction
- Anesthetic overdose
- Pneumothorax
- Hemorrhage
- Aspiration

ANAPHYLAXIS

Continued from previous page

TREATMENT

1. **Discontinue potential allergens: colloid solutions, blood products, latex products, antibiotics.**
2. **Discontinue volatile anesthetic** if hypotensive.
3. **Increase FiO$_2$** to 100%.
4. **Administer IV fluid bolus**. May require many liters!
5. **Administer epinephrine** IV in escalating doses every two minutes. Start at 10-100 mcg IV and increase dose every 2 minutes until clinical improvement is noted. May require large doses > 1 mg.
6. **Consider vasopressin** (start with 2–4 units IV).
7. Treat **bronchospasm** with **albuterol** and **epinephrine** (if severe).
8. Give **H$_1$ antagonist** (e.g. Diphenhydramine 25–50 mg IV).
9. Consider **corticosteroids** (e.g. Methylprednisolone 125 mg IV) to decrease bi–phasic response.
10. Consider **early intubation** to secure airway **prior to** development of **angioedema** of airway.
11. Consider **additional IV access** and **invasive monitors** (arterial line).

POST EVENT

Consider the following interventions following the event:
1. Send serum tryptase level (can be added for 6 hrs post-event)
2. If the event was moderate to severe, consider keeping patient intubated and sedated.
3. Refer the patient for postoperative allergy testing.
4. Can recur with biphasic response: Consider monitoring patient for 24 hours post-recovery.

MYOCARDIAL ISCHEMIA

By T. Kyle Harrison, MD • Larry F. Chu, MD • Sara Goldhaber-Fiebert, MD

SIGNS

Suspect myocardial ischemia if:
- Depression or elevation of **ST segment** from the isoelectric level.
- **Arrhythmias**, conduction abnormalities, **unexplained tachycardia, bradycardia, or hypotension.**
- Elevation of cardiac filling pressures
- Regional wall motion abnormalities or new onset mitral regurgitation on TEE.
- In the **awake patient** signs and symptoms may include: central chest pain radiating into the arms or throat, dyspnea, nausea and vomiting, heartburn, and/or altered level of consciousness.

INFORM SURGEON **CALL FOR HELP**

MYOCARDIAL ISCHEMIA

Continued from previous page

TREATMENT

1. Increase FiO$_2$ to **100%**.
2. Verify ischemia with 12 lead EKG if possible.
3. Consult cardiology- stat.
4. Treat hypotension or hypertension.
5. Slow heart rate with **beta-blocker** (esmolol or metoprolol). Hold for bradycardia or hypotension.
6. Consider **nitroglycerin** infusion (hold for hypotension).
7. Treat pain with narcotics (fentanyl or morphine).
8. Consider rectal or PO or NG/OG **aspirin**.
9. Place arterial line.
10. Check hematocrit/hemoglobin and treat anemia with packed red blood cells.
11. Consider central venous access.
12. Consider TEE for monitoring volume status and regional wall motion abnormalities.
13. Send ABG, hematocrit/hemoglobin, CK and troponin.
14. If hemodynamically unstable, consider intra aortic balloon pump.

**Be Prepared for Arrhythmias
Consider Code Cart at Bed Side**

HYPOTENSION

By Sara Goldhaber-Fiebert, MD • Larry F. Chu, MD
Geoff Lighthall, MD • T. Kyle Harrison, MD

SIGNS

1. Feel for **pulse**.
2. Check **heartrate**: if slow, treat and go to bradycardia cognitive aid.
3. Check **rhythm**: if abnormal, go to ACLS Protocol.

INFORM SURGEON CALL FOR HELP
INSPECT SURGICAL FIELD FOR BLOOD LOSS OR MANIPULATION

TREATMENT

1. Give **IV fluid** bolus.
2. Give **phenylephrine** or **ephedrine** to temporize.
3. Consider **Trendelenberg** or elevation of patient's legs.
4. Turn down or off **anesthetic agent**.
5. Consider **100% O$_2$**.
6. Consider code cart if severe.

RULE OUT

Consider and rule out other causes that might present in a similar fashion to hypotension:

1. Pneumothorax: listen to breath sounds.
2. Auto-PEEP: disconnect and reconnect circuit.
3. Hemorrhage: rule out occult blood loss.
4. Rule out anaphylaxis.

HYPOTENSION

Continued from previous page

SECONDARY

1. More **IV access**.
2. Call for **rapid infuser**.
3. Call for **blood**.
4. Place **arterial line**.
5. Send **labs**: ABG, Hgb, electrolytes, calcium, type & cross.
6. Consider **terminating surgical procedure** or get surgical help.
7. Consider **transesophageal echo** if unclear cause.
8. **Foley catheter** if not present.
9. Consider **hydrocortisone**.

DDX

MAP = CO x SVR; CO= SV x HR
SV from preload, afterload, contractility

1. **Decreased preload**
2. **Low SVR**
3. **Decreased Contractility**
4. **Low HR**
5. **Increased afterload**
6. **Low Stroke Volume**

HEMORRHAGE/MASSIVE TRANSFUSION

By Sara Goldhaber-Fiebert • MD, Larry F. Chu, MD • T. Kyle Harrison, MD

INFORM SURGEON **CALL FOR HELP**

TREATMENT

1. **Increase FiO$_2$** to 100%.
2. **Treat hypotension with IV fluid bolus**.
3. Consider **Trendelenberg** or **elevation of patient's legs**.
4. Call for **rapid infuser**.
5. Establish **additional IV access** as needed.
6. Use **vasopressors** (ephedrine, phenylephrine, epi) as **temporizing measure**. Consider accepting lower blood pressures until bleeding is controlled.
7. Mobilize blood bank to **prepare multiple units of pRBC** and begin to **prepare FFP, platelets, and cryoprecipitate.**
8. **Use O-negative blood** if patient **does not have type and crossed** units available. Use type and crossed units once available unless >10 units of O-negative blood have been given. If this has occurred, then continue with O-negative blood products (or use O+ in males).
9. **Maintain normothermia!** Use fluid warming devices for IV and blood products.
10. Place **arterial line** as indicated.
11. Follow patient's acid/base status by **ABG as indicator of adequate resuscitation. Monitor for hypocalcemia.**

HEMORRHAGE/MASSIVE TRANSFUSION

Continued from previous page

TREATMENT

As resuscitation continues: replace coagulation factors, platelets, fibrinogen as indicated by laboratory values **OR** when greater than 1-1.5X blood volumes have been replaced and laboratory values cannot be measured in a timely fashion.
CONSIDER EARLY REPLACEMENT!

COMPONENTS

PLATELETS: Transfuse for <50K or <50-100K with signs of ongoing bleeding. Dose: 1 pack per 10 kg body weight.

FRESH FROZEN PLASMA: Transfuse for INR (PT) or PTT >1.5X normal with signs of ongoing bleeding. Dose: 10-15 cc FFP per kg body weight.

CRYOPRECIPITATE: Transfuse for fibrinogen <80-100 mg/dL. Dose: 1 unit per 10 kg body weight.

VOLUMES

Estimated Blood Volume (EBV)
Adults: 7% total body weight (~5 L for 70 kg)
Chidren 9% total body weight
Infants 10% total body weight

EST. LOSS

$$\text{Est. Blood Loss} = \text{EBV} \times \frac{\text{HCT}_{starting} - \text{HCT}_{measured}}{\text{HCT}_{starting}}$$

VENOUS AIR EMBOLUS

By T. Kyle Harrison, MD • Larry F. Chu, MD • Sara Goldhaber-Fiebert, MD

SIGNS

OBSERVE SUDDEN:
- Decrease in blood pressure and $ETCO_2$.
- Decrease in SaO_2.
- Rise in CVP.
- Onset of dyspnea and respiratory distress in awake patient.
- Increase in ETN_2O (if monitoring).

INFORM SURGEON CALL FOR HELP
FLOOD SURGICAL FIELD WITH SALINE

TREATMENT

1. Go to 100% O_2.
2. Give rapid fluid bolus to increase CVP.
3. Turn down or off volatile anesthetic.
4. If possible, place patient in left lateral decubitus position and surgical site below heart.
5. Administer epi to maintain cardiac output.
6. If pulseless, start CPR.
7. Attempt to aspirate air from central line if present.
8. Consider TEE to assess RV function.
9. If severe event, terminate procedure if possible.
10. Monitor patient post operatively in ICU.

TOTAL SPINAL ANESTHESIA

By T. Kyle Harrison, MD • Larry F. Chu, MD • Sara Goldhaber-Fiebert, MD

SIGNS

AFTER NEURAXIAL ANESTHESIA BLOCK

1. Unexpected rapid rise in sensory levels
2. Numbness or weakness in upper extremities
3. Dyspnea
4. Bradycardia
5. Hypotension
6. Loss of consciousness
7. Apnea
8. Cardiac arrest

Most often occurs with dosing an epidural that has inadvertently become intrathecal.

INFORM SURGEON **CALL FOR HELP**

TREATMENT

1. Support ventilation and intubate trachea if necessary.
2. Support blood pressure with IV fluid bolus and vasopressors (may require epinephrine/ vasopressin).
3. Treat bradycardia with atropine but quickly move to epinephrine if patient is unstable.
4. If it is an OB patient, monitor fetal heart sounds, and prepare for possible emergent C-section.

LOCAL ANESTHETIC TOXICITY

By T. Kyle Harrison, MD • Larry F. Chu, MD • Sara Goldhaber-Fiebert, MD

SIGNS

1. Tinnitus
2. Altered mental status
3. Seizures
4. Hypotension
5. Bradycardia
6. Ventricular arrhythmias
7. Cardiovascular collapse

CALL FOR HELP **CODE CART**

TREATMENT

1. Stop local anesthetic injection and/or infusion.
2. Establish airway - ensure adequate ventilation and oxygenation. Consider endotracheal intubation.
3. Treat seizure activity with **propofol** (only if no hypotension) or **benzodiazepine.**
4. Monitor for hemodynamic instability - treat hypotension.

**If cardiovascular collapse occurs,
start CPR and proceed with ACLS cognitive aid**

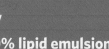

**Rapidly administer 20% lipid emulsion IV
1.5 cc/kg rapid bolus then start infusion at 0.25 cc/kg/min
May repeat loading dose (max 3 total doses) and may
increase infusion (max dose 12 cc/kg)**

SECONDARY

1. May require a prolonged resuscitation.
2. If refractory, consider cardiopulmonary bypass if available.
3. Monitor the patient post operatively in the ICU.

TRANSFUSION REACTIONS

By T. Kyle Harrison, MD • Larry F. Chu, MD • Sara Goldhaber-Fiebert, MD

In patients receiving blood products, monitor for the following signs that could indicate a possible transfusion reaction.

SIGNS

Hemolytic Reaction	Febrile	Anaphylactic
1. Tachycardia	1. Fever	1. Tachycardia
2. Tachypnea		2. Wheezing
3. Hypotension		3. Urticaria/ Hives
4. Disseminated Intravascular Coagulation		4. Hypotension
5. Dark Urine		

INFORM SURGEON **CALL FOR HELP**

TREATMENT

1. Stop transfusion. Save product for testing in blood bank.
2. Support blood pressure with IV fluids and vaso active medications if needed.
3. If severe **anaphylactic reaction** switch to anaphylaxis cognitive aid.
4. Consider antihistamine.
5. For **hemolytic reaction**, maintain urinary output with IV fluids, diuretics, renal dose dopamine.
6. Monitor for and treat disseminated intravascular coagulation if **hemolytic reaction**.
7. Monitor for lung injury and treat accordingly, may require post operative ventilation.

HYPOXEMIA

By Sara Goldhaber-Fiebert, MD • Larry F. Chu, MD •
Geoff Lighthall, MD • T. Kyle Harrison, MD

INFORM SURGEON **CALL FOR HELP**

TREATMENT

If low O$_2$ saturation, paO$_2$, or blue patient:

1. **100% O$_2$** with high flows.
2. Check gas analyzer to **rule out low FiO$_2$** or **high N$_2$O**. If concerned, go to oxygen failure cognitive aid.
3. Check other **vitals** (cycle NIBP) and PIP.
4. Check for **ETCO$_2$** (? extubated, disconnected, low BP).
5. Check surgical field and **feel for pulse**.
6. **Hand-ventilate** to check compliance/ leaks and decrease machine factors.
7. Listen for **breath sounds** (bilateral or clear).
8. **Soft suction** via ETT (to clear secretions and check obstructions).
9. Consider **Code Cart** if severe.
10. Consider **artifact** last (switch pulse ox machine or location).

CONSIDER

1. Nebulizers to **bronchodilate**- Arterial Blood Gas (ABG) - CXR.
2. Fiberoptic to **confirm ETT position** & check for mucus plugging.
3. **Additional neuromuscular blockade** if intubated and fighting ventilator.
4. Large recruitment breaths by **manual ventilation** (if ? atelectasis and patient not hypotensive).
5. **Artifacts**: check waveform, probe position, ambient light, cautery, dyes, location of probe, check ABG if still unclear.
6. Consider **terminating surgery**.
7. Plan for **postop care**: remain intubated? ICU bed?

DDX

1. Hypoventilation
2. Low FiO$_2$
3. V/Q mismatch or shunt
4. Diffusion problem
5. Artifacts

PNEUMOTHORAX

By T. Kyle Harrison, MD • Larry F. Chu, MD • Sara Goldhaber-Fiebert, MD

SIGNS

1. Increased peak inspiratory pressures
2. Tachycardia
3. Hypotension
4. Hypoxemia
5. Decreased breath sounds
6. Hyper resonance of chest to percussion
7. Tracheal deviation (late sign)
8. Increased JVD/CVP
9. Have **high index of suspicion** for pneumothorax in **trauma patients** and **COPD patients**.

INFORM SURGEON **CALL FOR HELP**

TREATMENT

1. **DO NOT WAIT FOR X-RAY TO TREAT IF HEMODYNAMICALLY UNSTABLE.**
2. Increase FiO_2 to 100%.
3. Rule out mainstem intubation.
4. Notify surgeon, call for stat portable CXR.
5. Hemodynamically unstable patients should have needle decompression or chest tube placed prior to CXR.
6. Place 14 or 16 gauge needle mid clavicular line 2nd intercostal space on affected side, should hear a whoosh of air if under tension.
7. Immediately follow up needle decompression with thoracostomy (chest tube).

BRONCHOSPASM

By T. Kyle Harrison, MD • Larry F. Chu, MD • Sara Goldhaber-Fiebert, MD

SIGNS

1. Increased peak airway pressures.
2. Wheezing on lung exam.
3. Increased expiratory time.
4. Increased ETCO$_2$ with upsloping ETCO$_2$ waveform.
5. Decreased tidal volumes if pressure control.

INFORM SURGEON ☠ CALL FOR HELP

Bronchospastic patients that develop sudden hypotension may be airtrapping - disconnect patient from circuit to allow for complete exhalation.

TREATMENT

1. Increase FiO$_2$ to 100%.
2. Deepen volatile anesthetic (sevoflurane = most bronchodilating).
3. Rule out mainstem intubation.
4. Suction ET tube.
5. Administer beta one agonist (albuterol).
6. Change I:E time to allow for adequate exhalation.
7. If severe consider epinephrine (start with 10 mcg IV and escalate, monitor for tachycardia and hypertension).
8. Consider ketamine: 0.2 - 1.0 mg/kg IV.
9. Rule out anaphylaxis (hypotension/tachycardia/rash) - if anaphylaxis, switch to anaphylaxis cognitive aid.
10. If severe or persistent, may require post operative ventilation.

DELAYED EMERGENCE

By T. Kyle Harrison, MD • Larry F. Chu, MD • Sara Goldhaber-Fiebert, MD

CHECK

Confirm that all anesthetic agents (inhalation/ IV) are **OFF.** Check for residual muscular paralysis with **Train of Four** if patient is asleep, and reverse accordingly.

CONSIDER

Consider:
1. Narcotic reversal: start with 40 mcg IV naloxone; repeat every 2 minutes up to 0.2 mg.
2. Benzodiazepine reversal: start with 0.2 mg flumazenil every 1 minute; max dose = 1 mg.
3. Reversal of scopolamine specifically, or many agents generally: 1 mg IV of physostigmine (watch for cholinergic crisis: bradycardia, bronchospasm, seizures, incontinence).

CHECK

Check:
1. Rule out hypoxemia (pulse ox).
2. Blood glucose level and **treat hypo- or hyperglycemia**.
3. Arterial blood gas plus electrolytes.
   Rule out: CO_2 narcosis from hypercarbia.
   Rule out: hypo- or hypernatremia.
4. Neuroexam if concerning, **obtain stat head CT scan** and consult neurology/ neurosurgery to rule out possible cerebral vascular accident.
5. Patient temperature and **warm patient** if <34 degrees Celsius.

TREATMENT

1. Correct any abnormalities in oxygenation, ventilation, laboratory values, or temperature.
2. **Perform complete neurological exam** if possible (pupils, asymmetric movement, gagging/ coughing, or focal neurological deficit).
3. If residual sedation persists, monitor the patient in the ICU with **neurological follow up**; repeat head CT scan in 6-8 hours.

OXYGEN FAILURE
O$_2$ CROSS OVER/ PIPELINE FAILURE

By Sara Goldhaber-Fiebert, MD • Larry F. Chu, MD • Steven K. Howard, MD
Seshadri C. Mudumbai, MD • T. Kyle Harrison, MD

IMMEDIATE LIVESAVING ACTIONS

1. **Disconnect the patient from the machine and ventilate with an Ambu™ bag on room air.**
   Do **not** connect the patient to auxiliary flowmeter on machine – comes from SAME central source!

2. Obtain full E cylinder of oxygen with a regulator, **OR** disconnect pipeline oxygen and open O$_2$ tank on back of anesthesia machine (check that it is not empty).

3. Connect Ambu™ bag or Jackson Rees circuit to oxygen tank and **ventilate**.

4. Connect adaptor to allow monitoring of respiratory gases:
   Is the patient receiving 100% oxygen?

5. Call for help & diagnose machine problem.

6. Maintain anesthesia (if necessary) with IV drugs.

POWER FAILURE

By Sara Goldhaber-Fiebert, MD • Larry F. Chu, MD • T. Kyle Harrison, MD

IMMEDIATE LIFESAVING ACTIONS

1. **Get additional light sources:**
   - Laryngoscopes, cell phones, flashlights, etc.

2. **Open doors and shades** to let in ambient light.

3. **Confirm ventilator is working** and **if not, ventilate patient with Ambu bag and switch to TIVA.**

4. If monitors fail, **check pulse and manual blood pressure.**

5. **Request Transport Monitor** or defibrillator monitor.

6. **Confirm adequate backup O_2 supply**.
   - Power failure may affect oxygen supply or alarms.

7. **Check extent of power failure.**
   - Call bio-med or engineering.
   - Is the problem in one OR, all ORs, or hospital-wide?
   - If only in your OR, check if circuit breaker has been tripped.

Page numbers in italics indicate figures and those followed by t indicate tables.